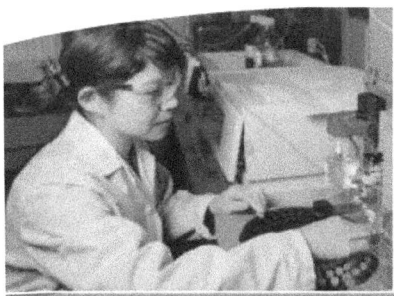
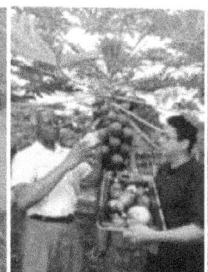
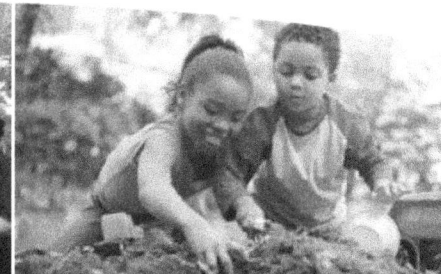
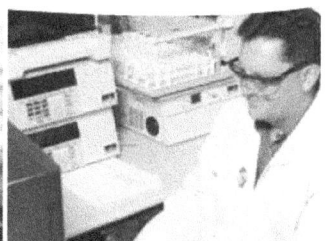

# 2009

# Fourth National Report on Human Exposure to Environmental Chemicals

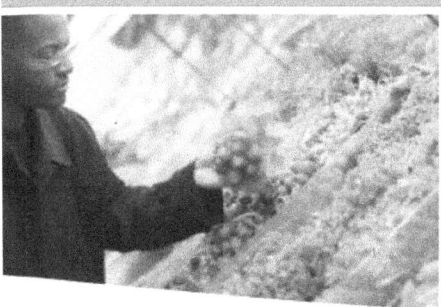
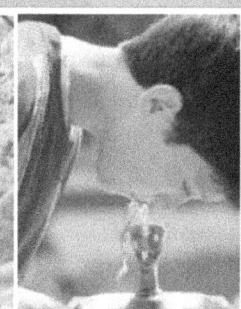
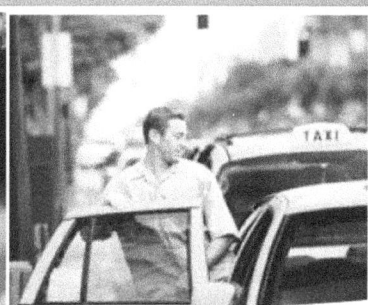
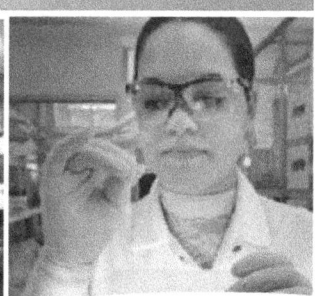

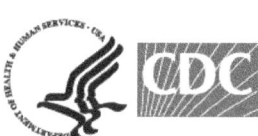

# Fourth National Report on Human Exposure to Environmental Chemicals

2009

**Department of Health and Human Services**
**Centers for Disease Control and Prevention**

# Contents

Contents

Contents

# Contents

# Introduction

The *Fourth National Report on Human Exposure to Environmental Chemicals, 2009* (the *Report*) provides an ongoing assessment of the exposure of the U.S. population to environmental chemicals by the use of biomonitoring. The *Report* is cumulative (containing all the results from previous *Reports*) and provides new data for years 2003-2004. Data for 75 new environmental chemicals are included for the survey period 2003-2004. The *Report* website http://www.cdc.gov/exposurereport is also the best source for the most recent update of available data.

In each survey period, most chemicals or their metabolites were measured in blood, serum, and urine samples from random subsamples of about 2500 participants from the National Health and Nutrition Examination Survey (NHANES) conducted by the Centers for Disease Control and Prevention's (CDC's) National Center for Health Statistics. NHANES is a series of surveys designed to collect data related to the health and nutritional status of the U.S. population. The blood, serum, and urine exposure measurements presented in the *Report* were made by CDC's Environmental Health Laboratory (Division of Laboratory Sciences, National Center for Environmental Health) using mass spectrometry methods.

The term *environmental chemical* refers to a chemical compound or chemical element present in air, water, food, soil, dust, or other environmental media (e.g., consumer products). Biomonitoring is the assessment of human exposure to chemicals by measuring the chemicals or their metabolites in such human specimens as blood or urine. A metabolite is a chemical alteration of the original compound produced by body tissues. Blood, serum, and urine levels reflect the amount of a chemical that actually gets into the body by all routes of exposure, including ingestion, inhalation, and dermal absorption. The measurement of an environmental chemical in a person's blood or urine is an indication of exposure; it does not by itself mean that the chemical causes disease or an adverse effect. Research studies, separate from these data, are required to determine which blood or urine levels are safe and which are associated with disease or an adverse effect. For blood, serum, and urine levels, the *Report* provides geometric means and percentiles of environmental chemicals by age group, gender and race/ethnicity. More in-depth statistical analysis, including multivariate analysis incorporating health endpoints and other predictive variables, is beyond the scope of this document. We encourage scientists to examine the data further through analysis of the raw data available at http://www.cdc.gov/nchs/nhanes.htm.

## Public Health Uses of the *Report*

The overall purpose of the *Report* is to provide unique exposure information to scientists, physicians, and health officials to help prevent exposure to some environmental chemicals. Specific public health uses of the exposure information in the *Report* are

- To determine which chemicals get into Americans and at what concentrations.
- For chemicals with a known toxicity level, to determine the prevalence of people with levels above those toxicity levels (e.g., a blood lead level greater than or equal to 10 micrograms per deciliter [$\geq 10$ µg/dL]).
- To establish reference values that can be used by physicians and scientists to determine whether a person or group has an unusually high exposure. This information is especially helpful to identify population groups that merit further assessment of exposure sources or health effects.
- To assess the effectiveness of public health efforts to reduce exposure of Americans to specific chemicals.
- To determine whether exposure levels are higher among such potentially vulnerable groups as minorities and children.
- To track, over time, trends in levels of exposure of the population.
- To set priorities for research on human health effects.

# What's New in this *Report*

In this *Fourth Report*, 75 new chemicals are added for the 2003-2004 survey period and are listed in Table 1. The process for selection is described at http://www.cdc.gov/exposurereport/chemical_selection.html.

**Table 1. Chemicals reported for the first time in the *Fourth National Report on Human Exposure to Environmental Chemicals, 2009***

**Acrylamide Adducts**
Acrylamide
Glycidamide

**Total and Speciated Arsenic**
Arsenic, Total
Arsenic (V) acid
Arsenobetaine
Arsenocholine
Arsenous (III) acid
Dimethylarsinic acid
Monomethylarsonic acid
Trimethylarsine oxide

**Disinfection By-Products (Trihalomethanes)**
Bromodichloromethane
Dibromochloromethane (Chlorodibromomethane)
Bromoform (Tribromomethane)
Chloroform (Trichloromethane)

**Environmental Phenols**
Benzophenone-3 (2-Hydroxy-4-methoxybenzophenone)
Bisphenol A (2,2-*bis*[4-Hydroxyphenyl] propane)
4-*tert*-Octyl phenol (4-[1,1,3,3-Tetramethylbutyl] phenol)
Triclosan (2,4,4'-Trichloro-2'-hydroxyphenyl ether)

**Non-dioxin-like Polychlorinated Biphenyls**
2,2'3,5'-Tetrachlorobiphenyl (PCB 44)
2,2'4,5'-Tetrachlorobiphenyl (PCB 49)
2,2',3,3',4,4',5,5',6,6'-Decachlorobiphenyl (PCB 209)

**Perchlorate**

**Perfluorinated Compounds**
Perfluorobutane sulfonic acid (PFBuS)
Perfluorodecanoic acid (PFDeA)
Perfluorododecanoic acid (PFDoA)
Perfluoroheptanoic acid (PFHpA)
Perfluorohexane sulfonic acid (PFHxS)
Perfluorononanoic acid (PFNA)
Perfluorooctane sulfonamide (PFOSA)
Perfluorooctane sulfonic acid (PFOS)
2-(N-Ethyl-Perfluorooctane sulfonamido) acetic acid
  (Et-PFOSA-AcOH)
2-(N-Methyl-perfluorooctane sulfonamido) acetic acid
  (Me-PFOSA-AcOH)
Perfluorooctanoic acid (PFOA)
Perfluoroundecanoic acid (PFUA)

**Phthalate Metabolite**
Mono-(2-ethyl-5-carboxypentyl) phthalate (MECPP)

**Polybrominated Diphenyl Ethers (PBDE) and**
  **Polybrominated Biphenyl**
2,2',4-Tribromodiphenyl ether (BDE 17)
2,4,4'-Tribromodiphenyl ether (BDE 28)
2,2',4,4'-Tetrabromodiphenyl ether (BDE 47)
2,3',4,4'-Tetrabromodiphenyl ether (BDE 66)
2,2',3,4,4'-Pentabromodiphenyl ether (BDE 85)
2,2',4,4',5-Pentabromodiphenyl ether (BDE 99)
2,2',4,4',6-Pentabromodiphenyl ether (BDE 100)
2,2',4,4',5,5'-Hexabromodiphenyl ether (BDE 153)
2,2',4,4',5,6'-Hexabromodiphenyl ether (BDE 154)
2,2',3,4,4',5',6-Heptabromodiphenyl ether (BDE 183)
2,2',4,4',5,5'-Hexabromobiphenyl (BB 153)

**Volatile Organic Compounds (VOCs)**
Benzene
Chlorobenzene (Monochlorobenzene)
1,2-Dibromo-3-chloropropane (DBCP)
Dibromomethane
1,2-Dichlorobenzene (*o*-Dichlorobenzene)
1,3-Dichlorobenzene (*m*-Dichlorobenzene)
1,4-Dichlorobenzene (*p*-Dichlorobenzene,
  Paradichlorobenzene)
1,1-Dichloroethane
1,2-Dichloroethane (Ethylene dichloride)
1,1-Dichloroethene (Vinylidene chloride)
*cis*-1,2-Dichloroethene
*trans*-1,2-Dichloroethene
Dichloromethane (Methylene chloride)
1,2-Dichloropropane
2,5-Dimethylfuran
Ethylbenzene
Hexachloroethane
Methyl-*tert*-butyl ether (MTBE)
Nitrobenzene
Styrene
1,1,2,2-Tetrachloroethane
Tetrachloroethene
Tetrachloromethane (Carbon tetrachloride)
Toluene
1,1,1-Trichloroethane (Methyl chloroform)
1,1,2-Trichloroethane
Trichloroethene (Trichloroethylene)
*m*- and *p*-Xylene
*o*-Xylene

# What's Different in this *Report*

The *Fourth Report* uses a new procedure to estimate percentiles when the percentile estimate falls on a value that is repeated multiple times (e.g., five results that all have the value 90.1). Percentiles for all three NHANES survey periods (1999-2000, 2001-2002, 2003-2004) have been re-computed by use of this improved procedure. Only slight differences should be noted when one compares the recomputations to previous releases of the *Report*. Details of this procedure are provided in Appendix A.

2003-2004 data for the organochlorine pesticides and the dialkyl phosphate organophosphorus insecticides are included in the *Report*. Data for other pesticides are included only for 1999-2000 and 2001-2002. 2003-2004 data for these other pesticides will be provided on this website as soon as they are available, and these data will be included in the next release of the *Report*.

Some results reported previously have been changed or removed due to improvements in analytical measurement or recognition of an analytical issue (e.g., the presence of an interference) that produced results of inadequate quality. Affected analytes were serum *beta*-hexachlorocyclohexane for the 2001-2002 survey period; urinary 2,4-dichlorophenol and 2,5-dichlorophenol for the 1999-2002 survey periods; and polycyclic aromatic hydrocarbons (PAHs) for one or more of the 1999-2002 survey periods. Explanations for each change are provided in Appendix B.

## Data Sources and Data Analysis

### Blood, serum, and urine samples from NHANES

Biomonitoring measurements for the *Report* were made in samples from participants in NHANES. NHANES is a series of surveys conducted by CDC's National Center for Health Statistics (NCHS). NHANES is designed to collect data on the health and nutritional status of the U.S. population. NHANES collects information about a wide range of health-related behaviors, performs physical examinations, and collects samples for laboratory tests. NHANES is unique in its ability to examine public health issues in the U.S. population, such as risk factors for cardiovascular disease. Beginning in 1999, NHANES became a continuous survey, sampling the U.S. population annually and releasing the data in 2-year cycles. The sampling plan follows a complex, stratified, multistage, probability-cluster design to select a representative sample of the civilian, noninstitutionalized population in the United States based on age, gender, and race/ethnicity.

The NHANES protocol includes a home interview followed by a standardized physical examination in a mobile examination center. As part of the examination component, blood is obtained by venipuncture from participants aged 1 year and older, and urine specimens are collected from participants aged 6 years and older. Additional detailed information on the design and conduct of the NHANES survey is available at http://www.cdc.gov/nchs/nhanes.htm.

Environmental chemicals were measured in blood, serum, or urine specimens collected as part of the examination component of NHANES. The participant ages for which a chemical was measured varied by chemical group. Most of the environmental chemicals were measured in randomly selected subsamples within specific age groups. Randomization of subsample selection is built into the NHANES design before sample collection begins. Different random subsamples include different participants. This subsampling was needed to ensure an adequate quantity of sample for analysis and to accommodate the throughput of the mass spectrometry analytical methods.

Age groups and sample sizes for each exposure measurement are provided in each of the data tables. Blood lead and blood cadmium were measured in all participants aged 1 year and older for all survey periods. Total blood mercury was measured in children aged 1-5 years and in women aged 16-49 years in 1999-2002. Total blood mercury and inorganic blood mercury were measured in all participants aged 1 year and older in 2003-2004. Urinary mercury was measured in women aged 16-49 years in 1999-2002. For the 2003-2004 survey, urinary mercury was measured in a random one-third subsample of participants aged 6 years and older. Serum cotinine and acrylamide adducts were measured in the entire NHANES sample for ages 3 years and older. Cotinine is reported only in nonsmokers.

Though most chemicals in urine were measured in a random one-third subsample of participants aged 6 years and older, there have been some exceptions. Urinary levels of herbicides, selected pesticides, and metabolites of organophosphate pesticides were measured in a random one-half subsample of children aged 6-11 years in 1999 and 2000; in a random one-quarter subsample of people aged 12-59 years in 1999; and in a random one-third subsample of people aged 12 years and older in 2000. Otherwise in 2001-2002 and 2003-2004, these chemicals were measured in a random one-third subsample of participants aged 6 years and older.

Dioxins, furans, polychlorinated biphenyls (PCBs), and organochlorine pesticides were measured in serum from a random one-third subsample of participants aged 12 years and older in 1999-2000 and 2003-2004. In 2001-2002, dioxins, furans, and coplanar PCBs were measured in a random one-third subsample of participants aged 20 years and older, while organochlorine pesticides and other PCBs were measured in a random one-third subsample of participants aged 12 years and older.

Chemicals in the *Report* were selected on the basis of scientific data that suggested exposure in the U.S. population; the seriousness of health effects known or suspected to result from some levels of exposure; the need to assess the effectiveness of public health actions to reduce exposure to a chemical; the availability of a biomonitoring analytical method with adequate accuracy, precision, sensitivity, specificity, and throughput; the availability of adequate blood or urine samples; and the incremental analytical cost to perform the biomonitoring analysis for the chemical. The availability of biomonitoring methods with adequate performance and acceptable cost was a major consideration. Details on the prioritization process for scoring nominated chemicals and the resulting scores are available at http://www.cdc.gov/exposurereport/chemical selection.html.

### Laboratory Analysis

The blood, serum and urine exposure measurements in the *Report* were made by CDC's Environmental Health Laboratory (Division of Laboratory Sciences, National Center for Environmental Health). The analytical methods used for measuring the environmental chemicals or their metabolites in blood, serum, and urine were based on isotope dilution mass spectrometry, inductively coupled plasma mass spectrometry, or graphite furnace atomic absorption spectrometry. Laboratory measurements underwent extensive quality control and quality assurance review, including tolerance limits for operational parameters, the measurement of quality control samples in each analytical run to detect unacceptable performance in accuracy or precision, and verification of traceable calibration materials. References for the analytical methods used to measure the different chemicals are provided in Appendix C.

## Data Analysis

Because the NHANES is a complex, stratified, multistage, probability-cluster design, sample weights must be used to adjust for the unequal probability of selection into the survey. Sample weights also are used to adjust for possible bias resulting from nonresponse and are post-stratified to U.S. Census Bureau estimates of the U.S. population. Data were analyzed using the statistical software package Statistical Analysis System (SAS) (SAS Institute Inc., 2002) and the statistical software package SUDAAN (SUDAAN Release 8.0, 2001). SUDAAN uses sample weights and calculates variance estimates that account for the complex survey design. This design does not permit straightforward analysis of exposure levels by non-targeted strata such as locality, state, or region; seasons of the year; proximity to sources of exposure; or by use of particular products. Guidelines for the analysis of NHANES data are provided by NCHS at http://www.cdc.gov/nchs/nhanes/nhanes2003-2004/analytical_guidelines.htm.

The *Report* presents descriptive statistics on the blood, serum, or urine levels for each environmental chemical. Statistics include unadjusted geometric means and percentiles with confidence intervals. In each table, results are given for the total population as well as by age group, gender, and race/ethnicity as defined in NHANES. For these analyses, race/ethnicity is categorized based on the sample design as Mexican American, non-Hispanic black, and non-Hispanic white. Other racial/ethnic groups are sampled, but the proportion of the total population represented by other racial/ethnic groups is not large enough to produce valid estimates. Other racial/ethnic groups are included in estimates that are based on the entire population sample. Age groups are as described for each chemical in each data table. Gender is coded as male or female.

**Units:** For chemicals measured in urine, levels are presented two ways: per volume of urine and per gram of creatinine. Urinary levels are expressed both ways in the literature and used for different purposes. Levels per gram of creatinine (i.e., creatinine corrected) adjust for urine dilution. For example, if one person has consumed more fluids than another person, his or her urine output is likely higher and the urine more dilute than that of the other person. Interpretation of creatinine corrected results should also recognize that creatinine correction can also partially adjust for differences in lean body mass or renal function among persons.

For dioxins, furans, PCBs, and organochlorine pesticides, serum levels are presented per gram of total lipid and per whole weight of serum. These compounds are lipophilic and concentrate in the body's lipid stores, including the lipid in serum. Serum levels reported per gram of total lipid reflect the amount of these compounds that are stored in body fat. Serum levels per whole weight of serum are also included to facilitate comparison with studies investigating exposure to these chemicals and reported levels in these units. Other mostly non-lipophilic chemicals measured in serum are expressed per liter of serum (e.g., micrograms per liter). Acrylamide and glycidamide adducts are expressed as the picomoles per gram of blood hemoglobin to which the adduct is bound.

Units of measurement are important. Results are reported here using standard units, generally conforming to those most commonly used in biomonitoring measurements. Useful unit conversions are shown in Table 2.

**Table 2. Units of Measurements and Abbreviations**

| Unit | Abbreviation | Value |
|------|--------------|-------|
| liter | L | |
| deciliter | dL | $10^{-1}$ liters |
| milliliter | mL | $10^{-3}$ liters |
| gram | g | |
| milligram | mg | $10^{-3}$ grams |
| microgram | μg | $10^{-6}$ grams |
| nanogram | ng | $10^{-9}$ grams |
| picogram | pg | $10^{-12}$ grams |
| femtogram | fg | $10^{-15}$ grams |

**Geometric means:** A geometric mean provides a better estimate of central tendency for data that are distributed with a long tail at the upper end of the distribution. This type of distribution is common in the measurement of environmental chemicals in blood or urine. The geometric mean is influenced less by high values than is the arithmetic mean. Geometric means were calculated by taking the log of each concentration and then computing the weighted mean of those log-transformed values using SUDAAN software. Ninety-five percent confidence intervals around this weighted mean were calculated by adding and subtracting an amount equal to the product of a Student's t-statistic and the standard error of the weighted mean estimate. The degrees of freedom of the t-statistic were determined by subtracting the number of strata from the number of primary sampling units (PSUs) according to the data available from the complex survey design. The standard error was computed with SUDAAN's Proc Descript (design=WR), which uses Taylor series linearization for variance estimation. The weighted geometric mean and its confidence limits were then obtained by taking the antilogs of this weighted mean and its upper and lower confidence limits.

**Limit of detection:** The limit of detection (LOD) is the level at which the measurement has a 95% probability of being greater than zero (Taylor, 1987). The LODs for each chemical and survey period are provided in each data table and collectively in Appendix D. Concentrations less than the LOD were assigned a value equal to the LOD divided by the square root of 2 for calculation of geometric means. Assigning a value of the LOD divided by 2 made little difference in geometric mean estimates. If the proportion of results below the LOD was greater than 40%, geometric means were not calculated. For the same chemical, LOD values may change over time as a result of improvements to analytical methods. One possible consequence is that results may be reported as "< LOD" in the 1999-2000 data but be reported as a concentration value above the LOD in 2001-2002 or 2003-2004 because the analytical method had improved. Thus, for proper interpretation of LODs in the data tables, care must be taken to use the LOD that applies to the survey period. Percentile estimates (see below) that are less than the LOD for the chemical analysis are reported as "< LOD."

For most chemicals, the LOD is constant for each individual specimen analyzed. For dioxins, furans, PCBs, organochlorine pesticides, and a few other pesticides, each individual sample has its own LOD. These analyses have an individual LOD for each sample, mostly because the sample volume used for analysis differed for each sample. A higher sample volume results in a lower LOD (i.e., a better ability to detect low levels). For these chemicals, the maximum LOD value is provided in each data table and in Appendix D. The maximum LOD was the highest LOD among all the individual samples analyzed — typically, the mean LOD was about 40-50% of the maximum LOD. The same procedure for imputing values below the LOD in calculations of geometric means was used for chemicals with individual LODs for each sample. That is, concentrations less than the individual LOD were assigned a value equal to the individual LOD divided by the square root of 2. For chemicals that had individual sample LODs,

a conservative rule was used for reporting percentiles: if any individual sample LOD in the demographic group was above the percentile estimate, the percentile estimate was not reported.

For chemicals measured in urine, separate tables are presented for the chemical concentration expressed per volume of urine (uncorrected table) and the chemical concentration expressed per gram of creatinine (creatinine corrected table). Geometric mean and percentile calculations were performed separately for each of these concentrations. LOD calculations were performed using the chemical concentration expressed per volume of urine, because this concentration determines the analytical sensitivity. For this reason, LOD results for urine measurements in each data table and in Appendix D are in units of weight per volume of urine. In the creatinine corrected tables, a result for a geometric mean or percentile was reported as < LOD if the corresponding geometric mean or percentile was < LOD in the table using weight per volume of urine. For example, if the 50th percentile for males was < LOD in the table using weight per volume of urine, it would also be < LOD in the creatinine corrected table.

For chemicals measured in serum lipid, separate tables are presented for the chemical concentration expressed per volume of serum (lipid unadjusted table) and the chemical concentration expressed per amount of lipid (lipid adjusted table). Geometric mean and percentile calculations were performed separately for each of these concentrations. LOD calculations were performed using the chemical concentration expressed per amount of lipid, because this concentration determines the analytical sensitivity. For this reason, LOD results for chemicals measured in each data table and in Appendix D are in weight per amount of lipid. In the lipid unadjusted tables, a result for a geometric mean or percentile was reported as < LOD if the corresponding geometric mean or percentile was < LOD in the lipid adjusted table.

**Percentiles:** Percentiles (50th, 75th, 90th, and 95th) are given to provide additional information about the shape of the distribution. Percentile estimates and 95% confidence interval estimates that are less than the limit of detection are indicated as <LOD in the data tables. In the *Third National Report on Human Exposure to Environmental Chemicals,* weighted percentile estimates for 1999-2000 and 2001-2002 data were calculated using SAS Proc Univariate and a proportions estimation procedure. A percentile estimate may fall on a value that is repeated multiple times in a particular demographic group defined by age, sex and race (e.g., in non-Hispanic white males 12-19 years old, five results that all have a value of 90.1). Since the *Third*

*Report*, we have improved the procedure for estimating percentiles to better handle this situation. This improved procedure makes each repeated value unique by adding a unique negligibly small number to each repeated value. All data from 1999-2004 have been reanalyzed using this new procedure to handle situations where the percentile falls on a repeating value. Therefore, occasional percentile estimates may differ slightly in the current *Fourth Report* than in the *Third Report*. Appendix A gives the details of the new procedure for estimating percentiles.

Taylor JK. Quality Assurance of Chemical Measurements. Lewis Publishers, Boca Raton (FL), 1987.

# Interpretation of *Report* Data: Important Factors

**Research studies, separate from the *Report*, are required for determining whether blood or urine levels are safe or are associated with disease or adverse effects.**

The measurement of an environmental chemical in a person's blood or urine does not by itself mean that the chemical causes disease. Advances in analytical methods allow us to measure low levels of environmental chemicals in people, but separate studies of varying exposure levels and health effects are needed to determine whether such blood or urine levels result in disease. These studies must also consider other factors such as duration of exposure. The *Fourth Report* does not present new data on health risks from different exposures.

For some environmental chemicals, such as lead, research studies have given us a good understanding of the health risks associated with different blood lead levels. However, for many environmental chemicals, we need more research to assess health risks from different blood or urine levels. The results shown in the *Fourth Report* should help prioritize and foster research on human health risks that result from exposure to environmental chemicals. For more information about exposure to environmental chemicals, see the section later in this *Report* titled "Chemical and Toxicological Information", which includes Internet reference sites.

## Persistent and nonpersistent chemicals; use of percentiles; comparison of levels between groups

In this *Report*, except for some metals, most measurements in urine quantify chemical metabolites of nonpersistent chemicals (those that do not stay in the body a long time). Persistent chemicals (those that stay in the body for a long time) are usually measured in serum as the parent chemical.

The higher percentiles (75th, 90th, 95th) provided for each chemical convey useful information about the upper distribution and range of levels in the population. The 95th percentile is helpful for determining whether levels observed in separate public health investigations or other studies are unusual.

Levels of chemicals are provided for the demographic groups as stratified by age, gender, and race/ethnicity. Demographic groups may not be equal in their composition with respect to other variables. CDC scientists publish separate scientific papers that make detailed comparisons of levels of chemicals in different demographic groups. See http://www.cdc.gov/exposurereport/ for a list of these papers.

Not all the chemicals in the *Report* are measured in the same individuals. Therefore, it is not possible to determine the fraction of all measured chemicals that were found at detectable levels in a given person.

**Blood, serum, and urine levels of a chemical should not be confused with levels of the chemical in air, water, food, soil, or dust.**

Concentrations of environmental chemicals in blood or urine are not the same as those in air, water, food, soil, or dust. For example, a chemical concentration of 10 µg/L in water does not produce a level of 10 µg/L in blood or urine. Blood or urine levels may reflect exposure from one or more sources, including air, water, food, soil, and dust.

Levels of a chemical in blood, serum, and urine are determined by how much of the chemical has entered the body through all routes of exposure, including ingestion, inhalation, and dermal absorption, and how the chemical is distributed in body tissues, transformed into metabolites, and eliminated from the body. Although the levels in the blood, serum and urine are measures of the amount of a chemical that has entered the body by all routes of exposure, the blood or urine level alone does not determine which exposure source or which route of exposure has occurred.

# Chemical and Toxicological Information

The *Fourth Report* presents biomonitoring data on the exposure of the U.S. population to environmental chemicals. The measurement of an environmental chemical in a person's blood or urine does not by itself mean that the chemical causes disease or adverse effects. Advances in analytical methods allow us to measure increasingly lower levels of environmental chemicals in people. Separate studies of varying exposure levels and health effects associated with these levels are required to determine whether blood, serum, and urine levels result in disease or adverse effects. The data and information in the *Fourth Report* do not establish health effects, nor do they create guidelines.

The *Fourth Report* provides descriptive information about each chemical or chemical group including uses, sources, and pathways of human exposure; disposition within the body; effects in animals or humans; and comparative blood or urine levels from other studies. The information in the text is provided as an overview, and it is not intended as a comprehensive review of each chemical. Generally, the information was compiled from many publicly available sources, including documents from national and international agencies and organizations, peer-reviewed scientific papers obtained from electronic searches, and public government documents. Statements are based on common general information, consensus agreement among experts, or concordance among multiple scientific papers and sources. Examples of common institutional sources of information include the Agency for Toxic Substances and Disease Registry, the U.S. Environmental Protection Agency, and the agencies of the World Health Organization.

If available, generally recognized guidelines for blood or urine levels are presented in the text. For most chemicals in this *Report*, such guidelines are not available. Some guidelines are from federal agencies. One exception is the American Conference of Governmental Industrial Hygienists (ACGIH), a private organization that publishes biological exposure indices (BEIs) that "generally indicate a concentration below which nearly all workers may be repeatedly exposed without adverse health effects" (ACGIH, 2007). BEIs can be the blood or urine levels of a chemical that correspond to air-exposure limits for workers set by ACGIH. This organization notes that these values are for workers and that it is not appropriate to apply them to the general population. Information about the BEI level is provided here for comparison, not to imply that the BEI is a safety level for general population exposure.

American Conference of Government Industrial Hygienists

(ACGIH). 2007 TLVs and BEIs. Cincinnati (OH). Signature Publications. 2007.

## Where can I find more information?

For more information about environmental chemicals, refer to the list of web links below and the references given in the text. Links to nonfederal organizations are provided solely as a service to our readers. These links do not constitute an endorsement of these organizations or their programs by CDC or the federal government. CDC is not responsible for the content of an individual organization's Web pages found at these links.

### U.S. Governmental Sources

### Centers for Disease Control and Prevention (CDC) Resources:
- National Center for Health Statistics (NCHS) (http://www.cdc.gov/nchs)
  - National Health and Nutrition Examination Survey (NHANES) (http://www.cdc.gov/nchs/nhanes.htm)
- National Institute for Occupational Safety and Health (NIOSH)
  - Databases and Information Resources (http://www.cdc.gov/niosh/database.html)
  - Registry of Toxic Effects of Chemical Substances (RTECS) (http://www.cdc.gov/niosh/rtecs)

### Agency for Toxic Substances and Disease Registry (ATSDR)
- Toxicological Profiles and ToxFAQs (http://www.atsdr.cdc.gov/toxpro2.html)
- Toxic Substances Portal (http://www.atsdr.cdc.gov/substances/index.asp)

### U.S. Food and Drug Administration (FDA)
- Center for Food Safety and Applied Nutrition (http://www.cfsan.fda.gov)
- National Center for Toxicological Research (http://www.fda.gov/nctr)

### U.S. Environmental Protection Agency (EPA)
- Integrated Risk-Information System (IRIS) (http://www.epa.gov/iris)
- Office of Prevention, Pesticides, and Toxic Substances (OPPTS) (http://www.epa.gov/opptsmnt/index.htm)

### U.S. Geological Survey (USGS)
- (http://www/usgs.gov)

**U.S. Department of Agriculture (USDA)**
- Food Safety and Inspection Service
  (http://www.fsis.usda.gov)

**National Institutes of Health (NIH)**
- National Institute for Environmental Health Sciences
  (NIEHS)
  (http://www.niehs.nih.gov)
- National Toxicology Program (NTP)
  (http://ntp.niehs.nih.gov)
- National Library of Medicine (NLM), Toxicology
  Data Network
  (http://toxnet.nlm.nih.gov)

## Professional and Academic Organizations

**American Conference of Governmental Industrial
Hygienists** (http://www.acgih.org/home.htm)

**Association of Public Health Laboratories**
(http://www.aphl.org)

**International Occupational Safety and Health
Information Center**
- International Chemical Safety Cards
  (http://www.ilo.org/public/english/protection/
  safework/cis/products/icsc/dtasht/index.htm)

**The EXtension TOXicology NETwork (EXTOXNET)**
- Pesticide Information Profiles
  (http://extoxnet.orst.edu/pips/ghindex.html)

## World Health Organization

**International Programme on Chemical Safety (IPCS)**
(http://www.who.int/pcs)
- Monographs of the Joint FAO/WHO Meeting on
  Pesticide Residues (http://www.inchem.org/pages/
  jmpr.html)

**International Agency for Research on Cancer (IARC)**
(www.iarc.fr)
- Monographs on the Evaluation of Carcinogenic
  Risks to Humans
  (http://monographs.iarc.fr/ENG/Monographs/
  allmonos90.php)

# Acrylamide

CAS No. 79-06-1

## General Information

Acrylamide is a small organic molecule existing as a white crystalline powder in its pure state. Commercially, acrylamide is synthesized and used in the production of polyacrylamide polymer, gels, and binding agents. Polyacrylamides are useful water-compatible polymers used in water treatment, mineral processing, pulp and paper production, and in the synthesis or compounding of dye materials, soil conditioners, and cosmetics (NTP-CERHR, 2005). Smaller scale applications of polyacrylamides include additives to paperboard used for food packaging, in permanent press fabrics, in some sealing grouts, as an absorbent in disposable diapers, and in some cosmetics. In 1997, 217 million pounds of acrylamide were produced commercially in the U.S. (NTP-CERHR, 2005). Since acrylamide has limited volatility and high water solubility, environmental releases of acrylamide can enter aquatic systems and soils where it degrades within days and does not bioaccumulate (U.S. EPA, 1994). Recently, it was discovered that acrylamide is formed when starch-rich foods, such as potatoes and some grains, are heated at temperatures used for frying and baking. Natural substances in the food are converted to acrylamide. Foods such as french fries and potato chips can contain acrylamide at levels up to 100 times greater than levels found in cooked fish or poultry (DiNovi and Howard, 2004; FAO/WHO, 2005; FDA, 2006; Tareke et al., 2002).

People may be exposed to acrylamide from foods, smoking, drinking water, and from dermal contact with products that contain residual acrylamide. In the general population, the main source of exposure is from the diet, and an average daily intake is estimated as 0.3-2.0 µg/kg for adults (FAO/WHO, 2005), although additional exposures from cosmetic products could add a similar amount (NTP-CERHR, 2005). Estimated intakes in children are about twice that of adults (DiNovi and Howard, 2004). These estimated intakes are hundreds of times lower than occupational exposures, and well below doses known to cause nerve damage or carcinogenicity in animals, but are generally above the U.S. EPA reference dose of 0.2 µg/kg/day (U.S. EPA, 2006). Animal studies indicate that acrylamide is well absorbed, widely distributed in tissues, and is either metabolized to the reactive epoxide, glycidamide, or to glutathione conjugates (Calleman et al., 1990; Fennell et al., 2005). Elimination occurs mainly in the urine as mercapturic acid conjugates. Acrylamide is not thought to accumulate in the body at environmental doses, but can covalently bind to form adducts with proteins.

In humans, acrylamide has produced upper airway irritation following inhalation of high levels, ocular and dermal irritation from direct contact with acrylamide containing materials, and peripheral neuropathy following chronic

## Acrylamide

Geometric mean and selected percentiles of hemoglobin adduct concentrations (in pmol/g hemoglobin) for the U.S. population from the National Health and Nutrition Examination Survey.

| | Survey years | Geometric mean (95% conf. interval) | Selected percentiles (95% confidence interval) | | | | Sample size |
|---|---|---|---|---|---|---|---|
| | | | 50th | 75th | 90th | 95th | |
| Total | 03-04 | 61.2 (58.1-64.4) | 54.8 (52.8-57.7) | 79.1 (73.5-85.6) | 141 (124-155) | 192 (168-217) | 7101 |
| **Age group** | | | | | | | |
| 3-5 years | 03-04 | 59.4 (53.6-65.7) | 58.6 (51.7-64.9) | 75.7 (63.4-83.6) | 90.6 (81.9-105) | 108 (86.2-118) | 350 |
| 6-11 years | 03-04 | 58.6 (56.1-61.2) | 57.3 (55.2-59.7) | 71.0 (67.4-76.3) | 86.8 (81.2-91.4) | 98.8 (91.0-104) | 769 |
| 12-19 years | 03-04 | 57.4 (54.4-60.5) | 54.5 (52.1-57.4) | 70.7 (65.6-75.7) | 100 (89.2-114) | 132 (115-151) | 1889 |
| 20-59 years | 03-04 | 66.2 (62.2-70.6) | 57.9 (54.6-61.1) | 96.1 (83.6-108) | 163 (147-191) | 223 (194-243) | 2570 |
| 60 years and older | 03-04 | 50.1 (47.9-52.3) | 46.5 (44.0-49.2) | 61.0 (57.6-66.0) | 96.1 (88.0-108) | 141 (120-152) | 1523 |
| **Gender** | | | | | | | |
| Males | 03-04 | 63.9 (60.2-67.9) | 57.0 (53.7-60.1) | 85.5 (79.2-93.7) | 152 (139-175) | 220 (189-237) | 3509 |
| Females | 03-04 | 58.7 (55.9-61.5) | 53.4 (51.8-55.9) | 73.9 (69.5-80.6) | 126 (111-142) | 164 (147-191) | 3592 |
| **Race/ethnicity** | | | | | | | |
| Mexican Americans | 03-04 | 61.7 (58.7-64.9) | 57.4 (54.4-60.4) | 73.0 (69.2-77.3) | 101 (95.0-115) | 149 (125-179) | 1792 |
| Non-Hispanic blacks | 03-04 | 63.8 (57.3-71.1) | 57.1 (52.1-64.1) | 86.5 (74.6-104) | 156 (120-203) | 218 (172-271) | 1874 |
| Non-Hispanic whites | 03-04 | 62.4 (59.0-66.0) | 55.3 (53.0-58.6) | 82.2 (75.4-89.1) | 146 (129-163) | 197 (172-223) | 2994 |

Limit of detection (LOD, see Data Analysis section) for Survey year 03-04 is 3 0.

occupational exposures. Axonal degeneration, presynaptic nerve terminal binding (LoPachin, 2005), and neuronal DNA reactivity (Doerge et al., 2005) have been demonstrated in animals. Animal studies have shown that acrylamide can cause nerve damage (neuropathy), reproductive effects (reduced litter size, fetal death, male germinal cell injury, dominant lethality), and cancer (mammary, adrenal, thyroid, scrotal, uterine, and other sites) (FAO/WHO, 2005; NTP-CERHR, 2005, Rice, 2005; U.S. EPA, 2006). Glycidamide has been shown to react with DNA (Doerge et al., 2005; Klaunig et al., 2005; Maniere et al., 2005; Puppel et al., 2005), to increase the unscheduled synthesis of DNA in tumor susceptible tissues (Klaunig et al., 2005), and to increase DNA reactivity when glutathione availability is reduced (Klaunig et al., 2005; Puppel et al., 2005). In addition, altered gene expression in testicular tissues (Yang et al., 2005) and sperm DNA adducts (Xie et al., 2006) have been demonstrated after acrylamide dosing. Acrylamide is clastogenic and can produce dominant lethal mutations, probably through its epoxide metabolite, glycidamide (NTP-CERHR, 2005; U.S. EPA, 2006). IARC classifies acrylamide as probably carcinogenic to humans. Additional information is available from U.S. EPA at: http://www.epa. gov/iris/ and from the Food and Agriculture Organization of the United Nations and WHO at: http://www.who.int/ ipcs/food/jecfa/summaries/summary_report_64_final.pdf.

**Biomonitoring Information**

Acrylamide and glycidamide hemoglobin adducts (AHA and GHA, respectively) are markers of integrated acrylamide exposure over the preceding few months. Adducts are formed when either acrylamide or glycidamide react to form a permanent covalent bond with hemoglobin in the blood. After exposure ceases, levels of AHA adducts decline but may remain detectable for several months (Hagmar et al., 2001). AHA levels have been shown to increase with dietary intake (Hagmar et al., 2005, Vesper 2005) and smoking (Bergmark, 1997; Schettgen et al., 2002, 2004).

Levels of AHA and GHA reported the NHANES 2003-2004 sample are generally similar to those seen in several previous studies of non-occupationally exposed subjects (Bergmark et al., 1997; Hagmar et al., 2005; Schettgen et al., 2002, 2003, 2004; Vesper et al., 2006, 2008), although different analytic methods can affect results. Several of these studies have shown that smokers have adduct levels that are three to fourfold higher than non-smokers; most non-smokers had levels less than about 100 pmol/gram hemoglobin. The degree of formation of the more toxic glycidamide and levels of GHA can be influenced by polymorphisms in several of the enzymes that metabolize acrylamide (Duale et al., 2009). Younger children may have slightly higher levels possibly due to increased intake of acrylamide-containing foods relative to body size (Dybing et al., 2005, Mucci et al., 2008).

## Glycidamide

Geometric mean and selected percentiles of hemoglobin adduct concentrations (in pmol/g hemoglobin) for the U.S. population from the National Health and Nutrition Examination Survey.

| | Survey years | Geometric mean (95% conf. interval) | Selected percentiles ( 95% confidence interval) 50th | 75th | 90th | 95th | Sample size |
|---|---|---|---|---|---|---|---|
| Total | 03-04 | 59.3 (56.7-62.1) | 59.9 (57.6-62 5) | 85.9 (81.6-90 5) | 130 (120-141) | 167 (153-181) | 7278 |
| Age group | | | | | | | |
| 3-5 years | 03-04 | 71.6 (66.9-76.7) | 71.1 (66.9-78 9) | 94.7 (87.3-101) | 118 (103-126) | 126 (119-135) | 411 |
| 6-11 years | 03-04 | 74.1 (70.3-78 2) | 75.0 (70.9-77 9) | 95.6 (90.4-103) | 121 (112-134) | 141 (126-157) | 784 |
| 12-19 years | 03-04 | 55.4 (51.1-60.1) | 59.2 (56.1-62.1) | 79.2 (72.7-86.7) | 113 (94.9-138) | 146 (123-169) | 1931 |
| 20-59 years | 03-04 | 62.5 (59.4-65 8) | 60.9 (58.7-64.4) | 90.7 (84.4-98 2) | 143 (130-159) | 187 (169-204) | 2623 |
| 60 years and older | 03-04 | 45.5 (42.8-48 3) | 46.8 (44.8-49 3) | 65.2 (63.5-66 9) | 96.4 (90.0-103) | 129 (111-141) | 1529 |
| Gender | | | | | | | |
| Males | 03-04 | 59.5 (56.9-62 3) | 59.4 (56.8-61 8) | 87.1 (82.5-92 3) | 136 (123-148) | 174 (157-197) | 3604 |
| Females | 03-04 | 59.1 (56.0-62 5) | 60.4 (57.5-64 0) | 85.0 (80.2-90 0) | 125 (116-135) | 159 (143-175) | 3674 |
| Race/ethnicity | | | | | | | |
| Mexican Americans | 03-04 | 64.7 (61.2-68.4) | 65.4 (61.1-70.1) | 87.4 (81.5-94.4) | 118 (110-129) | 152 (135-170) | 1841 |
| Non-Hispanic blacks | 03-04 | 53.8 (51.1-56.7) | 56.0 (52.4-59.7) | 83.0 (75.2-91 5) | 121 (108-140) | 159 (129-204) | 1954 |
| Non-Hispanic whites | 03-04 | 61.1 (57.6-64 9) | 60.7 (57.9-64 2) | 87.5 (83.0-93 5) | 136 (124-149) | 172 (157-194) | 3044 |

Limit of detection (LOD, see Data Analysis section) for Survey year 03-04 is 4.0.

In occupational settings, AHA levels were several fold to several hundredfold higher than levels in non-exposed non-smokers (Bergmark et al., 1993; Hagmar et al., 2001; Perez et al., 1999). AHA levels correlated with a neurologic symptom index and specific physiologic measures in an occupational setting and correlated better with clinical signs and symptoms than urinary excretion of the mercapturic acid metabolite (Calleman et al., 1994). In another study, symptoms of numbness or tingling in the extremities did not occur in exposed workers whose AHA levels were below 510 pmol/gram hemoglobin, and 39% of workers with levels above 1000 pmol/gram hemoglobin had these symptoms (Hagmar et al., 2001).

Finding a measurable amount of acrylamide or glycidamide hemoglobin adducts in blood does not mean that these levels of acrylamide or glycidamide hemoglobin adducts cause adverse health effects. Biomonitoring studies of acrylamide or glycidamide hemoglobin adducts provide physicians and public health officials with reference values so that they can determine whether people have been exposed to higher levels of acrylamide than are found in the general population. Biomonitoring data can also help scientists plan and conduct research on exposure and health effects.

## References

Bergmark E, Calleman CJ, He F, Costa LG. Determination of hemoglobin adducts in humans occupationally exposed to acrylamide. Toxicol Appl Pharmacol 1993;120(1):45-54.

Bergmark E. Hemoglobin adducts of acrylamide and acrylonitrile in laboratory workers, smokers and nonsmokers. Chem Res Toxicol 1997 Jan;10(1):78-84.

Calleman CJ, Bergmark E, Costa LG. Acrylamide is metabolized to glycidamide in the rat: evidence from hemoglobin adduct formation. Chem Res Toxicol 1990;3:406-412.

Calleman CJ, Wu Y, He F, Tian G, Bergmark E, Zhang S, et al. Relationships between biomarkers of exposure and neurological effects in a group of workers exposed to acrylamide. Toxicol Appl Pharmacol 1994;126(2):361-371.

DiNovi M and Howard D. The Updated Exposure Assessment for Acrylamide. 2004 Acrylamide in Food Workshop: Update - Scientific Issues, Uncertainties, and Research Strategies. April 13-15, 2004, Chicago, Illinois.

Doerge DR, da Costa GG, McDaniel LP, Churchwell MI, Twaddle NC, Beland FA. DNA adducts derived from administration of acrylamide and glycidamide to mice and rats. Mutat Res 2005;580(1-2):131-141.

Duale N, Bjellaas T, Alexander J, Becher G, Haugen M, Paulsen JE, et al. Biomarkers of human exposure to acrylamide and relation to polymorphisms in metabolizing genes. Toxicol Sci. 2009 Jan 8. [Epub ahead of print]

Dybing E, Farmer PB, Andersen M, Fennell TR, et al. Human exposure and internal dose assessments of acrylamide in food. Food Chem. Toxicol 2005;43:365–410.

Fennell TR, Summer SCJ, Snyder RW, Burgess J, Spicer R, Bridson WE, et al. Metabolism and hemoglobin adduct formation of acrylamide in humans. Toxicol Sci 2005;85:447-459.

Food and Drug Administration (FDA). Survey data on acrylamide in food: individual food products. CFSAN/Office of Plant and Dairy Foods. July, 2006. Available at URL: http://www.cfsan.fda.gov/~dms/acrydata.html#u1004. 2/3/09

Hagmar L, Tornqvist M, Nordander C, Rosen I, Bruze M, Kautiainen A, Magnusson AL, Malmberg B, Aprea P, Granath F, Axmon A. Health effects of occupational exposure to acrylamide using hemoglobin adducts as biomarkers of internal dose. Scand J Work Environ Health 2001;27(4):219-226.

Hagmar L, Wirfalt E, Paulsson B, Tornqvist M. Differences in hemoglobin adduct levels of acrylamide in the general population with respect to dietary intake, smoking habits and gender. Mutat Res 2005;580(1-2):157-165.

Joint FAO/WHO Expert Committee on Food Additives, 64th Meeting: Summary and Conclusions (FAO/WHO). Rome, Italy, 8-17 February 2005. Available at URL: http://www.who.int/ipcs/food/jecfa/summaries/summary_report_64_final.pdf. 2/3/09

Klaunig JE, Kamendulis LM. Mechanisms of acrylamide induced rodent carcinogenesis. Adv Exp Med Biol 2005;561:49-62.

LoPachin RM. Acrylamide neurotoxicity: neurological, morphological and molecular endpoints in animal models. Adv Exp Med Biol 2005;561:21-37.

Maniere I, Godard T, Doerge DR, Churchwell MI, Guffroy M, Laurentie M, et al. DNA damage and DNA adduct formation in rat tissues following oral administration of acrylamide. Mutat Res 2005;580(1-2):119-129.

Mucci LA, Wilson KM. Acrylamide intake through diet and human cancer risk. J Agric Food Chem 2008;56, 6013-6019.

National Toxicology Program, Center for the Evaluation of Risks to Human Reproduction (NTP-CERHR). Monograph on the Potential Human Reproductive and Developmental Effects of Acrylamide. February, 2005. NIH Publication No. 05-4472. Available at URL: http://cerhr.niehs.nih.gov/chemicals/acrylamide/Acrylamide_Monograph.pdf. 2/3/09

Perez HL, Cheong HK, Yang JS, Osterman-Golkar S. Simultaneous analysis of hemoglobin adducts of acrylamide and glycidamide by gas chromatography-mass spectrometry. Anal Biochem 1999;274(1):59-68.

Puppel N, Tjaden Z, Fueller F, Marko D. DNA strand breaking capacity of acrylamide and glycidamide in mammalian cells. Mutat Res 2005;580(1-2):71-80.

Rice JM. The carcinogenicity of acrylamide. Mutat Res 2005 Feb 7;580(1-2):3-20.

Schettgen T, Broding HC, Angerer J, Drexler H. Hemoglobin adducts of ethylene oxide, propylene oxide, acrylonitrile and acrylamide-biomarkers in occupational and environmental medicine. Toxicol Lett 2002;134(1-3):65-70.

Schettgen T, Rossbach B, Kutting B, Letzel S, Drexler H, Angerer J. Determination of haemoglobin adducts of acrylamide and glycidamide in smoking and non-smoking persons of the general population. Int J Hyg Environ Health 2004;207(6):531-9.

Schettgen T, Weiss T, Drexler H, Angerer J. A first approach to estimate the internal exposure to acrylamide in smoking and non-smoking adults from Germany. Int J Hyg Environ Health 2003;206(1):9-14.

Tareke E, Rydberg P, Karlsson P, Eriksson S, Tornqvist M. Analysis of acrylamide, a carcinogen formed in heated foodstuffs. J Agric Food Chem 2002;50(17):4998-5006.

U.S. Environmental Protection Agency (U.S. EPA). Acrylamide. Integrated Risk Information System (IRIS), revised 1/3/06. Available at URL: http://www.epa.gov/iris/subst/0286 htm, 2/3/09.

U.S. Environmental Protection Agency (U.S. EPA). Office of Pollution Prevention and Toxics. Chemical Summary for Acrylamide. Washington (DC), September, 1994. Available at URL: http://www.epa.gov/chemfact/s_acryla.txt. 2/3/09

Vesper HW, Ospina M, Meyers T, Ingham L, Smith A, Gray JG, et al. Automated method for measuring globin adducts of acrylamide and glycidamide at optimized Edman reaction conditions. Rapid Commun Mass Spectrom 2006;20(6):959-64.

Vesper HW, Licea-Perez H, Meyers T, Ospina M, Myers GL. Pilot study on the impact of potato chips consumption on biomarkers of acrylamide exposure. Adv Exp Med Biol 2005;561:89-96.

Vesper HW, Slimani N, Hallmans G, Tjønneland A, Agudo A, Benetou V, et al. Cross-sectional study on acrylamide hemoglobin adducts in subpopulations from the European Prospective Investigation into Cancer and Nutrition (EPIC) Study. J Agric Food Chem 2008;56(15):6046-53.

Xie Q, Sun H, Liu Y, Ding X, Fu D, Liu K. Adduction of biomacromolecules with acrylamide (AA) in mice at environmental dose levels studied by accelerator mass spectrometry. Toxicol Lett 2006;163(2):101-8.

Yang HJ, Lee SH, Jin Y, Choi JH, Han DU, Chae C, Lee MH, Han CH. Toxicological effects of acrylamide on rat testicular gene expression profile. Reprod Toxicol 2005;19(4):527-34.

# Cotinine

CAS No. 486-56-6

*Metabolite of nicotine (a component of tobacco smoke)*

## General Information

Tobacco use is the most important preventable cause of premature morbidity and mortality in the United States. The consequences of smoking and of using smokeless tobacco products are well known and include an increased risk for several types of cancer, emphysema, acute respiratory illness, cardiovascular disease, stroke, and various other disorders (U.S. DHHS, 2006). Persons exposed to secondhand tobacco smoke (environmental

tobacco smoke [ETS]) may have adverse health effects that include lung cancer and coronary heart disease; maternal exposure during pregnancy can result in lower birth weight. Children exposed to ETS are at increased risk for sudden infant death syndrome, acute respiratory infections, ear problems, and exacerbated asthma (U.S. DHHS, 2004). The smoke produced by burning tobacco contains at least 250 chemicals that are toxic or carcinogenic, and more than 50 compounds present in ETS are known or reasonably anticipated to be human carcinogens (NTP, 2004).

Cigarettes contain about 1.5% nicotine by weight (Kozlowski et al., 1998), producing roughly 1–2 mg of bioavailable nicotine per cigarette (Benowitz and Jacob,

## Serum Cotinine

*Metabolite of nicotine (component of tobacco smoke)*

Geometric mean and selected percentiles of serum concentrations (in ng/mL) for the **non-smoking** U.S. population from the National Health and Nutrition Examination Survey.

| | Survey years | Geometric mean (95% conf. interval) | 50th | 75th | 90th | 95th | Sample size |
|---|---|---|---|---|---|---|---|
| **Total** | 99-00 | * | .060 (<LOD- 080) | .240 (.190-.302) | 1.02 (.770-1 28) | 1.96 (1.60-2 62) | 5999 |
| | 01-02** | .062 (.050-.077) | < LOD | .160 (.120-.220) | .930 (.740-1.17) | 2.20 (1.83-2.44) | 6819 |
| | 03-04 | .071 (.057-.089) | .050 (.040-.070) | .210 (.140-.310) | .990 (.740-1 30) | 2.17 (1.81-2 54) | 6320 |
| **Age group** | | | | | | | |
| 3-11 years | 99-00 | .164 (.115-.234) | .110 (.066-.188) | .500 (.260-1.16) | 1.88 (.997-3.44) | 3.44 (1.42-4.79) | 1174 |
| | 01-02** | .110 (.076-.160) | .070 (<LOD-.130) | .570 (.310-1 00) | 2.23 (1.63-2.78) | 3.23 (2.53-4 01) | 1415 |
| | 03-04 | .137 (.088-.213) | .120 (.060-.220) | .620 (.310-1 20) | 2.04 (1.38-2 94) | 3.35 (2.12-4 68) | 1252 |
| 12-19 years | 99-00 | .163 (.142-.187) | .110 (.080-.163) | .540 (.428-.660) | 1.66 (1.50-1 95) | 2.62 (2.09-3 39) | 1773 |
| | 01-02** | .086 (.059-.126) | .050 (<LOD-.110) | .350 (.190-.580) | 1.53 (1.09-2.12) | 3.12 (2.47-3 99) | 1902 |
| | 03-04 | .110 (.087-.139) | .080 (.060-.120) | .510 (.350-.670) | 1.55 (1.21-1 93) | 2.68 (1.96-4 02) | 1783 |
| 20 years and older | 99-00 | * | .050 (<LOD- 061) | .167 (.140-.193) | .630 (.533-.820) | 1.50 (1.28-1 66) | 3052 |
| | 01-02** | .052 (<LOD- 063) | < LOD | .110 (.090-.150) | .630 (.470-.790) | 1.42 (1.14-1 89) | 3502 |
| | 03-04 | .058 (.047-.071) | .040 (.030-.050) | .140 (.100-.200) | .630 (.480-.840) | 1.54 (1.26-1 92) | 3285 |
| **Gender** | | | | | | | |
| Males | 99-00 | .124 (.106-.145) | .080 (.060-.110) | .308 (.220-.410) | 1.20 (.950-1.49) | 2.39 (1.66-3 22) | 2789 |
| | 01-02** | .075 (.059-.094) | .050 (<LOD- 070) | .230 (.160-.320) | 1.17 (.960-1.49) | 2.44 (2.23-2 99) | 3152 |
| | 03-04 | .087 (.070-.108) | .060 (.040-.080) | .280 (.190-.360) | 1.23 (.910-1 68) | 2.63 (2.09-3.19) | 2937 |
| Females | 99-00 | * | < LOD | .180 (.148-.230) | .850 (.600-1.14) | 1.85 (1.33-2.45) | 3210 |
| | 01-02** | .053 (<LOD- 066) | < LOD | .120 (.090-.180) | .710 (.540-.990) | 1.77 (1.32-2 20) | 3667 |
| | 03-04 | .060 (.047-.077) | .040 (.030-.060) | .160 (.110-.260) | .860 (.580-1.15) | 1.76 (1.32-2 22) | 3383 |
| **Race/ethnicity** | | | | | | | |
| Mexican Americans | 99-00 | * | < LOD | .140 (.110-.180) | .506 (.370-.726) | 1.21 (.900-1.70) | 2241 |
| | 01-02** | .060 (<LOD- 084) | < LOD | .160 (.080-.310) | .730 (.480-1.19) | 2.12 (1.19-2 96) | 1878 |
| | 03-04 | .054 (.043-.068) | .030 (.020-.050) | .120 (.080-.180) | .690 (.430-1 00) | 2.65 (1.87-3 57) | 1707 |
| Non-Hispanic blacks | 99-00 | .175 (.153-.201) | .131 (.111-.150) | .505 (.400-.625) | 1.43 (1.21-1.75) | 2.34 (1.84-3 50) | 1333 |
| | 01-02** | .164 (.137-.197) | .130 (.110-.160) | .580 (.450-.770) | 1.77 (1.55-2 05) | 3.15 (2.50-4 30) | 1602 |
| | 03-04 | .144 (.104-.198) | .120 (.080-.180) | .520 (.350-.770) | 1.54 (1.20-2.14) | 2.77 (2.18-3 54) | 1704 |
| Non-Hispanic whites | 99-00 | * | .050 (<LOD- 073) | .216 (.154-.312) | .950 (.621-1.40) | 1.92 (1.48-3 02) | 1950 |
| | 01-02** | .052 (<LOD- 068) | < LOD | .120 (.090-.180) | .800 (.570-1.11) | 1.88 (1.48-2 30) | 2847 |
| | 03-04 | .066 (.050-.087) | .040 (.030-.070) | .180 (.120-.300) | .920 (.620-1 32) | 2.01 (1.70-2.49) | 2500 |

Limit of detection (LOD, see Data Analysis section) for Survey years 99-00, and 03-04 are 0.05, and 0.015, respectively.

** In the 2001-2002 survey period, 83% of measurements had an LOD of 0.015 ng/mL, and 17% had an LOD of 0.05 ng/mL.

< LOD means less than the limit of detection, which may vary for some chemicals by year and by individual sample.

* Not calculated: proportion of results below limit of detection was too high to provide a valid result.

1994; Hukkanen et al., 2005). Inhaling tobacco smoke from either active or passive (ETS) smoking is the main source of nicotine exposure for the general population. Up to 90% of the nicotine delivered in tobacco smoke is absorbed rapidly from the lungs into the blood stream (Armitage et al., 1975; Iwase et al., 1991). Mean air concentrations of nicotine in public spaces where smoking is allowed range from 0.3 to 30 $\mu g/m^3$, with higher levels measured in restaurants and bars. In homes with one or more smokers, mean air concentrations typically range from 2 to 14 $\mu g/m^3$ (NTP, 2004). For an adult, the primary sources for ETS exposure are in a workplace where smoking occurs and in a residence shared with one or more smokers. Children are primarily exposed to ETS by parents and caregivers who smoke.

Nicotine can also be absorbed from the gastrointestinal tract and skin by using snuff, chewing tobacco, or chewing gum, nasal sprays, or skin patches that contain nicotine. Workers who harvest tobacco can be exposed to nicotine and become intoxicated as a result of the transdermal absorption of nicotine contained in the plant. The tobacco plant, *Nicotiana tabacum*, contains nicotine in larger amounts than other nicotine-containing plants, which include potatoes, tomatoes, eggplants, and peppers. Nicotine is also used commercially as an insecticide in its sulfate and alkaloid forms.

Once absorbed, nicotine has a half-life in blood plasma of several hours (Benowitz, 1996). Cotinine, the primary metabolite of nicotine, is currently regarded as the best biomarker in active smokers and in nonsmokers exposed to ETS. Measuring cotinine is preferred over measuring nicotine because cotinine persists longer in the body with a plasma half-life of about 16 hours (Benowitz and Jacob, 1994). However, non-Hispanic blacks metabolize cotinine more slowly than do non-Hispanic whites (Benowitz et al., 1999; Perez-Stable et al., 1998). Cotinine can be measured in serum, urine, saliva, and hair. Nonsmokers exposed to typical levels of ETS have serum cotinine levels of less than 1 ng/mL, with heavy exposure to ETS producing levels in the 1–10 ng/mL range. Active smokers almost always have levels higher than 10 ng/mL and sometimes higher than 500 ng/mL (Hukkanen et al., 2005).

Nicotine stimulates preganglionic cholinergic receptors within peripheral sympathetic autonomic ganglia and at cholinergic sites within the central nervous system. Acute tobacco or nicotine intoxication can produce dizziness, nausea, vomiting, diaphoresis, salivation, diarrhea, variable changes in blood pressure and heart rate, seizures, and death. Nicotine also indirectly causes a release of dopamine in the brain regions that control pleasure and motivation, a process involved in the development of addiction. Symptoms of nicotine withdrawal include irritability, craving, cognitive and sleep disturbances, and increased appetite.

The IARC and the NTP consider tobacco smoke to be a human carcinogen. NIOSH guidelines consider ETS to be a potential occupational carcinogen and recommend that exposure be reduced to the lowest feasible concentration. The Federal Aviation Administration has banned the smoking of tobacco products on both domestic and foreign air carrier flights in the United States. More information about the effects of smoking and nicotine can be found at: http://www.nida.nih.gov/researchreports/nicotine/nicotine.html.

**Biomonitoring Information**

Serum cotinine levels reflect recent exposure to nicotine in tobacco smoke. Nonsmoking is usually defined as a serum cotinine level of less than or equal to 10 ng/mL (Pirkle et al., 1996).

The serum cotinine levels seen in the NHANES 2003-2004 appear approximately similar to levels seen in the previous survey period (NHANES 2001-2002) for the total population estimates. Serum cotinine has been measured in many studies of nonsmoking populations, with levels showing similar or slightly higher results (depending on the degree of ETS exposure) than those reported in the previous NHANES (CDC 2005; NCI, 1999). Over the previous decade, levels of exposure to ETS appeared to decrease since geometric mean cotinine serum concentrations in nonsmokers had fallen by approximately 70% and the rate of detectable cotinine in nonsmokers fell from 88% to 43% when NHANES 1988–1991 was compared to NHANES 1999–2002, (CDC, 2005; Pirkle et al., 2006). The overall decline in population estimates of serum cotinine likely reflects decreased ETS exposure among nonsmokers in locations with smoke-free laws (Pickett et al., 2006; Soliman et al., 2004). During each previous NHANES survey, the adjusted geometric mean serum cotinine was higher in children (aged 4–11 years) than in adults among both non-Hispanic blacks and non-Hispanic whites (Pirkle et al., 2006). Non-Hispanic blacks had higher serum cotinine concentrations compared with either non-Hispanic whites or Mexican-Americans. Higher levels of cotinine have previously been reported for non-Hispanic black smokers (Caraballo et al., 1998). Differences in cotinine concentrations among race/ethnicity and age groups may be influenced by pharmacokinetic differences as well as by ETS exposure (Benowitz et al., 1999; Hukkanen et al., 2005; Wilson et al., 2005).

Biomonitoring studies of serum cotinine will help physicians and public health officials determine whether people have been exposed to higher levels of ETS than are found in the general population. Biomonitoring data can also help scientists plan and conduct research about exposure to ETS and about its health effects.

## References

Armitage AK, Dollery CT, George CF, Houseman TH, Lewis PJ, Turner DM. Absorption and metabolism of nicotine from cigarettes. BMJ 1975;4:313-316.

Benowitz NL. Cotinine as a biomarker of environmental tobacco smoke exposure. Epidemiol Rev 1996;18:188-204.

Benowitz NL, Jacob P. Metabolism of nicotine to cotinine studied by a dual stable isotope method. Clin Pharmacol Ther 1994;56:483-493.

Benowitz NL, Perez-Stable EJ, Fong I, Modin G, Herrera B, Jacob P III. Ethnic differences in N-glucuronidation of nicotine and cotinine. J Pharmacol Exp Ther 1999;291(3):1196-1203.

Caraballo R, Giovino G, Pechacek TF, Mowery PD, Richter PA, Strauss WJ, et al. Racial/ethnic differences in serum cotinine levels among adult U.S. cigarette smokers: the Third National Health and Nutrition Examination Survey, 1988-1991. JAMA 1998;280:135-140.

Centers for Disease Control, National Institute for Occupational Safety and Hygiene (NIOSH). Current Intelligence Bulletin 54: Environmental tobacco smoke in the workplace. June, 1991. available at URL: http://mtn.niosh.cdc.gov/eid/rmca/critdocs/criteriadoc/33.pdf. 4/13/09

Centers for Disease Control and Prevention (CDC). Third National Report on Human Exposure to Environmental Chemicals. Atlanta (GA): 2005.

Hukkanen J, Jacob III P, Benowitz NL. Metabolism and disposition kinetics of nicotine. Pharmacol Rev 2005;57(1):79-115.

International Agency for Research on Cancer. IARC Working Group on the Evaluation of Carcinogenic Risks to Humans. Tobacco Smoke. IARC Monogr Eval Carcinog Risks Hum. Vol 38. Summary of Data Reported and Evaluation [online] 1986. Available at URL: http://monographs.iarc.fr/ENG/Monographs/allmonos90.php. 4/13/09

International Agency for Research on Cancer. IARC Working Group on the Evaluation of Carcinogenic Risks to Humans. Tobacco Smoke and Involuntary Smoking. IARC Monogr Eval Carcinog Risks Hum. Vol 83. Summary of Data Reported and Evaluation [online] 2004. Available at URL: http://monographs.iarc.fr/ENG/Monographs/allmonos90.php. 4/13/09

Iwase A, Aiba M, Kira S. Respiratory nicotine absorption in non-smoking females during passive smoking. Int Arch Occup Environ Health 1991;63:139-43.

Kozlowski LT, Mehta NY, Sweeney CT, Schwartz SS, Vogler GP, Jarvis MJ, et al. Filter ventilation and nicotine content of tobacco in cigarettes from Canada, the United Kingdom, and the United States. Tob Control 1998;7:369-375.

National Toxicology Program (NTP). Tobacco related exposures. In Report on Carcinogens. 11th ed. [online]. 2004. Available at URL: http://ntp niehs nih.gov/ntp/roc/eleventh/profiles/s176toba.pdf. 4/13/09

National Cancer Institute (NCI). Health Effects of Exposure to Environmental Tobacco Smoke: The Report of the California Environmental Protection Agency. Smoking and Tobacco Control Monograph 10 [online]. 1999. Available at URL: http://cancercontrol.cancer.gov/tcrb/monographs/10/. 4/13/09

Perez-Stable EJ, Herrera B, Jacob P III, Benowitz NL. Nicotine metabolism and intake in black and white smokers. JAMA 1998;280:152-156.

Pickett MA, Schober SE, Brody DJ, Curtin LR, Giovino GA. Smoke-free laws and secondhand smoke exposure in US non-smoking adults, 1999-2002. Tob Control 2006;15:302-307.

Pirkle JL, Bernert JT, Caudill SP, Sosnoff CS, Pechacek TF. Trends in the exposure of nonsmokers in the U.S. population to secondhand smoke: 1988-2002. Environ Health Perspect 2006;114(6):853-858.

Pirkle JL, Flegal KM, Bernert JT, Brody DJ, Etzel RA, Maurer KR. Exposure of the U.S. population to environmental tobacco smoke: the Third National Health and Nutrition Examination Survey, 1988-1991. JAMA 1996;275:1233-1240.

Soliman S, Pollack HA, Warner K. Decrease in the prevalence of environmental tobacco smoke exposure in the home during the 1990s in families with children. Am J Public Health 2004;94(2):314-320.

U.S Department of Health and Human Services (U.S. DHHS). The Health Consequences of Involuntary Exposure to Tobacco Smoke: A Report of the Surgeon General — Executive Summary. U.S. Department of Heath and Human Services, Centers for Disease Control and Prevention, Coordinating Center for Health Promotion, National Center for Chronic Disease Prevention and Health Promotion, Office on Smoking and Health [online] 2006. Available at URL: http://www.surgeongeneral.gov/library/secondhandsmoke/. 4/13/09

U.S Department of Health and Human Services (U.S. DHHS). The Health Consequences of Smoking: The Surgeon General's Report—Executive Summary. U.S. Department of Heath and Human Services, Centers for Disease Control and Prevention, Coordinating Center for Health Promotion, National Center for

Chronic Disease Prevention and Health Promotion, Office on Smoking and Health. [online]. 2004. Available at URL: http://www.cdc.gov/tobacco/data_statistics/sgr/sgr_2004/index.htm#full. 4/13/09

Wilson SE, Kahn RS, Khoury J Lanphear BP. Racial differences in exposure to environmental tobacco smoke among children. Environ Health Perspect 2005;113(3):362-367.

# N,N-Diethyl-*meta*-toluamide (DEET)

CAS No. 134-62-3

## General Information

N,N-diethyl-*meta*-toluamide (DEET) is an insect repellent that was first marketed in 1957. DEET can be applied to clothing and the skin to repel biting insects. Its use is recommended for prevention of several vector-borne diseases. There are over 225 insect repellents brands containing DEET, and they range in concentration from 4% to 100%. DEET is also used in combination with dermal sun screens (U.S.EPA, 1998). DEET is not registered for use on agricultural commodities. One survey detected DEET in 74% of sampled streams in the U.S. (Kolpin et al., 2002).

General population exposure to DEET occurs from skin application and from inhalation of aerosol formulations. Exposure can also occur from consuming food contaminated by DEET on hands or that was sprayed nearby. About 3-8% of dermally applied DEET is absorbed, but higher DEET concentrations and different formulations may result in greater absorption (Sudakin and Trevathan, 2003). After absorption, DEET is metabolized via hydroxylation and dealkylation pathways and eliminated in the urine within approximately 24 hours (Selim et al., 1995; Sudakin and Trevathan, 2003). People in outdoor occupations may apply DEET more frequently or use higher concentration formulations resulting in higher levels of exposure.

Human health effects from DEET at low environmental doses or at biomonitored levels from low environmental exposures are unknown. DEET has low acute toxicity. Most reports of adverse effects from overexposure to DEET involve skin reactions (Bell et al., 2002). Neurological effects in humans, including seizures and encephalopathy, have been reported as result of self-poisoning by ingestion or excessive dermal application, (U.S. EPA, 1998). DEET is not a developmental or reproductive toxicant in animals (U.S.EPA, 2005). DEET is not genotoxic, and it has not been rated by IARC or NTP with respect to human carcinogenicity. Additional information is available from U.S.EPA at: http://www.epa.gov/pesticides/.

## Urinary N,N-Diethyl-*meta*-toluamide (DEET)

Geometric mean and selected percentiles of urine concentrations (in µg/L) for the U.S. population from the National Health and Nutrition Examination Survey.

| | Survey years | Geometric mean (95% conf. interval) | Selected percentiles ( 95% confidence interval) | | | | Sample size |
|---|---|---|---|---|---|---|---|
| | | | 50th | 75th | 90th | 95th | |
| Total | 99-00 | * | < LOD | < LOD | < LOD | < LOD | 1977 |
| | 01-02 | * | < LOD | < LOD | .110 (.100-.140) | .180 (.140-.220) | 2535 |
| **Age group** | | | | | | | |
| 6-11 years | 99-00 | * | < LOD | < LOD | < LOD | < LOD | 480 |
| | 01-02 | * | < LOD | < LOD | .130 (.100-.180) | .210 (.120-.560) | 580 |
| 12-19 years | 99-00 | * | < LOD | < LOD | < LOD | < LOD | 672 |
| | 01-02 | * | < LOD | < LOD | .130 (.110-.160) | .220 (.130-.520) | 829 |
| 20-59 years | 99-00 | * | < LOD | < LOD | < LOD | < LOD | 825 |
| | 01-02 | * | < LOD | < LOD | .110 (<LOD-.130) | .170 (.120-.210) | 1126 |
| **Gender** | | | | | | | |
| Males | 99-00 | * | < LOD | < LOD | < LOD | < LOD | 964 |
| | 01-02 | * | < LOD | < LOD | .110 (.100-.150) | .180 (.130-.250) | 1191 |
| Females | 99-00 | * | < LOD | < LOD | < LOD | < LOD | 1013 |
| | 01-02 | * | < LOD | < LOD | .110 (.100-.130) | .170 (.130-.210) | 1344 |
| **Race/ethnicity** | | | | | | | |
| Mexican Americans | 99-00 | * | < LOD | < LOD | < LOD | < LOD | 688 |
| | 01-02 | * | < LOD | < LOD | .110 (<LOD-.140) | .130 (.110-.190) | 678 |
| Non-Hispanic blacks | 99-00 | * | < LOD | < LOD | < LOD | < LOD | 518 |
| | 01-02 | * | < LOD | < LOD | .100 (<LOD-.140) | .140 (.100-.240) | 700 |
| Non-Hispanic whites | 99-00 | * | < LOD | < LOD | < LOD | < LOD | 598 |
| | 01-02 | * | < LOD | < LOD | .110 (.100-.140) | .180 (.130-.270) | 956 |

Limit of detection (LOD, see Data Analysis section) for Survey years 99-00 and 01-02 are 0.449 and 0.1.
< LOD means less than the limit of detection, which may vary for some chemicals by year and by individual sample.
* Not calculated: proportion of results below limit of detection was too high to provide a valid result.

## Biomonitoring Information

Urinary levels of DEET reflect recent exposure. Urinary levels of DEET were characterized only at the 90th and 95th percentiles of the U.S. representative subsamples from NHANES 2001-2002. In this survey period, the limit of detection was lower than for the NHANES 1999-2000 survey period (CDC, 2005). DEET was detected in 10% of 60 Latino children in eastern North Carolina farm worker households (Arcury et al., 2007). Urinary DEET levels as high as 5,690 µg/L were measured in eight park employees who applied 71% DEET once a day (Smallwood et al., 1992).

Finding a measurable amount of DEET in urine does not mean that the level of DEET causes an adverse health effect. Biomonitoring studies on levels of DEET provide physicians and public health officials with reference values so that they can determine whether people have been exposed to higher levels of DEET than are found in the general population. Biomonitoring data can also help scientists plan and conduct research on exposure and health effects.

### Urinary N,N-Diethyl-*meta*-toluamide (DEET) (creatinine corrected)

Geometric mean and selected percentiles of urine concentrations (in µg/g of creatinine) for the U.S. population from the National Health and Nutrition Examination Survey.

| | Survey years | Geometric mean (95% conf. interval) | Selected percentiles (95% confidence interval) | | | | Sample size |
|---|---|---|---|---|---|---|---|
| | | | 50th | 75th | 90th | 95th | |
| Total | 99-00 | * | < LOD | < LOD | < LOD | < LOD | 1977 |
| | 01-02 | * | < LOD | < LOD | .270 ( 240-.300) | .410 ( 350-.500) | 2534 |
| **Age group** | | | | | | | |
| 6-11 years | 99-00 | * | < LOD | < LOD | < LOD | < LOD | 480 |
| | 01-02 | * | < LOD | < LOD | .330 ( 230-.630) | .640 ( 280-1.93) | 580 |
| 12-19 years | 99-00 | * | < LOD | < LOD | < LOD | < LOD | 672 |
| | 01-02 | * | < LOD | < LOD | .190 (.150-.240) | .250 (.190-.490) | 828 |
| 20-59 years | 99-00 | * | < LOD | < LOD | < LOD | < LOD | 825 |
| | 01-02 | * | < LOD | < LOD | .270 (<LOD-.320) | .410 ( 370-.500) | 1126 |
| **Gender** | | | | | | | |
| Males | 99-00 | * | < LOD | < LOD | < LOD | < LOD | 964 |
| | 01-02 | * | < LOD | < LOD | .200 (.170-.250) | .320 ( 250-.440) | 1191 |
| Females | 99-00 | * | < LOD | < LOD | < LOD | < LOD | 1013 |
| | 01-02 | * | < LOD | < LOD | .330 ( 290-.370) | .500 (.410-.580) | 1343 |
| **Race/ethnicity** | | | | | | | |
| Mexican Americans | 99-00 | * | < LOD | < LOD | < LOD | < LOD | 688 |
| | 01-02 | * | < LOD | < LOD | .190 (<LOD-.230) | .280 ( 230-.350) | 678 |
| Non-Hispanic blacks | 99-00 | * | < LOD | < LOD | < LOD | < LOD | 518 |
| | 01-02 | * | < LOD | < LOD | .130 (<LOD-.150) | .190 (.140-.270) | 699 |
| Non-Hispanic whites | 99-00 | * | < LOD | < LOD | < LOD | < LOD | 598 |
| | 01-02 | * | < LOD | < LOD | .300 ( 270-.350) | .480 ( 390-.550) | 956 |

< LOD means less than the limit of detection for the urine levels not corrected for creatinine.
* Not calculated: proportion of results below limit of detection was too high to provide a valid result.

## References

Arcury TA, Grzywacz JG, Barr DB, Tapia J, Chen H, Quandt SA. Pesticide urinary metabolite levels of children in eastern North Carolina farmworker households. Environ Health Perspect 2007;115(8):1254-1260.

Bell JW, Veltri JC, Page BC. Human exposures to N,N-diethyl-*m*-toluamide insect repellents reported to the American Association of Poison Control Centers, 1993-1997. Int J Toxicol 2002;2:341-352.

Centers for Disease Control and Prevention (CDC). Third National Report on Human Exposure to Environmental Chemicals. Atlanta (GA). 2005

Kolpin DW, Furlong ET, Meyer MT, Thurman EM, Zaugg SD, Barber LB, et al. Pharmaceuticals, hormones, and other organic wastewater contaminants in U.S. streams, 1999-2000: a national reconnaissance. Environ Sci Technol 2002;36(6):1202-1211.

Selim S, Hartnagel RE Jr, Osimitz TG, Gabriel KL, Schoenig GP. Absorption, metabolism, and excretion of N,N-diethyl-*m*-toluamide following dermal application to human volunteers. Fundam Appl Toxicol 1995;25:95-100.

Smallwood AW, DeBord KE, Lowry LK. N,N'-diethyl-*m*-toluamide (*m*-DET): analysis of an insect repellent in human urine and serum by high-performance liquid chromatography. J Anal Toxicol 1992;16(1):10-13.

Sudakin DL, Trevathan WR. DEET: a review and update of safety and risk in the general population. J Toxicol Clin Toxicol 2003;41(6):831-839.

U.S. Environmental Protection Agency (U.S.EPA). Diethyltoluamide (DEET). Chemical Summary. U.S.EPA, Toxicity and Exposure Assessment in Children's Health. 2005. Available at URL: http://www.epa.gov/teach/chem_summ/DEET_summary.pdf. 4/9/09

U.S. Environmental Protection Agency (U.S.EPA). Reregistration Eligibility Decision (RED): DEET. EPA 738-R-98-010. Washington (DC): U.S. EPA; September 1998. pp. 1-118. Available at URL: http://www.epa.gov/oppsrrd1/REDs/0002red.pdf. 4/9/09

# Disinfection By-Products (Trihalomethanes)

**Bromodichloromethane** CAS No. 75-27-4

**Dibromochloromethane (Chlorodibromomethane)**
CAS No. 124-48-1

**Tribromomethane (Bromoform)** CAS No. 75-25-2

**Trichloromethane (Chloroform)** CAS No. 57-57-8

## General Information

Disinfection by-products (DBP) are a class of chemical by-products also referred to as trihalomethanes (THMs), formed when chlorine or bromine interacts with the natural organic materials found in water. DBPs also include other formed products, such as haloacetic acids, haloacetonitriles, haloketones, and chlorophenols. The composition and levels of specific DBPs are determined by water quality, water treatment conditions, and disinfectant type (IPCS, 2000). Primary sources of DBPs are chlorinated drinking water and recreational water bodies, such as swimming pools.

In drinking water, trichloromethane is the predominant DBP, usually found at much higher levels than bromodichloromethane; tribromomethane is the least abundant (Krasner et al., 1989). DBPs are volatile at room temperature and can be detected in ambient air during activities such as showering, bathing, dishwashing, and swimming (Backer, et al., 2000; Gordon et al., 2006). Trichloromethane has industrial applications and is used to produce refrigerants and feedstock. It may be released into the environment where chlorine-based chemicals are used for bleaching and disinfecting processes or disposed at hazardous waste sites (IPCS, 2004; LaRegina, et al. 1986). Tribromomethane has limited industrial uses, mainly in geological assaying, electronics manufacturing, and as a solvent in laboratory analyses (ATSDR, 2005). DBPs tend not to bioaccumulate in aquatic organisms or persist in open or surface waters or soils, but they can remain in water within closed pipe systems. Workplace exposure may occur during the production of trichloromethane or tribromomethane, or in workplaces where DBPs may be generated, such as pulp or paper manufacturing, swimming pools, and water treatment plants (IPCS, 2004).

General population exposure to DBPs occurs primarily through ingesting chlorinated water and inhaling the water

## Blood Bromodichloromethane

Geometric mean and selected percentiles of blood concentrations (in pg/mL) for the U.S. population from the National Health and Nutrition Examination Survey.

| | Survey years# | Geometric mean (95% conf. interval) | Selected percentiles (95% confidence interval) | | | | Sample size |
|---|---|---|---|---|---|---|---|
| | | | 50th | 75th | 90th | 95th | |
| **Total** | 01-02 | 2.21 (1.65-2 97) | 2.30 (1.56-3 21) | 4.63 (3.24-6 20) | 8.45 (5.86-12.0) | 12.0 (7.68-19.2) | 785 |
| | 03-04 | 1.50 (1.20-1 86) | 1.40 (1.10-1 90) | 3.40 (2.60-4 20) | 6.20 (5.30-7 00) | 9.50 (7.00-12.0) | 1322 |
| **Age group** | | | | | | | |
| 20-59 years | 01-02 | 2.21 (1.65-2 97) | 2.30 (1.56-3 21) | 4.63 (3.24-6 20) | 8.45 (5.86-12.0) | 12.0 (7.68-19.2) | 785 |
| | 03-04 | 1.50 (1.20-1 86) | 1.40 (1.10-1 90) | 3.40 (2.60-4 20) | 6.20 (5.30-7 00) | 9.50 (7.00-12.0) | 1322 |
| **Gender** | | | | | | | |
| Males | 01-02 | 2.19 (1.60-3 00) | 2.31 (1.63-3 21) | 4.64 (3.21-6 08) | 7.96 (5.74-15.3) | 13.0 (6.93-20.5) | 382 |
| | 03-04 | 1.48 (1.18-1 85) | 1.40 (.940-2 00) | 3.40 (2.60-4 30) | 6.60 (5.40-7 20) | 11.0 (7.20-14.0) | 650 |
| Females | 01-02 | 2.24 (1.66-3 01) | 2.28 (1.49-3 24) | 4.63 (3.09-7 01) | 8.62 (5.26-12.9) | 11.1 (7.68-25.0) | 403 |
| | 03-04 | 1.51 (1.21-1 90) | 1.50 (1.10-1 90) | 3.30 (2.50-4 20) | 6.10 (4.69-7 30) | 7.80 (6.40-12.0) | 672 |
| **Race/ethnicity** | | | | | | | |
| Mexican Americans | 01-02 | 3.28 (2.29-4.68) | 3.32 (2.19-4.70) | 6.81 (3.71-10.4) | 10.8 (8.24-14.7) | 14.7 (11.1-20.5) | 227 |
| | 03-04 | 1.65 (1.15-2 38) | 1.60 (.820-2 80) | 3.50 (2.60-4 90) | 7.30 (4.50-10.0) | 10.0 (7.30-11.0) | 244 |
| Non-Hispanic blacks | 01-02 | 2.32 (1.82-2 94) | 2.50 (1.56-3 55) | 4.57 (3.60-5 56) | 8.69 (5.63-9.49) | 10.0 (5.89-13.5) | 130 |
| | 03-04 | 1.56 (1.15-2.13) | 1.70 (1.10-2 20) | 2.90 (2.15-3 80) | 5.10 (3.80-6.60) | 6.60 (4.90-13.0) | 290 |
| Non-Hispanic whites | 01-02 | 2.02 (1.42-2 87) | 2.16 (1.36-3 09) | 4.34 (2.92-6 01) | 7.33 (4.72-15.3) | 11.1 (6.01-26.1) | 365 |
| | 03-04 | 1.42 (1.11-1 81) | 1.30 (.850-1 90) | 3.30 (2.30-4.40) | 6.20 (5.20-7 20) | 9.80 (6.70-13.0) | 684 |

Limits of detection (LOD, see Data Analysis section) for Survey years 01-02 and 03-04 are 0.233 and 0.62.
# Survey period 2001-2002 is a one-third subsample of 20-59 year olds; Survey period 2003-2004 is a one-half subsample of 20-59 year olds.

vapor. Dermal absorption also may occur during bathing and swimming (ATSDR, 1997, 2005; Dick, et al., 1995; Leavens et al., 2007). Each of the DBPs is rapidly absorbed and distributed widely throughout the body. In animals, these chemicals undergo hepatic metabolism to reactive chemicals, which can bind to cell macromolecules and be toxic in large amounts (IPCS, 2000). Ultimately, DBPs are metabolized to carbon dioxide, which is eliminated in exhaled air within a few hours. Only a small amount of each DBP is eliminated unchanged in urine. Elimination half-lives for these chemicals are less than four hours (ATSDR, 2005; Leavens et al., 2007).

Human health effects from DBPs at low environmental doses or at biomonitored levels from low environmental exposures are unclear or unknown. Humans exposed to massive levels of trichloromethane or tribromomethane develop central nervous system depression and hepatotoxicity (ATSDR, 2005, 1997). Acute animal toxicity studies of each of these chemicals have found central nervous system depression, liver and renal damage or necrosis, and occasionally, cardiac depression and arrhythmias (IPCS, 2000). In studies of rodents chronically fed high doses of either trichloromethane or bromodichloromethane, carcinomas occurred in the liver and kidney; large intestine tumors and

polyps were also noted with bromodichloromethane (NCI, 1976; NTP, 1987). Chronic feeding studies in rodents with either dibromochloromethane or tribromomethane showed inconsistent evidence of carcinogenicity across species and genders. The DBPs did not produce reproductive or developmental effects in animals unless maternal toxicity was present, but bromodichloromethane altered sperm motility (IPCS, 2000). Numerous epidemiologic studies of the relationships between chlorinated water source and various cancers, adverse reproductive outcomes, and cardiovascular disease have been inconclusive (IPCS, 2000). IARC classified trichloromethane and bromodichloromethane as possible human carcinogens, and NTP determined that these chemicals are reasonably anticipated to be human carcinogens. However, IARC found dibromochloromethane and tribromomethane to be unclassifiable regarding human carcinogenicity. The U.S. EPA has established drinking water and environmental standards for "total THMs." OSHA and ACGIH have established workplace standards and guidelines, respectively, for trichloromethane and tribromomethane. Information about external exposure (i.e., environmental levels) and health effects is available from ATSDR at: http://www.atsdr.cdc.gov/toxpro2.html.

## Blood Dibromochloromethane

Geometric mean and selected percentiles of blood concentrations (in pg/mL) for the U.S. population from the National Health and Nutrition Examination Survey.

| | Survey years# | Geometric mean (95% conf. interval) | Selected percentiles ( 95% confidence interval) | | | | Sample size |
|---|---|---|---|---|---|---|---|
| | | | 50th | 75th | 90th | 95th | |
| Total | 01-02 | .867 (.521-1.44) | .780 (.340-1.90) | 2.61 (1.22-4.38) | 5.46 (3.53-9.71) | 8.96 (5.04-12.9) | 781 |
| | 03-04 | * | < LOD | 1.30 (1.00-1.80) | 3.60 (2.70-4.80) | 7.20 (4.80-8.60) | 1333 |
| **Age group** | | | | | | | |
| 20-59 years | 01-02 | .867 (.521-1.44) | .780 (.340-1.90) | 2.61 (1.22-4.38) | 5.46 (3.53-9.71) | 8.96 (5.04-12.9) | 781 |
| | 03-04 | * | < LOD | 1.30 (1.00-1.80) | 3.60 (2.70-4.80) | 7.20 (4.80-8.60) | 1333 |
| **Gender** | | | | | | | |
| Males | 01-02 | .850 (.481-1.50) | .730 (.300-2.25) | 2.66 (.960-4.38) | 4.77 (3.33-9.20) | 8.06 (4.31-14.6) | 371 |
| | 03-04 | * | < LOD | 1.30 (1.00-1.90) | 3.70 (2.70-5.70) | 7.20 (5.20-8.60) | 657 |
| Females | 01-02 | .884 (.550-1.42) | .820 (.340-1.69) | 2.54 (1.37-4.31) | 6.30 (3.28-10.1) | 9.91 (5.02-13.0) | 410 |
| | 03-04 | * | < LOD | 1.30 (1.00-1.80) | 3.60 (2.50-4.80) | 6.60 (3.80-9.20) | 676 |
| **Race/ethnicity** | | | | | | | |
| Mexican Americans | 01-02 | 1.61 (.843-3.06) | 1.49 (.670-3.99) | 4.59 (1.93-8.89) | 9.26 (5.21-12.1) | 12.0 (9.63-16.1) | 233 |
| | 03-04 | 1.20 (.963-1.50) | 1.10 (.810-1.40) | 2.30 (1.50-4.10) | 5.20 (3.80-6.90) | 7.70 (5.20-11.0) | 256 |
| Non-Hispanic blacks | 01-02 | 1.03 (.505-2.09) | .930 (.530-2.03) | 2.03 (.770-7.06) | 4.22 (2.01-10.5) | 8.09 (2.80-16.5) | 128 |
| | 03-04 | * | < LOD | .970 (.650-1.60) | 1.90 (1.20-3.20) | 3.20 (1.80-5.20) | 288 |
| Non-Hispanic whites | 01-02 | .736 (.413-1.31) | .640 (<LOD-1.93) | 2.49 (.870-4.27) | 4.57 (3.00-7.12) | 6.98 (4.27-11.1) | 357 |
| | 03-04 | * | < LOD | 1.30 (.950-1.80) | 3.30 (2.50-4.60) | 6.60 (3.70-9.20) | 685 |

Limits of detection (LOD, see Data Analysis section) for Survey years 01-02 and 03-04 are 0.271 and 0.62.
\# Survey period 2001-2002 is a one-third subsample of 20-59 year olds; Survey period 2003-2004 is a one-half subsample of 20-59 year olds.
< LOD means less than the limit of detection, which may vary for some chemicals by year and by individual sample.
* Not calculated: proportion of results below limit of detection was too high to provide a valid result.

## Biomonitoring Information

Levels of blood DBPs reflect recent exposure. Geometric mean blood trichloromethane levels were 0.039 and 0.043 ng/mL among non-smoking and smoking adults, respectively, in a subsample of NHANES 1999-2000 participants (Lin et al., 2008), which were at least twice as high as comparable levels in NHANES 2001-2002 and 2003-2004. In a non-representative sample of NHANES III (1988-1994) participants, the geometric mean and median blood trichloromethane levels, respectively, were 0.043 and 0.023 µg/L (Churchill et al., 2001). Similar median blood trichloromethane levels were reported in smaller studies of U.S adults (Ashley et al., 2005; Backer et al., 2000; Buckley et al., 1997) and in this *Report*. Immediately following bathing or showering with chlorinated water, median blood levels of trichloromethane, dibromochloromethane, and bromodichloromethane can increase two to four times over baseline levels, and then return to baseline rapidly during the next one to two hours (Ashley et al., 2005; Backer et al., 2000).

Finding a measurable amount of one or more of these THMs in blood does not mean that the level of THMs causes an adverse health effect. Biomonitoring studies of blood THMs can provide physicians and public health officials with reference values so that they can determine whether or not people have been exposed to higher levels of THMs than levels found in the general population. Biomonitoring data can also help scientists plan and conduct research on exposure and health effects.

## Blood Tribromomethane (Bromoform)

Geometric mean and selected percentiles of blood concentrations (in pg/mL) for the U.S. population from the National Health and Nutrition Examination Survey.

| | Survey years# | Geometric mean (95% conf. interval) | Selected percentiles ( 95% confidence interval) | | | | Sample size |
|---|---|---|---|---|---|---|---|
| | | | 50th | 75th | 90th | 95th | |
| Total | 01-02 | 1.57 (1.07-2.31) | 1.39 (.960-2.02) | 2.78 (1.76-4.63) | 6.05 (2.92-29.2) | 15.5 (3.68-85.4) | 774 |
| | 03-04 | * | < LOD | 1.80 (<LOD-2.80) | 3.74 (2.30-7.10) | 6.40 (3.60-14.0) | 1310 |
| **Age group** | | | | | | | |
| 20-59 years | 01-02 | 1.57 (1.07-2.31) | 1.39 (.960-2.02) | 2.78 (1.76-4.63) | 6.05 (2.92-29.2) | 15.5 (3.68-85.4) | 774 |
| | 03-04 | * | < LOD | 1.80 (<LOD-2.80) | 3.74 (2.30-7.10) | 6.40 (3.60-14.0) | 1310 |
| **Gender** | | | | | | | |
| Males | 01-02 | 1.49 (.944-2.34) | 1.29 (.850-1.98) | 2.65 (1.49-5.05) | 6.12 (2.26-33.9) | 14.9 (2.79-69.9) | 374 |
| | 03-04 | * | < LOD | 1.90 (<LOD-2.87) | 4.00 (2.40-6.80) | 6.50 (4.00-13.0) | 645 |
| Females | 01-02 | 1.67 (1.17-2.39) | 1.46 (1.05-2.21) | 2.86 (1.89-4.57) | 5.69 (3.30-27.5) | 22.2 (5.09-49.6) | 400 |
| | 03-04 | * | < LOD | 1.72 (<LOD-2.65) | 3.20 (1.93-7.70) | 6.10 (3.10-31.0) | 665 |
| **Race/ethnicity** | | | | | | | |
| Mexican Americans | 01-02 | 2.34 (1.15-4.77) | 1.66 (.990-3.38) | 4.03 (1.42-36.5) | 28.3 (4.39-49.2) | 40.8 (31.5-57.9) | 234 |
| | 03-04 | * | 1.60 (<LOD-3.10) | 3.30 (<LOD-9.40) | 7.60 (3.60-14.0) | 11.0 (5.60-210) | 242 |
| Non-Hispanic blacks | 01-02 | 1.51 (.857-2.67) | 1.47 (.780-3.15) | 2.58 (1.39-4.64) | 4.34 (2.57-8.48) | 6.27 (3.28-15.2) | 121 |
| | 03-04 | * | < LOD | 1.60 (<LOD-2.30) | 2.50 (1.80-3.20) | 3.20 (2.40-6.10) | 289 |
| Non-Hispanic whites | 01-02 | 1.47 (.980-2.22) | 1.29 (.840-2.06) | 2.58 (1.51-4.91) | 5.69 (2.84-21.2) | 11.0 (3.30-69.9) | 362 |
| | 03-04 | * | < LOD | 1.70 (<LOD-2.90) | 3.50 (2.00-7.70) | 5.90 (3.30-21.0) | 680 |

Limits of detection (LOD, see Data Analysis section) for Survey years 01-02 and 03-04 are 0.596 and 1 5.
# Survey period 2001-2002 is a one-third subsample of 20-59 year olds; Survey period 2003-2004 is a one-half subsample of 20-59 year olds.
< LOD means less than the limit of detection, which may vary for some chemicals by year and by individual sample.
* Not calculated: proportion of results below limit of detection was too high to provide a valid result.

## Blood Trichloromethane (Chloroform)

Geometric mean and selected percentiles of blood concentrations (in pg/mL) for the U.S. population from the National Health and Nutrition Examination Survey.

| | Survey years# | Geometric mean (95% conf. interval) | Selected percentiles ( 95% confidence interval) | | | | Sample size |
|---|---|---|---|---|---|---|---|
| | | | 50th | 75th | 90th | 95th | |
| Total | 01-02 | 16.6 (13.0-21.1) | 16.1 (11.9-22.2) | 31.7 (23.9-40.4) | 55.5 (44.5-68.6) | 72.1 (57.3-105) | 744 |
| | 03-04 | 10.2 (8.56-12.2) | 10.0 (8.50-13.0) | 20.0 (17.0-24.0) | 35.0 (29.0-40.0) | 50.0 (37.0-65.0) | 1222 |
| **Age group** | | | | | | | |
| 20-59 years | 01-02 | 16.6 (13.0-21.1) | 16.1 (11.9-22.2) | 31.7 (23.9-40.4) | 55.5 (44.5-68.6) | 72.1 (57.3-105) | 744 |
| | 03-04 | 10.2 (8.56-12.2) | 10.0 (8.50-13.0) | 20.0 (17.0-24.0) | 35.0 (29.0-40.0) | 50.0 (37.0-65.0) | 1222 |
| **Gender** | | | | | | | |
| Males | 01-02 | 16.8 (12.0-23.5) | 16.1 (11.0-24.8) | 34.3 (22.4-48.7) | 57.0 (39.9-76.4) | 75.2 (54.5-156) | 358 |
| | 03-04 | 10.1 (8.43-12.1) | 10.0 (7.90-14.0) | 20.0 (17.0-25.0) | 36.8 (29.0-49.0) | 53.0 (36.8-69.0) | 599 |
| Females | 01-02 | 16.4 (13.4-20.1) | 16.6 (12.0-21.5) | 29.2 (24.0-36.5) | 53.5 (38.4-68.9) | 69.5 (53.3-104) | 386 |
| | 03-04 | 10.4 (8.41-12.7) | 10.0 (8.40-13.0) | 20.0 (16.0-23.9) | 33.0 (26.0-40.0) | 46.0 (35.0-65.0) | 623 |
| **Race/ethnicity** | | | | | | | |
| Mexican Americans | 01-02 | 17.0 (10.5-27.6) | 14.5 (10.0-32.7) | 35.1 (18.6-57.6) | 60.7 (41.5-100) | 93.0 (49.7-243) | 223 |
| | 03-04 | 9.17 (7.45-11.3) | 9.30 (7.60-11.0) | 19.0 (15.0-24.0) | 34.0 (24.0-44.4) | 44.4 (30.0-59.0) | 225 |
| Non-Hispanic blacks | 01-02 | 19.1 (12.9-28.1) | 20.9 (9.28-37.4) | 38.4 (27.7-46.0) | 55.9 (45.5-69.8) | 68.9 (51.9-74.0) | 116 |
| | 03-04 | 11.8 (9.54-14.6) | 12.0 (8.90-15.0) | 20.0 (15.0-30.0) | 35.0 (28.0-59.0) | 61.0 (34.0-100) | 272 |
| Non-Hispanic whites | 01-02 | 15.6 (12.0-20.2) | 15.2 (11.2-20.5) | 26.8 (20.4-39.5) | 53.5 (35.3-72.1) | 69.5 (53.5-105) | 348 |
| | 03-04 | 9.84 (8.09-12.0) | 10.0 (8.10-13.0) | 20.0 (16.0-23.0) | 33.8 (27.0-40.0) | 47.0 (35.0-67.0) | 630 |

Limits of detection (LOD, see Data Analysis section) for Survey years 01-02 and 03-04 are 2.37 and 2.11.
# Survey period 2001-2002 is a one-third subsample of 20-59 year olds; Survey period 2003-2004 is a one-half subsample of 20-59 year olds.

## References

Agency for Toxic Substances and Disease Registry (ATSDR). Toxicological profile for chloroform update. 1997 [online]. Available at URL: http://www.atsdr.cdc.gov/toxprofiles/tp6.html. 4/26/09

Agency for Toxic Substances and Disease Registry (ATSDR). Toxicological profile for bromoform and chlorodibromomethane. 2005 [online]. Available at URL: http://www.atsdr.cdc.gov/toxprofiles/tp130.html. 4/26/09

Ashley DL, Blount BC, Singer PC, Depaz E, Wilkes C, Gordon S, et al. Changes in blood trihalomethanes concentrations resulting from differences in water quality and water use activities. Arch Environ Occup Health 2005;60(1):7-15.

Backer LC, Ashley DL, Bonin MA, Cardinali FL, Kieszak SM, Wooten JV. Household exposures to drinking water disinfection by-products: whole blood trihalomethane levels. J Expo Anal Environ Epidemiol 2000;10(4):321-326.

Buckley TJ, Liddle J, Ashley DL, Paschal DC, Burse VW, Needham LL. Environmental and biomarker measurements in nine homes in the lower Rio Grande Valley: multimedia results for pesticides, metals, PAHs and VOCs. Environ Int 1997;23(5):705-732.

Churchill JE, Ashley DL, Kaye WE. Recent chemical exposures and blood volatile organic compound levels in a large population-based sample. Arch Environ Health 2001;56(2):157-166.

Dick D, Ng KM, Sauder DN, Chu I. *In vitro* and *in vivo* percutaneous absorption of $^{14}$C-chloroform in humans. Hum Exp Toxicol 1995;14: 260-265.

Gordon SM, Brinkman MC, Ashley DL, Blount BC, Lyu C, Masters J, Singer PC. Changes in breath trihalomethane levels resulting from household water-use activities. Environ Health Perspect 2006;114(4):514-521.

International Programme on Chemical Safety (IPCS). Environmental Health Criteria 216. Disinfectants and Disinfectant By-Products. 2000 [online]. Available at URL: http://www.inchem.org/documents/ehc/ehc/ehc216.htm.4/26/09

International Programme on Chemical Safety (IPCS). Concise International Chemical Assessment Document 58. Chloroform. 2004 [online]. Available at URL: http://www.inchem.org/documents/cicads/cicads/cicad58.htm. 4/26/09

Krasner SW, McGuire MJ, Jacaugelo JG, Patania NL, Reagan KM, Aieta EM. The occurrence of disinfection by-products in US drinking water. J Am Water Works Assoc 1989;81:41–53.

LaRegina J, Bozzelli JW, Harkov R, Gianti S. Volatility organic compounds at hazardous waste sites and a sanitary landfill in New Jersey. An up-to-date review of the present situation. Environ Prog 1986;5:18-27.

Leavens TL, Blount BC, De Marini DM, Madden MC, Valentine JL, Case MW, et al. Disposition of bromodichloromethane in humans following oral and dermal exposure. Toxicol Sci 2007;99(2):432-445.

Lin YS, Egeghy PP, Rappaport SM. Relationships between levels of volatile organic compounds in air and blood from the general population. J Expo Sci Environ Epidemiol 2008;18(4):421-9.

National Cancer Institute (NCI). Report on the carcinogenesis bioassay of chloroform (CAS No. 67-66-3). National Cancer Institute Carcinogenesis Technical Report Series March 1, 1976. [online]. Available at URL: http://ntp.niehs.nih.gov/ntp/htdocs/LT_rpts/trChloroform.pdf. 4/26/09

National Toxicology Program (NTP). Carcinogenesis studies of bromodichloromethane (CAS No. 75-27-4) in F344/N rats and B6C31F mice (gavage studies). Technical Report Series No. 321. 1987 [online]. Available at URL: http://ntp.niehs.nih.gov/ntp/htdocs/LT_rpts/tr321.pdf. 4/26/09

# Benzophenone-3

CAS No. 131-57-7

## General Information

Benzophenone-3 (2-hydroxy-4-methoxybenzophenone) occurs naturally in some flowering plants. It is commercially synthesized as a sunscreen for use in lotions, conditioners, and cosmetics. It is also used as a UV stabilizer in plastic surface coatings and polymers. Benzophenone-3 is a common ingredient in sun-blocking agents.

People may be exposed through dermal application of sunscreens and cosmetic products. Small amounts of benzophenone-3 can be absorbed through human skin and excreted in the urine, mostly as a glucuronidated conjugate (Gonzalez et al., 2006; Gustavsson et al., 2002; Janjua et al., 2004; Ye et al., 2005). After dermal application of a 4% lotion over the entire body daily for 5 days, one study found that 1.2-8.7% of the applied benzophenone-3 amount was recovered in the urine (Gonzalez et al., 2006).

Human health effects from benzophenone-3 at low environmental doses or at biomonitored levels from low environmental exposures are unknown. Following dermal application, some cases of photoallergy or allergy to benzophenone-3 have been reported. Male reproductive toxicity has been inconsistently reported in chronic high dose animal studies (Daston et al., 1993; French, 1992). Benzophenone-3 has weak estrogenic activity or weak anti-androgenic activity (French, 1992; Schlecht et al., 2004; Schlumpf et al., 2001; Schreurs et al., 2005). No human hormonal changes were observed during four days of application of 10% benzophenone-3 lotion (Janjua et al., 2004). Benzophenone-3 is not considered mutagenic (Robison et al., 1994). IARC and NTP have no ratings as to human carcinogenicity of benzophenone-3.

## Biomonitoring Information

Urinary benzophenone-3 levels include both conjugated and unconjugated forms and reflect recent exposure to the chemical. The NHANES 2003-2004 levels of urinary benzophenone-3 have been described by Calafat et al. (2008). The analysis showed that female participants had slightly higher urinary levels than males and that non-Hispanic whites were more likely than non-Hispanic blacks to have levels above the 95th percentile of the overall population. In a study of 90 U.S. females aged 6-8 years, the median urinary benzophenone-3 level of 14.7 µg/L was comparable to the median level of children 6-11 years of age (17.2 µg/L) in the NHANES 2003-2004 subsample (Calafat

et al., 2008; Wolff et al., 2007). Total benzophenone-3 urinary concentrations were detectable in 90% of a small sample of adults in whom the values ranged up to 3000 µg/L (Ye et al., 2005). Following short-term application of 10% benzophenone-3 lotion, men and women had mean urinary levels of 140 and 60 µg/L, respectively (Janjua et al., 2004).

Finding a measurable amount of benzophenone-3 in urine does not mean that the levels of benzophenone-3 cause an adverse health effect. Biomonitoring studies on levels of benzophenone-3 provide physicians and public health officials with reference values so that they can determine whether people have been exposed to higher levels of benzophenone-3 than are found in the general population. Biomonitoring data can also help scientists plan and conduct research on exposure and health effects.

## Urinary Benzophenone-3 (2-Hydroxy-4-methoxybenzophenone)

Geometric mean and selected percentiles of urine concentrations (in µg/L) for the U.S. population from the National Health and Nutrition Examination Survey.

| | Survey years | Geometric mean (95% conf. interval) | Selected percentiles ( 95% confidence interval) | | | | Sample size |
|---|---|---|---|---|---|---|---|
| | | | 50th | 75th | 90th | 95th | |
| Total | 03-04 | 22.9 (18.1-28 9) | 18.1 (15.5-23 2) | 94.0 (67.5-123) | 370 (225-570) | 1040 (698-1390) | 2517 |
| **Age group** | | | | | | | |
| 6-11 years | 03-04 | 21.2 (16.4-27 3) | 17.2 (14.9-25 9) | 66.7 (38.7-102) | 158 (106-246) | 246 (154-618) | 314 |
| 12-19 years | 03-04 | 22.9 (18.0-29 3) | 20.1 (16.1-25.1) | 67.1 (45.2-93 8) | 170 (137-240) | 407 (183-717) | 715 |
| 20 years and older | 03-04 | 23.1 (18.0-29 6) | 18.1 (14.7-23 3) | 109 (72.1-140) | 450 (315-733) | 1220 (769-1750) | 1488 |
| **Gender** | | | | | | | |
| Males | 03-04 | 16.8 (13.2-21 3) | 13.7 (11.4-16 8) | 55.3 (33.2-86 6) | 178 (134-324) | 567 (238-1350) | 1229 |
| Females | 03-04 | 30.7 (23.7-39 8) | 26.0 (20.2-34.1) | 137 (106-172) | 596 (403-769) | 1340 (776-1790) | 1288 |
| **Race/ethnicity** | | | | | | | |
| Mexican Americans | 03-04 | 16.5 (10.9-25.1) | 11.9 (8.50-18 3) | 45.5 (25.9-78 2) | 178 (76.4-412) | 412 (178-2180) | 613 |
| Non-Hispanic blacks | 03-04 | 12.8 (9.38-17.4) | 10.2 (7.40-14.4) | 34.3 (22.8-50 6) | 127 (90.8-176) | 247 (143-499) | 652 |
| Non-Hispanic whites | 03-04 | 27.7 (20.3-37 8) | 24.4 (16.8-32 0) | 121 (83.6-162) | 507 (316-769) | 1340 (733-2070) | 1092 |

Limit of detection (LOD, see Data Analysis section) for Survey year 03-04 is 0.3.

## Urinary Benzophenone-3 (2-Hydroxy-4-methoxybenzophenone) (creatinine corrected)

Geometric mean and selected percentiles of urine concentrations (in µg/g of creatinine) for the U.S. population from the National Health and Nutrition Examination Survey.

| | Survey years | Geometric mean (95% conf. interval) | Selected percentiles ( 95% confidence interval) | | | | Sample size |
|---|---|---|---|---|---|---|---|
| | | | 50th | 75th | 90th | 95th | |
| Total | 03-04 | 22.2 (17.6-28 0) | 16.2 (12.7-21 6) | 82.0 (58.7-108) | 415 (283-577) | 1080 (686-1600) | 2514 |
| **Age group** | | | | | | | |
| 6-11 years | 03-04 | 25.8 (19.5-34.1) | 22.4 (14.4-33.7) | 84.6 (41.0-131) | 171 (132-365) | 427 (171-710) | 314 |
| 12-19 years | 03-04 | 17.2 (13.7-21 5) | 12.9 (10.4-16 5) | 43.6 (29.5-57.7) | 136 (91.7-239) | 350 (173-646) | 713 |
| 20 years and older | 03-04 | 22.8 (17.8-29.1) | 16.2 (12.7-21 9) | 93.2 (66.0-130) | 491 (361-700) | 1330 (880-1880) | 1487 |
| **Gender** | | | | | | | |
| Males | 03-04 | 13.6 (10.8-17.1) | 10.3 (8.36-12 9) | 40.0 (24.9-62 5) | 169 (93.3-316) | 381 (229-685) | 1228 |
| Females | 03-04 | 35.5 (27.1-46.4) | 28.2 (20.2-37 0) | 144 (101-224) | 686 (491-1130) | 1850 (1220-2580) | 1286 |
| **Race/ethnicity** | | | | | | | |
| Mexican Americans | 03-04 | 15.1 (9.44-24 0) | 11.1 (6.95-16 0) | 40.7 (18.3-85 8) | 158 (87.4-362) | 595 (118-1860) | 612 |
| Non-Hispanic blacks | 03-04 | 8.78 (6.49-11 9) | 6.80 (5.27-9.00) | 19.7 (13.5-33.4) | 79.8 (46.8-139) | 185 (79.8-536) | 651 |
| Non-Hispanic whites | 03-04 | 28.3 (20.6-38 8) | 22.0 (14.6-32.7) | 116 (73.5-175) | 510 (380-760) | 1330 (852-2410) | 1091 |

## References

Calafat AM, Wong LY, Ye X, Reidy JA, Needham LL. Concentrations of the sunscreen agent benzophenone-3 in residents of the United States: National Health and Nutrition Examination Survey 2003--2004. Environ Health Perspect 2008;116(7):893-897.

Daston GP, Gettings SD, Carlton BD, Chudkowski M, Davis RA, Kraus AL, et al. Assessment of the reproductive toxic potential of dermally applied 2-hydroxy-4-methoxybenzophenone to male B6C3F1 mice. Fundam Appl Toxicol 1993;20(1):120-124.

French JE. NTP technical report on the toxicity studies of 2-hydroxy-4-methoxybenzophenone (CAS No. 131-57-7) Adminstered topically and in dosed feed to F344/N Rats and B6C3F1 mice. National Institutes of Health Publication No. 92-3344, October 1992 (also Toxic Rep Ser. 1992 Oct;21:1-E14).

Gonzalez H, Farbrot A, Larko O, Wennberg AM. Percutaneous absorption of the sunscreen benzophenone-3 after repeated whole-body applications, with and without ultraviolet irradiation. Br J Dermatol 2006;154(2):337-340.

Gustavsson Gonzalez H, Farbrot A, Larko O. Percutaneous absorption of benzophenone-3, a common component of topical sunscreens. Clin Exp Dermatol 2002;27(8):691-694.

Janjua NR, Mogensen B, Andersson AM, Petersen JH, Henriksen M, Skakkebaek NE, et al. Systemic absorption of the sunscreens benzophenone-3, octyl methoxycinnamate, and 3-(4-methyl-benzylidene) camphor after whole-body topical application and reproductive hormone levels in humans. J Invest Dermatol 2004;123(1):57-61.

Okereke CS, Barat SA, Abdel-Rahman MS. Safety evaluation of benzophenone-3 after dermal administration in rats. Toxicol Lett 1995;80(1-3):61-67.

Robison SH, Odio MR, Thompson ED, Aardema MJ, Kraus AL. Assessment of the in vivo genotoxicity of 2-hydroxy 4-methoxybenzophenone. Environ Mol Mutagen 1994;23(4):312-317.

Schlecht C, Klammer H, Jarry H, Wuttke W. Effects of estradiol, benzophenone-2 and benzophenone-3 on the expression pattern of the estrogen receptors (ER) alpha and beta, the estrogen receptor-related receptor 1 (ERR1) and the aryl hydrocarbon receptor (AhR) in adult ovariectomized rats. Toxicology 2004;205(1-2):123-130.

Schlumpf M, Cotton B, Conscience M, Haller V, Steinmann B, Lichtensteiger W. In vitro and in vivo estrogenicity of UV screens. Environ Health Perspect 2001;109(3):239-244. Erratum in: Environ Health Perspect 2001;109(11):A517.

Schreurs RH, Sonneveld E, Jansen JH, Seinen W, van der Burg B. Interaction of polycyclic musks and UV filters with the estrogen receptor (ER), androgen receptor (AR), and progesterone receptor (PR) in reporter gene bioassays. Toxicol Sci 2005;83(2):264-272.

Ye X, Kuklenyik Z, Needham LL, Calafat AM. Quantification of urinary conjugates of bisphenol A, 2,5-dichlorophenol, and 2-hydroxy-4-methoxybenzophenone in humans by online solid phase extraction-high performance liquid chromatography-tandem mass spectrometry. Anal Bioanal Chem 2005;383(4):638-644.

# Bisphenol A
CAS No. 80-05-7

## General Information

Bisphenol A is a phenolic chemical which has been used for over 50 years in the manufacture of polycarbonate plastics and epoxy resins; in thermal paper production; and as a polymerization inhibitor in the formation of some polyvinyl chloride plastics. Polycarbonates are used to make products such as compact discs, automobile parts, baby bottles, plastic dinnerware, eyeglass lenses, toys, and impact-resistant safety equipment. Epoxy resins containing bisphenol A are used in protective linings of some canned food containers, wine vat linings, epoxy resin-based paints, floorings, and some dental composites. In recent years, about 5-6 billion pounds of bisphenol were produced annually worldwide. Bisphenol A may enter the environment from industrial sources or from product leaching, disposal, and use. In 1999-2000, bisphenol A was detected in 41.2% of 139 U.S. streams in 30 states (Kolpin et al., 2002). Bisphenol A can be biodegraded and does not bioaccumulate significantly in aquatic organisms. Some invertebrates may be sensitive and show reproductive effects (European Commission, 2003).

General population exposure to bisphenol A may occur through ingestion of foods in contact with bisphenol A containing materials. For small children, hand-to-mouth and direct oral contact with materials containing bisphenol A are possible. Exposure from indoor air is a small component of total exposure estimates (Wilson et al., 2007. In animal and human studies, bisphenol A is well absorbed orally. In humans, little free bisphenol A circulates after oral absorption due to the high degree of glucuronidation by the liver. The glucuronidated bisphenol A is excreted in the urine within 24 hours with no evidence of accumulation (Volkel et al., 2002).

Human health effects from bisphenol A at low environmental doses or at biomonitored levels from low environmental exposures are unknown. Occupational exposure of epoxy workers to bisphenol A dust may produce eye irritation and skin sensitization. In animal studies, bisphenol A has low acute toxicity. It is not considered a teratogen (Kim et al., 2001). Bisphenol A is rated as weakly estrogenic (Matthews et al., 2001). Some reproductive or developmental changes are observed at high doses in standard experimental animal studies (e.g., delayed vaginal opening and preputial separation) (Ema et al., 2001; Tyl et al., 2002; NTP-CERHR, 2008). Reproductive and neurodevelopmental effects of bisphenol A at low doses in animals, including environmental doses potentially relevant to humans, have been the subject of ongoing scientific reviews and study (European Commission, 2002; Gray et al., 2004; NTP, 2001; NTP-CERHR, 2007 and 2008; vom Saal and Hughes, 2005 Welshons et al., 2006; Witorsch, 2002). Examples of recent animal studies which suggest possible low dose effects include altered development of the fetal prostate and mammary gland, inhibition of postnatal testosterone production, and changes in neurodevelopment (Akingbemi et al., 2004; Leranth et al., 2008; NTP-CERHR, 2007;

## Urinary Bisphenol A (2,2-bis[4-Hydroxyphenyl] propane)

Geometric mean and selected percentiles of urine concentrations (in µg/L) for the U.S. population from the National Health and Nutrition Examination Survey.

| | Survey years | Geometric mean (95% conf. interval) | Selected percentiles ( 95% confidence interval) | | | | Sample size |
|---|---|---|---|---|---|---|---|
| | | | 50th | 75th | 90th | 95th | |
| Total | 03-04 | 2.64 (2.38-2.94) | 2.80 (2.50-3.10) | 5.50 (5.00-6.20) | 10.6 (9.40-12 0) | 16.0 (14.4-17 2) | 2517 |
| Age group | | | | | | | |
| 6-11 years | 03-04 | 3.55 (2.95-4.29) | 3.80 (2.70-5.00) | 6.90 (6.00-8.30) | 12.6 (9.50-15.1) | 16.0 (11.5-23 3) | 314 |
| 12-19 years | 03-04 | 3.74 (3.31-4.22) | 4.30 (3.60-4.60) | 7.80 (6.50-9.00) | 13.5 (11.8-15 2) | 16.5 (15.2-20 9) | 715 |
| 20 years and older | 03-04 | 2.41 (2.15-2.72) | 2.60 (2.30-2.80) | 5.10 (4.50-5.70) | 9.50 (8.10-11 3) | 15.2 (12.4-18.1) | 1488 |
| Gender | | | | | | | |
| Males | 03-04 | 2.92 (2.63-3.24) | 3.20 (2.70-3.60) | 6.10 (5.40-6.60) | 10.4 (9.50-11 6) | 16.0 (12.7-17 6) | 1229 |
| Females | 03-04 | 2.41 (2.11-2.75) | 2.50 (2.20-2.80) | 5.00 (4.20-6.20) | 10.6 (8.70-12 5) | 15.9 (13.5-20.1) | 1288 |
| Race/ethnicity | | | | | | | |
| Mexican Americans | 03-04 | 2.58 (2.15-3.08) | 2.60 (2.10-3.20) | 5.20 (4.40-6.50) | 9.90 (7.30-13 9) | 15.4 (10.2-19.7) | 613 |
| Non-Hispanic blacks | 03-04 | 4.24 (3.73-4.82) | 4.30 (3.80-5.10) | 8.20 (7.10-9.80) | 14.2 (11.7-16 9) | 20.6 (14.9-25 2) | 652 |
| Non-Hispanic whites | 03-04 | 2.51 (2.26-2.79) | 2.70 (2.50-3.00) | 5.20 (4.70-5.80) | 9.60 (8.30-10 9) | 15.1 (12.6-16.7) | 1092 |

Limit of detection (LOD, see Data Analysis section) for Survey year 03-04 is 0.4.

Timms et al., 2005).

Bisphenol A is not considered mutagenic and is unlikely to be a carcinogen, although it may form DNA adducts *in vitro* and inhibit mitotic spindle activity (Haighton et al., 2002). IARC and NTP do not have ratings for bisphenol A with respect to human carcinogenicity. The epoxy resin oligomer, bisphenol A diglycidyl ether, has limited evidence of animal carcinogenicity and is not classifiable as a human carcinogen by IARC.

## Biomonitoring Information

Urinary levels of bisphenol A include both conjugated and unconjugated forms and reflect recent exposure to the chemical. In the participants of NHANES 2003-2004, prevalent exposure to bisphenol A in the U.S. population was demonstrated with children, females, and lower income strata having slightly higher urinary levels (Calafat et al., 2008). This study confirmed levels seen in an earlier smaller sample of 394 U.S. residents (Calafat et al., 2005). Several previous small studies in Japanese pregnant women, Japanese university students, and Korean residents have found mean urinary bisphenol A levels to be similar or up to several times higher than those in the U.S. representative NHANES 2003-2004 subsample (Fujimaki et al., 2004; Kim et al., 2003; Ouchi and Watanabe, 2002), although one study of 73 Koreans found levels that averaged seven times higher than median levels in the NHANES 2003-2004 subsample (Yang et al., 2003; Calafat et al., 2008). Applications of certain dental sealants were shown to increase urinary levels of bisphenol A for 24 hours (Joskow et al., 2006). Hanaoka et al. (2002) studied workers with exposure to bisphenol A diglycidyl ether and found mean urinary levels of bisphenol A about double that of unexposed workers.

Finding a measurable amount of bisphenol A in the urine does not mean that the levels of bisphenol A cause an adverse health effect. Biomonitoring studies on levels of bisphenol A provide physicians and public health officials with reference values so that they can determine whether people have been exposed to higher levels of bisphenol A than are found in the general population. Biomonitoring data can also help scientists plan and conduct research on exposure and health effects.

### Urinary Bisphenol A (2,2-*bis*[4-Hydroxyphenyl] propane) (creatinine corrected)

Geometric mean and selected percentiles of urine concentrations (in µg/g of creatinine) for the U.S. population from the National Health and Nutrition Examination Survey.

| | Survey years | Geometric mean (95% conf. interval) | Selected percentiles ( 95% confidence interval) | | | | Sample size |
|---|---|---|---|---|---|---|---|
| | | | 50th | 75th | 90th | 95th | |
| Total | 03-04 | 2.58 (2.36-2 82) | 2.50 (2.31-2 80) | 4.29 (3.88-4.75) | 7.67 (6.62-8 66) | 11.2 (9.78-12.4) | 2514 |
| **Age group** | | | | | | | |
| 6-11 years | 03-04 | 4.32 (3.63-5.14) | 4.29 (3.63-5 23) | 7.14 (5.83-9 56) | 12.2 (9.84-14.8) | 15.7 (12.2-23.2) | 314 |
| 12-19 years | 03-04 | 2.80 (2.52-3.11) | 2.74 (2.35-3 22) | 4.74 (4.21-5 09) | 7.79 (6.41-8 87) | 11.8 (8.05-14.2) | 713 |
| 20 years and older | 03-04 | 2.39 (2.17-2 64) | 2.36 (2.15-2 59) | 3.93 (3.44-4 33) | 6.64 (5.97-7.74) | 10.0 (9.01-11.4) | 1487 |
| **Gender** | | | | | | | |
| Males | 03-04 | 2.38 (2.15-2 63) | 2.31 (2.08-2.70) | 4.19 (3.81-4 64) | 7.10 (6.41-8 28) | 9.94 (9.06-11.7) | 1228 |
| Females | 03-04 | 2.78 (2.50-3 08) | 2.68 (2.40-2 94) | 4.41 (3.81-5.15) | 7.93 (6.48-10.2) | 12.4 (9.29-18.2) | 1286 |
| **Race/ethnicity** | | | | | | | |
| Mexican Americans | 03-04 | 2.34 (2.02-2.71) | 2.38 (2.00-2 65) | 3.85 (3.24-4 55) | 7.09 (5.00-9 04) | 10.9 (8.50-14.3) | 612 |
| Non-Hispanic blacks | 03-04 | 2.92 (2.58-3 32) | 2.95 (2.51-3 27) | 4.90 (4.07-6.13) | 8.64 (7.53-9 63) | 11.9 (10.2-13.3) | 651 |
| Non-Hispanic whites | 03-04 | 2.58 (2.37-2 81) | 2.55 (2.32-2 80) | 4.30 (3.93-4 67) | 7.58 (6.32-8 87) | 11.0 (9.34-12.4) | 1091 |

## References

Akingbemi BT, Sottas CM, Koulova AI, Klinefelter GR, and Hardy MP. Inhibition of testicular steroidogenesis by the xenoestrogen bisphenol A is associated with reduced pituitary luteinizing hormone secretion and decreased steroidogenic enzyme gene expression in rat Leydig cells. Endocrinology 2004;145:592-603.

Calafat AM, Kuklenyik Z, Reidy JA, Caudill SP, Ekong J, Needham LL. Urinary concentrations of bisphenol A and 4-nonylphenol in a human reference population. Environ Health Perspect 2005;113(4):391-395.

Calafat AM, Ye X, Wong LY, Reidy JA, Needham LL. Exposure of the U.S. population to bisphenol A and 4-tertiary-octylphenol: 2003-2004. Environ Health Perspect 2008;116(1):39-44.

Ema M, Fujii S, Furukawa M, Kiguchi M, Ikka T, Harazono A. Rat two-generation reproductive toxicity study of bisphenol A. Reprod Toxicol 2001; 5: 505-523.

European Commission. Bisphenol A. Human Health. Directorate-General Health and Consumer Protection.Scientific Committee on Toxicity, Ecotoxicity and the Environment (CSTEE). May 22, 2002. Brussels, Belgium. Available at URL: http://ec.europa.eu/health/ph_risk/committees/sct/documents/out156_en.pdf . 2/4/09

European Commission. 4,4'-Isopropylidenediphenol (Bisphenol-A) Summary Assessment Report. Joint Research Centre Institute of Health and Consumer Protection. 2003. Ispra, Italy. Available at URL: http://ecb.jrc.it/DOCUMENTS/Existing-Chemicals/RISK_ASSESSMENT/SUMMARY/bisphenolasum325.pdf. 2/4/09

Fujimaki K, Arakawa C, Yoshinaga J, Watanabe C, Serizawa S, Imai H, et al. Estimation of intake level of bisphenol A in Japanese pregnant women based on measurement of urinary excretion level of the metabolite. Nippon Eiseigaku Zasshi 2004;59(4):403-408.

Gray GM, Cohen JT, Cunha G, Hughes C, McConnell EE, Rhomberg et al. Weight of the evidence evaluation of low-dose reproductive and developmental effects of bisphenol A. Hum Ecol Risk Assess 2004;10:875-921.

Haighton LA, Hlywka JJ, Doull J, Kroes R, Lynch BS, Munro IC. An evaluation of the possible carcinogenicity of bisphenol A to humans. Regul Toxicol Pharmacol 2002;35(2 Pt 1):238-254.

Hanaoka T, Kawamura N, Hara K, Tsugane S. Urinary bisphenol A and plasma hormone concentrations in male workers exposed to bisphenol A diglycidyl ether and mixed organic solvents. Occup Environ Med 2002;59(9):625-628.

Joskow R, Barr DB, Barr JR, Calafat AM, Needham LL, Rubin C. Exposure to bisphenol A from bis-glycidyl dimethacrylate-based dental sealants. J Am Dent Assoc 2006;137(3):353-362.

Kim JC, Shin HC, Cha SW, Koh WS, Chung MK, Han SS. Evaluation of developmental toxicity in rats exposed to the environmental estrogen bisphenol A during pregnancy. Life Sci 2001;69(22):2611-2625.

Kim YH, Kim CS, Park S, Han SY, Pyo MY, Yang M. Gender differences in the levels of bisphenol A metabolites in urine. Biochem Biophys Res Commun 2003;312(2):441-448.

Kolpin DW, Furlong ET, Meyer MT, Thurman EM, Zaugg SD, Barber LB, et al. Pharmaceuticals, hormones, and other organic wastewater contaminants in U.S. streams, 1999-2000: a national reconnaissance. Environ Sci Technol 2002;36(6):1202-1211.

Leranth, C., Szigeti-Buck, K., MacLusky, N.J., and Hajszan, T. Bisphenol A prevents the synaptogenic response to testosterone in the brain of adult male rats. Endocrinology 2008;149:988-994.

Matthews JB, Twomey K, Zacharewski TR. In vitro and in vivo interactions of bisphenol A and its metabolite, bisphenol A glucuronide, with estrogen receptors alpha and beta. Chem Res Toxicol 2001;14(2):149-157.

National Toxicology Program Center for the Evaluation of Risks to Human Production (NTP-CERHR). NTP-CERHR Panel Report on Reproductive and Developmental Toxicity of Bisphenol A. November 26, 2007. Available at URL: http://cerhr.niehs.nih.gov/chemicals/bisphenol/BPAFinalEPVF112607.pdf. 2/4/09

National Toxicology Program Center for the Evaluation of Risks to Human Production (NTP-CERHR). NTP-CERHR Panel Report on Reproductive and Developmental Toxicity of Bisphenol A. September, 2008. Available at URL: http://cerhr.niehs.nih.gov/chemicals/bisphenol/bisphenol.pdf . 2/4/09

National Toxicology Program's Report of the Endocrine Disruptors Low-Dose Peer Review (NTP). August 2001. National Toxicology Program, U.S. Department of Health and Human Services. National Institute of Environmental Health Sciences, National Institutes of Health. Research Triangle Park, NC. Available at URL: http://ntp.niehs.nih.gov/ntp/htdocs/liason/LowDosePeerFinalRpt.pdf. 2/4/09

Ouchi K, Watanabe S. Measurement of bisphenol A in human urine using liquid chromatography with multi-channel coulometric electrochemical detection. J Chromatogr B Analyt Technol Biomed Life Sci 2002;780(2):365-370.

Timms BG, Howdeshell KL, Barton L, Bradley S, Richter CA, vom Saal FS. Estrogenic chemicals in plastic and oral contraceptives disrupt development of the fetal mouse prostate and urethra. Proc Natl Acad Sci USA 2005;102(19):7014-7019.

Tyl RW, Myers CB, Marr MC, Thomas BF, Keimowitz AR, Brine DR, et al. Three-generation reproductive toxicity study of dietary bisphenol A in CD Sprague-Dawley rats. Toxicol Sci 2002;68(1):121-146.

Volkel W, Colnot T, Csanady GA, Filser JG, Dekant W. Metabolism and kinetics of bisphenol A in humans at low doses following oral administration. Chem Res Toxicol 2002;15:1281-1287.

Vom Saal FS, Hughes C. An extensive new literature concerning low-dose effects of bisphenol A shows the need for a new risk assessment. Environ Health Perspect 2005;113(8):926-33.

Welshons WV, Nagel SC, vom Saal FS. Large effects from small exposures. III. Endocrine mechanisms mediating effects of bisphenol A at levels of human exposure. Endocrinology 2006;147(6 Suppl):S56-69.

Wilson NK, Chuang JC, Morgan MK, Lordo RA, Sheldon LS. An observational study of the potential exposures of preschool children to pentachlorophenol, bisphenol-A, and nonylphenol at home and daycare. Environ Res 2007;103(1):9-20.

Witorsch RJ. Low-dose in utero effects of xenoestrogens in mice and their relevance to humans: an analytical review of the literature. Food Chem Toxicol 2002;40(7):905-12.

Yang M, Kim SY, Lee SM, Chang SS, Kawamoto T, Jang JY, et al. Biological monitoring of bisphenol a in a Korean population. Arch Environ Contam Toxicol 2003;44(4):546-51.

# 4-*tert*-Octylphenol

CAS No. 140-66-9

## General Information

4-*tert*-Octyphenol, an alkylphenol, is used to manufacture alkylphenol ethoxylates, which are anionic surfactants used in detergents, industrial cleaners, and emulsifiers. Commercial formulations of alkylphenol ethoxylates usually contain a mixture of oligomers and isomers, and the polyethoxy chain may consist of up to 50 ethoxy units. Less frequently, the various alkylphenols have also been used as emulsifiers and modifiers in paints, pesticides, textiles, and some personal care products. Alkylphenols also have been used as plasticizers and antioxidants in plastics and resins. In the 1990s, over 500,000 tons of alkylphenol ethoxylates were produced annually worldwide. Nonylphenol ethoxylates are more commonly used than octylphenol ethoxylates. The alkylphenol ethoxylates enter the environment through human use of products containing them, through sewage, and through manufacturing waste streams (Warhurst, 1995; Ying et al., 2002). They are biodegraded to the corresponding alkylphenol (octylphenol or nonylphenol); to shorter chain alkylphenol ethoxylates; and to alkylphenoxycarboxylates. Octylphenols and nonylphenols can also enter the environment directly from manufacturing waste streams. During the 1980s and 1990s, several European nations banned the use of alkylphenol ethoxylates in domestic detergents and other uses. The alkylphenols can bioaccumulate in some fish, and some of their degradation products are toxic to aquatic life. In 1999-2000, 4-octylphenol monoethoxylate was detected in 43.5% of 139 U.S. streams in 30 states (Kolpin et al., 2002).

Human exposure to alkylphenols and alkylphenol ethoxylates may occur through ingestion of contaminated foods (e.g., fish) and drinking water, and from contact with some personal care products and detergents. Indoor and to a lesser extent, outdoor air may have detectable levels of 4-*tert*-octylphenol and 4-*tert*-octylphenol monoethoxylates, leading to inhalation as another potential exposure route (Rudel et al., 2003; Saito et al., 2004). In rats, orally administered 4-*tert*-octylphenol was well absorbed, did not bioaccumulate, and was quickly eliminated from the blood (Certa et al., 1996). Disposition in humans has not been studied sufficiently.

Human health effects from 4-*tert*-octylphenol or the corresponding octylphenol ethoxylates at low environmental doses or at biomonitored levels from low environmental exposures are unknown. Several alkylphenols, including 4-*tert*-octylphenol, have demonstrated estrogenic effects particularly when injected at high doses in animals. These high dose parenteral effects of 4-*tert*-octylphenol have included altered sex hormone levels and hypothalamic-pituitary suppression, impaired steroidogenesis, altered estrus cycles and reproductive outcomes, altered neonatal sexual development, testicular atrophy, and impaired spermatogenesis (e.g., Bian et al., 2006; Blake and Boockfor, 1997; Katsuda et al., 2000; Laws et al., 2000;

## Urinary 4-*tert*-Octylphenol (4-[1,1,3,3-Tetramethylbutyl] phenol)

Geometric mean and selected percentiles of urine concentrations (in µg/L) for the U.S. population from the National Health and Nutrition Examination Survey.

| | Survey years | Geometric mean (95% conf. interval) | Selected percentiles ( 95% confidence interval) | | | | Sample size |
|---|---|---|---|---|---|---|---|
| | | | 50th | 75th | 90th | 95th | |
| **Total** | 03-04 | * | .300 (<LOD-.500) | .900 ( 600-1.30) | 1.70 (1.20-2.40) | 2.30 (1.60-3.20) | 2517 |
| **Age group** | | | | | | | |
| 6-11 years | 03-04 | .357 ( 268-.477) | .400 ( 200-.500) | .900 ( 600-1.40) | 1.70 (1.20-2.10) | 2.10 (1.50-2.90) | 314 |
| 12-19 years | 03-04 | .369 ( 274-.497) | .400 ( 200-.600) | 1.10 ( 600-1.60) | 1.80 (1.20-2.50) | 2.40 (1.60-3.20) | 715 |
| 20 years and older | 03-04 | * | .300 (<LOD-.500) | .900 ( 500-1.30) | 1.70 (1.10-2.40) | 2.30 (1.60-3.20) | 1488 |
| **Gender** | | | | | | | |
| Males | 03-04 | * | .300 (<LOD-.500) | 1.00 ( 500-1.50) | 1.80 (1.20-2.40) | 2.20 (1.60-3.90) | 1229 |
| Females | 03-04 | * | .300 (<LOD-.400) | .900 ( 600-1.20) | 1.70 (1.20-2.30) | 2.30 (1.50-3.00) | 1288 |
| **Race/ethnicity** | | | | | | | |
| Mexican Americans | 03-04 | * | < LOD | .500 ( 300-.600) | .900 ( 600-1.40) | 1.30 ( 800-1.80) | 613 |
| Non-Hispanic blacks | 03-04 | .389 ( 299-.507) | .400 ( 300-.600) | 1.10 (.700-1.50) | 2.00 (1.30-2.60) | 2.50 (1.60-3.10) | 652 |
| Non-Hispanic whites | 03-04 | * | .300 (<LOD-.600) | 1.00 ( 600-1.50) | 1.80 (1.20-2.50) | 2.30 (1.60-3.60) | 1092 |

Limit of detection (LOD, see Data Analysis section) for Survey year 03-04 is 0.2.
< LOD means less than the limit of detection, which may vary for some chemicals by year and by individual sample.
* Not calculated: proportion of results below limit of detection was too high to provide a valid result.

Myllymaki et al., 2005; Nagao et al., 2001; Sweeney et al., 2000; Yoshida et al., 2001). It is unclear if estrogenic or other effects occur in animals through oral dosing, at lower or environmentally relevant doses (Blake et al., 2004; Tyl et al., 1999). 4-*tert*-Octylphenol is not considered directly genotoxic. IARC and NTP have not rated octylphenol, nonylphenol, or their corresponding ethoxylates with respect to human carcinogenicity.

## Biomonitoring Information

Urinary levels of 4-*tert*-octyphenol reflect recent exposure. Calafat et al. (2008) showed that urinary levels of 4-*tert*-octyphenol were detectable in slightly greater than half of the participants of the U.S. representative subsample of NHANES 2003-2004. In a small number of adult Japanese volunteers, the urinary concentrations of 4-*tert*-octyphenol were near or below the detection limit (Inoue et al. 2003; Kawaguchi et al. 2004).

Finding measurable amounts of 4-*tert*-octylphenol in the urine does not mean that the levels of 4-*tert*-octylphenol cause an adverse health effect. Biomonitoring studies on levels of 4-*tert*-octylphenol provide physicians and public health officials with reference values so that they can determine whether people have been exposed to higher levels of 4-*tert*-octylphenol than are found in the general population. Biomonitoring data can also help scientists plan and conduct research on exposure and health effects.

## Urinary 4-*tert*-Octylphenol (4-[1,1,3,3-Tetramethylbutyl] phenol) (creatinine corrected)

Geometric mean and selected percentiles of urine concentrations (in µg/g of creatinine) for the U.S. population from the National Health and Nutrition Examination Survey.

| | Survey years | Geometric mean (95% conf. interval) | Selected percentiles ( 95% confidence interval) | | | | Sample size |
|---|---|---|---|---|---|---|---|
| | | | 50th | 75th | 90th | 95th | |
| Total | 03-04 | * | .320 (<LOD-.470) | .860 (.550-1 25) | 1.85 (1.31-2 54) | 2.76 (2.02-4 00) | 2514 |
| **Age group** | | | | | | | |
| 6-11 years | 03-04 | .435 (.337-.560) | .460 (.280-.610) | 1.17 (.730-1 62) | 2.03 (1.67-2.15) | 2.50 (2.03-6 00) | 314 |
| 12-19 years | 03-04 | .276 (.199-.384) | .270 (.160-.450) | .740 (.470-1 22) | 1.62 (1.11-2 59) | 2.62 (1.53-3 68) | 713 |
| 20 years and older | 03-04 | * | .300 (<LOD-.450) | .850 (.540-1 25) | 1.81 (1.25-2.71) | 2.78 (1.96-4.14) | 1487 |
| **Gender** | | | | | | | |
| Males | 03-04 | * | .260 (<LOD-.420) | .740 (.470-1.11) | 1.59 (1.05-2 29) | 2.40 (1.65-3 33) | 1228 |
| Females | 03-04 | * | .370 (<LOD- 530) | 1.00 (.630-1.43) | 2.20 (1.43-3 00) | 3.33 (2.40-4.78) | 1286 |
| **Race/ethnicity** | | | | | | | |
| Mexican Americans | 03-04 | * | < LOD | .410 (.270-.620) | .910 (.640-1.43) | 1.64 (.890-2.73) | 612 |
| Non-Hispanic blacks | 03-04 | .269 (.207-.349) | .270 (.170-.400) | .770 (.500-1 08) | 1.60 (1.10-2.11) | 2.31 (1.68-2.78) | 651 |
| Non-Hispanic whites | 03-04 | * | .380 (<LOD- 570) | 1.00 (.620-1.41) | 2.03 (1.36-3 00) | 3.06 (2.18-4 24) | 1091 |

< LOD means less than the limit of detection for the urine levels not corrected for creatinine.
* Not calculated: proportion of results below limit of detection was too high to provide a valid result.

## References

Bian Q, Qian J, Xu L, Chen J, Song L, Wang X. The toxic effects of 4-*tert*-octylphenol on the reproductive system of male rats. Food Chem Toxicol 2006;44(8):1355-1361.

Blake CA, Boockfor FR, Nair-Menon JU, Millette CF, Raychoudhury SS, McCoy GL. Effects of 4-*tert*-octylphenol given in drinking water for 4 months on the male reproductive system of Fischer 344 rats. Reprod Toxicol 2004;18(1):43-51.

Blake CA, Boockfor FR. Chronic administration of the environmental pollutant 4-*tert*-octylphenol to adult male rats interferes with the secretion of luteinizing hormone,follicle-stimulating hormone, prolactin, and testosterone. Biol Reprod 1997;57(2):255-266.

Calafat AM, Ye X, Wong LY, Reidy JA, Needham LL. Exposure of the U.S. population to bisphenol A and 4-*tert*iary-octylphenol: 2003-2004. Environ Health Perspect 2008;116(1):39-44.

Certa H, Fedtke N, Wiegand HJ, Muller AM, Bolt HM. Toxicokinetics of p-*tert*-octylphenol in male Wistar rats. Arch Toxicol 1996;71(1-2):112-122.

Inoue K, Kawaguchi M, Okada F, Takai N, Yoshimura Y, Horie M, et al. 2003. Measurement of 4-nonylphenol and 4-*tert*-octylphenol in human urine by column-switching liquid chromatography-mass spectrometry. Anal Chim Acta 486:41-50.

Katsuda S, Yoshida M, Watanabe G, Taya K, Maekawa A. Irreversible effects of neonatal exposure to p-*tert*-octylphenol on the reproductive tract in female rats. Toxicol Appl Pharmacol 2000;165(3):217-226.

Kawaguchi M, Inoue K, Sakui N, Ito R, Izumi S, Makino T, et al. Stir bar sorptive extraction and thermal desorption-gas chromatography-mass spectrometry for the measurement of 4-nonylphenol and 4-*tert*-octylphenol in human biological samples. J Chromatogr B Analyt Technol Biomed Life Sci 2004;799(1):119-125.

Kolpin DW, Furlong ET, Meyer MT, Thurman EM, Zaugg SD, Barber LB, et al. Pharmaceuticals, hormones, and other organic wastewater contaminants in U.S. streams, 1999-2000: a national reconnaissance. Environ Sci Technol 2002;36(6):1202-1211.

Laws SC, Carey SA, Ferrell JM, Bodman GJ, Cooper RL. Estrogenic activity of octylphenol, nonylphenol, bisphenol A and methoxychlor in rats. Toxicol Sci 2000;54(1):154-167.

Myllymaki SA, Karjalainen M, Haavisto TE, Toppari J, Paranko J. Infantile 4-*tert*-octylphenol exposure transiently inhibits rat ovarian steroidogenesis and steroidogenic acute regulatory protein (StAR) expression. Toxicol Appl Pharmacol 2005;207(1):59-68.

Nagao T, Yoshimura S, Saito Y, Nakagomi M, Usumi K, Ono H. Reproductive effects in male and female rats from neonatal exposure to p-octylphenol. Reprod Toxicol 2001;15(6):683-692.

Rudel RA, Camann DE, Spengler JD, Korn LR, Brody JG. Phthalates, alkylphenols, pesticides, polybrominated diphenyl ethers, and other endocrine-disrupting compounds in indoor air and dust. Environ Sci Technol 2003;37(20):4543-53.

Saito I, Onuki A, Seto H. Indoor air pollution by alkylphenols in Tokyo. Indoor Air 2004;14(5):325-332.

Sweeney T, Nicol L, Roche JF, Brooks AN. Maternal exposure to octylphenol suppresses ovine fetal follicle-stimulating hormone secretion, testis size, and sertoli cell number. Endocrinology 2000;141(7):2667-2673.

Tyl RW, Myers CB, Marr MC, Brine DR, Fail PA, Seely JC, et al. Two-generation reproduction study with para-*tert*-octylphenol in rats. Regul Toxicol Pharmacol 1999;30(2 Pt 1):81-95.

Warhurst AM. An environmental assessment of alkylphenol ethoxylates and alkylphenols. 1995. Available at URL: http://www.foe.co.uk/resource/reports/ethoxylates_alkylphenols.pdf. 2/4/09

Ying GG, Williams B, Kookana R. Environmental fate of alkylphenols and alkylphenol ethoxylates--a review. Environ Int 2002;28(3):215-226.

Yoshida M, Katsuda S, Takenaka A, Watanabe G, Taya K, Maekawa A. Effects of neonatal exposure to a high-dose p-*tert*-octylphenol on the male reproductive tract in rats. Toxicol Lett 2001;121(1):21-33.

# Triclosan

CAS No. 3380-34-5

## General Information

Triclosan is a phenolic diphenyl ether used for over 30 years as a preservative and antiseptic agent. It acts by inhibiting bacterial fatty acid synthesis. Triclosan has been added to soaps, toothpastes, mouthwashes, acne medications, deodorants, and wound disinfection solutions, and has also been impregnated into some kitchen utensils, toys, and medical devices. Triclosan enters the aquatic environment mainly through residential wastewaters. It can be photochemically and biologically degraded, a process that can result in the formation of small amounts of 2,8-dichlorodibenzo-p-dioxin (Aranami et al., 2007; Mezcua et al., 2004). In 1999-2000, triclosan was found in 57.6% of 139 U.S. streams sampled in 30 states (Kolpin et al., 2002). Triclosan has a low bioaccumulation potential in fish. There is some concern that widespread use of triclosan and other biocides can alter antibiotic resistance in bacteria (Aiello et al., 2007).

General population exposure results from dermal and oral use of products containing triclosan. Triclosan can remain present in the oral saliva for several hours after the use of toothpaste containing triclosan (Gilbert et al., 1987). Triclosan can be absorbed across skin into the blood stream. In the body it is conjugated to glucuronides and sulfates (Bodey et al., 1976; Moss et al., 2000). In animal and human studies, it is excreted over several days in the feces and urine as primarily as unchanged triclosan (Kanetoshi et al., 1988; (Sandborgh-Englund et al., 2006).

Human health effects from triclosan at low environmental doses or at biomonitored levels from low environmental exposures are unknown. Triclosan formulations may rarely cause skin irritation. In animal studies, it has low acute toxicity. Some reports show endocrine effects are observed in amphibians and fish (Foran et al., 2000; Matsumura et al., 2005; Veldhoen et al., 2007). Triclosan is not considered teratogenic at maternally toxic doses, and has not been considered mutagenic or carcinogenic (Bhargava and Leonard, 1996; Lyman and Furia, 1969). IARC and NTP do not have ratings with respect to human carcinogenicity.

## Biomonitoring Information

Urinary triclosan levels reflect recent exposure. In a U.S. representative subsample of NHANES 2003-2004, Calafat et al., 2008 has shown higher levels during the third decade of life and among people with the highest household income, but not by race/ethnicity and sex. In a study of 90 U.S. young girls, the median urinary triclosan level of 7.2 µg/L was comparable to the median level (8.2 µg/L) of children 6-11 years of age who participated in NHANES 2003-2004 (Wolff et al., 2007; Calafat et al., 2008).

Finding measurable amounts of triclosan in the urine does not mean that the levels of triclosan cause an adverse health effect. Biomonitoring studies on levels of triclosan provide physicians and public health officials with a reference values so that they can determine whether people have been exposed to higher levels of triclosan than are found in the general population. Biomonitoring data can also help scientists plan and conduct research on exposure and health effects.

## Urinary Triclosan (2,4,4'-Trichloro-2'-hydroxyphenyl ether)

Geometric mean and selected percentiles of urine concentrations (in µg/L) for the U.S. population from the National Health and Nutrition Examination Survey.

| | Survey years | Geometric mean (95% conf. interval) | 50th | 75th | 90th | 95th | Sample size |
|---|---|---|---|---|---|---|---|
| | | | **Selected percentiles** ( 95% confidence interval) | | | | |
| Total | 03-04 | 13.0 (11.6-14 6) | 9.20 (7.90-10 9) | 47.4 (38.2-58.4) | 249 (188-304) | 461 (383-522) | 2517 |
| **Age group** | | | | | | | |
| 6-11 years | 03-04 | 8.16 (6.20-10 8) | 6.00 (4.00-8.50) | 20.7 (14.3-31 6) | 123 (36.4-163) | 157 (113-380) | 314 |
| 12-19 years | 03-04 | 14.5 (11.0-19.1) | 10.3 (8.20-13.1) | 39.0 (26.5-86.4) | 304 (134-566) | 655 (310-890) | 715 |
| 20 years and older | 03-04 | 13.6 (12.0-15 3) | 9.60 (8.20-11 5) | 51.7 (39.6-65.7) | 261 (198-317) | 472 (406-522) | 1488 |
| **Gender** | | | | | | | |
| Males | 03-04 | 16.2 (13.4-19 6) | 11.7 (9.30-14 8) | 84.9 (50.6-111) | 317 (231-433) | 574 (461-716) | 1229 |
| Females | 03-04 | 10.6 (9.29-12.1) | 7.60 (6.10-9.10) | 33.2 (27.1-39.4) | 144 (96.5-250) | 380 (258-430) | 1288 |
| **Race/ethnicity** | | | | | | | |
| Mexican Americans | 03-04 | 14.6 (10.6-20.1) | 8.80 (5.40-17 5) | 65.4 (32.8-127) | 357 (225-456) | 597 (372-992) | 613 |
| Non-Hispanic blacks | 03-04 | 14.4 (11.4-18 2) | 11.1 (8.70-16.1) | 37.6 (30.2-58 0) | 203 (87.5-341) | 450 (254-750) | 652 |
| Non-Hispanic whites | 03-04 | 12.9 (11.2-14 9) | 9.20 (7.40-11 0) | 49.2 (37.8-63.4) | 245 (163-334) | 461 (383-527) | 1092 |

Limit of detection (LOD, see Data Analysis section) for Survey year 03-04 is 2.3.

## Urinary Triclosan (2,4,4'-Trichloro-2'-hydroxyphenyl ether) (creatinine corrected)

Geometric mean and selected percentiles of urine concentrations (in µg/g of creatinine) for the U.S. population from the National Health and Nutrition Examination Survey.

| | Survey years | Geometric mean (95% conf. interval) | 50th | 75th | 90th | 95th | Sample size |
|---|---|---|---|---|---|---|---|
| | | | **Selected percentiles** ( 95% confidence interval) | | | | |
| Total | 03-04 | 12.7 (11.5-14.1) | 9.48 (8.22-10.4) | 43.9 (33.8-60 6) | 212 (172-241) | 368 (294-463) | 2514 |
| **Age group** | | | | | | | |
| 6-11 years | 03-04 | 9.93 (7.43-13 3) | 7.55 (4.72-13.4) | 25.1 (15.3-35 6) | 116 (39.9-236) | 236 (115-336) | 314 |
| 12-19 years | 03-04 | 10.9 (8.32-14 2) | 7.45 (5.48-10.7) | 31.8 (21.9-61.1) | 193 (90.7-318) | 356 (169-580) | 713 |
| 20 years and older | 03-04 | 13.4 (12.0-15.1) | 10.0 (8.89-11.4) | 50.0 (36.0-73 8) | 224 (186-272) | 385 (308-506) | 1487 |
| **Gender** | | | | | | | |
| Males | 03-04 | 13.2 (11.3-15 6) | 9.21 (6.86-12.1) | 73.1 (45.8-85 9) | 237 (175-294) | 384 (294-506) | 1228 |
| Females | 03-04 | 12.2 (10.6-14 2) | 9.54 (8.45-10.4) | 32.3 (26.2-46 6) | 182 (138-217) | 336 (225-480) | 1286 |
| **Race/ethnicity** | | | | | | | |
| Mexican Americans | 03-04 | 13.3 (9.38-18 8) | 9.18 (5.45-13 9) | 66.7 (28.8-112) | 292 (151-432) | 453 (263-1150) | 612 |
| Non-Hispanic blacks | 03-04 | 9.94 (7.92-12 5) | 7.74 (5.50-10 0) | 30.2 (25.6-37 3) | 132 (78.0-213) | 260 (127-513) | 651 |
| Non-Hispanic whites | 03-04 | 13.3 (11.6-15.1) | 9.82 (8.11-11 5) | 47.0 (34.3-67.7) | 213 (160-272) | 358 (276-480) | 1091 |

## References

Aiello AE, Larson EL, Levy SB. Consumer antibacterial soaps: effective or just risky? Clin Infect Dis 2007;45 Suppl 2:S137-S147.

Aranami K, Readman JW. Photolytic degradation of triclosan in freshwater and seawater. Chemosphere 2007;66:1052-1056.

Bhargava HN, Leonard PA.. Triclosan: applications and safety. Am J Infect Control 1996;24(3):209-218.

Bodey GP, Ebersole R, Hong HC. Randomized trial of a hexachlorophene preparation and P-300 bacteriostatic soaps. J Invest Dermatol 1976;67(4):532-537.

Calafat AM, Ye X, Wong LY, Reidy JA, Needham LL. Urinary concentrations of triclosan in the U.S. population: 2003-2004. Environ Health Perspect 2008;116(3):303-307.

Foran CM, Bennett ER, Benson WH. Developmental evaluation of a potential non-steroidal estrogen: triclosan. Mar Environ Res 2000;50(1-5):153-156.

Gilbert RJ, Williams PE. The oral retention and antiplaque efficacy of triclosan in human volunteers. Br J Clin Pharmacol 1987;23(5):579-583.

Kanetoshi A, Ogawa H, Katsura E, Okui T, Kaneshima H. Disposition and excretion of Irgasan DP300 and its chlorinated derivatives in mice. Arch Environ Contam Toxicol 1988;17(5):637-644.

Kolpin DW, Furlong ET, Meyer MT, Thurman EM, Zaugg SD, Barber LB, et al. Pharmaceuticals, hormones, and other organic wastewater contaminants in U.S. streams, 1999-2000: a national reconnaissance. Environ Sci Technol 2002;36(6):1202-1211.

Lyman FL, Furia T. Toxicology of 2, 4, 4'-trichloro-2'-hydroxy-diphenyl ether. IMS Ind Med Surg 1969;38(2):64-71.

Matsumura N, Ishibashi H, Hirano M, Nagao Y, Watanabe N, Shiratsuchi H, et al. Effects of nonylphenol and triclosan on production of plasma vitellogenin and testosterone in male South African clawed frogs (Xenopus laevis). Biol Pharm Bull 2005;28(9):1748-1751.

Mezcua M, Gomez MJ, Ferrer I, Aguera A, Hernando MD, Fernandez-Alba AR. Evidence of 2,7/2,8-dibenzodichloro-p-dioxin as a photodegradation product of triclosan in water and wastewater samples. Anal Chim Acta 1004;524:241-247.

Moss T, Howes D, Williams FM. Percutaneous penetration and dermal metabolism of triclosan (2,4,4'-trichloro-2'-hydroxydiphenyl ether). Food Chem Toxicol 2000;38(4):361-370.

Sandborgh-Englund G, Adolfsson-Erici M, Odham G, Ekstrand J. Pharmacokinetics of triclosan following oral ingestion in humans. J Toxicol Environ Health A 2006;69(20):1861-1873.

Veldhoen N, Skirrow RC, Osachoff H, Wigmore H, Clapson DJ, Gunderson MP, et al. The bactericidal agent triclosan modulates thyroid hormone-associated gene expression and disrupts postembryonic anuran development. Aquat Toxicol 2006;80(3):217-227. Erratum in: Aquat Toxicol 2007;83(1):84.

Wolff MS, Teitelbaum SL, Windham G, Pinney SM, Britton JA, Chelimo C, et al. Pilot study of urinary biomarkers of phytoestrogens, phthalates, and phenols in girls. Environ Health Perspect 2007;115:116-121.

# Pentachlorophenol

CAS No. 87-86-5

*Also a Metabolite of Several Organochlorine Insecticides*

## General Information

Pentachlorophenol (PCP) and its sodium salt were once widely used as a fungicide, bactericide, herbicide, mollusicide, algaecide and insecticide. Since 1984, PCP use in the U.S. has been restricted, and it is used primarily as a preservative for wood to be used outdoors (e.g., utility poles and fence posts). PCP cannot be used on wood in residential or agricultural buildings. PCP has been detected in soils, air, water and sediments because of the large amounts that were produced and used historically. In the environment, PCP is degraded by sunlight and metabolized rapidly by microorganisms, plants, and animals, so it is relatively non-persistent. General population exposure to PCP may occur by inhalation of contaminated air, ingestion of contaminated food or water, and dermal contact with PCP-treated products. Human exposure to PCP has become less common. Workers who manufacture or apply PCP may inhale it or absorb it through exposed skin.

PCP is absorbed rapidly and well by all exposure routes. After absorption, PCP is distributed to most tissues and is not extensively metabolized. The parent compound and conjugates, along with small amounts of tetrachlorohydroquinone and conjugates, are eliminated in the urine. After a single dose, PCP is eliminated over a few days (Braun et al., 1979); with repeated or chronic exposure, the elimination half-life may be a week or more (Uhl et al., 1986). PCP also may be eliminated in urine as a metabolite of hexachlorobenzene, other polychlorinated benzenes, and possibly of lindane (IPCS, 2002; Kohli et al., 1976; To-Figueras et al., 1997).

Human health effects from PCP at low environmental doses or at biomonitored levels from low environmental exposures are unknown. Acute, high dose exposure to PCP can induce a hypermetabolic state and excessive heat production as a result of uncoupling mitochondrial oxidative phosphorylation. Effects including hyperthermia, hypertension, and metabolic acidosis were observed in

## Urinary Pentachlorophenol

*Also a Metabolite of Several Organochlorine Insecticides*

Geometric mean and selected percentiles of urine concentrations (in µg/L) for the U.S. population from the National Health and Nutrition Examination Survey.

| | Survey years | Geometric mean (95% conf. interval) | 50th | 75th | 90th | 95th | Sample size |
|---|---|---|---|---|---|---|---|
| | | | Selected percentiles ( 95% confidence interval) | | | | |
| **Total** | 99-00 | * | .350 ( 350-.350) | .350 ( 350-.350) | .390 ( 350-.960) | 1.30 ( 500-2.10) | 1994 |
| | 01-02 | * | < LOD | < LOD | 1.23 ( 590-1.76) | 1.94 (1.58-2.53) | 2528 |
| **Age group** | | | | | | | |
| 6-11 years | 99-00 | * | .350 ( 350-.350) | .350 ( 350-.350) | .770 ( 350-1.51) | 1.65 ( 990-2.00) | 482 |
| | 01-02 | * | < LOD | < LOD | 1.37 ( 890-1.70) | 2.10 (1.58-2.75) | 577 |
| 12-19 years | 99-00 | * | .350 ( 350-.350) | .350 ( 350-.350) | .660 ( 350-2.60) | 2.00 ( 510-5.90) | 681 |
| | 01-02 | * | < LOD | < LOD | 1.48 ( 850-2.30) | 2.30 (1.47-5.04) | 826 |
| 20-59 years | 99-00 | * | .350 ( 350-.350) | .350 ( 350-.350) | .350 ( 350-.650) | 1.10 ( 350-2.00) | 831 |
| | 01-02 | * | < LOD | < LOD | 1.01 (<LOD-1.76) | 1.90 (1.45-2.53) | 1125 |
| **Gender** | | | | | | | |
| Males | 99-00 | * | .350 ( 350-.350) | .350 ( 350-.350) | .630 ( 350-1.30) | 1.40 (.480-2.60) | 973 |
| | 01-02 | * | < LOD | < LOD | 1.32 ( 680-1.80) | 1.94 (1.47-3.09) | 1190 |
| Females | 99-00 | * | .350 ( 350-.350) | .350 ( 350-.350) | .350 ( 350-.530) | .890 ( 350-2.00) | 1021 |
| | 01-02 | * | < LOD | < LOD | 1.10 (<LOD-1.78) | 1.98 (1.54-2.42) | 1338 |
| **Race/ethnicity** | | | | | | | |
| Mexican Americans | 99-00 | * | .350 ( 350-.350) | .350 ( 350-.350) | .350 ( 350-.350) | .650 ( 350-1.90) | 696 |
| | 01-02 | * | < LOD | < LOD | .990 (<LOD-2.37) | 1.62 ( 510-3.64) | 680 |
| Non-Hispanic blacks | 99-00 | * | .350 ( 350-.350) | .350 ( 350-.350) | .980 ( 350-2.50) | 1.65 ( 860-2.70) | 521 |
| | 01-02 | * | < LOD | < LOD | 1.73 (1.33-2.33) | 2.83 (2.08-3.67) | 696 |
| Non-Hispanic whites | 99-00 | * | .350 ( 350-.350) | .350 ( 350-.350) | .390 ( 350-1.10) | 1.30 ( 350-2.30) | 603 |
| | 01-02 | * | < LOD | < LOD | 1.18 (<LOD-1.76) | 1.91 (1.48-2.42) | 951 |

Limit of detection (LOD, see Data Analysis section) for Survey years 99-00 and 01-02 are 0.25 and 0.5.
< LOD means less than the limit of detection, which may vary for some chemicals by year and by individual sample.
* Not calculated: proportion of results below limit of detection was too high to provide a valid result.

adults and children severely exposed to PCP through ingestion, inhalation, or skin absorption. Death can result from seizures and cardiovascular collapse. In animals, chronically administered high doses of PCP were hepatotoxic, carcinogenic, and adversely affected thyroid function (U.S.EPA, 2004; van Raaij et al., 1991). Pentachlorophenol is not mutagenic or teratogenic. IARC has determined that pentachlorophenol is possibly carcinogenic to humans.

The U.S. EPA has developed standards for PCP in drinking water and the environment, and the FDA has established a standard for bottled water. OSHA has established an occupational standard. More information about external exposure (i.e., environmental levels) and health effects is available from the U.S. EPA at: http://www.epa.gov/pesticides/ and from ATSDR at: http://www.atsdr.cdc.gov/toxpro2.html.

## Biomonitoring Information

In NHANES 1999-2000 the median urinary PCP levels among children aged 6-11 and 12-19 years were as much as thirteen times lower compared to a sample of German children aged 6-14 years in 1990-1992 (4.6 and 14.9 µg/L, respectively) (Seifert et al., 2000). Among adults in the NHANES 1999-2000 subsample, the median and 95th percentile urinary PCP levels were approximately three times lower than comparable values in German adults (2.08 and 5.0 µg/L, respectively) (Becker et al., 2003). In NHANES 2001-2002 subsamples, urinary PCP levels at the 95th percentile were approximately fivefold lower than 95th percentile values measured in a nonrandom subsample from NHANES III (1988-1994) participants (Hill et al., 1995). Urinary PCP levels at the 95th percentile in this *Report* are approximately half the corresponding 95th percentile values found in German adults evaluated in 1998 (Becker et al., 2003). In a small sample of U.S. children in the 1980's, the 95th percentile of urinary PCP levels was about fiftyfold higher than that for 6-11 year olds in NHANES 2001-2002 (Hill et al., 1989). Urinary levels of pentachlorophenol in the general population are far below (hundreds of times lower than) urine levels reported for workplace exposure to PCP or among people living in PCP-treated log homes (Cline et al., 1989).

### Urinary Pentachlorophenol (creatinine corrected)
*Also a Metabolite of Several Organochlorine Insecticides*

Geometric mean and selected percentiles of urine concentrations (in µg/g of creatinine) for the U.S. population from the National Health and Nutrition Examination Survey.

| | Survey years | Geometric mean (95% conf. interval) | Selected percentiles ( 95% confidence interval) | | | | Sample size |
|---|---|---|---|---|---|---|---|
| | | | 50th | 75th | 90th | 95th | |
| **Total** | 99-00 | * | .300 (.290-.320) | .570 (.500-.650) | 1.16 (.950-1 35) | 1.67 (1.35-2.11) | 1994 |
| | 01-02 | * | < LOD | < LOD | 1.52 (1.25-1.75) | 2.26 (1.67-3 09) | 2527 |
| **Age group** | | | | | | | |
| 6-11 years | 99-00 | * | .370 (.340-.420) | .650 (.580-.780) | .990 (.900-1 30) | 1.83 (1.10-2 95) | 482 |
| | 01-02 | * | < LOD | < LOD | 1.84 (1.29-3.18) | 3.18 (1.84-4 52) | 577 |
| 12-19 years | 99-00 | * | .250 (.220-.290) | .400 (.330-.490) | .760 (.500-1.40) | 1.57 (.700-2 51) | 681 |
| | 01-02 | * | < LOD | < LOD | 1.21 (.910-1 56) | 1.82 (1.25-2 82) | 825 |
| 20-59 years | 99-00 | * | .300 (.270-.320) | .610 (.510-.730) | 1.25 (1.00-1.40) | 1.67 (1.30-2.19) | 831 |
| | 01-02 | * | < LOD | < LOD | 1.52 (<LOD-1.75) | 2.19 (1.67-2 99) | 1125 |
| **Gender** | | | | | | | |
| Males | 99-00 | * | .260 (.240-.280) | .470 (.380-.560) | .920 (.780-1 25) | 1.67 (1.16-1 84) | 973 |
| | 01-02 | * | < LOD | < LOD | 1.13 (.950-1.40) | 1.73 (1.25-2 92) | 1190 |
| Females | 99-00 | * | .360 (.310-.430) | .650 (.560-.830) | 1.26 (1.09-1 35) | 1.67 (1.35-2.19) | 1021 |
| | 01-02 | * | < LOD | < LOD | 1.75 (<LOD-2.06) | 2.69 (1.94-3 55) | 1337 |
| **Race/ethnicity** | | | | | | | |
| Mexican Americans | 99-00 | * | .300 (.270-.320) | .500 (.430-.560) | 1.06 (.710-1.40) | 1.57 (1.21-2 00) | 696 |
| | 01-02 | * | < LOD | < LOD | 1.09 (<LOD-2.36) | 1.94 (1.06-3 55) | 680 |
| Non-Hispanic blacks | 99-00 | * | .250 (.220-.310) | .440 (.360-.590) | .850 (.590-1 30) | 1.34 (.950-1 90) | 521 |
| | 01-02 | * | < LOD | < LOD | 1.30 (.800-1.78) | 1.94 (1.48-2.79) | 695 |
| Non-Hispanic whites | 99-00 | * | .320 (.290-.350) | .630 (.510-.800) | 1.25 (1.00-1.40) | 1.67 (1.40-2.19) | 603 |
| | 01-02 | * | < LOD | < LOD | 1.52 (<LOD-1.78) | 2.10 (1.67-3 08) | 951 |

< LOD means less than the limit of detection for the urine levels not corrected for creatinine.
* Not calculated: proportion of results below limit of detection was too high to provide a valid result.

Finding a measurable amount of PCP in urine does not mean that the level of PCP causes an adverse health effect. Biomonitoring studies on levels of PCP provide physicians and public health officials with reference values so that they can determine whether people have been exposed to higher levels of PCP than are found in the general population. Biomonitoring data can also help scientists plan and conduct research about PCP exposure and health effects.

## References

Becker K, Schulz C, Kaus S, Seiwert M, Seifert B. German environmental survey 1998 (GerES III): environmental pollutants in the urine of the German population. Int J Hyg Environ Health 2003; 206:15-24.

Braun WH, Blau GE, Chenoweth MB. The metabolism/ pharmacokinetics of pentachlorophenol in man and a comparison with the rat and monkey. Dev Toxicol Environ Sci 1979;4:289-296.

Cline RE, Hill RH, Phillips DL, Needham LL. Pentachlorophenol measurements in body fluids of people in log homes and workplaces. Arch Environ Contam Toxicol 1989;18:475-481.

Hill RH Jr, Head SL, Baker S, Gregg M, Shealy DB, Bailey SL, et al. Pesticide residues in urine of adults living in the United States: reference range concentrations. Environ Res 1995;71:99-108.

Hill RH Jr, To T, Holler JS, Fast DM, Smith SJ, Needham LL, et al. Residues of chlorinated phenols and phenoxy acid herbicides in the urine of Arkansas children. Arch Environ Contam Toxicol 1989;18(4):469-474.

International Programme on Chemical Safety (IPCS). Pesticide residues in food-2002-Joint FAO/WHO meeting on pesticide residues. Lindane. 2002. available at URL: http://www.inchem.org/documents/jmpr/jmpmono/2002pr08. htm. 4/21/09

Kohli J, Jones D, Safe A. The metabolism of higher chlorinated benzene isomers. Can J Biochem 1976;54(3):203-208.

Seifert B, Becker K, Helm D, Krause C, Schulz C, Seiwert M. The German Environmental Survey 1990/1992 (GerES II): reference concentrations of selected environmental pollutants in blood, urine, hair, house dust, drinking water and indoor air. J Expo Anal Environ Epidemiol 2000;10:552-65.

To-Figueras J, Sala M, Otero R, Barrot C, Santiago-Silva M, Rodamilans M, et al. Metabolism of hexachlorobenzene in humans: association between serum levels and urinary metabolites in a highly exposed population. Environ Health Perspect 1997;105(1):78-83.

Uhl S, Schmid P, Schlatter C. Pharmacokinetics of pentachlorophenol in man. Arch Toxicol 1986;58:182-186.

U.S. Environmental Protection Agency (U.S. EPA). PCP: Human Risk Characterization [online]. 11/30/2004. Available at URL: http://www.regulations.gov/fdmspublic/component/main?main=DocketDetail&d=EPA-HQ-OPP-2004-0402. 4/21/09

van Raaij JA, van den Berg KJ, Engel R, Bragt PC, Notten WR. Effects of hexachlorobenzene and its metabolites pentachlorophenol and tetrachlorohydroquinone on serum thyroid hormone levels in rats. Toxicology 1991: 67(1):107-16.

## *ortho*-Phenylphenol

CAS No. 90-43-7

### General Information

*Ortho*-phenylphenol (OPP, or 2-phenylphenol) and its water-soluble salt, sodium *ortho*-phenylphenate (SOPP), are antimicrobial agents used as bacteriostats, fungicides, and sanitizers. Both have been used in agriculture to control fungal and bacterial growth on stored crops, such as fruits and vegetables. SOPP is applied topically to the crop and then rinsed off, leaving the chemical residue OPP. Most agricultural food applications have been revoked, but OPP and SOPP are still used on pears and citrus (U.S.EPA, 2006). OPP is still used as a disinfectant fungicide for industrial applications, on ornamental plants and turfs, in paints, and as a wood preservative. In the past, it was used in home sanitizers for surfaces. OPP is volatile, and it has limited water solubility, whereas SOPP is not volatile and is more water soluble. Both chemicals degrade within hours to weeks in the environment (U.S. EPA, 2006).

General population exposure can occur via dermal, inhalational, or oral routes from residential use and by ingesting treated food or food that was in contact with treated surfaces or equipment. OPP was detected in 40 of 60 different canned beers at concentrations in the low parts per billion (Coelhan et al., 2006). Estimated human intakes have been below recommended intake limits (U.S.EPA, 2006). Workers who manufacture, formulate, or apply these chemicals may be more highly exposed than the general population. OPP is efficiently absorbed from the gastrointestinal tract and through the skin, and it is eliminated rapidly from the body as OPP glucuronide and sulfate conjugates (Bartels et al., 1998; Cnubben et al. 2002; Timchalk et al., 1998). Available evidence suggests that OPP does not accumulate in the body; however, small amounts of OPP have been measured in human adipose tissue (Onstot and Stanley, 1989).

Human health effects from OPP at low environmental doses or at biomonitored levels from low environmental exposures are unknown. OPP is considered to be moderately toxic after acute oral doses in animal studies. Chronic dosing in animals resulted in such systemic effects as weight loss and

### Urinary *ortho*-Phenylphenol

Geometric mean and selected percentiles of urine concentrations (in µg/L) for the U.S. population from the National Health and Nutrition Examination Survey.

| | Survey years | Geometric mean (95% conf. interval) | Selected percentiles ( 95% confidence interval) | | | | Sample size |
|---|---|---|---|---|---|---|---|
| | | | 50th | 75th | 90th | 95th | |
| **Total** | 99-00 | .497 (.390-.632) | .490 (<LOD- 600) | .850 (.600-1 30) | 1.50 (1.10-2.10) | 2.00 (1.60-3 80) | 1991 |
| | 01-02 | * | < LOD | < LOD | .570 (.370-.860) | 1.27 (.710-2 85) | 2529 |
| **Age group** | | | | | | | |
| 6-11 years | 99-00 | .509 (.402-.645) | .490 (<LOD- 630) | .890 (.610-1 50) | 1.90 (1.30-2.10) | 2.20 (1.80-3 90) | 480 |
| | 01-02 | * | < LOD | < LOD | 1.17 (.760-2 02) | 2.30 (1.28-3 61) | 577 |
| 12-19 years | 99-00 | .508 (.370-.696) | .490 (<LOD- 690) | .890 (.570-1 50) | 1.60 (1.20-3 50) | 2.10 (1.40-7 20) | 681 |
| | 01-02 | * | < LOD | < LOD | .740 (.480-1 34) | 2.33 (.800-3 09) | 827 |
| 20-59 years | 99-00 | .493 (.389-.624) | .490 (<LOD- 600) | .820 (.600-1 20) | 1.50 (1.10-1 90) | 2.00 (1.50-2 90) | 830 |
| | 01-02 | * | < LOD | < LOD | .450 (<LOD- 670) | .930 (.540-2 23) | 1125 |
| **Gender** | | | | | | | |
| Males | 99-00 | .498 (.389-.638) | .470 (<LOD- 640) | .830 (.600-1 30) | 1.60 (1.20-2 00) | 2.00 (1.50-3 90) | 973 |
| | 01-02 | * | < LOD | < LOD | .610 (.350-1 03) | 1.28 (.750-2 85) | 1190 |
| Females | 99-00 | .496 (.386-.636) | .490 (<LOD- 600) | .860 (.580-1 30) | 1.50 (1.00-2.10) | 2.10 (1.50-4 50) | 1018 |
| | 01-02 | * | < LOD | < LOD | .520 (.370-.790) | 1.22 (.590-2 91) | 1339 |
| **Race/ethnicity** | | | | | | | |
| Mexican Americans | 99-00 | .552 (.364-.836) | .420 (<LOD- 950) | 1.20 (.500-2 00) | 2.20 (1.40-5 80) | 3.80 (2.30-7.10) | 695 |
| | 01-02 | * | < LOD | < LOD | 1.14 (<LOD-3.88) | 2.92 (.560-8 22) | 680 |
| Non-Hispanic blacks | 99-00 | .567 (.433-.742) | .570 (.410-.780) | .970 (.690-1 50) | 1.60 (1.40-2 00) | 2.00 (1.60-2 30) | 520 |
| | 01-02 | * | < LOD | < LOD | .770 (.570-.890) | 1.19 (.840-1.76) | 695 |
| Non-Hispanic whites | 99-00 | .466 (.349-.621) | .450 (<LOD- 600) | .770 (.550-1 20) | 1.40 (.880-2.10) | 1.90 (1.40-5.10) | 603 |
| | 01-02 | * | < LOD | < LOD | .450 (<LOD-.710) | 1.07 (.570-2 23) | 953 |

Limit of detection (LOD, see Data Analysis section) for Survey years 99-00 and 01-02 are 0 3 and 0.3.
< LOD means less than the limit of detection, which may vary for some chemicals by year and by individual sample.
* Not calculated: proportion of results below limit of detection was too high to provide a valid result.

anemia, but no neurologic, reproductive, or developmental toxicity was observed (Bomhard et al., 2002; U.S.EPA 2006). OPP was not found to be mutagenic. Dermally applied OPP was not carcinogenic in a 2-year experimental study in animals (NTP, 1986). In high dose animal studies, OPP or SOPP produced carcinomas of the bladder only after phase II detoxification pathways were saturated, leading to production of two metabolites, *ortho*-phenylhydroquinone and *ortho*-phenylbenzoquinone. These metabolites may induce carcinogenicity via nongenotoxic regenerative hyperplasia of the bladder (Appel, 2000; Bomhard et al., 2002; Brusick, 2005; Kwok et al., 1999; Nakagawa et al., 1992; Smith et al., 1998; U.S.EPA 2006), or, less likely, by possible genotoxic mechanisms (Hagiwara et al., 1984; Ito et al., 1984; Murata et al., 1999; Pathak and Roy, 1993; Zhao et al., 2002). IARC has classified SOPP as a possible human carcinogen, and it has classified OPP as not classifiable with respect to human carcinogenicity. Additional information is available from U.S.EPA at: http:// www.epa.gov/pesticides/.

## Biomonitoring Information

Urinary OPP levels reflect recent exposure. Detectable levels were seen in over half the U.S. population in the subsamples from NHANES 1999-2000 and 2001-2002 (CDC, 2005). Volunteers exposed to 0.4 mg dermally had urinary levels of OPP that were several hundred times higher than median levels found in NHANES 1999-2000 and 2001-2002 (Bartels et al., 1997; CDC, 2005).

Finding a measurable amount of OPP in urine does not mean that the level of OPP causes an adverse health effect. Biomonitoring studies on levels of OPP provide physicians and public health officials with reference values so that they can determine whether people have been exposed to higher levels of OPP than are found in the general population. Biomonitoring data can also help scientists plan and conduct research on exposure and health effects.

## Urinary *ortho*-Phenylphenol (creatinine corrected)

Geometric mean and selected percentiles of urine concentrations (in µg/g of creatinine) for the U.S. population from the National Health and Nutrition Examination Survey.

| | Survey years | Geometric mean (95% conf. interval) | 50th | 75th | 90th | 95th | Sample size |
|---|---|---|---|---|---|---|---|
| **Total** | 99-00 | .444 ( 353-.558) | .410 (<LOD-.560) | .840 ( 620-1.11) | 1.84 (1.24-2.33) | 2.97 (2.04-4.29) | 1991 |
| | 01-02 | * | < LOD | < LOD | .980 ( 810-1.17) | 1.75 (1.21-2.33) | 2528 |
| **Age group** | | | | | | | |
| 6-11 years | 99-00 | .550 (.455-.666) | .510 (<LOD-.670) | 1.02 ( 800-1.27) | 1.96 (1.43-2.59) | 2.64 (2.09-3.58) | 480 |
| | 01-02 | * | < LOD | < LOD | 1.91 (1.08-2.53) | 2.69 (1.96-4.01) | 577 |
| 12-19 years | 99-00 | .343 ( 248-.473) | .320 (<LOD-.500) | .690 (.460-.950) | 1.17 ( 880-1.93) | 1.96 (1.09-6.32) | 681 |
| | 01-02 | * | < LOD | < LOD | .780 ( 640-1.21) | 1.52 ( 940-2.32) | 826 |
| 20-59 years | 99-00 | .453 ( 361-.568) | .420 (<LOD-.570) | .860 ( 620-1.12) | 1.89 (1.24-2.47) | 3.28 (2.06-4.93) | 830 |
| | 01-02 | * | < LOD | < LOD | .910 (<LOD-1.07) | 1.44 (1.05-2.30) | 1125 |
| **Gender** | | | | | | | |
| Males | 99-00 | .382 ( 301-.484) | .360 (<LOD-.470) | .750 ( 550-.990) | 1.43 (1.08-1.93) | 2.09 (1.51-3.29) | 973 |
| | 01-02 | * | < LOD | < LOD | .750 ( 580-1.17) | 1.61 (.750-2.43) | 1190 |
| Females | 99-00 | .514 (.403-.656) | .470 (<LOD-.580) | .910 ( 650-1.46) | 2.06 (1.38-3.38) | 3.78 (2.06-5.96) | 1018 |
| | 01-02 | * | < LOD | < LOD | 1.11 ( 910-1.38) | 1.75 (1.33-2.38) | 1338 |
| **Race/ethnicity** | | | | | | | |
| Mexican Americans | 99-00 | .496 ( 311-.791) | .420 (<LOD-.810) | 1.11 ( 560-2.31) | 3.00 (1.25-6.08) | 4.61 (2.40-13.4) | 695 |
| | 01-02 | * | < LOD | < LOD | 1.28 (<LOD-4.26) | 3.00 (.780-14 0) | 680 |
| Non-Hispanic blacks | 99-00 | .385 ( 291-.508) | .380 ( 270-.550) | .670 ( 510-.900) | 1.21 ( 900-1.62) | 1.74 (1.43-2.13) | 520 |
| | 01-02 | * | < LOD | < LOD | .670 (.480-.970) | 1.17 (.770-2.18) | 694 |
| Non-Hispanic whites | 99-00 | .440 ( 329-.590) | .410 (<LOD-.610) | .860 ( 600-1.20) | 1.86 (1.12-2.59) | 2.93 (1.88-4.81) | 603 |
| | 01-02 | * | < LOD | < LOD | .980 (<LOD-1.11) | 1.61 (1.11-1.91) | 953 |

< LOD means less than the limit of detection for the urine levels not corrected for creatinine.
* Not calculated: proportion of results below limit of detection was too high to provide a valid result.

## References

Appel KE. The carcinogenicity of the biocide *ortho*-phenylphenol. Arch Toxicol 2000;74(2):61-71.

Brusick D. Analysis of genotoxicity and the carcinogenic mode of action for *ortho*-phenylphenol. Environ Mol Mutagen 2005;45(5):460-481.

Bartels MJ, Brzak KA, Bormett GA. Determination of *ortho*-phenylphenol in human urine by gas chromatography-mass spectrometry. J Chromatogr B Biomed Sci Appl 1997;703(1-2):97-104.

Bartels MJ, McNett DA, Timchalk C, Mendrala AL, Christenson WR, Sangha GK, et al.. Comparative metabolism of *ortho*-phenylphenol in mouse, rat and man. Xenobiotica 1998;28(6):579-594.

Bomhard EM, Brendler-Schwaab SY, Freyberger A, Herbold BA, Leser KH, Richter M. O-phenylphenol and its sodium and potassium salts: a toxicological assessment. Crit Rev Toxicol 2002;32(6):551-625.

Centers for Disease Control and Prevention (CDC). Third National Report on Human Exposure to Environmental Chemicals. Atlanta (GA). 2005.

Cnubben NH, Elliott GR, Hakkert BC, Meuling WJ, van de Sandt JJ. Comparative in vitro-in vivo percutaneous penetration of the fungicide *ortho*-phenylphenol. Regul Toxicol Pharmacol 2002;35(2 Pt 1):198-208.

Coelhan M, Bromig KH, Glas K, Roberts AL. Determination and levels of the biocide *ortho*-phenylphenol in canned beers from different countries. J Agric Food Chem 2006;54(16):5731-5735.

Hagiwara A, Shibata M, Hirose M, Fukushima S, Ito N. Long-term toxicity and carcinogenicity study of sodium o-phenylphenate in B6C3F1 mice. Food Chem Toxicol 1984;22(10):809-814.

Ito N, Fukushima S, Shirai T, Hagiwara A, Imaida K. Drugs, food additives and natural products as promoters in rat urinary bladder carcinogenesis. IARC Sci Publ 1984;(56):399-407.

Kwok ES, Buchholz BA, Vogel JS, Turteltaub KW, Eastmond DA. Dose-dependent binding of *ortho*-phenylphenol to protein but not DNA in the urinary bladder of male F344 rats. Toxicol Appl Pharmacol 1999;159(1):18-24.

Murata M, Moriya K, Inoue S, Kawanishi S. Oxidative damage to cellular and isolated DNA by metabolites of a fungicide *ortho*-phenylphenol. Carcinogenesis 1999;20(5):851-857.

Nakagawa Y, Tayama S, Moore GA, Moldeus P. Relationship between metabolism and cytotoxicity of *ortho*-phenylphenol in isolated rat hepatocytes. Biochem Pharmacol 1992;43(7):1431-1437.

National Toxicology Program (NTP). NTP Technical report on the toxicology and carcinogenesis studies of *ortho*-phenylphenol (CAS No. 90-43-7) in Swiss CD-1 mice (dermal studies). March 1986. Available at URL: http://ntp.niehs.nih.gov/ntp/htdocs/LT_rpts/tr301.pdf. 4/13/09

Onstot JD, Stanley JS. Identification of SARA compounds in adipose tissue. U.S. Environmental Protection Agency (U.S. EPA), Office of Toxic Substances; 1989. EPA-560/5-89-003.

Pathak DN, Roy D. In vivo genotoxicity of sodium *ortho*-phenylphenol: phenylbenzoquinone is one of the DNA-binding metabolite(s) of sodium *ortho*-phenylphenol. Mutat Res 1993;286(2):309-319.

Smith RA, Christenson WR, Bartels MJ, Arnold LL, St John MK, Cano M, et al. Urinary physiologic and chemical metabolic effects on the urothelial cytotoxicity and potential DNA adducts of o-phenylphenol in male rats. Toxicol Appl Pharmacol 1998;150(2):402-413.

Timchalk C, Selim S, Sangha G, Bartels MJ. The pharmacokinetics and metabolism of 14C/13C-labeled *ortho*-phenylphenol formation following dermal application to human volunteers. Hum Exp Toxicol 1998;17(8):411-417.

U.S. Environmental Protection Agency (U.S.EPA). Reregistration Eligibility Decision (RED) for 2-phenylphenol and salts (Orthophenylphenol or OPP). July 28, 2006. EPA 739 R-06-004. Available at URL: http://www.epa.gov/oppsrrd1/REDs/phenylphenol_red.pdf. 4/9/09.

Zhao S, Narang A, Gierthy J, Eadon G. Detection and characterization of DNA adducts formed from metabolites of the fungicide *ortho*-phenylphenol. J Agric Food Chem 2002;50(11):3351-3358.

# Herbicides

Herbicides are used to control undesirable weeds and plants in agricultural, residential, and aquatic environments. More herbicides are used annually than insecticides, with about 553 million pounds of herbicides used in the U.S. during 2001 (U.S.EPA, 2004). The herbicides discussed in this *Report* can be classified into the following categories: chlorophenoxy acids, chloroacetanilides, and atrazine.

General population exposure may result from herbicides used in residential, forestal, or agricultural applications, from residues on food, or from contamination of drinking water. Workers who manufacture, formulate, or apply these chemicals have greater exposure to herbicides than others. The FDA, U.S.EPA, and OSHA have developed criteria for the allowable levels for many of these chemicals in foods, drinking water and other environmental media, and the workplace, respectively.

### Reference

U. S. Environmental Protection Agency (U.S.EPA). Office of Prevention Pesticides and Toxic Substances. Pesticide industry sales and usage - 2000 and 2001 market estimates. Washington (DC): U.S.EPA. May, 2004. Available at URL: http://www.epa. gov/oppbead1/pestsales/01pestsales/market_estimates2001.pdf.

3/17/09

# Acetochlor

CAS No. 34256-82-1

## General Information

Acetochlor is a chloroacetanilide type herbicide with restricted usage for preemergent control of grasses and broadleaf weeds on agricultural crop land, mainly corn. It is absorbed by plants and inhibits plant protein synthesis. Acetochlor is microbiologically degraded, remains in soils for up to 3 months, and has been detected in watersheds of agricultural lands (Battaglin et al., 2000; Hladik et al., 2005; Kolpin et al., 2000). Acetochlor degrades in water to acetochlor sulfonic acid and acetochlor oxanilic acid. Plants can degrade acetochlor to 2-ethyl-6-methylaniline, 2-hydroxyethyl-6-methylaniline, and hydroxymethyl ethyl aniline (U.S.EPA, 2006). Acetochlor is moderately toxic to fish and honey bees.

General population exposure to acetochlor may occur through diet or drinking water. Estimated human intakes of acetochlor have been below recommended limits (U.S.EPA, 2006). In animals, a major pathway for acetochlor metabolism involves mercapturate conjugation, but other pathways occur, including one that produces 2-methyl-6-ethylaniline and its reactive metabolite, the latter which may account for some observed effects (Coleman et al., 2000; Davison et al., 1994; Feng and Wratten, 1989; Jefferies et al., 1998). People exposed to acetochlor will excrete acetochlor mercapturate in their urine; however, this metabolite is not a marker of exposure to most plant metabolites or environmental degradates, which are often more prevalent in the environment.

Human health effects from acetochlor at low environmental doses or at biomonitored levels from low environmental exposures are unknown. Acetochlor has low acute toxicity. Acetochlor has not shown developmental or fetal toxicity in chronic animal studies, but it has produced testicular atrophy, renal injury, and neurologic movement abnormalities (U.S.EPA 2000, 2006). Acetochlor is not mutagenic, and it is unlikely to be genotoxic at relevant doses (Ashby et al., 1996). However, in some species and at doses above maximum tolerated doses, animals have demonstrated tumors of the lung, nasal epithelia, and thyroid (U.S.EPA, 2000, 2006). U.S.EPA considers acetochlor likely to be carcinogenic in humans; NTP and IARC do not have ratings regarding human carcinogenicity. Additional information about external exposure (i.e., environmental levels) is available from U.S. EPA at: http://www.epa.gov/pesticides/.

## Biomonitoring Information

Urinary levels of acetochlor mercapturate reflect recent exposure. Urinary levels of acetochlor mercapturate were generally not detectable in the NHANES 2001-2002 subsample (CDC, 2005). Acetochlor mercapturate was measured in the urine of farmers actively spraying the pesticide and the geometric mean was 8.0 µg/L (Curwin et al., 2005). Urinary acetochlor mercapturate levels of 0.5 to 449 µg/L were measured in commercial applicators within 24 hours following its application (Barr et al., 2007).

Finding measurable amounts of acetochlor mercapturate in the urine does not mean that the levels of acetochlor mercapturate cause an adverse health effect. Biomonitoring studies on levels of acetochlor mercapturate provide physicians and public health officials with reference values so that they can determine whether people have been exposed to higher levels of acetochlor than are found in the general population. Biomonitoring data can also help scientists plan and conduct research on exposure and health effects.

## Urinary Acetochlor mercapturate

*Metabolite of Acetochlor*

Geometric mean and selected percentiles of urine concentrations (in µg/L) for the U.S. population from the National Health and Nutrition Examination Survey.

| | Survey years | Geometric mean (95% conf. interval) | Selected percentiles ( 95% confidence interval) | | | | Sample size |
|---|---|---|---|---|---|---|---|
| | | | 50th | 75th | 90th | 95th | |
| Total | 01-02 | * | < LOD | < LOD | < LOD | < LOD | 2501 |
| Age group | | | | | | | |
| 6-11 years | 01-02 | * | < LOD | < LOD | < LOD | < LOD | 576 |
| 12-19 years | 01-02 | * | < LOD | < LOD | < LOD | < LOD | 820 |
| 20-59 years | 01-02 | * | < LOD | < LOD | < LOD | < LOD | 1105 |
| Gender | | | | | | | |
| Males | 01-02 | * | < LOD | < LOD | < LOD | < LOD | 1178 |
| Females | 01-02 | * | < LOD | < LOD | < LOD | < LOD | 1323 |
| Race/ethnicity | | | | | | | |
| Mexican Americans | 01-02 | * | < LOD | < LOD | < LOD | < LOD | 678 |
| Non-Hispanic blacks | 01-02 | * | < LOD | < LOD | < LOD | < LOD | 673 |
| Non-Hispanic whites | 01-02 | * | < LOD | < LOD | < LOD | < LOD | 952 |

Limit of detection (LOD, see Data Analysis section) for Survey year 01-02 is 0.1.
< LOD means less than the limit of detection, which may vary for some chemicals by year and by individual sample.
* Not calculated: proportion of results below limit of detection was too high to provide a valid result.

## Urinary Acetochlor mercapturate (creatinine corrected)

*Metabolite of Acetochlor*

Geometric mean and selected percentiles of urine concentrations (in µg/g of creatinine) for the U.S. population from the National Health and Nutrition Examination Survey.

| | Survey years | Geometric mean (95% conf. interval) | Selected percentiles ( 95% confidence interval) | | | | Sample size |
|---|---|---|---|---|---|---|---|
| | | | 50th | 75th | 90th | 95th | |
| Total | 01-02 | * | < LOD | < LOD | < LOD | < LOD | 2500 |
| Age group | | | | | | | |
| 6-11 years | 01-02 | * | < LOD | < LOD | < LOD | < LOD | 576 |
| 12-19 years | 01-02 | * | < LOD | < LOD | < LOD | < LOD | 819 |
| 20-59 years | 01-02 | * | < LOD | < LOD | < LOD | < LOD | 1105 |
| Gender | | | | | | | |
| Males | 01-02 | * | < LOD | < LOD | < LOD | < LOD | 1178 |
| Females | 01-02 | * | < LOD | < LOD | < LOD | < LOD | 1322 |
| Race/ethnicity | | | | | | | |
| Mexican Americans | 01-02 | * | < LOD | < LOD | < LOD | < LOD | 678 |
| Non-Hispanic blacks | 01-02 | * | < LOD | < LOD | < LOD | < LOD | 672 |
| Non-Hispanic whites | 01-02 | * | < LOD | < LOD | < LOD | < LOD | 952 |

< LOD means less than the limit of detection for the urine levels not corrected for creatinine.
* Not calculated: proportion of results below limit of detection was too high to provide a valid result.

## References

Ashby J, Kier L, Wilson AG, Green T, Lefevre PA, Tinwell H, et al. Evaluation of the potential carcinogenicity and genetic toxicity to humans of the herbicide acetochlor. Hum Exp Toxicol 1996;15(9):702-735.

Barr DB, Hines CJ, Olsson AO, Deddens JA, Bravo R, Striley CA, et al. Identification of human urinary metabolites of acetochlor in exposed herbicide applicators by high performance liquid chromatography-tandem mass spectrometry. J Expo Sci Environ Epidemiol 2007;17(6):559-566.

Battaglin WA, Furlong ET, Burkhardt MR, Peter CJ. Occurrence of sulfonylurea, sulfonamide, imidazolinone, and other herbicides in rivers, reservoirs and ground water in the Midwestern United States, 1998. Sci Total Environ 2000;248(2-3):123-133.

Centers for Disease Control and Prevention (CDC). Third National Report on Human Exposure to Environmental Chemicals. Atlanta (GA). 2005.

Coleman S, Linderman R, Hodgson E, Rose RL. Comparative metabolism of chloroacetamide herbicides and selected metabolites in human and rat liver microsomes. Environ Health Perspect 2000;108(12):1151-1157.

Curwin BD, Hein MJ, Sanderson WT, Barr DB, Heederik D, Reynolds SJ, Ward EM, Alavanja MC. Urinary and hand wipe pesticide levels among farmers and nonfarmers in Iowa. J Expo Anal Environ Epidemiol 2005;15(6):500-508.

Davison KL, Larsen GL, Feil VJ. Comparative metabolism and elimination of acetanilide compounds by rat. Xenobiotica 1994;24(10):1003-1012.

Feng PCC, Wratten SJ. In vitro transformation of chloroacetanilide herbicides by rat liver enzymes: A comparative study of metolachlor and alachlor. J Agri Food Chem 1989;37(4):1088-1093.

Hladik ML, Hsiao JJ, Roberts AL. Are neutral chloroacetamide herbicide degradates of potential environmental concern? Analysis and occurrence in the upper Chesapeake Bay. Environ Sci Technol 2005;39(17):6561-6574.

Jefferies PR, Quistad GB, Casida JE. Dialkylquinonimines validated as in vivo metabolites of alachlor, acetochlor, and metolachlor herbicides in rats. Chem Res Toxicol 1998;11(4):353-359.

Kolpin DW, Thurman EM, Linhart SM. Finding minimal herbicide concentrations in ground water? Try looking for their degradates. Sci Total Environ 2000;248(2-3):115-122.

U.S. Environmental Protection Agency (U.S. EPA). Acetochlor (Harness) Pesticide Petition Filing 1/00. Federal Register: January 24, 2000, Volume 65, Number 15, pages 3682-3690. Available at URL(non U.S.EPA): http://pmep.cce.cornell.edu/profiles/herb-growthreg/24-d-butylate/acetochlor/acetochlor_pet_100.html. 5/30/06

U.S. Environmental Protection Agency (U.S. EPA). Report of the Food Quality Protection Act (FQPA) Tolerance Reassessment Progress and Risk Management Decision (TRED) for Acetochlor. March 2006. EPA 738-R-00-009. Available at URL: http://www.epa.gov/oppsrrd1/reregistration/REDs/acetochlor_tred.pdf. 5/30/06.

Whyatt RM, Barr DB, Camann DE, Kinney PL, Barr JR, Andrews HF, et al. Contemporary-use pesticides in personal air samples during pregnancy and blood samples at delivery among urban minority mothers and newborns. Environ Health Perspect 2003;111(5):749-756.

# Alachlor

CAS No. 15972-60-8

## General Information

Alachlor is a chloroacetanilide type herbicide with restricted usage for preemergent control of grasses and broadleaf weeds on agricultural cropland, including corn, soybeans, peanuts and other crops, and on non-crop land for general weed control. Since the late 1980s alachlor use has been declining. In 1993-1995, about 20-25% of the U.S. corn cropland was treated with alachlor. It is absorbed by plants and inhibits plant protein synthesis. Alachlor has a soil half-life of a few weeks. It is both metabolized in plants and degraded microbiologically in agricultural soils into as many as 19 metabolites and degradates. Alachlor and its degradates are leachable from agricultural soils and have been detected in watersheds of agricultural land including ground and surface waters (Battaglin et al., 2000; Hladik et al., 2005; Kolpin et al., 2000; USGS, 1999 and 2007; WHO, 2003). Alachlor is highly toxic to freshwater fish and slightly toxic to birds and some invertebrates, but shows little bioaccumulation.

General population exposure to alachlor may occur through consumption of contaminated food or drinking water. Estimated human intakes have been below recommended limits (U.S.EPA, 1998). Because it can be absorbed through skin, the dermal exposure route is potentially significant for applicators, formulators, and field workers. In animal studies, alachlor is quickly absorbed after oral doses and mostly excreted as metabolites within a week (IPCS, 1996; U.S.EPA, 1998; WHO, 2003). In animals, mercapturate conjugates were predominant metabolites, but another metabolic pathway can produce 2,6-diethylaniline and its reactive metabolite; the latter may account for some observed effects (Davison et al., 1994; Feng and Wratten, 1989; Jefferies et al., 1998). People exposed to alachlor will excrete alachlor mercapturate in their urine (Driskell et al., 1996), but this metabolite is not a marker of exposure to most plant metabolites or environmental degradates which are often more prevalent in the environment.

Human health effects from alachlor at low environmental doses or at biomonitored levels from low environmental exposures are unknown. Alachlor has low potential for acute toxicity. In chronic animal testing, alachlor has demonstrated hepatotoxicity, hemosiderosis, and uveal degeneration, but has not shown developmental or reproductive toxicity in mammalian systems (U.S.EPA, 1998; WHO, 2003). Alachlor itself is not considered mutagenic, though positive genotoxic results are reported

for several metabolites of alachlor (Brown et al., 1988; Hill et al., 1997; Tessier and Clark, 1995; U.S.EPA, 1998). Animal carcinogenicity studies have demonstrated tumors of the nasal turbinates, stomach, and thyroid only at either maximum tolerated doses or related to species-specific pathways (Heydens et al., 1999; IPCS, 1996; U.S.EPA, 1998; WHO, 2003). U.S.EPA considers alachlor to be a probable human carcinogen at high doses, but not likely at low doses. NTP and IARC do not have ratings regarding human carcinogenicity. Additional information about is available from U.S. EPA at: http://www.epa.gov/pesticides/.

## Biomonitoring Information

Urinary levels of alachlor mercapturate reflect recent exposure. Urinary levels of alachlor mercapturate were generally not detectable in the NHANES 2001-2002 subsample (CDC, 2005). In a study of applicators and workers exposed to alachlor, mean values of urinary concentrations of alachlor metabolites, as measured through conversion to deethylamine, ranged from 0.1 to 1.1 mg/L at various collection times (Sanderson et al., 1995). Hines et al. (2003) showed that 2.2% of a reference population had detectable alachlor equivalents by immunoassay in their urine, whereas 60% of applicators had detectable amounts.

Finding measurable amounts of alachlor mercapturate in the urine does not mean that the levels of alachlor mercapturate cause an adverse health effect. Biomonitoring studies on levels of alachlor mercapturate provide physicians and public health officials with reference values so that they can determine whether people have been exposed to higher levels of alachlor than are found in the general population. Biomonitoring data can also help scientists plan and conduct research on exposure and health effects.

## Urinary Alachlor mercapturate

*Metabolite of Alachlor*

Geometric mean and selected percentiles of urine concentrations (in µg/L) for the U.S. population from the National Health and Nutrition Examination Survey.

| | Survey years | Geometric mean (95% conf. interval) | 50th | 75th | 90th | 95th | Sample size |
|---|---|---|---|---|---|---|---|
| Total | 99-00 | * | < LOD | < LOD | < LOD | < LOD | 1942 |
| **Age group** | | | | | | | |
| 6-11 years | 99-00 | * | < LOD | < LOD | < LOD | < LOD | 463 |
| 12-19 years | 99-00 | * | < LOD | < LOD | < LOD | < LOD | 662 |
| 20-59 years | 99-00 | * | < LOD | < LOD | < LOD | < LOD | 817 |
| **Gender** | | | | | | | |
| Males | 99-00 | * | < LOD | < LOD | < LOD | < LOD | 950 |
| Females | 99-00 | * | < LOD | < LOD | < LOD | < LOD | 992 |
| **Race/ethnicity** | | | | | | | |
| Mexican Americans | 99-00 | * | < LOD | < LOD | < LOD | < LOD | 679 |
| Non-Hispanic blacks | 99-00 | * | < LOD | < LOD | < LOD | < LOD | 507 |
| Non-Hispanic whites | 99-00 | * | < LOD | < LOD | < LOD | < LOD | 586 |

Limit of detection (LOD, see Data Analysis section) for Survey year 99-00 is 1.18.
< LOD means less than the limit of detection, which may vary for some chemicals by year and by individual sample.
* Not calculated: proportion of results below limit of detection was too high to provide a valid result.

## Urinary Alachlor mercapturate (creatinine corrected)

*Metabolite of Alachlor*

Geometric mean and selected percentiles of urine concentrations (in µg/g of creatinine) for the U.S. population from the National Health and Nutrition Examination Survey.

| | Survey years | Geometric mean (95% conf. interval) | 50th | 75th | 90th | 95th | Sample size |
|---|---|---|---|---|---|---|---|
| Total | 99-00 | * | < LOD | < LOD | < LOD | < LOD | 1942 |
| **Age group** | | | | | | | |
| 6-11 years | 99-00 | * | < LOD | < LOD | < LOD | < LOD | 463 |
| 12-19 years | 99-00 | * | < LOD | < LOD | < LOD | < LOD | 662 |
| 20-59 years | 99-00 | * | < LOD | < LOD | < LOD | < LOD | 817 |
| **Gender** | | | | | | | |
| Males | 99-00 | * | < LOD | < LOD | < LOD | < LOD | 950 |
| Females | 99-00 | * | < LOD | < LOD | < LOD | < LOD | 992 |
| **Race/ethnicity** | | | | | | | |
| Mexican Americans | 99-00 | * | < LOD | < LOD | < LOD | < LOD | 679 |
| Non-Hispanic blacks | 99-00 | * | < LOD | < LOD | < LOD | < LOD | 507 |
| Non-Hispanic whites | 99-00 | * | < LOD | < LOD | < LOD | < LOD | 586 |

< LOD means less than the limit of detection for the urine levels not corrected for creatinine.
* Not calculated: proportion of results below limit of detection was too high to provide a valid result.

## References

Battaglin WA, Furlong ET, Burkhardt MR, Peter CJ. Occurrence of sulfonylurea, sulfonamide, imidazolinone, and other herbicides in rivers, reservoirs and ground water in the Midwestern United States, 1998. Sci Total Environ 2000;248(2-3):123-133.

Brown MA, Kimmel EC, Casida JE. DNA adduct formation by alachlor metabolites. Life Sci 1988;43(25):2087-94. Erratum in: Life Sci 1989;44(18):1325.

Centers for Disease Control and Prevention (CDC). Third National Report on Human Exposure to Environmental Chemicals. Atlanta (GA). 2005.

Davison KL, Larsen GL, Feil VJ. Comparative metabolism and elimination of acetanilide compounds by rat. Xenobiotica 1994;24(10):1003-1012.

Driskell WJ, Hill RH Jr, Shealy DB, Hull RD, Hines CJ. Identification of a major human urinary metabolite of alachlor by LC-MS/MS. Bull Environ Contam Toxicol 1996;56(6):853-859.

Feng PCC, Wratten SJ. In vitro transformation of chloroacetanilide herbicides by rat liver enzymes: A comparative study of metolachlor and alachlor. J Agri Food Chem 1989;37(4):1088-1093.

Heydens WF, Wilson AG, Kier LD, Lau H, Thake DC, Martens MA. An evaluation of the carcinogenic potential of the herbicide alachlor to man. Hum Exp Toxicol. 1999;18(6):363-391.

Hill AB, Jefferies PR, Quistad GB, Casida JE. Dialkylquinoneimine metabolites of chloroacetanilide herbicides induce sister chromatid exchanges in cultured human lymphocytes. Mutat Res. 1997;395(2-3):159-171.

Hines CJ, Deddens JA, Striley CA, Biagini RE, Shoemaker DA, Brown KK, et al. Biological monitoring for selected herbicide biomarkers in the urine of exposed custom applicators: application of mixed-effect models. Ann Occup Hyg 2003;47(6):503-517.

Hladik ML, Hsiao JJ, Roberts AL. Are neutral chloroacetamide herbicide degradates of potential environmental concern? Analysis and occurrence in the upper Chesapeake Bay. Environ Sci Technol 2005;39(17):6561-6574.

International Programme on Chemical Safety (IPCS). WHO/FAO Data Sheets on Pesticides. No. 86. ALACHLOR. World Health Organization, Geneva, 1996. Available at URL: http://www.inchem.org/documents/pds/pds/pest86_e htm. 2/27/09

Jefferies PR, Quistad GB, Casida JE. Dialkylquinonimines validated as in vivo metabolites of alachlor, acetochlor, and metolachlor herbicides in rats. Chem Res Toxicol 1998;11(4):353-359.

Kolpin DW, Thurman EM, Linhart SM. Finding minimal herbicide concentrations in ground water? Try looking for their degradates. Sci Total Environ 2000;248(2-3):115-122.

Sanderson WT, Biagini R, Tolos W, Henningsen G, MacKenzie B. Biological monitoring of commercial pesticide applicators for urine metabolites of the herbicide alachlor. Am Ind Hyg Assoc J 1995;56(9):883-889.

Tessier DM, Clark JM. Quantitative assessment of the mutagenic potential of environmental degradative products of alachlor. J Ag Food Chem 1995;43(9):2504-2512.

U.S. Environmental Protection Agency (U.S. EPA). Reregistration Eligibility Decision (RED) Alachlor. December 1998. EPA 738-R-98-020. Available at URL: http://www.epa.gov/oppsrrd1/REDs/0063.pdf. 2/27/09

U.S. Geological Survey (USGS). The Quality of Our Nation's Waters Pesticides in the Nation's Streams and Ground Water, 1992-2001. Circular 1291. Supplemental Technical Information (available on-line only). March 2006, revised February 15, 2007. Available at URL: http://water.usgs.gov/nawqa/pnsp/pubs/circ1291/supporting_info.php. 4/2/09

U.S. Geological Survey (USGS). Water-Resources Investigations Report: Distribution of Major Herbicides in Ground Water of the United States Water Resource Investigations Report No. 98-4245 (by Barbash JE, Thelin GP, Kolpin DW, Gilliom RJ). Sacramento, California, 1999.

Whyatt RM, Barr DB, Camann DE, Kinney PL, Barr JR, Andrews HF, et al. Contemporary-use pesticides in personal air samples during pregnancy and blood samples at delivery among urban minority mothers and newborns. Environ Health Perspect 2003;111(5):749-756.

World Health Organization (WHO). Alachlor in Drinking-water. Background document for development of WHO Guidelines for Drinking-water Quality. 2003. Available at URL: http://www.who.int/water_sanitation_health/dwq/chemicals/en/alachlor.pdf. 2/27/00

# Atrazine

CAS No. 1912-24-9

## General Information

Atrazine is a widely used chlorotriazine herbicide that acts against broadleaf and grassy weeds. Related chlorotriazine herbicides include simazine, propazine, and cyanazine, all of which act by inhibiting plant photosynthesis. Atrazine is applied pre- and post-emergence to agricultural land for crops such as corn and sorghum. It is also used as a non-selective herbicide. Atrazine was first registered as an herbicide in 1958. More than 70 million pounds have been applied annually in recent years, with about 75% of corn cropland receiving treatment. Atrazine has limited water solubility and is not tightly bound to soil, but it is leachable into ground and surface waters. In regions where atrazine is used, it is one of the more commonly detected pesticides in surface and ground waters (USGS, 2007). In soils, atrazine is slowly degraded to dealkylated products, which have half-lives of several months. Bacteria and plants can metabolize atrazine to hydroxyatrazine. Atrazine does not

bioaccumulate. It has little toxicity in birds and moderate toxicity in some fish and aquatic invertebrates. Atrazine may alter the sexual development of frogs at environmental levels (Gammon et al., 2005; Hayes et al., 2002; U.S.EPA, 2003a).

For the general population, drinking water is an infrequent source of atrazine exposure, but estimates of seasonal intakes from drinking water in a small number of communities have exceeded the recommended limits (U.S.EPA, 2003b). As a result, atrazine use has progressively been restricted in an effort to reduce surface and ground water contamination. Applicators of atrazine may be exposed dermally and by inhalation. Atrazine is well absorbed orally, metabolized, and then eliminated in the urine over a few days (Bradway et al., 1982; Catenacci et al., 1993; Timchalk et al., 1990). In animals and humans, glutathione conjugation appeared to be the major route of biotransformation, resulting in atrazine mercapturate and N-dealkylation products (IPCS, 1996; U.S.EPA, 2003b). Atrazine mercapturate products accounted for a major proportion of human urinary metabolites (Lucas et al., 1993). The dealkylated chloroatrazine metabolites,

## Urinary Atrazine mercapturate

*Metabolite of Atrazine*

Geometric mean and selected percentiles of urine concentrations (in µg/L) for the U.S. population from the National Health and Nutrition Examination Survey.

| | Survey years | Geometric mean (95% conf. interval) | 50th | 75th | 90th | 95th | Sample size |
|---|---|---|---|---|---|---|---|
| Total | 99-00 | * | < LOD | < LOD | < LOD | < LOD | 1878 |
| | 01-02 | * | < LOD | < LOD | < LOD | < LOD | 2477 |
| **Age group** | | | | | | | |
| 6-11 years | 99-00 | * | < LOD | < LOD | < LOD | < LOD | 449 |
| | 01-02 | * | < LOD | < LOD | < LOD | < LOD | 568 |
| 12-19 years | 99-00 | * | < LOD | < LOD | < LOD | < LOD | 639 |
| | 01-02 | * | < LOD | < LOD | < LOD | < LOD | 809 |
| 20-59 years | 99-00 | * | < LOD | < LOD | < LOD | < LOD | 790 |
| | 01-02 | * | < LOD | < LOD | < LOD | < LOD | 1100 |
| **Gender** | | | | | | | |
| Males | 99-00 | * | < LOD | < LOD | < LOD | < LOD | 919 |
| | 01-02 | * | < LOD | < LOD | < LOD | < LOD | 1162 |
| Females | 99-00 | * | < LOD | < LOD | < LOD | < LOD | 959 |
| | 01-02 | * | < LOD | < LOD | < LOD | < LOD | 1315 |
| **Race/ethnicity** | | | | | | | |
| Mexican Americans | 99-00 | * | < LOD | < LOD | < LOD | < LOD | 667 |
| | 01-02 | * | < LOD | < LOD | < LOD | < LOD | 676 |
| Non-Hispanic blacks | 99-00 | * | < LOD | < LOD | < LOD | < LOD | 498 |
| | 01-02 | * | < LOD | < LOD | < LOD | < LOD | 684 |
| Non-Hispanic whites | 99-00 | * | < LOD | < LOD | < LOD | < LOD | 550 |
| | 01-02 | * | < LOD | < LOD | < LOD | < LOD | 918 |

Limit of detection (LOD, see Data Analysis section) for Survey years 99-00 and 01-02 are 0.791 and 0.3.
< LOD means less than the limit of detection, which may vary for some chemicals by year and by individual sample.
* Not calculated: proportion of results below limit of detection was too high to provide a valid result.

particularly diaminochloroatrazine (the main dealkylated product), may mediate some effects of atrazine (Laws et al., 2003). Dealkylated metabolites from atrazine can also result from metabolism of other chlorotriazine pesticides, including simazine, propazine, and cyanazine. In addition to being human metabolites of atrazine, the dealkylated atrazine metabolites and hydroxyatrazine can occur in the environment from the breakdown of the parent chemical. Thus, detection of these dealkylated metabolites in a person's urine may also reflect exposure to these degradates in the environment.

Human health effects of atrazine at environmental doses or at biomonitored levels from environmental exposure are unknown. In mammalian studies, atrazine is rated as having low acute toxicity. Atrazine product formulations can be mild skin sensitizers and irritants. Chronic high dose toxicity observed in animals includes decreased body weight, myocardial muscle degeneration, liver toxicity, developmental ossification defects, impaired fertility, altered estrus cycles, increased pituitary weight, delayed onset of puberty, and reduced levels of luteinizing hormone, prolactin, and testosterone (Gillis et al., 1994;

Laws et al., 2000 and 2003; Rayner et al., 2004; Stoker et al., 2000 and 2002; U.S.EPA, 2003b). Atrazine and the dealkylated chlorinated metabolites did not have estrogen receptor activity, but they reduced the pituitary secretion of luteinizing hormone and prolactin and also inhibited aromatase at high doses in some mammalian species (Cooper et al., 2000; Eldridge et al., 1994 and 1999; Gammon et al., 2005; Sanderson et al., 2002; Stevens et al., 1999). Estimated human exposures are thousands of times lower than doses that caused effects in animals (Gammon et al., 2005). Some human ecologic and epidemiologic studies of reproductive and cancer outcomes have shown either positive or no associations, but the effects are difficult to attribute due to lack of exposure markers or due to mixed chemical or pesticide exposures (ATSDR, 2003; Gammon et al., 2005; Sathiakumar and Delzell, 1997). Atrazine is not considered genotoxic. IARC considers atrazine not classifiable with respect to human carcinogenicity, and U.S.EPA considers atrazine unlikely to be a human carcinogen. Additional information is available from U.S. EPA at: http://www.epa.gov/pesticides/ and from ATSDR at: http://www.atsdr.cdc.gov/toxpro2.html.

## Urinary Atrazine mercapturate (creatinine corrected)
*Metabolite of Atrazine*

Geometric mean and selected percentiles of urine concentrations (in µg/g of creatinine) for the U.S. population from the National Health and Nutrition Examination Survey.

| | Survey years | Geometric mean (95% conf. interval) | Selected percentiles ( 95% confidence interval) | | | | Sample size |
|---|---|---|---|---|---|---|---|
| | | | 50th | 75th | 90th | 95th | |
| **Total** | 99-00 | * | < LOD | < LOD | < LOD | < LOD | 1878 |
| | 01-02 | * | < LOD | < LOD | < LOD | < LOD | 2476 |
| **Age group** | | | | | | | |
| 6-11 years | 99-00 | * | < LOD | < LOD | < LOD | < LOD | 449 |
| | 01-02 | * | < LOD | < LOD | < LOD | < LOD | 568 |
| 12-19 years | 99-00 | * | < LOD | < LOD | < LOD | < LOD | 639 |
| | 01-02 | * | < LOD | < LOD | < LOD | < LOD | 808 |
| 20-59 years | 99-00 | * | < LOD | < LOD | < LOD | < LOD | 790 |
| | 01-02 | * | < LOD | < LOD | < LOD | < LOD | 1100 |
| **Gender** | | | | | | | |
| Males | 99-00 | * | < LOD | < LOD | < LOD | < LOD | 919 |
| | 01-02 | * | < LOD | < LOD | < LOD | < LOD | 1162 |
| Females | 99-00 | * | < LOD | < LOD | < LOD | < LOD | 959 |
| | 01-02 | * | < LOD | < LOD | < LOD | < LOD | 1314 |
| **Race/ethnicity** | | | | | | | |
| Mexican Americans | 99-00 | * | < LOD | < LOD | < LOD | < LOD | 667 |
| | 01-02 | * | < LOD | < LOD | < LOD | < LOD | 676 |
| Non-Hispanic blacks | 99-00 | * | < LOD | < LOD | < LOD | < LOD | 498 |
| | 01-02 | * | < LOD | < LOD | < LOD | < LOD | 683 |
| Non-Hispanic whites | 99-00 | * | < LOD | < LOD | < LOD | < LOD | 550 |
| | 01-02 | * | < LOD | < LOD | < LOD | < LOD | 918 |

< LOD means less than the limit of detection for the urine levels not corrected for creatinine.
* Not calculated: proportion of results below limit of detection was too high to provide a valid result.

## Biomonitoring Information

Urinary levels of atrazine mercapturate reflect recent exposure. In the NHANES 2001-2002 subsample, levels of atrazine mercapturate were generally not detectable (CDC, 2005). In small studies of Maryland residents in 1995-1996 (MacIntosh et al., 1999) and 83 Minnesota children with multiple urine collections during 1997 (Adgate et al., 2001), atrazine mercapturate was infrequently detected at the detection limit of < 1 μg/L. In a study of 60 farm worker children, atrazine was detected in only four children (Arcury et al., 2007). Through immunoassay atrazine equivalents (detected mostly as atrazine mercapturate), the urinary geometric mean levels for herbicide applicators in Ohio and Wisconsin were about 6 μg/L (Hines et al., 2003; Perry et al., 2000). The geometric mean of urinary atrazine mercapturate was 1.2 μg/L in 15 farmers studied several days after spraying the pesticide (Curwin et al., 2005). In a small number of field workers, urinary concentrations ranged from 5-1756 μg/L (Lucas et al., 1993).

Finding measurable amounts of atrazine mercapturate in urine does not mean that the levels of atrazine mercapturate cause an adverse health effect. Biomonitoring studies on levels of atrazine mercapturate provide physicians and public health officials with reference values so that they can determine whether people have been exposed to higher levels of atrazine than are found in the general population. Biomonitoring data can also help scientists plan and conduct research on exposure and health effects.

## References

Adgate JL, Barr DB, Clayton CA, Eberly LE, Freeman NC, Lioy PJ, et al. Measurement of children's exposure to pesticides: analysis of urinary metabolite levels in a probability-based sample. Environ Health Perspect 2001;109(6):583-590.

Agency for Toxic Substances and Disease Registry (ATSDR). Toxicological profile for atrazine. 2001 [online]. Available at URL: http://www.atsdr.cdc.gov/toxprofiles/tp153.html. 3/11/09

Arcury TA, Grzywacz JG, Barr DB, Tapia J, Chen H, Quandt SA. Pesticide urinary metabolite levels of children in eastern North Carolina farmworker households. Environ Health Perspect 2007;115(8):1254-1260.

Bradway DE, Moseman RF. Determination of urinary residue levels of the N-dealkyl metabolites of triazine herbicides. J Agric Food Chem 1982;30(2):244-247.

Catenacci G, Barbieri F, Bersani M, Ferioli A, Cottica D, Maroni M. Biological monitoring of human exposure to atrazine. Toxicol Lett 1993;69(2):217-222.

Centers for Disease Control and Prevention (CDC). Third National Report on Human Exposure to Environmental Chemicals. Atlanta (GA). 2005.

Cooper RL, Stoker TE, Tyrey L, Goldman JM, McElroy WK. Atrazine disrupts the hypothalamic control of pituitary-ovarian function. Toxicol Sci 2000;53(2):297-307.

Curwin BD, Hein MJ, Sanderson WT, Barr DB, Heederik D, Reynolds SJ, et al. Urinary and hand wipe pesticide levels among farmers and nonfarmers in Iowa. J Expo Anal Environ Epidemiol 2005;15(6):500-508.

Eldridge JC, Wetzel LT, Stevens JT, Simpkins JW. The mammary tumor response in triazine-treated female rats: a threshold-mediated interaction with strain and species-specific reproductive senescence. Steroids 1999;64(9):672-678.

Eldridge JC, Fleenor-Heyser DG, Extrom PC, Wetzel LT, Breckenridge CB, Gillis JH, et al. Short-term effects of chlorotriazines on estrus in female Sprague-Dawley and Fischer 344 rats. J Toxicol Environ Health 1994;43(2):155-167.

Gammon DW, Aldous CN, Carr WC Jr, Sanborn JR, Pfeifer KF. A risk assessment of atrazine use in California: human health and ecological aspects. Pest Manag Sci 2005;61(4):331-355.

Gillis JH, et al. Short-term effects of chlorotriazines on estrus in female Sprague-Dawley and Fischer 344 rats. J Toxicol Environ Health 1994;43(2):155-167.

Hayes TB, Collins A, Lee M, Mendoza M, Noriega N, Stuart AA, Vonk A. Hermaphroditic, demasculinized frogs after exposure to the herbicide atrazine at low ecologically relevant doses. Proc Natl Acad Sci USA 2002;99(8):5476-5480.

Hines CJ, Deddens JA, Striley CA, Biagini RE, Shoemaker DA, Brown KK, et al. Biological monitoring for selected herbicide biomarkers in the urine of exposed custom applicators: application of mixed-effect models. Ann Occup Hyg 2003;47(6):503-517.

International Programme on Chemical Safety (IPCS). WHO/FAO Data Sheets on Pesticides. No. 82. ATRAZINE. World Health Organization, Geneva, 1996. Available at URL: http://www.inchem.org/documents/pds/pds/pest82_e.htm. 3/11/09

Laws SC, Ferrell JM, Stoker TE, Cooper RL. Pubertal development in female Wistar rats following exposure to propazine and atrazine biotransformation by-products, diamino-S-chlorotriazine and hydroxyatrazine. Toxicol Sci 2003;76(1):190-200.

Laws SC, Ferrell JM, Stoker TE, Schmid J, Cooper RL. The effects of atrazine on female wistar rats: an evaluation of the protocol for assessing pubertal development and thyroid function. Toxicol Sci 2000;58(2):366-376.

Lucas AD, Jones AD, Goodrow MH, Saiz SG, Blewett C, Seiber JN, et al. Determination of atrazine metabolites in human urine:

development of a biomarker of exposure. Chem Res Toxicol 1993;6(1):107-116.

MacIntosh DL, Needham LL, Hammerstrom KA, Ryan PB. A longitudinal investigation of selected pesticide metabolites in urine. J Expo Anal Environ Epidemiol 1999;9(5):494-501.

Perry M, Christiani D, Dagenhart D, Tortorelli J, Singzoni B. Urinary biomarkers of atrazine exposure among farm pesticide applicators. Ann Epidemiol 2000;10(7):479.

Rayner JL, Wood C, Fenton SE. Exposure parameters necessary for delayed puberty and mammary gland development in Long-Evans rats exposed in utero to atrazine. Toxicol Appl Pharmacol 2004;195(1):23-34.

Sanderson JT, Boerma J, Lansbergen GW, van den Berg M. Induction and inhibition of aromatase (CYP19) activity by various classes of pesticides in H295R human adrenocortical carcinoma cells. Toxicol Appl Pharmacol 2002;182(1):44-54.

Sathiakumar N, Delzell E. A review of epidemiologic studies of triazine herbicides and cancer. Crit Rev Toxicol 1997;27(6):599-612.

Stevens JT, Breckenridge CB, Wetzel L. A risk characterization for atrazine: oncogenicity profile. J Toxicol Environ Health A 1999;56(2):69-109.

Stoker TE, Laws SC, Guidici DL, Cooper RL. The effect of atrazine on puberty in male Wistar rats: an evaluation in the protocol for the assessment of pubertal development and thyroid function. Toxicol Sci 2000;58(1):50-59.

Stoker TE, Guidici DL, Laws SC, Cooper RL. The effects of atrazine metabolites on puberty and thyroid function in the male Wistar rat. Toxicol Sci 2002;67(2):198-206.

Timchalk C, Dryzga MD, Langvardt PW, Kastl PE, Osborne DW. Determination of the effect of tridiphane on the pharmacokinetics of [14C]-atrazine following oral administration to male Fischer 344 rats. Toxicology 1990;61(1):27-40.

U.S. Environmental Protection Agency (U.S. EPA). Office of Prevention, Pesticides and Toxic Substances, EPA Office of Pesticide Programs, Environmental Fate and Effects Division. White paper on potential developmental effects of atrazine on amphibians. Washington (DC). May 2003a. Available at URL: http://www.epa.gov/scipoly/sap/meetings/2003/june/finaljune2002telconfreport.pdf. 6/1/09

U.S. Environmental Protection Agency (U.S. EPA). Interim Reregistration Eligibility Decision For Atrazine. Case No. 0062. 2003b. Available at URL: http://www.epa.gov/oppsrrd1/REDs/atrazine_ired.pdf. 3/11/09

U.S. Geological Survey (USGS). The Quality of Our Nation's Waters. Pesticides in the Nation's Streams and Ground Water, 1992-2001. Circular 1291. Supplemental Technical Information (available on-line only). March 2006, revised February 15, 2007. Available at URL: http://water.usgs.gov/nawqa/pnsp/pubs/circ1291/supporting_info.php. 4/2/09

# 2,4-Dichlorophenoxyacetic Acid
CAS No. 94-75-7

## General Information

Widely used throughout the United States, the chlorophenoxy herbicide 2,4-dichlorophenoxyacetic acid (2,4-D) controls broadleaf weeds in residential, agricultural, and aquatic environments. It was first registered with U.S.EPA in 1948. Similar to other chlorophenoxy herbicides, it acts as a plant growth hormone. At low levels, these herbicides can enhance plant growth, but at higher levels they are herbicidal. 2,4-D can be applied either as an aqueous salt or as oil-soluble esters, and it is often mixed with other chlorophenoxy acid herbicides (such as dicamba, MCPA, and mecoprop). As much as 62 million pounds of 2,4-D were used in the U.S. in 2001 (U.S.EPA, 2004). It is poorly bound in soils, with a half-life of several days to several weeks. It is rarely detected in ground waters (USGS, 2007). Acid and salt forms are much less toxic to fish and aquatic invertebrates than the ester forms.

General population exposure to 2,4-D may occur during residential applications, by direct contact with agricultural and residential areas after applications, and by consuming food or drinking water contaminated with 2, 4-D. Recent estimates of chronic intakes of 2,4-D have been below recommended intake limits (U.S.EPA, 2005). 2,4-D is rapidly absorbed via oral and inhalation routes. It is not well absorbed through the skin, although dermal exposure may be significant for herbicide manufacturing plant workers exposed to high concentrations of 2,4-D or exposed for prolonged periods. Once absorbed, 2,4-D is eliminated mostly unchanged in the urine with an elimination half-life ranging from 10 to 33 hours (Arnold et al., 1989; Kohli et al., 1974; Sauerhoff et al., 1977).

Human health effects from 2,4-D at low environmental doses or at biomonitored levels from low environmental exposures are unknown. 2,4-D has low acute toxicity. Intentional overdoses and unintentional high dose exposures to chlorophenoxy acid herbicides have resulted in weakness, headache, dizziness, nausea, abdominal pain, myotonia, hypotension, renal and hepatic injury, and delayed

## Urinary 2,4-Dichlorophenoxyacetic acid

Geometric mean and selected percentiles of urine concentrations (in µg/L) for the U.S. population from the National Health and Nutrition Examination Survey.

| | Survey years | Geometric mean (95% conf. interval) | 50th | 75th | 90th | 95th | Sample size |
|---|---|---|---|---|---|---|---|
| Total | 99-00 | * | < LOD | < LOD | < LOD | < LOD | 1977 |
| | 01-02 | * | < LOD | .230 (<LOD- 320) | .690 (.560-.910) | 1.27 (1.02-1 37) | 2413 |
| **Age group** | | | | | | | |
| 6-11 years | 99-00 | * | < LOD | < LOD | < LOD | 1.30 (<LOD-2.40) | 477 |
| | 01-02 | * | < LOD | .310 (.210-.400) | .740 (.550-1.13) | 1.55 (1.00-2 21) | 546 |
| 12-19 years | 99-00 | * | < LOD | < LOD | < LOD | 1.10 (<LOD-1.60) | 677 |
| | 01-02 | * | < LOD | .250 (<LOD-.420) | .690 (.440-1.16) | 1.24 (.690-1 66) | 797 |
| 20-59 years | 99-00 | * | < LOD | < LOD | < LOD | < LOD | 823 |
| | 01-02 | * | < LOD | .210 (<LOD- 310) | .690 (.540-.910) | 1.27 (.930-1.49) | 1070 |
| **Gender** | | | | | | | |
| Males | 99-00 | * | < LOD | < LOD | < LOD | 1.10 (<LOD-1.80) | 962 |
| | 01-02 | * | < LOD | .330 (.230-.490) | .930 (.680-1 22) | 1.51 (1.27-2 08) | 1135 |
| Females | 99-00 | * | < LOD | < LOD | < LOD | < LOD | 1015 |
| | 01-02 | * | < LOD | < LOD | .490 (.370-.660) | .890 (.670-1 22) | 1278 |
| **Race/ethnicity** | | | | | | | |
| Mexican Americans | 99-00 | * | < LOD | < LOD | < LOD | < LOD | 695 |
| | 01-02 | * | < LOD | .260 (<LOD- 350) | .730 (.610-.910) | 1.20 (.960-1.43) | 659 |
| Non-Hispanic blacks | 99-00 | * | < LOD | < LOD | < LOD | 1.20 (<LOD-1.70) | 520 |
| | 01-02 | * | < LOD | < LOD | .610 (.420-.890) | 1.07 (.810-1.48) | 668 |
| Non-Hispanic whites | 99-00 | * | < LOD | < LOD | < LOD | < LOD | 589 |
| | 01-02 | * | < LOD | .250 (<LOD-.410) | .760 (.560-1.10) | 1.32 (1.05-2 03) | 892 |

Limit of detection (LOD, see Data Analysis section) for Survey years 99-00 and 01-02 are 0.952 and 0.2.
< LOD means less than the limit of detection, which may vary for some chemicals by year and by individual sample.
* Not calculated: proportion of results below limit of detection was too high to provide a valid result.

neuropathy (Bradberry et al., 2004). The acid and salt forms of 2,4-D are eye irritants. Acute high doses administered to laboratory animals produced ataxia, myotonia, and evidence of histological injury to the kidneys, liver, thyroid, eyes, adrenals and gonads (NTP, 2006; U.S.EPA, 2005). 2,4-D does not have significant reproductive, developmental, or teratogenic effects in chronic rodent studies (Charles et al., 2001; IPCS, 1996; U.S.EPA 2005). Epidemiological studies have reported associations of several types of cancer, such as soft tissue sarcoma and non-Hodgkin's lymphoma, with the exposure to chlorophenoxy herbicides as defoliants or contaminated herbicides. It is unclear whether these associations are related to the chlorophenoxy herbicides, other exposures, or to contaminants in the herbicide formulations (specifically 2,3,7,8-tetrachlorodibenzo-*p*-dioxin) (Garabrant and Philbert, 2002; IOM, 2003; IPCS, 1996; Pearce and McLean; 2005; U.S.EPA, 2005). 2,4-D was not found to be genotoxic or carcinogenic in animal studies (Garabrant and Philbert, 2002; IPCS, 1996; U.S.EPA, 2005). IARC considers the chlorophenoxyacetic acids group of chemicals as possibly carcinogenic to humans. Additional information is available from U.S.EPA at: http://www.epa.gov/pesticides/.

**Biomonitoring Information**

Urinary levels of 2,4-D reflect recent exposure. The 95th percentiles of the NHANES 1999-2000 and 2001-2002 subsamples were roughly similar to the 95th percentile values reported in a nonrandom subsample from NHANES III (1988-1994) (CDC, 2005; Hill et al., 1995). In previous samples of the U.S. population (Hill et al., 1995; Kutz et al., 1992), in small samples of children (Hill et al., 1989), and of adults and children (Baker et al., 2000), urinary 2,4-D levels were detectable in less than a quarter of the individuals studied.

2,4-D production plant workers and a few forestry workers spraying 2,4-D had urinary levels several hundred to several thousand times higher than the 95th percentiles of the NHANES subsamples (CDC, 2005; Frank et al., 1985; Kolmodin-Hedman and Erne, 1980; Knopp et al., 1994). Average post-application urinary levels of 2,4-D in farmers were more than 25-fold higher than the 95th percentiles in the NHANES 1999-2000 and 2001-2002 subsamples (Arbuckle et al., 2005; CDC, 2005). Post-application levels in farmers and home gardeners were dependent on

## Urinary 2,4-Dichlorophenoxyacetic acid (creatinine corrected)

Geometric mean and selected percentiles of urine concentrations (in µg/g of creatinine) for the U.S. population from the National Health and Nutrition Examination Survey.

| | Survey years | Geometric mean (95% conf. interval) | 50th | 75th | 90th | 95th | Sample size |
|---|---|---|---|---|---|---|---|
| **Total** | 99-00 | * | < LOD | < LOD | < LOD | < LOD | 1977 |
| | 01-02 | * | < LOD | .380 (<LOD-.410) | .670 ( 610-.780) | 1.08 ( 930-1.26) | 2412 |
| **Age group** | | | | | | | |
| 6-11 years | 99-00 | * | < LOD | < LOD | < LOD | 1.32 (<LOD-2.24) | 477 |
| | 01-02 | * | < LOD | .490 ( 380-.680) | 1.13 ( 820-1.35) | 1.41 (1.27-1.73) | 546 |
| 12-19 years | 99-00 | * | < LOD | < LOD | < LOD | .590 (<LOD-1.05) | 677 |
| | 01-02 | * | < LOD | .270 (<LOD-.380) | .480 ( 330-.660) | .660 ( 520-.920) | 796 |
| 20-59 years | 99-00 | * | < LOD | < LOD | < LOD | < LOD | 823 |
| | 01-02 | * | < LOD | .380 (<LOD-.410) | .670 ( 580-.790) | 1.08 ( 810-1.29) | 1070 |
| **Gender** | | | | | | | |
| Males | 99-00 | * | < LOD | < LOD | < LOD | .670 (<LOD-1.16) | 962 |
| | 01-02 | * | < LOD | .340 ( 270-.410) | .640 ( 560-.790) | 1.14 ( 890-1.39) | 1135 |
| Females | 99-00 | * | < LOD | < LOD | < LOD | < LOD | 1015 |
| | 01-02 | * | < LOD | < LOD | .700 ( 610-.780) | 1.08 ( 810-1.26) | 1277 |
| **Race/ethnicity** | | | | | | | |
| Mexican Americans | 99-00 | * | < LOD | < LOD | < LOD | < LOD | 695 |
| | 01-02 | * | < LOD | .350 (<LOD-.390) | .720 ( 560-.850) | 1.13 (.780-1.56) | 659 |
| Non-Hispanic blacks | 99-00 | * | < LOD | < LOD | < LOD | .590 (<LOD-1.19) | 520 |
| | 01-02 | * | < LOD | < LOD | .440 ( 340-.570) | .780 ( 550-.980) | 667 |
| Non-Hispanic whites | 99-00 | * | < LOD | < LOD | < LOD | < LOD | 589 |
| | 01-02 | * | < LOD | .410 (<LOD-.470) | .740 ( 620-.890) | 1.17 ( 990-1.40) | 892 |

< LOD means less than the limit of detection for the urine levels not corrected for creatinine.
* Not calculated: proportion of results below limit of detection was too high to provide a valid result.

the time since application, the amount of pesticide applied, the number of acres to which it was applied (Curwin et al., 2005), and the use of protective clothing or equipment (Arbuckle et al., 2005; Harris et al., 1992). In farm families, geometric mean urinary levels of 2,4-D were highest in the farmers who applied the 2,4-D; other family members had levels ranging only slightly higher than the 95th percentile levels in NHANES 1999-2000 and 2001-2002 subsamples (CDC, 2005; Mandel et al., 2005).

Finding a measurable amount of 2,4-D in urine does not mean that the level of the 2,4-D will result in an adverse health effect. Biomonitoring studies of 2,4-D in urine provide physicians and public health officials with reference values so that they can determine whether other people have been exposed to higher levels of 2,4-D than levels found in the general population. Biomonitoring data can also help scientists plan and conduct research on exposure and health effects.

## References

Arbuckle TE, Cole DC, Ritter L, Ripley BD. Biomonitoring of herbicides in Ontario farm applicators. Scand J Work Environ Health 2005;31 Suppl 1:90-97.

Arnold EK, Beasley VR. The pharmacokinetics of chlorinated phenoxy acid herbicides: a literature. Vet Hum Toxicol 1989;31(2):121-125.

Baker SE, Barr DB, Driskell WJ, Beeson MD, Needham LL. Quantification of selected pesticide metabolites in human urine using isotope dilution high-performance liquid chromatography/tandem mass spectrometry. J Expo Anal Environ Epidemiol 2000;10(6 Pt 2):789-798.

Centers for Disease Control and Prevention (CDC). Third National Report on Human Exposure to Environmental Chemicals. Atlanta (GA). 2005

Charles JM, Hanley TR Jr, Wilson RD, van Ravenzwaay B, Bus JS. Developmental toxicity studies in rats and rabbits on 2,4-dichlorophenoxyacetic acid and its forms. Toxicol Sci 2001;60(1):121-131.

Curwin BD, Hein MJ, Sanderson WT, Barr DB, Heederik D, Reynolds SJ, et al. Urinary and hand wipe pesticide levels among farmers and nonfarmers in Iowa. J Expo Anal Environ Epidemiol 2005 Nov;15(6):500-508.

Frank R, Campbell RA, Sirons G J. Forestry workers involved in aerial application of 2,4-dichlorophenoxyacetic acid (2,4-D): exposure and urinary excretion. Arch Environ Contam Toxicol 1985;4:427-435.

Garabrant DH, Philbert MA. Review of 2,4-dichlorophenoxyacetic acid (2,4-D) epidemiology and toxicology. Crit Rev Toxicol 2002;32(4):233-257.

Harris SA, Solomon KR, Stephenson GR. Exposure of homeowners and bystanders to 2,4 dichlorophenoxyacetic acid (2,4-D). J Environ Sci Health B 1992;27(1):23-38.

Hill RH Jr, To T, Holler JS, Fast DM, Smith SJ, Needham LL, et al. Residues of chlorinated phenols and phenoxy acid herbicides in the urine of Arkansas children. Arch Environ Contam Toxicol 1989;18(4):469-474.

Hill RH Jr, Head SL, Baker S, Gregg M, Shealy DB, Bailey SL, et al. Pesticide residues in urine of adults living in the United States: reference range concentrations. Environ Res 1995;71(2):99-108.

International Programme on Chemical Safety-INCHEM (IPCS). Pesticides residues in food: 1996 evaluations Part II Toxicology. 914. Dichlorophenoxyacetic acid, 2,4-. Available at URL: http://www.inchem.org/documents/jmpr/jmpmono/v96pr04.htm. 3/17/09

Institute of Medicine (IOM). Board on Health Promotion and Disease Prevention. Committee to Review the Health Effects in Vietnam Veterans of Exposure to Herbicides (Fourth Biennial Update. Veterans and Agent Orange: update 2002. Washington (DC): National Academies Press; 2003. Available at URL: http://www.nap.edu/catalog.php?record_id=10603. 3/17/09

Knopp D. Assessment of exposure to 2,4-dichlorophenoxyacetic acid in the chemical industry: results of a five year biological monitoring study. Occup Environ Med 1994;51(3):152-159.

Kohli JD, Khanna RN, Gupta BN, Dhar MM, Tandon JS, Sircar KP. Absorption and excretion of 2,4-dichlorophenoxyacetic acid in man. Xenobiotica 1974;4:97-100.

Kolmodin-Hedman B, Erne K. Estimation of occupational exposure to phenoxy acids (2,4-D and 2,4,5-T). Arch Toxicol Suppl 1980;4:318-321.

Kutz FW, Cook BT, Carter-Pokras OD, Brody D, Murphy RS. Selected pesticide residues and metabolites in urine from a survey of the U.S. general population. J Toxicol Environ Health 1992;37(2):277-291.

Mandel JS, Alexander BH, Baker BA, Acquavella JF, Chapman P, Honeycutt R. Biomonitoring for farm families in the farm family exposure study. Scand J Work Environ Health 2005;31 Suppl 1:98-104.

National Toxicology Program (NTP). TOX-63: TOXICITY REPORT CURVES. Tables, Survival and Growth Curves from NTP Toxicity Studies. TOX-63 Peroxisone Project (2,4-Dichlorophenoxyacetic Acid). Updated March 7, 2006. Available at URL: http://ntp.niehs.nih.gov/index.cfm?objectid=06FF8DA6-E5A1-90CD-3F26562CEC5CDDE5. 3/17/09

Sauerhoff MW, Braun WH, Blau GE, Gehring PJ. The fate of 2,4-dichlorophenoxyacetic acid (2,4-D) following oral administration to man. Toxicology 1977;8:3-1U.S. Environmental Protection Agency (U.S.EPA). 2,4-D RED Facts. June 2005. EPA 738 F-05-002. Available at URL: http://www.epa.gov/oppsrrd1/REDs/factsheets/24d_fs.htm. 3/17/09

U.S. Geological Survey (USGS). The Quality of Our Nation's Waters. Pesticides in the Nation's Streams and Ground Water, 1992-2001. Circular 1291. Supplemental Technical Information (available on-line only). March 2006, revised February 15, 2007. Available at URL: http://water.usgs.gov/nawqa/pnsp/pubs/circ1291/supporting_info.php. 4/2/09

U. S. Environmental Protection Agency (U.S.EPA). Office of Prevention Pesticides and Toxic Substances. Pesticide industry sales and usage - 2000 and 2001 market estimates. Washington (DC): U.S.EPA. May, 2004. Available at URL: http://www.epa.gov/oppbead1/pestsales/01pestsales/market_estimates2001.pdf. 3/17/09.

# Metolachlor

CAS No. 51218-45-2

## General Information

Metolachlor is a chloroacetanilide type herbicide that is applied for preemergent control of grasses and broadleaf weeds on agricultural crop land, including corn, soybeans, sorghum and other crops, and on non-crop land for general weed control. It is absorbed by plants and inhibits plant protein synthesis. Metolachlor has a soil half-life of a few weeks to three months and is degraded microbiologically and photochemically to at least five different products. Metolachlor or its degradates can leach from soils and have been detected in watersheds of agricultural land, in both ground and surface waters (Battaglin et al., 1999; Gilliom, 2007; Hladik et al., 2005; Kolpin et al., 2000; USGS, 2007; WHO, 2003). Occasionally in the past, metolachlor levels in water have exceeded lifetime human health advisory levels (U.S.EPA, 1995). Metolachlor shows little potential to bioaccumulate but is moderately toxic to fish.

General population exposure may occur through the consumption of contaminated food or drinking water. Estimated human intakes have been below recommended limits (U.S.EPA, 1995). Metolachlor is well absorbed dermally, so applicators, formulators, and field workers may have significant exposures via this route. In animal studies, metolachlor was quickly absorbed after dermal or oral doses, and eliminated in urine and feces over two to three days (WHO, 2003). In animals, mercapturate conjugates were the predominant metabolites, but another metabolic pathway can produce 2-methyl-6-ethylaniline and its reactive metabolite which may account for observed effects (Coleman et al., 2000; Davison et al., 1994; Feng and Wratten, 1989; Jefferies et al., 1998). People exposed to metolachlor will excrete metolachlor mercapturate in their urine. This metabolite is not a marker of exposure to either plant metabolites or environmental degradates of metolachlor which can be present in the environment.

Human health effects from metolachlor at low environmental doses or at biomonitored levels from low environmental exposures are unknown. Metolachlor has low potential for acute toxicity (U.S. EPA, 1995). Salivation, lacrimation, and convulsions were observed at lethal doses in animal studies. Metolachlor did not show developmental or reproductive toxicity in chronic animal studies, and it was not mutagenic in mammalian cells (U.S.EPA, 1995; WHO, 2003). U.S.EPA considers metolachlor to be a possible human carcinogen; NTP and IARC do not have ratings regarding human carcinogenicity. Additional information is available from U.S. EPA at: http://www.epa.gov/pesticides/.

## Biomonitoring Information

Urinary levels of metolachlor mercapturate reflect recent exposure. Urinary levels of metolachlor mercapturate were generally not detectable in the NHANES 2001-2002 subsample, though the 95th percentile for males was 0.200 µg/L (CDC, 2005). The geometric mean metolachlor mercapturate was 4.7 µg/L in the urine of farmers after they had sprayed metolachlor (Curwin et al., 2005). Hines et al. (2003) showed that 2.2% of a small reference population had detectable metolachlor equivalents by immunoassay in their urine, whereas 60% of applicators had detectable amounts.

Finding measurable amounts of metolachlor mercapturate in the urine does not mean that the levels of metolachlor mercapturate cause an adverse health effect. Biomonitoring studies on levels of metolachlor mercapturate provide physicians and public health officials with reference values so that they can determine whether people have been exposed to higher levels metolachlor than are found in the general population. Biomonitoring data can also help scientists plan and conduct research on exposure and health effects.

## Urinary Metolachlor mercapturate

*Metabolite of Metolachlor*

Geometric mean and selected percentiles of urine concentrations (in µg/L) for the U.S. population from the National Health and Nutrition Examination Survey.

| | Survey years | Geometric mean (95% conf. interval) | 50th | 75th | 90th | 95th | Sample size |
|---|---|---|---|---|---|---|---|
| | | | | Selected percentiles ( 95% confidence interval) | | | |
| Total | 01-02 | * | < LOD | < LOD | < LOD | < LOD | 2538 |
| **Age group** | | | | | | | |
| 6-11 years | 01-02 | * | < LOD | < LOD | < LOD | < LOD | 580 |
| 12-19 years | 01-02 | * | < LOD | < LOD | < LOD | < LOD | 831 |
| 20-59 years | 01-02 | * | < LOD | < LOD | < LOD | < LOD | 1127 |
| **Gender** | | | | | | | |
| Males | 01-02 | * | < LOD | < LOD | < LOD | .200 (<LOD-.220) | 1192 |
| Females | 01-02 | * | < LOD | < LOD | < LOD | < LOD | 1346 |
| **Race/ethnicity** | | | | | | | |
| Mexican Americans | 01-02 | * | < LOD | < LOD | < LOD | < LOD | 679 |
| Non-Hispanic blacks | 01-02 | * | < LOD | < LOD | < LOD | < LOD | 701 |
| Non-Hispanic whites | 01-02 | * | < LOD | < LOD | < LOD | .200 (<LOD-.240) | 957 |

Limit of detection (LOD, see Data Analysis section) for Survey year 01-02 is 0.2.
< LOD means less than the limit of detection, which may vary for some chemicals by year and by individual sample.
* Not calculated: proportion of results below limit of detection was too high to provide a valid result.

## Urinary Metolachlor mercapturate (creatinine corrected)

*Metabolite of Metolachlor*

Geometric mean and selected percentiles of urine concentrations (in µg/g of creatinine) for the U.S. population from the National Health and Nutrition Examination Survey.

| | Survey years | Geometric mean (95% conf. interval) | 50th | 75th | 90th | 95th | Sample size |
|---|---|---|---|---|---|---|---|
| | | | | Selected percentiles ( 95% confidence interval) | | | |
| Total | 01-02 | * | < LOD | < LOD | < LOD | < LOD | 2537 |
| **Age group** | | | | | | | |
| 6-11 years | 01-02 | * | < LOD | < LOD | < LOD | < LOD | 580 |
| 12-19 years | 01-02 | * | < LOD | < LOD | < LOD | < LOD | 830 |
| 20-59 years | 01-02 | * | < LOD | < LOD | < LOD | < LOD | 1127 |
| **Gender** | | | | | | | |
| Males | 01-02 | * | < LOD | < LOD | < LOD | .440 (<LOD-.500) | 1192 |
| Females | 01-02 | * | < LOD | < LOD | < LOD | < LOD | 1345 |
| **Race/ethnicity** | | | | | | | |
| Mexican Americans | 01-02 | * | < LOD | < LOD | < LOD | < LOD | 679 |
| Non-Hispanic blacks | 01-02 | * | < LOD | < LOD | < LOD | < LOD | 700 |
| Non-Hispanic whites | 01-02 | * | < LOD | < LOD | < LOD | .670 (<LOD-.740) | 957 |

< LOD means less than the limit of detection for the urine levels not corrected for creatinine.
* Not calculated: proportion of results below limit of detection was too high to provide a valid result.

## References

Battaglin WA, Furlong ET, Burkhardt MR, Peter CJ. Occurrence of sulfonylurea, sulfonamide, imidazolinone, and other herbicides in rivers, reservoirs and ground water in the Midwestern United States, 1998. Sci Total Environ 2000;248(2-3):123-133.

Centers for Disease Control and Prevention (CDC). Third National Report on Human Exposure to Environmental Chemicals. Atlanta (GA). 2005.

Coleman S, Linderman R, Hodgson E, Rose RL. Comparative metabolism of chloroacetamide herbicides and selected metabolites in human and rat liver microsomes. Environ Health Perspect 2000;108(12):1151-1157.

Curwin BD, Hein MJ, Sanderson WT, Barr DB, Heederik D, Reynolds SJ, Ward EM, Alavanja MC. Urinary and hand wipe pesticide levels among farmers and nonfarmers in Iowa. J Expo Anal Environ Epidemiol 2005;15(6):500-508.

Davison KL, Larsen GL, Feil VJ. Comparative metabolism and elimination of acetanilide compounds by rat. Xenobiotica 1994;24(10):1003-1012.

Feng PCC, Wratten SJ. In vitro transformation of chloroacetanilide herbicides by rat liver enzymes: A comparative study of metolachlor and alachlor. J Agri Food Chem 1989;37(4):1088-1093.

Gillion, R. Pesticides in U.S. streams and groundwater. Environ Sci Technol 2007;41:3409-3414. Available at URL: http://water.usgs.gov/nawqa/pnsp/pubs/files/051507.ESTfeature_gilliom.pdf 3/30/09

Hines CJ, Deddens JA, Striley CA, Biagini RE, Shoemaker DA, Brown KK, et al. Biological monitoring for selected herbicide biomarkers in the urine of exposed custom applicators: application of mixed-effect models. Ann Occup Hyg 2003;47(6):503-517.

Hladik ML, Hsiao JJ, Roberts AL. Are neutral chloroacetamide herbicide degradates of potential environmental concern? Analysis and occurrence in the upper Chesapeake Bay. Environ Sci Technol 2005;39(17):6561-6574.

Jefferies PR, Quistad GB, Casida JE. Dialkylquinonimines validated as in vivo metabolites of alachlor, acetochlor, and metolachlor herbicides in rats. Chem Res Toxicol 1998;11(4):353-359.

Kolpin DW, Thurman EM, Linhart SM. Finding minimal herbicide concentrations in ground water? Try looking for their degradates. Sci Total Environ 2000;248(2-3):115-122.

U.S. Environmental Protection Agency (U.S. EPA). Reregistration Eligibility Decision (RED) Metolachlor. April 1995. EPA 738-R-95-006. Available at URL: http://www.epa.gov/oppsrrd1/REDs/0001.pdf. 3/26/09

U.S. Geological Survey (USGS). The Quality of Our Nation's Waters Pesticides in the Nation's Streams and Ground Water, 1992-2001. Circular 1291. Supplemental Technical Information (available on-line only). March 2006, revised February 15, 2007. Available at URL: http://water.usgs.gov/nawqa/pnsp/pubs/circ1291/supporting_info.php. 4/2/09

U.S. Geological Survey (USGS). Water-Resources Investigations Report: Distribution of Major Herbicides in Ground Water of the United States Water Resource Investigations Report No. 98-4245 (by Barbash JE, Thelin GP, Kolpin DW, Gilliom RJ). Sacramento, California, 1999. Available at URL: http://water.usgs.gov/nawqa/pnsp/pubs/wrir984245/text.html. 6/1/09

Whyatt RM, Barr DB, Camann DE, Kinney PL, Barr JR, Andrews HF, et al. Contemporary-use pesticides in personal air samples during pregnancy and blood samples at delivery among urban minority mothers and newborns. Environ Health Perspect 2003;111(5):749-756.

World Health Organization (WHO). Metolachlor in Drinking-water. Background document for development of WHO Guidelines for Drinking-water Quality. 2003. Available at URL: http://www.who.int/water_sanitation_health/dwq/chemicals/metolachlor.pdf. 3/27/09

# 2,4,5-Trichlorophenoxyacetic Acid
CAS No. 93-76-5

## General Information

2,4,5-Trichlorophenoxyacetic acid (2,4,5-T) is a chlorophenoxy acid herbicide that is no longer registered for use in the United States. Chlorophenoxy herbicides act as plant growth hormones. At low levels, these herbicides can enhance plant growth, but higher levels are herbicidal. 2,4,5-T was once applied as either an aqueous salt or as an oil-soluble ester. Ester forms of 2,4,5-T and 2,4-D were used as defoliants in the Vietnam War (e.g., Agent Orange), and concern about contamination with 2,3,7,8-tetrachlorodibenzo-p-dioxin (TCDD) led to the discontinuation of 2,4,5-T use as a herbicide in 1985. The half-life of 2,4,5-T in soil varies with conditions, ranging from several weeks to many months. 2,4,5-T degrades to 2,4,5-trichlorophenol and other degradates. 2,4,5-T has been rarely detected in ground waters (USGS, 2007).

Given the commercial unavailability of 2,4,5-T, the general population is unlikely to be exposed to it. Although 2,4,5-T is rapidly absorbed via oral and inhalation routes, it is not well absorbed through the skin. Once absorbed into the body, 2,4,5-T is eliminated mostly unchanged in the urine, with an elimination half-life of approximately 19 hours (Arnold et al., 1989; Kohli et al., 1974).

Human health effects from 2,4,5-T at low environmental doses or at biomonitored levels from low environmental exposures are unknown. Intentional overdoses and unintentional high dose occupational exposures to chlorophenoxy acid herbicides have resulted in weakness, headache, dizziness, nausea, abdominal pain, myotonia, hypotension, renal and hepatic injury, and delayed neuropathy (Bradberry et al., 2004). Teratogenic and developmental effects have been reported in studies of multiple rodent strains treated with high doses of technical grade 2,4,5-T (Holson et al., 1992; Mohammad and St. Omer, 1986; Nelson et al., 1992). Epidemiological studies have reported associations of several types of cancer, such as soft tissue sarcoma and non-Hodgkin's lymphoma, with the exposure to chlorophenoxy herbicides as defoliants

## Urinary 2,4,5-Trichlorophenoxyacetic acid

Geometric mean and selected percentiles of urine concentrations (in µg/L) for the U.S. population from the National Health and Nutrition Examination Survey.

| | Survey years | Geometric mean (95% conf. interval) | 50th | 75th | 90th | 95th | Sample size |
|---|---|---|---|---|---|---|---|
| **Total** | 99-00 | * | < LOD | < LOD | < LOD | < LOD | 1814 |
| | 01-02 | * | < LOD | < LOD | < LOD | < LOD | 2538 |
| **Age group** | | | | | | | |
| 6-11 years | 99-00 | * | < LOD | < LOD | < LOD | < LOD | 430 |
| | 01-02 | * | < LOD | < LOD | < LOD | < LOD | 580 |
| 12-19 years | 99-00 | * | < LOD | < LOD | < LOD | < LOD | 618 |
| | 01-02 | * | < LOD | < LOD | < LOD | < LOD | 831 |
| 20-59 years | 99-00 | * | < LOD | < LOD | < LOD | < LOD | 766 |
| | 01-02 | * | < LOD | < LOD | < LOD | < LOD | 1127 |
| **Gender** | | | | | | | |
| Males | 99-00 | * | < LOD | < LOD | < LOD | < LOD | 891 |
| | 01-02 | * | < LOD | < LOD | < LOD | < LOD | 1192 |
| Females | 99-00 | * | < LOD | < LOD | < LOD | < LOD | 923 |
| | 01-02 | * | < LOD | < LOD | < LOD | < LOD | 1346 |
| **Race/ethnicity** | | | | | | | |
| Mexican Americans | 99-00 | * | < LOD | < LOD | < LOD | < LOD | 652 |
| | 01-02 | * | < LOD | < LOD | < LOD | < LOD | 679 |
| Non-Hispanic blacks | 99-00 | * | < LOD | < LOD | < LOD | < LOD | 483 |
| | 01-02 | * | < LOD | < LOD | < LOD | < LOD | 701 |
| Non-Hispanic whites | 99-00 | * | < LOD | < LOD | < LOD | < LOD | 531 |
| | 01-02 | * | < LOD | < LOD | < LOD | < LOD | 957 |

Limit of detection (LOD, see Data Analysis section) for Survey years 99-00 and 01-02 are 1.2 and 0.1.
< LOD means less than the limit of detection, which may vary for some chemicals by year and by individual sample.
* Not calculated: proportion of results below limit of detection was too high to provide a valid result.

or contaminated herbicides. It is unclear whether these associations are related to the chlorophenoxy herbicides, other exposures, or to contaminants in the herbicide formulations (specifically 2,3,7,8-tetrachlorodibenzo-*p*-dioxin) (Garabrant and Philbert, 2002; IOM, 2003; IPCS, 1996; Pearce and McLean, 2005; U.S.EPA, 2004). 2,4,5-T itself is not mutagenic. IARC considers the chlorophenoxyacetic acids group of chemicals as possibly carcinogenic to humans. Additional information is available from U.S.EPA at: http://www.epa.gov/pesticides/.

## Biomonitoring Information

Urinary levels of 2,4,5-T reflect recent exposure. In the NHANES 1999-2000 and 2001-2002 subsamples (CDC, 2005), urinary levels of 2,4,5-T were generally below the limit of detection, similar to results of NHANES II (1976-1980), in which urinary levels of 2,4,5-T also were below the limit of detection (Kutz et al., 1992). Mean urinary levels of 2,4,5-T measured after a day of exposure in a few asymptomatic herbicide applicators were 35,000 times higher than the detection limit for the NHANES 2001-2002 data (Kolmodin-Hedman and Erne, 1980).

Finding a measurable amount of 2,4,5-T does not mean that the level will result in an adverse health effect. Biomonitoring studies on 2,4,5-T in urine also provide physicians and public health officials with reference values so that they can determine whether other people have been exposed to higher levels of 2,4,5-T than levels found in the general population. Biomonitoring data can also help scientists plan and conduct research on exposure and health effects.

## Urinary 2,4,5-Trichlorophenoxyacetic acid (creatinine corrected)

Geometric mean and selected percentiles of urine concentrations (in µg/g of creatinine) for the U.S. population from the National Health and Nutrition Examination Survey.

| | Survey years | Geometric mean (95% conf. interval) | Selected percentiles ( 95% confidence interval) | | | | Sample size |
|---|---|---|---|---|---|---|---|
| | | | 50th | 75th | 90th | 95th | |
| Total | 99-00 | * | < LOD | < LOD | < LOD | < LOD | 1814 |
| | 01-02 | * | < LOD | < LOD | < LOD | < LOD | 2537 |
| **Age group** | | | | | | | |
| 6-11 years | 99-00 | * | < LOD | < LOD | < LOD | < LOD | 430 |
| | 01-02 | * | < LOD | < LOD | < LOD | < LOD | 580 |
| 12-19 years | 99-00 | * | < LOD | < LOD | < LOD | < LOD | 618 |
| | 01-02 | * | < LOD | < LOD | < LOD | < LOD | 830 |
| 20-59 years | 99-00 | * | < LOD | < LOD | < LOD | < LOD | 766 |
| | 01-02 | * | < LOD | < LOD | < LOD | < LOD | 1127 |
| **Gender** | | | | | | | |
| Males | 99-00 | * | < LOD | < LOD | < LOD | < LOD | 891 |
| | 01-02 | * | < LOD | < LOD | < LOD | < LOD | 1192 |
| Females | 99-00 | * | < LOD | < LOD | < LOD | < LOD | 923 |
| | 01-02 | * | < LOD | < LOD | < LOD | < LOD | 1345 |
| **Race/ethnicity** | | | | | | | |
| Mexican Americans | 99-00 | * | < LOD | < LOD | < LOD | < LOD | 652 |
| | 01-02 | * | < LOD | < LOD | < LOD | < LOD | 679 |
| Non-Hispanic blacks | 99-00 | * | < LOD | < LOD | < LOD | < LOD | 483 |
| | 01-02 | * | < LOD | < LOD | < LOD | < LOD | 700 |
| Non-Hispanic whites | 99-00 | * | < LOD | < LOD | < LOD | < LOD | 531 |
| | 01-02 | * | < LOD | < LOD | < LOD | < LOD | 957 |

< LOD means less than the limit of detection for the urine levels not corrected for creatinine.
* Not calculated: proportion of results below limit of detection was too high to provide a valid result.

## References

Arnold EK, Beasley VR. The pharmacokinetics of chlorinated phenoxy acid herbicides: a literature. Vet Hum Toxicol 1989;31(2):121-125.

Bradberry SM, Proudfoot AT, Vale JA. Poisoning due to chlorophenoxy herbicides. Toxicol Rev 2004;23(2):65-73.

Centers for Disease Control and Prevention (CDC). Third National Report on Human Exposure to Environmental Chemicals. Atlanta (GA). 2005.

Garabrant DH, Philbert MA. Review of 2,4-dichlorophenoxyacetic acid (2,4-D) epidemiology and toxicology. Crit Rev Toxicol 2002;32(4):233-257.

Holson JF, Gaines TB, Nelson CJ, LaBorde JB, Gaylor DW, Sheehan DM, et al. Developmental toxicity of 2,4,5-trichlorophenoxyacetic acid (2,4,5-T). I. Multireplicated dose-response studies in four inbred strains and one outbred stock of mice. Fundam Appl Toxicol 1992;19(2):286-297.

International Programme on Chemical Safety-INCHEM (IPCS). Pesticides residues in food: 1996 evaluations Part II Toxicology. 914. Dichlorophenoxyacetic acid, 2,4-. Available at URL: http://www.inchem.org/documents/jmpr/jmpmono/v96pr04.htm. 3/17/09

Institute of Medicine (IOM). Board on Health Promotion and Disease Prevention. Committee to Review the Health Effects in Vietnam Veterans of Exposure to Herbicides (Fourth Biennial Update. Veterans and Agent Orange: update 2002. Washington (DC): National Academies Press; 2003. Available at URL: http://www.nap.edu/catalog.php?record_id=10603. 3/17/09

Kohli JD, Khanna RN, Gupta BN, Dhar MM, Tandon JS, Sircar KP. Absorption and excretion of 2,4,5-trichlorophenoxy acetic acid in man. Arch Int Pharmacodyn Ther 1974; 210:250-255.

Kolmodin-Hedman B, Erne K. Estimation of occupational exposure to phenoxy acids (2,4-D and 2,4,5-T). Arch Toxicol Suppl 1980;4:318-21.

Kutz FW, Cook BT, Carter-Pokras OD, Brody D, Murphy RS. Selected pesticide residues and metabolites in urine from a survey of the U.S. general population. J Toxicol Environ Health 1992;37(2):277-91.

Mohammad FK, St Omer VE. Behavioral and developmental effects in rats following in utero exposure to 2,4-D/2,4,5-t mixture. Neurobehav Toxicol Teratol 1986;8(5):551-60.

Nelson CJ, Holson JF, Gaines TB, LaBorde JB, McCallum WF, Wolff GL, et al. Developmental toxicity of 2,4,5-trichlorophenoxyacetic acid (2,4,5-T). II. Multireplicated dose-response studies with technical and analytical grades of 2,4,5-T in four-way outcross mice. Fundam Appl Toxicol 1992;19(2):298-306.

Pearce N, McLean D. Agricultural exposures and non-Hodgkin's lymphoma. Scand J Work Environ Health 2005;31 Suppl 1:18-25; discussion 5-7.

U. S. Environmental Protection Agency (U.S.EPA). Office of Prevention Pesticides and Toxic Substances. Pesticide industry sales and usage - 2000 and 2001 market estimates. Washington (DC): U.S.EPA. May, 2004. Available at URL: http://www.epa.gov/oppbead1/pestsales/01pestsales/market_estimates2001.pdf. 3/17/09

# Carbamate Insecticides

## General Information

N-methyl carbamate insecticides (carbamates) have been widely used in the U.S. and throughout the world. In agricultural applications, the use of the carbamate insecticides has decreased, being replaced by pyrethroid and other insecticides. Carbamates have been used on residential lawns, ornamentals, in nurseries, and on golf courses. Carbamates do not persist in the environment and have a low potential for bioaccumulation. Some other chemical types of carbamates, thiocarbamates and dithiocarbamates, are used as herbicides and fungicides.

General population exposure to carbamates occurs during contact with residential uses and, less commonly, from ingesting contaminated foods. Agricultural workers can be exposed when they re-enter areas recently treated. Exposures of workers also can occur during the manufacture, formulation, or application of these chemicals. Carbamates can be absorbed through the skin, via inhalation, or by ingestion. Criteria for allowable levels of specific carbamates in food, the environment, and the workplace have been developed by the U.S. FDA, U.S. EPA, and OSHA, respectively.

Carbamate insecticides act by inhibiting acetylcholinesterase enzymes, leading to an increase of acetylcholine in the nervous system. At high doses, toxic symptoms include nausea, vomiting, cholinergic signs, weakness, paralysis, and seizures. The mechanism of toxicity of carbamate insecticides is similar to that of organophosphate pesticides; however, carbamate insecticides generally are reversible inhibitors of acetylcholinesterase activity, acting for a shorter time than organophosphate pesticides. Carbamate insecticides are rapidly eliminated from the body. Only two metabolites are measured in this *Report* (metabolites of carbofuran and propoxur), of the carbamate insecticides still used in the U.S.

# Carbofuran
CAS No. 1563-66-2

## General Information

Carbofuranphenol is a metabolite of four different carbamate insecticides: benfuracarb; carbofuran; carbosulfan; and furathiocarb. Only carbofuran is registered in the U.S. Carbofuran is a broad spectrum, restricted-use insecticide and nematicide applied to a variety of field, fruit, and vegetable crops for control of beetles, borers, nematodes, weevils, and similar pests. Recently, registered uses of carbofuran were cancelled except for the following: field corn; potatoes; pumpkins; sunflowers; pine seedlings; and spinach grown for seed (U.S.EPA, 2009). About 1 million pounds have been used annually (U.S.EPA, 2007). Carbofuran is not registered for use in residential settings or food-handling establishments. In soils of varying composition, carbofuran has a half-life ranging from one to three months. It can leach into ground waters, but it has been detected only infrequently in either surface or ground waters (Gilliom, 2007; USGS, 2007). Carbofuran

is very highly toxic to fish and aquatic invertebrates, and it is highly toxic to birds where granular applications are used, but such applications have been restricted since 1991 (U.S.EPA, 2007).

General population exposure can occur through consumption of food contaminated with carbofuran. Because estimated acute intakes from some dietary components in young children may exceed recommended intake limits, the U.S.EPA is in the process of revoking current regulations that allow carbofuran residues in food (U.S.EPA, 2009). Pesticide handlers and applicators are at greater risk for exposure and a number of incidents of systemic poisoning have been reported. After absorption, carbofuran is metabolized to phenolic metabolites and 3-hydroxycarbofuran, which are quickly eliminated in the urine.

Human health effects from carbofuran at low environmental doses or at biomonitored levels from low environmental exposures are unknown. Carbofuran was very highly acutely toxic in animal studies, causing effects related

## Urinary Carbofuranphenol
*Metabolite of Benfuracarb, Carbofuran, Carbosulfan, and Furathiocarb*
Geometric mean and selected percentiles of urine concentrations (in µg/L) for the U.S. population from the National Health and Nutrition Examination Survey.

| | Survey years | Geometric mean (95% conf. interval) | 50th | 75th | 90th | 95th | Sample size |
|---|---|---|---|---|---|---|---|
| **Total** | 99-00 | * | < LOD | < LOD | < LOD | .770 (<LOD-1.30) | 1994 |
| | 01-02 | * | < LOD | < LOD | < LOD | < LOD | 2530 |
| **Age group** | | | | | | | |
| 6-11 years | 99-00 | * | < LOD | < LOD | < LOD | .450 (<LOD-2.20) | 482 |
| | 01-02 | * | < LOD | < LOD | < LOD | < LOD | 578 |
| 12-19 years | 99-00 | * | < LOD | < LOD | < LOD | .570 (<LOD-1.20) | 681 |
| | 01-02 | * | < LOD | < LOD | < LOD | < LOD | 827 |
| 20-59 years | 99-00 | * | < LOD | < LOD | < LOD | .840 (<LOD-1.50) | 831 |
| | 01-02 | * | < LOD | < LOD | < LOD | < LOD | 1125 |
| **Gender** | | | | | | | |
| Males | 99-00 | * | < LOD | < LOD | < LOD | .740 (<LOD-1.50) | 973 |
| | 01-02 | * | < LOD | < LOD | < LOD | < LOD | 1190 |
| Females | 99-00 | * | < LOD | < LOD | < LOD | .840 (<LOD-1.50) | 1021 |
| | 01-02 | * | < LOD | < LOD | < LOD | < LOD | 1340 |
| **Race/ethnicity** | | | | | | | |
| Mexican Americans | 99-00 | * | < LOD | < LOD | .590 (<LOD-2.00) | 1.90 (<LOD-5.10) | 696 |
| | 01-02 | * | < LOD | < LOD | < LOD | < LOD | 680 |
| Non-Hispanic blacks | 99-00 | * | < LOD | < LOD | < LOD | .550 (<LOD-1.60) | 521 |
| | 01-02 | * | < LOD | < LOD | < LOD | < LOD | 696 |
| Non-Hispanic whites | 99-00 | * | < LOD | < LOD | < LOD | .740 (<LOD-1.50) | 603 |
| | 01-02 | * | < LOD | < LOD | < LOD | < LOD | 953 |

Limit of detection (LOD, see Data Analysis section) for Survey years 99-00 and 01-02 are 0.4 and 0.4.
< LOD means less than the limit of detection, which may vary for some chemicals by year and by individual sample.
* Not calculated: proportion of results below limit of detection was too high to provide a valid result.

to acetylcholinesterase enzyme inhibition. In contrast, carbofuranphenol is not an inhibitor of acetylcholinesterase enzymes. Carbofuran was not teratogenic, but high chronic doses in animals produced nonspecific developmental effects, such as reduced weight gain and pup survival (WHO, 2004). Testicular toxicity at subacute doses was reported in adult rats, rat pups, and dogs (Pant et al., 1995, 1997; WHO, 2004). Carbofuran was found not to be mutagenic or carcinogenic in animals (U.S.EPA, 2007). It is not rated by IARC with regard to human carcinogenicity. Additional information is available from U.S.EPA at: http://www.epa.gov/pesticides/.

## Biomonitoring Information

Urinary carbofuranphenol levels reflect recent exposure. The level of this metabolite in urine may reflect exposure to carbofuran or to carbofuranphenol as a degradation product in the environment or food. In representative subsamples from NHANES 1999-2000 and 2001-2002, most urinary levels of carbofuranphenol were below the limit of detection (CDC, 2005). In a nonrandom subsample from NHANES III (1988-1994), the 99th percentile level of carbofuranphenol

was 2.1µg/L (Hill et al., 1995). In a previous study of U.S. farmers and their families, carbofuranphenol was detected in 6.7% of urine samples (Shealy et al., 1997); the 95th percentile value in that study was 0.73 µg/L. Urinary levels of carbofuranphenol in two applicators were three and sixfold higher than the detection limit for the NHANES 2003-2004 subsample (Petropoulou et al., 2006).

Finding a measurable amount of carbofuranphenol in urine does not mean that the level of carbofuranphenol causes an adverse health effect. Biomonitoring studies on levels of carbofuranphenol provide physicians and public health officials with reference values so that they can determine whether people have been exposed to higher levels of carbofuran or related carbamates than are found in the general population. Biomonitoring data can also help scientists plan and conduct research on exposure and health effects.

## Urinary Carbofuranphenol (creatinine corrected)
*Metabolite of Benfuracarb, Carbofuran, Carbosulfan, and Furathiocarb*

Geometric mean and selected percentiles of urine concentrations (in µg/g of creatinine) for the U.S. population from the National Health and Nutrition Examination Survey.

| | Survey years | Geometric mean (95% conf. interval) | Selected percentiles (95% confidence interval) | | | | Sample size |
|---|---|---|---|---|---|---|---|
| | | | 50th | 75th | 90th | 95th | |
| Total | 99-00 | * | < LOD | < LOD | < LOD | .780 (<LOD-1.00) | 1994 |
| | 01-02 | * | < LOD | < LOD | < LOD | < LOD | 2529 |
| **Age group** | | | | | | | |
| 6-11 years | 99-00 | * | < LOD | < LOD | < LOD | .990 (<LOD-2.80) | 482 |
| | 01-02 | * | < LOD | < LOD | < LOD | < LOD | 578 |
| 12-19 years | 99-00 | * | < LOD | < LOD | < LOD | .480 (<LOD- 850) | 681 |
| | 01-02 | * | < LOD | < LOD | < LOD | < LOD | 826 |
| 20-59 years | 99-00 | * | < LOD | < LOD | < LOD | .880 (<LOD-1.06) | 831 |
| | 01-02 | * | < LOD | < LOD | < LOD | < LOD | 1125 |
| **Gender** | | | | | | | |
| Males | 99-00 | * | < LOD | < LOD | < LOD | .670 (<LOD-1.08) | 973 |
| | 01-02 | * | < LOD | < LOD | < LOD | < LOD | 1190 |
| Females | 99-00 | * | < LOD | < LOD | < LOD | .880 (<LOD-1.13) | 1021 |
| | 01-02 | * | < LOD | < LOD | < LOD | < LOD | 1339 |
| **Race/ethnicity** | | | | | | | |
| Mexican Americans | 99-00 | * | < LOD | < LOD | .780 (<LOD-1.94) | 1.83 (<LOD-4.16) | 696 |
| | 01-02 | * | < LOD | < LOD | < LOD | < LOD | 680 |
| Non-Hispanic blacks | 99-00 | * | < LOD | < LOD | < LOD | .700 (<LOD-1.08) | 521 |
| | 01-02 | * | < LOD | < LOD | < LOD | < LOD | 695 |
| Non-Hispanic whites | 99-00 | * | < LOD | < LOD | < LOD | .740 (<LOD- 930) | 603 |
| | 01-02 | * | < LOD | < LOD | < LOD | < LOD | 953 |

< LOD means less than the limit of detection for the urine levels not corrected for creatinine.
* Not calculated: proportion of results below limit of detection was too high to provide a valid result.

## References

Centers for Disease Control and Prevention (CDC). Third National Report on Human Exposure to Environmental Chemicals. Atlanta (GA). 2005.

Gillion, R. Pesticides in U.S. streams and groundwater. Environ Sci Technol 2007;41:3409-3414. Available at URL: http://water. usgs.gov/nawqa/pnsp/pubs/files/051507.ESTfeature_gilliom. pdf. 4/9/09

Hill RH Jr, Head SL, Baker S, Gregg M, Shealy DB, Bailey SL, et al. Pesticide residues in urine of adults living in the United States: reference range concentrations. Environ Res 1995;71(2):99-108.

Pant N, Prasad AK, Srivastava SC, Shankar R, Srivastava SP. Effect of oral administration of carbofuran on male reproductive system of rat. Hum Exp Toxicol 1995;14(11):889-894.

Pant N, Shankar R, Srivastava SP. In utero and lactational exposure of carbofuran to rats: effect on testes and sperm. Hum Exp Toxicol 1997;16(5):267-272.

Petropoulou SS, Gikas E, Tsarbopoulos A, Siskos PA. Gas chromatographic-tandem mass spectrometric method for the quantitation of carbofuran, carbaryl and their main metabolites in applicators' urine. J Chromatogr A 2006;1108(1):99-110.

Shealy DB, Barr JR., Ashley DL, Patterson DG Jr, Camann DE, Bond AE. Correlation of environmental carbaryl measurements with serum and urinary 1-naphthol measurements in a farmer applicator and his family. Environ Health Perspect 1997;105:510-513.

U.S. Environmental Protection Agency (U.S.EPA) Carbofuran cancellation process. March 28, 2009. Available at URL: http://www.epa.gov/pesticides/reregistration/carbofuran/carbofuran_noic htm. 4/10/09

U.S. Environmental Protection Agency (U.S.EPA). Reregistration Eligibility Decision for Carbofuran. September 2007. Available at URL: http://www.epa.gov/pesticides/reregistration/REDs/carbofuran_red.pdf. 4/10/09

U.S.Geological Survey (USGS). The Quality of Our Nation's Waters: Pesticides in the Nation's Streams and Ground Water, 1992-2001. Circular 1291. Supplemental Technical Information (available on-line only). March 2006, revised February 15, 2007. Available at URL: http://water.usgs.gov/nawqa/pnsp/pubs/circ1291/supporting_info.php. 4/2/09

World Health Organization (WHO). Carbofuran in Drinking-Water. Background document for development of WHO Guidelines for Drinking-water Quality. 2004. Available at URL: http://www.who.int/water_sanitation_health/dwq/chemicals/carbofuran.pdf. 4/9/09

# Propoxur

CAS No. 114-26-1

## General Information

2-Isopropoxyphenol is a metabolite of propoxur, a carbamate used to control ants, roaches, hornets, and similar pests in residential areas and around commercial food-handling establishments. Propoxur has also been used in pest strips and pet flea collars. Like several other pesticides, propoxur has been used outside the U.S. as a replacement for DDT in malaria vector control. Propoxur may remain in the environment for weeks to several months, longer than most carbamates (U.S.EPA, 1997b). Despite its mobility in soil and its potential for leaching into groundwater, propoxur has been rarely detected in U.S. surface or ground waters (Gilliom, 2007; USGS, 2007). Although propoxur is toxic to birds and aquatic life, ecologic exposures are unlikely due to current outdoor use restrictions.

General population exposure to propoxur through the diet is likely to be limited because of usage restrictions (U.S. EPA, 1997a). Estimated human intakes have been below recommended intake limits (U.S.EPA, 1997b). Pesticide applicators are likely to have the highest exposures. Propoxur can be absorbed through the skin, lungs, and gastrointestinal tract. Propoxur does not accumulate in blood or tissues and is eliminated rapidly from the body (Leenheers et al., 1992; WHO, 2003). In animal and human studies, 2-isopropoxyphenol was one of several urine metabolites (U.S.EPA, 1997b).

Human health effects from propoxur at low environmental doses or at biomonitored levels from low environmental exposures are unknown. In animal studies, propoxur has moderate acute toxicity consisting of anticholinesterase effects (U.S.EPA, 1997b). 2-Isopropoxyphenol does not inhibit acetylcholinesterase enzymes. Propoxur is not considered mutagenic, embryotoxic, or teratogenic (WHO, 2003). U.S. EPA considers propoxur to be a probable human carcinogen, based on bladder tumors in male rats (U.S. EPA, 1997b). The human carcinogenic potential of propoxur has not been evaluated by IARC or NTP. Additional information is available from U.S.EPA at: http://www.epa.gov/pesticides/.

## Biomonitoring Information

Urinary 2-isopropoxyphenol levels reflect recent exposure. The level of this metabolite in urine may reflect exposure to propoxur or to 2-isopropoxyphenol as a degradation product in the environment or food (U.S.EPA, 1997b). In the U.S. representative subsamples from NHANES 1999-2000 and 2001-2002, most 2-isopropoxyphenol levels in urine were below the limit of detection (CDC, 2005). In a nonrandom subsample from NHANES III (1988-1994), the 95th percentile level of 2-isopropoxyphenol was 1.7 µg/L (Hill et al., 1995). Higher urinary levels of 2-isopropoxyphenol have been measured in a few pesticide applicators, with a range of 45-306 µg/g creatinine (Hardt and Angerer, 1999).

Finding a measurable amount of 2-isopropoxyphenol in urine does not mean that the level of 2-isopropoxyphenol causes an adverse health effect. Biomonitoring studies on levels of 2-isopropoxyphenol provide physicians and public health officials with reference values so that they can determine whether people have been exposed to higher levels of propoxur than are found in the general population. Biomonitoring data can also help scientists plan and conduct research on exposure and health effects.

## Urinary 2-Isopropoxyphenol
*Metabolite of Propoxur*

Geometric mean and selected percentiles of urine concentrations (in µg/L) for the U.S. population from the National Health and Nutrition Examination Survey.

| | Survey years | Geometric mean (95% conf. interval) | 50th | 75th | 90th | 95th | Sample size |
|---|---|---|---|---|---|---|---|
| **Total** | 99-00 | * | < LOD | < LOD | < LOD | < LOD | 1917 |
| | 01-02 | * | < LOD | < LOD | < LOD | < LOD | 2503 |
| **Age group** | | | | | | | |
| 6-11 years | 99-00 | * | < LOD | < LOD | < LOD | < LOD | 456 |
| | 01-02 | * | < LOD | < LOD | < LOD | < LOD | 574 |
| 12-19 years | 99-00 | * | < LOD | < LOD | < LOD | < LOD | 655 |
| | 01-02 | * | < LOD | < LOD | < LOD | < LOD | 820 |
| 20-59 years | 99-00 | * | < LOD | < LOD | < LOD | < LOD | 806 |
| | 01-02 | * | < LOD | < LOD | < LOD | < LOD | 1109 |
| **Gender** | | | | | | | |
| Males | 99-00 | * | < LOD | < LOD | < LOD | < LOD | 936 |
| | 01-02 | * | < LOD | < LOD | < LOD | < LOD | 1178 |
| Females | 99-00 | * | < LOD | < LOD | < LOD | < LOD | 981 |
| | 01-02 | * | < LOD | < LOD | < LOD | < LOD | 1325 |
| **Race/ethnicity** | | | | | | | |
| Mexican Americans | 99-00 | * | < LOD | < LOD | < LOD | < LOD | 664 |
| | 01-02 | * | < LOD | < LOD | < LOD | < LOD | 677 |
| Non-Hispanic blacks | 99-00 | * | < LOD | < LOD | < LOD | < LOD | 500 |
| | 01-02 | * | < LOD | < LOD | < LOD | < LOD | 696 |
| Non-Hispanic whites | 99-00 | * | < LOD | < LOD | < LOD | < LOD | 585 |
| | 01-02 | * | < LOD | < LOD | < LOD | < LOD | 931 |

Limit of detection (LOD, see Data Analysis section) for Survey years 99-00 and 01-02 are 1.1 and 0.4.
< LOD means less than the limit of detection, which may vary for some chemicals by year and by individual sample.
* Not calculated: proportion of results below limit of detection was too high to provide a valid result.

## Urinary 2-Isopropoxyphenol (creatinine corrected)
*Metabolite of Propoxur*

Geometric mean and selected percentiles of urine concentrations (in µg/g of creatinine) for the U.S. population from the National Health and Nutrition Examination Survey.

| | Survey years | Geometric mean (95% conf. interval) | 50th | 75th | 90th | 95th | Sample size |
|---|---|---|---|---|---|---|---|
| | | | | Selected percentiles ( 95% confidence interval) | | | |
| **Total** | 99-00 | * | < LOD | < LOD | < LOD | < LOD | 1917 |
| | 01-02 | * | < LOD | < LOD | < LOD | < LOD | 2502 |
| **Age group** | | | | | | | |
| 6-11 years | 99-00 | * | < LOD | < LOD | < LOD | < LOD | 456 |
| | 01-02 | * | < LOD | < LOD | < LOD | < LOD | 574 |
| 12-19 years | 99-00 | * | < LOD | < LOD | < LOD | < LOD | 655 |
| | 01-02 | * | < LOD | < LOD | < LOD | < LOD | 819 |
| 20-59 years | 99-00 | * | < LOD | < LOD | < LOD | < LOD | 806 |
| | 01-02 | * | < LOD | < LOD | < LOD | < LOD | 1109 |
| **Gender** | | | | | | | |
| Males | 99-00 | * | < LOD | < LOD | < LOD | < LOD | 936 |
| | 01-02 | * | < LOD | < LOD | < LOD | < LOD | 1178 |
| Females | 99-00 | * | < LOD | < LOD | < LOD | < LOD | 981 |
| | 01-02 | * | < LOD | < LOD | < LOD | < LOD | 1324 |
| **Race/ethnicity** | | | | | | | |
| Mexican Americans | 99-00 | * | < LOD | < LOD | < LOD | < LOD | 664 |
| | 01-02 | * | < LOD | < LOD | < LOD | < LOD | 677 |
| Non-Hispanic blacks | 99-00 | * | < LOD | < LOD | < LOD | < LOD | 500 |
| | 01-02 | * | < LOD | < LOD | < LOD | < LOD | 695 |
| Non-Hispanic whites | 99-00 | * | < LOD | < LOD | < LOD | < LOD | 585 |
| | 01-02 | * | < LOD | < LOD | < LOD | < LOD | 931 |

< LOD means less than the limit of detection for the urine levels not corrected for creatinine.
* Not calculated: proportion of results below limit of detection was too high to provide a valid result.

## References

Centers for Disease Control and Prevention (CDC). Third National Report on Human Exposure to Environmental Chemicals. Atlanta (GA). 2005.

Gillion, R. Pesticides in U.S. streams and groundwater. Environ Sci Technol 2007;41:3409-3414. Available at URL: http://water. usgs.gov/nawqa/pnsp/pubs/files/051507.ESTfeature_gilliom. pdf. 4/9/09

Hardt J, Angerer J. Gas chromatographic method with mass-selective detection for the determination of 2-isopropoxyphenol in human urine. J Chromatogr B Biomed Sci Appl 1999;723(1-2):139-145.

Hill RH Jr, Head SL, Baker S, Gregg M, Shealy DB, Bailey SL, et al. Pesticide residues in urine of adults living in the United States: reference range concentrations. Environ Res 1995;71(2):99-108.

Leenheers LH, van Breugel DC, Ravensberg JC, Meuling WJ, Jongen MJ. Determination of 2-isopropoxyphenol in urine by capillary gas chromatography and mass-selective detection. J Chromatogr 1992;578(2):189-194.

U.S. Environmental Protection Agency (U.S.EPA). RED Facts. Propoxur. August 1997a. EPA 738 F-97-009. Available at URL: http://www.epa.gov/oppsrrd1/REDs/factsheets/2555fact.pdf. 4/9/09

U.S. Environmental Protection Agency (U.S.EPA). Reregistration Eligibility Decision (RED) Propoxur. August 1997b. EPA 738-R-97-009. Available at URL: http://www.epa.gov/pesticides/reregistration/REDs/2555red.pdf. 4/9/09

U.S. Geological Survey (USGS). The Quality of Our Nation's Waters. Pesticides in the Nation's Streams and Ground Water, 1992-2001. Circular 1291. Supplemental Technical Information (available on-line only). March 2006, revised February 15, 2007. Available at URL: http://water.usgs.gov/nawqa/pnsp/pubs/circ1291/supporting_info.php. 4/2/09

World Health Organization (WHO). WHO Specifications and Evaluations for Public Health Pesticides. Propoxur. FAO/WHO Evaluation Report 80/2003. 2003. Available at URL: http://www.who.int/whopes/quality/en/propoxur_eval_spec_WHO_October_2005.pdf. 4/9/09

# Organochlorine Pesticides

## General Information

Organochlorine pesticides, an older class of pesticides, are effective against a variety of insects. These chemicals were introduced in the 1940s, and many of their uses have been cancelled or restricted by the U.S. EPA because of their environmental persistence and potential adverse effects on wildlife and human health. Many organochlorines are no longer used widely in the U.S., but other countries continue to use them. Hexachlorobenzene has been used primarily as a fungicide or biocide.

Organochlorine pesticides can enter the environment after pesticide applications, disposal of contaminated wastes into landfills, and releases from manufacturing plants that produce these chemicals. Some organochlorines are volatile, and some can adhere to soil or particles in the air. In aquatic systems, sediments adsorb organochlorines, which can then bioaccumulate in fish and other aquatic mammals. These chemicals are fat soluble, so they are found at higher concentrations in fatty foods. In the general population, diet is the main source of exposure, primarily through the ingestion of fatty foods such as dairy products and fish. Usage restrictions have been associated with a general decrease in serum organochlorine levels in the U.S. population and other developed countries (Hagmar et al., 2006; Kutz et al., 1991). Contaminated drinking water and air are usually minor exposure sources. Infants can be exposed through breast milk, and the fetus can be exposed *in utero* via the placenta. Workers can be exposed to organochlorines in the manufacture, formulation, or application of these chemicals. The FDA, U.S. EPA, and OSHA have developed standards for allowable levels of certain organochlorines in foods, the environment, and the workplace, respectively. Attributing human health effects to specific organochlorine chemicals is difficult because exposure to multiple organochlorine chemicals occurs often and these chemicals may have similar actions.

The table shows selected parent organochlorines and their metabolites that can be measured in serum or urine. Measurements of these chemicals can reflect either recent or cumulative exposures, or both. Some of the metabolites can be produced from more than one pesticide. The level of a metabolite in a person's blood or urine may indicate exposure to the parent pesticide as well as to the metabolite itself.

## Organochlorine Pesticides and Metabolites in this *Report*

| Organochlorine Pesticide (CAS number) | Serum pesticide or metabolite(s) (CAS number) | Urinary pesticide or metabolite(s) (CAS number) |
|---|---|---|
| Aldrin (309-00-02) | Aldrin (309-00-02) Dieldrin (60-57-1) | |
| Chlordane (12789-03-6) | Oxychlordane (27304-13-8) *trans*-Nonachlor (3734-49-4) | |
| Dichlorodiphenyltrichloroethanes | *p,p*'-DDT (50-29-3) *p,p*'-DDE (72-55-9) *o,p*'-DDT (789-02-6) | |
| Dieldrin (60-57-1) | Dieldrin (60-57-1) | |
| Endrin (72-20-8) | Endrin (72-20-8) | |
| Heptachlor (76-44-8) | Heptachlor epoxide (1024-57-3) | |
| Hexachlorobenzene (118-74-1) | Hexachlorobenzene (118-74-1) | Pentachlorophenol (87-86-5) 2,4,6-Trichlorophenol (88-06-2) 2,4,5-Trichlorophenol (95-95-4) |
| Hexachlorocyclohexanes | *beta*-Hexachlorocyclohexane (319-85-7) *gamma*-Hexachlorocyclohexane (58-89-9) | Pentachlorophenol (87-86-5) 2,4,6-Trichlorophenol (88-06-2) 2,4,5-Trichlorophenol (95-95-4) |
| Mirex (2385-85-5) | Mirex (2385-85-5) | |
| 2,4,5-Trichlorophenol (95-95-4) 2,4,6-Trichlorophenol (88-06-2) | | 2,4,5-Trichlorophenol (95-95-4) 2,4,6-Trichlorophenol (88-06-2) |

## References

Hagmar L, Wallin E, Vessby B, Jonsson BA, Bergman A, Rylander L. Intra-individual variations and time trends 1991-2001 in human serum levels of PCB, DDE and hexachlorobenzene. Chemosphere 2006;64(9):507-513.

Kutz FW, Wood PH, Bottimore DP. Organochlorine pesticides and polychlorinated biphenyls in human adipose tissue. Rev Environ Contam Toxicol 1991;120:1-82.

# Aldrin

CAS No. 309-00-02

# Dieldrin

CAS No. 60-57-1
*Also a Metabolite of Aldrin*

## General Information

Aldrin and dieldrin are no longer produced or used in the U.S. From the 1950s to 1970, both chemicals were applied mainly as a soil insecticide or seed dressing for food and commodity crops. Dieldrin was also used for mothproofing clothes and carpets. In tropical countries, dieldrin was used as a residual spray in residential dwellings to control vector-borne diseases such as malaria. The U.S. EPA cancelled agricultural uses of both pesticides in 1970; termiticide uses were cancelled in 1987. Aldrin is readily converted to dieldrin in the environment and in plants that take up the chemical. Aldrin volatilizes after agricultural soil applications or is converted to dieldrin, which volatilizes more slowly. These chemicals persist in the environment and bioaccumulate in foods (Jorgenson 2001; USGS, 2007). Aldrin is rarely detected in plants or animal tissues,

but dieldrin has been detected in meats, dairy products, and in crops grown in soils that have been contaminated, usually by application, manufacturing, or disposal.

General population exposure to these chemicals occurs through the diet, and detection of dieldrin residue in foods has decreased over time (FDA, 2008). Inhalation exposure may occur among people living in residences where aldrin was applied historically as a pesticide. Aldrin and dieldrin are absorbed following ingestion, inhalation, and dermal application. After absorption, aldrin is metabolized to dieldrin so rapidly that aldrin is rarely detected. Dieldrin accumulates in fatty tissues, and its metabolites are excreted in bile and feces (ATSDR, 2002). It is also excreted in breast milk and can cross the placenta. The elimination half-life of dieldrin is approximately 1 year (IPCS, 1989; Jorgenson 2001).

Human health effects from aldrin and dieldrin at low environmental doses or at biomonitored levels from low environmental exposures are unknown. At high doses, aldrin and dieldrin block inhibitory neurotransmitters in the central nervous system (Narahashi et al., 1992). This blocking action can cause abnormal excitation of the brain, leading to symptoms such as headache, confusion, muscle

## Serum Aldrin (lipid adjusted)

Geometric mean and selected percentiles of serum concentrations (in ng/g of lipid or parts per billion on a lipid-weight basis) for the U.S. population from the National Health and Nutrition Examination Survey.

| | Survey years | Geometric mean (95% conf. interval) | Selected percentiles ( 95% confidence interval) | | | | Sample size |
|---|---|---|---|---|---|---|---|
| | | | 50th | 75th | 90th | 95th | |
| Total | 01-02 | * | < LOD | < LOD | < LOD | < LOD | 2275 |
| | 03-04 | * | < LOD | < LOD | < LOD | < LOD | 1946 |
| **Age group** | | | | | | | |
| 12-19 years | 01-02 | * | < LOD | < LOD | < LOD | < LOD | 756 |
| | 03-04 | * | < LOD | < LOD | < LOD | < LOD | 588 |
| 20 years and older | 01-02 | * | < LOD | < LOD | < LOD | < LOD | 1519 |
| | 03-04 | * | < LOD | < LOD | < LOD | < LOD | 1358 |
| **Gender** | | | | | | | |
| Males | 01-02 | * | < LOD | < LOD | < LOD | < LOD | 1057 |
| | 03-04 | * | < LOD | < LOD | < LOD | < LOD | 946 |
| Females | 01-02 | * | < LOD | < LOD | < LOD | < LOD | 1218 |
| | 03-04 | * | < LOD | < LOD | < LOD | < LOD | 1000 |
| **Race/ethnicity** | | | | | | | |
| Mexican Americans | 01-02 | * | < LOD | < LOD | < LOD | < LOD | 559 |
| | 03-04 | * | < LOD | < LOD | < LOD | < LOD | 456 |
| Non-Hispanic blacks | 01-02 | * | < LOD | < LOD | < LOD | < LOD | 512 |
| | 03-04 | * | < LOD | < LOD | < LOD | < LOD | 485 |
| Non-Hispanic whites | 01-02 | * | < LOD | < LOD | < LOD | < LOD | 1045 |
| | 03-04 | * | < LOD | < LOD | < LOD | < LOD | 881 |

Limit of detection (LOD, see Data Analysis section) for Survey years 01-02 and 03-04 are 5.94 and 7.8.
< LOD means less than the limit of detection, which may vary for some chemicals by year and by individual sample.
* Not calculated: proportion of results below limit of detection was too high to provide a valid result.

twitching, nausea, vomiting, and seizures. When fed to experimental animals, both aldrin and dieldrin caused liver enlargement and liver tumors; dieldrin at higher doses caused irritability, tremors, and occasionally, seizures (Smith, 1991). When dieldrin was fed to pregnant rodents, the offspring had altered CNS neurotransmitter levels (Sanchez-Ramos et al., 1998) and behavioral changes (Carlson and Rosellini, 1987). Studies done *in vitro* showed that dieldrin binds to estrogen receptors (Soto et al., 1995), but no estrogenic effect was noted in a study that used cultured cells (Tully et al., 2000). Epidemiologic and animal studies have not conclusively associated dieldrin exposure with risk for developing Parkinson's disease (Corrigan et al., 2000; Kanthasamy et al., 2005; Li et al., 2005).

The U.S. EPA has established environmental standards for aldrin and dieldrin, and the FDA monitors foods for pesticide residues. OSHA has established workplace exposure standards for aldrin and dieldrin. IARC has determined that aldrin and dieldrin are not classifiable with regard to human carcinogenicity. Information about external exposure (i.e., environmental levels) and health effects is available from ATSDR at: http://www.atsdr.cdc.gov/toxpro2.html.

## Biomonitoring Information

In the NHANES 2001-2002 and 2003-2004 subsamples, serum aldrin levels were below the limit of detection, similar to results in a subsample of NHANES II (1976-1980) (Stehr-Green, 1989). Levels of aldrin also were not detectable in 1996-1997 pooled samples from New Zealand adults (Bates et al., 2004).

Serum dieldrin levels at the 95th percentile in NHANES 2001-2002 and 2003-2004 subsamples were approximately ten times lower than the corresponding percentile measured in NHANES II (1976-1980), in which only 10.6% of the subsample had dieldrin levels above the limit of detection (Stehr-Green 1989). The median level in pooled samples from New Zealand adults obtained in 1996-1997 was generally similar to the 90th percentile for adults in this *Report* (Bates et al., 2004). In samples obtained between 1973 and 1991 from Norwegian women, the median serum dieldrin level was generally similar to the 90th percentile for females in this *Report* (Ward et al., 2000). Danish women whose serum was collected in 1976 had a median dieldrin level near the 95th percentile for females in this *Report* (Hoyer et al., 1998). In a study of pesticide applicators with occupational exposure to aldrin, median levels of dieldrin were more than thirtyfold higher than the 95th percentile

## Serum Aldrin (whole weight)

Geometric mean and selected percentiles of serum concentrations (in ng/g of serum or parts per billion) for the U.S. population from the National Health and Nutrition Examination Survey.

| | Survey years | Geometric mean (95% conf. interval) | Selected percentiles ( 95% confidence interval) | | | | Sample size |
|---|---|---|---|---|---|---|---|
| | | | 50th | 75th | 90th | 95th | |
| **Total** | 01-02 | * | < LOD | < LOD | < LOD | < LOD | 2275 |
| | 03-04 | * | < LOD | < LOD | < LOD | < LOD | 1946 |
| **Age group** | | | | | | | |
| 12-19 years | 01-02 | * | < LOD | < LOD | < LOD | < LOD | 756 |
| | 03-04 | * | < LOD | < LOD | < LOD | < LOD | 588 |
| 20 years and older | 01-02 | * | < LOD | < LOD | < LOD | < LOD | 1519 |
| | 03-04 | * | < LOD | < LOD | < LOD | < LOD | 1358 |
| **Gender** | | | | | | | |
| Males | 01-02 | * | < LOD | < LOD | < LOD | < LOD | 1057 |
| | 03-04 | * | < LOD | < LOD | < LOD | < LOD | 946 |
| Females | 01-02 | * | < LOD | < LOD | < LOD | < LOD | 1218 |
| | 03-04 | * | < LOD | < LOD | < LOD | < LOD | 1000 |
| **Race/ethnicity** | | | | | | | |
| Mexican Americans | 01-02 | * | < LOD | < LOD | < LOD | < LOD | 559 |
| | 03-04 | * | < LOD | < LOD | < LOD | < LOD | 456 |
| Non-Hispanic blacks | 01-02 | * | < LOD | < LOD | < LOD | < LOD | 512 |
| | 03-04 | * | < LOD | < LOD | < LOD | < LOD | 485 |
| Non-Hispanic whites | 01-02 | * | < LOD | < LOD | < LOD | < LOD | 1045 |
| | 03-04 | * | < LOD | < LOD | < LOD | < LOD | 881 |

< LOD means less than the limit of detection for the lipid adjusted serum level, which may vary for some chemicals by year and by individual sample.
* Not calculated: proportion of results below limit of detection was too high to provide a valid result.

## Serum Dieldrin (lipid adjusted)

*Also a Metabolite of Aldrin*

Geometric mean and selected percentiles of serum concentrations (in ng/g of lipid or parts per billion on a lipid-weight basis) for the U.S. population from the National Health and Nutrition Examination Survey.

| | Survey years | Geometric mean (95% conf. interval) | 50th | 75th | 90th | 95th | Sample size |
|---|---|---|---|---|---|---|---|
| | | | | **Selected percentiles** ( 95% confidence interval) | | | |
| **Total** | 01-02 | * | < LOD | < LOD | **15.3** (14.5-17.4) | **20.3** (18.7-22.4) | 2159 |
| | 03-04 | * | < LOD | **9.00** (8.40-9.90) | **14.4** (12.1-16.4) | **19.0** (15.8-24.2) | 1952 |
| **Age group** | | | | | | | |
| 12-19 years | 01-02 | * | < LOD | < LOD | < LOD | < LOD | 716 |
| | 03-04 | * | < LOD | < LOD | < LOD | **9.10** (<LOD-16.4) | 587 |
| 20 years and older | 01-02 | * | < LOD | **10.5** (<LOD-11.6) | **16.6** (15.1-18.2) | **21.3** (19.1-24.0) | 1443 |
| | 03-04 | * | < LOD | **9.50** (8.80-10.4) | **14.9** (12.8-17.0) | **19.5** (16.0-25.7) | 1365 |
| **Gender** | | | | | | | |
| Males | 01-02 | * | < LOD | < LOD | **15.7** (14.4-18.7) | **20.3** (18.6-24.0) | 1007 |
| | 03-04 | * | < LOD | **9.30** (8.40-10.8) | **15.1** (13.1-19.1) | **21.9** (14.9-38.5) | 954 |
| Females | 01-02 | * | < LOD | < LOD | **15.3** (13.4-17.2) | **19.8** (18.0-21.6) | 1152 |
| | 03-04 | * | < LOD | **8.70** (7.80-9.50) | **12.8** (11.2-15.4) | **16.9** (13.9-22.4) | 998 |
| **Race/ethnicity** | | | | | | | |
| Mexican Americans | 01-02 | * | < LOD | < LOD | **11.7** (<LOD-15.1) | **15.4** (12.7-19.1) | 539 |
| | 03-04 | * | < LOD | < LOD | **10.8** (9.00-14.1) | **14.0** (10.6-24.1) | 456 |
| Non-Hispanic blacks | 01-02 | * | < LOD | < LOD | **15.0** (11.8-19.1) | **20.6** (15.8-25.2) | 484 |
| | 03-04 | * | < LOD | **8.80** (<LOD-10.1) | **13.0** (10.5-15.8) | **15.9** (13.3-21.5) | 487 |
| Non-Hispanic whites | 01-02 | * | < LOD | < LOD | **15.6** (14.8-17.8) | **21.1** (18.9-23.6) | 980 |
| | 03-04 | * | < LOD | **9.30** (8.60-10.2) | **14.9** (12.5-17.5) | **19.7** (15.6-33.4) | 885 |

Limits of detection (LOD, see Data Analysis section) for survey years 01-02 and 03-04 are 10.5 and 7.8.
< LOD means less than the limit of detection, which may vary for some chemicals by year and by individual sample.
* Not calculated: proportion of results below limit of detection was too high to provide a valid result.


## Serum Dieldrin (whole weight)

*Also a Metabolite of Aldrin*

Geometric mean and selected percentiles of serum concentrations (in ng/g of serum or parts per billion) for the U.S. population from the National Health and Nutrition Examination Survey.

| | Survey years | Geometric mean (95% conf. interval) | 50th | 75th | 90th | 95th | Sample size |
|---|---|---|---|---|---|---|---|
| | | | | **Selected percentiles** ( 95% confidence interval) | | | |
| **Total** | 01-02 | * | < LOD | < LOD | **.110** (.100-.120) | **.150** (.130-.170) | 2159 |
| | 03-04 | * | < LOD | **.059** (.054-.064) | **.098** (.083-.112) | **.138** (.109-.177) | 1952 |
| **Age group** | | | | | | | |
| 12-19 years | 01-02 | * | < LOD | < LOD | < LOD | < LOD | 716 |
| | 03-04 | * | < LOD | < LOD | < LOD | **.048** (<LOD-.093) | 587 |
| 20 years and older | 01-02 | * | < LOD | **.070** (<LOD-.080) | **.120** (.110-.130) | **.160** (.140-.180) | 1443 |
| | 03-04 | * | < LOD | **.062** (.056-.069) | **.102** (.088-.117) | **.139** (.112-.182) | 1365 |
| **Gender** | | | | | | | |
| Males | 01-02 | * | < LOD | < LOD | **.120** (.100-.130) | **.160** (.130-.190) | 1007 |
| | 03-04 | * | < LOD | **.064** (.054-.075) | **.109** (.084-.138) | **.147** (.108-.242) | 954 |
| Females | 01-02 | * | < LOD | < LOD | **.100** (.090-.110) | **.140** (.120-.160) | 1152 |
| | 03-04 | * | < LOD | **.055** (.049-.060) | **.089** (.077-.100) | **.110** (.096-.147) | 998 |
| **Race/ethnicity** | | | | | | | |
| Mexican Americans | 01-02 | * | < LOD | < LOD | **.090** (<LOD-.100) | **.120** (.090-.140) | 539 |
| | 03-04 | * | < LOD | < LOD | **.077** (.062-.116) | **.113** (.073-.158) | 456 |
| Non-Hispanic blacks | 01-02 | * | < LOD | < LOD | **.090** (.070-.110) | **.130** (.090-.190) | 484 |
| | 03-04 | * | < LOD | **.053** (<LOD-.058) | **.080** (.063-.101) | **.103** (.080-.149) | 487 |
| Non-Hispanic whites | 01-02 | * | < LOD | < LOD | **.110** (.100-.130) | **.150** (.130-.180) | 980 |
| | 03-04 | * | < LOD | **.062** (.054-.070) | **.103** (.086-.124) | **.139** (.109-.202) | 885 |

< LOD means less than the limit of detection for the lipid adjusted serum level, which may vary for some chemicals by year and by individual sample.
* Not calculated: proportion of results below limit of detection was too high to provide a valid result.

in the NHANES 2001-2002 and 2003-2004 subsamples (Edwards and Priestly 1994).

Finding a measurable amount of aldrin or dieldrin in serum does not mean that the level of aldrin or dieldrin causes an adverse health effect. Biomonitoring studies on levels of aldrin and dieldrin provide physicians and public health officials with reference values so that they can determine whether people have been exposed to higher levels of aldrin or dieldrin than are found in the general population. Biomonitoring data can also help scientists plan and conduct research on exposure and health effects.

## References

Agency for Toxic Substances and Disease Registry (ATSDR). Toxicological profile for aldrin/dieldrin [online]. September 2002. Available at URL: http://www.atsdr.cdc.gov/toxprofiles/tp1.html. 4/21/09

Bates MN, Buckland SJ, Garrett N, Ellis H, Needham LL, Patterson DG Jr, et al. Persistent organochlorines in the serum of the non-occupationally exposed New Zealand population. Chemosphere 2004;54:1431-1443.

Carlson JN, Rosellini RA. Exposure to low doses of the environmental chemical dieldrin causes behavioral deficits in animals prevented from coping with stress. Psychopharmacology (Berl) 1987;91(1):122-126.

Corrigan FM, Wienburg CL, Shore RF, Daniel SE, Mann D. Organochlorine insecticides in substantia nigra in Parkinson's disease. J Toxicol Environ Health, Part A 2000;59:229-234.

Edwards JW, Priestly BG. Effect of occupational exposure to aldrin on urinary D-glucaric acid, plasma dieldrin, and lymphocyte sister chromatid exchange. Int Arch Occup Environ Health 1994;66(4):229-234.

Food and Drug Administration (FDA). Center for Food Safety and Applied Nutrition/Office of Plant and Dairy Foods. FDA Pesticide Program Residue Monitoring 1993-2006 [online]. August 2008. Available at URL: http://www.cfsan.fda.gov/~dms/pesrpts html. 4/21/09

Hoyer AP, Grandjean P, Jorgensen T, Brock JW, Hartvig HB. Organochlorine exposure and risk of breast cancer. Lancet 1998;352:1816-1820.

International Programme on Chemical Safety (IPCS). Environmental Health Criteria 91. Aldrin and Dieldrin [online]. 1989. Available at URL: http://www.inchem.org/documents/ehc/ehc/ehc91 htm. 4/21/09

Jorgenson JL. Aldrin and dieldrin: A review of research on their production environmental deposition and fate, bioaccumulation,

toxicology, and epidemiology in the United States. Environ Health Perspect 2001;109(Supp1):113-139.

Kanthasamy AG, Kitzazwa M, Kanthasamy A, Anantharam V. Dieldrin-induced neurotoxicity: relevance to Parkinson's disease pathogenesis. Neurotoxicol 2005;26:701-719.

Li AA, Mink PJ, McIntosh LJ, Teta MJ, Finley B. Evaluation of epidemiologic and animal data associating pesticides with Parkinson's disease. J Occup Environ Med 2005;47:1059-1087.

Narahashi T, Frey JM, Ginsburg KS, Roy ML. Sodium and GABA-activated channels as the targets of pyrethroids and cyclodienes. Toxicol Lett 1992;64-65 Spec. No:429-436.

Sanchez-Ramos J, Facca A, Basit A, Song S. Toxicity of dieldrin for dopaminergic neurons in mesencephalic cultures. Exp Neurol 1998;150:263-271.

Smith AG. Chlorinated Hydrocarbon Insecticides. In Hayes WJ, Jr and Laws ER, Jr, Eds. Handbook of Pesticide Toxicology, Vol. 2 Classes of Pesticides. New York, Academic Press, Inc. 1991, pp. 731-915.

Soto AM, Sonnenschein C, Chung KL, Fernandez MG, Olea N, Serrano FO. The E-SCREEN assay as a tool to identify estrogens: an update on estrogenic environmental pollutants. Environ Health Perspect 1995;103(Suppl 7):113-122.

Stehr-Green, PA. Demographic and seasonal influences on human serum pesticide residue levels. J Toxicol Environ Health 1989;27:405-421.

Tully DB, Cox, VT, Mumtaz MM, David VL, Chapin RE. Six high-priority organochlorine pesticides, either singly or in combination, are nonestrogenic in transfected HeLa cells. Reprod Toxicol 2000;14:95-102.

United States Geological Survey (USGS). Pesticides in the Nation's Stream and Ground Water, 1992-2001. Revised Feb. 15, 2007 [online]. Available at URL: http://pubs.usgs.gov/circ/2005/1291/. 6/1/09

Ward EM, Schulte P, Grajewski B, Andersen A, Patterson DG Jr, Turner W, et al. Serum organochlorine levels and breast cancer: a nested case-control study of Norwegian women. Cancer Epidemiol Biomarkers Prev 2000;9:1357-1367.

# Chlordane
CAS No. 57-74-9

# Heptachlor
CAS No. 76-44-8

## General Information

Chlordane and heptachlor are structurally related organochlorine pesticides and were used in the U.S. from the early 1950's until the mid-1980's. As a result of the manufacturing process, the technical grade product of each chemical contains 10%-20% of the other chemical, in addition to trace amounts of numerous other related compounds (ATSDR, 2007). Technical grade chlordane had contained 7% *trans*-nonachlor. Chlordane is not currently produced or used in the U.S. Since 1992, heptachlor use has been limited to treatment of fire ants near power transformers. Until 1988, chlordane was used to kill termites and other insects on agricultural crops, lawns, buildings, and in soil. Heptachlor was used as a soil and seed treatment and for termite control in and around buildings until 1988. Both pesticides are persistent in soils and sediments and have been detected in water from agricultural run-off and near production and disposal facilities (ATSDR, 1994, 2007). Heptachlor and chlordane are somewhat volatile and may be detected in the air and dust of buildings long after treatment for termite or insect control (Whitemore et al., 1994).

Heptachlor and chlordane and their metabolites bioaccumulate in fatty animal tissues. Consequently, foods high in fat such as meat, fish, and dairy products are the usual sources of exposure to these chemicals in the general population. Both of these chemicals and their metabolites can cross the placenta and are excreted into breast milk, which results in exposure to the fetus and nursing infant

## Serum Oxychlordane (lipid adjusted)
*Metabolite of Chlordane*

Geometric mean and selected percentiles of serum concentrations (in ng/g of lipid or parts per billion on a lipid-weight basis) for the U.S. population from the National Health and Nutrition Examination Survey.

| | Survey years | Geometric mean (95% conf. interval) | Selected percentiles ( 95% confidence interval) | | | | Sample size |
|---|---|---|---|---|---|---|---|
| | | | 50th | 75th | 90th | 95th | |
| **Total** | 99-00 | * | < LOD | 20.8 (17 8-23.0) | 34.4 (30.5-38.6) | 44.8 (40.2-49 6) | 1661 |
| | 01-02 | 11.4 (<LOD-12 5) | 11.1 (<LOD-12 5) | 21.7 (19 3-24.4) | 36.4 (31.5-41.4) | 49.7 (42.0-61 2) | 2249 |
| | 03-04 | 9.37 (8.69-10.1) | 10.3 (9.20-11.0) | 18.0 (16 8-20.1) | 29.0 (26.8-32.1) | 37.7 (34.8-43 8) | 1978 |
| **Age group** | | | | | | | |
| 12-19 years | 99-00 | * | < LOD | < LOD | < LOD | < LOD | 663 |
| | 01-02 | * | < LOD | < LOD | < LOD | 11.5 (<LOD-12.6) | 752 |
| | 03-04 | * | < LOD | < LOD | 9.20 (<LOD-11.5) | 11.5 (8.10-18 9) | 595 |
| 20 years and older | 99-00 | * | < LOD | 23.3 (21 0-25.9) | 37.7 (32.3-43.5) | 47.7 (43.1-50 8) | 998 |
| | 01-02 | 12.9 (11.7-14.3) | 13.3 (11.4-14.9) | 23.9 (21 2-26.7) | 38.5 (33.4-45.9) | 53.1 (44.1-65 9) | 1497 |
| | 03-04 | 10.6 (9.82-11.5) | 11.4 (10.6-12.4) | 19.9 (17 9-21.5) | 31.3 (28.8-33.2) | 39.2 (36.5-44 8) | 1383 |
| **Gender** | | | | | | | |
| Males | 99-00 | * | < LOD | 18.1 (16.1-19.6) | 31.3 (25.9-38.2) | 42.4 (35.3-49 6) | 793 |
| | 01-02 | 11.1 (<LOD-12 6) | 11.1 (<LOD-12 6) | 20.6 (16 6-24.9) | 33.1 (27.5-43.8) | 48.1 (40.2-56 9) | 1049 |
| | 03-04 | 9.10 (8.20-10.1) | 9.90 (8.30-11.2) | 17.1 (15 6-18.4) | 27.6 (25.3-32.2) | 36.0 (32.7-39 2) | 963 |
| Females | 99-00 | * | < LOD | 22.3 (20.1-25.9) | 36.9 (31.5-40.3) | 46.2 (39.1-51 8) | 868 |
| | 01-02 | 11.7 (10.7-12.7) | 11.0 (<LOD-12 9) | 23.1 (20.7-25.0) | 37.5 (34.5-42.1) | 52.8 (42.7-70 0) | 1200 |
| | 03-04 | 9.63 (8.89-10.4) | 10.6 (9.10-11.3) | 20.1 (17.4-21.7) | 30.3 (27.5-32.7) | 41.9 (36.3-45 5) | 1015 |
| **Race/ethnicity** | | | | | | | |
| Mexican Americans | 99-00 | * | < LOD | 16.3 (<LOD-19.9) | 28.9 (18.8-42.0) | 39.9 (26.8-61 0) | 628 |
| | 01-02 | * | < LOD | 13.9 (11 0-18.4) | 27.2 (21.0-33.1) | 37.9 (29.9-42 0) | 557 |
| | 03-04 | * | < LOD | 12.8 (10.1-15.8) | 22.9 (15.8-31.4) | 31.4 (22.4-51 6) | 462 |
| Non-Hispanic blacks | 99-00 | * | < LOD | 18.7 (<LOD-32.2) | 39.9 (26.5-47.3) | 48.6 (43.5-65 5) | 350 |
| | 01-02 | 11.7 (<LOD-13 6) | < LOD | 22.8 (17 2-28.3) | 41.4 (30.6-53.7) | 56.5 (41.8-73 5) | 501 |
| | 03-04 | 8.74 (<LOD-10 2) | 8.70 (<LOD-10 6) | 18.9 (15 9-21.5) | 35.1 (25.4-40.2) | 44.2 (37.7-56 8) | 493 |
| Non-Hispanic whites | 99-00 | * | < LOD | 21.8 (18 6-24.6) | 34.2 (28.9-40.9) | 44.0 (37.2-49 8) | 559 |
| | 01-02 | 12.1 (11.0-13.3) | 11.8 (10.5-13.9) | 23.0 (20.1-25.7) | 37.5 (31.6-45.1) | 52.2 (41.0-67.4) | 1031 |
| | 03-04 | 10.2 (9.36-11.1) | 11.2 (10.0-12.1) | 19.7 (17 2-21.7) | 30.3 (26.8-33.6) | 37.7 (34.3-45 5) | 898 |

Limit of detection (LOD, see Data Analysis section) for Survey years 99-00, 01-02, and 03-04 are 14 5, 10.5, and 7 8, respectively.
< LOD means less than the limit of detection, which may vary for some chemicals by year and by individual sample.
* Not calculated: proportion of results below limit of detection was too high to provide a valid result.

(Dallaire et al., 2002; Rogan, 1996; Takahashi et al., 1981). Chlordane and heptachlor are absorbed after oral, dermal, and inhalation exposure. Chlordane is metabolized primarily to oxychlordane and to a lesser extent, to heptachlor. The major metabolite of heptachlor is heptachlor epoxide, which is also persistent in the body (ATSDR, 2007). Elimination of all these chemicals from the body occurs over months to years, and breast milk is a major excretion route in lactating women.

Human health effects from either chlordane or heptachlor at low environmental doses or at biomonitored levels from low environmental exposures are unknown. Acute, high doses of either chlordane or heptachlor block inhibitory neurotransmitters and result in central nervous system toxicity, characterized by seizures and paralysis. In laboratory animal studies, chronic doses of heptachlor have produced liver enlargement and injury; both chlordane and heptachlor induced hepatic cytochrome P450 enzymes

and increased the incidence of liver tumors (NTP, 1977a, 1977b; Smith, 1991). Chronic feeding studies with either chlordane or heptachlor have demonstrated reduced fertility, neonatal mortality, and alterations in immune function of offspring. Subtle neurodevelopmental effects have been observed rodents after prenatal exposure to heptachlor (IPCS, 2006). Epidemiologic studies have not demonstrated teratogenic or developmental effects (Baker et al., 1991; Le Marchand et al., 1986). No clear evidence of excessive cancer rates was demonstrated in human epidemiologic studies (ATSDR, 2007; IARC, 2001; Shindell and Ulrich, 1986). IARC considers chlordane and heptachlor as possibly carcinogenic to humans. OSHA has established occupational exposure criteria, and NIOSH and ACGIH have recommended workplace exposure levels for each pesticide. The U.S. EPA has established environmental criteria for chlordane and heptachlor, and the U.S. FDA established allowable residues of chlordane, heptachlor, and heptachlor epoxide in foods and bottled water. Information

## Serum Oxychlordane (whole weight)
*Metabolite of Chlordane*

Geometric mean and selected percentiles of serum concentrations (in ng/g of serum or parts per billion) for the U.S. population from the National Health and Nutrition Examination Survey.

| | Survey years | Geometric mean (95% conf. interval) | Selected percentiles (95% confidence interval) 50th | 75th | 90th | 95th | Sample size |
|---|---|---|---|---|---|---|---|
| **Total** | 99-00 | * | < LOD | .140 (.120-.150) | .260 (.200-.290) | .310 ( .290-.340) | 1661 |
| | 01-02 | .070 (<LOD-.077) | .070 (<LOD-.080) | .140 (.130-.160) | .250 (.220-.300) | .350 ( .290-.440) | 2249 |
| | 03-04 | .057 (.053- 062) | .063 (.058-.068) | .119 (.106-.133) | .204 (.189-.213) | .269 ( .246-.291) | 1978 |
| **Age group** | | | | | | | |
| 12-19 years | 99-00 | * | < LOD | < LOD | < LOD | < LOD | 663 |
| | 01-02 | * | < LOD | < LOD | < LOD | .060 (<LOD-.070) | 752 |
| | 03-04 | * | < LOD | < LOD | .047 (<LOD- 063) | .066 ( 048-.092) | 595 |
| 20 years and older | 99-00 | * | < LOD | .150 (.140-.180) | .280 (.230-.300) | .330 ( 300-.400) | 998 |
| | 01-02 | .082 (.074- 091) | .080 (.070-.090) | .160 (.140-.180) | .270 (.230-.320) | .370 ( 310-.450) | 1497 |
| | 03-04 | .067 (.061- 073) | .073 (.066-.079) | .130 (.115-.146) | .210 (.203-.227) | .286 ( 258-.320) | 1383 |
| **Gender** | | | | | | | |
| Males | 99-00 | * | < LOD | .120 (.100-.140) | .220 (.180-.280) | .300 ( 260-.340) | 793 |
| | 01-02 | .069 (<LOD-.079) | .070 (<LOD-.080) | .130 (.120-.160) | .230 (.190-.300) | .320 ( 250-.430) | 1049 |
| | 03-04 | .056 (.050- 063) | .063 (.055-.076) | .115 (.100-.126) | .189 (.168-.207) | .258 ( 216-.302) | 963 |
| Females | 99-00 | * | < LOD | .140 (.130-.170) | .270 (.200-.310) | .320 ( 290-.400) | 868 |
| | 01-02 | .071 (.065- 077) | .070 (<LOD-.080) | .150 (.130-.160) | .260 (.230-.310) | .370 ( 280-.510) | 1200 |
| | 03-04 | .058 (.053- 064) | .063 (.057-.068) | .126 (.104-.146) | .208 (.199-.231) | .286 ( 245-.331) | 1015 |
| **Race/ethnicity** | | | | | | | |
| Mexican Americans | 99-00 | * | < LOD | .100 (<LOD-.130) | .210 (.130-.320) | .290 (.190-.410) | 628 |
| | 01-02 | * | < LOD | .100 (.070-.130) | .200 (.150-.240) | .280 ( 210-.360) | 557 |
| | 03-04 | * | < LOD | .083 (.066-.104) | .149 (.108-.230) | .230 (.148-.373) | 462 |
| Non-Hispanic blacks | 99-00 | * | < LOD | .110 (<LOD-.170) | .240 (.170-.290) | .320 ( 240-.430) | 350 |
| | 01-02 | .066 (<LOD-.077) | < LOD | .130 (.090-.170) | .260 (.180-.350) | .350 ( 240-.560) | 501 |
| | 03-04 | .049 (<LOD-.057) | .050 (<LOD-.062) | .112 (.087-.136) | .225 (.165-.287) | .315 ( 253-.348) | 493 |
| Non-Hispanic whites | 99-00 | * | < LOD | .140 (.120-.170) | .270 (.200-.300) | .320 ( 280-.380) | 559 |
| | 01-02 | .075 (.068- 083) | .080 (.070-.090) | .150 (.130-.170) | .250 (.220-.310) | .370 ( 280-.450) | 1031 |
| | 03-04 | .063 (.058- 070) | .070 (.063-.077) | .128 (.110-.148) | .207 (.190-.223) | .271 ( 242-.315) | 898 |

< LOD means less than the limit of detection for the lipid adjusted serum level, which may vary for some chemicals by year and by individual sample.
* Not calculated: proportion of results below limit of detection was too high to provide a valid result.

about external exposure (i.e., environmental levels) and health effects of chlordane and heptachlor is available from ATSDR at: http://www.atsdr.cdc.gov/toxpro2.html. A recent assessment of heptachlor is available at: http://www.inchem.org/documents/cicads/cicads/cicad70.htm#ref.

**Biomonitoring Information**

Serum oxychlordane and *trans*-nonachlor levels in NHANES 1999-2000, 2001-2002, and 2003-2004 subsamples were comparable to levels measured in Swedish women from 1996-1997 (Glynn et al., 2003). In serum samples obtained in between 1994 and 1997 from Inuit women in different Arctic countries, the reported oxychlordane and *trans*-nonachlor geometric mean levels from Canada and Greenland groups were about threefold to fivefold higher than among females in this *Report* (van Oostdam et al., 2004). A small sample of Polish women had mean levels of oxychlordane and *trans*-nonachlor that were about fivefold lower than in females in the NHANES 2001-2002 subsample (Jaraczweska et al., 2006). Serum *trans*-nonachlor levels among females in the NHANES 1999-2001 subsample were about one half the levels obtained between 1994 and 1996 from women in New York (Wolff et al., 2000).

Levels of heptachlor epoxide among females in this *Report* were approximately one tenth of the corresponding 90th percentile for a cohort of pregnant women in California studied from 1963 to 1967 (James et al., 2002). Two episodes (one each in Arkansas and Hawaii) of inadvertent heptachlor contamination of dairy cattle feed occurred in the early-to-mid 1980's, resulting in human exposure to heptachlor epoxide that was excreted into the milk. For the exposed persons drinking milk in the Arkansas episode, mean serum heptachlor epoxide and oxychlordane levels were about sevenfold and threefold higher, respectively, than the 90th percentile values of NHANES 1999-2000 (Stehr-Green et al., 1988). In the Hawaii episode, the mean serum heptachlor epoxide and oxychlordane levels were more than twice as high, respectively, than the 90th percentile values of NHANES 1999-2000 (Baker, 1993).

Finding a measurable amount of oxychlordane, *trans*-nonachlor, or heptachlor epoxide in serum does not mean that the level of oxychlordane, *trans*-nonachlor, or heptachlor epoxide causes an adverse health effect. Biomonitoring studies on levels of oxychlordane, *trans*-nonachlor, and heptachlor epoxide provide physicians and public health officials with reference ranges so that they can determine whether people have been exposed to higher levels of heptachlor and chlordane than are found in the general population. Biomonitoring data can also help

scientists plan and conduct research on exposure and health effects.

## Serum Heptachlor epoxide (lipid adjusted)
*Metabolite of Heptachlor*

Geometric mean and selected percentiles of serum concentrations (in ng/g of lipid or parts per billion on a lipid-weight basis) for the U.S. population from the National Health and Nutrition Examination Survey.

| | Survey years | Geometric mean (95% conf. interval) | Selected percentiles ( 95% confidence interval) | | | | Sample size |
|---|---|---|---|---|---|---|---|
| | | | 50th | 75th | 90th | 95th | |
| **Total** | 99-00 | * | < LOD | < LOD | 15.4 (<LOD-19 8) | 24.0 (15.1-38.8) | 1589 |
| | 01-02 | * | < LOD | < LOD | 14.8 (13.0-17.8) | 21.8 (18 2-27.3) | 2259 |
| | 03-04 | * | < LOD | < LOD | 13.4 (11.1-15.9) | 18.9 (15 9-23.0) | 1963 |
| **Age group** | | | | | | | |
| 12-19 years | 99-00 | * | < LOD | < LOD | < LOD | < LOD | 638 |
| | 01-02 | * | < LOD | < LOD | < LOD | < LOD | 741 |
| | 03-04 | * | < LOD | < LOD | < LOD | < LOD | 592 |
| 20 years and older | 99-00 | * | < LOD | < LOD | 17.8 (<LOD-23 9) | 27.1 (16 8-46.1) | 951 |
| | 01-02 | * | < LOD | < LOD | 15.7 (13.7-18.8) | 23.1 (19.1-29.1) | 1518 |
| | 03-04 | * | < LOD | 8.20 (<LOD-9.50) | 14.5 (11.6-17.6) | 20.6 (16 8-24.0) | 1371 |
| **Gender** | | | | | | | |
| Males | 99-00 | * | < LOD | < LOD | < LOD | 19.6 (<LOD-27.2) | 760 |
| | 01-02 | * | < LOD | < LOD | 13.9 (12.0-17.8) | 20.8 (15 9-25.3) | 1047 |
| | 03-04 | * | < LOD | < LOD | 13.4 (11.2-16.4) | 18.6 (16 6-21.3) | 956 |
| Females | 99-00 | * | < LOD | < LOD | 18.2 (<LOD-25 2) | 27.7 (16 0-54.3) | 829 |
| | 01-02 | * | < LOD | < LOD | 15.6 (13.3-18.2) | 23.2 (18 9-29.8) | 1212 |
| | 03-04 | * | < LOD | < LOD | 13.5 (11.0-16.8) | 19.6 (14 8-24.5) | 1007 |
| **Race/ethnicity** | | | | | | | |
| Mexican Americans | 99-00 | * | < LOD | < LOD | 15.3 (<LOD-25 6) | 22.2 (<LOD-62.3) | 598 |
| | 01-02 | * | < LOD | < LOD | 13.2 (<LOD-16 3) | 16.8 (13 8-23.1) | 553 |
| | 03-04 | * | < LOD | < LOD | 10.6 (8.10-13.5) | 13.7 (10 9-16.5) | 460 |
| Non-Hispanic blacks | 99-00 | * | < LOD | < LOD | < LOD | 19.5 (<LOD-32.4) | 336 |
| | 01-02 | * | < LOD | < LOD | 14.6 (11.7-19.0) | 21.5 (18 2-27.3) | 503 |
| | 03-04 | * | < LOD | < LOD | 13.5 (10.1-16.8) | 18.6 (12.7-25.2) | 490 |
| Non-Hispanic whites | 99-00 | * | < LOD | < LOD | 16.5 (<LOD-21 8) | 26.4 (<LOD-54.3) | 539 |
| | 01-02 | * | < LOD | < LOD | 15.3 (13.0-19.6) | 22.8 (18 9-29.8) | 1041 |
| | 03-04 | * | < LOD | 7.90 (<LOD-9.40) | 14.0 (11.2-17.6) | 20.4 (15 8-24.5) | 888 |

Limit of detection (LOD, see Data Analysis section) for Survey years 99-00, 01-02, and 03-04 are 14.6, 10 5, and 7.8, respectively.
< LOD means less than the limit of detection, which may vary for some chemicals by year and by individual sample.
* Not calculated: proportion of results below limit of detection was too high to provide a valid result.

## Serum Heptachlor epoxide (whole weight)
*Metabolite of Heptachlor*

Geometric mean and selected percentiles of serum concentrations (in ng/g of serum or parts per billion) for the U.S. population from the National Health and Nutrition Examination Survey.

| | Survey years | Geometric mean (95% conf. interval) | 50th | 75th | 90th | 95th | Sample size |
|---|---|---|---|---|---|---|---|
| | | | | Selected percentiles ( 95% confidence interval) | | | |
| Total | 99-00 | * | < LOD | < LOD | .110 (<LOD-.140) | .180 (.110-.220) | 1589 |
| | 01-02 | * | < LOD | < LOD | .100 (.090-.120) | .150 (.130-.180) | 2259 |
| | 03-04 | * | < LOD | < LOD | .094 (.076-.108) | .128 (.108-.161) | 1963 |
| **Age group** | | | | | | | |
| 12-19 years | 99-00 | * | < LOD | < LOD | < LOD | < LOD | 638 |
| | 01-02 | * | < LOD | < LOD | < LOD | < LOD | 741 |
| | 03-04 | * | < LOD | < LOD | < LOD | < LOD | 592 |
| 20 years and older | 99-00 | * | < LOD | < LOD | .130 (<LOD-.170) | .190 (.130-.270) | 951 |
| | 01-02 | * | < LOD | < LOD | .110 (.090-.140) | .170 (.140-.190) | 1518 |
| | 03-04 | * | < LOD | .057 (<LOD-.063) | .101 (.082-.116) | .135 (.113-.173) | 1371 |
| **Gender** | | | | | | | |
| Males | 99-00 | * | < LOD | < LOD | < LOD | .150 (<LOD-.180) | 760 |
| | 01-02 | * | < LOD | < LOD | .100 (.090-.120) | .150 (.110-.180) | 1047 |
| | 03-04 | * | < LOD | < LOD | .094 (.077-.111) | .126 (.106-.149) | 956 |
| Females | 99-00 | * | < LOD | < LOD | .120 (<LOD-.190) | .200 (.120-.310) | 829 |
| | 01-02 | * | < LOD | < LOD | .100 (.090-.130) | .170 (.130-.200) | 1212 |
| | 03-04 | * | < LOD | < LOD | .096 (.071-.108) | .133 (.107-.173) | 1007 |
| **Race/ethnicity** | | | | | | | |
| Mexican Americans | 99-00 | * | < LOD | < LOD | .100 (<LOD-.170) | .170 (<LOD-.380) | 598 |
| | 01-02 | * | < LOD | < LOD | .090 (<LOD-.110) | .120 (.100-.240) | 553 |
| | 03-04 | * | < LOD | < LOD | .069 (.053-.097) | .098 (.074-.113) | 460 |
| Non-Hispanic blacks | 99-00 | * | < LOD | < LOD | < LOD | .110 (<LOD-.200) | 336 |
| | 01-02 | * | < LOD | < LOD | .090 (.070-.110) | .130 (.100-.180) | 503 |
| | 03-04 | * | < LOD | < LOD | .087 (.067-.104) | .110 (.090-.157) | 490 |
| Non-Hispanic whites | 99-00 | * | < LOD | < LOD | .120 (<LOD-.170) | .180 (<LOD-.310) | 539 |
| | 01-02 | * | < LOD | < LOD | .100 (.090-.130) | .170 (.130-.190) | 1041 |
| | 03-04 | * | < LOD | .055 (<LOD-.063) | .101 (.077-.117) | .135 (.111-.180) | 888 |

< LOD means less than the limit of detection for the lipid adjusted serum level, which may vary for some chemicals by year and by individual sample.
* Not calculated: proportion of results below limit of detection was too high to provide a valid result.

## Serum *trans*-Nonachlor (lipid adjusted)
*Metabolite of Chlordane*

Geometric mean and selected percentiles of serum concentrations (in ng/g of lipid or parts per billion on a lipid-weight basis) for the U.S. population from the National Health and Nutrition Examination Survey.

| | Survey years | Geometric mean (95% conf. interval) | Selected percentiles ( 95% confidence interval) | | | | Sample size |
|---|---|---|---|---|---|---|---|
| | | | 50th | 75th | 90th | 95th | |
| **Total** | 99-00 | 18.3 (16.7-20 0) | 17.9 (16.1-20.1) | 31.9 (28.9-36.0) | 55.1 (48.4-62.6) | 79.4 (67 6-88.1) | 1933 |
| | 01-02 | 17.0 (15.2-18 9) | 17.9 (15.5-20 5) | 33.7 (30.2-37.2) | 56.3 (49.6-66.0) | 78.2 (64 0-113) | 2286 |
| | 03-04 | 14.7 (13.1-16 5) | 14.8 (13.5-17 0) | 30.2 (26.7-32.5) | 49.0 (42.6-54.7) | 68.3 (58 6-82.3) | 1955 |
| **Age group** | | | | | | | |
| 12-19 years | 99-00 | * | < LOD | < LOD | 18.8 (<LOD-20 6) | 25.2 (19.1-28.4) | 664 |
| | 01-02 | * | < LOD | < LOD | 13.4 (11.8-16.4) | 19.2 (15 2-23.5) | 758 |
| | 03-04 | * | < LOD | 8.70 (<LOD-12 5) | 16.1 (10.7-23.7) | 22.6 (16.1-34.6) | 589 |
| 20 years and older | 99-00 | 20.8 (19.0-22 8) | 20.7 (18.0-23 5) | 35.4 (30.9-40.3) | 59.9 (51.8-67.6) | 82.7 (74 9-89.6) | 1269 |
| | 01-02 | 19.8 (17.6-22 3) | 20.9 (19.0-23.1) | 36.6 (32.8-41.1) | 60.6 (52.5-69.9) | 84.9 (66 0-123) | 1528 |
| | 03-04 | 16.9 (15.1-18 9) | 17.3 (14.6-20 0) | 31.8 (28.9-35.3) | 51.4 (45.9-58.6) | 74.7 (59 8-90.0) | 1366 |
| **Gender** | | | | | | | |
| Males | 99-00 | 17.7 (16.5-19.1) | 17.2 (14.9-20.1) | 30.2 (27.7-34.2) | 51.1 (47.3-58.6) | 78.2 (60 2-88.1) | 922 |
| | 01-02 | 17.0 (14.8-19 5) | 18.3 (14.8-21.1) | 34.4 (28.3-39.3) | 54.8 (45.0-68.9) | 78.2 (59.7-113) | 1062 |
| | 03-04 | 14.8 (12.7-17 3) | 14.6 (12.2-18 0) | 30.8 (26.7-35.3) | 51.0 (42.0-59.4) | 68.6 (56 0-93.8) | 955 |
| Females | 99-00 | 18.8 (16.7-21.1) | 18.4 (16.1-22 2) | 32.9 (29.0-38.3) | 59.0 (48.4-67.6) | 80.8 (71 5-95.5) | 1011 |
| | 01-02 | 17.0 (15.4-18.7) | 17.6 (15.0-20 3) | 32.8 (30.4-36.7) | 56.9 (51.9-65.5) | 78.1 (65 5-111) | 1224 |
| | 03-04 | 14.5 (13.1-16.1) | 15.0 (13.8-16 3) | 28.2 (25.3-32.8) | 48.1 (41.4-52.7) | 68.3 (56 8-79.9) | 1000 |
| **Race/ethnicity** | | | | | | | |
| Mexican Americans | 99-00 | * | < LOD | 25.1 (22.7-29.5) | 40.7 (35.1-51.8) | 56.3 (45 8-77.2) | 650 |
| | 01-02 | 11.9 (<LOD-14.6) | 10.6 (<LOD-14.5) | 26.0 (19.3-30.4) | 47.9 (36.3-57.2) | 59.8 (49 3-74.1) | 558 |
| | 03-04 | 10.2 (7.86-13 2) | 9.10 (<LOD-11.1) | 20.7 (11.1-34.7) | 39.5 (25.9-65.5) | 62.2 (36 0-93.4) | 457 |
| Non-Hispanic blacks | 99-00 | 20.3 (17.0-24.1) | 17.5 (15.4-23 5) | 35.7 (28.9-45.5) | 77.0 (60.8-90.7) | 107 (84 0-143) | 404 |
| | 01-02 | 18.8 (15.4-22 9) | 19.2 (14.7-22 0) | 36.8 (28.3-50.5) | 73.6 (50.8-110) | 112 (68.7-160) | 514 |
| | 03-04 | 14.4 (12.2-17 0) | 13.8 (11.2-16 3) | 30.8 (26.5-36.1) | 59.9 (47.7-77.7) | 86.6 (56 8-129) | 486 |
| Non-Hispanic whites | 99-00 | 19.1 (17.2-21.1) | 19.0 (16.9-22 2) | 32.8 (28.0-37.6) | 52.5 (44.9-64.4) | 74.0 (62 3-86.7) | 722 |
| | 01-02 | 17.5 (15.6-19.7) | 19.0 (16.3-21.1) | 34.0 (29.7-38.1) | 55.5 (45.9-69.4) | 78.7 (59.1-126) | 1052 |
| | 03-04 | 15.8 (13.7-18 2) | 16.0 (13.8-19 3) | 30.8 (26.4-35.0) | 48.8 (42.1-55.7) | 67.6 (57 5-87.3) | 889 |

Limit of detection (LOD, see Data Analysis section) for Survey years 99-00, 01-02, and 03-04 are 14.5, 10 5, and 7.8, respectively.
< LOD means less than the limit of detection, which may vary for some chemicals by year and by individual sample.
* Not calculated: proportion of results below limit of detection was too high to provide a valid result.

## Serum *trans*-Nonachlor (whole weight)
*Metabolite of Chlordane*

Geometric mean and selected percentiles of serum concentrations (in ng/g of serum or parts per billion) for the U.S. population from the National Health and Nutrition Examination Survey.

| | Survey years | Geometric mean (95% conf. interval) | Selected percentiles ( 95% confidence interval) | | | | Sample size |
|---|---|---|---|---|---|---|---|
| | | | 50th | 75th | 90th | 95th | |
| **Total** | 99-00 | .109 (.099-.119) | .110 (.090-.120) | .210 (.190-.240) | .370 (.330-.420) | .550 (.470- 630) | 1933 |
| | 01-02 | .104 (.093-.116) | .110 (.100-.120) | .220 (.190-.250) | .390 (.330-.480) | .590 (.430- 800) | 2286 |
| | 03-04 | .089 (.080-.100) | .094 (.084-.108) | .191 (.171-.211) | .324 (.290-.371) | .470 (.410- 558) | 1955 |
| **Age group** | | | | | | | |
| 12-19 years | 99-00 | * | < LOD | < LOD | .090 (<LOD-.110) | .120 (.100-.130) | 664 |
| | 01-02 | * | < LOD | < LOD | .070 (.060-.080) | .090 (.080-.130) | 758 |
| | 03-04 | * | < LOD | .041 (<LOD-.060) | .081 (.054-.117) | .109 (.081-.161) | 589 |
| 20 years and older | 99-00 | .128 (.116-.141) | .130 (.110-.150) | .230 ( 210-.260) | .400 (.360-.460) | .580 (.490- 690) | 1269 |
| | 01-02 | .125 (.111-.141) | .130 (.120-.150) | .240 ( 210-.280) | .420 (.350-.540) | .640 (.470- 840) | 1528 |
| | 03-04 | .106 (.095-.119) | .112 (.096-.127) | .210 (.186-.237) | .355 (.301-.405) | .520 (.430- 594) | 1366 |
| **Gender** | | | | | | | |
| Males | 99-00 | .106 (.098-.114) | .100 (.090-.120) | .210 (.180-.220) | .350 (.310-.400) | .520 (.400- 630) | 922 |
| | 01-02 | .105 (.091-.122) | .110 (.090-.130) | .220 (.190-.260) | .380 (.310-.500) | .580 (.390- 830) | 1062 |
| | 03-04 | .092 (.079-.108) | .098 (.085-.126) | .202 (.177-.232) | .343 (.285-.395) | .458 (.395-.594) | 955 |
| Females | 99-00 | .111 (.099-.125) | .110 (.090-.130) | .220 (.190-.250) | .390 (.310-.460) | .580 (.460- 690) | 1011 |
| | 01-02 | .103 (.093-.113) | .110 (.090-.120) | .220 (.180-.240) | .400 (.340-.450) | .590 (.430- 830) | 1224 |
| | 03-04 | .087 (.078-.097) | .092 (.079-.098) | .183 (.161-.210) | .317 (.286-.367) | .470 (.409-.565) | 1000 |
| **Race/ethnicity** | | | | | | | |
| Mexican Americans | 99-00 | * | < LOD | .170 (.120-.210) | .310 (.240-.340) | .390 (.320- 520) | 650 |
| | 01-02 | .071 (<LOD- 091) | .060 (<LOD- 090) | .160 (.120-.210) | .330 (.270-.390) | .470 (.360- 590) | 558 |
| | 03-04 | .062 (.047-.082) | .055 (<LOD- 069) | .135 ( 069-.237) | .288 (.158-.559) | .414 (.279- 651) | 457 |
| Non-Hispanic blacks | 99-00 | .112 (.093-.134) | .100 (.080-.130) | .220 (.180-.300) | .490 (.340-.600) | .760 (.510- 960) | 404 |
| | 01-02 | .106 (.085-.131) | .110 (.080-.130) | .220 (.160-.310) | .490 (.320-.680) | .680 (.410-1.20) | 514 |
| | 03-04 | .080 (.068-.096) | .078 (.061-.093) | .186 (.145-.242) | .417 (.272-.565) | .573 (.497- 684) | 486 |
| Non-Hispanic whites | 99-00 | .116 (.104-.129) | .120 (.100-.140) | .220 (.190-.240) | .370 (.300-.440) | .510 (.440- 630) | 722 |
| | 01-02 | .108 (.096-.122) | .120 (.100-.130) | .220 (.190-.250) | .390 (.310-.490) | .600 (.400- 930) | 1052 |
| | 03-04 | .098 (.085-.113) | .103 (.090-.124) | .205 (.173-.234) | .327 (.288-.390) | .461 (.397- 576) | 889 |

< LOD means less than the limit of detection for the lipid adjusted serum level, which may vary for some chemicals by year and by individual sample.
* Not calculated: proportion of results below limit of detection was too high to provide a valid result.

## References

Agency for Toxic Substances and Disease Registry (ATSDR). Toxicological profile for chlordane [online]. May 1994. Available at URL: http://www.atsdr.cdc.gov/toxprofiles/tp31.html. 4/21/09

Agency for Toxic Substances and Disease Registry (ATSDR). Toxicological profile for heptachlor and heptachlor epoxide [online]. August 2007. Available at URL: http://www.atsdr.cdc.gov/toxprofiles/tp12.html. 4/21/09

Baker DB, Loo S, Barker J. Evaluation of human exposure to the heptachlor epoxide contamination of milk in Hawaii. Hawaii Med J 1991;50(3):108-118.

Baker DB. Estimation of Human Exposure to Heptachlor Epoxide and Related Pesticides in Hawaii. A Report to the Hawaii Heptachlor Research and Education Foundation. 1993. Available at URL: http://www.heptachlor.org/site/foundation/research/projects2.htm. 4/21/09

Dallaire F, Dewailly E, Laliberte C, Muckle G, Ayotte P. Temporal trends of organochlorine concentrations in umbilical cord blood of newborns from the lower north shore of the St. Lawrence River (Quebec, Canada). Environ Health Perspect 2002;110(8):835-838.

Glynn AW, Granath F, Aune M, Atuma S, Darnerud PO, Bjerselius R, et al. Organochlorines in Swedish women: determinants of serum concentrations. Environ Health Perspect 2003;111:349-355.

International Agency for Research on Cancer (IARC). International Agency for Research on Cancer (IARC) - Summaries & Evaluations. Chlordane and heptachlor [online]. Vol. 79, 2001. Available at URL: http://www.inchem.org/documents/iarc/vol79/79-12.html. 9/25/07

International Programme in Chemical Safety (IPCS). Concise International Chemical Assessment Document 70 Heptachlor [online]. 2006. Available at URL: http://www.inchem.org/documents/cicads/cicads/cicad70.htm. 4/21/09

James RA, Hertz-Picciotto I, Willman E, Keller JA, Charles MJ. Determinants of serum polychlorinated biphenyls and organochlorine pesticides measured in women from the child health and development study cohort, 1963-1967. Environ Health Perspect 2002;110:617-624.

Jaraczewska K, Lulek J, Covaci A, Voorspoels S, Kaluba-Skotarczak A, Drews K, et al. Distribution of polychlorinated biphenyls, organochlorine pesticides and polybrominated diphenyl ethers in human umbilical cord serum, maternal serum and milk from Wielkopolska region, Poland. Sci Tot Environ 2006;372:20-31.

LeMarchand L, Kolonel LN, Siegel BZ, Dendle WH. Trends in birth defects for a Hawaiian population exposed to heptachlor and for the United States. Arch Environ Health, 1986;41:145–148.

National Toxicology Program (NTP). Bioassay of chlordane for possible carcinogenicity. Natl Cancer Inst Carcinog Tech Rep Ser 1977a;8:1-123. Available at URL: http://ntp.niehs.nih.gov/ntp/htdocs/LT_rpts/tr008.pdf. 6/1/09

National Toxicology Program (NTP). Bioassay of heptachlor for possible carcinogenicity. Natl Cancer Inst Carcinog Tech Rep Ser 1977b;9:1-109. Available at URL: http://ntp.niehs.nih.gov/ntp/htdocs/LT_rpts/tr009.pdf. 6/1/09

Rogan WJ. Pollutants in breast milk. Arch Pediatr Adolesc Med 1996;150:981-990.

Shindell S and Ulrich S. Mortality of workers employed in the manufacture of chlordane: an update. J Occup Med 1986;28:497-501.

Smith AG. Chlorinated Hydrocarbon Insecticides. In Hayes WJ, Jr and Laws ER, Jr, Eds. Handbook of Pesticide Toxicology, Vol. 2 Classes of Pesticides. New York, Academic Press, Inc. 1991 pp. 731-915.

Stehr-Green P, Wohlleb JC, Royce W, Head SL. An evaluation of serum pesticide residue levels and liver function in persons exposed to dairy products contaminated with heptachlor. JAMA 1988;259(3):374-377.

Takahashi W, Saidein D, Takei G, Wong L. Organochloride pesticide residues in human milk in Hawaii, 1979-1980. Bull Environ Contam Toxicol 1981:27:506-511.

Van Oostdam JC, Dewailly E, Gilman A, Hansen JC, Odland JO, Chashchin V, et al. Circumpolar maternal blood contaminant survey, 1994-1997 organochlorine compounds. Sci Total Environ 2004;330:55-70.

Wolff MS, Berkowitz GS, Brower S, Senie R, Bleiweiss IJ, Tartter P, et al. Organochlorine exposures and breast cancer risk in New York City women. Environ Res 2000;84:151-161.

# Dichlorodiphenyltrichloroethane (DDT)
CAS No. 50-29-3

## General Information

Dichlorodiphenyltrichloroethane (DDT) has been used widely as a broad spectrum insecticide in agriculture and for control of vector-borne diseases. It was produced and used in the U.S. after World War II until 1972, when virtually all use of it was banned. It is still used in some countries, particularly for endemic vector and malaria control. DDT was used at one time as a treatment for head and body lice. DDT usually refers to the technical product, which is a mixture containing p,p'-DDT (65%-80%), o,p'-DDT (15%-21%), p,p'-DDD (4% or less), and trace amounts of several related compounds. DDT is converted in the environment to other more stable chemical forms, including 1,1'-(2,2-dichloroethenylidene)-bis[4-chlorobenzene]

(DDE) and 1,1'-dichloro-(2,2-bis(p-chlorophenyl) ethane (DDD). These chemicals are highly persistent in soil, sediments, air, and water, as well as in plant and animal tissues. The biodegradation half-life of DDT in soil varies from 2 to 15 years, depending on conditions.

In the general U.S. population, food, particularly meat, fish, and dairy products, continues to be the primary source of DDT exposure, although DDT and DDE intakes have decreased over time (FDA, 2008; Gunderson, 1988). Food imported from countries that still use DDT may contain the chemical or its residues. DDT can be absorbed after ingestion, inhalation, or dermal exposure. In the body, DDT is converted to DDE and several other metabolites. DDT and DDE are distributed to all body tissues with the highest concentrations found in adipose tissues (ATSDR, 2002; Smith, 1991). Only a small proportion of DDT is metabolized and excreted (Smith, 1991). DDT and DDE can cross the placenta, resulting in fetal exposure. Both

## Serum p,p'-Dichlorodiphenyltrichloroethane (DDT) (lipid adjusted)

Geometric mean and selected percentiles of serum concentrations (in ng/g of lipid or parts per billion on a lipid-weight basis) for the U.S. population from the National Health and Nutrition Examination Survey.

| | Survey years | Geometric mean (95% conf. interval) | 50th | 75th | 90th | 95th | Sample size |
|---|---|---|---|---|---|---|---|
| **Total** | 99-00 | * | < LOD | < LOD | < LOD | 28.0 (21.9-34 0) | 1679 |
| | 01-02 | * | < LOD | < LOD | < LOD | 26.6 (22.5-36 0) | 2305 |
| | 03-04 | * | < LOD | < LOD | 11.9 (10.0-15.1) | 19.5 (15.1-27 5) | 1965 |
| **Age group** | | | | | | | |
| 12-19 years | 99-00 | * | < LOD | < LOD | < LOD | < LOD | 677 |
| | 01-02 | * | < LOD | < LOD | < LOD | < LOD | 756 |
| | 03-04 | * | < LOD | < LOD | < LOD | 9.10 (<LOD-12.2) | 595 |
| 20 years and older | 99-00 | * | < LOD | < LOD | < LOD | 30.5 (23.0-37 3) | 1002 |
| | 01-02 | * | < LOD | < LOD | < LOD | 28.1 (23.8-39 0) | 1549 |
| | 03-04 | * | < LOD | < LOD | 12.9 (10.3-16.5) | 20.7 (15.9-28.7) | 1370 |
| **Gender** | | | | | | | |
| Males | 99-00 | * | < LOD | < LOD | < LOD | 25.1 (<LOD-39.3) | 799 |
| | 01-02 | * | < LOD | < LOD | < LOD | 21.6 (<LOD-25.8) | 1073 |
| | 03-04 | * | < LOD | < LOD | 10.6 (9.10-13.7) | 15.2 (11.8-26 9) | 959 |
| Females | 99-00 | * | < LOD | < LOD | < LOD | 29.4 (23.0-35 8) | 880 |
| | 01-02 | * | < LOD | < LOD | 18.3 (<LOD-21.9) | 36.6 (25.5-54 3) | 1232 |
| | 03-04 | * | < LOD | < LOD | 14.0 (10.8-17.5) | 21.0 (18.0-27 8) | 1006 |
| **Race/ethnicity** | | | | | | | |
| Mexican Americans | 99-00 | * | < LOD | < LOD | 61.3 (27.0-155) | 155 (59.3-590) | 635 |
| | 01-02 | * | < LOD | < LOD | 83.1 (33.3-236) | 293 (104-541) | 566 |
| | 03-04 | * | < LOD | 8.90 (<LOD-12.9) | 24.0 (18.6-33.3) | 48.6 (31.1-71.1) | 461 |
| Non-Hispanic blacks | 99-00 | * | < LOD | < LOD | 22.3 (<LOD-31.5) | 31.5 (23.2-65 0) | 356 |
| | 01-02 | * | < LOD | < LOD | 23.2 (<LOD-40.9) | 40.9 (21.2-95 8) | 514 |
| | 03-04 | * | < LOD | 9.00 (<LOD-10.4) | 17.5 (14.8-23.2) | 30.7 (19.0-53.4) | 490 |
| Non-Hispanic whites | 99-00 | * | < LOD | < LOD | < LOD | < LOD | 564 |
| | 01-02 | * | < LOD | < LOD | < LOD | 17.9 (<LOD-20.7) | 1061 |
| | 03-04 | * | < LOD | < LOD | 9.70 (8.50-11.2) | 12.9 (10.7-16 6) | 890 |

Limit of detection (LOD, see Data Analysis section) for Survey years 99-00, 01-02, and 03-04 are 20.7, 17.4, and 7 8, respectively.
< LOD means less than the limit of detection, which may vary for some chemicals by year and by individual sample.
* Not calculated: proportion of results below limit of detection was too high to provide a valid result.

chemicals are excreted in breast milk, resulting in exposure to nursing infants (Rogan, 1996).

Human health effects from DDT at low environmental doses or at biomonitored levels from low environmental exposures are unknown. In high dose, accidental exposures, overt signs of acute human toxicity include vomiting, tremor, and seizures. Experimental human dosing studies conducted over an 18 month period and during which doses well above environmental levels were given did not demonstrate overt clinical abnormalities (ATSDR, 2002; Hayes et al., 1956). In laboratory animals, both DDT and DDE may induce specific cytochrome P450 isozymes (Nims et al., 1998). DDT may bind to estrogen receptors (Chen et al., 1997); and $o,p'$-DDD and $p,p'$-DDE can produce anti-androgenic effects (Gray et al., 2001). Animal studies reported reduced fertility, premature delivery, reproductive organ abnormalities, and altered behavior after neonatal exposure (Eriksson and Talts, 2000; Gray et al., 2001). Reproductive effects in humans affecting

birth weight, fertility, and duration of lactation, have not been consistently demonstrated (Beard, 2006; Gladen and Rogan, 1995; Jusko et al., 2006), although the risk for preterm delivery may be related to maternal DDE levels (Longnecker et al., 2001). Epidemiologic studies of children with environmental exposure to DDT and DDE have not demonstrated neurologic or developmental abnormalities (Gladen et al., 2004; Jusko et al., 2006; Longnecker et al., 2002; Mariussen and Fonnum, 2006). Several reviews of cancer epidemiologic studies have concluded that a link between DDT and breast cancer is inconclusive (Beard, 2006; Calle et al., 2002; Snedeker, 2001). Studies of DDT exposure and pancreatic cancer, lung cancer, and leukemia have also been inconclusive (ADSDR, 2002; Beard, 2006). It is difficult to attribute outcomes in human studies solely to DDT because of potential co-exposure to other persistent organohalogen chemicals (e.g., polychlorinated biphenyls, other organochlorines, dioxins and furans).

A workplace standard for DDT has been established by

### Serum $p,p'$-Dichlorodiphenyltrichloroethane (DDT) (whole weight)

Geometric mean and selected percentiles of serum concentrations (in ng/g of serum or parts per billion) for the U.S. population from the National Health and Nutrition Examination Survey.

| | Survey years | Geometric mean (95% conf. interval) | Selected percentiles ( 95% confidence interval) | | | | Sample size |
|---|---|---|---|---|---|---|---|
| | | | 50th | 75th | 90th | 95th | |
| **Total** | 99-00 | * | < LOD | < LOD | < LOD | .170 (.130-.220) | 1679 |
| | 01-02 | * | < LOD | < LOD | < LOD | .180 (.160-.220) | 2305 |
| | 03-04 | * | < LOD | < LOD | .078 (.065-.097) | .128 ( 098-.167) | 1965 |
| **Age group** | | | | | | | |
| 12-19 years | 99-00 | * | < LOD | < LOD | < LOD | < LOD | 677 |
| | 01-02 | * | < LOD | < LOD | < LOD | < LOD | 756 |
| | 03-04 | * | < LOD | < LOD | < LOD | .048 (<LOD-.069) | 595 |
| 20 years and older | 99-00 | * | < LOD | < LOD | < LOD | .190 (.150-.230) | 1002 |
| | 01-02 | * | < LOD | < LOD | < LOD | .200 (.170-.260) | 1549 |
| | 03-04 | * | < LOD | < LOD | .084 (.068-.106) | .142 (.105-.189) | 1370 |
| **Gender** | | | | | | | |
| Males | 99-00 | * | < LOD | < LOD | < LOD | .150 (<LOD-.240) | 799 |
| | 01-02 | * | < LOD | < LOD | < LOD | .150 (<LOD-.180) | 1073 |
| | 03-04 | * | < LOD | < LOD | .071 (.059-.095) | .108 ( 078-.180) | 959 |
| Females | 99-00 | * | < LOD | < LOD | < LOD | .190 (.150-.230) | 880 |
| | 01-02 | * | < LOD | < LOD | .130 (<LOD-.150) | .240 (.180-.400) | 1232 |
| | 03-04 | * | < LOD | < LOD | .087 (.071-.106) | .146 (.106-.207) | 1006 |
| **Race/ethnicity** | | | | | | | |
| Mexican Americans | 99-00 | * | < LOD | < LOD | .400 (.190-1 00) | 1.00 ( 330-4.26) | 635 |
| | 01-02 | * | < LOD | < LOD | .530 (.250-1 34) | 1.62 ( 570-4.01) | 566 |
| | 03-04 | * | < LOD | .063 (<LOD- 079) | .146 (.114-.203) | .313 (.189-.627) | 461 |
| Non-Hispanic blacks | 99-00 | * | < LOD | < LOD | .120 (<LOD-.170) | .180 (.140-.420) | 356 |
| | 01-02 | * | < LOD | < LOD | .130 (<LOD- 290) | .250 (.120-.530) | 514 |
| | 03-04 | * | < LOD | .051 (<LOD- 061) | .112 (.080-.143) | .201 (.132-.343) | 490 |
| Non-Hispanic whites | 99-00 | * | < LOD | < LOD | < LOD | < LOD | 564 |
| | 01-02 | * | < LOD | < LOD | < LOD | .130 (<LOD-.140) | 1061 |
| | 03-04 | * | < LOD | < LOD | .064 (.054-.075) | .086 ( 074-.107) | 890 |

< LOD means less than the limit of detection for the lipid adjusted serum level, which may vary for some chemicals by year and by individual sample.
* Not calculated: proportion of results below limit of detection was too high to provide a valid result.

OSHA and a guidance established by ACGIH. IARC classifies DDT (*p,p'*-DDT) as a possible human carcinogen. NTP considers DDT as being reasonably anticipated to be a human carcinogen. More information about external exposure (i.e., environmental levels) and health effects is available from the U.S. EPA at: http://www.epa.gov/pestcides/ and from ATSDR at: http://www.atsdr.cdc.gov/toxpro2.html.

## Biomonitoring Information

DDE persists in the body longer than DDT, so serum DDE levels may be an indicator of historic exposure and may be higher than DDT levels in the same person. In general, levels of DDT and DDE increase as a person ages as a result of cumulative exposure (ATSDR, 2002; Smith, 1991). Since the 1970's, mean serum levels of DDT and DDE in the U.S. population declined by about fivefold to tenfold, compared to levels observed in this *Report* (Anderson et al., 1998; Stehr-Green, 1989). Declining DDE levels over time have

also been observed in the German population, and the most recent median levels for German adults and children are similar to levels in this *Report* (Becker et al., 2002; Heudorf et al., 2003; Link et al., 2005). Median DDE levels among a population-based sample of Swedish women in 1996-1997 were similar to females in the NHANES 1999-2000 subsample (Glynn et al., 2003). A study of New Zealand adults sampled in 1996-1997 reported median DDE levels that were about threefold higher than the median for adults in the NHANES 1999-2000 subsample (Bates et al., 2004). In a population-based sample of men and women from eastern Slovakia, the lipid-adjusted geometric mean levels of DDT and DDE were each fivefold to tenfold higher than the 95th percentile and geometric mean levels, respectively, for males and females in the NHANES 1999-2000 subsample (Pavuk et al., 2004).

Compared to females in the NHANES 1999-2000 subsample, mean DDE levels were about fivefold higher among women of southern Spain exposed by virtue of

## Serum *p,p'*-Dichlorodiphenyldichloroethene (DDE) (lipid adjusted)
*Metabolite of Dichlorodiphenyltrichloroethane*

Geometric mean and selected percentiles of serum concentrations (in ng/g of lipid or parts per billion on a lipid-weight basis) for the U.S. population from the National Health and Nutrition Examination Survey.

| | Survey years | Geometric mean (95% conf. interval) | Selected percentiles (95% confidence interval) 50th | 75th | 90th | 95th | Sample size |
|---|---|---|---|---|---|---|---|
| **Total** | 99-00 | 260 (226-298) | 226 (184-278) | 537 (476-631) | 1150 (976-1350) | 1830 (1410-2300) | 1964 |
| | 01-02 | 295 (267-327) | 251 (228-278) | 598 (521-699) | 1410 (1210-1500) | 2320 (1830-2780) | 2298 |
| | 03-04 | 238 (195-292) | 203 (163-275) | 509 (376-655) | 1170 (836-1570) | 1860 (1400-2380) | 1956 |
| **Age group** | | | | | | | |
| 12-19 years | 99-00 | 118 (102-135) | 108 (97.7-119) | 185 (141-237) | 339 (243-479) | 528 (339-812) | 686 |
| | 01-02 | 124 (106-146) | 113 (100-140) | 213 (172-253) | 319 (282-389) | 456 (343-722) | 758 |
| | 03-04 | 105 (84.7-129) | 93.6 (81.0-114) | 167 (123-240) | 341 (211-586) | 522 (313-1430) | 588 |
| 20 years and older | 99-00 | 297 (256-344) | 269 (213-323) | 608 (530-693) | 1260 (1030-1550) | 2020 (1520-2730) | 1278 |
| | 01-02 | 338 (303-376) | 285 (249-337) | 695 (595-798) | 1480 (1310-1700) | 2550 (1980-3080) | 1540 |
| | 03-04 | 268 (217-332) | 233 (175-314) | 557 (420-734) | 1270 (877-1800) | 1990 (1500-2470) | 1368 |
| **Gender** | | | | | | | |
| Males | 99-00 | 249 (220-283) | 223 (182-262) | 494 (380-578) | 1010 (789-1130) | 1430 (1080-2160) | 937 |
| | 01-02 | 285 (252-323) | 248 (222-285) | 520 (441-627) | 1160 (937-1360) | 1900 (1580-2490) | 1069 |
| | 03-04 | 235 (193-288) | 200 (164-262) | 466 (331-653) | 1000 (763-1400) | 1610 (1210-2320) | 955 |
| Females | 99-00 | 270 (226-322) | 234 (184-302) | 601 (492-711) | 1350 (1040-1720) | 2210 (1570-2810) | 1027 |
| | 01-02 | 305 (273-341) | 256 (219-297) | 708 (567-844) | 1480 (1410-1710) | 2670 (1940-3300) | 1229 |
| | 03-04 | 241 (193-301) | 207 (161-281) | 539 (386-735) | 1250 (813-1900) | 2010 (1500-2450) | 1001 |
| **Race/ethnicity** | | | | | | | |
| Mexican Americans | 99-00 | 674 (574-792) | 624 (545-701) | 1350 (1090-1660) | 3090 (2040-4950) | 4950 (3070-9350) | 657 |
| | 01-02 | 652 (569-747) | 561 (455-690) | 1400 (1050-1950) | 4110 (2520-6550) | 7080 (3080-15600) | 566 |
| | 03-04 | 444 (362-545) | 373 (283-522) | 875 (608-1170) | 2150 (1520-2470) | 3290 (2380-9240) | 457 |
| Non-Hispanic blacks | 99-00 | 295 (241-362) | 251 (199-313) | 668 (492-874) | 1850 (1040-2220) | 2300 (1560-5680) | 416 |
| | 01-02 | 324 (262-400) | 248 (223-296) | 762 (583-999) | 1620 (1180-2980) | 3260 (1270-6900) | 515 |
| | 03-04 | 262 (233-295) | 216 (173-267) | 589 (453-747) | 1620 (1130-2310) | 2860 (1880-3440) | 487 |
| Non-Hispanic whites | 99-00 | 217 (189-249) | 194 (162-238) | 438 (355-507) | 825 (647-1010) | 1160 (1010-1350) | 732 |
| | 01-02 | 253 (226-284) | 225 (203-254) | 463 (402-558) | 1150 (878-1340) | 1640 (1410-1940) | 1053 |
| | 03-04 | 208 (165-263) | 177 (148-238) | 417 (302-564) | 907 (574-1480) | 1490 (909-2300) | 888 |

Limit of detection (LOD, see Data Analysis section) for Survey years 99-00, 01-02, and 03-04 are 18 6, 8.3, and 7 8, respectively.

nearby agriculture (Botella et al., 2004). A small study of Indian men with background exposure reported mean serum DDT and DDE levels that were around fiftyfold higher than the 95th percentile for DDT and tenfold to twentyfold higher than the geometric mean DDE levels among males in this *Report* (Bhatnagar et al., 2004). Consumers of Great Lakes sport fish had mean serum DDE levels that were only slightly higher than nonconsumers, 309 versus 268 ng/g lipid, which is similar to the overall geometric mean of 260 ng/g lipid in the NHANES 1999-2000 subsample (Bloom et al., 2005). High mean levels of whole blood DDT (about 3,860 ng/L) and DDE (about 14,490 ng/L) were found many years ago in a study of pesticide workers in Argentina (Radomski et al., 1971). Workers involved in production or application of DDT developed neurologic abnormalities associated with blood levels around 100-300 μg/L, considerably higher than levels in this *Report* (Smith, 1991).

In the NHANES 1999-2000, 2001-2002 and 2003-2004 subsamples, serum levels of *o,p'*-DDT were below the limits of detection. In a subsample of NHANES II (1976-1980) participants, less than one percent had detectable serum levels of *o,p'*-DDT (Stehr-Green, 1989).

Finding a measurable amount of *p,p'*-DDT, *o,p'*-DDT, or *p,p'*-DDE in serum does not mean that the level of the chemical causes an adverse health effect. Biomonitoring studies on levels of DDT and DDE provide physicians and public health officials with reference values so that they can determine whether people have been exposed to higher levels of DDT or DDE than are found in the general population. Biomonitoring data can also help scientists plan and conduct research on exposure and health effects.

## Serum *p,p'*-Dichlorodiphenyldichloroethene (DDE) (whole weight)

*Metabolite of Dichlorodiphenyltrichloroethane*

Geometric mean and selected percentiles of serum concentrations (in ng/g of serum or parts per billion) for the U.S. population from the National Health and Nutrition Examination Survey.

| | Survey years | Geometric mean (95% conf. interval) | Selected percentiles ( 95% confidence interval) 50th | 75th | 90th | 95th | Sample size |
|---|---|---|---|---|---|---|---|
| **Total** | 99-00 | 1.54 (1.33-1.79) | 1.31 (1 09-1.66) | 3.50 (2.97-4.27) | 7.49 (6.14-9 25) | 11.6 (9.25-14.8) | 1964 |
| | 01-02 | 1.81 (1.64-2.01) | 1.57 (1 37-1.72) | 3.97 (3.43-4.59) | 8.81 (7.85-10.1) | 15.4 (12 9-17.6) | 2298 |
| | 03-04 | 1.45 (1.18-1.79) | 1.26 (1 00-1.58) | 3.16 (2.40-4.21) | 7.07 (5.55-9 80) | 12.1 (8.37-16.0) | 1956 |
| **Age group** | | | | | | | |
| 12-19 years | 99-00 | .561 (.488- 646) | .520 (.430-.600) | .870 (.680-1.18) | 1.52 (1.13-2 25) | 2.32 (1.76-3.56) | 686 |
| | 01-02 | .623 (.534-.726) | .590 (.500-.730) | 1.00 (.820-1.22) | 1.65 (1.39-2 07) | 2.30 (1.91-3.14) | 758 |
| | 03-04 | .516 (.419- 635) | .456 (.385-.557) | .796 (.611-1.19) | 1.69 (.994-2 69) | 2.51 (1.56-6.71) | 588 |
| 20 years and older | 99-00 | 1.83 (1.56-2.14) | 1.61 (1 26-2.07) | 4.17 (3.48-4.66) | 8.12 (6.37-10.6) | 12.3 (9.87-16.7) | 1278 |
| | 01-02 | 2.14 (1.91-2.39) | 1.77 (1 61-2.05) | 4.59 (4.10-5.26) | 9.75 (8.34-11.5) | 16.8 (13.7-19.1) | 1540 |
| | 03-04 | 1.69 (1.36-2.10) | 1.46 (1.12-1.96) | 3.68 (2.66-4.96) | 7.91 (6.01-11.0) | 12.8 (9.25-16.8) | 1368 |
| **Gender** | | | | | | | |
| Males | 99-00 | 1.49 (1.30-1.70) | 1.25 (1.10-1.44) | 3.02 (2.57-3.80) | 6.43 (5.40-8 00) | 9.63 (6.63-15.6) | 937 |
| | 01-02 | 1.77 (1.57-2.01) | 1.59 (1 36-1.76) | 3.40 (3.03-4.10) | 7.48 (6.43-8.75) | 13.1 (9.66-17.6) | 1069 |
| | 03-04 | 1.46 (1.18-1.80) | 1.30 (1 04-1.58) | 2.80 (2.18-4.13) | 6.71 (5.51-8 54) | 9.93 (7.51-15.4) | 955 |
| Females | 99-00 | 1.59 (1.32-1.92) | 1.38 (1 03-1.99) | 4.05 (3.15-4.79) | 8.18 (6.36-11.5) | 13.2 (9.81-18.5) | 1027 |
| | 01-02 | 1.85 (1.66-2.06) | 1.49 (1 32-1.75) | 4.57 (3.81-5.47) | 10.2 (9.01-11.9) | 16.8 (13.4-19.7) | 1229 |
| | 03-04 | 1.45 (1.16-1.82) | 1.25 (.965-1.66) | 3.55 (2.43-4.59) | 7.87 (5.41-12.6) | 13.7 (8.50-17.3) | 1001 |
| **Race/ethnicity** | | | | | | | |
| Mexican Americans | 99-00 | 3.92 (3.40-4.51) | 3.52 (3.17-3.91) | 8.22 (7.26-10.4) | 22.0 (12.2-32.2) | 32.2 (19.7-48.1) | 657 |
| | 01-02 | 3.92 (3.37-4.57) | 3.53 (2 68-4.34) | 9.34 (7.31-12.5) | 26.6 (17.9-38.3) | 40.9 (26 8-90.5) | 566 |
| | 03-04 | 2.69 (2.18-3.32) | 2.24 (1.70-3.24) | 5.78 (4.54-7.21) | 13.0 (9.53-15.6) | 22.9 (15 3-43.4) | 457 |
| Non-Hispanic blacks | 99-00 | 1.63 (1.31-2.02) | 1.37 (1.11-1.66) | 3.84 (3.01-5.69) | 11.2 (6.57-13.3) | 14.6 (8.88-35.2) | 416 |
| | 01-02 | 1.82 (1.46-2.28) | 1.38 (1 22-1.72) | 4.39 (3.52-6.06) | 10.6 (7.24-17.6) | 19.4 (8.51-49.3) | 515 |
| | 03-04 | 1.47 (1.30-1.65) | 1.20 (.963-1.51) | 3.76 (2.85-4.75) | 9.23 (7.19-14.9) | 16.8 (14.7-20.6) | 487 |
| Non-Hispanic whites | 99-00 | 1.32 (1.14-1.53) | 1.13 (1 01-1.35) | 2.88 (2.34-3.36) | 5.75 (4.62-6 53) | 8.04 (6.32-9.81) | 732 |
| | 01-02 | 1.57 (1.39-1.76) | 1.41 (1 27-1.58) | 3.11 (2.56-3.68) | 7.00 (6.02-8 34) | 11.3 (8.60-13.7) | 1053 |
| | 03-04 | 1.29 (1.01-1.64) | 1.12 (.890-1.49) | 2.63 (1.84-3.90) | 6.36 (3.90-8.71) | 9.71 (6.01-15.0) | 888 |

## Serum *o,p'*-Dichlorodiphenyltrichloroethane (lipid adjusted)

Geometric mean and selected percentiles of serum concentrations (in ng/g of lipid or parts per billion on a lipid-weight basis) for the U.S. population from the National Health and Nutrition Examination Survey.

| | Survey years | Geometric mean (95% conf. interval) | Selected percentiles ( 95% confidence interval) | | | | Sample size |
|---|---|---|---|---|---|---|---|
| | | | 50th | 75th | 90th | 95th | |
| **Total** | 99-00 | * | < LOD | < LOD | < LOD | < LOD | 1669 |
| | 01-02 | * | < LOD | < LOD | < LOD | < LOD | 2279 |
| | 03-04 | * | < LOD | < LOD | < LOD | < LOD | 1946 |
| **Age group** | | | | | | | |
| 12-19 years | 99-00 | * | < LOD | < LOD | < LOD | < LOD | 667 |
| | 01-02 | * | < LOD | < LOD | < LOD | < LOD | 756 |
| | 03-04 | * | < LOD | < LOD | < LOD | < LOD | 588 |
| 20 years and older | 99-00 | * | < LOD | < LOD | < LOD | < LOD | 1002 |
| | 01-02 | * | < LOD | < LOD | < LOD | < LOD | 1523 |
| | 03-04 | * | < LOD | < LOD | < LOD | < LOD | 1358 |
| **Gender** | | | | | | | |
| Males | 99-00 | * | < LOD | < LOD | < LOD | < LOD | 796 |
| | 01-02 | * | < LOD | < LOD | < LOD | < LOD | 1059 |
| | 03-04 | * | < LOD | < LOD | < LOD | < LOD | 949 |
| Females | 99-00 | * | < LOD | < LOD | < LOD | < LOD | 873 |
| | 01-02 | * | < LOD | < LOD | < LOD | < LOD | 1220 |
| | 03-04 | * | < LOD | < LOD | < LOD | < LOD | 997 |
| **Race/ethnicity** | | | | | | | |
| Mexican Americans | 99-00 | * | < LOD | < LOD | < LOD | < LOD | 632 |
| | 01-02 | * | < LOD | < LOD | < LOD | < LOD | 565 |
| | 03-04 | * | < LOD | < LOD | < LOD | < LOD | 458 |
| Non-Hispanic blacks | 99-00 | * | < LOD | < LOD | < LOD | < LOD | 354 |
| | 01-02 | * | < LOD | < LOD | < LOD | < LOD | 507 |
| | 03-04 | * | < LOD | < LOD | < LOD | < LOD | 486 |
| Non-Hispanic whites | 99-00 | * | < LOD | < LOD | < LOD | < LOD | 560 |
| | 01-02 | * | < LOD | < LOD | < LOD | < LOD | 1045 |
| | 03-04 | * | < LOD | < LOD | < LOD | < LOD | 880 |

Limit of detection (LOD, see Data Analysis section) for Survey years 99-00, 01-02, and 03-04 are 20.7, 17.4, and 7 8, respectively.
< LOD means less than the limit of detection, which may vary for some chemicals by year and by individual sample.
* Not calculated: proportion of results below limit of detection was too high to provide a valid result.

## Serum *o,p'*-Dichlorodiphenyltrichloroethane (whole weight)

Geometric mean and selected percentiles of serum concentrations (in ng/g of serum or parts per billion) for the U.S. population from the National Health and Nutrition Examination Survey.

| | Survey years | Geometric mean (95% conf. interval) | Selected percentiles ( 95% confidence interval) | | | | Sample size |
|---|---|---|---|---|---|---|---|
| | | | 50th | 75th | 90th | 95th | |
| **Total** | 99-00 | * | < LOD | < LOD | < LOD | < LOD | 1669 |
| | 01-02 | * | < LOD | < LOD | < LOD | < LOD | 2279 |
| | 03-04 | * | < LOD | < LOD | < LOD | < LOD | 1946 |
| **Age group** | | | | | | | |
| 12-19 years | 99-00 | * | < LOD | < LOD | < LOD | < LOD | 667 |
| | 01-02 | * | < LOD | < LOD | < LOD | < LOD | 756 |
| | 03-04 | * | < LOD | < LOD | < LOD | < LOD | 588 |
| 20 years and older | 99-00 | * | < LOD | < LOD | < LOD | < LOD | 1002 |
| | 01-02 | * | < LOD | < LOD | < LOD | < LOD | 1523 |
| | 03-04 | * | < LOD | < LOD | < LOD | < LOD | 1358 |
| **Gender** | | | | | | | |
| Males | 99-00 | * | < LOD | < LOD | < LOD | < LOD | 796 |
| | 01-02 | * | < LOD | < LOD | < LOD | < LOD | 1059 |
| | 03-04 | * | < LOD | < LOD | < LOD | < LOD | 949 |
| Females | 99-00 | * | < LOD | < LOD | < LOD | < LOD | 873 |
| | 01-02 | * | < LOD | < LOD | < LOD | < LOD | 1220 |
| | 03-04 | * | < LOD | < LOD | < LOD | < LOD | 997 |
| **Race/ethnicity** | | | | | | | |
| Mexican Americans | 99-00 | * | < LOD | < LOD | < LOD | < LOD | 632 |
| | 01-02 | * | < LOD | < LOD | < LOD | < LOD | 565 |
| | 03-04 | * | < LOD | < LOD | < LOD | < LOD | 458 |
| Non-Hispanic blacks | 99-00 | * | < LOD | < LOD | < LOD | < LOD | 354 |
| | 01-02 | * | < LOD | < LOD | < LOD | < LOD | 507 |
| | 03-04 | * | < LOD | < LOD | < LOD | < LOD | 486 |
| Non-Hispanic whites | 99-00 | * | < LOD | < LOD | < LOD | < LOD | 560 |
| | 01-02 | * | < LOD | < LOD | < LOD | < LOD | 1045 |
| | 03-04 | * | < LOD | < LOD | < LOD | < LOD | 880 |

< LOD means less than the limit of detection for the lipid adjusted serum level, which may vary for some chemicals by year and by individual sample.
* Not calculated: proportion of results below limit of detection was too high to provide a valid result.

## References

Agency for Toxic Substances and Disease Registry (ATSDR). Toxicological profile for DDT, DDE, and DDD [online]. September 2002. Available at URL: http://www.atsdr.cdc.gov/toxprofiles/tp35.html. 4/21/09

Anderson HA, Falk C, Hanrahan L, Olson J, Burse VW, Needham LL, et al. Profiles of Great Lakes critical pollutants: a sentinel analysis of human blood and urine. The Great Lakes Consortium. Environ Health Perspect 1998;106(5):279-289.

Bates MN, Buckland SJ, Garrett N, Ellis H, Needham LL, Patterson DG Jr, et al. Persistent organochlorines in the serum of the non-occupationally exposed New Zealand population. Chemosphere 2004;54:1431-1443.

Beard J. DDT and human health. Sci Tot Environ 2006;355:78-89.

Becker K, Kaus S, Krause C, Lepom P, Schulz C, Seiwert M, et al. German Environmental Survey 1998 (GerES III): environmental pollutants in blood of the German population. Int J Hyg Environ Health 2002;205:297-308.

Bhatnagar VK, Kashyap R, Zaidi SS, Kulkarni PK, Saiyed HN. Levels of DDT, HCH, and HCB residues in human blood in Ahmedabad, India. Bull Environ Contam Toxicol 2004;72:261-265.

Bloom MS, Vena JE, Swanson MK, Moysich KB, Olson JR. Profiles of ortho-polychlorinated biphenyl congeners, dichlorodiphenyldichloroethylene, hexachlorobenzene, and Mirex among male Lake Ontario sportfish consumers: the New York State Angler cohort study. Environ Res 2005;97(2):178-192.

Botella B, Crespo J, Rivas A, Cerrillo I, Olea-Serrano MF, Olea N. Exposure of women to organochlorine pesticides in Southern Spain. Environ Res 2004;96:34-40.

Calle EE, Frumkin H, Henley SJ, Savitz DA, Thun MJ. Organochlorines and breast cancer risk. CA Cancer J Clin 2002;52:301-309.

Chen CW, Hurd C, Vorojeikina DP, Arnold SF, Notides AC. Transcriptional activation of the human estrogen receptor by DDT isomers and metabolites in yeast and MCF-7 cells. Biochem Pharmacol 1997;53(8):1161-1172.

Eriksson P, Talts U. Neonatal exposure to neurotoxic pesticides increases adult susceptibility: a review of current findings. Neurotoxicol 2000;21(1-2)37-48.

Food and Drug Administration (FDA). Center for Food Safety and Applied Nutrition/Office of Plant and Dairy Foods. FDA Pesticide Program Residue Monitoring 1993-2006 [online]. August 2008. Available at URL: http://www.cfsan.fda.gov/~dms/pesrpts.html. 4/21/09

Gladen BC, Rogan WJ. DDE and shortened duration of lactation in a northern Mexican town. Am J Public Health 1995;85:504-508.

Gladen BC, Klebanoff MA, Hediger ML, Katz SH, Barr DB, Davis MD, et al. Prenatal DDT exposure in relation to anthropometric and pubertal measures in adolescent males. Environ Health Perspect 2004;112(17):1761-1767.

Glynn AW, Granath F, Aune M, Atuma S, Darnerud PO, Bjerselius R, et al. Organochlorines in Swedish women: determinants of serum concentrations. Environ Health Perspect 2003;111:349-355.

Gray LE Jr, Ostby J, Furr J, Wolf CJ, Lambright C, Parks L, et al. Effects of environmental antiandrogens on reproductive development in experimental animals. Hum Reprod Updat 2001;7(3):248-264.

Gunderson EL. FDA total diet study, April 1982 to 1984, dietary intakes of pesticides, selected elements, and other chemicals. J Assoc Off Anal Chem 1988;71(6):1200-1209.

Hayes WJ, Jr., Durham WF, Cueto C, Jr. The effect of known repeated oral doses of chlorophenothane (DDT) in man. JAMA 1956;162:890-897.

Heudorf U, Angerer J, Drexler H. Current internal exposure to pesticides in children and adolescents in Germany: blood plasma levels of pentachlorophenol (PCP), lindane ($\gamma$–HCH), and dichloro(diphenyl)ethylene (DDE), a biostable metabolite of dichloro(diphenyl)trichloroethane (DDT). Int J Hyg Environ Health 2003;206:485-491.

Jusko TA, Koepsell TD, Baker RJ, Greenfield TA, Willman EJ, Charles MJ, et al. Maternal DDT exposures in relation to fetal and 5-year growth. Epidemiology 2006;17(6):692-700.

Link B, Gabrio T, Zoellner I, Piechotowski I, Paepke O, Herrman T, et al. Biomonitoring of persistent organochlorine pesticides, PCD/PCDFs and dioxin-like PCBs in blood of children from South West Germany (Baden-Wuerttemberg) from 1993-2003. Chemosphere 2005;58:1185-1201.

Longnecker MP, Klebanoff MA, Zhou H, Brock JW. Association between maternal serum concentration of the DDT metabolite DDE and preterm and small-for-gestational-age babies at birth. Lancet 2001;358:110-114.

Longnecker MP, Klebanoff MA, Brock JW, Zhou H, Gray KA, Needham LL, et al. Maternal serum level of 1,1-dichloro-2,2-bi(p-chlorophenyl)ethylene and risk of cryptorchidism, hypospadias, and polythelia among male offspring. Am J Epidemiol 2002;155(4):313-322.

Mariussen E, Fonnum F. Neurochemical targets and behavioral effects of organohalogen compounds: an update. Crit Rev Toxicol 2006;36:253-589.

Nims R, Lubet R, Fox S, Jones CR, Thomas PE, Reddy AB, et al. Comparative pharmacodynamics of CYP2B induction by DDT, DDE, and DDD in male rat liver and cultured rat hepatocytes. J Toxicol Environ Health Part A 1998;53:455-477.

Pavuk M, Cerhan JR, Lynch CF, Schecter A, Petrik J, Chovancova J, et al. Environmental exposure to PCBs and cancer incidence in eastern Slovakia. Chemosphere 2004;54:1509-520.

Radomski JL, Astolfi E, Deichmann WB, Rey AA. Blood levels of organochlorine pesticides in Argentina: occupationally and nonoccupationally exposed adults, children and newborn infants. Toxicol Appl Pharmacol 1971;20(2):186-193.

Rogan WJ. Pollutants in breast milk. Arch Pediatr Adolesc Med 1996;150:981-990.

Smith AG. Chlorinated Hydrocarbon Insecticides. In Hayes WJ, Jr and Laws ER, Jr, Eds. Handbook of Pesticide Toxicology, Vol. 2 Classes of Pesticides. New York, Academic Press, Inc. 1991 pp. 731-915.

Snedeker SM. Pesticides and breast cancer risk: a review of DDT, DDE, and dieldrin. Environ Health Perspect 2001;109:35-47.

Stehr-Green, PA. Demographic and seasonal influences on human serum pesticide residue levels. J Toxicol Environ Health 1989;27:405-421.

# Endrin

CAS No. 72-20-8

## General Information

Endrin, a stereoisomer of dieldrin, is no longer manufactured in the U.S. All uses of the pesticide in the U.S. have been cancelled by the U.S. EPA. Endrin was used as an insecticide, rodenticide and avicide. Endrin was not widely used as a termiticide, unlike aldrin and dieldrin. Depending on soil conditions, endrin can persist for years. Ketoendrin is a major photodegradation product (IPCS, 1992). Endrin has been detected in soils, and occasionally at low levels in sediment and surface waters, largely the result of historical agricultural application or run off from contaminated soils (ATSDR, 1996; IPCS, 1992).

General population exposure can occur after ingestion of endrin residues on food items imported from countries where endrin is still used, or from contact with contaminated soils and sediments in areas where endrin was applied, manufactured, or discarded. Over time, endrin has been detected with declining frequency in U.S. total diet surveys (FDA, 2008). Endrin is absorbed rapidly after ingestion, inhalation or dermal exposure routes. In the body, endrin is converted rapidly to its major metabolite, *anti*-12-hydroxyendrin. Further conversion occurs to 12-ketoendrin and various conjugated metabolites which are excreted in urine and feces. Because it is metabolized so rapidly, endrin usually is not detected in serum of exposed individuals, unless the dose is high and the exposure is very recent. Endrin does not accumulate in body tissues (IPCS, 1992; Smith, 1991).

Human health effects from endrin at low environmental doses or at biomonitored levels from low environmental exposures are unknown. At high doses, endrin blocks inhibitory neurotransmitters in the central nervous system resulting in excitation and seizures (Narahashi et al., 1992). An epidemic of acute endrin poisoning, characterized by generalized seizures in previously healthy persons occurred in Pakistan when sugar contaminated with endrin was ingested (Rowley et al., 1987). High doses produced renal tubular necrosis and diffuse kidney degeneration in animals. Hepatic effects of endrin exposure have included necrosis, fatty infiltration, and inflammation (Smith, 1991). Skeletal abnormalities and cleft palate in the offspring were associated with endrin when it was fed to pregnant laboratory rodents (Chernoff et al., 1979; Kavlock et al., 1981).

## Serum Endrin (lipid adjusted)

Geometric mean and selected percentiles of serum concentrations (in ng/g of lipid or parts per billion on a lipid-weight basis) for the U.S. population from the National Health and Nutrition Examination Survey.

| | Survey years | Geometric mean (95% conf. interval) | Selected percentiles (95% confidence interval) | | | | Sample size |
|---|---|---|---|---|---|---|---|
| | | | 50th | 75th | 90th | 95th | |
| **Total** | 01-02 | * | < LOD | < LOD | < LOD | 5.10 (<LOD-5.40) | 2187 |
| | 03-04 | * | < LOD | < LOD | < LOD | < LOD | 1825 |
| **Age group** | | | | | | | |
| 12-19 years | 01-02 | * | < LOD | < LOD | 5.20 (<LOD-5 50) | 5.60 (5.40-5.70) | 730 |
| | 03-04 | * | < LOD | < LOD | < LOD | < LOD | 539 |
| 20 years and older | 01-02 | * | < LOD | < LOD | < LOD | < LOD | 1457 |
| | 03-04 | * | < LOD | < LOD | < LOD | < LOD | 1286 |
| **Gender** | | | | | | | |
| Males | 01-02 | * | < LOD | < LOD | < LOD | 5.20 (<LOD-5.40) | 1022 |
| | 03-04 | * | < LOD | < LOD | < LOD | < LOD | 885 |
| Females | 01-02 | * | < LOD | < LOD | < LOD | < LOD | 1165 |
| | 03-04 | * | < LOD | < LOD | < LOD | < LOD | 940 |
| **Race/ethnicity** | | | | | | | |
| Mexican Americans | 01-02 | * | < LOD | < LOD | < LOD | 5.30 (<LOD-6.50) | 547 |
| | 03-04 | * | < LOD | < LOD | < LOD | < LOD | 433 |
| Non-Hispanic blacks | 01-02 | * | < LOD | < LOD | < LOD | 5.40 (<LOD-6.30) | 487 |
| | 03-04 | * | < LOD | < LOD | < LOD | < LOD | 446 |
| Non-Hispanic whites | 01-02 | * | < LOD | < LOD | < LOD | 5.10 (<LOD-5.40) | 1000 |
| | 03-04 | * | < LOD | < LOD | < LOD | < LOD | 831 |

Limit of detection (LOD, see Data Analysis section) for Survey years 01-02 and 03-04 are 5 09 and 7.8.
< LOD means less than the limit of detection, which may vary for some chemicals by year and by individual sample.
* Not calculated: proportion of results below limit of detection was too high to provide a valid result.

The U.S. EPA has established environmental standards for endrin, and the FDA monitors foods for pesticide residues. Workplace exposure standards for endrin have been established by OSHA. IARC has determined that endrin is not classifiable with regard to human carcinogenicity. Information about external exposure (i.e., environmental levels) and health effects of endrin is available from ATSDR at: http://www.atsdr.cdc.gov/toxpro2.html.

## Biomonitoring Information

In the NHANES 2001-2002 and 2003-2004 subsamples, serum levels of endrin were below the limit of detection. This finding is consistent with other general population studies (Bates et al., 2004; Ward et al., 2000). In a small study of Spanish women hospitalized for elective surgery, endrin was detected in 9% of serum samples, with the highest value 6.24 ng/mL (about 6.24 ng/g of serum) (Botella et al., 2004).

Finding a measurable amount of endrin in serum does not mean that the level of endrin causes an adverse health effect. Biomonitoring studies on levels of endrin provide physicians and public health officials with reference values so that they can determine whether people have been exposed to higher levels of endrin than are found in the general population. Biomonitoring data can also help scientists plan and conduct research on exposure and health effects.

### Serum Endrin (whole weight)

Geometric mean and selected percentiles of serum concentrations (in ng/g of serum or parts per billion) for the U.S. population from the National Health and Nutrition Examination Survey.

| | Survey years | Geometric mean (95% conf. interval) | 50th | 75th | 90th | 95th | Sample size |
|---|---|---|---|---|---|---|---|
| **Total** | 01-02 | * | < LOD | < LOD | < LOD | .020 (<LOD-.020) | 2187 |
| | 03-04 | * | < LOD | < LOD | < LOD | < LOD | 1825 |
| **Age group** | | | | | | | |
| 12-19 years | 01-02 | * | < LOD | < LOD | .020 (<LOD- 020) | .020 ( 020-.020) | 730 |
| | 03-04 | * | < LOD | < LOD | < LOD | < LOD | 539 |
| 20 years and older | 01-02 | * | < LOD | < LOD | < LOD | < LOD | 1457 |
| | 03-04 | * | < LOD | < LOD | < LOD | < LOD | 1286 |
| **Gender** | | | | | | | |
| Males | 01-02 | * | < LOD | < LOD | < LOD | .020 (<LOD-.020) | 1022 |
| | 03-04 | * | < LOD | < LOD | < LOD | < LOD | 885 |
| Females | 01-02 | * | < LOD | < LOD | < LOD | < LOD | 1165 |
| | 03-04 | * | < LOD | < LOD | < LOD | < LOD | 940 |
| **Race/ethnicity** | | | | | | | |
| Mexican Americans | 01-02 | * | < LOD | < LOD | < LOD | .020 (<LOD-.020) | 547 |
| | 03-04 | * | < LOD | < LOD | < LOD | < LOD | 433 |
| Non-Hispanic blacks | 01-02 | * | < LOD | < LOD | < LOD | .020 (<LOD-.020) | 487 |
| | 03-04 | * | < LOD | < LOD | < LOD | < LOD | 446 |
| Non-Hispanic whites | 01-02 | * | < LOD | < LOD | < LOD | .020 (<LOD-.020) | 1000 |
| | 03-04 | * | < LOD | < LOD | < LOD | < LOD | 831 |

< LOD means less than the limit of detection for the lipid adjusted serum level, which may vary for some chemicals by year and by individual sample.
* Not calculated: proportion of results below limit of detection was too high to provide a valid result.

## References

Agency for Toxic Substances and Disease Registry (ATSDR). Toxicological profile for endrin [online]. August 1996. Available at URL: http://www.atsdr.cdc.gov/toxprofiles/tp89.html. 4/21/09

Bates MN, Buckland SJ, Garrett N, Ellis H, Needham LL, Patterson DG Jr, et al. Persistent organochlorines in the serum of the non-occupationally exposed New Zealand population. Chemosphere 2004;54:1431-1443.

Botella B, Crespo J, Rivas A, Cerrillo I, Olea-Serrano MF, Olea N. Exposure of women to organochlorine pesticides in Southern Spain. Environ Res 2004;96:34-40.

Chernoff N, Kavlock RJ, Hanisch RC, Whitehouse DA, Gray JA, Gray LE, et al. Perinatal toxicity of endrin in rodents. I. Fetotoxic effects of prenatal exposure in hamsters. Toxicology 1979;13:155-165.

Food and Drug Administration (FDA). Center for Food Safety and Applied Nutrition/Office of Plant and Dairy Foods. FDA Pesticide Program Residue Monitoring 1993-2006 [online]. August 2008. Available at URL: http://www.cfsan.fda.gov/~dms/pesrpts.html. 4/21/09

International Programme on Chemical Safety (IPCS). Environmental Health Criteria 130. Endrin [online]. 1992. Available at URL: http://www.inchem.org/documents/ehc/ehc/ehc130.htm. 4/21/09

Kavlock RJ, Chernoff H, Hanisch RC, Gray J, Rogers E, Gray LE. Perinatal toxicity of endrin in rodents. II. Fetotoxic effects of prenatal exposure in rats and mice. Toxicology 1981;21:141-150.

Narahashi T, Frey JM, Ginsburg KS, Roy ML. Sodium and GABA-activated channels as the targets of pyrethroids and cyclodienes. Toxicol Lett 1992;64-65 Spec. No:429-436.

Rowley DL, Rab MA, Hardjotanojo W, Liddle J, Burse VW, Saleem M, Sokal D, et al. Convulsions caused by endrin poisoning in Pakistan. Pediatrics 1987;79(6):928-934.

Smith AG. Chlorinated Hydrocarbon Insecticides. In Hayes WJ, Jr and Laws ER, Jr, Eds. Handbook of Pesticide Toxicology, Vol. 2 Classes of Pesticides. New York, Academic Press, Inc. 1991, pp. 731-915.

Ward EM, Schulte P, Grajewski B, Andersen A, Patterson DG Jr, Turner W, et al. Serum organochlorine levels and breast cancer: a nested case-control study of Norwegian women. Cancer Epidemiol Biomarkers Prev 2000;9:1357-136.

# Hexachlorobenzene
CAS No. 118-74-1

## General Information

Hexachlorobenzene (HCB) was used from the 1930's to the 1970's in the U.S. primarily as a fungicide and seed treatment until the U.S. EPA cancelled its use in 1984. Although it is not manufactured as an end-product in the U.S., HCB may be created as either a byproduct or an impurity in the manufacturing process for certain chemicals and pesticides.

Hexachlorobenzene has entered the environment as a result of industrial activities and pesticide applications, and has been detected in soil, air, water, and sediment (Barber et al., 2005). It is a persistent chemical and bioaccumulates in both aquatic and terrestrial food chains (ATSDR, 2002). The general population may be exposed to HCB through diet, particularly by consuming fish, wildfowl, or game taken from areas with HCB contamination, and foods with a high fat content. The FDA dietary surveys have shown that over time, HCB has been detected in fewer foods since the 1980s (FDA, 2008; Gunderson, 1988). Workers in chemical manufacturing industries may be exposed to HCB via inhalation or dermal pathways.

HCB is well absorbed after oral administration, distributes widely throughout the body, and accumulates in fatty tissues where it persists for years. HCB is slowly metabolized, and elimination occurs by renal and fecal routes; breast milk is an additional route of elimination in nursing women. Urinary metabolites include pentachlorophenol (PCP), 2,4,5-trichlorophenol (2,4,5-TCP) and 2,4,6-trichlorophenol (2,4,6-TCP) (To-Figueras et al., 1997); these metabolites can also be produced after exposure to other chlorinated compounds (Kohli et al., 1976). Therefore, measuring HCB in serum is a specific indicator of exposure to the parent

## Serum Hexachlorobenzene (lipid adjusted)

Geometric mean and selected percentiles of serum concentrations (in ng/g of lipid or parts per billion on a lipid-weight basis) for the U.S. population from the National Health and Nutrition Examination Survey.

| | Survey years | Geometric mean (95% conf. interval) | Selected percentiles (95% confidence interval) | | | | Sample size |
|---|---|---|---|---|---|---|---|
| | | | 50th | 75th | 90th | 95th | |
| **Total** | 99-00 | * | < LOD | < LOD | < LOD | < LOD | 1702 |
| | 01-02 | * | < LOD | < LOD | < LOD | < LOD | 2277 |
| | 03-04 | 15.2 (14.5-15 9) | 14.9 (14.2-15.7) | 19.0 (18.1-20.3) | 24.4 (22.6-26.4) | 28.9 (25 6-32.8) | 1961 |
| **Age group** | | | | | | | |
| 12-19 years | 99-00 | * | < LOD | < LOD | < LOD | < LOD | 591 |
| | 01-02 | * | < LOD | < LOD | < LOD | < LOD | 747 |
| | 03-04 | 13.3 (12.5-14.1) | 13.4 (11.5-14 9) | 16.7 (15.5-18.4) | 20.7 (19.7-22.7) | 25.3 (22.7-30.2) | 588 |
| 20 years and older | 99-00 | * | < LOD | < LOD | < LOD | < LOD | 1111 |
| | 01-02 | * | < LOD | < LOD | < LOD | < LOD | 1530 |
| | 03-04 | 15.5 (14.7-16 2) | 15.1 (14.5-15 9) | 19.4 (18.3-20.9) | 24.8 (22.7-26.6) | 29.0 (25 6-33.6) | 1373 |
| **Gender** | | | | | | | |
| Males | 99-00 | * | < LOD | < LOD | < LOD | < LOD | 807 |
| | 01-02 | * | < LOD | < LOD | < LOD | < LOD | 1058 |
| | 03-04 | 14.5 (13.8-15 3) | 14.2 (13.4-15 0) | 18.1 (17.0-19.3) | 23.6 (21.0-25.6) | 26.9 (25 2-31.3) | 957 |
| Females | 99-00 | * | < LOD | < LOD | < LOD | < LOD | 895 |
| | 01-02 | * | < LOD | < LOD | < LOD | < LOD | 1219 |
| | 03-04 | 15.8 (15.0-16 6) | 15.7 (15.1-16.4) | 20.0 (18.7-21.4) | 24.9 (23.0-28.6) | 29.8 (26 5-33.7) | 1004 |
| **Race/ethnicity** | | | | | | | |
| Mexican Americans | 99-00 | * | < LOD | < LOD | < LOD | < LOD | 583 |
| | 01-02 | * | < LOD | < LOD | < LOD | < LOD | 554 |
| | 03-04 | 16.2 (14.9-17.7) | 15.3 (14.7-16.4) | 20.4 (18.3-22.5) | 27.6 (24.7-29.4) | 33.7 (27 6-44.6) | 460 |
| Non-Hispanic blacks | 99-00 | * | < LOD | < LOD | < LOD | < LOD | 350 |
| | 01-02 | * | < LOD | < LOD | < LOD | < LOD | 511 |
| | 03-04 | 14.5 (13.9-15 0) | 14.1 (13.7-15.1) | 18.3 (16.6-19.9) | 22.3 (20.9-24.0) | 26.6 (23 9-30.9) | 488 |
| Non-Hispanic whites | 99-00 | * | < LOD | < LOD | < LOD | < LOD | 636 |
| | 01-02 | * | < LOD | < LOD | < LOD | < LOD | 1052 |
| | 03-04 | 15.1 (14.4-16 0) | 15.0 (14.2-15 9) | 19.2 (17.9-20.8) | 24.3 (22.3-26.4) | 28.2 (24 9-32.8) | 888 |

Limit of detection (LOD, see Data Analysis section) for Survey years 99-00, 01-02, and 03-04 are 118.0, 31.4, and 7 8, respectively.
< LOD means less than the limit of detection, which may vary for some chemicals by year and by individual sample.
* Not calculated: proportion of results below limit of detection was too high to provide a valid result.

chemical.

Human health effects from HCB at low environmental doses or at biomonitored levels from low environmental exposures are unknown. Chronic feeding studies in animals have demonstrated kidney injury, immunologic abnormalities, reproductive and developmental toxicities, and liver and thyroid cancers (ATSDR, 2002). In humans, very high, acute doses produce central nervous system depression and seizures. HCB interferes with normal heme synthesis, which is manifested by increased delta-aminolevulinic acid synthase activity and decreased uroporphyrinogen decarboxylase activity. With chronic exposure, a consequence of these heme abnormalities is a condition known as acquired porphyria cutanea tarda. This condition, as well as hypertrichosis, arthritis, thyromegaly, anorexia, and weakness, were seen in an epidemic of poisoning in Turkey that occurred from 1955 to 1959 when HCB-treated seed grain was diverted for bread production.

Infants were exposed transplacentally and through breast milk, and many died before 2 years of age (Peters et al., 1982; Schmid, 1960).

IARC classifies hexachlorobenzene as possibly carcinogenic to humans, and NTP classifies hexachlorobenzene as reasonably anticipated to be a human carcinogen. ACGIH has developed workplace exposure limits for HCB. The U.S. EPA has established a drinking water standard, and the FDA has established a bottled water standard for HCB. More information about external exposure (i.e., environmental levels) and health effects is available from the U.S. EPA at: http://www.epa.gov/pesticides/ and from ATSDR at: http://www.atsdr.cdc.gov/toxpro2.html.

**Biomonitoring Information**

Serum concentrations reflect the body burden of HCB. HCB levels were generally below the limits of detection

### Serum Hexachlorobenzene (whole weight)

Geometric mean and selected percentiles of serum concentrations (in ng/g of serum or parts per billion) for the U.S. population from the National Health and Nutrition Examination Survey.

| | Survey years | Geometric mean (95% conf. interval) | 50th | 75th | 90th | 95th | Sample size |
|---|---|---|---|---|---|---|---|
| **Total** | 99-00 | * | < LOD | < LOD | < LOD | < LOD | 1702 |
| | 01-02 | * | < LOD | < LOD | < LOD | < LOD | 2277 |
| | 03-04 | .092 (.088-.097) | .090 (.086-.095) | .120 (.113-.126) | .157 (.145-.167) | .186 (.169-.212) | 1961 |
| **Age group** | | | | | | | |
| 12-19 years | 99-00 | * | < LOD | < LOD | < LOD | < LOD | 591 |
| | 01-02 | * | < LOD | < LOD | < LOD | < LOD | 747 |
| | 03-04 | .065 (.062-.069) | .064 (.060-.069) | .079 (.072-.086) | .102 (.091-.111) | .123 (.111-.141) | 588 |
| 20 years and older | 99-00 | * | < LOD | < LOD | < LOD | < LOD | 1111 |
| | 01-02 | * | < LOD | < LOD | < LOD | < LOD | 1530 |
| | 03-04 | .097 (.092-.102) | .095 (.090-.099) | .123 (.118-.130) | .160 (.147-.175) | .191 (.174-.223) | 1373 |
| **Gender** | | | | | | | |
| Males | 99-00 | * | < LOD | < LOD | < LOD | < LOD | 807 |
| | 01-02 | * | < LOD | < LOD | < LOD | < LOD | 1058 |
| | 03-04 | .090 (.085-.095) | .087 (.082-.094) | .115 (.107-.122) | .147 (.135-.163) | .179 (.159-.203) | 957 |
| Females | 99-00 | * | < LOD | < LOD | < LOD | < LOD | 895 |
| | 01-02 | * | < LOD | < LOD | < LOD | < LOD | 1219 |
| | 03-04 | .095 (.089-.100) | .092 (.088-.099) | .123 (.118-.132) | .163 (.148-.176) | .190 (.176-.226) | 1004 |
| **Race/ethnicity** | | | | | | | |
| Mexican Americans | 99-00 | * | < LOD | < LOD | < LOD | < LOD | 583 |
| | 01-02 | * | < LOD | < LOD | < LOD | < LOD | 554 |
| | 03-04 | .098 (.089-.109) | .090 (.081-.107) | .125 (.114-.152) | .171 (.157-.203) | .225 (.178-.258) | 460 |
| Non-Hispanic blacks | 99-00 | * | < LOD | < LOD | < LOD | < LOD | 350 |
| | 01-02 | * | < LOD | < LOD | < LOD | < LOD | 511 |
| | 03-04 | .081 (.077-.085) | .078 (.073-.083) | .104 (.095-.118) | .140 (.127-.155) | .167 (.145-.196) | 488 |
| Non-Hispanic whites | 99-00 | * | < LOD | < LOD | < LOD | < LOD | 636 |
| | 01-02 | * | < LOD | < LOD | < LOD | < LOD | 1052 |
| | 03-04 | .094 (.088-.099) | .092 (.086-.097) | .121 (.114-.129) | .156 (.143-.173) | .182 (.163-.218) | 888 |

< LOD means less than the limit of detection for the lipid adjusted serum level, which may vary for some chemicals by year and by individual sample.
* Not calculated: proportion of results below limit of detection was too high to provide a valid result.

in the NHANES 1999-2000 and 2001-2002 subsamples. As a result of the lower limit of detection in NHANES 2003-2004, more HCB levels were quantified. Age-related increases of HCB in body fat and serum have been consistently noted in general population studies (Becker et al., 2002; Bertram et al., 1986; Glynn et al., 2003). In a representative sample of the 1998 German adult population, HCB levels were directly related to age, and the geometric mean concentration of HCB in whole blood was 0.44 µg/L, lower than the limit of detection (on a lipid adjusted basis) in NHANES 1999-2000 and 2001-2002, but approximately five times higher than the overall geometric mean level in 2003-2004 (Becker et al., 2002). In the 1976-1980 NHANES subsample, HCB detection in serum also was proportional to age, but overall, only 4.9% of participants had quantifiable levels (Stehr-Green, 1989). In Spain, factory workers chronically exposed to HCB and residents near the factory had serum HCB levels that were 150 to 50 times higher, respectively, than the limits of detection (on a whole weight basis) in NHANES 1999-2000 and 2001-2002 (Herrero et al., 1999). Residency near industrial or agricultural areas has been associated with higher serum HCB levels (Barber et al., 2005; Bradman et al., 2006). Over the past two decades, however, declines in background HCB levels ranging from around 50%-90% have been documented in studies using cord blood (Dallaire et al., 2002; Lackman, 2002) and among children (Link et al., 2005); the more recent values in these studies were similar to the lipid adjusted limit of detection in NHANES 1999-2000 and 2001-2002 (Dallaire et al., 2002; Lackmann, 2002; Link et al., 2005).

Finding a measurable amount of hexachlorobenzene in serum does not mean that the level of the hexachlorobenzene causes an adverse health effect. Biomonitoring studies on levels of HCB provide physicians and public health officials with reference values so that they can determine whether people have been exposed to higher levels of hexachlorobenzene than are found in the general population. Biomonitoring data can also help scientists plan and conduct research on exposure and health effects.

## References

Agency for Toxic Substances and Disease Registry (ATSDR). Toxicological profile for hexachlorobenzene update [online]. September 2002. Available at URL: http://www.atsdr.cdc.gov/toxprofiles/tp90 html. 4/21/09

Barber JL, Sweetman AJ, van Wijk D, Jones KC. Hexachlorobenzene in the global environment: emissions, levels, distribution, trends and processes. Sci Tot Environ 2005;349:1-44.

Becker K, Kaus S, Krause C, Lepom P, Schulz C, Seiwert M, et al. German Environmental Survey 1998 (GerES III): environmental pollutants in blood of the German population. Int J Hyg Environ Health 2002;205:297-308.

Bertram HP, Kemper FH, Muller C. Hexachlorobenzene content in human whole blood and adipose tissue: experiences in environmental specimen banking. IARC Sci Publ 1986;77:173-182.

Bradman A, Schwartz JM. Fenster L, Barr DB, Holland NT, Eskenazi B. Factors predicting organochlorine pesticide levels in pregnant Latina women living in a United States agricultural area. J Exp Sci Environ Epidemiol 2007;17:388–399.

Dallaire F, Dewailly E, Laliberte C, Muckle G, Ayotte P. Temporal trends of organochlorine concentrations in umbilical cord blood of newborns from the lower north shore of the St. Lawrence River (Quebec, Canada). Environ Health Perspect 2002;110(8):835-838.

Food and Drug Administration (FDA). Center for Food Safety and Applied Nutrition/Office of Plant and Dairy Foods. FDA Pesticide Program Residue Monitoring 1993-2006 [online]. August 2008. Available at URL: http://www.cfsan fda.gov/~dms/pesrpts.html. 4/21/09

Glynn AW, Granath F, Aune M, Atuma S, Darnerud PO, Bjerselius R, et al. Organochlorines in Swedish women: determinants of serum concentrations. Environ Health Perspect 2003;111:349-355.

Gunderson EL. FDA total diet study, April 1982 to 1984, dietary intakes of pesticides, selected elements, and other chemicals. J Assoc Off Anal Chem 1988;71(6):1200-1209.

Herrero C, Ozalla D, Sala M, Otero R, Santiago-Silva M, Lecha M, et al. Urinary porphyrin excretion in a human population highly exposed to hexachlorobenzene. Arch Dermatol 1999;135(4):400-404.

Kohli J, Jones D, Safe A. The metabolism of higher chlorinated benzene isomers. Can J Biochem 1976;54(3):203-208.

Lackmann GM. Polychlorinated biphenyls and hexachlorobenzene in full-term neonates. Reference values updated. Biol Neonate 2002;81(2):82-85.

Link B, Gabrio T, Zoellner I, Piechotowski I, Paepke O, Herrman T, et al. Biomonitoring of persistent organochlorine pesticides, PCD/PCDFs and dioxin-like PCBs in blood of children from South West Germany (Baden-Wuerttemberg) from 1993-2003. Chemosphere 2005;58:1185-1201.

Peters HA, Gocmen A, Cripps DJ, Bryan GT, Dogramaci I. Epidemiology of hexachlorobenzene-induced porphyria in Turkey: clinical and laboratory follow-up after 25 years. Arch Neurol 1982;39(12):744-749.

Schmid R. Cutaneous porphyria in Turkey. N Engl J Med 1960;263:397-398.

Stehr-Green, PA. Demographic and seasonal influences on human serum pesticide residue levels. J Toxicol Environ Health 1989;27:405-421.

To-Figueras J, Sala M, Otero R, Barrot C, Santiago-Silva M, Rodamilans M, et al. Metabolism of hexachlorobenzene in humans: association between serum levels and urinary metabolites in a highly exposed population. Environ Health Perspect 1997;105(1):78-83.

# Hexachlorocyclohexane
CAS No. 608-73-1

## *beta*-Hexachlorocyclohexane
CAS No. 319-85-7

## *gamma*-Hexachlorocyclohexane
CAS No. 58-89-9

### General Information

Hexachlorocyclohexane (HCH), formerly referred to as benzene hexachloride, exists in several isomeric forms, including *alpha*, *beta*, *gamma*, and *delta*. The *gamma* isomer, commonly known as lindane, can be used as an insecticide and has been used to kill soil-dwelling and plant-eating insects. The other isomers can be formed during the synthesis of lindane, and have been used either as fungicides or to synthesize other chemicals. Technical grade HCH is a mixture of all four isomers, containing about 64% *alpha* and 10%-15% *gamma* isomers. It is no longer produced or sold in the U.S. In 2006, the U.S. EPA cancelled agricultural uses of lindane (ATSDR, 2005). Lindane (1%) lotion and shampoo are available by prescription for single-use application to treat human scabies and head lice.

HCH isomers, particularly *alpha* and *gamma* have been detected widely in air, soil, water, and sediment as a result of historic production and use. As pesticide applications of HCH were increasingly restricted or eliminated, environmental levels declined. Lindane has a half-life of about two weeks in soils and water. HCH does not bioaccumulate to an appreciable extent in plants (ATSDR, 2005). However, HCH isomers are lipophilic, so they can accumulate in fatty tissues of animals. General population

## Serum *beta*-Hexachlorocyclohexane (lipid adjusted)

Geometric mean and selected percentiles of serum concentrations (in ng/g of lipid or parts per billion on a lipid-weight basis) for the U.S. population from the National Health and Nutrition Examination Survey.

| | Survey years | Geometric mean (95% conf. interval) | 50th | 75th | 90th | 95th | Sample size |
|---|---|---|---|---|---|---|---|
| **Total** | 99-00 | 9.68 (<LOD-10.9) | < LOD | 19.1 (16.0-21.6) | 42.0 (33.4-50.6) | 68.9 (50.6-89.5) | 1893 |
| | 01-02** | * | < LOD | 16.0 (14.2-17.3) | 36.7 (30.4-45.7) | 67.2 (50.3-85.7) | 2291 |
| | 03-04 | * | < LOD | 14.1 (12.1-16.5) | 32.1 (27.1-37.8) | 56.5 (43.7-69.4) | 1959 |
| **Age group** | | | | | | | |
| 12-19 years | 99-00 | * | < LOD | < LOD | < LOD | 11.7 (<LOD-16.1) | 653 |
| | 01-02** | * | < LOD | < LOD | < LOD | 13.1 (9.70-19.0) | 758 |
| | 03-04 | * | < LOD | < LOD | < LOD | 8.80 (<LOD-14.7) | 589 |
| 20 years and older | 99-00 | 10.9 (9.61-12.4) | < LOD | 21.1 (18.9-24.0) | 46.0 (35.9-56.8) | 73.4 (52.7-96.0) | 1240 |
| | 01-02** | 9.87 (9.04-10.8) | 7.80 (6 90-8.90) | 17.4 (16.0-20.5) | 39.6 (33.2-52.0) | 71.7 (53.7-96.2) | 1533 |
| | 03-04 | 7.89 (<LOD-9.09) | < LOD | 16.3 (13.6-18.4) | 35.2 (29.6-42.5) | 62.2 (48.2-87.6) | 1370 |
| **Gender** | | | | | | | |
| Males | 99-00 | * | < LOD | 14.6 (10.8-19.1) | 29.8 (23.3-38.7) | 44.9 (32.8-68.9) | 901 |
| | 01-02** | * | < LOD | 12.9 (11.1-15.7) | 27.5 (24.0-34.4) | 45.7 (35.2-55.6) | 1067 |
| | 03-04 | * | < LOD | 10.4 (8.70-12.5) | 21.6 (17.7-26.4) | 35.3 (26.1-49.9) | 952 |
| Females | 99-00 | 11.1 (9.56-12.8) | < LOD | 22.0 (19.1-27.6) | 51.3 (42.2-67.6) | 81.8 (64.4-111) | 992 |
| | 01-02** | 10.2 (9.46-11.0) | 7.70 (6 90-8.50) | 18.5 (16.2-22.7) | 47.5 (37.6-62.0) | 84.7 (62.0-111) | 1224 |
| | 03-04 | 8.43 (<LOD-9.45) | < LOD | 18.6 (16.9-21.5) | 41.8 (33.9-51.4) | 70.3 (62.2-98.4) | 1007 |
| **Race/ethnicity** | | | | | | | |
| Mexican Americans | 99-00 | 16.7 (13.7-20.2) | 15.5 (11.6-20.4) | 37.7 (29.6-47.3) | 97.9 (62.6-135) | 142 (99.8-199) | 632 |
| | 01-02** | 13.1 (11.6-14.7) | 11.8 (9.60-13.4) | 25.8 (21.1-32.7) | 69.4 (50.8-87.6) | 134 (85.7-166) | 563 |
| | 03-04 | 10.5 (8.66-12.8) | 10.0 (<LOD-12.7) | 23.8 (17.5-29.9) | 50.1 (30.0-70.3) | 70.3 (42.5-123) | 460 |
| Non-Hispanic blacks | 99-00 | * | < LOD | 15.4 (12.0-23.1) | 37.9 (30.2-42.2) | 49.9 (40.9-81.1) | 403 |
| | 01-02** | * | < LOD | 12.0 (8.20-16.2) | 36.2 (18.4-73.4) | 71.2 (31.9-178) | 513 |
| | 03-04 | * | < LOD | 9.70 (8.30-11.9) | 27.1 (21.1-36.3) | 48.2 (34.8-54.3) | 487 |
| Non-Hispanic whites | 99-00 | * | < LOD | 17.5 (14.2-20.5) | 34.7 (25.2-46.1) | 51.6 (40.0-70.8) | 702 |
| | 01-02** | * | < LOD | 14.4 (11.8-16.8) | 31.9 (26.6-37.8) | 52.0 (37.7-69.5) | 1051 |
| | 03-04 | * | < LOD | 12.8 (10.9-14.7) | 27.6 (22.1-32.2) | 40.8 (32.3-56.5) | 887 |

Limits of detection (LOD, see Data Analysis section) for survey years 99-00, 01-02, and 03-04 are 9.36, 6.76, and 7 8, respectively.
< LOD means less than the limit of detection, which may vary for some chemicals by year and by individual sample.
* Not calculated: proportion of results below limit of detection was too high to provide a valid result.
**In survey period 2001-2002, each result has been multiplied by 1.5528. See the section "What's New" at the beginning of this *Report* for details.

exposure to HCH is through the diet. The U.S. FDA pesticide monitoring program has shown a temporal decline in the detection of lindane, from 6% of samples in 1982-1984 to 2% in 1994 (FDA, 2008; Gunderson 1988). Pesticide applicators or agricultural workers could be exposed to HCH by inhalation and dermal pathways.

HCH isomers are absorbed after inhalation, ingestion, or dermal exposure. Distribution is mainly to fatty tissues. After dermal application of lindane 1% lotion, the serum half-life was about 20 hours among children (Ginsburg et al., 1977). The *beta* isomer accumulates in fatty tissues and is metabolized more slowly, resulting in a half-life of about seven years. HCH isomers are metabolized to chlorophenol metabolites that are excreted in the urine (Angerer et al., 1983). HCH crosses the placenta and is also excreted in breast milk (Radomski et al., 1971; Rogan, 1996; Saxena et al., 1981).

Human health effects from HCH isomers at low environmental doses or at biomonitored levels from low environmental exposures are unknown. Acute high dose toxicity in rodents affects the central nervous system producing decreased activity, ataxia, and seizures. When animals were chronically fed lindane at high doses, enlarged livers, hepatic enzyme induction, and nephropathy developed (IPCS, 2002). Acute high doses of lindane after ingestion or excessive skin application of the 1% lotion have produced seizures in humans, probably by blocking inhibitory neurotransmitters in the central nervous system. Workers who directly handled HCH have complained of headache, paresthesias, tremors, and memory loss (Nigam et al., 1986). OSHA and ACGIH have established workplace standards and guidelines, respectively, for lindane. U.S. EPA has established a drinking water standard, and FDA has established a bottled water standard and food residue tolerances for lindane. IARC classifies

## Serum *beta*-Hexachlorocyclohexane (whole weight)

Geometric mean and selected percentiles of serum concentrations (in ng/g of serum or parts per billion) for the U.S. population from the National Health and Nutrition Examination Survey.

| | Survey years | Geometric mean (95% conf. interval) | 50th | 75th | 90th | 95th | Sample size |
|---|---|---|---|---|---|---|---|
| **Total** | 99-00 | .058 (<LOD-.066) | < LOD | .120 (.100-.150) | .290 (.220-.360) | .450 (.360-.560) | 1893 |
| | 01-02** | * | < LOD | .100 (.090-.120) | .250 (.210-.310) | .460 (.340-.600) | 2291 |
| | 03-04 | * | < LOD | .092 (.081-.103) | .216 (.173-.254) | .372 (.294-.442) | 1959 |
| **Age group** | | | | | | | |
| 12-19 years | 99-00 | * | < LOD | < LOD | < LOD | .050 (<LOD-.070) | 653 |
| | 01-02** | * | < LOD | < LOD | < LOD | .080 (.050-.100) | 758 |
| | 03-04 | * | < LOD | < LOD | < LOD | .048 (<LOD-.064) | 589 |
| 20 years and older | 99-00 | .067 (.059-.077) | < LOD | .140 (.120-.160) | .330 (.240-.410) | .480 (.410-.620) | 1240 |
| | 01-02** | .062 (.057-.069) | .050 (.050-.060) | .120 (.100-.140) | .270 (.230-.350) | .480 (.370-.690) | 1533 |
| | 03-04 | .050 (<LOD-.058) | < LOD | .103 (.089-.125) | .234 (.191-.290) | .412 (.308-.587) | 1370 |
| **Gender** | | | | | | | |
| Males | 99-00 | * | < LOD | .090 (.080-.120) | .210 (.160-.250) | .290 (.220-.470) | 901 |
| | 01-02** | * | < LOD | .080 (.070-.100) | .200 (.150-.260) | .310 (.250-.400) | 1067 |
| | 03-04 | * | < LOD | .072 (.056-.089) | .144 (.118-.174) | .222 (.170-.305) | 952 |
| Females | 99-00 | .065 (.056-.077) | < LOD | .150 (.120-.190) | .380 (.300-.450) | .560 (.420-.680) | 992 |
| | 01-02** | .062 (.057-.067) | .050 (.040-.050) | .130 (.110-.150) | .320 (.260-.400) | .570 (.450-.710) | 1224 |
| | 03-04 | .051 (<LOD-.057) | < LOD | .118 (.103-.130) | .290 (.244-.319) | .442 (.382-.661) | 1007 |
| **Race/ethnicity** | | | | | | | |
| Mexican Americans | 99-00 | .098 (.080-.119) | .090 (.070-.110) | .240 (.200-.310) | .580 (.390-.840) | .910 (.580-1.37) | 632 |
| | 01-02** | .078 (.068-.091) | .070 (.050-.080) | .160 (.130-.210) | .470 (.330-.700) | 1.01 (.620-1.32) | 563 |
| | 03-04 | .064 (.051-.080) | .057 (<LOD-.086) | .139 (.124-.190) | .331 (.191-.501) | .521 (.297-.814) | 460 |
| Non-Hispanic blacks | 99-00 | * | < LOD | .100 (.070-.140) | .250 (.190-.290) | .360 (.280-.460) | 403 |
| | 01-02** | * | < LOD | .070 (.050-.110) | .220 (.120-.410) | .410 (.190-1.05) | 513 |
| | 03-04 | * | < LOD | .065 (.047-.083) | .167 (.131-.214) | .281 (.200-.404) | 487 |
| Non-Hispanic whites | 99-00 | * | < LOD | .120 (.100-.140) | .250 (.170-.340) | .390 (.280-.510) | 702 |
| | 01-02** | * | < LOD | .090 (.080-.110) | .210 (.180-.260) | .350 (.250-.480) | 1051 |
| | 03-04 | * | < LOD | .083 (.073-.096) | .175 (.146-.220) | .287 (.221-.372) | 887 |

< LOD means less than the limit of detection for the lipid adjusted serum level, which may vary for some chemicals by year and by individual sample.
* Not calculated: proportion of results below limit of detection was too high to provide a valid result.
**In survey period 2001-2002, each result has been multiplied by 1.5528. See the section "What's New" at the beginning of this *Report* for details.

hexachlorocyclohexane isomers as possibly carcinogenic to humans, and NTP classifies hexachlorocyclohexane isomers as reasonably anticipated to be human carcinogens. More information about external exposure (i.e., environmental levels) and health effects is available from the U.S. EPA at: http://www.epa.gov/pesticides/ and from ATSDR at: http://www.atsdr.cdc.gov/toxpro2.html.

## Biomonitoring Information

Because of its longer half-life, *beta*-HCH may be detected in a higher percentage of the general population than are the other HCH isomers. Studies of general populations have shown declining *beta*-HCH levels since the 1970s (ATSDR, 2005; Kutz et al., 1991; Link et al., 2005; Radomski et al., 1971; Stehr-Green, 1989; Sturgeon et al., 1998). Additional factors associated with higher *beta*-HCH levels include rural residence, older age, male sex, and a diet that includes

meat (Becker et al., 2002; Kutz et al., 1991; Stehr-Green, 1989).

In NHANES 1999-2000, 2001-2002, and 2003-2004, serum levels of lindane were generally below the limits of detection, which were considerably lower (as much as twentyfold) than mean levels reported in small studies of adults in Spain (Botella et al., 2004) and India (Bhatnagar et al., 2004). In recent years, studies in populations with environmental exposure have reported lindane levels below the limit of detection in most persons (Anderson et al., 1998; Bates et al., 2004; Becker et al., 2002). In population-based studies of New Zealand adults and German adults and children, the maximum and 95th percentile *beta*-HCH values, respectively, were similar to the 95th percentiles in this *Report*. In an earlier (1996-1997) sample of German children, aged 9-11 years, the 95th percentile of *beta*-HCH levels was twofold to threefold higher than the 95th percentile of 12-19 year olds in the comparable NHANES

## Serum *gamma*-Hexachlorocyclohexane (Lindane) (lipid adjusted)

Geometric mean and selected percentiles of serum concentrations (in ng/g of lipid or parts per billion on a lipid-weight basis) for the U.S. population from the National Health and Nutrition Examination Survey.

| | Survey years | Geometric mean (95% conf. interval) | Selected percentiles ( 95% confidence interval) | | | | Sample size |
|---|---|---|---|---|---|---|---|
| | | | 50th | 75th | 90th | 95th | |
| **Total** | 99-00 | * | < LOD | < LOD | < LOD | < LOD | 1799 |
| | 01-02 | * | < LOD | < LOD | < LOD | < LOD | 2280 |
| | 03-04 | * | < LOD | < LOD | < LOD | < LOD | 1960 |
| **Age group** | | | | | | | |
| 12-19 years | 99-00 | * | < LOD | < LOD | < LOD | < LOD | 660 |
| | 01-02 | * | < LOD | < LOD | < LOD | < LOD | 758 |
| | 03-04 | * | < LOD | < LOD | < LOD | < LOD | 593 |
| 20 years and older | 99-00 | * | < LOD | < LOD | < LOD | < LOD | 1139 |
| | 01-02 | * | < LOD | < LOD | < LOD | < LOD | 1522 |
| | 03-04 | * | < LOD | < LOD | < LOD | < LOD | 1367 |
| **Gender** | | | | | | | |
| Males | 99-00 | * | < LOD | < LOD | < LOD | < LOD | 863 |
| | 01-02 | * | < LOD | < LOD | < LOD | < LOD | 1060 |
| | 03-04 | * | < LOD | < LOD | < LOD | < LOD | 952 |
| Females | 99-00 | * | < LOD | < LOD | < LOD | < LOD | 936 |
| | 01-02 | * | < LOD | < LOD | < LOD | < LOD | 1220 |
| | 03-04 | * | < LOD | < LOD | < LOD | < LOD | 1008 |
| **Race/ethnicity** | | | | | | | |
| Mexican Americans | 99-00 | * | < LOD | < LOD | < LOD | < LOD | 631 |
| | 01-02 | * | < LOD | < LOD | < LOD | < LOD | 563 |
| | 03-04 | * | < LOD | < LOD | < LOD | < LOD | 461 |
| Non-Hispanic blacks | 99-00 | * | < LOD | < LOD | < LOD | < LOD | 380 |
| | 01-02 | * | < LOD | < LOD | < LOD | < LOD | 509 |
| | 03-04 | * | < LOD | < LOD | < LOD | < LOD | 490 |
| Non-Hispanic whites | 99-00 | * | < LOD | < LOD | < LOD | < LOD | 646 |
| | 01-02 | * | < LOD | < LOD | < LOD | < LOD | 1045 |
| | 03-04 | * | < LOD | < LOD | < LOD | < LOD | 884 |

Limit of detection (LOD, see Data Analysis section) for Survey years 99-00, 01-02, and 03-04 are 14.5, 10.5, and 7.8, respectively.
< LOD means less than the limit of detection, which may vary for some chemicals by year and by individual sample.
* Not calculated: proportion of results below limit of detection was too high to provide a valid result.

2001-2002 survey period (Link et al., 2005). In a small study of adults who consumed sport fish from the Great Lakes, the median *beta*-HCH levels were similar or slightly higher than the 95th percentile in this *Report* (Anderson et al., 1998). A study of Swedish women aged 54 years and older reported a median *beta*-HCH level that was slightly higher than the geometric mean for women reported in the NHANES 1999-2000 survey period (Glynn et al., 2003). *Beta*-HCH and lindane levels in workers involved in HCH production have been more than 1000-fold higher than the 95th percentile and limit of detection (lipid adjusted), respectively, in this *Report* (Nigam et al., 1986; Radomski et al., 1971).

Finding a measurable amount of HCH isomers in serum does not mean that the level of HCH isomers causes an adverse health effect. Biomonitoring studies on levels of HCH isomers provide physicians and public health officials with reference values so that they can determine whether

people have been exposed to higher levels of HCH isomers than are found in the general population. Biomonitoring data can also help scientists plan and conduct research on exposure and health effects.

## Serum *gamma*-Hexachlorocyclohexane (Lindane) (whole weight)

Geometric mean and selected percentiles of serum concentrations (in ng/g of serum or parts per billion) for the U.S. population from the National Health and Nutrition Examination Survey.

| | Survey years | Geometric mean (95% conf. interval) | Selected percentiles ( 95% confidence interval) 50th | 75th | 90th | 95th | Sample size |
|---|---|---|---|---|---|---|---|
| **Total** | 99-00 | * | < LOD | < LOD | < LOD | < LOD | 1799 |
| | 01-02 | * | < LOD | < LOD | < LOD | < LOD | 2280 |
| | 03-04 | * | < LOD | < LOD | < LOD | < LOD | 1960 |
| **Age group** | | | | | | | |
| 12-19 years | 99-00 | * | < LOD | < LOD | < LOD | < LOD | 660 |
| | 01-02 | * | < LOD | < LOD | < LOD | < LOD | 758 |
| | 03-04 | * | < LOD | < LOD | < LOD | < LOD | 593 |
| 20 years and older | 99-00 | * | < LOD | < LOD | < LOD | < LOD | 1139 |
| | 01-02 | * | < LOD | < LOD | < LOD | < LOD | 1522 |
| | 03-04 | * | < LOD | < LOD | < LOD | < LOD | 1367 |
| **Gender** | | | | | | | |
| Males | 99-00 | * | < LOD | < LOD | < LOD | < LOD | 863 |
| | 01-02 | * | < LOD | < LOD | < LOD | < LOD | 1060 |
| | 03-04 | * | < LOD | < LOD | < LOD | < LOD | 952 |
| Females | 99-00 | * | < LOD | < LOD | < LOD | < LOD | 936 |
| | 01-02 | * | < LOD | < LOD | < LOD | < LOD | 1220 |
| | 03-04 | * | < LOD | < LOD | < LOD | < LOD | 1008 |
| **Race/ethnicity** | | | | | | | |
| Mexican Americans | 99-00 | * | < LOD | < LOD | < LOD | < LOD | 631 |
| | 01-02 | * | < LOD | < LOD | < LOD | < LOD | 563 |
| | 03-04 | * | < LOD | < LOD | < LOD | < LOD | 461 |
| Non-Hispanic blacks | 99-00 | * | < LOD | < LOD | < LOD | < LOD | 380 |
| | 01-02 | * | < LOD | < LOD | < LOD | < LOD | 509 |
| | 03-04 | * | < LOD | < LOD | < LOD | < LOD | 490 |
| Non-Hispanic whites | 99-00 | * | < LOD | < LOD | < LOD | < LOD | 646 |
| | 01-02 | * | < LOD | < LOD | < LOD | < LOD | 1045 |
| | 03-04 | * | < LOD | < LOD | < LOD | < LOD | 884 |

< LOD means less than the limit of detection for the lipid adjusted serum level, which may vary for some chemicals by year and by individual sample.
* Not calculated: proportion of results below limit of detection was too high to provide a valid result.

## References

Agency for Toxic Substances and Disease Registry (ATSDR). Toxicological profile for hexachlorocyclohexanes update [online]. August 2005. Available at URL: http://www.atsdr.cdc. gov/toxprofiles/tp43.html. 4/21/09

Anderson HA, Falk C, Hanrahan L, Olson J, Burse VW, Needham LL, et al. Profiles of Great Lakes critical pollutants: a sentinel analysis of human blood and urine. The Great Lakes Consortium. Environ Health Perspect 1998;106(5):279-289.

Angerer J, Maass R, Heinrich R. Occupational exposure to hexachlorocyclohexane. VI. Metabolism of *gamma*-hexachlorocyclohexane in man. Int Arch Occup Environ Health 1983;52(1):59-67.

Bates MN, Buckland SJ, Garrett N, Ellis H, Needham LL, Patterson DG Jr, et al. Persistent organochlorines in the serum of the non-occupationally exposed New Zealand population. Chemosphere 2004;54:1431-1443.

Becker K, Kaus S, Krause C, Lepom P, Schulz C, Seiwert M, et al. German Environmental Survey 1998 (GerES III): environmental pollutants in blood of the German population. Int J Hyg Environ Health 2002;205:297-308.

Bhatnagar VK, Kashyap R, Zaidi SS, Kulkarni PK, Saiyed HN. Levels of DDT, HCH, and HCB residues in human blood in Ahmedabad, India. Bull Environ Contam Toxicol 2004;72:261-265.

Botella B, Crespo J, Rivas A, Cerrillo I, Olea-Serrano MF, Olea N. Exposure of women to organochlorine pesticides in Southern Spain. Environ Res 2004;96:34-4Food and Drug Administration (FDA). Center for Food Safety and Applied Nutrition/Office of Plant and Dairy Foods. FDA Pesticide Program Residue Monitoring 1993-2006 [online]. August 2008. Available at URL: http://www.cfsan fda.gov/~dms/pesrpts html. 4/21/09

Ginsburg CM, Lowry W, Reisch JS. Absorption of lindane ($\gamma$ benzene hexachloride) in infants and children. J Pediatr 1977;91:998-1000.

Glynn AW, Granath F, Aune M, Atuma S, Darnerud PO, Bjerselius R, et al. Organochlorines in Swedish women: determinants of serum concentrations. Environ Health Perspect 2003;111:349-355.

Gunderson EL. FDA total diet study, April 1982 to 1984, dietary intakes of pesticides, selected elements, and other chemicals. J Assoc Off Anal Chem 1988;71(6):1200-1209.

International Programme on Chemical Safety (IPCS). Pesticide residues in food-2002-Joint FAO/WHO meeting on pesticide residues. Lindane. 2002. available at URL: http://www.inchem. org/documents/jmpr/jmpmono/2002pr08 htm. 4/21/09

Kutz FW, Wood PH, Bottimore DP. Organochlorine pesticides and polychlorinated biphenyls in human adipose tissue. Rev Environ Contam Toxicol 1991;120:1-82.

Link B, Gabrio T, Zoellner I, Piechotowski I, Paepke O, Herrman T, et al. Biomonitoring of persistent organochlorine pesticides, PCD/PCDFs and dioxin-like PCBs in blood of children from South West Germany (Baden-Wuerttemberg) from 1993-2003. Chemosphere 2005;58:1185-1201.

Nigam SK, Karnik AB, Majumder SK, Visweswariah K, Raju GS, Bai KM, et al. Serum hexachlorocyclohexane residues in workers engaged at a HCH manufacturing plant. Int Arch Occup Environ Health 1986;57(4):315-320.

Radomski JL, Astolfi E, Deichmann WB, Rey AA. Blood levels of organochlorine pesticides in Argentina: occupationally and nonoccupationally exposed adults, children and newborn infants. Toxicol Appl Pharmacol 1971;20(2):186-193.

Rogan WJ. Pollutants in breast milk. Arch Pediatr Adolesc Med 1996;150:981-990.

Saxena MC, Siddiqui MKJ, Bhargava AK, Krishna Murti CR, Kutty D. Placental transfer of pesticides in humans. Arch Toxicol 1981;48:127-134.

Stehr-Green, PA. Demographic and seasonal influences on human serum pesticide residue levels. J Toxicol Environ Health 1989;27:405-421.

Sturgeon SR, Brock JW, Potischman N, Needham LL, Rothman N, Brinton LA, et al. Serum concentrations of organochlorine compounds and endometrial cancer risk (United States). Cancer Causes and Control 1998;9(4):417-424.

# Mirex

CAS No. 2385-85-5

## General Information

Mirex has not been produced or used in the U.S. since 1977. Formerly, its major uses were as a flame retardant additive and as a pesticide to kill fire ants and yellow jackets in the southeastern U.S., where it was applied directly to soil and by aerial spraying. Mirex binds strongly to soil, where it has a half-life of 12 years; it is a highly persistent chemical in the environment. Mirex has been detected in air, soil, sediments, water, aquatic organisms, animals, and foods. Mirex contamination of Lake Ontario and adjacent waterways has been well documented (ATSDR, 1995). The most likely sources of human exposure to mirex are eating fish from contaminated water or living in areas with soil contaminated by historic mirex manufacturing, disposal,

or pesticide application. Some states and the U.S. EPA have issued public health advisories or warnings that fish from contaminated lakes and rivers may contain mirex. Occupational exposure is limited to workers at sites where mirex contamination is present.

Mirex is absorbed through the skin and from the gastrointestinal tract, after which it is widely distributed in the body and stored in fat. Ingested mirex that is not absorbed is eliminated in the feces within about 48 hours. Mirex is not metabolized in the body. In studies conducted in the 1970's and 1980's, mirex was detected in human adipose samples, especially those from persons living in the southeastern U.S. (Kutz et al., 1985, 1991). Mirex can cross the placenta and be excreted in breast milk, resulting in exposure to newborns and nursing infants.

Human health effects from mirex at low environmental doses or at biomonitored levels from low environmental

## Serum Mirex (lipid adjusted)

Geometric mean and selected percentiles of serum concentrations (in ng/g of lipid or parts per billion on a lipid-weight basis) for the U.S. population from the National Health and Nutrition Examination Survey.

| | Survey years | Geometric mean (95% conf. interval) | Selected percentiles ( 95% confidence interval) | | | | Sample size |
|---|---|---|---|---|---|---|---|
| | | | 50th | 75th | 90th | 95th | |
| Total | 99-00 | * | < LOD | < LOD | < LOD | < LOD | 1853 |
| | 01-02 | * | < LOD | < LOD | 15.8 (<LOD-73.7) | 57.1 (13.2-230) | 2257 |
| | 03-04 | * | < LOD | < LOD | 8.40 (<LOD-13.0) | 13.2 (7.90-29 6) | 1951 |
| **Age group** | | | | | | | |
| 12-19 years | 99-00 | * | < LOD | < LOD | < LOD | < LOD | 659 |
| | 01-02 | * | < LOD | < LOD | < LOD | < LOD | 728 |
| | 03-04 | * | < LOD | < LOD | < LOD | < LOD | 592 |
| 20 years and older | 99-00 | * | < LOD | < LOD | < LOD | < LOD | 1194 |
| | 01-02 | * | < LOD | < LOD | 19.6 (<LOD-108) | 71.0 (14.6-305) | 1529 |
| | 03-04 | * | < LOD | < LOD | 9.10 (<LOD-15.6) | 15.4 (8.10-37.1) | 1359 |
| **Gender** | | | | | | | |
| Males | 99-00 | * | < LOD | < LOD | < LOD | < LOD | 887 |
| | 01-02 | * | < LOD | < LOD | 16.1 (<LOD-65.6) | 50.8 (12.3-225) | 1052 |
| | 03-04 | * | < LOD | < LOD | 9.70 (<LOD-15.4) | 15.5 (9.70-24.4) | 949 |
| Females | 99-00 | * | < LOD | < LOD | < LOD | < LOD | 966 |
| | 01-02 | * | < LOD | < LOD | 15.0 (<LOD-108) | 63.0 (12.0-374) | 1205 |
| | 03-04 | * | < LOD | < LOD | < LOD | 11.6 (<LOD-31.3) | 1002 |
| **Race/ethnicity** | | | | | | | |
| Mexican Americans | 99-00 | * | < LOD | < LOD | < LOD | < LOD | 617 |
| | 01-02 | * | < LOD | < LOD | < LOD | < LOD | 548 |
| | 03-04 | * | < LOD | < LOD | < LOD | < LOD | 459 |
| Non-Hispanic blacks | 99-00 | * | < LOD | < LOD | 15.5 (<LOD-42.2) | 39.5 (<LOD-115) | 398 |
| | 01-02 | * | < LOD | 13.7 (<LOD-47.3) | 51.3 (15.4-230) | 153 (30.5-425) | 500 |
| | 03-04 | * | < LOD | < LOD | 18.1 (8.70-40.8) | 40.3 (15.5-82.7) | 484 |
| Non-Hispanic whites | 99-00 | * | < LOD | < LOD | < LOD | < LOD | 688 |
| | 01-02 | * | < LOD | < LOD | 15.1 (<LOD-104) | 66.7 (12.5-291) | 1049 |
| | 03-04 | * | < LOD | < LOD | < LOD | 11.6 (<LOD-23.4) | 884 |

Limit of detection (LOD, see Data Analysis section) for Survey years 99-00, 01-02, and 03-04 are 14 6, 10.5, and 7 8, respectively.
< LOD means less than the limit of detection, which may vary for some chemicals by year and by individual sample.
* Not calculated: proportion of results below limit of detection was too high to provide a valid result.

exposures are unknown. Laboratory animals fed high doses developed liver enlargement and liver tumors; reproductive toxicity included decreased fertility and testicular damage. In addition, developmental abnormalities including cataracts and edema in the offspring have been reported (ATSDR, 1995; Smith, 1991). The U.S. EPA has established environmental standards for mirex, and the FDA monitors foods for pesticide residue and has established an action level for mirex in fish tissue. IARC classifies mirex as possibly carcinogenic to humans, and NTP classifies mirex as reasonably anticipated to be a human carcinogen. More information about external exposure (i.e., environmental levels) and health effects is available from the ATSDR at: http://www.atsdr.cdc.gov/toxpro2.html.

## Biomonitoring Information

In the NHANES 1999-2000, 2001-2002, and 2003-2004 subsamples, as well as in a subsample of NHANES

II (1976-1980) participants, serum mirex levels were generally below the limits of detection (Stehr-Green, 1989). Fishermen in New York who consumed Great Lakes sport fish had median levels of lipid-adjusted serum mirex that were lower than the 95th percentile value among males the NHANES 2001-2002 subsample (Bloom et al., 2005). In samples obtained between 1994 and 1997, Inuit mothers from three Arctic areas had geometric mean serum mirex levels that were threefold to sevenfold higher than non-Inuit mother from other Arctic regions. The geometric mean mirex levels of the Inuit mothers were 8, 7.8, and 4.7 ng/g of lipid, which is approximately twofold to threefold lower than the 90th percentile for females in the NHANES 2001-2002 subsample but similar to 95th percentile for females in the NHANES 2003-2004 subsample (Van Oostdam et al., 2004).

Finding a measurable amount of mirex in serum does not mean that the level of mirex causes an adverse health

### Serum Mirex (whole weight)

Geometric mean and selected percentiles of serum concentrations (in ng/g of serum or parts per billion) for the U.S. population from the National Health and Nutrition Examination Survey.

| | Survey years | Geometric mean (95% conf. interval) | Selected percentiles (95% confidence interval) | | | | Sample size |
|---|---|---|---|---|---|---|---|
| | | | 50th | 75th | 90th | 95th | |
| **Total** | 99-00 | * | < LOD | < LOD | < LOD | < LOD | 1853 |
| | 01-02 | * | < LOD | < LOD | .100 (<LOD-.470) | .410 ( 080-1.73) | 2257 |
| | 03-04 | * | < LOD | < LOD | .054 (<LOD- 084) | .093 ( 052-.170) | 1951 |
| **Age group** | | | | | | | |
| 12-19 years | 99-00 | * | < LOD | < LOD | < LOD | < LOD | 659 |
| | 01-02 | * | < LOD | < LOD | < LOD | < LOD | 728 |
| | 03-04 | * | < LOD | < LOD | < LOD | < LOD | 592 |
| 20 years and older | 99-00 | * | < LOD | < LOD | < LOD | < LOD | 1194 |
| | 01-02 | * | < LOD | < LOD | .140 (<LOD- 690) | .470 ( 090-1.92) | 1529 |
| | 03-04 | * | < LOD | < LOD | .059 (<LOD-.102) | .106 ( 053-.215) | 1359 |
| **Gender** | | | | | | | |
| Males | 99-00 | * | < LOD | < LOD | < LOD | < LOD | 887 |
| | 01-02 | * | < LOD | < LOD | .110 (<LOD-.470) | .370 ( 090-1.37) | 1052 |
| | 03-04 | * | < LOD | < LOD | .064 (<LOD-.106) | .108 ( 062-.170) | 949 |
| Females | 99-00 | * | < LOD | < LOD | < LOD | < LOD | 966 |
| | 01-02 | * | < LOD | < LOD | .090 (<LOD- 510) | .430 ( 070-1.79) | 1205 |
| | 03-04 | * | < LOD | < LOD | < LOD | .077 (<LOD-.170) | 1002 |
| **Race/ethnicity** | | | | | | | |
| Mexican Americans | 99-00 | * | < LOD | < LOD | < LOD | < LOD | 617 |
| | 01-02 | * | < LOD | < LOD | < LOD | < LOD | 548 |
| | 03-04 | * | < LOD | < LOD | < LOD | < LOD | 459 |
| Non-Hispanic blacks | 99-00 | * | < LOD | < LOD | .090 (<LOD-.220) | .220 (<LOD-.450) | 398 |
| | 01-02 | * | < LOD | .090 (<LOD- 240) | .310 (.090-1.41) | 1.08 (.170-3.02) | 500 |
| | 03-04 | * | < LOD | < LOD | .112 (.055-.268) | .256 ( 089-.635) | 484 |
| Non-Hispanic whites | 99-00 | * | < LOD | < LOD | < LOD | < LOD | 688 |
| | 01-02 | * | < LOD | < LOD | .100 (<LOD- 610) | .450 ( 080-1.79) | 1049 |
| | 03-04 | * | < LOD | < LOD | < LOD | .079 (<LOD-.174) | 884 |

< LOD means less than the limit of detection for the lipid adjusted serum level, which may vary for some chemicals by year and by individual sample.
* Not calculated: proportion of results below limit of detection was too high to provide a valid result.

effect. Biomonitoring studies on levels of mirex provide physicians and public health officials with reference values so that they can determine whether people have been exposed to higher levels of mirex than are found in the general population. Biomonitoring data can also help scientists plan and conduct research on exposure and health effects.

## References

Agency for Toxic Substances and Disease Registry (ATSDR). Toxicological profile for mirex and chlordecone [online]. August 1995. Available at URL: http://www.atsdr.cdc.gov/toxprofiles/tp66 html. 4/21/09

Bloom MS, Vena JE, Swanson MK, Moysich KB, Olson JR. Profiles of ortho-polychlorinated biphenyl congeners, dichlorodiphenyldichloroethylene, hexachlorobenzene, and Mirex among male Lake Ontario sportfish consumers: the New York State Angler cohort study. Environ Res 2005;97(2):178-192.

Kutz FW, Strassman SC, Stroup CR, Carra JS, Leininger CC, Watts DL, et al. The human body burden of mirex in the southeastern United States. J Toxicol Environ Health 1985;15:385-394.

Kutz FW, Wood PH, Bottimore DP. Organochlorine pesticides and polychlorinated biphenyls in human adipose tissue. Rev Environ Contam Toxicol 1991;120:1-82.

Smith AG. Chlorinated Hydrocarbon Insecticides. In Hayes WJ, Jr and Laws ER, Jr, Eds. Handbook of Pesticide Toxicology, Vol. 2 Classes of Pesticides. New York, Academic Press, Inc. 1991 pp. 731-915.

Stehr-Green, PA. Demographic and seasonal influences on human serum pesticide residue levels. J Toxicol Environ Health 1989;27:405-421.

Van Oostdam JC, Dewailly E, Gilman A, Hansen JC, Odland JO, Chashchin V, et al. Circumpolar maternal blood contaminant survey, 1994-1997 organochlorine compounds. Sci Total Environ 2004;330:55-70.

# 2,4,5-Trichlorophenol
CAS No. 95-95-4

# 2,4,6-Trichlorophenol
CAS No. 88-06-2

*Metabolites of Organochlorine Pesticides and Other Environmental Chemicals*

## General Information

The chlorophenols, 2,4,5-trichlorophenol (2,4,5-TCP) and 2,4,6-trichlorophenol (2,4,6-TCP), are metabolites of several organochlorine chemicals, including hexachlorobenzene and hexachlorocyclohexanes. Historically, 2,4,5-TCP and 2,4,6-TCP were used as intermediates in the production of certain pesticides; 2,4,6-TCP was also used as a wood preservative and may still be used in production of some fungicides (ATSDR, 1999). Trichlorophenols are no longer manufactured commercially, but they may be produced as by-products during manufacturing of other chlorinated aromatic compounds. Formation of

2,3,7,8-tetrachlorodibenzo-*p*-dioxin occurs during the synthesis of 2,4,5-trichlorophenol. Small amounts of trichlorophenols also can be produced during combustion of natural materials and the chlorination of drinking water or waste water that contains phenols. Environmental sources of these compounds include industrial discharges or run off from pesticide facilities or disposal sites. Both chemicals have been detected in air, surface water, soils, and sediments; however, recent sampling of U.S. public drinking water systems did not detect 2,4,6-TCP in any of the samples (U.S. EPA, 2006). Trichlorophenols have been detected in fish taken from waters near waste water treatment and industrial discharges (ATSDR, 1999).

General population exposure may occur by ingesting contaminated food or water and by inhaling contaminated air. Exposure to trichlorophenols also may result from metabolism of lindane, hexachlorobenzene, other organochlorines, and polychlorinated benzenes (Kohil et al., 1976). Occupational exposures, usually at herbicide production or waste incineration facilities, may occur by inhalation or dermal routes. Such workers would probably

## Urinary 2,4,5-Trichlorophenol
*Metabolite of Several Organochlorine Insecticides*
Geometric mean and selected percentiles of urine concentrations (in µg/L) for the U.S. population from the National Health and Nutrition Examination Survey.

| | Survey years | Geometric mean (95% conf. interval) | 50th | 75th | 90th | 95th | Sample size |
|---|---|---|---|---|---|---|---|
| **Total** | 99-00 | * | < LOD | 1.40 (1.00-3.20) | 5.40 (2.50-16 0) | 16.0 (4.30-40 0) | 1994 |
| | 01-02 | * | < LOD | < LOD | < LOD | 2.42 (<LOD-8.27) | 2497 |
| **Age group** | | | | | | | |
| 6-11 years | 99-00 | * | < LOD | 1.40 (1.10-3.40) | 4.80 (2.30-11 0) | 11.0 (4.20-36 0) | 482 |
| | 01-02 | * | < LOD | < LOD | < LOD | 2.42 (<LOD-12.7) | 570 |
| 12-19 years | 99-00 | * | < LOD | 1.60 ( 940-3.72) | 5.40 (2.50-25 0) | 24.0 (3.80-41 0) | 681 |
| | 01-02 | * | < LOD | < LOD | < LOD | 2.19 (<LOD-6.63) | 815 |
| 20-59 years | 99-00 | * | < LOD | 1.40 ( 980-3.30) | 5.40 (2.40-18 0) | 18.0 (4.30-44 0) | 831 |
| | 01-02 | * | < LOD | < LOD | < LOD | 2.71 (<LOD-8.27) | 1112 |
| **Gender** | | | | | | | |
| Males | 99-00 | * | < LOD | 1.40 ( 980-3.80) | 5.40 (2.60-8.40) | 11.0 (5.30-27 0) | 973 |
| | 01-02 | * | < LOD | < LOD | < LOD | 5.57 (<LOD-15.8) | 1178 |
| Females | 99-00 | * | < LOD | 1.50 (1.00-3.20) | 6.50 (2.30-27 0) | 21.0 (3.20-71 0) | 1021 |
| | 01-02 | * | < LOD | < LOD | < LOD | < LOD | 1319 |
| **Race/ethnicity** | | | | | | | |
| Mexican Americans | 99-00 | * | .950 (<LOD-1.30) | 1.80 (1.30-3.50) | 8.60 (4.60-18 0) | 21.0 (8.90-33 0) | 696 |
| | 01-02 | * | < LOD | < LOD | < LOD | 14.9 (<LOD-121) | 661 |
| Non-Hispanic blacks | 99-00 | * | < LOD | 1.30 ( 900-2.20) | 5.00 (2.00-8.40) | 9.00 (3.50-63 0) | 521 |
| | 01-02 | * | < LOD | < LOD | < LOD | 2.31 (<LOD-9.03) | 696 |
| Non-Hispanic whites | 99-00 | * | < LOD | 1.50 ( 920-3.60) | 4.60 (2.40-11 0) | 9.20 (4.30-27 0) | 603 |
| | 01-02 | * | < LOD | < LOD | < LOD | 2.71 (<LOD-8.27) | 939 |

Limit of detection (LOD, see Data Analysis section) for Survey years 99-00 and 01-02 are 0.9 and 0 9.
< LOD means less than the limit of detection, which may vary for some chemicals by year and by individual sample.
* Not calculated: proportion of results below limit of detection was too high to provide a valid result.

be exposed to mixtures of chlorophenols, in addition to dioxins, furans, and other chlorinated compounds. However, recent small studies have not demonstrated increased exposure to trichlorophenols in workers who dredged contaminated soils or incinerated waste materials (Agramunt et al., 2003; Radon et al., 2004).

Human health effects from 2,4,5-TCP or 2,4,6-TCP at low environmental doses or at biomonitored levels from low environmental exposures are unknown. Laboratory animals chronically fed high doses of 2,4,6-TCP had increased rates of hepatic tumors, leukemias, and lymphomas. At lower doses, animals showed hepatocellular abnormalities. Neither 2,4,5-TCP nor 2,4,6-TCP were developmental or reproductive toxicants in animals (ATSDR 1999). IARC classifies combined exposures to polychlorophenols, which includes trichlorophenols, as being possibly carcinogenic to humans. IARC considers the experimental evidence for animal carcinogenicity inadequate for 2,4,5-TCP and limited for 2,4,6-TCP. NTP classifies 2,4,6-TCP as reasonably anticipated to be a human carcinogen. More information about external exposure (i.e., environmental levels) and health effects is available from ATSDR at:

http://www.atsdr.cdc.gov/toxpro2.html.

## Biomonitoring Information

In the NHANES 1999-2000 and 2001-2002 subsamples, urinary 2,4,6-TCP levels at the 95th percentile were up to eight times higher than 3.3 µg/L in a nonrandom subsample from NHANES III (Hill et al., 1995) and up to 19 times higher than the 95th percentile value of 1.3 µg/L reported in German adults aged 18-69 years (Becker et al., 2003). Among 6-11 year old children in NHANES 1999-2000, the 95th percentile urinary 2,4,6-TCP level was approximately eight times higher than the corresponding percentile in a small group of 2-6 year old children living near an herbicide manufacturing facility: 33 versus 4 µg/L (Hill et al., 1989). In the same 2-6 year old children, the 95th percentile urinary 2,4,5-TCP, 7.0 µg/L, was similar to the corresponding percentile for 6-11 year olds in NHANES 1999-2000 (Hill et al., 1989). The 95th percentiles for 2,4,5-TCP among adults in this *Report* and in a nonrandom subsample from NHANES III (Hill et al., 1995) were similar, but almost twenty times higher than 95th percentile values reported in German adults aged 18-69 years (Becker et al., 2003).

## Urinary 2,4,5-Trichlorophenol (creatinine corrected)
*Metabolite of Several Organochlorine Insecticides*
Geometric mean and selected percentiles of urine concentrations (in µg/g of creatinine) for the U.S. population from the National Health and Nutrition Examination Survey.

| | Survey years | Geometric mean (95% conf. interval) | Selected percentiles ( 95% confidence interval) | | | | Sample size |
|---|---|---|---|---|---|---|---|
| | | | 50th | 75th | 90th | 95th | |
| Total | 99-00 | * | < LOD | 2.36 (1.53-3.16) | 5.57 (3.24-11.2) | 11.9 (5.00-19.6) | 1994 |
| | 01-02 | * | < LOD | < LOD | < LOD | 4.57 (<LOD-7.11) | 2496 |
| **Age group** | | | | | | | |
| 6-11 years | 99-00 | * | < LOD | 2.29 (1.19-4.78) | 5.86 (3.83-12.4) | 12.8 (5.28-25.4) | 482 |
| | 01-02 | * | < LOD | < LOD | < LOD | 5.82 (<LOD-32.5) | 570 |
| 12-19 years | 99-00 | * | < LOD | 1.44 (.920-2 50) | 3.80 (1.93-11.2) | 11.2 (2.62-20.1) | 681 |
| | 01-02 | * | < LOD | < LOD | < LOD | 2.75 (<LOD-6.74) | 814 |
| 20-59 years | 99-00 | * | < LOD | 2.46 (1.60-3 24) | 5.75 (3.37-11.5) | 11.7 (4.78-19.6) | 831 |
| | 01-02 | * | < LOD | < LOD | < LOD | 4.57 (<LOD-7.11) | 1112 |
| **Gender** | | | | | | | |
| Males | 99-00 | * | < LOD | 1.67 (1.02-3.15) | 4.24 (3.05-8 02) | 9.55 (4.13-13.6) | 973 |
| | 01-02 | * | < LOD | < LOD | < LOD | 4.68 (<LOD-8.37) | 1178 |
| Females | 99-00 | * | < LOD | 2.67 (1.79-4 00) | 7.95 (3.05-17.8) | 16.3 (5.00-29.3) | 1021 |
| | 01-02 | * | < LOD | < LOD | < LOD | < LOD | 1318 |
| **Race/ethnicity** | | | | | | | |
| Mexican Americans | 99-00 | * | .980 (<LOD-1.33) | 2.49 (1.68-4 24) | 6.90 (4.19-12.4) | 12.4 (6.88-16.9) | 696 |
| | 01-02 | * | < LOD | < LOD | < LOD | 12.1 (<LOD-58.0) | 661 |
| Non-Hispanic blacks | 99-00 | * | < LOD | 1.16 (.820-2 31) | 3.43 (2.20-6 32) | 7.69 (2.69-18.2) | 521 |
| | 01-02 | * | < LOD | < LOD | < LOD | 2.81 (<LOD-9.17) | 695 |
| Non-Hispanic whites | 99-00 | * | < LOD | 2.44 (1.53-3 24) | 4.78 (3.47-8.43) | 9.64 (4.27-17.8) | 603 |
| | 01-02 | * | < LOD | < LOD | < LOD | 4.73 (<LOD-8.37) | 939 |

< LOD means less than the limit of detection for the urine levels not corrected for creatinine.
* Not calculated: proportion of results below limit of detection was too high to provide a valid result.

A small study of adults who ate Great Lakes sport fish reported a mean urine 2,4,5-TCP level of 0.7 µg/L, similar to the limit of detection for this *Report* (Anderson et al., 1998). Urinary 2,4,5-TCP and 2,4,6-TCP were monitored in a group of hazardous waste incinerator workers from 1999-2002. Mean values of 2,4,5-TCP (0.2-0.6 µg/g creatinine) and 2,4,6-TCP (0.7-3.5 µg/g creatinine) were similar to the limit of detection for 2,4,5-TCP and to the median 2,4,6-TCP values, respectively, for males in NHANES 1999-2002 (Agramunt et al., 2003). In harbor workers exposed to chlorophenol-contaminated river silt, the median urinary 2,4,6-TCP level, 0.36 µg/g creatinine, was about six times lower than the median urinary levels for males in this *Report* (Radon et al., 2004). Sawmill workers exposed to chlorophenol wood preservatives had urinary 2,4,6-TCP levels that were as much as 450 times higher than the median level among adults in the NHANES 1999-2000 subsample (Pekari et al., 1991).

Finding a measurable amount of 2,4,5-TCP or 2,4,6-TCP in urine does not mean that the level of 2,4,5-TCP or 2,4,6-TCP causes an adverse health effect. Biomonitoring studies on levels of 2,4,5-TCP and 2,4,6-TCP provide physicians and public health officials with reference values so that they can determine whether people have been exposed to higher levels of 2,4,5-TCP or 2,4,6-TCP than are found in the general population. Biomonitoring data will also help scientists plan and conduct research about 2,4,5-TCP or 2,4,6-TCP exposure and health effects.

## Urinary 2,4,6-Trichlorophenol
*Metabolite of Several Organochlorine Insecticides*
Geometric mean and selected percentiles of urine concentrations (in µg/L) for the U.S. population from the National Health and Nutrition Examination Survey.

| | Survey years | Geometric mean (95% conf. interval) | 50th | 75th | 90th | 95th | Sample size |
|---|---|---|---|---|---|---|---|
| **Total** | 99-00 | 2.85 (2.55-3.18) | 2.50 (2.40-2.70) | 4.90 (3.80-7.70) | 15.0 (7.80-25 0) | 25.0 (15.0-44 0) | 1989 |
| | 01-02 | * | 1.68 (<LOD-2.44) | 5.95 (4.89-6.63) | 10.8 (9.98-11.7) | 14.9 (13.4-17 9) | 2503 |
| **Age group** | | | | | | | |
| 6-11 years | 99-00 | 4.47 (3.36-5.95) | 3.80 (2.70-6.40) | 11.0 (4.80-20 0) | 24.0 (14.0-38 0) | 33.0 (20.5-46 0) | 481 |
| | 01-02 | 3.08 (2.52-3.76) | 3.00 (1.91-4.32) | 7.79 (5.73-9.99) | 13.4 (10.6-17 3) | 19.2 (14.1-25 3) | 574 |
| 12-19 years | 99-00 | 3.56 (3.00-4.23) | 3.00 (2.60-3.70) | 6.00 (4.30-11 0) | 20.4 (9.60-37 0) | 37.0 (20.0-54 0) | 678 |
| | 01-02 | 3.24 (2.74-3.84) | 3.26 (2.33-4.40) | 7.49 (6.45-9.40) | 13.6 (11.0-18 2) | 19.4 (17.3-26 6) | 820 |
| 20-59 years | 99-00 | 2.52 (2.23-2.85) | 2.40 (2.10-2.45) | 4.20 (3.50-5.30) | 12.0 (6.00-21 0) | 21.0 (11.0-41 0) | 830 |
| | 01-02 | * | < LOD | 4.89 (3.70-6.28) | 9.66 (8.72-10.7) | 13.3 (11.8-15 2) | 1109 |
| **Gender** | | | | | | | |
| Males | 99-00 | 2.92 (2.58-3.31) | 2.60 (2.40-2.90) | 5.20 (3.90-8.10) | 15.0 (8.48-26 0) | 26.0 (15.0-38 0) | 970 |
| | 01-02 | * | 2.36 (1.70-3.04) | 6.65 (5.98-7.53) | 12.1 (10.8-13.1) | 17.0 (13.6-22 2) | 1178 |
| Females | 99-00 | 2.78 (2.35-3.28) | 2.40 (2.30-2.60) | 4.80 (3.40-7.59) | 16.0 (6.40-32 0) | 25.0 (14.0-50 0) | 1019 |
| | 01-02 | * | < LOD | 4.69 (3.59-6.09) | 9.75 (8.25-11 6) | 13.3 (11.7-16 6) | 1325 |
| **Race/ethnicity** | | | | | | | |
| Mexican Americans | 99-00 | 2.70 (2.20-3.32) | 2.70 (2.10-3.10) | 4.90 (4.20-6.70) | 15.0 (8.20-23 0) | 23.0 (14.0-43 0) | 694 |
| | 01-02 | * | 2.07 (<LOD-3.23) | 5.31 (3.95-6.54) | 11.4 (8.51-12 8) | 15.6 (12.6-19 8) | 677 |
| Non-Hispanic blacks | 99-00 | 3.14 (2.40-4.12) | 2.80 (2.10-3.40) | 6.60 (3.40-14 0) | 18.0 (9.30-33 0) | 32.0 (16.0-68 0) | 519 |
| | 01-02 | 2.78 (2.18-3.53) | 2.58 (1.32-4.02) | 6.45 (5.09-7.67) | 11.1 (8.87-14 9) | 17.9 (11.8-24.7) | 696 |
| Non-Hispanic whites | 99-00 | 2.74 (2.46-3.06) | 2.45 (2.30-2.80) | 4.60 (3.80-6.60) | 13.0 (6.60-21 0) | 21.0 (12.0-37 0) | 602 |
| | 01-02 | * | 1.57 (<LOD-2.20) | 6.10 (5.01-6.65) | 10.7 (9.67-12 3) | 14.7 (13.3-17 9) | 931 |

Limit of detection (LOD, see Data Analysis section) for Survey years 99-00 and 01-02 are 1.0 and 1 3.
< LOD means less than the limit of detection, which may vary for some chemicals by year and by individual sample.
* Not calculated: proportion of results below limit of detection was too high to provide a valid result.

## Urinary 2,4,6-Trichlorophenol (creatinine corrected)

*Metabolite of Several Organochlorine Insecticides*

Geometric mean and selected percentiles of urine concentrations (in µg/g of creatinine) for the U.S. population from the National Health and Nutrition Examination Survey.

| | Survey years | Geometric mean (95% conf. interval) | Selected percentiles ( 95% confidence interval) | | | | Sample size |
|---|---|---|---|---|---|---|---|
| | | | 50th | 75th | 90th | 95th | |
| **Total** | 99-00 | 2.54 (2.30-2 81) | 2.38 (2.14-2 68) | 4.91 (3.83-6.49) | 12.1 (8.67-17.0) | 21.2 (13.6-31.5) | 1989 |
| | 01-02 | * | 2.43 (<LOD-2.75) | 4.38 (4.18-4.78) | 8.33 (7.10-9 26) | 11.6 (9.25-15.6) | 2502 |
| **Age group** | | | | | | | |
| 6-11 years | 99-00 | 4.82 (3.87-6 00) | 4.71 (3.41-6 53) | 11.5 (7.63-15.3) | 22.7 (14.1-32.6) | 32.6 (22.7-36.8) | 481 |
| | 01-02 | 4.00 (3.28-4 87) | 4.01 (3.29-4 81) | 8.26 (6.16-10.4) | 13.9 (9.51-21.5) | 21.2 (12.9-64.1) | 574 |
| 12-19 years | 99-00 | 2.40 (2.08-2.78) | 2.33 (1.95-2 68) | 4.35 (3.13-6 00) | 11.6 (6.94-13.6) | 14.4 (11.3-23.6) | 678 |
| | 01-02 | 2.51 (2.18-2 90) | 2.78 (2.09-3.17) | 4.52 (3.83-5 92) | 8.29 (6.81-9 89) | 12.5 (8.73-22.8) | 819 |
| 20-59 years | 99-00 | 2.32 (2.04-2 63) | 2.22 (1.89-2 56) | 4.25 (3.38-5 63) | 10.0 (6.72-16.9) | 19.6 (10.9-34.4) | 830 |
| | 01-02 | * | < LOD | 4.05 (3.66-4 38) | 7.10 (6.43-7.72) | 9.82 (8.53-11.9) | 1109 |
| **Gender** | | | | | | | |
| Males | 99-00 | 2.24 (1.99-2 53) | 2.15 (1.82-2.42) | 4.41 (3.56-5 88) | 10.8 (7.04-16.4) | 18.0 (11.5-28.5) | 970 |
| | 01-02 | * | 2.23 (1.91-2 65) | 4.22 (3.77-4.73) | 8.05 (6.70-9.17) | 12.2 (8.79-17.7) | 1178 |
| Females | 99-00 | 2.88 (2.49-3 33) | 2.63 (2.25-2 96) | 5.53 (3.88-7 23) | 13.3 (9.65-21.9) | 25.1 (13.3-37.0) | 1019 |
| | 01-02 | * | < LOD | 4.58 (4.19-5.11) | 8.40 (7.27-9 51) | 10.9 (9.26-13.6) | 1324 |
| **Race/ethnicity** | | | | | | | |
| Mexican Americans | 99-00 | 2.43 (2.06-2 87) | 2.50 (2.22-2 82) | 5.44 (3.87-7.10) | 10.8 (8.46-14.9) | 18.4 (12.1-21.8) | 694 |
| | 01-02 | * | 2.22 (<LOD-2.88) | 4.25 (3.47-5.76) | 8.15 (6.21-11.1) | 11.6 (9.63-13.9) | 677 |
| Non-Hispanic blacks | 99-00 | 2.13 (1.65-2.76) | 1.90 (1.60-2 52) | 4.00 (2.76-8 02) | 11.6 (5.32-19.7) | 19.5 (10.9-29.5) | 519 |
| | 01-02 | 1.98 (1.55-2 52) | 2.02 (1.48-2.76) | 3.83 (3.17-4 88) | 6.52 (5.50-8 06) | 9.91 (7.14-13.2) | 695 |
| Non-Hispanic whites | 99-00 | 2.59 (2.33-2 88) | 2.42 (2.20-2.77) | 4.87 (3.83-6 06) | 11.2 (7.62-15.5) | 19.6 (12.9-32.8) | 602 |
| | 01-02 | * | 2.63 (<LOD-2.88) | 4.60 (4.29-4 98) | 8.56 (7.22-9 65) | 12.0 (9.25-17.1) | 931 |

< LOD means less than the limit of detection for the urine levels not corrected for creatinine.
* Not calculated: proportion of results below limit of detection was too high to provide a valid result.

## References

Agency for Toxic Substances and Disease Registry (ATSDR). Toxicological profile for chlorophenols [online]. July 1999. Available at URL: http://www.atsdr.cdc.gov/toxprofiles/tp107.html. 4/21/09

Agramunt MC, Domingo A, Domingo JL, Corbella J. Monitoring internal exposure to metals and organic substances in workers at a hazardous waste incinerator after 3 years of operation. Toxicol Lett 2003;146:83-91.

Anderson HA, Falk C, Hanrahan L, Olson J, Burse VW, Needham LL, et al. Profiles of Great Lakes critical pollutants: a sentinel analysis of human blood and urine. The Great Lakes Consortium. Environ Health Perspect 1998;106(5):279-289.

Becker K, Schulz C, Kaus S, Seiwert M, Seifert B. German environmental survey 1998 (GerES III): environmental pollutants in the urine of the German population. Int J Hyg Environ Health 2003; 206:15-24.

Hill RH Jr, Head SL, Baker S, Gregg M, Shealy DB, Bailey SL, et al. Pesticide residues in urine of adults living in the United States: reference range concentrations. Environ Res 1995;71:99-108.

Hill RH Jr, To T, Holler JS, Fast DM, Smith SJ, Needham LL, et al. Residues of chlorinated phenols and phenoxy acid herbicides in the urine of Arkansas children. Arch Environ Contam Toxicol 1989;18(4):469-474.

Kohli J, Jones D, Safe A. The metabolism of higher chlorinated benzene isomers. Can J Biochem 1976;54(3):203-208.

Pekari K, Luotamo M, Jarvisalo J, Lindroos L, Aitio A. Urinary excretion of chlorinated phenols in saw-mill workers. Int Arch Occup Environ Health 1991;63:57-62.

Radon K, Wegner R, Heinrich-Ramm R, Baur X, Poschadel B, Szadkowski D. Chlorophenol exposure in harbor workers exposed to river silt aerosols. Am J Ind Med 2004;45:440-445.

U. S. Environmental Protection Agency (U.S.EPA). The analysis of occurrence data from the first unregulated contaminant monitoring regulation (UCMR 1) in support of regulatory determinations for the second drinking water contaminant candidate list [online]. December 2006 Draft. Available at URL: http://www.epa.gov/safewater/ccl/pdfs/reg_determine2/report_ccl2-reg2_ucmr1_occurrencereport.pdf. 5/19/09

# Organophosphorus Insecticides: Dialkyl Phosphate Metabolites

## General Information

Organophosphorus insecticides, which are active against a broad spectrum of insects, have accounted for a large share of all insecticides used in the United States. Although organophosphorus insecticides are still used for insect control on many food crops, most residential uses have been phased out in the United States as a result of implementation of the Food Quality Protection Act of 1996. Certain organophosphorus insecticides (e.g., malathion, naled) are also registered for public health applications (e.g., mosquito control) in the United States. An estimated 73 million pounds of organophosphorus insecticides (70% of all insecticides) were used in the United States in 2001, with usage declining 45% since 1980 (U.S. EPA, 2004). Approximately 40 organophosphorus insecticides in a wide variety of formulations are registered for use in the United States by the U.S. EPA. In general, the various organophosphorus insecticides demonstrate low vapor pressures (with some exceptions), slight to moderate water solubility, moderate to high soil binding, widely varying degrees of soil leaching or runoff potential, and a low persistence in the environment.

General population exposure to organophosphorus insecticides may occur by ingesting contaminated food and from hand-to-mouth contact with surfaces containing organophosphorus insecticides; less common routes include inhalation and dermal contact. In general, the organophosphorus insecticides have better gastrointestinal than dermal absorption. Mammalian elimination half-lives can range from hours to weeks. The thiophosphate type organophosphorus insecticides (e.g., chlorpyriphos) are initially metabolized to the more toxic "oxon" form. Most organophosphorus insecticides undergo hydrolysis with excretion of major hydrolytic metabolites in the urine. Estimated intakes by the general population are usually considered below regulatory thresholds though concerns have been raised about some organophosphrus insecticides because of unique routes of exposures and intakes in infants and children (NRC, 1993). Farm workers, gardeners, florists, pesticide applicators, and manufacturers of these insecticides may have greater exposure than the general population. Many states have programs to monitor

| Pesticide (CAS number) | Dimethyl-phosphate (813-79-5) | Dimethylthio-phosphate (1112-38-5) | Dimethyldithio-phosphate (756-80-9) | Diethyl-phosphate (598-02-7) | Diethylthio-phosphate (2465-65-8) | Diethyldithio-phosphate (298-06-6) |
|---|---|---|---|---|---|---|
| Azinphos methyl | • | • | • | | | |
| Chlorethoxyphos | | | | • | • | |
| Chlorpyrifos | | | | • | • | |
| Chlorpyrifos methyl | • | • | | | | |
| Coumaphos | | | | • | • | |
| Dichlorvos (DDVP) | • | | | | | |
| Diazinon | | | | • | • | |
| Dicrotophos | • | | | | | |
| Dimethoate | • | • | • | | | |
| Disulfoton | | | | • | • | • |
| Ethion | | | | • | • | • |
| Fenitrothion | • | • | | | | |
| Fenthion | • | • | | | | |
| Isazaphos-methyl | • | • | | | | |
| Malathion | • | • | • | | | |
| Methidathion | • | • | • | | | |
| Methyl parathion | • | • | | | | |
| Naled | • | | | | | |
| Oxydemeton-methyl | • | • | | | | |
| Parathion | | | | • | • | |
| Phorate | | | | • | • | • |
| Phosmet | • | • | • | | | |
| Pirimiphos-methyl | • | • | | | | |
| Sulfotepp | | | | • | • | |
| Temephos | • | • | | | | |
| Terbufos | | | | • | • | • |
| Tetrachlorvinphos | • | | | | | |

cholinesterase activity in the blood of pesticide applicators as part of monitoring exposure to organophosphorus insecticides. The U.S. FDA, USDA, U.S. EPA, and OSHA have developed criteria on allowable levels of these chemicals in foods, the environment, and the workplace.

The acute high dose effects of the organophosphorus insecticides from intentional and unintentional overdoses or from high-dose worker exposures are well known and include neurological dysfunction that results from the inhibition of the enzyme acetylcholinesterase leading to excess acetylcholine in the central and peripheral nervous systems. Acute symptoms include nausea, vomiting, cholinergic effects, weakness, paralysis, and seizures. Mild to severe peripheral neuropathies and residual deficits in neurocognitive functioning can persist following acute poisonings (London et al., 1998; Rosenstock et al., 1991; Savage et al., 1988). Chronic exposures studied in farmers and insecticide applicators, who have neither past acute poisoning or significant reduction in blood cholinesterase activity, have shown possible subtle or subclinical neurological effects, though various study results are inconsistent (Albers et al., 2004; Daniell et al., 1992.; Engel et al., 1998; Farahat et al., 2003; Fiedler et al., 1997; Jamal et al., 2002; Maizlish et al., 1987; Peiris-John et al., 2002; Pilkington et al., 2001; Rodnitzky et al., 1975; Rothlein et al., 2006; Stephens et al., 1995; Stokes et al., 1995; Young et al., 2005). Animal studies at high doses generally demonstrate the effects of inhibition of acetylcholinesterase mentioned above for acute poisoning in humans, as well as mechanistically-related neurodevelopmental and reproductive effects (Astroff et al., 1998a and 1998b; Prendergast et al., 1998). Few animal studies have addressed the potential for low environmental doses to produce non-cholinergic effects (i.e., without inhibition of acetylcholinesterase). Additional information about insecticides is available from U.S. EPA at: http://www.epa.gov/pesticides/ and from ATSDR at: http://www.atsdr.cdc.gov/toxpro2.html.

About 75% of registered organophosphorus insecticides are metabolized in the body to measurable dialkyl phosphate metabolites. The dialkyl phosphate metabolites do not inhibit acetylcholinesterase and are not considered toxic, but are regarded as markers of exposure to organophosphorus insecticides. Dialkyl phosphate metabolites can be present in urine after low level exposures to organophosphorus insecticides that do not cause clinical symptoms or inhibition of cholinesterase activity (Davies and Peterson, 1997; Franklin et al., 1981). Measurement of these metabolites reflects recent exposure, predominantly in the previous few days. Dialkyl phosphates may also occur in the environment as a result of degradation of organophosphorus insecticides

(Lu et al., 2005), and therefore, the presence in a person's urine may reflect exposure to the metabolite itself.

Generally, six urinary dialkyl phosphate metabolites of organophosphorus insecticides are measured in this *Report* and other research studies: dimethylphosphate (DMP); dimethylthiophosphate (DMTP); dimethyldithiophosphate (DMDTP); diethylphosphate (DEP); diethylthiophosphate (DETP); and diethyldithiophosphate (DEDTP). The table shows the six urinary metabolites and the parent organophosphorus insecticides responsible for these metabolites. For example, chlorpyrifos is metabolized to both diethylphosphate and diethythiophosphate. Each of the six urinary dialkyl phosphate metabolites can be produced from the metabolism of more than one organophosphorus insecticide. Therefore, the presence of one or more dialkyl phosphate metabolites without additional information cannot be linked to exposure to a specific organophosphorus insecticide.

**Biomonitoring Information**

Urinary dialkyl phosphate levels reflect recent exposure. In nationally representative subsamples of the U.S. population from NHANES 1999-2000 and 2001-2002 (CDC, 2005), geometric mean urinary dialkyl phosphate levels were generally lower than levels reported in smaller studies of children and adults in Italy and Germany (Aprea et al., 2000; Aprea et al., 1996; Heudorf and Angerer, 2001; Saieva et al., 2004). In these studies and the NHANES subsamples, children have slightly higher levels than adults. Diet influences the measured levels of urinary dialkyl phosphates. For example, subjects ingesting "organically-grown" foods were shown to have lower levels of urinary dialkyl phosphates than subjects eating a conventional diet (Curl et al., 2003). Also, urinary levels in children of farm workers and non-farm workers have been reported to correlate weakly with environmental dust levels of particular insecticides in some, but not all, studies (Bouvier et al., 2006; Curl et al., 2003; Rothlein et al., 2006).

Measurements of dialkyl phosphates in urine have been used to document exposure of farmers, agricultural workers, pest-control workers, and others to organophosphorus insecticides (Davies and Peterson, 1997; Franklin et al., 1981; Krieger and Dinoff, 2000; Takamiya, 1994). In some of these occupational studies, reported levels of urinary dialkyl phosphates may exceed levels seen in the general population by up to fiftyfold, though in general, worker levels are only moderately higher. Urinary levels of dialkyl phosphate metabolites vary with the type of field application, seasonal use of the parent insecticide, and demonstrate substantial variability when measured over multiple times of day and over multiple days, which may reflect changes in exposure, collection timing, and elimination kinetics (Kissel et al., 2005; Koch et al., 2002; Lambert et al., 2005; Petchuay et al., 2006).

Children and pregnant family members of farm workers were reported to have median levels of many urinary dialkyl phosphates that were either similar or slightly higher (Arcury et al., 2006; Bradman et al., 2005) than those presented in U.S. representative subsamples from NHANES 1999-2000 and 2001-2002 (CDC, 2005), except for one study in which DMTP levels were up to fourteenfold higher depending on the season and the type of crop application (Lambert et al., 2005). Also, estimates of dose or intake calculated from urinary dialkyl phosphate levels in studies of pregnant women in one agricultural community (Castorina et al., 2003) and in another study of workers exposed on reentry to treated orchards (Fenske et al., 2003) generally did not exceed doses considered to be safe. Estimates of dose or intake for the general U.S. population as calculated from urinary dialkyl phosphate measurements were below environmental dose estimates based on multiple routes of exposure (Duggan et al., 2003).

Information is limited with regard to associations between levels of urinary dialkyl phosphates and any health effects. Summed levels of urinary dialkyl phosphates in prenatal samples from mothers of neonates living in an agricultural community were associated with subtle changes in one of seven domains of neurophysiologic neonatal testing during one restricted postnatal period of time (Young et al., 2005). In a study of farm workers, median urinary levels of DMTP and DMDTP were more than twentyfold higher than median levels in the U.S. population (CDC, 2005), and these higher levels were associated with a few subtle neurobehavioral test results (Rothlein et al., 2006).

Finding a measurable amount of dialkyl phosphate metabolites in urine does not mean that the level of dialkyl phosphate metabolites causes an adverse health effect. Biomonitoring studies of dialkyl phosphate metabolites provide physicians and public health officials with reference values so that they can determine whether or not people have been exposed to higher levels of organophosphorus pesticides than are found in the general population. Biomonitoring data can also help scientists plan and conduct research on exposure and health effects.

# Urinary Diethylphosphate (DEP)

*Metabolite of Several Organophosphorus Insecticides*

Geometric mean and selected percentiles of urine concentrations (in µg/L) for the U.S. population from the National Health and Nutrition Examination Survey.

| | Survey years | Geometric mean (95% conf. interval) | Selected percentiles ( 95% confidence interval) | | | | Sample size |
|---|---|---|---|---|---|---|---|
| | | | 50th | 75th | 90th | 95th | |
| **Total** | 99-00 | **1.03** (.670-1.58) | **1.20** (.750-1.70) | **3.20** (2.30-4.80) | **7.60** (5.00-12.0) | **13.0** (7.70-23.0) | 1949 |
| | 01-02 | * | < LOD | **2.76** (2.42-3.16) | **6.33** (5.68-7.46) | **11.4** (9.15-12.5) | 2520 |
| | 03-04 | * | < LOD | **4.54** (3.38-5.97) | **10.2** (9.00-12.1) | **15.7** (14.1-17.2) | 1931 |
| **Age group** | | | | | | | |
| 6-11 years | 99-00 | **1.32** (.757-2.29) | **1.50** (.860-2.60) | **4.50** (2.10-7.90) | **11.0** (4.80-24.0) | **16.0** (8.50-36.0) | 471 |
| | 01-02 | * | **.290** (<LOD-1.04) | **3.45** (2.36-4.47) | **9.56** (6.33-18.0) | **20.0** (9.44-38.2) | 576 |
| | 03-04 | * | < LOD | **5.13** (2.48-7.94) | **10.9** (8.08-15.9) | **16.1** (10.9-18.5) | 308 |
| 12-19 years | 99-00 | **1.21** (.758-1.94) | **1.40** (.970-2.10) | **3.70** (2.40-5.50) | **8.00** (4.70-19.0) | **20.0** (8.00-27.0) | 664 |
| | 01-02 | * | < LOD | **2.86** (1.96-3.95) | **7.58** (5.71-9.15) | **11.0** (9.35-12.4) | 822 |
| | 03-04 | * | **.530** (<LOD-2.32) | **5.80** (4.34-7.67) | **14.8** (9.12-19.8) | **20.8** (14.8-32.7) | 701 |
| 20-59 years | 99-00 | **.955** (.623-1.47) | **1.10** (.700-1.60) | **3.00** (1.80-4.80) | **7.30** (4.70-11.0) | **11.0** (6.80-22.0) | 814 |
| | 01-02 | * | < LOD | **2.71** (2.34-3.12) | **5.79** (5.05-7.21) | **10.4** (7.43-12.3) | 1122 |
| | 03-04 | * | < LOD | **4.37** (3.02-5.81) | **9.74** (8.35-11.3) | **14.2** (11.5-16.2) | 922 |
| **Gender** | | | | | | | |
| Males | 99-00 | **1.11** (.717-1.73) | **1.20** (.810-1.70) | **3.80** (2.50-5.00) | **8.00** (5.00-19.0) | **19.0** (7.20-30.0) | 952 |
| | 01-02 | * | < LOD | **3.13** (2.44-3.53) | **6.99** (5.79-7.80) | **11.5** (8.98-12.4) | 1187 |
| | 03-04 | * | < LOD | **4.85** (3.26-6.51) | **11.1** (9.56-13.8) | **17.2** (14.2-20.8) | 928 |
| Females | 99-00 | **.954** (.599-1.52) | **1.20** (.620-1.70) | **2.90** (1.90-4.80) | **7.50** (4.60-11.0) | **11.0** (7.40-16.0) | 997 |
| | 01-02 | * | **.290** (<LOD-.780) | **2.58** (2.17-3.02) | **5.93** (4.55-8.19) | **10.4** (7.27-15.1) | 1333 |
| | 03-04 | * | < LOD | **4.39** (3.23-5.97) | **9.39** (8.07-10.8) | **13.5** (11.3-15.9) | 1003 |
| **Race/ethnicity** | | | | | | | |
| Mexican Americans | 99-00 | **1.22** (.740-2.01) | **1.20** (.840-1.80) | **4.10** (2.20-7.00) | **11.0** (6.40-19.0) | **18.0** (12.0-27.0) | 672 |
| | 01-02 | * | **.600** (<LOD-1.63) | **3.10** (2.27-3.72) | **6.26** (5.00-7.82) | **11.2** (7.82-12.3) | 678 |
| | 03-04 | * | **1.08** (<LOD-2.81) | **5.58** (3.57-7.61) | **10.8** (8.35-16.1) | **17.7** (12.0-28.4) | 473 |
| Non-Hispanic blacks | 99-00 | **1.56** (1.13-2.14) | **1.60** (1.40-1.80) | **4.30** (2.90-5.80) | **10.0** (5.60-18.0) | **18.0** (8.00-27.0) | 509 |
| | 01-02 | * | **.890** (<LOD-2.42) | **4.61** (3.30-6.52) | **10.2** (7.40-14.0) | **15.4** (9.93-24.2) | 696 |
| | 03-04 | * | **.830** (<LOD-3.28) | **6.83** (5.26-8.80) | **12.2** (9.86-15.6) | **16.2** (14.1-23.2) | 578 |
| Non-Hispanic whites | 99-00 | **.981** (.579-1.66) | **1.10** (.490-2.10) | **3.30** (2.20-4.90) | **7.70** (4.70-14.0) | **14.0** (7.60-25.0) | 595 |
| | 01-02 | * | < LOD | **2.44** (2.08-2.91) | **5.56** (4.55-6.89) | **10.2** (7.52-11.9) | 948 |
| | 03-04 | * | < LOD | **4.16** (2.98-5.81) | **9.74** (8.40-11.6) | **14.8** (12.5-17.2) | 752 |

Limit of detection (LOD, see Data Analysis section) for Survey years 99-00, 01-02, and 03-04 are 0 2, 0.2, and 0.1, respectively.
< LOD means less than the limit of detection, which may vary for some chemicals by year and by individual sample.
* Not calculated: proportion of results below limit of detection was too high to provide a valid result.

## Urinary Diethylphosphate (DEP) (creatinine corrected)
*Metabolite of Several Organophosphorus Insecticides*

Geometric mean and selected percentiles of urine concentrations (in µg/g of creatinine) for the U.S. population from the National Health and Nutrition Examination Survey.

| | Survey years | Geometric mean (95% conf. interval) | 50th | 75th | 90th | 95th | Sample size |
|---|---|---|---|---|---|---|---|
| **Total** | 99-00 | .924 (.608-1.41) | .920 (.570-1.40) | 2.73 (1.68-4.60) | 7.94 (4.40-12.2) | 12.2 (8.00-19.6) | 1949 |
| | 01-02 | * | < LOD | 2.39 (2.06-2.69) | 5.23 (4.64-5.98) | 8.53 (6.94-10.2) | 2519 |
| | 03-04 | * | < LOD | 4.42 (3.45-5.74) | 9.02 (7.45-11.2) | 13.2 (10.5-16.1) | 1928 |
| **Age group** | | | | | | | |
| 6-11 years | 99-00 | 1.43 (.870-2.34) | 1.47 (1.02-2.41) | 3.94 (2.20-8.57) | 10.5 (4.55-20.8) | 16.6 (10.5-32.7) | 471 |
| | 01-02 | * | .890 (<LOD-1.76) | 4.02 (2.87-5.25) | 8.85 (6.88-15.6) | 18.4 (9.40-28.8) | 576 |
| | 03-04 | * | < LOD | 6.10 (3.79-9.03) | 11.9 (9.54-15.2) | 16.1 (11.9-28.3) | 308 |
| 12-19 years | 99-00 | .818 (.533-1.26) | .790 (.560-1.25) | 2.35 (1.37-3.75) | 5.44 (2.82-14.4) | 12.4 (4.66-34.2) | 664 |
| | 01-02 | * | < LOD | 2.05 (1.54-2.67) | 4.40 (3.40-5.28) | 7.28 (5.28-9.75) | 821 |
| | 03-04 | * | .440 (<LOD-2.05) | 4.47 (3.90-5.43) | 10.1 (7.10-13.5) | 14.7 (9.82-26.5) | 699 |
| 20-59 years | 99-00 | .883 (.574-1.36) | .860 (.500-1.35) | 2.66 (1.54-4.95) | 7.37 (4.32-12.1) | 12.1 (8.00-17.5) | 814 |
| | 01-02 | * | < LOD | 2.28 (2.01-2.56) | 4.75 (3.92-5.83) | 7.37 (5.93-9.72) | 1122 |
| | 03-04 | * | < LOD | 4.29 (2.98-5.71) | 8.34 (6.09-11.3) | 11.9 (9.02-14.7) | 921 |
| **Gender** | | | | | | | |
| Males | 99-00 | .855 (.566-1.29) | .820 (.510-1.34) | 2.61 (1.76-4.03) | 7.69 (4.41-12.1) | 12.2 (6.94-23.8) | 952 |
| | 01-02 | * | < LOD | 2.04 (1.71-2.52) | 4.31 (3.62-5.00) | 6.88 (5.60-9.42) | 1187 |
| | 03-04 | * | < LOD | 4.03 (2.81-5.30) | 8.34 (6.69-10.2) | 12.1 (9.31-14.8) | 927 |
| Females | 99-00 | .996 (.620-1.60) | .960 (.540-1.62) | 2.81 (1.45-5.85) | 8.00 (4.00-13.0) | 12.1 (6.67-19.6) | 997 |
| | 01-02 | * | .750 (<LOD-1.27) | 2.66 (2.24-3.23) | 6.28 (4.75-7.37) | 9.57 (6.61-13.6) | 1332 |
| | 03-04 | * | < LOD | 4.87 (3.82-6.50) | 9.83 (7.54-11.9) | 13.8 (10.5-20.3) | 1001 |
| **Race/ethnicity** | | | | | | | |
| Mexican Americans | 99-00 | 1.09 (.633-1.89) | 1.05 (.650-1.98) | 3.78 (2.11-6.46) | 9.84 (5.66-15.7) | 15.7 (8.61-29.0) | 672 |
| | 01-02 | * | .890 (<LOD-1.38) | 2.38 (1.79-3.13) | 5.00 (4.04-6.53) | 7.66 (5.88-10.9) | 678 |
| | 03-04 | * | .960 (<LOD-2.67) | 4.43 (3.03-6.69) | 9.80 (7.56-13.3) | 16.6 (9.94-22.5) | 472 |
| Non-Hispanic blacks | 99-00 | 1.07 (.773-1.47) | 1.18 (.830-1.54) | 2.61 (1.89-3.47) | 5.98 (3.94-9.56) | 11.9 (5.98-22.2) | 509 |
| | 01-02 | * | .780 (<LOD-1.56) | 2.80 (2.40-3.40) | 7.19 (4.90-8.84) | 9.75 (7.82-14.9) | 695 |
| | 03-04 | * | .710 (<LOD-1.98) | 4.14 (3.46-5.09) | 7.77 (6.57-10.5) | 11.7 (10.5-13.4) | 577 |
| Non-Hispanic whites | 99-00 | .932 (.549-1.58) | .900 (.430-1.68) | 2.87 (1.51-5.88) | 8.57 (4.40-14.4) | 13.0 (8.21-23.8) | 595 |
| | 01-02 | * | < LOD | 2.30 (1.92-2.74) | 4.95 (3.93-5.93) | 7.80 (6.15-10.7) | 948 |
| | 03-04 | * | < LOD | 4.47 (3.37-5.80) | 9.03 (7.53-11.3) | 12.1 (10.1-15.7) | 751 |

< LOD means less than the limit of detection for the urine levels not corrected for creatinine.
* Not calculated: proportion of results below limit of detection was too high to provide a valid result.

# Urinary Dimethylphosphate (DMP)
*Metabolite of Several Organophosphorus Insecticides*
Geometric mean and selected percentiles of urine concentrations (in µg/L) for the U.S. population from the National Health and Nutrition Examination Survey.

| | Survey years | Geometric mean (95% conf. interval) | Selected percentiles ( 95% confidence interval) | | | | Sample size |
|---|---|---|---|---|---|---|---|
| | | | 50th | 75th | 90th | 95th | |
| **Total** | 99-00 | * | .740 (<LOD-1.40) | 2.90 (2.10-4.00) | 7.90 (6.20-8.90) | 14.0 (10.0-19.0) | 1949 |
| | 01-02 | * | < LOD | 3.25 (2.77-3.67) | 8.22 (6.95-9.27) | 13.4 (10.9-15.6) | 2519 |
| | 03-04 | * | < LOD | 3.99 (3.29-4.96) | 9.17 (7.33-11.9) | 14.8 (12.4-17.8) | 1965 |
| **Age group** | | | | | | | |
| 6-11 years | 99-00 | 1.58 (1.15-2.18) | 1.10 (.580-2.20) | 4.40 (2.80-6.80) | 10.0 (7.80-21.0) | 22.0 (15.0-33.0) | 471 |
| | 01-02 | * | .970 (<LOD-2.00) | 5.04 (3.31-7.66) | 12.2 (9.10-15.1) | 18.3 (12.6-41.7) | 576 |
| | 03-04 | * | < LOD | 4.53 (3.34-5.96) | 11.0 (5.62-17.9) | 16.2 (7.46-28.3) | 310 |
| 12-19 years | 99-00 | * | .670 (<LOD-1.80) | 3.80 (2.50-4.90) | 9.90 (6.20-18.0) | 22.0 (13.0-29.0) | 664 |
| | 01-02 | * | .670 (<LOD-1.31) | 4.27 (3.41-5.35) | 9.27 (7.80-12.3) | 14.7 (11.8-21.3) | 822 |
| | 03-04 | * | 1.20 (<LOD-2.27) | 4.61 (3.47-6.72) | 10.9 (7.90-15.0) | 20.9 (12.5-26.8) | 717 |
| 20-59 years | 99-00 | * | .680 (<LOD-1.30) | 2.70 (1.80-3.70) | 6.60 (5.70-8.10) | 9.70 (8.80-14.0) | 814 |
| | 01-02 | * | < LOD | 2.95 (2.35-3.41) | 6.95 (5.80-8.82) | 11.5 (9.66-13.7) | 1121 |
| | 03-04 | * | < LOD | 3.75 (2.84-4.88) | 8.52 (6.86-10.7) | 14.1 (10.8-17.5) | 938 |
| **Gender** | | | | | | | |
| Males | 99-00 | * | .670 (<LOD-1.30) | 2.90 (2.20-4.00) | 7.90 (6.00-9.30) | 18.0 (10.0-24.0) | 952 |
| | 01-02 | * | < LOD | 3.40 (2.49-4.30) | 8.22 (6.67-10.3) | 12.6 (10.9-14.7) | 1187 |
| | 03-04 | * | < LOD | 3.89 (2.97-4.89) | 8.14 (6.34-10.4) | 15.1 (10.8-20.4) | 946 |
| Females | 99-00 | * | .790 (<LOD-1.60) | 2.90 (2.00-4.20) | 7.80 (5.70-9.00) | 11.0 (9.00-18.0) | 997 |
| | 01-02 | * | < LOD | 3.06 (2.59-3.67) | 8.34 (6.70-9.64) | 13.7 (10.9-17.2) | 1332 |
| | 03-04 | * | < LOD | 4.18 (3.24-5.73) | 10.3 (7.39-13.6) | 14.8 (12.6-19.6) | 1019 |
| **Race/ethnicity** | | | | | | | |
| Mexican Americans | 99-00 | * | 1.10 (<LOD-1.80) | 3.80 (2.70-5.30) | 9.60 (6.00-16.0) | 16.0 (8.90-31.0) | 672 |
| | 01-02 | * | .670 (<LOD-1.51) | 3.24 (2.46-4.27) | 9.28 (7.10-10.7) | 14.4 (10.7-21.0) | 678 |
| | 03-04 | * | < LOD | 4.37 (3.15-6.88) | 10.3 (6.92-17.8) | 23.3 (9.61-32.5) | 498 |
| Non-Hispanic blacks | 99-00 | 1.42 (1.16-1.74) | 1.00 (.650-1.50) | 3.60 (2.50-5.50) | 8.90 (6.90-15.0) | 21.0 (14.0-24.0) | 509 |
| | 01-02 | * | .910 (<LOD-2.29) | 5.45 (3.81-6.78) | 11.5 (8.77-14.9) | 19.4 (14.1-23.3) | 695 |
| | 03-04 | * | < LOD | 5.12 (4.11-6.37) | 10.5 (8.31-12.0) | 14.3 (11.7-19.6) | 579 |
| Non-Hispanic whites | 99-00 | * | < LOD | 2.90 (1.80-4.20) | 7.90 (5.90-9.00) | 11.0 (9.00-18.0) | 595 |
| | 01-02 | * | < LOD | 3.01 (2.34-3.50) | 7.39 (5.98-9.22) | 12.3 (9.63-14.6) | 948 |
| | 03-04 | * | < LOD | 3.75 (3.00-4.92) | 8.35 (6.22-12.9) | 14.6 (10.8-20.4) | 757 |

Limit of detection (LOD, see Data Analysis section) for Survey years 99-00, 01-02, and 03-04 are 0 58, 0.5, and 0.5, respectively.
< LOD means less than the limit of detection, which may vary for some chemicals by year and by individual sample.
* Not calculated: proportion of results below limit of detection was too high to provide a valid result.

# Urinary Dimethylphosphate (DMP) (creatinine corrected)

*Metabolite of Several Organophosphorus Insecticides*

Geometric mean and selected percentiles of urine concentrations (in µg/g of creatinine) for the U.S. population from the National Health and Nutrition Examination Survey.

| | Survey years | Geometric mean (95% conf. interval) | Selected percentiles ( 95% confidence interval) | | | | Sample size |
|---|---|---|---|---|---|---|---|
| | | | 50th | 75th | 90th | 95th | |
| **Total** | 99-00 | * | .810 (<LOD-1.15) | 2.93 (2.11-3.92) | 8.50 (6.96-10.4) | 16.1 (13.3-17.6) | 1949 |
| | 01-02 | * | < LOD | 3.00 (2.59-3.33) | 7.83 (6.47-9.04) | 12.7 (10.3-15.0) | 2518 |
| | 03-04 | * | < LOD | 3.86 (3.02-4.95) | 9.54 (7.93-10.6) | 14.6 (12.5-17.6) | 1962 |
| **Age group** | | | | | | | |
| 6-11 years | 99-00 | 1.71 (1.29-2.27) | 1.38 (.890-2.38) | 4.48 (2.88-7.89) | 16.7 (8.21-21.2) | 22.1 (19.2-30.1) | 471 |
| | 01-02 | * | 1.93 (<LOD-2.97) | 5.99 (4.32-8.28) | 12.9 (9.34-18.5) | 20.6 (13.3-34.9) | 576 |
| | 03-04 | * | < LOD | 6.87 (3.79-9.00) | 13.9 (9.68-19.4) | 19.6 (13.9-25.9) | 310 |
| 12-19 years | 99-00 | * | .590 (<LOD-.950) | 2.28 (1.70-2.80) | 7.78 (4.16-14.4) | 16.0 (8.70-35.3) | 664 |
| | 01-02 | * | .910 (<LOD-1.27) | 3.29 (2.75-3.78) | 6.29 (5.51-7.30) | 9.83 (7.94-14.2) | 821 |
| | 03-04 | * | 1.00 (<LOD-1.68) | 4.16 (3.37-5.07) | 8.81 (7.78-10.2) | 12.7 (10.3-17.7) | 715 |
| 20-59 years | 99-00 | * | .760 (<LOD-1.12) | 2.88 (1.89-3.99) | 8.11 (5.89-10.3) | 14.6 (10.4-16.8) | 814 |
| | 01-02 | * | < LOD | 2.55 (2.05-3.03) | 6.92 (5.85-8.00) | 11.5 (9.38-13.6) | 1121 |
| | 03-04 | * | < LOD | 3.77 (2.72-4.55) | 8.78 (6.68-10.5) | 13.5 (11.2-15.6) | 937 |
| **Gender** | | | | | | | |
| Males | 99-00 | * | .620 (<LOD-.940) | 2.38 (1.86-3.18) | 7.58 (4.64-11.6) | 15.2 (9.74-19.5) | 952 |
| | 01-02 | * | < LOD | 2.61 (2.07-3.07) | 6.25 (4.82-8.42) | 10.5 (8.28-12.7) | 1187 |
| | 03-04 | * | < LOD | 2.95 (2.23-3.91) | 7.93 (6.33-10.4) | 12.5 (10.4-15.4) | 945 |
| Females | 99-00 | * | 1.00 (<LOD-1.71) | 3.63 (2.30-5.19) | 9.12 (7.82-11.7) | 16.4 (11.7-19.7) | 997 |
| | 01-02 | * | < LOD | 3.43 (2.74-4.27) | 9.00 (7.51-10.1) | 15.0 (11.9-17.8) | 1331 |
| | 03-04 | * | < LOD | 5.00 (3.79-6.30) | 10.1 (8.27-13.4) | 16.0 (13.0-19.6) | 1017 |
| **Race/ethnicity** | | | | | | | |
| Mexican Americans | 99-00 | * | 1.06 (<LOD-1.55) | 3.89 (2.54-5.45) | 9.41 (7.69-11.5) | 16.7 (11.7-23.6) | 672 |
| | 01-02 | * | .920 (<LOD-1.27) | 3.03 (2.52-3.72) | 8.03 (6.09-11.3) | 14.6 (11.4-16.2) | 678 |
| | 03-04 | * | < LOD | 4.14 (2.44-6.30) | 12.3 (7.39-17.6) | 19.5 (15.3-21.8) | 497 |
| Non-Hispanic blacks | 99-00 | .973 (.780-1.21) | .690 (.530-1.06) | 2.67 (1.89-3.77) | 7.07 (5.09-11.4) | 14.0 (10.6-19.1) | 509 |
| | 01-02 | * | .850 (<LOD-1.34) | 3.36 (2.68-4.29) | 7.63 (6.25-9.45) | 13.2 (9.50-17.2) | 694 |
| | 03-04 | * | < LOD | 3.38 (2.75-3.95) | 6.94 (5.53-8.42) | 10.8 (8.42-19.2) | 578 |
| Non-Hispanic whites | 99-00 | * | < LOD | 3.15 (1.97-4.32) | 8.73 (5.89-13.3) | 15.8 (10.0-21.2) | 595 |
| | 01-02 | * | < LOD | 2.77 (2.20-3.37) | 8.00 (5.91-9.86) | 12.9 (9.85-17.7) | 948 |
| | 03-04 | * | < LOD | 3.89 (3.01-5.54) | 9.67 (7.96-11.2) | 14.6 (11.4-18.2) | 756 |

< LOD means less than the limit of detection for the urine levels not corrected for creatinine.
* Not calculated: proportion of results below limit of detection was too high to provide a valid result.

## Urinary Diethylthiophosphate (DETP)
*Metabolite of Several Organophosphorus Insecticides*

Geometric mean and selected percentiles of urine concentrations (in µg/L) for the U.S. population from the National Health and Nutrition Examination Survey.

| | Survey years | Geometric mean (95% conf. interval) | Selected percentiles ( 95% confidence interval) | | | | Sample size |
|---|---|---|---|---|---|---|---|
| | | | 50th | 75th | 90th | 95th | |
| **Total** | 99-00 | * | .500 (<LOD-.690) | .760 (.620-1.10) | 1.40 (1.10-1.80) | 2.20 (1.70-2.80) | 1949 |
| | 01-02 | .457 (.353-.592) | .570 (.390-.880) | 1.50 (1.25-1.79) | 2.48 (2.22-3.04) | 3.94 (3.17-4.95) | 2519 |
| | 03-04 | * | < LOD | .830 (.690-.950) | 1.77 (1.42-2.31) | 2.80 (2.31-3.78) | 1905 |
| **Age group** | | | | | | | |
| 6-11 years | 99-00 | * | .600 (<LOD-.810) | .910 (.720-1.30) | 1.70 (1.20-3.20) | 3.20 (1.70-7.30) | 471 |
| | 01-02 | .453 (.350-.585) | .550 (.350-.850) | 1.58 (1.33-2.04) | 2.75 (2.22-3.38) | 4.08 (2.95-5.16) | 575 |
| | 03-04 | * | < LOD | .820 (.580-.970) | 1.45 (1.05-2.16) | 2.18 (1.45-4.13) | 296 |
| 12-19 years | 99-00 | * | .210 (<LOD-.710) | .780 (.600-1.20) | 1.50 (1.20-2.30) | 2.30 (1.60-4.30) | 664 |
| | 01-02 | .505 (.388-.657) | .690 (.440-.960) | 1.61 (1.32-1.94) | 2.57 (2.23-3.39) | 4.08 (2.73-5.86) | 822 |
| | 03-04 | * | .260 (<LOD-.400) | .930 (.750-1.13) | 2.14 (1.75-2.89) | 3.27 (2.69-4.83) | 690 |
| 20-59 years | 99-00 | * | .490 (<LOD-.670) | .740 (.600-.930) | 1.30 (.990-1.80) | 2.00 (1.50-2.60) | 814 |
| | 01-02 | .449 (.340-.592) | .540 (.380-.880) | 1.45 (1.19-1.79) | 2.46 (2.11-3.17) | 3.83 (2.96-5.34) | 1122 |
| | 03-04 | * | < LOD | .800 (.650-.960) | 1.76 (1.37-2.32) | 2.65 (2.31-3.89) | 919 |
| **Gender** | | | | | | | |
| Males | 99-00 | * | .510 (<LOD-.700) | .790 (.680-1.10) | 1.50 (1.20-2.20) | 2.70 (1.90-4.10) | 952 |
| | 01-02 | .459 (.359-.587) | .570 (.390-.860) | 1.50 (1.30-1.78) | 2.54 (2.16-3.34) | 3.83 (2.76-6.15) | 1187 |
| | 03-04 | * | < LOD | .880 (.720-1.01) | 2.20 (1.54-2.50) | 2.95 (2.36-4.29) | 907 |
| Females | 99-00 | * | < LOD | .720 (.570-1.00) | 1.30 (.910-1.60) | 1.70 (1.30-3.20) | 997 |
| | 01-02 | .455 (.336-.618) | .550 (.380-.940) | 1.48 (1.14-1.89) | 2.45 (2.11-3.35) | 3.94 (2.68-5.49) | 1332 |
| | 03-04 | * | < LOD | .780 (.590-.970) | 1.47 (1.22-2.00) | 2.57 (1.87-3.78) | 998 |
| **Race/ethnicity** | | | | | | | |
| Mexican Americans | 99-00 | * | .570 (<LOD-.780) | .840 (.740-.980) | 1.50 (1.20-1.90) | 2.20 (2.00-2.90) | 672 |
| | 01-02 | .549 (.398-.759) | .710 (.460-.960) | 1.40 (1.01-1.98) | 2.63 (1.98-3.47) | 3.98 (2.74-5.21) | 678 |
| | 03-04 | * | .240 (<LOD-.380) | .960 (.680-1.54) | 2.22 (1.46-3.83) | 3.97 (2.22-8.80) | 478 |
| Non-Hispanic blacks | 99-00 | .343 (.201-.584) | .570 (<LOD-.750) | .820 (.690-1.20) | 1.80 (1.30-3.20) | 3.60 (2.00-4.80) | 509 |
| | 01-02 | .749 (.592-.949) | 1.18 (.740-1.49) | 1.86 (1.77-2.03) | 3.55 (3.01-3.91) | 5.27 (3.89-6.74) | 695 |
| | 03-04 | .467 (.382-.570) | .450 (<LOD-.730) | 1.09 (.930-1.26) | 2.32 (1.59-2.88) | 3.26 (2.41-5.46) | 553 |
| Non-Hispanic whites | 99-00 | * | .160 (<LOD-.700) | .740 (.580-1.10) | 1.30 (.960-1.90) | 1.90 (1.50-2.80) | 595 |
| | 01-02 | .425 (.303-.597) | .510 (.280-.930) | 1.46 (1.10-1.83) | 2.41 (2.05-3.17) | 3.73 (2.59-6.15) | 948 |
| | 03-04 | * | < LOD | .710 (.560-.910) | 1.73 (1.29-2.31) | 2.64 (1.96-3.89) | 745 |

Limit of detection (LOD, see Data Analysis section) for Survey years 99-00, 01-02, and 03-04 are 0 09, 0.1, and 0.2, respectively.
< LOD means less than the limit of detection, which may vary for some chemicals by year and by individual sample.
* Not calculated: proportion of results below limit of detection was too high to provide a valid result.

# Urinary Diethylthiophosphate (DETP) (creatinine corrected)

*Metabolite of Several Organophosphorus Insecticides*

Geometric mean and selected percentiles of urine concentrations (in µg/g of creatinine) for the U.S. population from the National Health and Nutrition Examination Survey.

| | Survey years | Geometric mean (95% conf. interval) | Selected percentiles ( 95% confidence interval) | | | | Sample size |
|---|---|---|---|---|---|---|---|
| | | | 50th | 75th | 90th | 95th | |
| **Total** | 99-00 | * | .250 (<LOD-.480) | .710 (.460-1.07) | 1.72 (1.17-2.32) | 2.64 (2.08-3.06) | 1949 |
| | 01-02 | .453 (.348-.590) | .520 (.330-.760) | 1.33 (1.04-1.66) | 2.84 (2.22-3.76) | 4.61 (3.42-6.65) | 2518 |
| | 03-04 | * | < LOD | .700 (.580-.830) | 1.47 (1.16-2.04) | 2.62 (2.00-3.72) | 1903 |
| **Age group** | | | | | | | |
| 6-11 years | 99-00 | * | .470 (<LOD-.870) | 1.08 (.800-1.32) | 1.75 (1.44-2.36) | 2.45 (2.04-5.32) | 471 |
| | 01-02 | .591 (.471-.742) | .640 (.400-1.05) | 1.63 (1.31-1.94) | 3.22 (2.72-4.16) | 5.70 (3.84-6.80) | 575 |
| | 03-04 | * | < LOD | .870 (.590-1.09) | 1.57 (1.08-2.67) | 2.67 (1.57-4.05) | 296 |
| 12-19 years | 99-00 | * | .180 (<LOD-.400) | .510 (.320-.820) | 1.07 (.720-1.61) | 1.97 (1.07-3.92) | 664 |
| | 01-02 | .393 (.300-.515) | .530 (.310-.740) | 1.23 (.980-1.53) | 2.19 (1.61-3.07) | 3.14 (2.25-3.97) | 821 |
| | 03-04 | * | .300 (<LOD-.350) | .640 (.560-.730) | 1.49 (1.16-1.60) | 1.97 (1.57-2.43) | 689 |
| 20-59 years | 99-00 | * | .250 (<LOD-.460) | .680 (.440-1.08) | 1.79 (1.08-2.39) | 2.75 (2.02-3.22) | 814 |
| | 01-02 | .447 (.335-.597) | .490 (.320-.740) | 1.32 (.990-1.71) | 2.87 (2.08-3.95) | 4.69 (3.20-7.81) | 1122 |
| | 03-04 | * | < LOD | .700 (.550-.880) | 1.47 (1.11-2.23) | 2.82 (2.02-3.80) | 918 |
| **Gender** | | | | | | | |
| Males | 99-00 | * | .270 (<LOD-.470) | .670 (.520-.840) | 1.34 (1.08-2.17) | 2.67 (1.67-3.23) | 952 |
| | 01-02 | .372 (.285-.485) | .460 (.270-.690) | 1.11 (.940-1.33) | 2.05 (1.55-3.11) | 3.38 (2.47-4.71) | 1187 |
| | 03-04 | * | < LOD | .590 (.500-.760) | 1.42 (.950-2.07) | 2.62 (1.61-3.97) | 906 |
| Females | 99-00 | * | < LOD | .790 (.380-1.50) | 1.89 (1.07-2.52) | 2.52 (1.89-3.75) | 997 |
| | 01-02 | .552 (.412-.739) | .580 (.370-.910) | 1.60 (1.18-2.42) | 3.70 (2.77-4.99) | 6.57 (3.92-8.82) | 1331 |
| | 03-04 | * | < LOD | .750 (.660-.900) | 1.50 (1.22-2.23) | 2.60 (2.08-3.98) | 997 |
| **Race/ethnicity** | | | | | | | |
| Mexican Americans | 99-00 | * | .330 (<LOD-.790) | .830 (.550-1.20) | 1.69 (1.20-2.43) | 2.71 (1.75-3.78) | 672 |
| | 01-02 | .509 (.377-.688) | .560 (.380-.840) | 1.28 (1.03-1.67) | 2.55 (1.77-3.72) | 3.72 (2.58-6.30) | 678 |
| | 03-04 | * | .310 (<LOD-.390) | .750 (.480-1.22) | 1.92 (1.22-3.43) | 3.66 (2.02-6.17) | 478 |
| Non-Hispanic blacks | 99-00 | .234 (.136-.403) | .310 (<LOD-.580) | .720 (.510-.850) | 1.39 (1.03-2.10) | 2.91 (1.49-4.24) | 509 |
| | 01-02 | .535 (.444-.645) | .710 (.550-.920) | 1.43 (1.32-1.60) | 2.73 (2.30-2.98) | 4.00 (3.05-4.99) | 694 |
| | 03-04 | .305 (.253-.368) | .280 (<LOD-.380) | .640 (.540-.820) | 1.41 (.930-1.79) | 2.13 (1.38-3.90) | 552 |
| Non-Hispanic whites | 99-00 | * | .230 (<LOD-.550) | .710 (.390-1.22) | 1.88 (1.05-2.58) | 2.64 (2.08-3.07) | 595 |
| | 01-02 | .448 (.318-.630) | .510 (.270-.800) | 1.38 (1.00-1.88) | 3.08 (2.29-4.23) | 5.77 (3.42-8.44) | 948 |
| | 03-04 | * | < LOD | .700 (.560-.840) | 1.45 (1.06-2.08) | 2.58 (1.73-3.97) | 744 |

< LOD means less than the limit of detection for the urine levels not corrected for creatinine.
* Not calculated: proportion of results below limit of detection was too high to provide a valid result.

# Urinary Dimethylthiophosphate (DMTP)
*Metabolite of Several Organophosphorus Insecticides*

Geometric mean and selected percentiles of urine concentrations (in µg/L) for the U.S. population from the National Health and Nutrition Examination Survey.

| | Survey years | Geometric mean (95% conf. interval) | 50th | 75th | 90th | 95th | Sample size |
|---|---|---|---|---|---|---|---|
| **Total** | 99-00 | 1.82 (1.36-2.44) | 2.70 (1.40-4.10) | 11.0 (8.40-16.0) | 38.0 (25.0-41.0) | 48.0 (38.0-62.0) | 1948 |
| | 01-02 | * | .470 (<LOD-1.41) | 4.02 (2.92-5.70) | 16.2 (12.4-22.9) | 32.6 (26.6-45.3) | 2518 |
| | 03-04 | 2.10 (1.83-2.40) | 1.90 (1.61-2.26) | 5.65 (4.63-6.80) | 17.3 (14.5-20.1) | 31.1 (26.5-40.0) | 1965 |
| **Age group** | | | | | | | |
| 6-11 years | 99-00 | 2.72 (1.93-3.85) | 4.20 (2.50-7.20) | 20.0 (13.0-29.0) | 40.0 (38.0-52.0) | 62.0 (40.0-92.0) | 471 |
| | 01-02 | * | 1.46 (.600-2.69) | 8.33 (5.75-14.0) | 28.4 (19.7-41.4) | 45.7 (28.5-74.5) | 575 |
| | 03-04 | 2.79 (2.25-3.45) | 2.67 (1.81-3.88) | 6.95 (5.64-8.58) | 19.4 (10.5-27.4) | 30.9 (19.4-76.5) | 310 |
| 12-19 years | 99-00 | 2.53 (1.64-3.92) | 3.70 (1.70-6.80) | 16.0 (11.0-31.0) | 38.0 (33.0-58.0) | 69.0 (38.0-260) | 664 |
| | 01-02 | * | 1.04 (<LOD-2.12) | 4.83 (3.35-6.48) | 20.8 (12.2-27.9) | 34.9 (23.6-54.7) | 822 |
| | 03-04 | 2.21 (1.81-2.70) | 1.83 (1.46-2.16) | 5.91 (4.04-8.78) | 18.7 (12.2-33.9) | 47.1 (22.2-80.8) | 717 |
| 20-59 years | 99-00 | 1.59 (1.17-2.16) | 2.30 (.830-3.80) | 9.10 (7.10-13.0) | 38.0 (19.0-39.0) | 39.0 (38.0-58.0) | 813 |
| | 01-02 | * | < LOD | 3.32 (2.29-4.96) | 13.6 (9.50-20.0) | 30.0 (20.5-45.3) | 1121 |
| | 03-04 | 1.98 (1.71-2.30) | 1.78 (1.48-2.18) | 5.11 (4.31-6.53) | 16.7 (12.1-20.8) | 28.5 (24.1-40.0) | 938 |
| **Gender** | | | | | | | |
| Males | 99-00 | 2.10 (1.48-2.98) | 3.50 (2.20-4.80) | 14.0 (8.00-24.0) | 38.0 (21.0-49.0) | 42.0 (38.0-53.0) | 952 |
| | 01-02 | * | .610 (<LOD-1.42) | 4.21 (3.07-5.97) | 18.3 (12.2-27.2) | 31.1 (25.0-43.3) | 1187 |
| | 03-04 | 2.13 (1.80-2.53) | 1.94 (1.49-2.44) | 6.09 (4.44-7.23) | 16.1 (10.9-21.1) | 26.8 (22.0-41.6) | 946 |
| Females | 99-00 | 1.59 (1.23-2.06) | 2.00 (.690-3.60) | 9.70 (7.30-14.0) | 38.0 (26.0-39.0) | 52.0 (38.0-110) | 996 |
| | 01-02 | * | < LOD | 3.76 (2.50-5.71) | 15.9 (10.6-22.0) | 34.3 (23.2-47.3) | 1331 |
| | 03-04 | 2.06 (1.74-2.44) | 1.86 (1.58-2.18) | 5.21 (4.27-6.77) | 19.8 (12.8-24.0) | 33.8 (26.1-47.8) | 1019 |
| **Race/ethnicity** | | | | | | | |
| Mexican Americans | 99-00 | 1.79 (1.05-3.05) | 2.00 (.530-4.40) | 11.0 (6.70-17.0) | 39.0 (32.0-62.0) | 140 (46.0-230) | 671 |
| | 01-02 | * | < LOD | 3.76 (2.66-5.18) | 15.1 (11.1-19.1) | 35.2 (19.1-46.0) | 678 |
| | 03-04 | 2.41 (1.86-3.11) | 2.54 (1.41-4.04) | 6.52 (4.90-8.13) | 18.6 (11.7-22.3) | 28.9 (19.2-39.8) | 498 |
| Non-Hispanic blacks | 99-00 | 2.13 (1.57-2.88) | 3.60 (2.10-4.70) | 12.0 (8.80-18.0) | 38.0 (20.0-41.0) | 41.0 (37.0-110) | 509 |
| | 01-02 | 1.61 (1.19-2.19) | 1.26 (.660-2.05) | 5.54 (3.29-9.41) | 20.6 (15.6-27.7) | 42.9 (27.2-62.8) | 695 |
| | 03-04 | 2.10 (1.83-2.41) | 1.85 (1.50-2.29) | 5.12 (3.87-7.90) | 20.4 (15.2-26.1) | 32.0 (24.9-51.9) | 579 |
| Non-Hispanic whites | 99-00 | 1.77 (1.23-2.53) | 2.70 (.830-4.40) | 11.0 (7.50-17.0) | 38.0 (17.0-53.0) | 48.0 (38.0-69.0) | 595 |
| | 01-02 | * | < LOD | 3.99 (2.46-6.14) | 17.3 (10.1-25.0) | 33.1 (25.0-50.2) | 947 |
| | 03-04 | 2.10 (1.79-2.45) | 1.90 (1.57-2.30) | 5.71 (4.43-7.10) | 17.3 (12.8-21.1) | 31.3 (24.0-47.8) | 757 |

Limit of detection (LOD, see Data Analysis section) for Survey years 99-00, 01-02, and 03-04 are 0.18, 0.4, and 0.5, respectively.
< LOD means less than the limit of detection, which may vary for some chemicals by year and by individual sample.
* Not calculated: proportion of results below limit of detection was too high to provide a valid result.

# Urinary Dimethylthiophosphate (DMTP) (creatinine corrected)

*Metabolite of Several Organophosphorus Insecticides*

Geometric mean and selected percentiles of urine concentrations (in µg/g of creatinine) for the U.S. population from the National Health and Nutrition Examination Survey.

| | Survey years | Geometric mean (95% conf. interval) | 50th | 75th | 90th | 95th | Sample size |
|---|---|---|---|---|---|---|---|
| **Total** | 99-00 | 1.64 (1.22-2.20) | 2.12 (1.22-3.35) | 9.57 (6.59-15.8) | 32.0 (23.9-41.1) | 51.0 (39.0-70.1) | 1948 |
| | 01-02 | * | .860 (<LOD-1.33) | 3.79 (2.50-5.19) | 13.3 (10.9-18.8) | 27.2 (21.7-37.7) | 2517 |
| | 03-04 | 1.97 (1.71-2.27) | 1.75 (1.54-2.06) | 5.21 (4.46-5.95) | 15.7 (11.7-19.7) | 30.4 (25.4-34.2) | 1962 |
| **Age group** | | | | | | | |
| 6-11 years | 99-00 | 2.95 (2.25-3.86) | 5.32 (3.75-6.33) | 19.1 (12.2-28.0) | 47.0 (32.1-60.3) | 66.1 (50.9-95.0) | 471 |
| | 01-02 | * | 2.16 (1.32-3.12) | 10.6 (7.84-13.6) | 28.7 (18.8-45.0) | 48.1 (33.4-71.1) | 575 |
| | 03-04 | 3.40 (2.70-4.28) | 3.41 (2.40-4.17) | 7.91 (6.43-12.2) | 25.2 (16.8-34.2) | 36.1 (25.4-67.7) | 310 |
| 12-19 years | 99-00 | 1.71 (1.07-2.75) | 2.14 (.890-4.83) | 13.5 (6.46-22.6) | 36.0 (25.6-51.4) | 61.5 (41.7-109) | 664 |
| | 01-02 | * | .930 (<LOD-1.56) | 3.56 (2.38-5.57) | 12.2 (8.96-16.0) | 22.5 (13.2-34.7) | 821 |
| | 03-04 | 1.66 (1.37-2.03) | 1.52 (1.18-1.82) | 4.38 (3.29-5.66) | 13.3 (9.94-20.5) | 26.5 (15.5-36.0) | 715 |
| 20-59 years | 99-00 | 1.47 (1.07-2.02) | 1.90 (.870-3.11) | 8.09 (5.19-14.6) | 27.0 (19.8-37.6) | 47.5 (34.2-70.1) | 813 |
| | 01-02 | * | < LOD | 3.16 (1.99-4.62) | 11.9 (7.79-17.2) | 25.2 (15.9-37.0) | 1121 |
| | 03-04 | 1.88 (1.61-2.19) | 1.67 (1.45-1.94) | 4.88 (4.20-5.68) | 13.9 (10.3-19.7) | 30.4 (19.7-38.2) | 937 |
| **Gender** | | | | | | | |
| Males | 99-00 | 1.61 (1.11-2.34) | 2.39 (1.27-3.51) | 9.27 (6.00-16.9) | 28.9 (19.0-40.4) | 41.1 (34.9-52.9) | 952 |
| | 01-02 | * | .750 (<LOD-1.08) | 3.35 (2.26-4.60) | 12.5 (8.54-15.9) | 24.0 (14.6-38.9) | 1187 |
| | 03-04 | 1.70 (1.43-2.02) | 1.67 (1.38-1.96) | 4.47 (3.63-5.36) | 12.3 (8.47-17.7) | 24.5 (17.6-32.5) | 945 |
| Females | 99-00 | 1.66 (1.26-2.18) | 2.01 (.870-3.33) | 10.0 (6.67-16.2) | 34.9 (26.2-47.1) | 70.1 (39.0-118) | 996 |
| | 01-02 | * | < LOD | 4.22 (2.40-7.00) | 15.6 (11.3-22.6) | 29.6 (24.8-43.8) | 1330 |
| | 03-04 | 2.28 (1.91-2.72) | 1.88 (1.59-2.44) | 6.00 (4.80-8.30) | 19.4 (12.8-26.2) | 32.6 (27.3-42.0) | 1017 |
| **Race/ethnicity** | | | | | | | |
| Mexican Americans | 99-00 | 1.60 (.899-2.86) | 1.83 (.680-4.23) | 10.4 (5.95-16.9) | 37.0 (23.1-63.1) | 112 (40.5-190) | 671 |
| | 01-02 | * | < LOD | 3.55 (2.52-4.93) | 13.2 (9.61-22.7) | 30.2 (22.7-47.7) | 678 |
| | 03-04 | 2.16 (1.58-2.94) | 2.24 (1.67-3.00) | 5.88 (4.14-8.71) | 15.7 (10.7-20.1) | 23.7 (18.9-36.9) | 497 |
| Non-Hispanic blacks | 99-00 | 1.45 (1.03-2.06) | 1.75 (1.17-3.06) | 8.48 (4.36-13.4) | 25.5 (15.4-39.3) | 54.4 (25.5-97.6) | 509 |
| | 01-02 | 1.15 (.888-1.48) | 1.02 (.670-1.35) | 3.62 (2.33-5.18) | 13.4 (9.69-18.8) | 23.0 (17.5-43.8) | 694 |
| | 03-04 | 1.37 (1.23-1.53) | 1.19 (1.06-1.31) | 3.50 (2.69-5.07) | 11.8 (7.95-16.2) | 23.9 (13.3-27.1) | 578 |
| Non-Hispanic whites | 99-00 | 1.68 (1.16-2.43) | 2.22 (.870-3.51) | 9.40 (5.58-17.0) | 33.3 (20.6-49.4) | 52.9 (39.0-71.1) | 595 |
| | 01-02 | * | < LOD | 3.82 (2.19-6.38) | 14.3 (10.1-22.1) | 27.4 (21.7-43.8) | 947 |
| | 03-04 | 2.08 (1.76-2.46) | 1.80 (1.59-2.27) | 5.36 (4.46-6.23) | 17.4 (11.4-21.6) | 31.7 (24.2-38.2) | 756 |

< LOD means less than the limit of detection for the urine levels not corrected for creatinine.
* Not calculated: proportion of results below limit of detection was too high to provide a valid result.

## Urinary Diethyldithiophosphate (DEDTP)
*Metabolite of Several Organophosphorus Insecticides*
Geometric mean and selected percentiles of urine concentrations (in μg/L) for the U.S. population from the National Health and Nutrition Examination Survey.

| | Survey years | Geometric mean (95% conf. interval) | 50th | 75th | 90th | 95th | Sample size |
|---|---|---|---|---|---|---|---|
| **Total** | 99-00 | * | .090 (<LOD-.140) | .210 (.140-.290) | .470 (.380-.640) | .870 (.640-1.10) | 1949 |
| | 01-02 | * | < LOD | < LOD | .610 (.410-.770) | .850 (.700-1.30) | 2516 |
| | 03-04 | * | < LOD | < LOD | < LOD | .320 (.170-.540) | 1965 |
| **Age group** | | | | | | | |
| 6-11 years | 99-00 | * | .090 (<LOD-.160) | .190 (.130-.280) | .430 (.300-.650) | .850 (.470-1.00) | 471 |
| | 01-02 | * | < LOD | < LOD | .630 (.380-.870) | .940 (.690-1.42) | 576 |
| | 03-04 | * | < LOD | < LOD | < LOD | .540 (<LOD-.650) | 310 |
| 12-19 years | 99-00 | * | .080 (<LOD-.180) | .260 (.120-.350) | .640 (.420-.840) | .930 (.720-1.30) | 664 |
| | 01-02 | * | < LOD | < LOD | .560 (.330-.730) | .820 (.610-.990) | 822 |
| | 03-04 | * | < LOD | < LOD | .150 (<LOD-.350) | .450 (.370-.570) | 717 |
| 20-59 years | 99-00 | * | .090 (<LOD-.130) | .210 (.130-.290) | .450 (.360-.640) | .900 (.610-1.10) | 814 |
| | 01-02 | * | < LOD | < LOD | .620 (.430-.760) | .830 (.700-1.32) | 1118 |
| | 03-04 | * | < LOD | < LOD | < LOD | .220 (<LOD-.580) | 938 |
| **Gender** | | | | | | | |
| Males | 99-00 | * | .090 (<LOD-.150) | .220 (.140-.310) | .490 (.380-.680) | .870 (.680-1.10) | 952 |
| | 01-02 | * | < LOD | < LOD | .600 (.370-.740) | .770 (.680-1.03) | 1187 |
| | 03-04 | * | < LOD | < LOD | < LOD | .390 (.130-.540) | 946 |
| Females | 99-00 | * | .090 (<LOD-.130) | .190 (.110-.310) | .460 (.320-.840) | .870 (.440-1.40) | 997 |
| | 01-02 | * | < LOD | < LOD | .660 (.460-.850) | .990 (.700-1.42) | 1329 |
| | 03-04 | * | < LOD | < LOD | < LOD | .240 (<LOD-.700) | 1019 |
| **Race/ethnicity** | | | | | | | |
| Mexican Americans | 99-00 | .130 (.099-.171) | .100 (.050-.200) | .310 (.230-.390) | .650 (.530-.860) | 1.10 (.860-1.60) | 672 |
| | 01-02 | * | < LOD | < LOD | .720 (.410-1.13) | 1.12 (.700-1.58) | 678 |
| | 03-04 | * | < LOD | < LOD | .120 (<LOD-.550) | .680 (.300-1.15) | 498 |
| Non-Hispanic blacks | 99-00 | .117 (.084-.162) | .090 (<LOD-.230) | .270 (.140-.410) | .560 (.400-.830) | .870 (.650-1.20) | 509 |
| | 01-02 | * | < LOD | < LOD | .630 (.410-.830) | .820 (.730-.990) | 694 |
| | 03-04 | * | < LOD | < LOD | < LOD | .310 (.160-.540) | 579 |
| Non-Hispanic whites | 99-00 | * | .080 (<LOD-.160) | .190 (.120-.290) | .450 (.310-.720) | .870 (.510-1.30) | 595 |
| | 01-02 | * | < LOD | < LOD | .610 (.360-.780) | .830 (.650-1.36) | 947 |
| | 03-04 | * | < LOD | < LOD | < LOD | .290 (<LOD-.540) | 757 |

Limit of detection (LOD, see Data Analysis section) for Survey years 99-00, 01-02, and 03-04 are 0 05, 0.1, and 0.1, respectively.
< LOD means less than the limit of detection, which may vary for some chemicals by year and by individual sample.
* Not calculated: proportion of results below limit of detection was too high to provide a valid result.

# Urinary Diethyldithiophosphate (DEDTP) (creatinine corrected)
*Metabolite of Several Organophosphorus Insecticides*
Geometric mean and selected percentiles of urine concentrations (in µg/g of creatinine) for the U.S. population from the National Health and Nutrition Examination Survey.

| | Survey years | Geometric mean (95% conf. interval) | Selected percentiles ( 95% confidence interval) | | | | Sample size |
|---|---|---|---|---|---|---|---|
| | | | 50th | 75th | 90th | 95th | |
| **Total** | 99-00 | * | .070 (<LOD-.110) | .200 (.140-.290) | .550 (.390-.700) | .860 (.670-1.14) | 1949 |
| | 01-02 | * | < LOD | < LOD | .580 (.390-.750) | 1.01 (.710-1.43) | 2515 |
| | 03-04 | * | < LOD | < LOD | < LOD | .410 (.330-.510) | 1962 |
| **Age group** | | | | | | | |
| 6-11 years | 99-00 | * | .100 (<LOD-.140) | .190 (.150-.270) | .570 (.410-.760) | 1.03 (.570-1.58) | 471 |
| | 01-02 | * | < LOD | < LOD | .780 (.610-1.12) | 1.36 (1.02-1.86) | 576 |
| | 03-04 | * | < LOD | < LOD | < LOD | .470 (<LOD-.970) | 310 |
| 12-19 years | 99-00 | * | .050 (<LOD-.080) | .170 (.100-.220) | .440 (.230-.730) | .730 (.380-1.09) | 664 |
| | 01-02 | * | < LOD | < LOD | .360 (.250-.540) | .670 (.380-.990) | 821 |
| | 03-04 | * | < LOD | < LOD | .230 (<LOD-.260) | .330 (.240-.600) | 715 |
| 20-59 years | 99-00 | * | .080 (<LOD-.110) | .210 (.140-.310) | .550 (.360-.730) | .860 (.650-1.20) | 814 |
| | 01-02 | * | < LOD | < LOD | .580 (.380-.740) | 1.03 (.700-1.60) | 1118 |
| | 03-04 | * | < LOD | < LOD | < LOD | .400 (<LOD-.540) | 937 |
| **Gender** | | | | | | | |
| Males | 99-00 | * | .070 (<LOD-.110) | .190 (.140-.230) | .410 (.340-.500) | .720 (.520-.940) | 952 |
| | 01-02 | * | < LOD | < LOD | .380 (.300-.650) | .740 (.580-1.03) | 1187 |
| | 03-04 | * | < LOD | < LOD | < LOD | .330 (.260-.410) | 945 |
| Females | 99-00 | * | .090 (<LOD-.120) | .220 (.140-.360) | .670 (.410-.870) | .890 (.660-1.62) | 997 |
| | 01-02 | * | < LOD | < LOD | .700 (.490-1.00) | 1.24 (.800-1.86) | 1328 |
| | 03-04 | * | < LOD | < LOD | < LOD | .500 (<LOD-.640) | 1017 |
| **Race/ethnicity** | | | | | | | |
| Mexican Americans | 99-00 | .116 (.084-.161) | .090 (.060-.170) | .300 (.190-.410) | .810 (.570-.990) | 1.19 (.860-2.66) | 672 |
| | 01-02 | * | < LOD | < LOD | .850 (.440-1.24) | 1.29 (.880-1.78) | 678 |
| | 03-04 | * | < LOD | < LOD | .320 (<LOD-.450) | .540 (.330-.940) | 497 |
| Non-Hispanic blacks | 99-00 | .080 (.057-.111) | .070 (<LOD-.110) | .170 (.110-.280) | .450 (.300-.580) | .700 (.500-1.02) | 509 |
| | 01-02 | * | < LOD | < LOD | .460 (.330-.580) | .720 (.510-.960) | 693 |
| | 03-04 | * | < LOD | < LOD | < LOD | .270 (.180-.400) | 578 |
| Non-Hispanic whites | 99-00 | * | .070 (<LOD-.120) | .200 (.140-.310) | .560 (.380-.730) | .880 (.600-1.38) | 595 |
| | 01-02 | * | < LOD | < LOD | .540 (.360-.780) | 1.03 (.640-1.67) | 947 |
| | 03-04 | * | < LOD | < LOD | < LOD | .370 (<LOD-.520) | 756 |

< LOD means less than the limit of detection for the urine levels not corrected for creatinine.
* Not calculated: proportion of results below limit of detection was too high to provide a valid result.

## Urinary Dimethyldithiophosphate (DMDTP)
*Metabolite of Several Organophosphorus Insecticides*

Geometric mean and selected percentiles of urine concentrations (in μg/L) for the U.S. population from the National Health and Nutrition Examination Survey.

| | Survey years | Geometric mean (95% conf. interval) | 50th | 75th | 90th | 95th | Sample size |
|---|---|---|---|---|---|---|---|
| **Total** | 99-00 | * | < LOD | 2.30 (1.30-3.90) | 13.0 (5.00-17.0) | 19.0 (17.0-38.0) | 1949 |
| | 01-02 | * | < LOD | .890 (.210-1.30) | 2.49 (1.88-3.40) | 5.10 (3.55-8.35) | 2518 |
| | 03-04 | * | < LOD | .640 (.480-.800) | 1.99 (1.38-3.30) | 5.05 (3.30-7.16) | 1930 |
| **Age group** | | | | | | | |
| 6-11 years | 99-00 | .691 (.425-1.12) | .740 (.080-1.80) | 4.30 (2.40-8.60) | 17.0 (6.90-37.0) | 32.0 (17.0-44.0) | 471 |
| | 01-02 | * | < LOD | 1.30 (.750-2.11) | 3.53 (2.20-4.50) | 7.33 (4.32-9.74) | 575 |
| | 03-04 | * | < LOD | .900 (.620-1.14) | 2.94 (1.14-5.48) | 5.48 (2.94-8.53) | 306 |
| 12-19 years | 99-00 | * | < LOD | 2.30 (1.40-4.50) | 13.0 (5.40-20.0) | 20.0 (17.0-38.0) | 664 |
| | 01-02 | * | < LOD | .830 (.400-1.14) | 2.52 (1.85-3.07) | 4.63 (3.59-5.83) | 821 |
| | 03-04 | * | < LOD | .580 (.350-.770) | 1.46 (1.12-1.99) | 2.67 (1.82-4.49) | 699 |
| 20-59 years | 99-00 | * | < LOD | 2.10 (.840-3.60) | 11.0 (4.00-17.0) | 17.0 (7.70-50.0) | 814 |
| | 01-02 | * | < LOD | .840 (<LOD-1.31) | 2.32 (1.70-3.40) | 4.90 (2.90-9.52) | 1122 |
| | 03-04 | * | < LOD | .610 (.350-.800) | 2.00 (1.36-3.63) | 5.07 (3.62-8.62) | 925 |
| **Gender** | | | | | | | |
| Males | 99-00 | * | .110 (<LOD-.610) | 2.30 (1.20-4.90) | 16.0 (5.70-17.0) | 19.0 (17.0-38.0) | 952 |
| | 01-02 | * | < LOD | .840 (.190-1.28) | 2.40 (1.83-3.28) | 5.13 (3.53-7.86) | 1187 |
| | 03-04 | * | < LOD | .600 (.260-.910) | 1.76 (1.07-3.35) | 4.45 (2.24-7.97) | 935 |
| Females | 99-00 | * | < LOD | 2.20 (1.10-3.90) | 11.0 (4.20-17.0) | 20.0 (13.0-40.0) | 997 |
| | 01-02 | * | < LOD | .960 (.170-1.39) | 2.52 (1.94-3.68) | 5.10 (3.31-10.6) | 1331 |
| | 03-04 | * | < LOD | .690 (.510-.850) | 2.40 (1.43-4.15) | 5.07 (3.35-10.3) | 995 |
| **Race/ethnicity** | | | | | | | |
| Mexican Americans | 99-00 | * | .250 (<LOD-.870) | 1.90 (1.10-3.00) | 5.80 (4.10-9.70) | 12.0 (5.90-28.0) | 672 |
| | 01-02 | * | < LOD | 1.03 (.750-1.37) | 2.67 (2.07-3.42) | 4.47 (3.70-7.01) | 678 |
| | 03-04 | * | < LOD | .730 (.360-1.21) | 2.07 (1.36-3.15) | 5.26 (2.30-6.99) | 498 |
| Non-Hispanic blacks | 99-00 | * | .330 (<LOD-1.20) | 3.20 (1.40-7.00) | 14.0 (5.70-30.0) | 19.0 (17.0-39.0) | 509 |
| | 01-02 | * | < LOD | .770 (<LOD-1.67) | 2.11 (1.55-4.18) | 4.39 (2.51-8.66) | 695 |
| | 03-04 | * | < LOD | .590 (.370-.720) | 1.61 (1.05-3.11) | 4.51 (2.23-6.97) | 552 |
| Non-Hispanic whites | 99-00 | * | < LOD | 2.00 (.800-4.00) | 13.0 (3.90-20.0) | 20.0 (16.0-40.0) | 595 |
| | 01-02 | * | < LOD | .960 (<LOD-1.42) | 2.49 (1.83-3.65) | 5.74 (3.28-9.87) | 947 |
| | 03-04 | * | < LOD | .640 (.380-.880) | 1.96 (1.21-3.87) | 5.05 (2.29-10.6) | 752 |

Limit of detection (LOD, see Data Analysis section) for Survey years 99-00, 01-02, and 03-04 are 0 08, 0.1, and 0.1, respectively.
< LOD means less than the limit of detection, which may vary for some chemicals by year and by individual sample.
* Not calculated: proportion of results below limit of detection was too high to provide a valid result.

## Urinary Dimethyldithiophosphate (DMDTP) (creatinine corrected)

*Metabolite of Several Organophosphorus Insecticides*

Geometric mean and selected percentiles of urine concentrations (in µg/g of creatinine) for the U.S. population from the National Health and Nutrition Examination Survey.

| | Survey years | Geometric mean (95% conf. interval) | Selected percentiles ( 95% confidence interval) | | | | Sample size |
|---|---|---|---|---|---|---|---|
| | | | 50th | 75th | 90th | 95th | |
| **Total** | 99-00 | * | < LOD | 1.88 (.970-3.86) | 10.1 (5.31-18.3) | 21.7 (12.8-33.7) | 1949 |
| | 01-02 | * | < LOD | .670 (.330-1.08) | 2.60 (1.85-3.69) | 5.83 (4.23-7.75) | 2517 |
| | 03-04 | * | < LOD | .500 (.340-.650) | 2.14 (1.21-3.18) | 5.27 (2.69-7.61) | 1927 |
| **Age group** | | | | | | | |
| 6-11 years | 99-00 | .748 (.474-1.18) | .790 (.190-1.60) | 4.07 (2.31-7.18) | 16.2 (8.22-27.0) | 30.8 (20.2-38.9) | 471 |
| | 01-02 | * | < LOD | 1.36 (.800-2.31) | 4.10 (2.67-6.24) | 6.98 (4.40-12.8) | 575 |
| | 03-04 | * | < LOD | .960 (.580-1.57) | 3.38 (2.28-6.15) | 7.12 (4.48-7.55) | 306 |
| 12-19 years | 99-00 | * | < LOD | 1.52 (.620-3.47) | 9.48 (4.04-16.8) | 21.5 (9.48-42.3) | 664 |
| | 01-02 | * | < LOD | .540 (.310-.770) | 2.02 (1.49-2.40) | 3.13 (2.51-4.67) | 820 |
| | 03-04 | * | < LOD | .360 (.240-.580) | 1.02 (.630-1.57) | 2.45 (1.33-3.39) | 697 |
| 20-59 years | 99-00 | * | < LOD | 1.71 (.850-3.56) | 8.50 (4.00-19.1) | 20.5 (8.57-40.7) | 814 |
| | 01-02 | * | < LOD | .600 (<LOD-1.05) | 2.56 (1.64-4.03) | 6.33 (3.96-8.17) | 1122 |
| | 03-04 | * | < LOD | .450 (.340-.580) | 2.17 (1.10-3.64) | 5.71 (2.47-10.1) | 924 |
| **Gender** | | | | | | | |
| Males | 99-00 | * | .150 (<LOD-.370) | 1.79 (.840-3.97) | 11.0 (4.62-17.4) | 18.1 (7.51-44.7) | 952 |
| | 01-02 | * | < LOD | .580 (.270-.820) | 2.01 (1.40-2.67) | 4.67 (2.90-6.80) | 1187 |
| | 03-04 | * | < LOD | .370 (.260-.590) | 1.57 (.730-3.32) | 3.74 (2.14-6.53) | 934 |
| Females | 99-00 | * | < LOD | 2.06 (.940-4.00) | 9.30 (4.96-25.5) | 27.0 (9.66-47.5) | 997 |
| | 01-02 | * | < LOD | .820 (.370-1.43) | 2.92 (2.29-4.56) | 7.73 (4.44-11.9) | 1330 |
| | 03-04 | * | < LOD | .560 (.390-.790) | 2.62 (1.33-4.41) | 5.88 (2.82-11.6) | 993 |
| **Race/ethnicity** | | | | | | | |
| Mexican Americans | 99-00 | * | .270 (<LOD-.660) | 1.35 (.860-2.53) | 6.55 (3.83-11.8) | 16.7 (6.25-38.8) | 672 |
| | 01-02 | * | < LOD | .830 (.540-1.11) | 2.59 (1.88-3.22) | 4.86 (3.32-6.37) | 678 |
| | 03-04 | * | < LOD | .650 (.320-1.10) | 2.04 (1.09-3.84) | 4.50 (2.11-5.88) | 497 |
| Non-Hispanic blacks | 99-00 | * | .250 (<LOD-.700) | 2.40 (.690-5.44) | 9.41 (4.81-17.8) | 17.9 (11.5-40.7) | 509 |
| | 01-02 | * | < LOD | .430 (<LOD-.930) | 1.80 (.830-3.50) | 3.65 (2.33-5.91) | 694 |
| | 03-04 | * | < LOD | .340 (.260-.430) | .890 (.740-1.50) | 2.33 (1.12-4.55) | 551 |
| Non-Hispanic whites | 99-00 | * | < LOD | 1.77 (.780-4.02) | 11.4 (4.07-21.5) | 21.5 (11.4-34.8) | 595 |
| | 01-02 | * | < LOD | .710 (<LOD-1.31) | 2.85 (1.91-4.96) | 7.29 (4.25-9.47) | 947 |
| | 03-04 | * | < LOD | .470 (.340-.700) | 2.25 (1.02-4.03) | 5.89 (2.47-10.1) | 751 |

< LOD means less than the limit of detection for the urine levels not corrected for creatinine.
* Not calculated: proportion of results below limit of detection was too high to provide a valid result.

## References

Albers JW, Berent S, Garabrant DH, Giordani B, Schweitzer SJ, Garrison RP, Richardson RJ. The effects of occupational exposure to chlorpyrifos on the neurologic examination of central nervous system function: a prospective cohort study. J Occup Environ Med 2004;46(4):367-378.

Aprea C, Sciarra G, Orsi D, Boccalon P, Sartorelli P, Sartorelli E. Urinary excretion of alkylphosphates in the general population (Italy). Sci Total Environ 1996;177:37-41.

Aprea C, Strambi M, Novelli MT, Lunghini L, Bozzi N. Biologic monitoring of exposure to organophosphorus pesticides in 195 Italian children. Environ Health Perspect 2000;108:521-525.

Arcury TA, Grzywacz JG, Davis SW, Barr DB, Quandt SA. Organophosphorus pesticide urinary metabolite levels of children in farmworker households in eastern North Carolina. Am J Ind Med 2006;49(9):751-760.

Astroff AB, Freshwater KJ, Eigenberg DA. Comparative organophosphate-induced effects observed in adult and neonatal Sprague-Dawley rats during the conduct of multigeneration toxicity studies. Reprod Toxicol 1998a;12(6):619-645.

Astroff AB, Young AD. The relationship between maternal and fetal effects following maternal organophosphate exposure during gestation in the rat. Toxicol Ind Health 1998b;14(6):869-889.

Bouvier G, Blanchard O, Momas I, Seta N. Environmental and biological monitoring of exposure to organophosphorus pesticides: application to occupationally and non-occupationally exposed adult populations. J Expo Sci Environ Epidemiol 2006;16(5):417-426.

Bradman A, Eskenazi B, Barr DB, Bravo R, Castorina R, Chevrier J, et al. Organophosphate urinary metabolite levels during pregnancy and after delivery in women living in an agricultural community. Environ Health Perspect 2005;113(12):1802-1807.

Castorina R, Bradman A, McKone TE, Barr DB, Harnly ME, Eskenazi B. Cumulative organophosphate pesticide exposure and risk assessment among pregnant women living in an agricultural community: a case study from the CHAMACOS cohort. Environ Health Perspect 2003;111(13):1640-1648.

Centers for Disease Control and Prevention (CDC). Third National Report on Human Exposure to Environmental Chemicals. Atlanta (GA). 2005.

Curl CL, Fenske RA, Elgethun K. Organophosphorus pesticide exposure of urban and suburban preschool children with organic and conventional diets. Environ Health Perspect 2003;111(3):377-382.

Daniell W, Barnhart S, Demers P, Costa LG, Eaton DL, Miller M, et al. Neuropsychological performance among agricultural pesticide applicators. Environ Res 1992;59(1):217-228.

Davies JE, Peterson JC. Surveillance of occupational, accidental, and incidental exposure to organophosphate pesticides using urine alkyl phosphate and phenolic metabolite measurements. Ann NY Acad Sci 1997;837:257-268.

Duggan A, Charnley G, Chen W, Chukwudebe A, Hawk R, Krieger RI, et al. Di-alkyl phosphate biomonitoring data: assessing cumulative exposure to organophosphate pesticides. Regul Toxicol Pharmacol 2003;37(3):382-395.

Engel LS, Keifer MC, Checkoway H, Robinson LR, Vaughan TL. Neurophysiological function in farm workers exposed to organophosphate pesticides. Arch Environ Health 1998;53(1):7-14.

Farahat TM, Abdelrasoul GM, Amr MM, Shebl MM, Farahat FM, Anger WK. Neurobehavioural effects among workers occupationally exposed to organophosphorous pesticides. Occup Environ Med 2003;60(4):279-286.

Fenske RA, Curl CL, Kissel JC. The effect of the 14-day agricultural restricted entry interval on azinphosmethyl exposures in a group of apple thinners in Washington State. Regul Toxicol Pharmacol 2003;38(1):91-97.

Fiedler N, Kipen H, Kelly-McNeil K, Fenske R. Long-term use of organophosphates and neuropsychological performance. Am J Ind Med 1997;32(5):487-496.

Franklin CA, Fenske RA, Greenhalgh R, Mathieu L, Denley HV, Leffingwell JT, et al. Correlation of urinary pesticide metabolite excretion with estimated dermal contact in the course of occupational exposure to Guthion. J Toxicol Environ Health 1981;7(5):715-731.

Heudorf U, Angerer J. Metabolites of organophosphorous insecticides in urine specimens from inhabitants of a residential area. Environ Res 2001; 86:80-87.

Jamal GA, Hansen S, Pilkington A, Buchanan D, Gillham RA, Abdel-Azis M, et al. A clinical neurological, neurophysiological, and neuropsychological study of sheep farmers and dippers exposed to organophosphate pesticides. Occup Environ Med 2002;59(7):434-441.

Kissel JC, Curl CL, Kedan G, Lu C, Griffith W, Barr DB, et al. Comparison of organophosphorus pesticide metabolite levels in single and multiple daily urine samples collected from preschool children in Washington State. J Expo Anal Environ Epidemiol 2005;15(2):164-171.

Koch D, Lu C, Fisker-Andersen J, Jolley L, Fenske RA. Temporal association of children's pesticide exposure and agricultural spraying: report of a longitudinal biological monitoring study. Environ Health Perspect 2002;110(8):829-833.

Krieger RI, Dinoff TM. Malathion deposition, metabolite clearance, and cholinesterase status of date dusters and harvesters in California. Arch Environ Contam Toxicol 2000;38(4):546-563.

Lambert WE, Lasarev M, Muniz J, Scherer J, Rothlein J, Santana J, et al. Variation in organophosphate pesticide metabolites in urine of children living in agricultural communities. Environ Health Perspect 2005;113(4):504-508.

London L, Nell V, Thompson ML, Myers JE. Effects of long-term organophosphate exposures on neurological symptoms, vibration sense and tremor among South African farm workers. Scand J Work Environ Health 1998;24(1):18-29.

Lu C, Bravo R, Caltabiano LM, Irish RM, Weerasekera G, Barr DB. The presence of dialkylphosphates in fresh fruit juices: implication for organophosphorus pesticide exposure and risk assessments. J Toxicol Environ Health A 2005;68(3):209-227

Maizlish N, Schenker M, Weisskopf C, Seiber J, Samuels S. A behavioral evaluation of pest control workers with short-term, low-level exposure to the organophosphate diazinon. Am J Ind Med 1987;12(2):153-172.

National Research Council (NRC). Pesticides in the Diets of Infants and Children. National Academy of Sciences. Washington (DC). 1993 [online]. Available at URL: http://books.nap.edu/openbook.php?record_id=2126&page=1. 1/12/09

Peiris-John RJ, Ruberu DK, Wickremasinghe AR, Smit LA, van der Hoek W. Effects of occupational exposure to organophosphate pesticides on nerve and neuromuscular function. J Occup Environ Med 2002;44(4):352-357.

Petchuay C, Visuthismajarn P, Vitayavirasak B, Hore P, Robson MG. Biological monitoring of organophosphate pesticides in preschool children in an agricultural community in Thailand. Int J Occup Environ Health 2006;12(2):134-141.

Pilkington A, Buchanan D, Jamal GA, Gillham R, Hansen S, Kidd M, et al. An epidemiological study of the relations between exposure to organophosphate pesticides and indices of chronic peripheral neuropathy and neuropsychological abnormalities in sheep farmers and dippers. Occup Environ Med 2001;58(11):702-710.

Prendergast MA, Terry AV Jr, Buccafusco JJ. Effects of chronic, low-level organophosphate exposure on delayed recall, discrimination, and spatial learning in monkeys and rats. Neurotoxicol Teratol 1998;20(2):115-22.

Rodnitzky RL. Occupational exposure to organophosphate pesticides: a neurobehavioral study. Arch Environ Health 1975;30(2):98-103.

Rosenstock L, Keifer M, Daniell WE, McConnell R, Claypoole K. Chronic central nervous system effects of acute organophosphate pesticide intoxication. The Pesticide Health Effects Study Group.

Lancet. 1991;338(8761):223-227.

Rothlein J, Rohlman D, Lasarev M, Phillips J, Muniz J, McCauley L. Organophosphate pesticide exposure and neurobehavioral performance in agricultural and non-agricultural Hispanic workers. Environ Health Perspect 2006;114(5):691-696.

Saieva C, Aprea C, Tumino R, Masala G, Salvini S, Frasca G, et al. Twenty-four-hour urinary excretion of ten pesticide metabolites in healthy adults in two different areas of Italy (Florence and Ragusa). Sci Total Environ 2004;332(1-3):71-80.

Savage EP, Keefe TJ, Mounce LM, Heaton RK, Lewis JA, Burcar PJ. Chronic neurological sequelae of acute organophosphate pesticide poisoning. Arch Environ Health 1988;43(1):38-45.

Steenland K, Jenkins B, Ames RG, O'Malley M, Chrislip D, Russo J. Chronic neurological sequelae to organophosphate pesticide poisoning. Am J Public Health 1994;84(5):731-736.

Stephens R, Spurgeon A, Calvert IA, Beach J, Levy LS, Berry H, et al. Neuropsychological effects of long-term exposure to organophosphates in sheep dip. Lancet 1995;345(8958):1135-1139.

Stokes L, Stark A, Marshall E, Narang A. Neurotoxicity among pesticide applicators exposed to organophosphates. Occup Environ Med 1995;52(10):648-653.

Takamiya K. Monitoring of urinary alkyl phosphates in pest-control operators exposed to various organophosphorus insecticides. Bull Environ Contam Toxicol 1994;52(2):190-195.

U. S. Environmental Protection Agency (U.S. EPA). Office of Prevention Pesticides and Toxic Substances. Pesticide industry sales and usage - 2000 and 2001 market estimates. Washington (DC): U.S. EPA; May, 2004. Available at URL: http://www.epa.gov/oppbead1/pestsales/01pestsales/market_estimates2001.pdf. 4/7/09

Young JG, Eskenazi B, Gladstone EA, Bradman A, Pedersen L, Johnson C, et al. Association between in utero organophosphate pesticide exposure and abnormal reflexes in neonates. Neurotoxicology 2005;26(2):199-209.

# Organophosphorus Insecticides: Specific Metabolites

## General Information

The specific metabolites of the organophosphorus insecticides discussed in this section are those that are often measured in biomonitoring studies. These metabolites differ from the dialkyl phosphate metabolites because each specific metabolite derives from one or only a few parent insecticides. The table below shows the parent organophosphorus insecticides and their metabolites measured in this *Report*. For example, malathion is metabolized to malathion dicarboxylic acid; parathion and methyl parathion are metabolized to para-nitrophenol. In addition to reflecting exposure to the parent insecticide, the level may reflect exposure to the environmental degradation products of these pesticides. For general information about the organophosphorus class of insecticides, see the section titled "Organophosphorus Insecticides: Dialkyl Phosphate Metabolites."

| Organophosphorus insecticide (CAS number) | Primary urinary metabolite (CAS number) |
|---|---|
| Chlorpyrifos (2921-88-2) Chlorpyrifos-methyl (5598-13-0) | 3,5,6-Trichloro-2-pyridinol (6515-38-4) |
| Coumaphos (56-72-4) | 3-Chloro-7-hydroxy-4-methyl-2H-chromen-2-one/ol |
| Diazinon (333-41-5) | 2-Isopropyl-4-methyl-6-hydroxypyrimidine (2814-20-2) |
| Malathion (121-75-5) | Malathion dicarboxylic acid (1190-28-9) |
| Ethyl parathion (56-38-2) Methyl parathion (298-00-0) | para-Nitrophenol (100-02-7) |
| Pirimiphos-methyl (29232-93-7) | 2-(Diethylamino)-6-methylpyrimidin-4-ol/one |

# Chlorpyrifos
CAS No. 2921-88-2

# Chlorpyrifos-methyl
CAS No. 5598-13-0

## General Information

The chemical 3,5,6-trichloro-2-pyridinol (TCPy) is a metabolite of chlorpyrifos and chlorpyrifos-methyl. Chlorpyrifos is a broad spectrum organophosphorus insecticide that has been widely used to control insects on food crops such as corn. It also has been applied directly on animals to kill mites, applied to structures to kill termites, and sprayed to kill mosquitoes. Approximately 21-24 million pounds per year were used domestically from 1987-1998. After 2001, chlorpyrifos was no longer registered for indoor residential uses in the United States; pre- and post-construction structural applications for termite control were to be phased out by 2005 (U.S.EPA, 2002). Chlorpyrifos-methyl is an organophosphorus insecticide also used in agriculture and not registered for residential use. Approximately 80,000 pounds are used

per year. Chlorpyrifos is degraded in agricultural soils with a half-life of several months, and on plants for days to several weeks. It has low leachability, staying bound to soil particles, and is infrequently detected in ground water (IPCS, 1999; USGS, 2007), but can be detected in streams receiving runoff from application sites. Chlorpyrifos is very toxic to fish and aquatic invertebrates and shows modest degrees of bioconcentration.

The general population may be exposed to chlorpyrifos via oral, dermal, and inhalation routes. Estimated intakes from diet and water have not exceeded recommended intake limits, although some tolerances for specific food crops have been reduced in the past to avoid exceeding recommended intake limits for total dietary intake in special groups (U.S.EPA, 2002). Exposure can also result from contact with contaminated surfaces, air, and dust. For instance, in 142 urban homes and preschools in North Carolina, chlorpyrifos and TCPy were detected in all indoor air and dust samples (Morgan et al., 2005). Chlorpyrifos is not well absorbed through the skin but dermal exposure can be significant when other routes of exposure are low. Inhalational and dermal routes of exposure are important in pesticide formulators and applicators. Chlorpyrifos is

## Urinary 3,5,6-Trichloro-2-pyridinol
*Metabolite of Chlorpyrifos and Chlorpyrifos-methyl*

Geometric mean and selected percentiles of urine concentrations (in µg/L) for the U.S. population from the National Health and Nutrition Examination Survey.

| | Survey years | Geometric mean (95% conf. interval) | 50th | 75th | 90th | 95th | Sample size |
|---|---|---|---|---|---|---|---|
| Total | 99-00 | 1.77 (1.46-2.14) | 1.70 (1.40-2 20) | 3.50 (2.50-5 20) | 7.30 (4.80-10.0) | 10.0 (7.70-15.0) | 1994 |
| | 01-02 | 1.76 (1.52-2 03) | 2.22 (1.90-2 61) | 4.95 (4.55-5 29) | 8.80 (7.74-9.77) | 12.4 (10.4-15.3) | 2509 |
| **Age group** | | | | | | | |
| 6-11 years | 99-00 | 2.88 (1.99-4.16) | 2.80 (1.60-4 90) | 7.09 (3.40-10.0) | 12.0 (7.70-17.0) | 16.0 (10.0-28.0) | 481 |
| | 01-02 | 2.67 (2.13-3 35) | 3.09 (2.50-4 22) | 6.36 (4.97-7 97) | 10.9 (7.98-15.3) | 15.3 (11.5-24.0) | 573 |
| 12-19 years | 99-00 | 2.37 (1.89-2 97) | 2.10 (1.60-3 00) | 4.50 (2.90-7.10) | 8.10 (5.50-14.0) | 12.5 (8.00-24.0) | 681 |
| | 01-02 | 2.71 (2.19-3 35) | 3.57 (2.66-4 34) | 6.60 (5.61-7 59) | 11.3 (8.66-15.1) | 18.0 (13.7-23.7) | 823 |
| 20-59 years | 99-00 | 1.53 (1.29-1 83) | 1.50 (1.30-1 80) | 2.90 (2.20-4 30) | 5.90 (3.90-8 90) | 8.90 (6.70-11.0) | 832 |
| | 01-02 | 1.51 (1.32-1.72) | 1.91 (1.44-2 26) | 4.44 (3.90-4 80) | 7.78 (7.00-8 91) | 10.9 (9.52-12.4) | 1113 |
| **Gender** | | | | | | | |
| Males | 99-00 | 1.92 (1.60-2 32) | 1.90 (1.50-2.40) | 3.60 (2.70-5 60) | 7.40 (5.04-10.0) | 10.0 (7.70-16.0) | 972 |
| | 01-02 | 2.13 (1.81-2 51) | 2.67 (2.20-3 25) | 5.37 (4.87-6 25) | 9.63 (8.20-11.5) | 14.9 (10.9-18.9) | 1183 |
| Females | 99-00 | 1.63 (1.31-2 02) | 1.50 (1.20-2 00) | 3.30 (2.30-5 30) | 7.20 (4.30-12.0) | 11.0 (7.20-16.0) | 1022 |
| | 01-02 | 1.45 (1.24-1.70) | 1.74 (1.39-2 21) | 4.38 (3.72-4 95) | 7.71 (6.30-9 20) | 10.4 (8.47-13.2) | 1326 |
| **Race/ethnicity** | | | | | | | |
| Mexican Americans | 99-00 | 1.61 (1.31-2 00) | 1.67 (1.30-2 20) | 3.20 (2.60-3 80) | 5.10 (3.80-8.40) | 7.40 (5.10-17.0) | 697 |
| | 01-02 | 2.02 (1.79-2 28) | 2.63 (2.24-3 01) | 4.60 (4.05-5 39) | 9.02 (7.04-10.8) | 12.2 (10.8-15.7) | 660 |
| Non-Hispanic blacks | 99-00 | 2.17 (1.59-2 97) | 1.90 (1.43-2 80) | 4.30 (2.50-8 30) | 9.40 (6.40-13.7) | 13.0 (9.40-26.0) | 521 |
| | 01-02 | 2.19 (1.68-2 84) | 2.89 (2.28-3.47) | 5.47 (4.77-6 96) | 9.27 (7.47-11.6) | 12.3 (10.1-16.8) | 701 |
| Non-Hispanic whites | 99-00 | 1.76 (1.51-2 05) | 1.70 (1.50-2.10) | 3.50 (2.50-4 86) | 7.10 (4.30-11.0) | 10.0 (7.20-14.0) | 602 |
| | 01-02 | 1.71 (1.43-2 03) | 2.15 (1.62-2 64) | 4.94 (4.44-5 37) | 8.68 (7.47-9 97) | 12.4 (9.77-15.9) | 947 |

Limit of detection (LOD, see Data Analysis section) for Survey years 99-00 and 01-02 are 0.4 and 0.4.

rapidly absorbed following ingestion. Once absorbed, phosphorothioates such as chlorpyrifos are metabolically activated to the "oxon" form which has greater toxicity than the parent insecticide. Metabolic hydrolysis leads to the formation of TCPy, dialkyl phosphate metabolites (see section titled "Organophosphorus Insecticides: Dialkyl Phosphate Metabolites"), and other metabolites. Chlorpyrifos is eliminated from the body primarily in the urine with a half-life of approximately 27 hours (Nolan et al., 1984). In addition to being a metabolite of chlorpyrifos and chlorpyrifos-methyl in the body, TCPy can also occur in the environment from the breakdown of the parent compounds. TCPy is more persistent in the environment than chlorpyrifos itself (U.S.EPA, 2002). Thus, the detection of TCPy in a person's urine may reflect exposure to the environmental degradates.

Human health effects from chlorpyrifos or chlorpyrifos-methyl at low environmental doses or at biomonitored levels from low environmental exposures are unknown. Chlorpyrifos and chlorpyrifos-methyl both demonstrate moderate acute toxicity in animal studies. These organophosphorus insecticides share a mechanism of toxicity: inhibition of the activity of acetylcholinesterase enzymes in the nervous system, resulting in excess acetylcholine at nerve terminals, and producing acute symptoms such as nausea, vomiting, cholinergic effects, weakness, paralysis, and seizures. The metabolite TCPy does not inhibit acetylcholinesterase enzymes. Overt cholinergic toxicity from chlorpyrifos has been described following suicidal ingestion and unintentional high level occupational exposure. Based on animal data and human cholinesterase monitoring during occupational exposure, ubiquitous low-level environmental exposures in humans would not be expected to result in inhibition of cholinesterase activity. Recent *in vitro* and *in vivo* animal studies suggest that effects on neuronal morphogenesis, neurotransmission, and behavior may occur at systemically nontoxic doses or at doses of chlorpyrifos that do not result in cholinergic signs (Aldridge et al., 2005; Betancourt et al., 2006; Howard et al., 2005; Ricceri et al., 2006; Roy et al., 2005; Slotkin et al., 2006a, 2006b). In pesticide applicators, chronic exposure to chlorpyrifos may be associated with slight alterations in some components of neurophysiologic testing (Steenland et al., 2000). Two observational studies of pregnant women and their offspring exposed to chlorpyrifos at environmental levels have found inconsistent relationships with birth outcomes of weight and length (Eskenazi et al.,

## Urinary 3,5,6-Trichloro-2-pyridinol (creatinine corrected)
*Metabolite of Chlorpyrifos and Chlorpyrifos-methyl*
Geometric mean and selected percentiles of urine concentrations (in µg/g of creatinine) for the U.S. population from the National Health and Nutrition Examination Survey.

| | Survey years | Geometric mean (95% conf. interval) | Selected percentiles ( 95% confidence interval) | | | | Sample size |
|---|---|---|---|---|---|---|---|
| | | | 50th | 75th | 90th | 95th | |
| **Total** | 99-00 | 1.58 (1.35-1.85) | 1.47 (1.24-1.74) | 2.85 (2.12-3.59) | 5.43 (4.22-6.68) | 8.42 (6.25-11 6) | 1994 |
| | 01-02 | 1.73 (1.49-2.01) | 1.88 (1.64-2.24) | 3.76 (2.91-4.62) | 6.15 (4.99-8.31) | 9.22 (6.94-12 3) | 2508 |
| **Age group** | | | | | | | |
| 6-11 years | 99-00 | 3.11 (2.31-4.19) | 3.20 (2.05-4.80) | 6.39 (4.14-8.19) | 10.1 (7.26-14 0) | 14.1 (10.1-21 0) | 481 |
| | 01-02 | 3.48 (2.80-4.32) | 3.76 (3.17-4.36) | 6.22 (4.88-8.57) | 12.2 (7.24-24.4) | 16.9 (12.1-38 0) | 573 |
| 12-19 years | 99-00 | 1.60 (1.34-1.91) | 1.45 (1.21-1.81) | 2.58 (1.97-3.92) | 4.82 (3.44-6.16) | 6.16 (4.43-10 6) | 681 |
| | 01-02 | 2.09 (1.72-2.55) | 2.24 (1.92-2.66) | 3.97 (3.30-4.72) | 6.33 (5.62-7.89) | 10.3 (7.65-15 2) | 822 |
| 20-59 years | 99-00 | 1.41 (1.23-1.62) | 1.33 (1.12-1.58) | 2.37 (1.87-3.01) | 4.29 (3.53-5.56) | 6.42 (5.11-9.02) | 832 |
| | 01-02 | 1.49 (1.30-1.71) | 1.64 (1.39-1.88) | 3.11 (2.60-3.91) | 5.50 (4.33-7.23) | 7.44 (5.80-11 0) | 1113 |
| **Gender** | | | | | | | |
| Males | 99-00 | 1.48 (1.27-1.72) | 1.44 (1.19-1.68) | 2.54 (2.05-3.38) | 4.95 (3.84-6.54) | 7.63 (5.65-11 0) | 972 |
| | 01-02 | 1.71 (1.47-2.00) | 1.88 (1.57-2.22) | 3.46 (2.82-4.28) | 5.93 (4.90-9.24) | 10.5 (6.94-14 3) | 1183 |
| Females | 99-00 | 1.69 (1.42-2.01) | 1.51 (1.25-1.85) | 2.97 (2.24-4.01) | 5.63 (4.27-7.39) | 8.44 (5.79-13 3) | 1022 |
| | 01-02 | 1.75 (1.49-2.07) | 1.93 (1.59-2.33) | 3.91 (3.06-4.85) | 6.47 (5.00-8.11) | 8.98 (6.83-11 8) | 1325 |
| **Race/ethnicity** | | | | | | | |
| Mexican Americans | 99-00 | 1.46 (1.20-1.77) | 1.44 (1.05-1.93) | 2.39 (2.09-2.96) | 3.86 (3.24-5.08) | 5.85 (3.88-9.57) | 697 |
| | 01-02 | 1.86 (1.63-2.12) | 2.06 (1.83-2.35) | 3.81 (3.17-4.56) | 6.52 (5.64-7.58) | 9.00 (7.66-11 8) | 660 |
| Non-Hispanic blacks | 99-00 | 1.47 (1.09-1.99) | 1.33 ( 940-1.91) | 2.86 (1.58-5.05) | 5.91 (4.05-8.93) | 9.02 (5.91-13.7) | 521 |
| | 01-02 | 1.56 (1.19-2.03) | 1.92 (1.57-2.40) | 3.53 (2.85-4.28) | 5.58 (4.80-6.07) | 7.06 (5.88-8.82) | 700 |
| Non-Hispanic whites | 99-00 | 1.66 (1.45-1.91) | 1.55 (1.31-1.83) | 2.93 (2.09-3.97) | 5.56 (4.21-6.75) | 8.44 (6.25-12 3) | 602 |
| | 01-02 | 1.78 (1.49-2.14) | 1.95 (1.56-2.35) | 3.82 (2.70-4.97) | 6.55 (4.88-10 5) | 9.98 (7.00-13.7) | 947 |

2004; Perera et al., 2003; Whyatt et al., 2004).

Some reproductive and teratogenic effects in animal testing were only observed at high doses of chlorpyrifos that caused overt maternal toxicity. Chlorpyrifos is not considered to be mutagenic or carcinogenic (NTP, 1992; U.S.EPA, 2002). Additional information about external exposure (i.e., environmental levels) and health effects is available from ATSDR at: http://www.atsdr.cdc.gov/toxpro2.html and from U.S. EPA at: http://www.epa.gov/pesticides/.

## Biomonitoring Information

Urinary TCPy levels reflect recent exposure. Levels of TCPy in the U.S. subsamples of NHANES 1999-2000 and 2001-2002 (CDC, 2005) appear roughly similar to values reported for a nonrandom subsample of NHANES III (1988-1994) participants (Hill et al., 1995) and were similar to levels reported in studies of healthy adults in Germany (Koch et al., 2001) and Italy (Aprea et al., 1999). In a probability-based sample of 102 Minnesota children aged 3-13 years, the weighted population mean of TCPy measurements was approximately three times higher (Adgate, 2001) than the corresponding values reported for the group aged 6-11 years from the NHANES 1999-2000 subsample (CDC, 2005). MacIntosh et al. (1999) reported mean urinary TCPy levels in a sample of Maryland adults that were about three times higher than adults in the U.S. population (CDC, 2005). Of 482 pregnant women living in an agricultural community, 76% had detectable levels of TCPy and levels were similar to those reported for NHANES 1999-2000 (Eskenazi et al., 2004). Other small studies of environmentally-exposed persons have shown a high frequency of detecting low levels of TCPy.

Following crack-and-crevice application of chlorpyrifos in their homes, urinary TCPy levels in children were reported not to have increased (Hore et al., 2005). Chlorpyrifos levels in house dust and hand rinses did not correlate with levels of TCPy in urine (Lioy et al., 2000). Replacing conventional diets with organic diets in 23 children led to about a fourfold decrease in urinary levels of chlorpyrifos; median urinary levels on the conventional diet were several fold higher than those in the NHANES 1999-2000 subsample (Lu et al., 2006). Measurements of urinary TCPy in single spot urine collections show variability over time in environmentally exposed individuals and are poorly correlated between collections, suggesting changing low-level exposure and variance in collection timing with respect to exposure (Meeker et al., 2005). Estimation of dose or intake based on the urinary excretion of TCPy indicates that environmental doses are generally below recommended limits (Hore et al., 2005; Koch et al., 2001).

In Iowa farm families using several different pesticides, but not chlorpyrifos, the geometric mean urinary TCPy levels were similar in parents and children, but levels were roughly four to six times higher than the geometric means in the U.S. representative subsample of NHANES 1999-2000 (CDC, 2005; Curwin et al., 2007). In Minnesota and South Carolina farmers who used chlorpyrifos, urinary TCPy levels averaged about sixfold higher than those in the NHANES 1999-2000 subsample (Mandel et al., 2005; CDC, 2005). Urinary levels of TCPy have been found to be hundredsfold higher for chlorpyrifos manufacturing workers (Burns et al., 2006) and episodically many times higher for pesticide applicators than median levels from NHANES 1999-2000 (CDC, 2005).

Finding a measurable amount of TCPy in urine does not mean that the level will result in an adverse health effect. Biomonitoring studies of TCPy provide physicians and public health officials with reference values so that they can determine whether people have been exposed to higher levels of chlorpyrifos or chlorpyrifos-methyl than are found in the general population. Biomonitoring data can also help scientists plan and conduct research on exposure and health effects.

## References

Adgate JL, Barr DB, Clayton CA, Eberly LE, Freeman NC, Lioy PJ, et al. Measurement of children's exposure to pesticides: analysis of urinary metabolite levels in a probability-based sample. Environ Health Perspect 2001;109(6):583-590.

Aldridge JE, Meyer A, Seidler FJ, Slotkin TA. Alterations in central nervous system serotonergic and dopaminergic synaptic activity in adulthood after prenatal or neonatal chlorpyrifos exposure. Environ Health Perspect 2005;113(8):1027-1031.

Aprea C, Betta A, Catenacci G, Lotti A, Magnaghi S, Barisano A, et al.Reference values of urinary 3,5,6-trichloro-2-pyridinol in the Italian population—validation of analytical method and preliminary results (multicentric study). J AOAC Int 1999;82(2):305-312.

Betancourt AM, Burgess SC, Carr RL. Effect of developmental exposure to chlorpyrifos on the expression of neurotrophin growth factors and cell-specific markers in neonatal rat brain. Toxicol Sci 2006;92(2):500-506.

Burns CJ, Garabrant D, Albers JW, Berent S, Giordani B, Haidar S, et al. Chlorpyrifos exposure and biological monitoring among manufacturing workers. Occup Environ Med 2006;63(3):218-220.

Centers for Disease Control and Prevention (CDC). Third National Report on Human Exposure to Environmental Chemicals. Atlanta (GA). 2005.

Curwin BD, Hein MJ, Sanderson WT, Striley C, Heederik D, Kromhout H, et al. Urinary pesticide concentrations among children, mothers and fathers living in farm and non-farm households in Iowa. Ann Occup Hyg 2007;51(1):53-65.

Eskenazi B, Harley K, Bradman A, Weltzien E, Jewell NP, Barr DB, et al. Association of in utero organophosphate pesticide exposure and fetal growth and length of gestation in an agricultural population. Environ Health Perspect 2004;112(10):1116-1124.

Hill RH Jr, Head SL, Baker S, Gregg M, Shealy DB, Bailey SL, et al. Pesticide residues in urine of adults living in the United States: reference range concentrations. Environ Res 1995;71:99-108.

Hore P, Robson M, Freeman N, Zhang J, Wartenberg D, Ozkaynak H, et al. Chlorpyrifos accumulation patterns for child-accessible surfaces and objects and urinary metabolite excretion by children for 2 weeks after crack-and-crevice application. Environ Health Perspect 2005;113(2):211-219.

Howard AS, Bucelli R, Jett DA, Bruun D, Yang D, Lein PJ. Chlorpyrifos exerts opposing effects on axonal and dendritic growth in primary neuronal cultures. Toxicol Appl Pharmacol 2005;207(2):112-124.

International Programme on Chemical Safety-INCHEM (IPCS). Environmental Health Criteria 198. Chlorpyrifos. 1999. Available at URL: http://www.inchem.org/documents/jmpr/jmpmono/v99pr03.htm. 4/7/09

Koch HM, Hardt J, Angerer J. Biological monitoring of exposure of the general population to the organophosphorus pesticides chlorpyrifos and chlorpyrifos-methyl by determination of their specific metabolite 3,5,6-trichloro-2-pyridinol. Int J Hyg Environ Health 2001;204(2-3):175-180.

Lioy PJ, Edwards RD, Freeman N, Gurunathan S, Pellizzari E, Adgate JL, et al. House dust levels of selected insecticides and a herbicide measured by the EL and LWW samplers and comparisons to hand rinses and urine metabolites. J Expo Anal Environ Epidemiol 2000;10(4):327-340.

Lu C, Toepel K, Irish R, Fenske RA, Barr DB, Bravo R. Organic diets significantly lower children's dietary exposure to organophosphorus pesticides. Environ Health Perspect 2006;114(2):260-263.

MacIntosh DL, Needham LL, Hammerstrom KA, Ryan PB. A longitudinal investigation of selected pesticide metabolites in urine. J Expo Anal Environ Epidemiol 1999;9(5):494-501.

Mandel JS, Alexander BH, Baker BA, Acquavella JF, Chapman P, Honeycutt R. Biomonitoring for farm families in the farm family exposure study. Scand J Work Environ Health 2005;31 Suppl 1:98-104.

Meeker JD, Barr DB, Ryan L, Herrick RF, Bennett DH, Bravo R, et al. Temporal variability of urinary levels of nonpersistent insecticides in adult men. J Expo Anal Environ Epidemiol 2005;15(3):271-281.

Morgan MK, Sheldon LS, Croghan CW, Jones PA, Robertson GL, Chuang JC, et al. Exposures of preschool children to chlorpyrifos and its degradation product 3,5,6-trichloro 2-pyridinol in their everyday environments. J Expo Anal Environ Epidemiol 2005;15(4):297-309.

Nolan RJ, Rick DL, Freshour NL, Saunders JH. Chlorpyrifos: pharmacokinetics in human volunteers. Toxicol Appl Pharmacol 1984;73:8-15.

National Toxicology Program (NTP). Executive summary of safety and toxicity information. chlorpyrifos. 2921-88-2. February 5, 1992. Available at URL: http://ntp.niehs.nih.gov/ntpweb/index.cfm?objectid=6F5E95EB-F1F6-975E-7C20F4211536F46F. 4/7/09

Perera FP, Rauh V, Tsai WY, Kinney P, Camann D, Barr D, et al. Effects of transplacental exposure to environmental pollution on birth outcomes in a multiethnic population. Environ Health Perspect 2003;111(2):201-205.

Ricceri L, Venerosi A, Capone F, Cometa MF, Lorenzini P, Fortuna S, et al. Developmental neurotoxicity of organophosphorous pesticides: fetal and neonatal exposure to chlorpyrifos alters sex specific behaviors at adulthood in mice. Toxicol Sci 2006;93(1):105-113.

Roy TS, Sharma V, Seidler FJ, Slotkin TA. Quantitative morphological assessment reveals neuronal and glial deficits in hippocampus after a brief subtoxic exposure to chlorpyrifos in neonatal rats. Brain Res Dev Brain Res 2005;155(1):71-80.

Slotkin TA, Levin ED, Seidler FJ. Comparative developmental neurotoxicity of organophosphate insecticides: effects on brain development are separable from systemic toxicity. Environ Health Perspect 2006a;114(5):746-751.

Slotkin TA, Tate CA, Ryde IT, Levin ED, Seidler FJ. Organophosphate insecticides target the serotonergic system in developing rat brain regions: disparate effects of diazinon and parathion at doses spanning the threshold for cholinesterase inhibition. Environ Health Perspect 2006b;114(10):1542-1546.

Steenland K, Dick RB, Howell RJ, Chrislip DW, Hines CJ, Reid TM, et al. Neurologic function among termiticide applicators exposed to chlorpyrifos. Environ Health Perspect 2000;108(4):293-300.

U.S. Environmental Protection Agency (U.S. EPA). Interim registration eligibility decision for chlorpyrifos. EPA 738-R-

01-007. February 2002. Available at URL: http://www.epa.gov/oppsrrd1/REDs/chlorpyrifos_ired.pdf. 1/14/09

U.S. Geological Survey (USGS). The Quality of Our Nation's Waters. Pesticides in the Nation's Streams and Ground Water, 1992-2001. March 2006, revised February 15, 2007 [online]. Available at URL: http://pubs.usgs.gov/circ/2005/1291/. 6/1/09

Whyatt RM, Barr DB, Camann DE, Kinney PL, Barr JR, Andrews HF, et al. Contemporary-use pesticides in personal air samples during pregnancy and blood samples at delivery among urban minority mothers and newborns. Environ Health Perspect 2003;111(5):749-56.

## Coumaphos
CAS No. 56-72-4

### General Information

The chemical 3-chloro-7-hydroxy-4-methyl-2H-chromen-2-one/ol is a metabolite of coumaphos. First registered in 1958, coumaphos is an organophosphorus insecticide that is used to control ticks, lice, mites, and arthropod pests on beef cattle, dairy cows, swine, and certain other farm animals. Also, it has limited use in controlling mites in honeybee hives. It is not registered for uses on food crops, ornamentals, or for residential use. Coumaphos may enter the environment from spillage of animal dipping and spraying solutions (U.S.EPA, 2000). Coumaphos is generally immobile in soils and can persist for up to a year in some types of soils. It degrades to chlorferon, 6-hydroxyl-3-methylbenzofuran, and alkyl phosphates. Coumaphos is highly toxic to birds and aquatic invertebrates and moderately toxic to fish.

General population exposure to coumaphos is unlikely, though exposure through dietary meat and milk intake is possible. Estimated intakes from diet and water have not exceeded recommended intake limits (U.S.EPA, 2000). Farm and animal workers may have higher exposures as a result of absorption through dermal and inhalational routes. Once absorbed, phosphorothioates such as coumaphos are metabolically activated to the "oxon" form which has greater toxicity than the parent insecticide. Metabolic hydrolysis leads to the formation of 3-chloro-7-hydroxy-4-methyl-2H-chromen-2-one/ol, dialkyl phosphate metabolites (see section titled "Organophosphorus Insecticides: Dialkyl Phosphate Metabolites"), and other metabolites. Animal studies indicate elimination in the urine over a period of a week.

Human health effects from coumaphos at low environmental doses or at biomonitored levels from low environmental exposures are unknown. Coumaphos is considered to be an organophosphorus insecticide of moderate-to-high acute toxicity in animal studies. At high doses, coumaphos and other organophosphorus insecticides share a mechanism of toxicity: inhibition of the activity of acetylcholinesterase enzymes in the nervous system, resulting in excess acetylcholine at nerve terminals, and producing acute symptoms such as nausea, vomiting, cholinergic effects, weakness, paralysis, and seizures. Toxic effects below doses that cause inhibition of acetylcholinesterase are unknown, e.g., reproductive effects such as decrease litter size are unlikely at doses that do not inhibit acetylcholinesterase (Astroff et al., 1998). Coumaphos is not considered mutagenic and rated by the U.S.EPA as not likely to be carcinogenic in humans (U.S.EPA, 2000). Additional information about pesticides is available from U.S. EPA at: http://www.epa.gov/pesticides/.

### Biomonitoring Information

Urinary levels of 3-chloro-7-hydroxy-4-methyl-2H-chromen-2-one/ol reflect recent exposure. In the NHANES 2001-2002 subsample, most of the measurements of 3-chloro-7-hydroxy-4-methyl-2H-chromen-2-one/ol in urine were below the limit of detection, though the 95th percentile was 0.200 µg/L for the non-Hispanic black subsample (CDC, 2005). In a nonrandom study of 140 adults and children in the United States, Olsson et al. (2003) found that urinary levels of 3-chloro-7-hydroxy-4-methyl-2H-chromen-2-one/ol were below the limit of detection.

Finding a measurable amount of 3-chloro-7-hydroxy-4-methyl-2H-chromen-2-one/ol in urine does not mean that the level will result in an adverse health effect. Biomonitoring studies of 3-chloro-7-hydroxy-4-methyl-2H-chromen-2-one/ol provide physicians and public health officials with reference values so that they can determine whether people have been exposed to higher levels of coumaphos than are found in the general population. Biomonitoring data can also help scientists plan and conduct research on exposure and health effects.

## Urinary 3-Chloro-7-hydroxy-4-methyl-2H-chromen-2-one/ol
*Metabolite of Coumaphos*

Geometric mean and selected percentiles of urine concentrations (in µg/L) for the U.S. population from the National Health and Nutrition Examination Survey.

| | Survey years | Geometric mean (95% conf. interval) | Selected percentiles ( 95% confidence interval) | | | | Sample size |
|---|---|---|---|---|---|---|---|
| | | | 50th | 75th | 90th | 95th | |
| Total | 01-02 | * | < LOD | < LOD | < LOD | < LOD | 2481 |
| **Age group** | | | | | | | |
| 6-11 years | 01-02 | * | < LOD | < LOD | < LOD | .200 (<LOD- 210) | 567 |
| 12-19 years | 01-02 | * | < LOD | < LOD | < LOD | < LOD | 815 |
| 20-59 years | 01-02 | * | < LOD | < LOD | < LOD | < LOD | 1099 |
| **Gender** | | | | | | | |
| Males | 01-02 | * | < LOD | < LOD | < LOD | < LOD | 1169 |
| Females | 01-02 | * | < LOD | < LOD | < LOD | < LOD | 1312 |
| **Race/ethnicity** | | | | | | | |
| Mexican Americans | 01-02 | * | < LOD | < LOD | < LOD | < LOD | 659 |
| Non-Hispanic blacks | 01-02 | * | < LOD | < LOD | < LOD | .200 (<LOD- 270) | 701 |
| Non-Hispanic whites | 01-02 | * | < LOD | < LOD | < LOD | < LOD | 920 |

Limit of detection (LOD, see Data Analysis section) for Survey year 01-02 is 0 2.
< LOD means less than the limit of detection, which may vary for some chemicals by year and by individual sample.
* Not calculated: proportion of results below limit of detection was too high to provide a valid result.

## Urinary 3-Chloro-7-hydroxy-4-methyl-2H-chromen-2-one/ol (creatinine corrected)
*Metabolite of Coumaphos*

Geometric mean and selected percentiles of urine concentrations (in µg/g of creatinine) for the U.S. population from the National Health and Nutrition Examination Survey.

| | Survey years | Geometric mean (95% conf. interval) | Selected percentiles ( 95% confidence interval) | | | | Sample size |
|---|---|---|---|---|---|---|---|
| | | | 50th | 75th | 90th | 95th | |
| Total | 01-02 | * | < LOD | < LOD | < LOD | < LOD | 2480 |
| **Age group** | | | | | | | |
| 6-11 years | 01-02 | * | < LOD | < LOD | < LOD | .670 (<LOD-1.27) | 567 |
| 12-19 years | 01-02 | * | < LOD | < LOD | < LOD | < LOD | 814 |
| 20-59 years | 01-02 | * | < LOD | < LOD | < LOD | < LOD | 1099 |
| **Gender** | | | | | | | |
| Males | 01-02 | * | < LOD | < LOD | < LOD | < LOD | 1169 |
| Females | 01-02 | * | < LOD | < LOD | < LOD | < LOD | 1311 |
| **Race/ethnicity** | | | | | | | |
| Mexican Americans | 01-02 | * | < LOD | < LOD | < LOD | < LOD | 659 |
| Non-Hispanic blacks | 01-02 | * | < LOD | < LOD | < LOD | .380 (<LOD- 560) | 700 |
| Non-Hispanic whites | 01-02 | * | < LOD | < LOD | < LOD | < LOD | 920 |

< LOD means less than the limit of detection for the urine levels not corrected for creatinine.
* Not calculated: proportion of results below limit of detection was too high to provide a valid result.

## References

Astroff AB, Freshwater KJ, Eigenberg DA. Comparative organophosphate-induced effects observed in adult and neonatal Sprague-Dawley rats during the conduct of multigeneration toxicity studies. Reprod Toxicol 1998;12(6):619-645.

Centers for Disease Control and Prevention (CDC). Third National Report on Human Exposure to Environmental Chemicals. Atlanta (GA). 2005.

Olsson AO, Nguyen JV, Sadowski MA, Barr DB. A liquid chromatography/electrospray ionization tandem mass spectrometry method for quantification of specific organophosphorus pesticide biomarkers in human urine. Anal Bioanal Chem 2003;376(6):808-815.

U.S. Environmental Protection Agency (U.S. EPA). Reregistration eligibility decision (RED) addendum and FPQA tolerance reassessment progress report: Coumaphos. September 2000. EPA 738-R-00-010. Available at URL: http://www.epa.gov/oppsrrd1/REDs/0018tred.pdf. 1/14/09

# Diazinon

CAS No. 333-41-5

## General Information

The chemical 2-isopropyl-4-methyl-6-hydroxypyrimidine is a metabolite of diazinon, an organophosphorus insecticide that is used to control insects on nuts, fruits, vegetable, and forage crops. It is also used for cattle ear tag applications to control flies and ticks and, in the past, in some pest strips. Most granular formulations, aerial, seed and foliar applications are planned to be phased out (U.S.EPA, 2004). Prior to 2000, diazinon was widely used in residential and garden application, but these uses have been phased out; since 2004, diazinon cannot be sold for residential use. Before these restrictions, about 13 million pounds of diazinon were used annually on agricultural sites in the United States. Diazinon is biologically and chemically degraded in soils with a half-life of about a few weeks. It has been infrequently detected in general groundwater sampling but has been detected in streams receiving runoff from application sites (IPCS, 1998; USGS, 2007). It is

toxic to birds, and particularly when it was ingested in granular form, diazinon produced wild bird kills before use restrictions were in place. Fish and aquatic invertebrates show modest degrees of bioconcentration and are very sensitive to toxic effects.

Human exposure to diazinon from dietary sources is expected to be low due to its limited applications to food crops and due to its rapid degradation. Estimated intakes from diet and water do not exceed recommended intake limits (U.S.EPA, 2004). Inhalational and dermal routes of exposure can be significant for pesticide applicators. Diazinon is not well-absorbed through the skin, but is rapidly absorbed orally (IPCS, 1998). Once absorbed, phosphorothioates such as diazinon are metabolically activated to the "oxon" form which has greater toxicity. Metabolic hydrolysis leads to the formation of 2-isopropyl-4-methyl-6-hydroxypyrimidine, dialkyl phosphate metabolites (see section titled "Organophosphorus Insecticides: Dialkyl Phosphate Metabolites"), and other metabolites. Experimental diazinon exposure in people has demonstrated its rapid elimination into urine, as inferred

### Urinary 2-Isopropyl-4-methyl-6-hydroxypyrimidine

*Metabolite of Diazinon*

Geometric mean and selected percentiles of urine concentrations (in µg/L) for the U.S. population from the National Health and Nutrition Examination Survey.

| | Survey years | Geometric mean (95% conf. interval) | Selected percentiles ( 95% confidence interval) | | | | Sample size |
|---|---|---|---|---|---|---|---|
| | | | 50th | 75th | 90th | 95th | |
| **Total** | 99-00 | * | < LOD | < LOD | < LOD | < LOD | 1842 |
| | 01-02 | * | < LOD | < LOD | < LOD | < LOD | 2535 |
| **Age group** | | | | | | | |
| 6-11 years | 99-00 | * | < LOD | < LOD | < LOD | < LOD | 454 |
| | 01-02 | * | < LOD | < LOD | < LOD | 1.45 (<LOD-3.11) | 580 |
| 12-19 years | 99-00 | * | < LOD | < LOD | < LOD | < LOD | 632 |
| | 01-02 | * | < LOD | < LOD | < LOD | < LOD | 829 |
| 20-59 years | 99-00 | * | < LOD | < LOD | < LOD | < LOD | 756 |
| | 01-02 | * | < LOD | < LOD | < LOD | < LOD | 1126 |
| **Gender** | | | | | | | |
| Males | 99-00 | * | < LOD | < LOD | < LOD | < LOD | 894 |
| | 01-02 | * | < LOD | < LOD | < LOD | < LOD | 1191 |
| Females | 99-00 | * | < LOD | < LOD | < LOD | < LOD | 948 |
| | 01-02 | * | < LOD | < LOD | < LOD | < LOD | 1344 |
| **Race/ethnicity** | | | | | | | |
| Mexican Americans | 99-00 | * | < LOD | < LOD | < LOD | < LOD | 644 |
| | 01-02 | * | < LOD | < LOD | < LOD | < LOD | 678 |
| Non-Hispanic blacks | 99-00 | * | < LOD | < LOD | < LOD | < LOD | 484 |
| | 01-02 | * | < LOD | < LOD | < LOD | 1.49 (<LOD-2.05) | 700 |
| Non-Hispanic whites | 99-00 | * | < LOD | < LOD | < LOD | < LOD | 554 |
| | 01-02 | * | < LOD | < LOD | < LOD | < LOD | 956 |

Limit of detection (LOD, see Data Analysis section) for Survey years 99-00 and 01-02 are 7.2 and 0.7.
< LOD means less than the limit of detection, which may vary for some chemicals by year and by individual sample.
* Not calculated: proportion of results below limit of detection was too high to provide a valid result.

from dialkyl phosphate metabolite excretion (Garfitt et al., 2002). In animals, diazinon does not accumulate in tissues (IPCS, 1998). In addition to being a human metabolite of diazinon, 2-isopropyl-4-methyl-6-hydroxypyrimidine can also occur in the environment from the breakdown of the parent compound. Thus, the detection of 2-isopropyl-4-methyl-6-hydroxypyrimidine in a person's urine may reflect exposure to the environmental degradate.

Human health effects from diazinon at low environmental doses or at biomonitored levels from low environmental exposures are unknown. Diazinon has moderate acute toxicity in animal studies. At high doses, diazinon and other organophosphorus insecticides share a mechanism of toxicity: inhibition of the activity of acetylcholinesterase enzymes in the nervous system, resulting in excess acetylcholine at nerve terminals, and producing acute symptoms such as nausea, vomiting, cholinergic effects, weakness, paralysis, and seizures. Intoxications in humans from intentional overdose, agricultural, and indoor applications have been documented. There has been only limited study of diazinon at systemically non-toxic doses that do not result in cholinergic signs (Anthony et al., 1986

Rajendra et al., 1986; Seifert and Pewnim, 1992). Diazinon is not considered to be a mutagen, animal carcinogen, teratogen, or reproductive toxicant (IPCS, 1998). The U.S.EPA considers diazinon unlikely to be carcinogenic in humans. Additional information about external exposure (i.e., environmental levels) and health effects is available from ATSDR at: http://www.atsdr.cdc.gov/toxpro2.html and from U.S. EPA at: http://www.epa.gov/pesticides/.

**Biomonitoring Information**

Urinary levels of 2-isopropyl-4-methyl-6-hydroxypyrimidine reflect recent exposure. In two nonrandom samples of United States adults and children, 2-isopropyl-4-methyl-6-hydroxypyrimidine was detectable in 57% and 43% of the 130 and 140 participants, respectively (Baker et al., 2000; Olsson et al., 2003). In the U.S. subsamples of NHANES 1999-2000 and 2001-2002, most of the measurements of 2-isopropyl-4-methyl-6-hydroxypyrimidine in urine were below the limit of detection, although the 95th percentiles for children 6-11 years old and for non-Hispanic blacks were 1.45 and 1.49 μg/L, respectively, in the 2001-2002 subsample (CDC,

## Urinary 2-Isopropyl-4-methyl-6-hydroxypyrimidine (creatinine corrected)
*Metabolite of Diazinon*

Geometric mean and selected percentiles of urine concentrations (in μg/g of creatinine) for the U.S. population from the National Health and Nutrition Examination Survey.

| | Survey years | Geometric mean (95% conf. interval) | Selected percentiles ( 95% confidence interval) | | | | Sample size |
|---|---|---|---|---|---|---|---|
| | | | 50th | 75th | 90th | 95th | |
| **Total** | 99-00 | * | < LOD | < LOD | < LOD | < LOD | 1842 |
| | 01-02 | * | < LOD | < LOD | < LOD | < LOD | 2534 |
| **Age group** | | | | | | | |
| 6-11 years | 99-00 | * | < LOD | < LOD | < LOD | < LOD | 454 |
| | 01-02 | * | < LOD | < LOD | < LOD | 2.72 (<LOD-4.45) | 580 |
| 12-19 years | 99-00 | * | < LOD | < LOD | < LOD | < LOD | 632 |
| | 01-02 | * | < LOD | < LOD | < LOD | < LOD | 828 |
| 20-59 years | 99-00 | * | < LOD | < LOD | < LOD | < LOD | 756 |
| | 01-02 | * | < LOD | < LOD | < LOD | < LOD | 1126 |
| **Gender** | | | | | | | |
| Males | 99-00 | * | < LOD | < LOD | < LOD | < LOD | 894 |
| | 01-02 | * | < LOD | < LOD | < LOD | < LOD | 1191 |
| Females | 99-00 | * | < LOD | < LOD | < LOD | < LOD | 948 |
| | 01-02 | * | < LOD | < LOD | < LOD | < LOD | 1343 |
| **Race/ethnicity** | | | | | | | |
| Mexican Americans | 99-00 | * | < LOD | < LOD | < LOD | < LOD | 644 |
| | 01-02 | * | < LOD | < LOD | < LOD | < LOD | 678 |
| Non-Hispanic blacks | 99-00 | * | < LOD | < LOD | < LOD | < LOD | 484 |
| | 01-02 | * | < LOD | < LOD | < LOD | 1.76 (<LOD-3.48) | 699 |
| Non-Hispanic whites | 99-00 | * | < LOD | < LOD | < LOD | < LOD | 554 |
| | 01-02 | * | < LOD | < LOD | < LOD | < LOD | 956 |

< LOD means less than the limit of detection for the urine levels not corrected for creatinine.
* Not calculated: proportion of results below limit of detection was too high to provide a valid result.

2005). In 23 children, urinary 2-isopropyl-4-methyl-6-hydroxypyrimidine was detected in less than 14% of multiple samples collected during varied diets (Lu et al., 2006). In a small number of men visiting fertility clinics in Missouri and Minnesota, Swan et al. (2003) found that 2-isopropyl-4-methyl-6-hydroxypyrimidine was detectable in 96% and 58% of the subjects. In 54 Canadian greenhouse workers, urinary 2-isopropyl-4-methyl-6-hydroxypyrimidine levels were below the limit of detection (Bouchard et al., 2006).

Finding a measurable amount of 2-isopropyl-4-methyl-6-hydroxypyrimidine in urine does not mean that the level will result in an adverse health effect. Biomonitoring studies of 2-isopropyl-4-methyl-6-hydroxypyrimidine provide physicians and public health officials with reference values so that they can determine whether people have been exposed to higher levels of diazinon than are found in the general population. Biomonitoring data can also help scientists plan and conduct research on exposure and health effects.

### References

Anthony J, Banister E, Oloffs PC. Effect of sublethal levels of diazinon: histopathology of liver. Bull Environ Contam Toxicol 1986;37(4):501-507.

Baker SE, Barr DB, Driskell WJ, Beeson MD, Needham LL. Quantification of selected pesticide metabolites in human urine using isotope dilution high-performance liquid chromatography/tandem mass spectrometry. J Expo Anal Environ Epidemiol 2000;10(6 Pt 2):789-798.

Bouchard M, Carrier G, Brunet RC, Dumas P, Noisel N. Biological monitoring of exposure to organophosphorus insecticides in a group of horticultural greenhouse workers. Ann Occup Hyg 2006;50(5):505-515.

Centers for Disease Control and Prevention (CDC). Third National Report on Human Exposure to Environmental Chemicals. Atlanta (GA). 2005.

Garfitt SJ, Jones K, Mason HJ, Cocker J. Exposure to the organophosphate diazinon: data from a human volunteer study with oral and dermal doses. Toxicol Lett 2002;134(1-3):105-113.

International Programme on Chemical Safety-INCHEM (IPCS). Environmental Health Criteria 198. Diazinon. 1998. Available at URL: http://www.inchem.org/documents/ehc/ehc/ehc198.htm. 4/7/09

Lu C, Toepel K, Irish R, Fenske RA, Barr DB, Bravo R. Organic diets significantly lower children's dietary exposure to organophosphorus pesticides. Environ Health Perspect 2006;114(2):260-263.

Olsson AO, Nguyen JV, Sadowski MA, Barr DB. A liquid chromatography/electrospray ionization tandem mass spectrometry method for quantification of specific organophosphorus pesticide biomarkers in human urine. Anal Bioanal Chem 2003;376(6):808-815.

Rajendra W, Oloffs PC, Banister EW. Effects of chronic intake of diazinon on blood and brain monoamines and amino acids. Drug Chem Toxicol 1986;9(2):117-131.

Seifert J, Pewnim T. Alteration of mice L-tryptophan metabolism by the organophosphorous acid triester diazinon. Biochem Pharmacol 1992;44(11):2243-2250.

Swan SH, Kruse RL, Liu F, Barr DB, Drobnis EZ, Redmon JB, et al. Study for Future Families Research Group. Semen quality in relation to biomarkers of pesticide exposure. Environ Health Perspect 2003;111(12):1478-1484.

U.S. Environmental Protection Agency (U.S. EPA). Interim reregistration eligibility decision (IRED. Diazinon. May 2004. EPA 738-R-04-006. Available at URL: http://www.epa.gov/oppsrrd1/REDs/diazinon_ired.pdf. 1/14/09

U.S. Geological Survey (USGS). The Quality of Our Nation's Waters. Pesticides in the Nation's Streams and Ground Water, 1992-2001. March 2006, revised February 15, 2007 [online]. Available at URL: http://pubs.usgs.gov/circ/2005/1291/. 6/1/09

# Malathion
CAS No. 121-75-5

## General Information

Malathion dicarboxylic acid is a metabolite of malathion, which is an organophosphorus insecticide that is used on a wide variety of agricultural crops, as well as lawns, gardens, ornamental trees, shrubs, and plants. It is registered for use in public health mosquito control, in fruit fly control, and in government programs such as the USDA's Boll Weevil Eradication Program. Most of the estimated 15 million pounds used annually are applied to cotton (U.S.EPA, 2006). When malathion is used on food or feed crops, usually only a small fraction of the crop is treated. It has a short half-life in soils and water and is not considered persistent in the environment. Malathion is infrequently detected in groundwater sampling (USGS, 2007). It is moderately to highly toxic to fish, depending on the species. It is highly toxic to aquatic invertebrates and rare fish kills have been reported from wide area applications onto surface waters and runoff into waters. Malathion is also used medically in lotion form (0.5%) to kill body lice.

Limited general population exposure occurs through the diet. Estimated intakes for the general population have not exceeded recommended intake limits. Pesticide applicators and agricultural workers can have higher exposures via dermal, inhalational, or oral routes (U.S.EPA, 2006). Malathion is slowly absorbed through the skin, but is more rapidly and efficiently absorbed via ingestion. Once they are absorbed, phosphorothioates such as malathion are metabolically activated to the "oxon" forms which have greater toxicity than the parent insecticide. Metabolism of malathion leads to the formation of malathion monocarboxylic acid, malathion dicarboxylic acid, dialkyl phosphate metabolites (see section titled "Organophosphorus Insecticides: Dialkyl Phosphate Metabolites"), and other metabolites. Malathion is rapidly eliminated from the body within 12-24 hours (Bouchard et al., 2003). About 31-35% of oral doses of malathion are excreted in the urine as malathion monocarboxylic acid (Krieger and Dinoff, 2000). In addition to being a metabolite of malathion, malathion dicarboxylic acid can also occur in the environment from the breakdown of the parent compound. Thus, the detection of malathion dicarboxylic acid in a person's urine may also reflect exposure to the environmental degradate.

Human health effects from malathion at low environmental doses or at biomonitored levels from low environmental exposures are unknown. At high doses, malathion and other organophosphorus insecticides share a common mechanism of toxicity: inhibition of the activity of acetylcholinesterase enzymes in the nervous system, resulting in excess acetylcholine at nerve terminals, and producing acute symptoms such as nausea, vomiting, cholinergic effects, weakness, paralysis, and seizures. Compared with other organophosphorus insecticides, malathion has low acute toxicity. Severe toxicity or deaths have been reported from

## Urinary Malathion dicarboxylic acid
*Metabolite of Malathion*

Geometric mean and selected percentiles of urine concentrations (in µg/L) for the U.S. population from the National Health and Nutrition Examination Survey.

| | Survey years | Geometric mean (95% conf. interval) | Selected percentiles ( 95% confidence interval) | | | | Sample size |
|---|---|---|---|---|---|---|---|
| | | | 50th | 75th | 90th | 95th | |
| **Total** | 99-00 | * | < LOD | < LOD | < LOD | < LOD | 1920 |
| **Age group** | | | | | | | |
| 6-11 years | 99-00 | * | < LOD | < LOD | < LOD | 2.80 (<LOD-5.50) | 453 |
| 12-19 years | 99-00 | * | < LOD | < LOD | < LOD | < LOD | 660 |
| 20-59 years | 99-00 | * | < LOD | < LOD | < LOD | < LOD | 807 |
| **Gender** | | | | | | | |
| Males | 99-00 | * | < LOD | < LOD | < LOD | < LOD | 937 |
| Females | 99-00 | * | < LOD | < LOD | < LOD | < LOD | 983 |
| **Race/ethnicity** | | | | | | | |
| Mexican Americans | 99-00 | * | < LOD | < LOD | < LOD | < LOD | 680 |
| Non-Hispanic blacks | 99-00 | * | < LOD | < LOD | < LOD | < LOD | 498 |
| Non-Hispanic whites | 99-00 | * | < LOD | < LOD | < LOD | < LOD | 580 |

Limit of detection (LOD, see Data Analysis section) for Survey year 99-00 is 2.64.
< LOD means less than the limit of detection, which may vary for some chemicals by year and by individual sample.
* Not calculated: proportion of results below limit of detection was too high to provide a valid result.

direct ingestion of agricultural strength solutions. Toxicity from unprotected bystander exposure during applications is rare (U.S.EPA, 2006). Human studies of single oral doses between 0.5 and 5.0 mg/kg/day have shown no acetylcholinesterase inhibition or other short term effects (IPCS, 2003). Malathion does not appear to produce human reproductive or teratogenic effects at environmental levels of exposure (Grether et al., 1987; Thomas et al., 1990), and it is not considered an animal teratogen or a reproductive toxicant. Malathion itself has not been considered genotoxic (U.S.EPA, 2006), but isomalathion, a malaoxon metabolite and a technical grade impurity tested positive in some chromosomal tests (Blasiak et al., 1999; Flessel et al., 1993; Giri et al., 2002; Pluth et al., 1996. IARC considers malathion not classifiable as a human carcinogen. Additional information about external exposure (i.e., environmental levels) and health effects is available from ATSDR at: http://www.atsdr.cdc.gov/toxpro2.html and from U.S. EPA at: http://www.epa.gov/pesticides/.

**Biomonitoring Information**

Levels of urinary malathion dicarboxylic acid reflect recent exposure. The 95th percentile urinary levels of malathion dicarboxylic acid in both urban and nonurban Minnesota children aged 3-13 years (adjusted for sociodemographic variables) in 1997 were several-fold higher than the analytical detection limits reported for children aged 6-11 years in the U.S. representative subsample from NHANES 1999-2000 (Adgate, 2001; CDC, 2005). Malathion dicarboxylic acid was infrequently detected in multiple samples from 80

Maryland residents in 1995-96 (MacIntosh et al., 1999). Of 382 pregnant women living in an agricultural community, 30% had detectable levels of malathion dicarboxylic acid at a detection limit about tenfold lower than the detection limit in the NHANES 1999-2000 analyses (Eskenazi et al., 2004). A study of 13 children from an agricultural region of Washington State reported median levels that were below the detection limit in the NHANES 1999-2000 subsample (Kissel et al., 2005). Replacing conventional diets with organic diets in 23 children led to a tenfold decrease in urinary levels of malathion dicarboxylic acid; median urinary levels on the conventional diet were similar to the detection limit in the NHANES 1999-2000 subsample (CDC, 2005; Lu et al., 2006). A study of agricultural workers reported preshift urinary levels of malathion dicarboxylic acid that were twofold to eightfold higher than detection limits in the NHANES 1999-2000 subsample (Krieger and Dinoff, 2000); some of the postshift urine levels in duster-applicators were thousandsfold higher than the detection limits in the NHANES 1999-2000 subsample, but cholinesterase activity was not affected.

Finding a measurable amount of malathion dicarboxylic acid in urine does not mean that the level will result in an adverse health effect. Biomonitoring studies of malathion dicarboxylic acid provide physicians and public health officials with reference values so that they can determine whether people have been exposed to higher levels of malathion than are found in the general population. Biomonitoring data can also help scientists plan and conduct research on exposure and health effects.

**Urinary Malathion dicarboxylic acid (creatinine corrected)**
*Metabolite of Malathion*
Geometric mean and selected percentiles of urine concentrations (in µg/g of creatinine) for the U.S. population from the National Health and Nutrition Examination Survey.

| | Survey years | Geometric mean (95% conf. interval) | Selected percentiles ( 95% confidence interval) | | | | Sample size |
|---|---|---|---|---|---|---|---|
| | | | 50th | 75th | 90th | 95th | |
| Total | 99-00 | * | < LOD | < LOD | < LOD | < LOD | 1920 |
| **Age group** | | | | | | | |
| 6-11 years | 99-00 | * | < LOD | < LOD | < LOD | 3.74 (<LOD-5.50) | 453 |
| 12-19 years | 99-00 | * | < LOD | < LOD | < LOD | < LOD | 660 |
| 20-59 years | 99-00 | * | < LOD | < LOD | < LOD | < LOD | 807 |
| **Gender** | | | | | | | |
| Males | 99-00 | * | < LOD | < LOD | < LOD | < LOD | 937 |
| Females | 99-00 | * | < LOD | < LOD | < LOD | < LOD | 983 |
| **Race/ethnicity** | | | | | | | |
| Mexican Americans | 99-00 | * | < LOD | < LOD | < LOD | < LOD | 680 |
| Non-Hispanic blacks | 99-00 | * | < LOD | < LOD | < LOD | < LOD | 498 |
| Non-Hispanic whites | 99-00 | * | < LOD | < LOD | < LOD | < LOD | 580 |

< LOD means less than the limit of detection for the urine levels not corrected for creatinine.
* Not calculated: proportion of results below limit of detection was too high to provide a valid result.

## References

Adgate JL, Barr DB, Clayton CA, Eberly LE, Freeman NC, Lioy PJ, et al. Measurement of children's exposure to pesticides: analysis of urinary metabolite levels in a probability-based sample. Environ Health Perspect 2001;109(6):583-590.

Blasiak J, Jaloszynski P, Trzeciak A, Szyfter K. In vitro studies on the genotoxicity of the organophosphorus insecticide malathion and its two analogues. Mutat Res 1999;445(2):275-283.

Bouchard M, Gosselin NH, Brunet RC, Samuel O, Dumoulin MJ, Carrier G. A toxicokinetic model of malathion and its metabolites as a tool to assess human exposure and risk through measurements of urinary biomarkers. Toxicol Sci 2003 May;73(1):182-94. Erratum in: Toxicol Sci 2003 Aug;74(2):following table of contents.

Centers for Disease Control and Prevention (CDC). Third National Report on Human Exposure to Environmental Chemicals. Atlanta (GA). 2005.

Eskenazi B, Harley K, Bradman A, Weltzien E, Jewell NP, Barr DB, et al. Association of in utero organophosphate pesticide exposure and fetal growth and length of gestation in an agricultural population. Environ Health Perspect 2004;112(10):1116-1124.

Flessel P, Quintana PJ, Hooper K. Genetic toxicity of malathion: a review. Environ Mol Mutagen 1993;22(1):7-17.

Giri S, Prasad SB, Giri A, Sharma GD. Genotoxic effects of malathion: an organophosphorus insecticide using three mammalian bioassays in vivo. Mutat Res 2002;514(1-2):223-231.

Grether JK, Harris JA, Neutra R, Kizer KW: Exposure to aerial malathion application and the occurrence of congenital anomalies and low birthweight. Am J Public Health 1987;77:1009-1010.

International Programme on Chemical Safety-INCHEM (IPCS). Pesticides residues in food: 2003 FAO/WHO Meeting on Pesticide Residues. Malathion (addendum). Available at URL: http://www.inchem.org/documents/jmpr/jmpmono/v2003pr06. htm. 4/7/09

Kissel JC, Curl CL, Kedan G, Lu C, Griffith W, Barr DB, et al. Comparison of organophosphorus pesticide metabolite levels in single and multiple daily urine samples collected from preschool children in Washington State. J Expo Anal Environ Epidemiol 2005;15(2):164-171.

Krieger RI, Dinoff TM. Malathion deposition, metabolite clearance, and cholinesterase status of date dusters and harvesters in California. Arch Environ Contam Toxicol 2000;38(4):546-553.

Lu C, Toepel K, Irish R, Fenske RA, Barr DB, Bravo R. Organic diets significantly lower children's dietary exposure to organophosphorus pesticides. Environ Health Perspect 2006;114(2):260-263.

MacIntosh DL, Needham LL, Hammerstrom KA, Ryan PB. A longitudinal investigation of selected pesticide metabolites in urine. J Expo Anal Environ Epidemiol 1999;9(5):494-501.

Pluth JM, Nicklas JA, O'Neill JP, Albertini RJ. Increased frequency of specific genomic deletions resulting from in vitro malathion exposure. Cancer Res 1996;56(10):2393-2399.

Thomas D, Goldhaber M, Petitti D, Swan SH, Rappaport E, Hertz-Picciotto I. Reproductive outcome in women exposed to malathion. Am J Epidemiol 1990;132(4):794-795.

U.S. Environmental Protection Agency (U.S. EPA). Reregistration eligibility decision (RED) Malathion. July 2006. EPA 738-R-06-030. Available at URL: http://www.epa.gov/oppsrrd1/REDs/malathion_red.pdf. 6/1/09

U.S. Geological Survey (USGS). The Quality of Our Nation's Waters. Pesticides in the Nation's Streams and Ground Water, 1992-2001. March 2006, revised February 15, 2007 [online]. Available at URL: http://pubs.usgs.gov/circ/2005/1291/. 6/1/09

# Methyl Parathion
CAS No.298-00-0

# Ethyl Parathion
CAS No. 56-38-2

## General Information

Para-nitrophenol is a metabolite of the insecticides methyl parathion, ethyl parathion, O-ethyl-O-(4-nitrophenyl) phenylphosphonothioate, and of the chemical nitrobenzene. Methyl parathion use is highly restricted, with limited applications in agriculture. Many previous registered agricultural uses of methyl parathion have been cancelled (U.S.EPA, 2003). It had been applied to cotton, and to a lesser extent, on cereal grains. In the 1990s, peak domestic use was as high as 5-6 million pounds per year. Methyl parathion is not registered for residential use in the United States. Ethyl parathion, first registered in 1948, was once a restricted-use insecticide with limited applications on certain agricultural crops, but by 2003, all registered uses were voluntarily cancelled (U.S.EPA, 2000). Methyl

parathion has low water solubility, binds tightly to soils resulting in low leachability, and has a short half-life in soils and on plants. Ethyl and methyl parathion are infrequently detected in groundwater sampling (USGS, 2007). Both are toxic to birds, fish, and aquatic invertebrates.

Given its limited use, the potential for human exposure to either ethyl or methyl parathion through the diet or drinking water is low. Estimated intakes from diet and drinking water have been below recommended limits. Increased risk of exposure via dermal, pulmonary, and oral routes can occur in pesticide and agricultural workers (Muttray et al., 2006). In animal studies, methyl parathion was rapidly absorbed after ingestion, more slowly absorbed through the skin, and eliminated rapidly from the body after absorption (Kramer et al., 2002; Morgan et al., 1977). Once absorbed, phosphorothioates such as methyl and ethyl parathion are metabolically activated to the "oxon" forms which have greater toxicity than the parent insecticides. Metabolism of ethyl or methyl parathion leads to the formation of para-nitrophenol, dialkyl phosphate metabolites (see section titled "Organophosphorus Insecticides: Dialkyl Phosphate

## Urinary *para*-Nitrophenol
*Metabolite of Ethyl Parathion, Methyl Parathion, and Nitrobenzene*
Geometric mean and selected percentiles of urine concentrations (in µg/L) for the U.S. population from the National Health and Nutrition Examination Survey.

| | Survey years | Geometric mean (95% conf. interval) | Selected percentiles ( 95% confidence interval) | | | | Sample size |
|---|---|---|---|---|---|---|---|
| | | | 50th | 75th | 90th | 95th | |
| Total | 99-00 | * | < LOD | < LOD | 2.50 (1.40-4 50) | 5.00 (2.90-11.0) | 1989 |
| | 01-02 | * | < LOD | 1.33 (1.21-1.48) | 2.70 (2.40-3 02) | 3.71 (3.41-4 00) | 2477 |
| Age group | | | | | | | |
| 6-11 years | 99-00 | * | < LOD | .940 (<LOD-2.40) | 2.67 (1.70-3 80) | 4.30 (2.70-6.40) | 479 |
| | 01-02 | * | .790 (<LOD- 910) | 1.49 (1.36-1 61) | 2.89 (2.22-3 58) | 4.10 (3.01-4.74) | 565 |
| 12-19 years | 99-00 | * | < LOD | < LOD | 3.40 (1.60-5.70) | 5.70 (2.60-19.0) | 680 |
| | 01-02 | * | .730 (<LOD- 910) | 1.45 (1.32-1 61) | 2.66 (2.15-3.11) | 3.34 (3.11-4 01) | 813 |
| 20-59 years | 99-00 | * | < LOD | < LOD | 2.30 (1.20-5.70) | 4.50 (2.30-16.0) | 830 |
| | 01-02 | * | < LOD | 1.28 (1.09-1.47) | 2.69 (2.32-3.10) | 3.72 (3.37-4 24) | 1099 |
| Gender | | | | | | | |
| Males | 99-00 | * | < LOD | < LOD | 2.50 (1.40-4 50) | 4.50 (2.50-14.0) | 971 |
| | 01-02 | * | .770 (.300-.910) | 1.50 (1.32-1 67) | 3.00 (2.70-3 27) | 4.10 (3.37-4 92) | 1164 |
| Females | 99-00 | * | < LOD | < LOD | 2.50 (1.30-5.70) | 5.70 (2.90-9 50) | 1018 |
| | 01-02 | * | < LOD | 1.19 (.990-1 37) | 2.26 (1.92-2 69) | 3.46 (3.18-3.71) | 1313 |
| Race/ethnicity | | | | | | | |
| Mexican Americans | 99-00 | * | < LOD | 1.70 (<LOD-3.50) | 5.80 (2.60-24.0) | 22.0 (3.60-36.0) | 695 |
| | 01-02 | * | .700 (<LOD- 850) | 1.32 (1.10-1 57) | 2.62 (1.91-3.44) | 3.85 (2.70-6 05) | 660 |
| Non-Hispanic blacks | 99-00 | * | < LOD | 1.20 (<LOD-2.60) | 2.90 (1.70-6 00) | 4.80 (2.50-9 20) | 518 |
| | 01-02 | * | .860 (<LOD-1.12) | 1.80 (1.37-2.16) | 3.21 (2.57-4.40) | 5.60 (4.02-6.79) | 679 |
| Non-Hispanic whites | 99-00 | * | < LOD | < LOD | 2.10 (<LOD-6.33) | 4.20 (2.10-11.0) | 603 |
| | 01-02 | * | < LOD | 1.28 (1.13-1.45) | 2.71 (2.30-3.10) | 3.70 (3.28-4 01) | 941 |

Limit of detection (LOD, see Data Analysis section) for Survey years 99-00 and 01-02 are 0 8 and 0.1.
< LOD means less than the limit of detection, which may vary for some chemicals by year and by individual sample.
* Not calculated: proportion of results below limit of detection was too high to provide a valid result.

Metabolites"), and other metabolites. In addition to being a metabolite of methyl and ethyl parathion, para-nitrophenol can also occur in the environment from the breakdown of the parent these organophosphorus pesticides and from nitrobenzene. Thus, the detection of para-nitrophenol in a person's urine may also reflect exposure to the environmental degradate.

Human health effects from parathion or ethyl parathion at low environmental doses or at biomonitored levels from low environmental exposures are unknown. Parathion and methyl parathion have high acute toxicity in animal testing. In large doses, methyl parathion, ethyl parathion, and other organophosphorus insecticides share a common mechanism of toxicity: inhibition of the activity of acetylcholinesterase enzymes in the nervous system, resulting in excess acetylcholine at nerve terminals, and producing acute symptoms such as nausea, vomiting, cholinergic effects, weakness, paralysis, and seizures. The metabolite, para-nitrophenol, does not inhibit acetylcholinesterase enzymes. At high animal doses of methyl parathion, retinal atrophy and sciatic nerve degeneration have also been observed (IPCS, 1995; WHO, 2004). Recent *in vitro* and *in vivo* animal

studies suggest that parathion may have additional neuronal and glial cell effects at lower doses (Guizzetti et al., 2005; Karanth and Pope et al., 2003; Slotkin et al., 2006; Zurich et al., 2004). Overt cholinergic toxicity and death from methyl and ethyl parathion have been described following suicidal ingestion, accidental exposure, and unintentional acute or chronic high-level occupational exposure (Hill et al., 1990; Jaga and Dharmani, 2006; Lores et al., 1978; Orsorio et al., 1991). Methyl parathion is not considered genotoxic, teratogenic, or generally to have reproductive toxicity at doses below those causing acetylcholinesterase inhibition in most animal studies (IPCS, 1995). IARC does not consider ethyl parathion and methyl parathion classifiable as human carcinogens. U.S.EPA considers methyl parathion unlikely to be carcinogenic to humans, but lists ethyl parathion as a possible human carcinogen. Additional information about external exposure (i.e., environmental levels) and health effects is available from ATSDR at: http://www.atsdr.cdc. gov/toxpro2.html and from U.S. EPA at: http://www.epa. gov/pesticides/.

## Urinary *para*-Nitrophenol (creatinine corrected)
*Metabolite of Ethyl Parathion, Methyl Parathion, and Nitrobenzene*

Geometric mean and selected percentiles of urine concentrations (in µg/g of creatinine) for the U.S. population from the National Health and Nutrition Examination Survey.

| | Survey years | Geometric mean (95% conf. interval) | 50th | 75th | 90th | 95th | Sample size |
|---|---|---|---|---|---|---|---|
| **Total** | 99-00 | * | < LOD | < LOD | 2.08 (1.33-3.91) | 4.25 (2.15-10 2) | 1989 |
| | 01-02 | * | < LOD | .970 ( 830-1.10) | 1.91 (1.72-2.03) | 2.89 (2.44-3.23) | 2476 |
| **Age group** | | | | | | | |
| 6-11 years | 99-00 | * | < LOD | .940 (<LOD-1.95) | 2.80 (1.94-4.00) | 4.20 (3.33-6.70) | 479 |
| | 01-02 | * | .720 (<LOD-.870) | 1.60 (1.30-1.82) | 2.78 (2.31-3.11) | 3.67 (3.11-4.61) | 565 |
| 12-19 years | 99-00 | * | < LOD | < LOD | 1.80 (1.08-3.04) | 4.00 (1.57-7.29) | 680 |
| | 01-02 | * | .370 (<LOD-.500) | .840 (.790-.950) | 1.59 (1.37-1.78) | 2.10 (1.78-2.43) | 812 |
| 20-59 years | 99-00 | * | < LOD | < LOD | 2.00 (1.17-4.25) | 4.29 (2.13-12 3) | 830 |
| | 01-02 | * | < LOD | .880 ( 690-1.07) | 1.79 (1.56-2.05) | 2.89 (2.35-3.33) | 1099 |
| **Gender** | | | | | | | |
| Males | 99-00 | * | < LOD | < LOD | 1.90 (1.01-3.39) | 3.39 (1.77-7.55) | 971 |
| | 01-02 | * | .430 ( 310-.530) | .980 ( 850-1.08) | 1.87 (1.57-2.09) | 2.97 (2.14-3.57) | 1164 |
| Females | 99-00 | * | < LOD | < LOD | 2.26 (1.48-4.88) | 6.92 (2.76-14.1) | 1018 |
| | 01-02 | * | < LOD | .930 (.730-1.23) | 1.96 (1.78-2.15) | 2.82 (2.44-3.06) | 1312 |
| **Race/ethnicity** | | | | | | | |
| Mexican Americans | 99-00 | * | < LOD | 1.55 (<LOD-3.17) | 4.86 (2.21-21 9) | 17.4 (3.94-47.7) | 695 |
| | 01-02 | * | .400 (<LOD-.540) | .930 (.720-1.20) | 1.88 (1.41-2.60) | 3.04 (2.38-3.84) | 660 |
| Non-Hispanic blacks | 99-00 | * | < LOD | .680 (<LOD-1.79) | 2.07 (1.33-3.71) | 3.71 (1.98-7.20) | 518 |
| | 01-02 | * | .440 (<LOD-.640) | 1.01 ( 800-1.31) | 1.73 (1.60-2.21) | 3.01 (2.16-4.30) | 678 |
| Non-Hispanic whites | 99-00 | * | < LOD | < LOD | 1.97 (<LOD-4.29) | 3.83 (1.97-10 2) | 603 |
| | 01-02 | * | < LOD | .970 (.790-1.13) | 1.96 (1.67-2.26) | 2.93 (2.35-3.45) | 941 |

< LOD means less than the limit of detection for the urine levels not corrected for creatinine.
* Not calculated: proportion of results below limit of detection was too high to provide a valid result.

## Biomonitoring Information

Urinary levels of para-nitrophenol reflect recent exposure. Levels of para-nitrophenol in the NHANES 1999-2000 and 2001-2002 subsamples were similar or slightly lower than those in a nonrandom subsample of NHANES III (1988-1994) participants (CDC, 2005; Hill et al., 1995), and levels were similar or slightly lower that those in a small convenience sample of the U.S. population (Olsson et al., 2003) and in 482 pregnant females from an agricultural region of California (Eskenazi et al., 2004). A study of 13 children from an agricultural region of Washington State reported median levels that were more than threefold higher than median levels in the NHANES 1999-2000 subsample (Kissel et al., 2005). Children and adults living in residences where methyl parathion was applied indoors had urinary levels of para-nitrophenol which were several hundred times higher than those in the NHANES 1999-2000 subsample, and many residents were symptomatic (Barr et al., 2002; CDC, 2005; McCann et al., 2002; Rubin et al., 2002).

Pesticide workers may have much higher levels following pesticide applications. ACGIH recommends a BEI of 0.5 mg (500 µg)/g creatinine for workers at the end of shift. In a study of workers who handle parathion, end-of-shift urinary para-nitrophenol levels ranged from 190 to 410 µg/gram of creatinine (Leng and Lewalter, 1999), a range of values several hundred times higher than levels found in the U.S. general population (CDC, 2005).

Finding a measurable amount of para-nitrophenol in urine does not mean that the level will result in an adverse health effect. Biomonitoring studies of para-nitrophenol can provide physicians and public health officials with reference values so that they can determine whether people have been exposed to higher levels of parathion than are found in the general population. Biomonitoring data can also help scientists plan and conduct research on exposure and health effects.

## References

Barr DB, Turner WE, DiPietro E, McClure PC, Baker SE, Barr JR, et al. Measurement of p-nitrophenol in the urine of residents whose homes were contaminated with methyl parathion. Environ Health Perspect 2002;110 Suppl 6:1085-1091.

Centers for Disease Control and Prevention (CDC). Third National Report on Human Exposure to Environmental Chemicals. Atlanta (GA). 2005.

Eskenazi B, Harley K, Bradman A, Weltzien E, Jewell NP, Barr DB, et al. Association of in utero organophosphate pesticide exposure and fetal growth and length of gestation in an agricultural population. Environ Health Perspect 2004;112(10):1116-1124.

Guizzetti M, Pathak S, Giordano G, Costa LG. Effect of organophosphorus insecticides and their metabolites on astroglial cell proliferation. Toxicology 2005;215(3):182-190.

Hill RH Jr, Alley CC, Ashley DL, Cline RE, Head SL, Needham LL, et al. Laboratory investigation of a poisoning epidemic in Sierra Leone. J Anal Toxicol 1990;14(4):213-216.

Hill RH Jr, Head SL, Baker S, Gregg M, Shealy DB, Bailey SL, et al. Pesticide residues in urine of adults living in the United States: reference range concentrations. Environ Res 1995;71:99-108.

International Programme on Chemical Safety-INCHEM (IPCS). Parathion-Methyl (addendum). 1995. Available at URL: http://www.inchem.org/documents/jmpr/jmpmono/v95pr14.htm. 4/7/09

Jaga K, Dharmani C. Methyl parathion: an organophosphate insecticide not quite forgotten. Rev Environ Health 2006;21(1):57-67.

Karanth S, Pope C. Age-related effects of chlorpyrifos and parathion on acetylcholine synthesis in rat striatum. Neurotoxicol Teratol 2003;25(5):599-606.

Kissel JC, Curl CL, Kedan G, Lu C, Griffith W, Barr DB, et al. Comparison of organophosphorus pesticide metabolite levels in single and multiple daily urine samples collected from preschool children in Washington State. J Expo Anal Environ Epidemiol 2005;15(2):164-171.

Kramer RE, Wellman SE, Rockhold RW, Baker RC. Pharmacokinetics of methyl parathion: a comparison following single intravenous, oral or dermal administration. J Biomed Sci 2002;9:311-320.

Leng G, Lewalter J. Role of individual susceptibility in risk assessment of pesticides. Occup Environ Med 1999;56(7):449-553.

Lores EM, Bradway DE, Moseman RF. Organophosphorus pesticide poisonings in humans: determination of residues and metabolites in tissues and urine. Arch Environ Health 1978;33(5):270-276.

McCann KG, Moomey CM, Runkle KD, Hryhorczuk DO, Clark JM, Barr DB. Chicago area methyl parathion response. Environ Health Perspect 2002;110 Suppl 6:1075-1078.

Morgan DP, Hetzler HL, Slach EF, Lin LI. Urinary excretion of paranitrophenol and alkyl phosphates following ingestion of methyl or ethyl parathion by human subjects. Arch Environ Contam Toxicol 1977;6(2-3):159-173.

Muttray A, Backer G, Jung D, Hill G, Letzel S. External and internal exposure of wine growers spraying methyl parathion. Toxicol Lett 2006;162(2-3):219-224.

Olsson AO, Nguyen JV, Sadowski MA, Barr DB. A liquid chromatography/electrospray ionization tandem mass spectrometry method for quantification of specific organophosphorus pesticide biomarkers in human urine. Anal Bioanal Chem 2003;376(6):808-815.

Osorio AM, Ames RG, Rosenberg J, Mengle DC. Investigation of a fatality among parathion applicators in California. Am J Ind Med 1991;20(4):533-546.

Rubin C, Esteban E, Kieszak S, Hill RH Jr, Dunlop B, Yacovac R, et al. Assessment of human exposure and human health effects after indoor application of methyl parathion in Lorain County, Ohio, 1995-1996. Environ Health Perspect 2002;110 Suppl 6:1047-1051.

Slotkin TA, Tate CA, Ryde IT, Levin ED, Seidler FJ. Organophosphate insecticides target the serotonergic system in developing rat brain regions: disparate effects of diazinon and parathion at doses spanning the threshold for cholinesterase inhibition. Environ Health Perspect 2006;114(10):1542-1546.

U.S. Environmental Protection Agency (U.S. EPA). R.E.D. Facts. Ethyl parathion. September 2000. EPA-738-FOO-009. Available at URL: http://www.epa.gov/oppsrrd1/REDs/factsheets/0155fct.pdf. 1/14/09

U.S. Environmental Protection Agency (U.S. EPA). Interim reregistration eligibility decision (IRED) for Methyl Parathion. Case No. 0153. May 2003. Available at URL: http://www.epa.gov/oppsrrd1/REDs/methylparathion_ired.pdf. 1/12/07

U.S. Geological Survey (USGS). The Quality of Our Nation's Waters. Pesticides in the Nation's Streams and Ground Water, 1992-2001. March 2006, revised February 15, 2007 [online]. Available at URL: http://pubs.usgs.gov/circ/2005/1291/. 6/1/09

World Health Organization (WHO). Methyl parathion in drinking water. WHO/SDE/WSH/03.04/106. 2004. Available at URL: http://www.who.int/water_sanitation_health/dwq/chemicals/methylparathion.pdf. 5/19/09

Zurich MG, Honegger P, Schilter B, Costa LG, Monnet-Tschudi F. Involvement of glial cells in the neurotoxicity of parathion and chlorpyrifos. Toxicol Appl Pharmacol 2004;201(2):97-104.

# Pirimiphos-methyl

CAS No. 29232-93-7

## General Information

The chemical 2-(diethylamino)-6-methylpyrimidin-4-ol/one is a metabolite of the organophosphorus insecticide pirimiphos-methyl, which has limited applications for control of beetles, weevils, and moths on stored grain products such as corn, sorghum, and seed. It has a lesser use as a cattle ear tag application to control flies. Pirimiphos-methyl is not registered for residential use in the United States. It easily hydrolyzes in the environment to 2-(diethylamino)-6-methylpyrimidine and other breakdown products, and it is not considered persistent. Though considered moderately-to-highly toxic in birds, fish, and aquatic invertebrates, occurrence of such toxicity is mitigated by its rapid degradation and its use in closed storage systems.

In the general population, infrequent dietary exposure to pirimiphos-methyl residues may occur from ingestion of food products containing stored corn or other treated grain (FDA, 2003). Estimated intakes from diet and water have not exceeded recommended intake limits (U.S.EPA, 2006). In animal studies, pirimiphos-methyl is rapidly absorbed and metabolized to 12 metabolites, which are mainly excreted in the urine (IPCS, 1992). Once absorbed, phosphorothioates such as pirimiphos-methyl are metabolically activated to the "oxon" form which has greater toxicity than the parent insecticide. Metabolic hydrolysis leads to the formation of 2-(diethylamino)-6-methylpyrimidin-4-ol/one, dialkyl phosphate metabolites (see section titled "Organophosphorus Insecticides: Dialkyl Phosphate Metabolites"), and other metabolites. In addition to being a human metabolite of pirimiphos-methyl in the body, 2-(diethylamino)-6-methylpyrimidin-4-ol/one can also occur in the environment. Thus, the detection of 2-(diethylamino)-6-methylpyrimidin-4-ol/one may also reflect exposure to the environmental degradate.

Human health effects from pirimiphos-methyl at low environmental doses or at biomonitored levels from low environmental exposures are unknown. Pirimiphos-methyl has low acute toxicity in animal studies. At high doses, pirimiphos-methyl and other organophosphorus insecticides share a mechanism of toxicity: inhibition of the activity of acetylcholinesterase enzymes in the nervous system, resulting in excess acetylcholine at nerve terminals, and producing acute symptoms such as nausea, vomiting, cholinergic effects, weakness, paralysis, and seizures. The metabolite 2-(diethylamino)-6-methylpyrimidin-4-ol/one

does not inhibit acetylcholinesterase enzymes. Toxic effects below doses that cause inhibition of acetylcholinesterase are unknown. Pirimiphos-methyl is not considered mutagenic, teratogenic, or known to cause delayed neurotoxicity, or reproductive toxicity (IPCS, 1992; U.S.EPA, 2006). Additional information about pesticides is available from U.S. EPA at: http://www.epa.gov/pesticides/.

## Biomonitoring Information

Urinary levels of 2-(diethylamino)-6-methylpyrimidin-4-ol/one reflect recent exposure. In the U.S. subsample of NHANES 2001-2002, most of the urinary measurements of 2-(diethylamino)-6-methylpyrimidin-4-ol/one were below the limit of detection, although the 95th percentile was characterized at 0.47 µg/L for the total population (CDC, 2005). In a nonrandom sample of 140 urine specimens obtained from adults and children in the United States, Olsson et al. (2003) detected 2-(diethylamino)-6-methylpyrimidin-4-ol/one in 7.1% of the sampled population.

Finding a measurable amount of 2-(diethylamino)-6-methylpyrimidin-4-ol/one in urine does not mean that the level will result in an adverse health effect. Biomonitoring studies of 2-(diethylamino)-6-methylpyrimidin-4-ol/one provide physicians and public health officials with reference values so that they can determine whether people have been exposed to higher levels of pirimiphos-methyl than are found in the general population. Biomonitoring data can also help scientists plan and conduct research on exposure and health effects.

## Urinary 2-(Diethylamino)-6-methylpyrimidin-4-ol/one
*Metabolite of Pirimiphos-methyl*

Geometric mean and selected percentiles of urine concentrations (in µg/L) for the U.S. population from the National Health and Nutrition Examination Survey.

| | Survey years | Geometric mean (95% conf. interval) | Selected percentiles ( 95% confidence interval) | | | | Sample size |
|---|---|---|---|---|---|---|---|
| | | | 50th | 75th | 90th | 95th | |
| Total | 01-02 | * | < LOD | < LOD | < LOD | .470 ( 210-.770) | 2481 |
| **Age group** | | | | | | | |
| 6-11 years | 01-02 | * | < LOD | < LOD | .250 (<LOD-.820) | .840 ( 210-1.64) | 567 |
| 12-19 years | 01-02 | * | < LOD | < LOD | < LOD | .610 (<LOD-1.94) | 810 |
| 20-59 years | 01-02 | * | < LOD | < LOD | < LOD | .430 (<LOD-.670) | 1104 |
| **Gender** | | | | | | | |
| Males | 01-02 | * | < LOD | < LOD | < LOD | .850 ( 300-1.55) | 1165 |
| Females | 01-02 | * | < LOD | < LOD | < LOD | .210 (<LOD-.460) | 1316 |
| **Race/ethnicity** | | | | | | | |
| Mexican Americans | 01-02 | * | < LOD | < LOD | < LOD | .410 (<LOD-1.15) | 669 |
| Non-Hispanic blacks | 01-02 | * | < LOD | < LOD | < LOD | < LOD | 687 |
| Non-Hispanic whites | 01-02 | * | < LOD | < LOD | < LOD | .500 ( 200-.840) | 929 |

Limit of detection (LOD, see Data Analysis section) for Survey year 01-02 is 0.2.
< LOD means less than the limit of detection, which may vary for some chemicals by year and by individual sample.
* Not calculated: proportion of results below limit of detection was too high to provide a valid result.

## Urinary 2-(Diethylamino)-6-methylpyrimidin-4-ol/one (creatinine corrected)
*Metabolite of Pirimiphos-methyl*

Geometric mean and selected percentiles of urine concentrations (in µg/g of creatinine) for the U.S. population from the National Health and Nutrition Examination Survey.

| | Survey years | Geometric mean (95% conf. interval) | Selected percentiles ( 95% confidence interval) | | | | Sample size |
|---|---|---|---|---|---|---|---|
| | | | 50th | 75th | 90th | 95th | |
| Total | 01-02 | * | < LOD | < LOD | < LOD | .780 (.700-.930) | 2481 |
| **Age group** | | | | | | | |
| 6-11 years | 01-02 | * | < LOD | < LOD | .680 (<LOD-.950) | 1.17 (.740-1.27) | 567 |
| 12-19 years | 01-02 | * | < LOD | < LOD | < LOD | .670 (<LOD-1.31) | 810 |
| 20-59 years | 01-02 | * | < LOD | < LOD | < LOD | .760 (<LOD-.880) | 1104 |
| **Gender** | | | | | | | |
| Males | 01-02 | * | < LOD | < LOD | < LOD | .740 ( 580-1.07) | 1165 |
| Females | 01-02 | * | < LOD | < LOD | < LOD | .780 (<LOD-1.08) | 1316 |
| **Race/ethnicity** | | | | | | | |
| Mexican Americans | 01-02 | * | < LOD | < LOD | < LOD | .780 (<LOD-1.21) | 669 |
| Non-Hispanic blacks | 01-02 | * | < LOD | < LOD | < LOD | < LOD | 687 |
| Non-Hispanic whites | 01-02 | * | < LOD | < LOD | < LOD | .780 (.700-1.00) | 929 |

< LOD means less than the limit of detection for the urine levels not corrected for creatinine.
* Not calculated: proportion of results below limit of detection was too high to provide a valid result.

## References

Centers for Disease Control and Prevention (CDC). Third National Report on Human Exposure to Environmental Chemicals. Atlanta (GA). 2005.

Food and Drug Administration (FDA). Total Diet Study: Summary of Residues Found Ordered by Pesticide, Market Baskets 91-3-01-4. June 2003. Available at URL: http://www. cfsan.fda.gov/~acrobat/tds1byps.pdf. 4/7/09

International Programme on Chemical Safety-INCHEM (IPCS). Pesticides residues in food: 1992 evaluations Part II Toxicology. 850. Pirimiphos-methyl. Available at URL: http://www.inchem. org/documents/jmpr/jmpmono/v92pr16.htm. 4/7/09

Olsson AO, Nguyen JV, Sadowski MA, Barr DB. A liquid chromatography/electrospray ionization tandem mass spectrometry method for quantification of specific organophosphorus pesticide biomarkers in human urine. Anal Bioanal Chem 2003;376(6):808-815.

U.S. Environmental Protection Agency (U.S. EPA). Finalization of interim registration eligibility decision for pirimiphos-methyl. Case No. 2535. July 2006. Available at URL: http://www.epa. gov/oppsrrd1/REDs/pirimiphos-methyl_ired.pdf. 1/14/09

# Pyrethroid Pesticides

## General Information

Pyrethroid pesticides are synthetic analogues of pyrethrins, which are natural chemicals found in chrysanthemum flowers. Pyrethroid pesticides are used to control a wide range of insects in public and commercial buildings, animal facilities, warehouses, agricultural fields, and greenhouses. They are also applied on livestock to control insects. In agriculture, cypermethrin, cyfluthrin, and deltamethrin have been used frequently on cotton. Pyrethroid insecticides are the most common active ingredient in commercially available insect sprays and are also used as structural termiticides. Certain pyrethroid insecticides (such as permethrin, resmethrin, and sumithrin) are also registered for use in mosquito-control programs in the United States. Outside the U.S., deltamethrin has been used for indoor protection against mosquitoes that carry malaria, in some situations replacing the use of DDT. About two million pounds of permethrin and one million pounds of cypermethrin have been applied annually (U.S. EPA, 2006a, 2006b). Permethrin is also used in skin lotions and shampoos as medical treatments for lice and scabies. Pyrethroid pesticides are generally formulated as complex mixtures of different chemical isomers, solvent oils, and synergists, such as piperonyl butoxide. Pyrethroid pesticides have low volatility, bind to soils, and are rarely detected in ground waters (USGS, 2007). Generally, they are not persistent in the environment due to their rapid degradation within days to several months. This class of pesticides has low toxicity in birds and mammals, but pyrethroids are highly toxic to fish and some aquatic invertebrates, so usage is restricted near water (U.S.EPA, 2002). There are about 30 different pyrethroid pesticides in use. The table shows the urinary pyrethroid metabolites measured in this *Report*.

The general population may be exposed to pyrethroid insecticides primarily from the ingestion of food or from residential use. Estimated intakes from diet and drinking water are below recommended limits. Dermal exposure with the potential for inadvertent ingestion may occur when lotions or shampoos are applied to treat lice or scabies. Pesticide applicators can be exposed to pyrethroid pesticides via dermal and inhalation routes from powders and liquid formulations. Pyrethroids are not well absorbed through the skin (ATSDR, 2003; Woollen et al., 1992). After absorption from inhalation or ingestion, pyrethroids are rapidly metabolized, by either ester hydrolysis or hydroxylation, followed by conjugation, and then eliminated over several days in urine and bile (Kuhn et al., 1999; Leng et al., 1997; Soderlund et al., 2002; Woollen et al., 1992). Unmetabolized pyrethroids have been measured in breast milk, but may be poorly transferred across the placenta (ATSDR, 2003; WHO, 2005).

Human health effects from pyrethroid pesticides at low environmental doses or at biomonitored levels from low environmental exposures are unknown. Compared with other classes of insecticides such as organochlorines, organophosphorus, or carbamate pesticides, pyrethroid pesticides have less acute toxicity in animals and people. They are ranked as having moderate acute oral toxicity. Adverse effects from large doses are related to the action of pyrethroids on the nervous system, where these chemicals prolong sodium channel opening when a nerve cell is depolarized (Shafer et al., 2005; Soderlund et al., 2002). Possible other additional actions on neuroreceptors

## Pyrethroid Insecticides Metabolites in this *Report*

| Pyrethroid (CAS number) | Urinary metabolite (CAS number) |
| --- | --- |
| Cyfluthrin (68359-37-5) | 4-Fluoro-3-phenoxybenzoic acid (77279-89-1) |
| Cypermethrin (52315-07-8) Cyfluthrin (68359-37-5) and Permethrin (52645-53-1) | *cis*-3-(2,2-Dichlorovinyl)-2,2-dimethylcyclopropane carboxylic acid (55701-05-8 ) *trans*-3-(2,2-Dichlorovinyl)-2,2-dimethylcyclopropane carboxylic acid (55701-03-6) |
| Deltamethrin (52918-63-5) | *cis*-3-(2,2-Dibromovinyl)-2,2-dimethylcyclopropane carboxylic acid |
| Cyhalothrin (68359-37-5) Cypermethrin (52315-07-8) Deltamethrin (52918-63-5) Fenpropathrin (39515-41-8) Permethrin (52645-53-1) Tralomethrin (66841-25-6) | 3-Phenoxybenzoic acid (3739-38-6) |

and other ion channels may also explain some pyrethroid effects. Human cases of systemic poisoning are rare and usually result from accidental exposure or intentional ingestion of pyrethroid insecticides. Signs and symptoms of acute pyrethroid poisoning after massive ingestions include agitation, hypersensitivity, tremor, salivation, choreoathetosis, and seizures (ATSDR, 2003; Ray et al., 2000; Soderlund et al., 2002). Concomitant exposure to organophosphorus insecticides may increase pyrethroid toxicity by slowing metabolic clearance of the pyrethroid. In California, cyfluthrin was the most frequent pyrethroid associated with symptomatic effects (irritant respiratory and dermal effects, paresthesias) reported in agricultural workers from 1996 to 2002 (Spencer and O'Malley, 2006). Transient dermal paresthesias have been reported among pesticide applicators after direct contact with certain types of pyrethroid pesticides. No relationship of indoor air or housedust concentrations of permethrin and irritant symptoms was found in a study of urban residents in 80 private homes (Berger-Preiss et al., 2002).

In developing rodents, neurochemical changes in cholinergic, dopaminergic, and catecholaminergic pathways and behavioral changes have been demonstrated at subacute and subchronic doses for some pyrethroid pesticides (Aziz et al., 2001; Elwan et al., 2006; Eriksson and Fredriksson, 1991; Lazarini et al., 2001; Shafer, et al., 2005). The pyrethroids in general use are not considered teratogenic or to have significant reproductive toxicity (ATSDR, 2003; WHO, 2005), though a few pyrethroid pesticides and some metabolites have shown weak or inconsistent estrogenic effects on standardized assays (ATSDR, 2003; Garey and Wolff, 1998; Go et al., 1999; Hu et al., 2003; Kim et al., 2004; Kunimatsu et al., 2002; McCarthy et al., 2006; Moniz et al., 2005). Generally, the pyrethroids are not considered genotoxic in *in vitro* testing or carcinogenic in animal testing (WHO, 2005). IARC considers deltamethrin and permethrin as not classifiable as to their human carcinogenicity. Additional information about pesticides is available from U.S. EPA at: http://www. epa.gov/pesticides/ and from ATSDR at: http://www.atsdr. cdc.gov/toxpro2.html.

**References**

Agency for Toxic Substances and Disease Registry (ATSDR). Toxicological profile for pyrethrins and pyrethroids. September 2003. Available from URL: http://www.atsdr.cdc.gov/toxprofiles/ tp155.html.1/15/09

Aziz MH, Agrawal AK, Adhami VM, Shukla Y, Seth PK. Neurodevelopmental consequences of gestational exposure (GD14-GD20) to low dose deltamethrin in rats. Neurosci Lett 2001;300(3):161-165.

Berger-Preiss E, Levsen K, Leng G, Idel H, Sugiri D, Ranft U. Indoor pyrethroid exposure in homes with woollen textile floor coverings. Int J Hyg Environ Health 2002;205(6):459-472.

Elwan MA, Richardson JR, Guillot TS, Caudle WM, Miller GW. Pyrethroid pesticide-induced alterations in dopamine transporter function. Toxicol Appl Pharmacol 2006;211(3):188-197.

Eriksson P, Fredriksson A. Neurotoxic effects of two different pyrethroids, bioallethrin and deltamethrin, on immature and adult mice: changes in behavioral and muscarinic receptor variables. Toxicol Appl Pharmacol 1991;108(1):78-85.

Garey J, Wolff MS. Estrogenic and antiprogestagenic activities of pyrethroid insecticides. Biochem Biophys Res Commun 1998;251(3):855-859.

Go V, Garey J, Wolff MS, Pogo BG. Estrogenic potential of certain pyrethroid compounds in the MCF-7 human breast carcinoma cell line. Environ Health Perspect 1999;107(3):173-177.

Hu JY, Wang SL, Zhao RC, Yang J, Chen JH, Song L, et al. [Effects of fenvalerate on reproductive and endocrine systems of male rats] Zhonghua Nan Ke Xue 2002;8(1):18-21.

Kim IY, Shin JH, Kim HS, Lee SJ, Kang IH, Kim TS, et al. Assessing estrogenic activity of pyrethroid insecticides using in vitro combination assays. J Reprod Dev 2004;50(2):245-255.

Kuhn K, Wieseler B, Leng G, Idel H. Toxicokinetics of pyrethroids in humans: consequences for biological monitoring. Bull Environ Contam Toxicol 1999;62:101-108.

Kunimatsu T, Yamada T, Ose K, Sunami O, Kamita Y, Okuno Y, et al. Lack of (anti-) androgenic or estrogenic effects of three pyrethroids (esfenvalerate, fenvalerate, and permethrin) in the Hershberger and uterotrophic assays. Regul Toxicol Pharmacol 2002;35(2 Pt 1):227-237.

Lazarini CA, Florio JC, Lemonica IP, Bernardi MM. Effects of prenatal exposure to deltamethrin on forced swimming behavior, motor activity, and striatal dopamine levels in male and female rats. Neurotoxicol Teratol 2001;23(6):665-673.

Leng G, Leng A, Kuhn KH, Lewalter J, Pauluhn J. Human dose-excretion studies with the pyrethroid insecticide cyfluthrin: urinary metabolite profile following inhalation. Xenobiotica 1997;27(12):1273-1283.

McCarthy AR, Thomson BM, Shaw IC, Abell AD. Estrogenicity of pyrethroid insecticide metabolites. J Environ Monit 2006;8(1):197-202.

Moniz AC, Cruz-Casallas PE, Salzgeber SA, Varoli FM, Spinosa HS, Bernardi MM. Behavioral and endocrine changes induced by perinatal fenvalerate exposure in female rats. Neurotoxicol Teratol 2005;27(4):609-614.

Ray DE, Forshaw PJ. Pyrethroid insecticides: poisoning syndromes, synergies, and therapy. J Toxicol Clin Toxicol 2000;38:95-101.

Shafer TJ, Meyer DA, Crofton KM. Developmental neurotoxicity of pyrethroid insecticides: critical review and future research needs. Environ Health Perspect 2005;113(2):123-136.

Soderlund DM, Clark JM, Sheets LP, Mullin LS, Piccirillo VJ, Sargent D, et al. Mechanisms of pyrethroid neurotoxicity: implications for cumulative risk assessment. Toxicology 2002;171:3-59.

Spencer J, O'Malley M. Pyrethroid illnesses in California, 1996-2002. Rev Environ Contam Toxicol 2006;186:57-72.

U.S. Environmental Protection Agency (U.S. EPA). Permethrin, resmethrin, sumithrin synthetic pyrethroids for mosquito control. April 2002. Available at URL: http://www.epa.gov/pesticides/health/mosquitoes/pyrethroids4mosquitoes.htm. 5/26/09

U.S. Environmental Protection Agency (U.S. EPA). Permethrin Facts (Reregistration Eligibility Decision Fact Sheet). June 2006a. Available at URL: http://www.epa.gov/oppsrrd1/REDs/factsheets/permethrin_fs.htm. 5/26/09

U.S. Environmental Protection Agency (U.S. EPA). Reregistration Eligibility Decision for Cypermethrin. June 2006b. Available at URL: http://www.epa.gov/oppsrrd1/REDs/cypermethrin_red.pdf. 5/26/09

U.S. Geological Survey (USGS). Pesticides in the Nation's Streams and Ground Water, 1992–2001. March 2006, Revised February 25, 2007. Available at URL: http://pubs.usgs.gov/circ/2005/1291/. 5/26/09

Woollen BH, Marsh JR, Laird WJ, Lesser JE. The metabolism of cypermethrin in man: differences in urinary metabolite profiles following oral and dermal administration. Xenobiotica 1992;22(8):983-991.

World Health Organization (WHO). Pesticide and Evaluation Scheme. Safety of pyrethroids for public health use. 2005. Available at URL: http://whqlibdoc.who.int/hq/2005/WHO_CDS_WHOPES_GCDPP_2005.10.pdf. 5/26/09

# Cyfluthrin

CAS No.68359-37-5

## General Information

The chemical 4-fluoro-3-phenoxybenzoic acid is a specific metabolite of the pyrethroid insecticide cyfluthrin. Cyfluthrin accounted for one-third of pyrethroid-related worker illnesses reported in California from 1996-2002; most of which were dermal and respiratory irritations (Spencer and O'Malley, 2006). Cyfluthrin is rapidly metabolized and eliminated from the body. Following an indoor application exposure, the mean elimination half-life of cyfluthrin from the plasma was 16 hours (Williams et al., 2003).

Degradation of cyfluthrin to 4-fluoro-3-phenoxybenzoic acid occurs in the environment. Thus, the presence of 4-fluoro-3-phenoxybenzoic acid in urine not only reflects the metabolic transformation of cyfluthrin, but it can also reflect direct exposure to 4-fluoro-3-phenoxybenzoic acid formed in the environment.

## Biomonitoring Information

Urinary levels of 4-fluoro-3-phenoxybenzoic acid reflect recent exposure to cyfluthrin or its environmental degradate. Urinary levels of 4-fluoro-3-phenoxybenzoic acid were generally below the limit of detection (0.2 µg/L) in the U.S. representative subsample in NHANES 2001-2002 (CDC, 2005). In an analysis of 217 urine specimens from a nonrandom sample of United States residents, Baker et al. (2004) reported a geometric mean concentration of 4-fluoro-3-phenoxybenzoic acid of 0.95 µg/L. Studies in Germany of 396 children and adolescents (Becker et al., 2006) and 1177 urban adults and children (Heudorf et al., 2001) showed that urinary levels of 4-fluoro-3-phenoxybenzoic acid at the 95th percentile ranged from either slightly higher or lower than the detection limit in the U.S. representative 2001-2002 NHANES subsample (CDC, 2005). Urinary levels for adults and children in these studies were similar (Heudorf et al., 2001, 2006) and estimated daily intakes based on urinary levels in children were considered to be below acceptable daily intakes (Heudorf et al., 2004).

In 57 volunteers entering areas previously spot-sprayed with various pyrethroid pesticides (including cyfluthrin), median urinary levels of 4-fluoro-3-phenoxybenzoic acid were slightly less than the limit of detection in the NHANES 2001-2002 subsample (CDC, 2005; Leng et al., 2003). Seven individuals participating in floor exercises on cyfluthrin treated carpet demonstrated a rise in the urinary excretion of 4-fluoro-3-phenoxybenzoic acid in the 72 hours following the activity (Williams et al., 2003).

Finding a measurable amount of 4-fluoro-3-phenoxybenzoic acid in urine does not mean that the level will result in an adverse health effect. Biomonitoring studies of 4-fluoro-3-phenoxybenzoic acid in urine provide physicians and public health officials with reference values so that they can determine whether other people have been exposed to higher levels of cyfluthrin than levels found in the general population. Biomonitoring data can also help scientists plan and conduct research on exposure and health effects.

## Urinary 4-Fluoro-3-phenoxybenzoic acid
*Metabolite of Cyfluthrin*

Geometric mean and selected percentiles of urine concentrations (in µg/L) for the U.S. population from the National Health and Nutrition Examination Survey.

| | Survey years | Geometric mean (95% conf. interval) | Selected percentiles ( 95% confidence interval) | | | | Sample size |
|---|---|---|---|---|---|---|---|
| | | | 50th | 75th | 90th | 95th | |
| **Total** | 99-00 | * | < LOD | < LOD | < LOD | < LOD | 1949 |
| | 01-02 | * | < LOD | < LOD | < LOD | < LOD | 2539 |
| **Age group** | | | | | | | |
| 6-11 years | 99-00 | * | < LOD | < LOD | < LOD | < LOD | 473 |
| | 01-02 | * | < LOD | < LOD | < LOD | < LOD | 580 |
| 12-19 years | 99-00 | * | < LOD | < LOD | < LOD | < LOD | 662 |
| | 01-02 | * | < LOD | < LOD | < LOD | < LOD | 831 |
| 20-59 years | 99-00 | * | < LOD | < LOD | < LOD | < LOD | 814 |
| | 01-02 | * | < LOD | < LOD | < LOD | < LOD | 1128 |
| **Gender** | | | | | | | |
| Males | 99-00 | * | < LOD | < LOD | < LOD | < LOD | 950 |
| | 01-02 | * | < LOD | < LOD | < LOD | < LOD | 1193 |
| Females | 99-00 | * | < LOD | < LOD | < LOD | < LOD | 999 |
| | 01-02 | * | < LOD | < LOD | < LOD | < LOD | 1346 |
| **Race/ethnicity** | | | | | | | |
| Mexican Americans | 99-00 | * | < LOD | < LOD | < LOD | < LOD | 666 |
| | 01-02 | * | < LOD | < LOD | < LOD | < LOD | 680 |
| Non-Hispanic blacks | 99-00 | * | < LOD | < LOD | < LOD | < LOD | 517 |
| | 01-02 | * | < LOD | < LOD | < LOD | < LOD | 701 |
| Non-Hispanic whites | 99-00 | * | < LOD | < LOD | < LOD | < LOD | 594 |
| | 01-02 | * | < LOD | < LOD | < LOD | < LOD | 957 |

Limit of detection (LOD, see Data Analysis section) for Survey years 99-00 and 01-02 are 0.2 and 0 2.
< LOD means less than the limit of detection, which may vary for some chemicals by year and by individual sample.
* Not calculated: proportion of results below limit of detection was too high to provide a valid result.

# Urinary 4-Fluoro-3-phenoxybenzoic acid (creatinine corrected)
*Metabolite of Cyfluthrin*

Geometric mean and selected percentiles of urine concentrations (in µg/g of creatinine) for the U.S. population from the National Health and Nutrition Examination Survey.

| | Survey years | Geometric mean (95% conf. interval) | Selected percentiles ( 95% confidence interval) | | | | Sample size |
|---|---|---|---|---|---|---|---|
| | | | 50th | 75th | 90th | 95th | |
| Total | 99-00 | * | < LOD | < LOD | < LOD | < LOD | 1949 |
| | 01-02 | * | < LOD | < LOD | < LOD | < LOD | 2538 |
| **Age group** | | | | | | | |
| 6-11 years | 99-00 | * | < LOD | < LOD | < LOD | < LOD | 473 |
| | 01-02 | * | < LOD | < LOD | < LOD | < LOD | 580 |
| 12-19 years | 99-00 | * | < LOD | < LOD | < LOD | < LOD | 662 |
| | 01-02 | * | < LOD | < LOD | < LOD | < LOD | 830 |
| 20-59 years | 99-00 | * | < LOD | < LOD | < LOD | < LOD | 814 |
| | 01-02 | * | < LOD | < LOD | < LOD | < LOD | 1128 |
| **Gender** | | | | | | | |
| Males | 99-00 | * | < LOD | < LOD | < LOD | < LOD | 950 |
| | 01-02 | * | < LOD | < LOD | < LOD | < LOD | 1193 |
| Females | 99-00 | * | < LOD | < LOD | < LOD | < LOD | 999 |
| | 01-02 | * | < LOD | < LOD | < LOD | < LOD | 1345 |
| **Race/ethnicity** | | | | | | | |
| Mexican Americans | 99-00 | * | < LOD | < LOD | < LOD | < LOD | 666 |
| | 01-02 | * | < LOD | < LOD | < LOD | < LOD | 680 |
| Non-Hispanic blacks | 99-00 | * | < LOD | < LOD | < LOD | < LOD | 517 |
| | 01-02 | * | < LOD | < LOD | < LOD | < LOD | 700 |
| Non-Hispanic whites | 99-00 | * | < LOD | < LOD | < LOD | < LOD | 594 |
| | 01-02 | * | < LOD | < LOD | < LOD | < LOD | 957 |

< LOD means less than the limit of detection for the urine levels not corrected for creatinine.
* Not calculated: proportion of results below limit of detection was too high to provide a valid result.

## References

Baker SE, Olsson AO, Barr DB. Isotope dilution high-performance liquid chromatography-tandem mass spectrometry method for quantifying urinary metabolites of synthetic pyrethroid insecticides. Arch Environ Contam Toxicol 2004;46(3):281-288.

Becker K, Seiwert M, Angerer J, Kolossa-Gehring M, Hoppe HW, Ball M, et al. GerES IV pilot study: assessment of the exposure of German children to organophosphorus and pyrethroid pesticides. Int J Hyg Environ Health 2006;209(3):221-233.

Centers for Disease Control and Prevention (CDC). Third National Report on Human Exposure to Environmental Chemicals. Atlanta (GA). 2005.

Heudorf U, Angerer J, Drexler H. Current internal exposure to pesticides in children and adolescents in Germany: urinary levels of metabolites of pyrethroid and organophosphorus insecticides. Int Arch Occup Environ Health 2004;77(1):67-72.

Heudorf U, Angerer J. Metabolites of pyrethroid insecticides in urine specimens: current exposure in an urban population in Germany. Environ Health Perspect 2001;109(3):213-217.

Heudorf U, Butte W, Schulz C, Angerer J. Reference values for metabolites of pyrethroid and organophosphorous insecticides in urine for human biomonitoring in environmental medicine. Int J Hyg Environ Health 2006;209(3):293-299.

Leng G, Ranft U, Sugiri D, Hadnagy W, Berger-Preiss E, Idel H. Pyrethroids used indoors—biological monitoring of exposure to pyrethroids following an indoor pest control operation. Int J Hyg Environ Health 2003;206(2):85-92.

Spencer J, O'Malley M. Pyrethroid illnesses in California, 1996-2002. Rev Environ Contam Toxicol 2006;186:57-72.

Williams RL, Bernard CE, Krieger RI. Human exposure to indoor residential cyfluthrin residues during a structured activity program. J Expo Anal Environ Epidemiol 2003;13(2):112-119.

# Cyfluthrin
CAS No.68359-37-5

# Cypermethrin
CAS No. 52315-07-8

# Permethrin
CAS No.52645-53-1

## General Information

Several pyrethroid pesticides are formulated as a mixture of *cis*- and *trans*-isomers. In the body, *cis*-3-(2,2-dichlorovinyl)-2,2-dimethylcyclopropane carboxylic acid is a metabolite formed from *cis*-permethrin, *cis*-cypermethrin and *cis*-cyfluthrin. The chemical *trans*-3-(2,2-dichlorovinyl)-2,2-dimethylcyclopropane carboxylic acid is a metabolite formed from *trans*-permethrin, *trans*-cypermethrin and *trans*-cyfluthrin. The *cis*-isomer of permethrin has more potent insecticidal activity than *trans*-permethrin. Generally, more of the *trans*-metabolite than

the *cis*-metabolite is found in the urine.

The presence of *cis*-3-(2,2-dichlorovinyl)-2,2-dimethylcyclopropane carboxylic acid in urine not only reflects the metabolic transformation of any of the three pesticides, *cis*-permethrin, *cis*-cypermethrin, and *cis*-cyfluthrin, but it can also reflect exposure to *cis*-3-(2,2-dichlorovinyl)-2,2-dimethylcyclopropane carboxylic acid that is formed in the environment from the degradation of these pesticides (George, 1985; Kuhn et al., 1999). Similarly, the presence of *trans*-3-(2,2-dichlorovinyl)-2,2-dimethylcyclopropane carboxylic acid in urine not only reflects the metabolic transformation of any of the three pesticides, *trans*-permethrin, *trans*-cypermethrin, and *trans*-cyfluthrin, but can also reflect exposure to *trans*-3-(2,2-dichlorovinyl)-2,2-dimethylcyclopropane carboxylic acid formed in the environment from the degradation of these pesticides (George, 1985; Kuhn et al., 1999).

## Biomonitoring Information

Urinary levels of *cis*- or *trans*-3-(2,2-dichlorovinyl)-

## Urinary *cis*-3-(2,2-Dichlorovinyl)-2,2-dimethylcyclopropane carboxylic acid
*Metabolite of cis-Permethrin, Cyfluthrin, and cis-Cypermethrin*
Geometric mean and selected percentiles of urine concentrations (in µg/L) for the U.S. population from the National Health and Nutrition Examination Survey.

| | Survey years | Geometric mean (95% conf. interval) | Selected percentiles ( 95% confidence interval) | | | | Sample size |
|---|---|---|---|---|---|---|---|
| | | | 50th | 75th | 90th | 95th | |
| Total | 99-00 | * | < LOD | .270 (.220-.340) | .600 (.490-.710) | 1.12 (.770-1 68) | 1951 |
| | 01-02 | * | < LOD | .160 (.120-.210) | .500 (.380-.680) | .890 (.740-1.10) | 2539 |
| Age group | | | | | | | |
| 6-11 years | 99-00 | * | < LOD | .330 (.210-.550) | .740 (.580-1 53) | 1.77 (.680-3.15) | 468 |
| | 01-02 | * | < LOD | .110 (<LOD- 200) | .370 (.280-.610) | .730 (.490-.870) | 580 |
| 12-19 years | 99-00 | * | < LOD | .300 (.200-.410) | .670 (.460-1.11) | 1.44 (.670-2 21) | 667 |
| | 01-02 | * | < LOD | .160 (<LOD- 210) | .440 (.300-.630) | .730 (.630-.920) | 831 |
| 20-59 years | 99-00 | * | < LOD | .260 (.200-.330) | .570 (.430-.690) | 1.07 (.670-1 80) | 816 |
| | 01-02 | * | < LOD | .170 (.120-.230) | .510 (.400-.740) | .960 (.790-1 28) | 1128 |
| Gender | | | | | | | |
| Males | 99-00 | * | < LOD | .250 (.200-.310) | .530 (.420-.600) | .790 (.600-1 50) | 947 |
| | 01-02 | * | < LOD | .150 (.110-.200) | .470 (.380-.630) | .880 (.650-1 35) | 1193 |
| Females | 99-00 | * | < LOD | .280 (.220-.380) | .680 (.490-1 08) | 1.47 (.950-2 54) | 1004 |
| | 01-02 | * | < LOD | .180 (.120-.240) | .510 (.370-.770) | .890 (.790-1 08) | 1346 |
| Race/ethnicity | | | | | | | |
| Mexican Americans | 99-00 | * | < LOD | .200 (.110-.240) | .460 (.300-.610) | .730 (.470-1 32) | 671 |
| | 01-02 | * | < LOD | .140 (.110-.180) | .300 (.250-.410) | .510 (.380-.580) | 680 |
| Non-Hispanic blacks | 99-00 | .202 (.155-.262) | .160 (.120-.200) | .380 (.270-.520) | .820 (.490-1 68) | 1.68 (.910-5.43) | 518 |
| | 01-02 | * | < LOD | .270 (.220-.350) | .640 (.570-.700) | .850 (.710-1 24) | 701 |
| Non-Hispanic whites | 99-00 | * | < LOD | .270 (.220-.340) | .630 (.460-.780) | 1.13 (.740-2 35) | 591 |
| | 01-02 | * | < LOD | .140 (<LOD- 220) | .500 (.340-.790) | .900 (.670-1 28) | 957 |

Limit of detection (LOD, see Data Analysis section) for Survey years 99-00 and 01-02 are 0.1 and 0.1.
< LOD means less than the limit of detection, which may vary for some chemicals by year and by individual sample.
* Not calculated: proportion of results below limit of detection was too high to provide a valid result.

2,2-dimethylcyclopropane carboxylic acid reflect recent exposure to either their parent pyrethroid pesticides or their environmental degradates. Studies in Germany of 396 children and adolescents (Becker et al., 2006) and 1177 urban adults and children (Heudorf et al., 2001) showed urinary levels of *cis-* and *trans*-3-(2,2-dichlorovinyl)-2,2-dimethylcyclopropane carboxylic acids at the 95th percentile that were similar or slightly less than the 95th percentiles in the U.S. representative NHANES 2001-2002 subsample (CDC, 2005). Urinary levels of the two chemicals in adults were similar to those in children in these studies (Heudorf et al., 2001, 2006). Estimated daily pyrethroid intakes based on urinary levels in the German children were below the acceptable daily tolerances (Heudorf et al., 2004). These studies indicated that intake is mainly from the diet and that dermal absorption contributes little to intake (Heudorf et al., 2004, 2006; Schettgen et al., 2002). Other studies have provided evidence that urinary levels of *cis-* and *trans*-3-(2,2-dichlorovinyl)-2,2-dimethylcyclopropane carboxylic acids in children were related to residential pesticide use and house dust levels (Becker et al., 2006; Lu et al., 2006).

In a study of urban residents in Germany (Berger-Preiss et

al., 2002), urinary levels of *cis*-3-(2,2-dichlorovinyl)-2,2-dimethylcyclopropane carboxylic acid at the 95th percentile were about half the 95th percentile in the NHANES 2001-2002 subsample (CDC, 2005). In the same residents, urinary *trans*-3-(2,2-dichlorovinyl)-2,2-dimethylcyclopropane carboxylic acid levels at the 95th percentile were about one-third of the 95th percentile in the NHANES 2001-2002 subsample (CDC, 2005). In a study of volunteers, the median and 95th percentile of urinary levels of *cis*-3-(2,2-dichlorovinyl)-2,2-dimethylcyclopropane carboxylic acid did not increase at 24-72 hours after exposure to nearby pest control operations (Leng et al., 2003); the levels at 24-72 hours were slightly less than the 95th percentile in the NHANES 2001-2002 subsample (CDC, 2005). In these volunteers, median urinary levels of *trans*-3-(2,2-dichlorovinyl)-2,2-dimethylcyclopropane carboxylic acid did not increase, though the 95th percentile levels increased several fold after exposure to nearby pest control operations (Leng et al., 2003); the levels at 24-72 hours were slightly less than the 95th percentile in the NHANES 2001-2002 subsample (CDC, 2005)

In a small group of indoor pest-control operators, post-

## Urinary *cis*-3-(2,2-Dichlorovinyl)-2,2-dimethylcyclopropane carboxylic acid (creatinine corrected)
*Metabolite of cis-Permethrin, Cyfluthrin, and cis-Cypermethrin*

Geometric mean and selected percentiles of urine concentrations (in µg/g of creatinine) for the U.S. population from the National Health and Nutrition Examination Survey.

| | Survey years | Geometric mean (95% conf. interval) | 50th | 75th | 90th | 95th | Sample size |
|---|---|---|---|---|---|---|---|
| | | | | Selected percentiles ( 95% confidence interval) | | | |
| **Total** | 99-00 | * | < LOD | .260 ( 230-.290) | .540 (.440-.700) | 1.12 ( 690-1.59) | 1951 |
| | 01-02 | * | < LOD | .220 ( 200-.250) | .440 ( 370-.520) | .780 ( 640-1.03) | 2538 |
| **Age group** | | | | | | | |
| 6-11 years | 99-00 | * | < LOD | .400 ( 250-.550) | .900 ( 550-1.67) | 1.67 (.700-2.31) | 468 |
| | 01-02 | * | < LOD | .250 (<LOD-.320) | .600 (.430-.700) | .750 ( 640-.890) | 580 |
| 12-19 years | 99-00 | * | < LOD | .200 (.150-.270) | .430 ( 320-.590) | .810 (.430-1.49) | 667 |
| | 01-02 | * | < LOD | .160 (<LOD-.200) | .300 ( 250-.380) | .530 ( 370-.780) | 830 |
| 20-59 years | 99-00 | * | < LOD | .260 ( 230-.290) | .530 ( 380-.830) | 1.11 ( 680-1.59) | 816 |
| | 01-02 | * | < LOD | .230 ( 210-.250) | .440 ( 390-.560) | .890 ( 640-1.08) | 1128 |
| **Gender** | | | | | | | |
| Males | 99-00 | * | < LOD | .220 (.180-.250) | .420 ( 340-.570) | .800 ( 510-1.11) | 947 |
| | 01-02 | * | < LOD | .170 (.150-.190) | .350 ( 300-.410) | .680 (.450-1.03) | 1193 |
| Females | 99-00 | * | < LOD | .290 ( 270-.340) | .640 (.470-1.33) | 1.59 (1.12-2.21) | 1004 |
| | 01-02 | * | < LOD | .270 ( 230-.300) | .500 (.440-.580) | .920 (.750-1.11) | 1345 |
| **Race/ethnicity** | | | | | | | |
| Mexican Americans | 99-00 | * | < LOD | .190 (.130-.260) | .380 ( 280-.540) | .710 (.400-1.24) | 671 |
| | 01-02 | * | < LOD | .170 (.150-.190) | .300 ( 260-.350) | .540 ( 370-.640) | 680 |
| Non-Hispanic blacks | 99-00 | .138 (.104-.182) | .120 ( 080-.170) | .260 ( 200-.340) | .590 ( 360-1.11) | 1.29 (.710-3.37) | 518 |
| | 01-02 | * | < LOD | .180 (.140-.220) | .390 ( 290-.550) | .840 ( 550-1.11) | 700 |
| Non-Hispanic whites | 99-00 | * | < LOD | .280 ( 250-.300) | .550 (.450-.880) | 1.33 ( 680-1.80) | 591 |
| | 01-02 | * | < LOD | .240 (<LOD-.270) | .450 ( 390-.560) | .840 ( 580-1.14) | 957 |

< LOD means less than the limit of detection for the urine levels not corrected for creatinine.
* Not calculated: proportion of results below limit of detection was too high to provide a valid result.

application median urinary levels of summed *cis-* and *trans*-3-(2,2-dichlorovinyl)-2,2-dimethylcyclopropane carboxylic acid (Hardt and Angerer, 2003) were similar to the 95th percentiles for adults in the NHANES 2001-2002 subsample (CDC, 2005). The maximum post-application urinary levels, however, were up to 27 times higher than the 95th percentile for adults in the NHANES 2001-2002 subsample (CDC, 2005).

Finding a measurable amount of *cis-* or *trans*-3-(2,2-dichlorovinyl)-2,2-dimethylcyclopropane carboxylic acid in urine does not mean that the level causes an adverse health effect. Biomonitoring studies on urinary levels of *cis-* or *trans*-3-(2,2-dichlorovinyl)-2,2-dimethylcyclopropane carboxylic acid provide physicians and public health officials with reference values so that they can determine whether people have been exposed to higher levels of pyrethroid pesticides than are found in the general population. Biomonitoring data can also help scientists plan and conduct research on exposure and health effects.

## Urinary *trans*-3-(2,2-Dichlorovinyl)-2,2-dimethylcyclopropane carboxylic acid

*Metabolite of Cyfluthrin, trans-Cypermethrin, and trans-Permethrin*

Geometric mean and selected percentiles of urine concentrations (in µg/L) for the U.S. population from the National Health and Nutrition Examination Survey.

| | Survey years | Geometric mean (95% conf. interval) | 50th | 75th | 90th | 95th | Sample size |
|---|---|---|---|---|---|---|---|
| **Total** | 99-00 | * | < LOD | .560 (.480-.700) | 1.40 (1.17-1.77) | 3.42 (2.39-5 56) | 1976 |
| | 01-02 | * | < LOD | .420 (<LOD- 570) | 1.20 (.910-1.77) | 2.54 (1.68-3.70) | 2525 |
| **Age group** | | | | | | | |
| 6-11 years | 99-00 | * | < LOD | .970 (.700-1 66) | 2.91 (1.76-4.19) | 4.19 (2.97-11.7) | 478 |
| | 01-02 | * | < LOD | .470 (<LOD-.760) | 1.39 (1.03-1 68) | 2.50 (1.55-3 54) | 576 |
| 12-19 years | 99-00 | * | < LOD | .710 (.520-.860) | 2.07 (1.25-3.42) | 4.28 (2.12-6 23) | 675 |
| | 01-02 | * | < LOD | .490 (<LOD- 670) | 1.20 (.800-1 60) | 2.01 (1.49-3.77) | 826 |
| 20-59 years | 99-00 | * | < LOD | .500 (.400-.620) | 1.17 (.910-1 68) | 2.94 (1.49-5 56) | 823 |
| | 01-02 | * | < LOD | < LOD | 1.17 (.850-1 85) | 2.56 (1.64-4 66) | 1123 |
| **Gender** | | | | | | | |
| Males | 99-00 | * | < LOD | .560 (.500-.670) | 1.28 (1.11-1 63) | 2.25 (1.55-5.10) | 961 |
| | 01-02 | * | < LOD | .410 (<LOD- 500) | 1.09 (.810-1 63) | 2.37 (1.55-4.48) | 1184 |
| Females | 99-00 | * | < LOD | .550 (.410-.820) | 1.77 (1.07-3 08) | 4.19 (3.08-6 81) | 1015 |
| | 01-02 | * | < LOD | .440 (<LOD- 660) | 1.26 (.920-1 95) | 2.56 (1.76-3 58) | 1341 |
| **Race/ethnicity** | | | | | | | |
| Mexican Americans | 99-00 | * | < LOD | .470 (.410-.530) | 1.23 (.830-1 60) | 1.87 (1.49-3 35) | 691 |
| | 01-02 | * | < LOD | .410 (<LOD- 520) | .940 (.680-1.16) | 1.59 (1.11-2 01) | 680 |
| Non-Hispanic blacks | 99-00 | * | < LOD | .780 (.490-1.13) | 1.84 (1.08-4 69) | 4.69 (1.41-14.5) | 518 |
| | 01-02 | * | < LOD | .580 (.460-.750) | 1.27 (1.03-1 68) | 2.22 (1.68-2 95) | 690 |
| Non-Hispanic whites | 99-00 | * | < LOD | .560 (.460-.730) | 1.41 (1.14-2.14) | 3.89 (2.14-6.43) | 595 |
| | 01-02 | * | < LOD | .400 (<LOD- 610) | 1.20 (.840-1 90) | 2.62 (1.60-4 66) | 954 |

Limit of detection (LOD, see Data Analysis section) for Survey years 99-00 and 01-02 are 0.4 and 0.4.
< LOD means less than the limit of detection, which may vary for some chemicals by year and by individual sample.
* Not calculated: proportion of results below limit of detection was too high to provide a valid result.

## Urinary *trans*-3-(2,2-Dichlorovinyl)-2,2-dimethylcyclopropane carboxylic acid (creatinine corrected)
*Metabolite of Cyfluthrin, trans-Cypermethrin, and trans-Permethrin*

Geometric mean and selected percentiles of urine concentrations (in µg/g of creatinine) for the U.S. population from the National Health and Nutrition Examination Survey.

| | Survey years | Geometric mean (95% conf. interval) | 50th | 75th | 90th | 95th | Sample size |
|---|---|---|---|---|---|---|---|
| | | | | Selected percentiles ( 95% confidence interval) | | | |
| **Total** | 99-00 | * | < LOD | .700 ( 610-.780) | 1.56 (1.33-1.87) | 2.65 (2.15-3.89) | 1976 |
| | 01-02 | * | < LOD | .720 (<LOD-.780) | 1.45 (1.22-1.88) | 2.55 (2.15-3.10) | 2524 |
| **Age group** | | | | | | | |
| 6-11 years | 99-00 | * | < LOD | 1.31 (.720-1.74) | 2.37 (1.56-5.07) | 5.60 (1.91-11 3) | 478 |
| | 01-02 | * | < LOD | .900 (<LOD-1.13) | 2.16 (1.40-2.61) | 2.86 (2.34-3.44) | 576 |
| 12-19 years | 99-00 | * | < LOD | .530 (.440-.730) | 1.42 ( 820-2.19) | 2.19 (1.34-4.31) | 675 |
| | 01-02 | * | < LOD | .530 (<LOD-.660) | .970 ( 800-1.29) | 1.57 (1.07-2.60) | 825 |
| 20-59 years | 99-00 | * | < LOD | .700 ( 570-.770) | 1.33 (1.12-1.87) | 2.39 (1.87-3.36) | 823 |
| | 01-02 | * | < LOD | < LOD | 1.47 (1.22-2.00) | 2.55 (2.07-3.11) | 1123 |
| **Gender** | | | | | | | |
| Males | 99-00 | * | < LOD | .560 (.480-.670) | 1.26 (1.07-1.42) | 2.15 (1.47-2.74) | 961 |
| | 01-02 | * | < LOD | .520 (<LOD-.580) | 1.08 ( 880-1.35) | 2.20 (1.45-2.57) | 1184 |
| Females | 99-00 | * | < LOD | .880 (.720-1.11) | 1.91 (1.48-2.39) | 3.67 (2.30-6.28) | 1015 |
| | 01-02 | * | < LOD | .880 (<LOD-1.00) | 1.75 (1.47-2.15) | 2.81 (2.30-3.19) | 1340 |
| **Race/ethnicity** | | | | | | | |
| Mexican Americans | 99-00 | * | < LOD | .580 ( 500-.750) | 1.35 (1.02-1.65) | 2.00 (1.56-2.80) | 691 |
| | 01-02 | * | < LOD | .570 (<LOD-.640) | 1.08 ( 930-1.22) | 1.87 (1.27-2.15) | 680 |
| Non-Hispanic blacks | 99-00 | * | < LOD | .570 (.470-.740) | 1.70 ( 850-3.13) | 3.36 (1.87-8.91) | 518 |
| | 01-02 | * | < LOD | .470 (.410-.540) | 1.12 ( 800-1.41) | 1.98 (1.20-2.68) | 689 |
| Non-Hispanic whites | 99-00 | * | < LOD | .760 (.700-.850) | 1.64 (1.33-2.00) | 3.31 (2.00-5.60) | 595 |
| | 01-02 | * | < LOD | .780 (<LOD-.850) | 1.48 (1.27-2.07) | 2.55 (2.15-3.11) | 954 |

< LOD means less than the limit of detection for the urine levels not corrected for creatinine.
* Not calculated: proportion of results below limit of detection was too high to provide a valid result.

## References

Becker K, Seiwert M, Angerer J, Kolossa-Gehring M, Hoppe HW, Ball M, et al. GerES IV pilot study: assessment of the exposure of German children to organophosphorus and pyrethroid pesticides. Int J Hyg Environ Health 2006;209(3):221-233.

Berger-Preiss E, Levsen K, Leng G, Idel H, Sugiri D, Ranft U. Indoor pyrethroid exposure in homes with woollen textile floor coverings. Int J Hyg Environ Health 2002;205(6):459-472.

Centers for Disease Control and Prevention (CDC). Third National Report on Human Exposure to Environmental Chemicals. Atlanta (GA). 2005.

George DA. Permethrin and its two metabolite residues in seven agricultural crops. J AOAC 1985;68(6):1160-1163.

Hardt J, Angerer J. Biological monitoring of workers after the application of insecticidal pyrethroids. Int Arch Occup Environ Health 2003;76(7):492-498.

Heudorf U, Angerer J, Drexler H. Current internal exposure to pesticides in children and adolescents in Germany: urinary levels of metabolites of pyrethroid and organophosphorus insecticides. Int Arch Occup Environ Health 2004;77(1):67-72.

Heudorf U, Angerer J. Metabolites of pyrethroid insecticides in urine specimens: current exposure in an urban population in Germany. Environ Health Perspect 2001;109(3):213-217.

Heudorf U, Butte W, Schulz C, Angerer J. Reference values for metabolites of pyrethroid and organophosphorous insecticides in urine for human biomonitoring in environmental medicine. Int J Hyg Environ Health 2006;209(3):293-299.

Kuhn K, Wieseler B, Leng G, Idel H. Toxicokinetics of pyrethroids in humans: consequences for biological monitoring. Bull Environ Contam Toxicol 1999;62:101-108.

Leng G, Ranft U, Sugiri D, Hadnagy W, Berger-Preiss E, Idel H. Pyrethroids used indoors—biological monitoring of exposure to pyrethroids following an indoor pest control operation. Int J Hyg Environ Health 2003;206(2):85-92.

Lu C, Barr DB, Pearson M, Bartell S, Bravo R. A longitudinal approach to assessing urban and suburban children's exposure to pyrethroid pesticides. Environ Health Perspect 2006;114(9):1419-1423.

Schettgen T, Heudorf U, Drexler H, Angerer J. Pyrethroid exposure of the general population-is this due to diet? Toxicol Lett 2002;134(1-3):141-145.

# Deltamethrin

CAS No. 52918-63-5

## General Information

*Cis*-3-(2,2-dibromovinyl)-2,2-dimethylcyclopropane carboxylic acid is a metabolite of the pyrethroid insecticide deltamethrin. Outside the U.S., deltamethrin has been used against mosquitoes that carry malaria, in some situations replacing the use of DDT. Deltamethrin can degrade to *cis*-3-(2,2-dibromovinyl)-2,2-dimethylcyclopropane carboxylic acid in the environment (IPCS, 1990). Thus, in detection of *cis*-3-(2,2-dibromovinyl)-2,2-dimethylcyclopropane carboxylic acid in the urine may reflect exposure to deltamethrin or to *cis*-3-(2,2-dibromovinyl)-2,2-dimethylcyclopropane carboxylic acid formed in the environment.

## Biomonitoring Information

Urinary levels of *cis*-3-(2,2-dibromovinyl)-2,2-dimethylcyclopropane carboxylic acid reflect recent exposure to deltamethrin or its environmental degradate. In the NHANES 2001-2002 subsample, urinary levels of *cis*-3-(2,2-dibromovinyl)-2,2-dimethylcyclopropane carboxylic acid were below the limit of detection (CDC, 2005). In an analysis of 217 urine specimens from a nonrandom sample of United States residents, Baker et al. (2004) reported a geometric mean concentration of *cis*-3-(2,2-dibromovinyl)-2,2-dimethylcyclopropane carboxylic acid of 0.39 µg/L. Studies in Germany of 396 children and adolescents (Becker et al., 2006) and 1177 urban adults and children (Heudorf et al., 2001) showed that urinary levels of *cis*-3-(2,2-dibromovinyl)-2,2-dimethylcyclopropane carboxylic acid at the 95th percentile ranged slightly higher (0.3-0.5 µg/L) than the detection limit (0.1 µg/L) for the NHANES 2001-2002 subsample (CDC, 2005). Urinary levels for adults and children in these studies were similar (Heudorf et al., 2001, 2006) and estimated daily intakes based on urinary levels in children were considered to be below acceptable daily intakes (Heudorf et al., 2004).

Following residential spraying with deltamethrin for malaria protection in Mexico, mean peak urinary levels of *cis*-3-(2,2-dibromovinyl)-2,2-dimethylcyclopropane carboxylic acid in children increased at least 450-fold relative to the non-detectable background levels for several days and mean levels remained slightly above background levels 45 days after the spraying (Ortiz-Perez et al., 2005). The peak mean levels in these children were more than 800-fold higher than the detection limit in the 2001-2002 NHANES subsample.

Finding a measurable amount of *cis*-3-(2,2-dibromovinyl)-2,2-dimethylcyclopropane carboxylic acid in urine does not mean that the level will result in an adverse health effect. Biomonitoring studies provide physicians and public health officials with reference values so that they can determine whether other people have been exposed to higher levels of deltamethrin than levels found in the general population. Biomonitoring data can also help scientists plan and conduct research on exposure and health effects.

# Urinary *cis*-3-(2,2-Dibromovinyl)-2,2-dimethylcyclopropane carboxylic acid
*Metabolite of Deltamethrin*

Geometric mean and selected percentiles of urine concentrations (in µg/L) for the U.S. population from the National Health and Nutrition Examination Survey.

| | Survey years | Geometric mean (95% conf. interval) | Selected percentiles ( 95% confidence interval) | | | | Sample size |
|---|---|---|---|---|---|---|---|
| | | | 50th | 75th | 90th | 95th | |
| Total | 99-00 | * | < LOD | < LOD | < LOD | < LOD | 1698 |
| | 01-02 | * | < LOD | < LOD | < LOD | < LOD | 2539 |
| **Age group** | | | | | | | |
| 6-11 years | 99-00 | * | < LOD | < LOD | < LOD | < LOD | 415 |
| | 01-02 | * | < LOD | < LOD | < LOD | < LOD | 580 |
| 12-19 years | 99-00 | * | < LOD | < LOD | < LOD | < LOD | 570 |
| | 01-02 | * | < LOD | < LOD | < LOD | < LOD | 831 |
| 20-59 years | 99-00 | * | < LOD | < LOD | < LOD | < LOD | 713 |
| | 01-02 | * | < LOD | < LOD | < LOD | < LOD | 1128 |
| **Gender** | | | | | | | |
| Males | 99-00 | * | < LOD | < LOD | < LOD | < LOD | 818 |
| | 01-02 | * | < LOD | < LOD | < LOD | < LOD | 1193 |
| Females | 99-00 | * | < LOD | < LOD | < LOD | < LOD | 880 |
| | 01-02 | * | < LOD | < LOD | < LOD | < LOD | 1346 |
| **Race/ethnicity** | | | | | | | |
| Mexican Americans | 99-00 | * | < LOD | < LOD | < LOD | < LOD | 578 |
| | 01-02 | * | < LOD | < LOD | < LOD | < LOD | 680 |
| Non-Hispanic blacks | 99-00 | * | < LOD | < LOD | < LOD | < LOD | 445 |
| | 01-02 | * | < LOD | < LOD | < LOD | < LOD | 701 |
| Non-Hispanic whites | 99-00 | * | < LOD | < LOD | < LOD | < LOD | 527 |
| | 01-02 | * | < LOD | < LOD | < LOD | < LOD | 957 |

Limit of detection (LOD, see Data Analysis section) for Survey years 99-00 and 01-02 are 0.1 and 0.1.
< LOD means less than the limit of detection, which may vary for some chemicals by year and by individual sample.
* Not calculated: proportion of results below limit of detection was too high to provide a valid result.

## Urinary *cis*-3-(2,2-Dibromovinyl)-2,2-dimethylcyclopropane carboxylic acid (creatinine corrected)
*Metabolite of Deltamethrin*

Geometric mean and selected percentiles of urine concentrations (in µg/g of creatinine) for the U.S. population from the National Health and Nutrition Examination Survey.

| | Survey years | Geometric mean (95% conf. interval) | Selected percentiles ( 95% confidence interval) | | | | Sample size |
|---|---|---|---|---|---|---|---|
| | | | 50th | 75th | 90th | 95th | |
| **Total** | 99-00 | * | < LOD | < LOD | < LOD | < LOD | 1698 |
| | 01-02 | * | < LOD | < LOD | < LOD | < LOD | 2538 |
| **Age group** | | | | | | | |
| 6-11 years | 99-00 | * | < LOD | < LOD | < LOD | < LOD | 415 |
| | 01-02 | * | < LOD | < LOD | < LOD | < LOD | 580 |
| 12-19 years | 99-00 | * | < LOD | < LOD | < LOD | < LOD | 570 |
| | 01-02 | * | < LOD | < LOD | < LOD | < LOD | 830 |
| 20-59 years | 99-00 | * | < LOD | < LOD | < LOD | < LOD | 713 |
| | 01-02 | * | < LOD | < LOD | < LOD | < LOD | 1128 |
| **Gender** | | | | | | | |
| Males | 99-00 | * | < LOD | < LOD | < LOD | < LOD | 818 |
| | 01-02 | * | < LOD | < LOD | < LOD | < LOD | 1193 |
| Females | 99-00 | * | < LOD | < LOD | < LOD | < LOD | 880 |
| | 01-02 | * | < LOD | < LOD | < LOD | < LOD | 1345 |
| **Race/ethnicity** | | | | | | | |
| Mexican Americans | 99-00 | * | < LOD | < LOD | < LOD | < LOD | 578 |
| | 01-02 | * | < LOD | < LOD | < LOD | < LOD | 680 |
| Non-Hispanic blacks | 99-00 | * | < LOD | < LOD | < LOD | < LOD | 445 |
| | 01-02 | * | < LOD | < LOD | < LOD | < LOD | 700 |
| Non-Hispanic whites | 99-00 | * | < LOD | < LOD | < LOD | < LOD | 527 |
| | 01-02 | * | < LOD | < LOD | < LOD | < LOD | 957 |

< LOD means less than the limit of detection for the urine levels not corrected for creatinine.
* Not calculated: proportion of results below limit of detection was too high to provide a valid result.

## References

Becker K, Seiwert M, Angerer J, Kolossa-Gehring M, Hoppe HW, Ball M, et al. GerES IV pilot study: assessment of the exposure of German children to organophosphorus and pyrethroid pesticides. Int J Hyg Environ Health 2006;209(3):221-233.

Centers for Disease Control and Prevention (CDC). Third National Report on Human Exposure to Environmental Chemicals. Atlanta (GA). 2005.

Heudorf U, Angerer J, Drexler H. Current internal exposure to pesticides in children and adolescents in Germany: urinary levels of metabolites of pyrethroid and organophosphorus insecticides. Int Arch Occup Environ Health 2004;77(1):67-72.

Heudorf U, Angerer J. Metabolites of pyrethroid insecticides in urine specimens: current exposure in an urban population in Germany. Environ Health Perspect 2001;109(3):213-217.

Heudorf U, Butte W, Schulz C, Angerer J. Reference values for metabolites of pyrethroid and organophosphorous insecticides in urine for human biomonitoring in environmental medicine. Int J Hyg Environ Health 2006;209(3):293-299.

International Programme On Chemical Safety (IPCS). Environmental Health Criteria 97. Deltamethrin. [online] 1990. Available at URL: http://www.inchem.org/documents/ehc/ehc/ehc97 htm. 5/26/09

Ortiz-Perez MD, Torres-Dosal A, Batres LE, Lopez-Guzman OD, Grimaldo M, Carranza C, et al. Environmental health assessment of deltamethrin in a malarious area of Mexico: environmental persistence, toxicokinetics, and genotoxicity in exposed children. Environ Health Perspect 2005;113(6):782-786.

# Cyhalothrin
CAS No. 68359-37-5

# Cypermethrin
CAS No.52315-07-8

# Deltamethrin
CAS No. 52918-63-5

# Fenpropathrin
CAS No. 39515-41-8

# Permethrin
CAS No. 52645-53-1

# Tralomethrin
CAS No. 66841-25-6

## General Information

The chemical 3-phenoxybenzoic acid is a metabolite and an environmental degradate of the six pyrethroid pesticides listed above. Thus, the presence of 3-phenoxybenzoic acid in urine not only reflects the metabolic transformation of any of the six pesticides listed above, but can reflect direct exposure to 3-phenoxybenzoic acid formed in the environment from the degradation of these pesticides.

## Biomonitoring Information

Urinary levels of 3-phenoxybenzoic acid reflect recent exposure to the parent pyrethroid pesticides. In an analysis of 217 urine specimens from a nonrandom sample of United States residents, Baker et al. (2004) reported geometric mean levels of 3-phenoxybenzoic acid that were approximately sixfold higher than levels for adults in the NHANES 2001-2002 subsample (CDC, 2005). Median levels of urinary 3-phenoxybenzoic acid were 67-fold higher in 307 pregnant New York City women who used indoor pesticides compared with the median levels for adults in the NHANES 2001-2002 subsample (Berkowitz et al., 2003; CDC, 2005). In the New York City study, a temporal variation in levels was observed and considered to correspond to seasonal spraying of pesticides. A study of 396 German children (Becker et al., 2006) showed that urinary levels of 3-phenoxybenzoic acid at the 95th percentile were similar to levels at the 95th percentile for children in the U.S. representative NHANES 2001-2002 subsample (CDC, 2005). Urinary levels of 3-phenoxybenzoic acid in children were found to be related to residential pesticide

use and house dust levels (Lu et al., 2006; Becker et al., 2006). A small sample of occupationally unexposed Italian residents had median levels of urinary 3-phenoxybenzoic acid that were about fourfold higher than for adults in the NHANES 2001-2002 subsample (CDC, 2005; Saieva et al., 2004). In one study of 145 urban residents in 80 private homes in Germany, urinary 3-phenoxybenzoic acid levels at the 95th percentile were about threefold lower than the levels at the 95th percentile in the 2001-2002 NHANES subsample (Berger-Preiss et al., 2002; CDC, 2005).

In 57 volunteers entering areas previously spot-sprayed with various pyrethroid pesticides, median urinary levels of 3-phenoxybenzoic acid were slightly less than median levels in the NHANES 2001-2002 subsample (Leng et al., 2003; CDC, 2005). Following residential spraying with deltamethrin for malaria protection in Mexico, mean peak urinary levels of 3-phenoxybenzoic acid in children increased at least sixtyfold over non-detectable background levels for several days and mean levels remained slightly above background levels 45 days after the spraying (Ortiz-Perez et al., 2005). The mean peak levels in these children were 83-fold higher than the geometric mean for children in the NHANES 2001-2002 subsample (CDC, 2005). In a small group of indoor pest-control operators, the post-application median urinary levels of 3-phenoxybenzoic acid were 24-fold higher than those for adults in the NHANES 2001-2002 subsample (CDC, 2005; Hardt and Angerer, 2003).

Finding a measurable amount in urine does not mean that the level will result in an adverse health effect. Biomonitoring studies of 3-phenoxybenzoic acid provide physicians and public health officials with reference values so that they can determine whether other people have been exposed to higher levels of pyrethroids than levels found in the general population. Biomonitoring data can also help scientists plan and conduct research on exposure and health effects.

## Urinary 3-Phenoxybenzoic acid
*Metabolite of Cypermethrin, Deltamethrin, and Permethrin*

Geometric mean and selected percentiles of urine concentrations (in µg/L) for the U.S. population from the National Health and Nutrition Examination Survey.

| | Survey years | Geometric mean (95% conf. interval) | 50th | 75th | 90th | 95th | Sample size |
|---|---|---|---|---|---|---|---|
| | | | \[Selected percentiles (95% confidence interval)\] | | | | |
| Total | 99-00 | .292 (.247-.345) | .250 (.190-.320) | .730 (.590-.850) | 1.75 (1.49-2.16) | 4.33 (2.62-6 30) | 1998 |
| | 01-02 | .321 (.276-.374) | .280 (.230-.340) | .700 (.560-.830) | 1.69 (1.41-2 33) | 3.32 (2.52-5 25) | 2539 |
| **Age group** | | | | | | | |
| 6-11 years | 99-00 | .417 (.292-.595) | .320 (.210-.490) | 1.12 (.700-1 60) | 4.18 (2.02-6 54) | 8.63 (3.89-71.1) | 483 |
| | 01-02 | .325 (.260-.406) | .300 (.200-.420) | .760 (.570-1 05) | 1.81 (1.42-2.78) | 3.38 (2.25-4.12) | 580 |
| 12-19 years | 99-00 | .336 (.265-.427) | .290 (.200-.440) | .870 (.620-1 04) | 1.93 (1.49-2 90) | 4.33 (1.83-11.1) | 682 |
| | 01-02 | .353 (.288-.434) | .300 (.250-.390) | .800 (.560-1.13) | 1.86 (1.48-2 35) | 3.45 (2.14-6 69) | 831 |
| 20-59 years | 99-00 | .267 (.227-.314) | .230 (.160-.300) | .640 (.510-.820) | 1.49 (1.25-1.78) | 3.21 (2.04-5.41) | 833 |
| | 01-02 | .314 (.271-.364) | .270 (.220-.340) | .670 (.530-.780) | 1.65 (1.27-2 34) | 3.25 (2.51-6.16) | 1128 |
| **Gender** | | | | | | | |
| Males | 99-00 | .273 (.226-.330) | .250 (.180-.330) | .710 (.570-.820) | 1.49 (1.29-1.73) | 2.41 (1.92-3.79) | 974 |
| | 01-02 | .328 (.277-.387) | .300 (.230-.370) | .680 (.560-.750) | 1.55 (1.26-2 35) | 3.23 (2.56-5.78) | 1193 |
| Females | 99-00 | .311 (.253-.384) | .250 (.190-.340) | .740 (.510-.990) | 2.30 (1.63-3 36) | 6.03 (3.27-11.8) | 1024 |
| | 01-02 | .315 (.266-.373) | .260 (.210-.320) | .740 (.550-.940) | 1.76 (1.48-2 39) | 3.38 (2.34-6.16) | 1346 |
| **Race/ethnicity** | | | | | | | |
| Mexican Americans | 99-00 | .260 (.230-.295) | .230 (.190-.270) | .600 (.430-.750) | 1.35 (1.16-1 53) | 2.18 (1.53-3 26) | 697 |
| | 01-02 | .297 (.238-.369) | .260 (.200-.360) | .650 (.490-.810) | 1.30 (.830-2 26) | 2.71 (1.51-3.44) | 680 |
| Non-Hispanic blacks | 99-00 | .454 (.352-.586) | .450 (.350-.610) | 1.13 (.750-1.46) | 2.32 (1.45-5 35) | 5.35 (2.32-21.1) | 524 |
| | 01-02 | .507 (.428-.601) | .520 (.430-.630) | .960 (.840-1.12) | 2.01 (1.65-2 28) | 3.25 (2.52-4 62) | 701 |
| Non-Hispanic whites | 99-00 | .288 (.233-.355) | .240 (.160-.320) | .710 (.530-.850) | 1.78 (1.41-3 05) | 5.34 (2.62-8.43) | 603 |
| | 01-02 | .298 (.246-.362) | .240 (.190-.320) | .590 (.470-.800) | 1.72 (1.27-2.46) | 3.50 (2.25-7 64) | 957 |

Limit of detection (LOD, see Data Analysis section) for Survey years 99-00 and 01-02 are 0.1 and 0.1.

## Urinary 3-Phenoxybenzoic acid (creatinine corrected)
*Metabolite of Cypermethrin, Deltamethrin, and Permethrin*

Geometric mean and selected percentiles of urine concentrations (in µg/g of creatinine) for the U.S. population from the National Health and Nutrition Examination Survey.

| | Survey years | Geometric mean (95% conf. interval) | Selected percentiles ( 95% confidence interval) | | | | Sample size |
|---|---|---|---|---|---|---|---|
| | | | 50th | 75th | 90th | 95th | |
| **Total** | 99-00 | .261 ( 224-.304) | .250 ( 200-.280) | .550 (.460-.630) | 1.40 (1.13-1.73) | 3.19 (2.16-4.55) | 1998 |
| | 01-02 | .316 ( 274-.365) | .280 ( 240-.330) | .580 (.490-.720) | 1.48 (1.13-1.91) | 3.10 (2.21-4.88) | 2538 |
| **Age group** | | | | | | | |
| 6-11 years | 99-00 | .450 ( 299-.677) | .370 ( 240-.590) | 1.13 (.730-1.62) | 3.96 (1.75-8.07) | 9.91 (2.43-64 0) | 483 |
| | 01-02 | .423 ( 335-.534) | .380 ( 300-.500) | .860 ( 590-1.35) | 2.21 (1.61-2.95) | 3.32 (2.64-5.40) | 580 |
| 12-19 years | 99-00 | .227 (.178-.290) | .210 (.160-.270) | .490 ( 380-.730) | 1.37 (1.03-1.62) | 2.52 (1.41-4.44) | 682 |
| | 01-02 | .274 ( 229-.328) | .240 (.190-.310) | .540 (.420-.730) | 1.11 ( 860-1.63) | 2.35 (1.36-6.19) | 830 |
| 20-59 years | 99-00 | .246 ( 216-.278) | .240 ( 200-.270) | .510 (.400-.590) | 1.11 ( 860-1.49) | 2.53 (1.73-4.09) | 833 |
| | 01-02 | .311 ( 271-.357) | .280 ( 240-.330) | .550 (.440-.670) | 1.44 (1.02-1.91) | 3.22 (1.91-4.92) | 1128 |
| **Gender** | | | | | | | |
| Males | 99-00 | .210 (.173-.253) | .190 (.150-.250) | .510 ( 390-.580) | 1.09 ( 840-1.41) | 1.72 (1.49-2.52) | 974 |
| | 01-02 | .264 ( 226-.309) | .240 ( 200-.280) | .490 (.410-.570) | 1.17 ( 960-1.60) | 2.81 (1.60-4.00) | 1193 |
| Females | 99-00 | .323 ( 270-.387) | .270 ( 240-.330) | .610 (.480-.740) | 1.94 (1.35-3.00) | 5.04 (3.19-6.90) | 1024 |
| | 01-02 | .378 ( 321-.446) | .330 ( 290-.400) | .720 ( 530-.930) | 1.67 (1.25-2.37) | 3.43 (2.25-5.19) | 1345 |
| **Race/ethnicity** | | | | | | | |
| Mexican Americans | 99-00 | .234 ( 202-.272) | .220 (.190-.230) | .480 ( 370-.590) | 1.04 (.700-1.39) | 1.67 (1.06-3.00) | 697 |
| | 01-02 | .275 ( 230-.329) | .240 ( 210-.320) | .510 (.400-.650) | 1.03 (.750-1.67) | 1.83 (1.15-2.74) | 680 |
| Non-Hispanic blacks | 99-00 | .309 ( 238-.401) | .270 ( 220-.350) | .640 (.460-.930) | 1.49 (1.05-3.43) | 3.86 (1.51-7.25) | 524 |
| | 01-02 | .362 ( 300-.437) | .350 ( 280-.410) | .640 ( 530-.760) | 1.36 (1.17-1.83) | 2.84 (1.63-3.80) | 700 |
| Non-Hispanic whites | 99-00 | .272 ( 225-.329) | .250 ( 200-.290) | .550 (.440-.670) | 1.55 (1.09-2.27) | 4.02 (2.07-5.49) | 603 |
| | 01-02 | .312 ( 261-.372) | .280 ( 230-.330) | .560 (.440-.810) | 1.54 (1.09-2.35) | 3.43 (1.88-5.48) | 957 |

# References

Baker SE, Olsson AO, Barr DB. Isotope dilution high-performance liquid chromatography-tandem mass spectrometry method for quantifying urinary metabolites of synthetic pyrethroid insecticides. Arch Environ Contam Toxicol 2004;46(3):281-288.

Becker K, Seiwert M, Angerer J, Kolossa-Gehring M, Hoppe HW, Ball M, et al. GerES IV pilot study: assessment of the exposure of German children to organophosphorus and pyrethroid pesticides. Int J Hyg Environ Health 2006;209(3):221-233.

Berger-Preiss E, Levsen K, Leng G, Idel H, Sugiri D, Ranft U. Indoor pyrethroid exposure in homes with woollen textile floor coverings. Int J Hyg Environ Health 2002;205(6):459-472.

Berkowitz GS, Obel J, Deych E, Lapinski R, Godbold J, Liu Z, et al. Exposure to indoor pesticides during pregnancy in a multiethnic, urban cohort. Environ Health Perspect 2003;111(1):79-84.

Centers for Disease Control and Prevention (CDC). Third National Report on Human Exposure to Environmental Chemicals. Atlanta (GA). 2005.

Hardt J, Angerer J. Biological monitoring of workers after the application of insecticidal pyrethroids. Int Arch Occup Environ Health 2003;76(7):492-498.

Leng G, Ranft U, Sugiri D, Hadnagy W, Berger-Preiss E, Idel H. Pyrethroids used indoors—biological monitoring of exposure to pyrethroids following an indoor pest control operation. Int J Hyg Environ Health 2003;206(2):85-92.

Lu C, Barr DB, Pearson M, Bartell S, Bravo R. A longitudinal approach to assessing urban and suburban children's exposure to pyrethroid pesticides. Environ Health Perspect 2006;114(9):1419-1423.

Ortiz-Perez MD, Torres-Dosal A, Batres LE, Lopez-Guzman OD, Grimaldo M, Carranza C, et al. Environmental health assessment of deltamethrin in a malarious area of Mexico: environmental persistence, toxicokinetics, and genotoxicity in exposed children. Environ Health Perspect 2005;113(6):782-786.

# Antimony
CAS No. 7440-36-0

## General Information

Antimony is found in ores or other minerals, often combined with oxygen to form antimony trioxide or with sulfur to form stibnite. Antimony can exist in one of four valences in its various chemical and physical forms: -3, 0, +3, and +5. It is used in metal alloys, storage batteries, solder, sheet and pipe metal, ammunition, metal bearings, castings, and pewter. It is also used in paints, ceramics, fireworks, enamels, and glass, and as a fire-retardant in textiles and plastics. Stibine is a metal hydride form of antimony used in the semiconductor industry. Two antimony compounds (sodium stibogluconate and antimony potassium tartrate) have been used as antiparasitic medications.

Antimony enters the environment from natural sources and from its use in industry. People are exposed to antimony primarily through food and, to a lesser extent, from air and drinking water. Workplace exposures can occur at smelters, coal-fired plants, and refuse incinerators that process or release antimony. Dermal contact with soil, water, or other substances containing antimony is another means of exposure. The absorption, distribution, and excretion of antimony vary depending on its oxidation state. Urinary excretion appears to be greater for pentavalent antimony

## Urinary Antimony

Geometric mean and selected percentiles of urine concentrations (in μg/L) for the U.S. population from the National Health and Nutrition Examination Survey.

| | Survey years | Geometric mean (95% conf. interval) | 50th | 75th | 90th | 95th | Sample size |
|---|---|---|---|---|---|---|---|
| **Total** | 99-00 | .132 (.120-.145) | .130 (.120-.150) | .220 (.200-.230) | .330 (.300-.350) | .430 (.390-.470) | 2276 |
| | 01-02 | .134 (.126-.142) | .130 (.130-.140) | .190 (.180-.200) | .270 (.250-.310) | .350 (.320-.400) | 2690 |
| | 03-04 | * | .080 (<LOD-.090) | .130 (.120-.150) | .200 (.190-.220) | .280 (.250-.320) | 2558 |
| **Age group** | | | | | | | |
| 6-11 years | 99-00 | .176 (.154-.200) | .190 (.160-.210) | .260 (.230-.280) | .350 (.300-.400) | .440 (.320-.600) | 316 |
| | 01-02 | .146 (.134-.160) | .150 (.130-.160) | .200 (.180-.210) | .270 (.240-.330) | .340 (.280-.440) | 368 |
| | 03-04 | .099 (.087-.114) | .100 (.070-.120) | .160 (.120-.200) | .240 (.190-.310) | .310 (.230-.330) | 290 |
| 12-19 years | 99-00 | .158 (.141-.178) | .170 (.150-.180) | .240 (.210-.270) | .350 (.290-.420) | .460 (.350-.510) | 663 |
| | 01-02 | .169 (.156-.184) | .160 (.150-.180) | .240 (.220-.260) | .350 (.320-.410) | .460 (.400-.500) | 762 |
| | 03-04 | .105 (.095-.115) | .100 (.090-.120) | .150 (.140-.160) | .230 (.200-.270) | .290 (.250-.370) | 725 |
| 20 years and older | 99-00 | .123 (.112-.137) | .120 (.110-.130) | .200 (.180-.220) | .310 (.290-.350) | .430 (.390-.470) | 1297 |
| | 01-02 | .128 (.119-.136) | .130 (.120-.130) | .180 (.170-.190) | .250 (.220-.300) | .330 (.280-.390) | 1560 |
| | 03-04 | * | .070 (<LOD-.080) | .120 (.100-.140) | .190 (.170-.210) | .270 (.220-.320) | 1543 |
| **Gender** | | | | | | | |
| Males | 99-00 | .143 (.131-.157) | .150 (.130-.160) | .240 (.220-.260) | .350 (.330-.390) | .470 (.390-.570) | 1132 |
| | 01-02 | .145 (.136-.154) | .140 (.130-.150) | .200 (.190-.210) | .310 (.280-.330) | .390 (.350-.440) | 1335 |
| | 03-04 | .095 (.088-.103) | .090 (.080-.100) | .140 (.130-.160) | .220 (.200-.250) | .320 (.270-.350) | 1281 |
| Females | 99-00 | .122 (.109-.137) | .120 (.110-.140) | .200 (.180-.220) | .300 (.280-.340) | .400 (.350-.460) | 1144 |
| | 01-02 | .125 (.117-.133) | .120 (.120-.130) | .180 (.160-.190) | .240 (.220-.280) | .320 (.260-.360) | 1355 |
| | 03-04 | * | < LOD | .120 (.090-.140) | .180 (.150-.220) | .230 (.190-.330) | 1277 |
| **Race/ethnicity** | | | | | | | |
| Mexican Americans | 99-00 | .132 (.108-.161) | .140 (.120-.170) | .210 (.180-.240) | .300 (.260-.390) | .430 (.330-.560) | 787 |
| | 01-02 | .142 (.130-.154) | .130 (.130-.150) | .200 (.170-.230) | .260 (.240-.320) | .360 (.300-.400) | 683 |
| | 03-04 | .093 (.079-.110) | .090 (<LOD-.120) | .140 (.120-.160) | .190 (.160-.260) | .270 (.210-.330) | 618 |
| Non-Hispanic blacks | 99-00 | .175 (.148-.207) | .180 (.150-.200) | .260 (.230-.300) | .400 (.310-.490) | .490 (.410-.710) | 554 |
| | 01-02 | .180 (.164-.197) | .170 (.160-.190) | .250 (.220-.280) | .360 (.320-.410) | .460 (.370-.530) | 667 |
| | 03-04 | .108 (.098-.119) | .110 (.100-.120) | .160 (.150-.190) | .230 (.200-.280) | .310 (.250-.360) | 723 |
| Non-Hispanic whites | 99-00 | .128 (.115-.144) | .130 (.110-.140) | .210 (.190-.230) | .330 (.280-.350) | .400 (.360-.500) | 768 |
| | 01-02 | .126 (.117-.135) | .130 (.120-.130) | .180 (.170-.190) | .250 (.230-.300) | .340 (.310-.390) | 1132 |
| | 03-04 | * | .070 (<LOD-.080) | .130 (.110-.140) | .190 (.170-.210) | .280 (.230-.320) | 1074 |

Limit of detection (LOD, see Data Analysis section) for Survey years 99-00, 01-02, and 03-04 are 0 04, 0.04, and 0.07, respectively.
< LOD means less than the limit of detection, which may vary for some chemicals by year and by individual sample.
* Not calculated: proportion of results below limit of detection was too high to provide a valid result.

than for trivalent compounds (Elinder and Friberg, 1986). An elimination half-life of approximately 95 hours has been estimated after occupational exposures (Kentner et al., 1995).

Human health effects from antimony at low environmental doses or at biomonitored levels from low environmental exposures are unknown. Inorganic antimony salts irritate the mucous membranes, skin, and eyes. Acute inhalation of antimony has been associated with irritation of the respiratory tract and impaired pulmonary function (Renes, 1953). Pulmonary edema may occur in severe cases of inhalation exposure (Cordasco et al., 1973). Dysrhythmias and T-wave changes on electrocardiogram have also been

noted after both therapeutic (Berman, 1988; Ming-Hsin et al., 1958) and occupational exposures (Briegner et al., 1954). Histopathologic inflammatory and degenerative changes in the lung, myocardium, liver, and kidney have been demonstrated in high dose animal studies depending on the dose, species, and route of exposure (Elinder and Friberg, 1986). Acute antimony poisoning may cause a metallic taste, and gastrointestinal symptoms such as vomiting, diarrhea, abdominal pain, and ulcers (Werrin, 1962). The toxicity of stibine after acute inhalational exposure is similar to that of arsine, resulting in hemolysis with abdominal and back pain (Dernehl et al., 1944).

Workplace standards and recommendations for air exposure

## Urinary Antimony (creatinine corrected)

Geometric mean and selected percentiles of urine concentrations (in µg/g of creatinine) for the U.S. population from the National Health and Nutrition Examination Survey.

| | Survey years | Geometric mean (95% conf. interval) | Selected percentiles ( 95% confidence interval) 50th | 75th | 90th | 95th | Sample size |
|---|---|---|---|---|---|---|---|
| **Total** | 99-00 | .124 (.108-.143) | .119 (.102-.143) | .185 (.164-.214) | .276 (.233-.333) | .385 (.333-.430) | 2276 |
| | 01-02 | .126 (.119-.134) | .120 (.115-.126) | .173 (.162-.188) | .267 (.242-.300) | .364 (.320-.414) | 2689 |
| | 03-04 | * | .080 (<LOD-.086) | .135 (.119-.143) | .208 (.192-.230) | .277 (.250-.294) | 2558 |
| **Age group** | | | | | | | |
| 6-11 years | 99-00 | .191 (.147-.248) | .185 (.156-.220) | .250 (.200-.417) | .447 (.271-.741) | .741 (.333-1.30) | 316 |
| | 01-02 | .178 (.159-.200) | .173 (.150-.193) | .228 (.200-.272) | .338 (.265-.480) | .471 (.313-.727) | 368 |
| | 03-04 | .116 (.103-.130) | .118 (.098-.136) | .167 (.146-.187) | .256 (.194-.317) | .333 (.250-.500) | 290 |
| 12-19 years | 99-00 | .121 (.104-.140) | .120 (.095-.146) | .176 (.146-.207) | .259 (.206-.310) | .310 (.228-.421) | 663 |
| | 01-02 | .121 (.112-.131) | .115 (.106-.127) | .160 (.138-.186) | .224 (.199-.245) | .266 (.244-.310) | 762 |
| | 03-04 | .075 (.068-.082) | .068 (.061-.077) | .100 (.092-.113) | .156 (.126-.173) | .193 (.172-.255) | 725 |
| 20 years and older | 99-00 | .118 (.104-.135) | .111 (.097-.135) | .175 (.149-.209) | .263 (.227-.320) | .352 (.320-.391) | 1297 |
| | 01-02 | .122 (.115-.129) | .115 (.108-.121) | .167 (.153-.181) | .265 (.241-.300) | .364 (.318-.405) | 1559 |
| | 03-04 | * | .079 (<LOD-.087) | .135 (.116-.145) | .209 (.195-.233) | .278 (.250-.294) | 1543 |
| **Gender** | | | | | | | |
| Males | 99-00 | .112 (.099-.127) | .109 (.095-.127) | .164 (.146-.181) | .226 (.204-.268) | .320 (.235-.391) | 1132 |
| | 01-02 | .114 (.107-.123) | .108 (.103-.115) | .153 (.138-.171) | .228 (.205-.250) | .333 (.281-.438) | 1334 |
| | 03-04 | .080 (.076-.084) | .075 (.069-.081) | .122 (.111-.132) | .192 (.173-.209) | .253 (.230-.278) | 1281 |
| Females | 99-00 | .137 (.117-.161) | .131 (.108-.164) | .213 (.176-.247) | .320 (.263-.417) | .429 (.357-.485) | 1144 |
| | 01-02 | .139 (.131-.148) | .132 (.124-.140) | .196 (.178-.211) | .295 (.267-.317) | .371 (.333-.444) | 1355 |
| | 03-04 | * | < LOD | .143 (.125-.161) | .225 (.188-.261) | .288 (.250-.333) | 1277 |
| **Race/ethnicity** | | | | | | | |
| Mexican Americans | 99-00 | .120 (.107-.135) | .114 (.105-.129) | .167 (.148-.203) | .250 (.209-.315) | .333 (.280-.357) | 787 |
| | 01-02 | .138 (.128-.149) | .130 (.117-.143) | .182 (.159-.203) | .269 (.229-.308) | .338 (.308-.429) | 682 |
| | 03-04 | .086 (.076-.098) | .082 (<LOD-.092) | .129 (.107-.151) | .189 (.154-.238) | .238 (.185-.321) | 618 |
| Non-Hispanic blacks | 99-00 | .114 (.099-.133) | .112 (.098-.130) | .163 (.144-.183) | .236 (.195-.338) | .343 (.255-.425) | 554 |
| | 01-02 | .123 (.113-.134) | .115 (.106-.127) | .163 (.150-.181) | .233 (.208-.267) | .300 (.248-.373) | 667 |
| | 03-04 | .078 (.071-.085) | .074 (.069-.082) | .109 (.096-.124) | .170 (.148-.192) | .222 (.179-.257) | 723 |
| Non-Hispanic whites | 99-00 | .129 (.109-.152) | .125 (.102-.152) | .195 (.167-.225) | .298 (.239-.352) | .400 (.333-.444) | 768 |
| | 01-02 | .127 (.117-.138) | .120 (.113-.130) | .176 (.159-.198) | .280 (.241-.317) | .380 (.318-.471) | 1132 |
| | 03-04 | * | .081 (<LOD-.089) | .139 (.124-.147) | .217 (.200-.238) | .286 (.253-.333) | 1074 |

< LOD means less than the limit of detection for the urine levels not corrected for creatinine.
* Not calculated: proportion of results below limit of detection was too high to provide a valid result.

to antimony have been established by OSHA and ACGIH, respectively, and a drinking water standard has been established by the U.S. EPA. Antimony trioxide is rated by IARC as a possible human carcinogen. Information about external exposure (i.e., environmental levels) and health effects is available from ATSDR at: http://www.atsdr.cdc.gov/toxpro2.html.

## Biomonitoring Information

Levels of urinary antimony reflect recent exposure. Earlier measurements in general populations (Minoia et al., 1990; Paschal et al., 1998) or compiled reference ranges (Hamilton et al., 1994) have reported values slightly higher than those in this *Report,* which may be due to methodologic, population, or exposure differences. Levels of urinary antimony in infants appeared to be similar to those reported by CDC (2005) for young children (Cullen et al., 1998; Dezateux et al., 1997). Urinary antimony was not associated with locally elevated soil levels in a study of more than 200 German residents (Gebel et al., 1998). Several investigations of airborne antimony exposures in workers have found urinary levels that are many times higher than those seen in NHANES 1999-2000, 2001-2002, and 2003-2004, even when exposure levels were below workplace air standards (Bailly et al., 1991; Iavicoli et al., 2002; Kentner et al., 1995; Liao Y-H et al., 2004; Ludersdorf et al., 1987).

Finding a measurable amount of antimony in urine does not mean that the level of antimony causes an adverse health effect. Biomonitoring studies on levels of urinary antimony can provide physicians and public health officials with reference values so that they can determine whether people have been exposed to higher levels of antimony than are found in the general population. Biomonitoring data can also help scientists plan and conduct research on exposure and health effects.

## References

Berman JD. Chemotherapy for leishmaniasis: Biochemical mechanisms, clinical efficacy, and future strategies. Rev Infect Dis 1988;10(3):560-586.

Bailly R, Lauwerys R, Buchet JP, Mahieu P, Konings J. Experimental and human studies on antimony metabolism: their relevance for the biological monitoring of workers exposed to inorganic antimony. Br J Ind Med 1991;48:93-97.

Briegner H, Semisch CW, Stasney J, Piatnek DA. Industrial antimony poisoning. Industrial Medicine and Surgery (Dec.)1954;521-523.

Centers for Disease Control and Prevention (CDC). Third National Report on Human Exposure to Environmental Chemicals. Atlanta (GA). 2005.

Cordasco EM, Stone FD. Pulmonary edema of environmental origin. Chest 1973;64(2):182-185.

Cullen A, Kiberd B, Matthews T, Mayne P, Delves HT, O'Regan M. Antimony in blood and urine of infants. J Clin Pathol 1998;51:238-240.

Dernehl CU, Stead FM, Nau CA. Arsine, stibine, and hydrogen sulfide. Industrial Medicine 1944;13:361-362.

Dezateux C, Delves HT, Stocks J, Wade A, Pilgrim L, Costeloe K. Urinary antimony in infancy. Arch Dis Child 1997;76:432-436.

Elinder CG, Friberg L. Antimony. In: Friberg L, Nordberg GF, Vouk VB, eds. Handbook on the toxicology of metals. 2nd ed. New York: Elsevier; 1986. pp. 26-42.

Gebel TW, Roland H, Suchenwirth R, Bolten C, Dunkelberg, HH. Human biomonitoring of arsenic and antimony in case of an elevated geogenic exposure. Environ Health Perspect 1998;106:33-39.

Hamilton EI, Sabbioni E, Van der Venne MT. Element reference values in tissues from inhabitants of the European community. VI. Review of elements in blood, plasma and urine and a critical evaluation of reference values for the United Kingdom population. Sci Total Environ 1994;158:165-190.

Iavicoli I, Caroli S, Alimonti A, Petrucci F, Carelli G. Biomonitoring of a worker population exposed to low antimony trioxide levels. J Trace Elem Med Biol 2002;16: 33-39.

Kentner M, Leinemann M, Schaller KH, Weltle D, Lenert G. External and internal antimony exposure in starter battery production. Int Arch Occup Environ Health 1995;67:119-123.

Liao Y-H, Yu H-S, Ho C-K, Wu M-T, Yang C-Y, Chen J-R, et al. Biological monitoring of exposures to aluminum, gallium, indium, arsenic, and antimony in optoelectronic industry workers. J Occup Environ Med 2004;46:931-936.

Luedersdorf R, Fuchs A, Mayer P, Skulsukai G, Schacke G. Biological assessment of exposure to antimony and lead in the glass-producing industry. Int Arch Occup Environ Health 1987;59:469-474.

Ming-Hsin H, Shao-Chi C, Ju-Sun P, Kuo-Juie Y, Cheng-Wei L, Chia-Yu H, et al. Mechanism and treatment of cardiac arrhythmias in tartar emetic intoxication. Chin Med J 1958;76(2):103-115.

Minoia C, Sabbioni E, Apostoli P, Pietra R, Pozzoli L, Gallorini M, et al. Trace element reference values in tissues from inhabitants of the European community I. A study of 46 elements in urine, blood, and serum of Italian subjects. Sci Total Environ 1990;95:89-105.

Paschal DC, Ting BG, Morrow JC, Pirkle JL, Jackson RJ, Sampson EJ, et al. Trace metals in urine of United States residents: reference range concentrations. Environ Res 1998;76(1):53-59.

Renes LE. Antimony poisoning in industry. Industrial Hygiene and Occupational Medicine 1953;99-108.

Werrin M. Chemical food poisoning. Quarterly Bulletin of the Association of Food and Drug Officials 1962; 27:38-45.

# Arsenic
CAS No. 7440-38-2

## General Information

Arsenic is an element that is widely distributed in the earth's surface in small amounts. In nature, it is found in over 200 crystalline or mineral forms, such as arsenopyrite (FeAsS) and realgar (As$_4$S$_4$), or rarely as elemental metalloids (yellow, black, and gray forms). Arsenic can combine with such non-carbon chemicals as sulfur and oxygen to form arsenides, arsenites, and arsenates (oxidation states of -3, +3 and +5), referred to as inorganic arsenic compounds. Arsenic trioxide (As$_2$O$_3$, a trivalent compound known as white arsenic) is a common natural and commercial form that can be released into the air during volcanic action; the smelting of copper, lead, and other metals; and, to a lesser extent, from coal burning. The United States no longer produces arsenic from mining but imports about 22,000 metric tons annually, mostly for use in wood preservation (ATSDR, 2005). Various forms of inorganic arsenic can occur in groundwater from natural sources or as a result of soil application or industrial waste. Arsenic can also combine with organic substances in nature to form such organic arsenic compounds as arsenobetaine, arsenocholine, trimethylarsine oxide, and arsenosugars. Arsine (AsH$_3$) is a reactive, gaseous hydride manufactured in small quantities for use in the semiconductor industry.

Arsenic and its compounds have had many uses in the past and present as medicines, pesticides, alloys, semiconductors, and as homicidal poisons. Before the 20th century, arsenic compounds, particularly arsenic trioxide, were used as treatments for syphilis, psoriasis, cancers, mental disorders, and as a cosmetic to lighten complexion. Various arsenic compounds were used in paint pigments and for tanning animal hides. In the last century, lead hydrogen arsenate, copper arsenates, sodium arsenite, cacodylic acid, and monosodium methyl arsenate were used as pesticides but contemporary uses are restricted. Roxarsone and other organic arsenicals are anticoccidial agents added to poultry feed. Since the 1940s, chromated copper arsenate (CCA) has been used to treat outdoor timbers and pressure-treated woods to prevent wood rot. Although it is still widely used in the United States, CCA-treated wood has been restricted since 2003 and no longer can be used in residential applications such as decks, retaining walls, and play sets. Arsenic trioxide is approved to treat acute promyelocytic leukemia. Gallium, aluminum, and indium arsenides are used in the semiconductor industry. Also, arsenic as elemental metalloids may be used in some ammunition, solders, as alloy in metal bearings, and in lead-acid storage battery grids.

General population exposure to inorganic arsenic can occur through consumption of drinking water and, to a lesser extent, meats, grain, and produce. Arsenic is measurable in most soils, ocean and fresh waters, and foods. Water sources contain mostly inorganic arsenate, though in some locations arsenite may be prevalent (WHO, 2001). Groundwater

## Urinary Total Arsenic

Geometric mean and selected percentiles of urine concentrations (in µg/L) for the U.S. population from the National Health and Nutrition Examination Survey.

| | Survey years | Geometric mean (95% conf. interval) | Selected percentiles (95% confidence interval) | | | | Sample size |
|---|---|---|---|---|---|---|---|
| | | | 50th | 75th | 90th | 95th | |
| Total | 03-04 | 8.30 (7.19-9.57) | 7.70 (6.90-8.90) | 16.0 (14.1-18.7) | 37.4 (31.6-43.5) | 65.4 (48.7-83.3) | 2557 |
| **Age group** | | | | | | | |
| 6-11 years | 03-04 | 7.08 (5.66-8.84) | 6.80 (5.90-7.70) | 10.9 (8.90-14.2) | 24.6 (13.8-61.8) | 46.9 (17.5-178) | 290 |
| 12-19 years | 03-04 | 8.55 (7.34-9.97) | 8.10 (6.80-9.40) | 15.2 (12.2-17.8) | 30.5 (23.1-40.4) | 46.1 (32.9-62.5) | 725 |
| 20 years and older | 03-04 | 8.41 (7.25-9.77) | 7.90 (7.00-9.10) | 17.0 (15.0-19.7) | 40.5 (34.9-46.2) | 66.2 (51.2-93.1) | 1542 |
| **Gender** | | | | | | | |
| Males | 03-04 | 9.50 (8.34-10.8) | 8.90 (7.70-9.80) | 17.6 (15.2-20.1) | 41.6 (32.5-52.8) | 65.8 (48.7-95.4) | 1281 |
| Females | 03-04 | 7.30 (6.02-8.84) | 6.90 (5.90-8.30) | 15.0 (11.3-19.5) | 33.4 (26.5-41.7) | 60.5 (40.8-77.1) | 1276 |
| **Race/ethnicity** | | | | | | | |
| Mexican Americans | 03-04 | 9.29 (8.12-10.6) | 9.20 (8.10-10.3) | 16.2 (13.5-19.9) | 34.4 (24.0-60.5) | 68.2 (41.3-111) | 618 |
| Non-Hispanic blacks | 03-04 | 11.6 (9.50-14.1) | 10.4 (7.90-11.8) | 21.5 (14.9-34.4) | 43.5 (36.2-61.8) | 78.0 (43.6-141) | 722 |
| Non-Hispanic whites | 03-04 | 7.12 (6.13-8.27) | 7.00 (6.10-7.90) | 13.7 (11.3-15.8) | 29.0 (22.6-35.9) | 53.1 (38.4-65.6) | 1074 |

Limit of detection (LOD, see Data Analysis section) for Survey year 03-04 is 0.74.

sources of drinking water often have measurable arsenic and several regions of the United States have naturally higher arsenic levels than the U.S. EPA's maximum contaminant level (Hughes, 2006; U.S. EPA, 2001). Extremely high groundwater arsenic levels, as observed in Bangladesh where millions of people have been exposed, have caused clinical arsenic poisoning. Though modest bioconcentration occurs in some aquatic life, arsenic does not show biomagnification in the food chain (WHO, 2001). Children may have additional exposures from ingestion of contaminated soils (e.g., mine tailings), dust, and contact with CCA-preserved wood structures. Smelter workers can have significant inhalational exposures to airborne arsenic trioxide for which air standards have been established. Smoking tobacco is also a source of inorganic arsenic. The semiconductor dopants, gallium arsenide and indium arsenide, are used in enclosed ultraclean operations within the semiconductor industry, so exposure to the general population is extremely limited.

Inorganic arsenic is well absorbed from the gastrointestinal tract and absorbed to a lesser degree through inhalation, but is poorly absorbed dermally (WHO, 2001). After absorption, inorganic arsenic is widely distributed within the body. Arsenate is reduced in the body to arsenite (oxidation state +3), though some reduction may occur in the gut prior to absorption. Arsenite is then oxidatively methylated to the monomethylarsonic acid (MMA) and dimethylarsinic acid (DMA) with subsequent excretion primarily in the urine (NRC, 2001). Inorganic arsenic and

its metabolites have elimination half-lives of approximately 2–4 days (Lauwerys and Hoet, 2001; NRC, 2001). Some studies suggest that variation in the degree of methylation among persons is related to the susceptibility of arsenic-induced disease and may involve consideration of genetic polymorphisms, dose level, age, selenium, and folate status (Chen et al., 2007; Chowdhury et al., 2003; Gamble et al., 2006; Steinmaus et al., 2007; Tseng, 2007; WHO, 2001). Direct exposure to DMA and MMA may result from use of the two pesticides, cacodylic acid and monosodium methyl arsenate.

Fish, shellfish, kelp, and some other seafood can contain organic forms of arsenic including arsenobetaine, arsenocholine, trimethylarsine oxide (TMAO), and arsenosugars. In aquatic organisms, arsenocholine is converted to arsenobetaine and also to small amounts of TMAO (Christakopoulos et al., 1988). TMAO is also formed in the environment from microbiological action and is a metabolite of arsenic in certain mammals. In aquatic sediments, organic arsenic can be converted back to methylated and inorganic arsenic. Ingestion of arsenosugars in kelp and algae can also lead to the excretion of DMA. These organic forms of arsenic from seafood are absorbed and quickly excreted in the urine (WHO, 2001).

Inorganic forms of arsenic demonstrate high acute toxicity, with trivalent inorganic arsenic (arsenite) being more toxic than pentavalent inorganic arsenic (arsenate) (NRC, 2001, WHO, 2001). The reduced form of MMA (oxidation state

## Urinary Total Arsenic (creatinine corrected)

Geometric mean and selected percentiles of urine concentrations (in µg/g of creatinine) for the U.S. population from the National Health and Nutrition Examination Survey.

| | Survey years | Geometric mean (95% conf. interval) | Selected percentiles ( 95% confidence interval) | | | | Sample size |
|---|---|---|---|---|---|---|---|
| | | | 50th | 75th | 90th | 95th | |
| Total | 03-04 | 8.24 (7.07-9.59) | 7.04 (5.93-8.51) | 14.1 (11.6-17.2) | 30.4 (26.0-38.7) | 50.4 (40.3-64.5) | 2557 |
| **Age group** | | | | | | | |
| 6-11 years | 03-04 | 8.25 (6.58-10.3) | 7.18 (5.93-9.45) | 11.7 (9.10-16.3) | 22.2 (12.0-69.5) | 40.1 (14.7-188) | 290 |
| 12-19 years | 03-04 | 6.11 (5.23-7.13) | 5.06 (4.47-6.04) | 9.66 (7.44-11.2) | 17.8 (12.0-26.0) | 27.8 (20.7-35.9) | 725 |
| 20 years and older | 03-04 | 8.64 (7.38-10.1) | 7.47 (6.20-9.01) | 15.4 (12.7-18.8) | 33.8 (27.3-41.2) | 53.9 (45.4-64.5) | 1542 |
| **Gender** | | | | | | | |
| Males | 03-04 | 8.00 (6.81-9.40) | 6.75 (5.66-8.35) | 13.7 (11.0-18.0) | 28.7 (25.1-36.4) | 45.6 (35.3-62.1) | 1281 |
| Females | 03-04 | 8.47 (7.12-10.1) | 7.33 (6.10-8.75) | 14.4 (11.7-17.7) | 32.3 (24.2-46.6) | 58.4 (42.8-75.0) | 1276 |
| **Race/ethnicity** | | | | | | | |
| Mexican Americans | 03-04 | 8.61 (7.33-10.1) | 7.76 (6.30-9.44) | 12.6 (10.2-15.9) | 24.0 (17.7-34.8) | 42.4 (24.8-62.4) | 618 |
| Non-Hispanic blacks | 03-04 | 8.31 (6.99-9.88) | 6.88 (5.66-8.41) | 13.8 (11.5-17.0) | 27.6 (17.9-56.0) | 54.3 (27.5-120) | 722 |
| Non-Hispanic whites | 03-04 | 7.50 (6.25-9.01) | 6.32 (5.28-7.96) | 12.5 (9.86-17.1) | 26.8 (21.8-32.0) | 40.0 (31.3-53.9) | 1074 |

+3) shows greater toxicity than arsenite itself (Aposhian et al., 2000; Bredfeldt et al., 2006; Cohen et al., 2006) and newly discovered thioarsenic metabolites may also be as toxic (Naranmandura et al., 2007; Raml et al., 2007). Arsenic has many actions demonstrated in cellular studies, including inhibition of numerous enzymes, substitution in phosphate metabolism, interference in signal transduction pathways, and altered gene expression. Such actions may lead to decreased energy production, increased oxidative stress, apoptosis, cytotoxicity, and endothelial injury (Kumagai and Sumi, 2007; NRC; 2001). Acutely, arsenite will inhibit cellular pyruvate dehydrogenase by binding to the sulfhydryl groups of dihydrolipoamide, and it also will inhibit succinate dehydrogenase, leading to a decrease in adenosine triphosphate energy production. Cellular glucose uptake, gluconeogenesis, fatty acid oxidation, and production of glutathione may be affected as well. Although arsenate is reduced in the body to arsenite, it may have its own separate toxic action by substituting for phosphate in glycolysis and other pathways, and by uncoupling oxidative phosphorylation (NRC, 2001; WHO, 2001).

Acute toxicity resulting from the ingestion of large amounts of trivalent arsenic (e.g., arsenic trioxide) includes hemorrhagic gastritis with nausea, vomiting, and diarrhea, which can lead to dehydration and shock. Cardiac arrhythmias, hepatotoxicity, renal failure, and peripheral neuropathy may also occur with large doses or after surviving an acute overdose. Chronic human intake of arsenic at less than acutely toxic doses, including drinking water sources with elevated arsenic levels (e.g., Bangladesh, Taiwan, Chile), can cause peripheral sensorimotor neuropathies, peripheral vascular disease, noncirrhotic portal hypertension, hematocytopenias, hyperkeratosis, and hyperpigmentation of the skin (NRC, 2001; WHO, 2001). With chronic exposure, some of these effects may take years to develop. Chronic elevated arsenic intakes have been associated with diabetes, hypertension, and childhood neurodevelopmental effects in observational human studies, but additional or confirmatory research is needed (Kapaj et al., 2006; WHO, 2001). The organic forms of arsenic occurring in seafood have little known toxicity. Acute unintentional inhalation of arsine gas can produce hemolysis of red blood cells.

Chronic arsenic exposure in humans is considered to be a cause of skin, lung, and bladder cancer (IARC, 2004; NRC, 2001). The risk of lung cancer appears more pronounced when large environmental exposures start in childhood (Smith et al., 2006) or when exposure occurs in smokers (Chen et al., 2004). Studies of arsenic at levels typical of U.S. drinking water have not been associated with increased cancer rates (Schoen et al., 2004). Laboratory studies using inorganic arsenic have shown chromosomal aberrations, cell transformations, and DNA repair inhibition (Cohen et al., 2006; U.S.EPA, 1998; WHO, 2001). OSHA and ACGIH have established workplace standards and guidelines for arsenic exposure and monitoring, respectively. The U.S.EPA has established drinking water, food residue, and environmental standards for arsenic and arsenic

## Urinary Arsenic (V) Acid

Geometric mean and selected percentiles of urine concentrations (in µg/L) for the U.S. population from the National Health and Nutrition Examination Survey.

| | Survey years | Geometric mean (95% conf. interval) | Selected percentiles ( 95% confidence interval) | | | | Sample size |
|---|---|---|---|---|---|---|---|
| | | | 50th | 75th | 90th | 95th | |
| **Total** | 03-04 | * | < LOD | < LOD | < LOD | 1.10 (<LOD-1.50) | 2568 |
| **Age group** | | | | | | | |
| 6-11 years | 03-04 | * | < LOD | < LOD | < LOD | 1.10 (<LOD-1.30) | 292 |
| 12-19 years | 03-04 | * | < LOD | < LOD | < LOD | 1.20 (<LOD-1.60) | 728 |
| 20 years and older | 03-04 | * | < LOD | < LOD | < LOD | 1.10 (<LOD-1.50) | 1548 |
| **Gender** | | | | | | | |
| Males | 03-04 | * | < LOD | < LOD | < LOD | 1.20 (<LOD-1.50) | 1284 |
| Females | 03-04 | * | < LOD | < LOD | < LOD | 1.10 (<LOD-1.30) | 1284 |
| **Race/ethnicity** | | | | | | | |
| Mexican Americans | 03-04 | * | < LOD | < LOD | < LOD | 1.20 (<LOD-1.60) | 621 |
| Non-Hispanic blacks | 03-04 | * | < LOD | < LOD | < LOD | 1.20 (<LOD-1.80) | 725 |
| Non-Hispanic whites | 03-04 | * | < LOD | < LOD | < LOD | 1.10 (<LOD-1.50) | 1078 |

Limit of detection (LOD, see Data Analysis section) for Survey year 03-04 is 1.0.
< LOD means less than the limit of detection, which may vary for some chemicals by year and by individual sample.
* Not calculated: proportion of results below limit of detection was too high to provide a valid result.

compounds, and the FDA has established a bottled drinking water standard. IARC and NTP recognize inorganic arsenic and arsenic compounds as human carcinogens. DMA produced bladder cancer in some chronic rat studies (Cohen et al., 2006). In animal studies, arsenic has been fetotoxic and teratogenic, but generally only at maternally toxic doses (WHO, 2001). Additional information about external exposure (i.e., environmental levels) and health effects is available from ATSDR at: http://www.atsdr.cdc.gov/toxpro2.html.

## Biomonitoring Information

Urinary arsenic levels reflect recent exposures and are moderately to highly correlated with arsenic intakes from drinking water and dietary sources (Ahsan et al., 2000; Calderon et al., 1999; Pellizzari and Clayton, 2006; WHO, 2001). Daily variation in creatinine-corrected urinary arsenic is relatively small when intake is constant (Calderon et al., 1999). Urinary arsenic levels were a better predictor for risk of arsenical skin lesions than were arsenic levels in drinking water in Bangladesh (Ahsan et al., 2000). Consequently, urinary arsenic levels have been accepted as a good biomarker of dose (WHO, 2001). Several studies have shown that urinary arsenic levels are not correlated with low levels of arsenic measured in house dust or in washings taken from hands (Hysong et al., 2003; Pellizzari and Clayton, 2006; Shalat et al., 2006), though air levels of arsenic fume and dust are correlated with urinary arsenic levels at higher occupational inhalational exposures

(Jakubowski et al., 1998; Offergelt et al., 1992; Vahter et al., 1986). Though CCA-treated wood contains several thousand times more arsenic than untreated wood, hand washings from children playing on CCA-treated wood compared to children playing on non-CCA-treated wood playground equipment were slightly to fivefold higher (Kwon et al., 2004; Shalat et al., 2006), although urinary arsenic levels were not associated with CCA contact (Shalat et al., 2006).

Levels of total urinary arsenic in the U.S. population in the National Health and Nutrition Examination Survey (NHANES) 2003–2004 were similar to levels reported in the National Human Exposure Assessment Survey (NHEXAS) 1995–1996 for about 80 children residing in the Great Lakes region (Caldwell et al., 2008; Pellizzari and Clayton 2006). In the German Environmental Survey III of 1998, median urinary total arsenic levels in 4052 adults varied with seafood intake, had decreased since the prior 1990–1992 survey, and were about two-fold lower than those for the U.S. population in NHANES 2003–2004 (Schulz et al., 2007; Caldwell et al., 2008). In a Nevada town where groundwater levels were naturally elevated, the median total urinary arsenic in about 200 people was approximately four times higher than that of the U.S. population (Rubin et al., 2007; Caldwell et al., 2008). Compared with this *Report,* higher mean or median total urinary arsenic levels have been reported among people living in specific western areas of North America (Calderon et al., 1999; Josyula et al., 2006; Meza et al., 2004; Valenzuela et al., 2005) and

## Urinary Arsenic (V) Acid (creatinine corrected)

Geometric mean and selected percentiles of urine concentrations (in µg/g of creatinine) for the U.S. population from the National Health and Nutrition Examination Survey.

| | Survey years | Geometric mean (95% conf. interval) | 50th | 75th | 90th | 95th | Sample size |
|---|---|---|---|---|---|---|---|
| **Total** | 03-04 | * | < LOD | < LOD | < LOD | 3.04 (<LOD-3.50) | 2568 |
| **Age group** | | | | | | | |
| 6-11 years | 03-04 | * | < LOD | < LOD | < LOD | 2.80 (<LOD-4.00) | 292 |
| 12-19 years | 03-04 | * | < LOD | < LOD | < LOD | 1.75 (<LOD-2.41) | 728 |
| 20 years and older | 03-04 | * | < LOD | < LOD | < LOD | 3.18 (<LOD-3.70) | 1548 |
| **Gender** | | | | | | | |
| Males | 03-04 | * | < LOD | < LOD | < LOD | 2.61 (<LOD-3.18) | 1284 |
| Females | 03-04 | * | < LOD | < LOD | < LOD | 3.33 (<LOD-3.89) | 1284 |
| **Race/ethnicity** | | | | | | | |
| Mexican Americans | 03-04 | * | < LOD | < LOD | < LOD | 2.69 (<LOD-3.50) | 621 |
| Non-Hispanic blacks | 03-04 | * | < LOD | < LOD | < LOD | 1.75 (<LOD-2.19) | 725 |
| Non-Hispanic whites | 03-04 | * | < LOD | < LOD | < LOD | 3.33 (<LOD-3.95) | 1078 |

< LOD means less than the limit of detection for the urine levels not corrected for creatinine.
* Not calculated: proportion of results below limit of detection was too high to provide a valid result.

other areas of the world (Ahsan et al., 2000; Aposhian et al., 2000; Caceres et al., 2005; Sun et al., 2007) with higher levels of arsenic in the drinking water. Median and mean total urinary arsenic levels for residents in some districts in Bangladesh were reported to be about 50-fold higher than respective levels in the U.S. population (Ahsan et al., 2000; Caldwell et al., 2008; Chowdhury et al., 2003). For residents of Inner Mongolia, China, geometric mean levels were about 70-fold higher than for the U.S. population (Sun et al., 2007). Some noncancer effects of arsenic (e.g., dermal keratosis, vasospasm, and peripheral neuropathy) have been associated with urinary levels as low as 50–100 µg/L in chronically exposed populations (ACGIH, 2001; Blom et al., 1985; Tseng et al., 2005; Valenzuela et al., 2005; WHO, 2001). These associations are stronger at higher urinary levels, and other factors such as nutrition, methylation capacity, and duration of exposure are also considered important.

Total arsenic measured in the urine includes all species of inorganic and organic arsenic. Individually measurable species resulting from inorganic arsenic exposure are arsenate, arsenite, and two methylated metabolic products, DMA and MMA. Measurable organic arsenic species in this *Report* are three biologically generated environmental forms, arsenobetaine, arsenocholine, and TMAO. Arsenate, arsenite, arsenocholine, and TMAO were detected in only 7.6, 4.6, 1.8, and 0.3% of a representative sample of the U.S. population in the NHANES 2003–2004 subsample, respectively, with DMA, MMA, and arsenobetaine being

the main contributors to the total urinary arsenic levels (Caldwell et al., 2008). When seafood intake is avoided, as evidenced by trace or nondetectable levels of arsenobetaine and arsenocholine in the urine, DMA and MMA compose most (about 75%) of the total arsenic species measured in urine. After recent seafood ingestion, arsenobetaine and arsenocholine will greatly increase the level of total urinary arsenic and comprise the highest percentage of the total urinary arsenic level. The higher percentiles of total urinary arsenic levels in the U.S. population showed a higher contribution of arsenobetaine (Caldwell et al., 2008). In most human studies, DMA has been the predominant metabolite composing the majority of measurable inorganic-related arsenic in the urine (i.e., when seafood organic arsenic is subtracted). Levels of DMA and MMA increase in approximate proportion to the intake of inorganic arsenic. In the late 1980s, a control population of 696 Tacoma residents had median urinary DMA levels similar to those for NHANES 2003–2004 (Kalman et al., 1990; Caldwell et al., 2008). Also, in NHEXAS 1995–1996, Great Lakes region residents had median urinary DMA levels that were slightly less than median levels in NHANES 2003-2004 (Caldwell et al., 2008; Pellizzari and Clayton, 2006). In the residents of a Chilean town who consumed water with high levels of arsenic, median levels of urinary DMA were about 40-fold higher than the adult median reported in NHANES 2003–2004, and urinary DMA represented about 67% of the total urinary arsenic (Hopenhayn-Rich et al., 1996; Caldwell et al., 2008). Detectable levels of MMA reported in NHANES 2003–2004 were found only at the upper percentiles and,

## Urinary Arsenobetaine

Geometric mean and selected percentiles of urine concentrations (in µg/L) for the U.S. population from the National Health and Nutrition Examination Survey.

| | Survey years | Geometric mean (95% conf. interval) | 50th | 75th | 90th | 95th | Sample size |
|---|---|---|---|---|---|---|---|
| **Total** | 03-04 | **1.55** (1.31-1.83) | **1.00** (.800-1.40) | **5.20** (4.00-6.50) | **16.8** (12.7-22.3) | **35.0** (27.6-44.6) | 2568 |
| **Age group** | | | | | | | |
| 6-11 years | 03-04 | * | < LOD | **1.80** (.800-4.00) | **8.80** (3.90-29.9) | **29.9** (6.20-190) | 292 |
| 12-19 years | 03-04 | * | **.600** (.400-.800) | **3.20** (2.00-4.70) | **13.9** (7.20-25.1) | **31.8** (17.2-35.8) | 728 |
| 20 years and older | 03-04 | **1.74** (1.48-2.05) | **1.30** (1.00-1.60) | **6.10** (4.90-7.10) | **18.5** (14.0-23.5) | **35.5** (26.8-50.5) | 1548 |
| **Gender** | | | | | | | |
| Males | 03-04 | **1.66** (1.43-1.93) | **1.20** (.900-1.50) | **5.80** (4.40-7.10) | **18.6** (13.9-23.7) | **35.0** (26.8-40.5) | 1284 |
| Females | 03-04 | **1.45** (1.17-1.80) | **.900** (.700-1.40) | **4.70** (3.40-6.20) | **15.6** (11.1-25.3) | **32.7** (21.1-51.3) | 1284 |
| **Race/ethnicity** | | | | | | | |
| Mexican Americans | 03-04 | **1.19** (.871-1.62) | **.800** (.500-1.30) | **3.20** (1.80-5.20) | **10.2** (6.70-21.4) | **31.4** (16.3-39.1) | 621 |
| Non-Hispanic blacks | 03-04 | **2.29** (1.60-3.28) | **2.00** (1.20-3.50) | **7.70** (5.00-12.0) | **23.7** (13.2-38.7) | **45.6** (25.1-94.0) | 725 |
| Non-Hispanic whites | 03-04 | **1.37** (1.11-1.68) | **.800** (.700-1.20) | **4.30** (2.50-6.30) | **13.3** (9.70-21.4) | **29.3** (21.4-35.5) | 1078 |

Limit of detection (LOD, see Data Analysis section) for Survey year 03-04 is 0.4.
< LOD means less than the limit of detection, which may vary for some chemicals by year and by individual sample.
* Not calculated: proportion of results below limit of detection was too high to provide a valid result.

as with DMA, these levels were much lower than those found in other studies where environmental exposures were highly elevated (Chowdhury et al., 2003; Sun et al., 2007).

In recent years, occupational monitoring and research studies have focused on the sum of inorganic-related species (arsenate + arsenite + DMA + MMA) as a measure of inorganic arsenic intake. Studies of small groups of metal and sulfuric acid smelter workers with varying industrial hygiene conditions have reported urinary inorganic arsenic levels (arsenate + arsenite + DMA + MMA) ranging as high as several hundreds of µg/L during or after work exposure (Jakubowski et al., 1998; Offergelt et al., 1992; Vahter et al., 1986; WHO, 2001). Timber treatment workers had median urinary DMA levels that were about 15-fold higher than the general adult median levels reported in NHANES 2003–2004 (Morton et al., 2006; Caldwell et al., 2008). The American Conference of Governmental Industrial Hygienists (ACGIH) provides an occupational biologic effect index (BEI) for urinary inorganic arsenic plus metabolites equal to 35 µg/L (ACGIH, 2001). The 95th percentile of the U.S. population for the sum of inorganic related species was 18.9 µg/L, which is below the ACGIH BEI (Caldwell et al., 2008). Information about the biological exposure indices is provided here for comparison, not to imply a safety level for general population exposure.

Finding a measurable amount of arsenic in urine does not mean that the level of arsenic causes an adverse health effect. Biomonitoring studies of urinary arsenic can provide physicians and public health officials with reference values so that they can determine whether people have been exposed to higher levels of arsenic than are found in the general population. Biomonitoring data can also help scientists plan and conduct research on exposure and health effects.

## Urinary Arsenobetaine (creatinine corrected)

Geometric mean and selected percentiles of urine concentrations (in µg/g of creatinine) for the U.S. population from the National Health and Nutrition Examination Survey.

| | Survey years | Geometric mean (95% conf. interval) | 50th | 75th | 90th | 95th | Sample size |
|---|---|---|---|---|---|---|---|
| Total | 03-04 | 1.54 (1.30-1.82) | 1.16 (.959-1.43) | 5.00 (3.62-6.91) | 16.2 (12.5-20.3) | 29.4 (24.0-36.4) | 2568 |
| Age group | | | | | | | |
| 6-11 years | 03-04 | * | < LOD | 2.00 (1.15-4.83) | 12.2 (4.13-39.7) | 29.6 (6.80-153) | 292 |
| 12-19 years | 03-04 | * | .531 (.400-.638) | 2.14 (1.39-3.51) | 9.29 (4.29-14.7) | 17.3 (10.4-28.7) | 728 |
| 20 years and older | 03-04 | 1.79 (1.51-2.12) | 1.47 (1.15-1.88) | 5.91 (4.32-7.72) | 17.2 (13.4-21.8) | 30.1 (26.1-36.4) | 1548 |
| Gender | | | | | | | |
| Males | 03-04 | 1.40 (1.18-1.67) | 1.11 (.909-1.28) | 4.78 (3.61-6.70) | 14.4 (11.1-18.5) | 26.5 (18.6-29.9) | 1284 |
| Females | 03-04 | 1.68 (1.37-2.05) | 1.25 (.938-1.67) | 5.58 (3.50-7.43) | 17.2 (12.3-24.5) | 32.9 (25.6-46.3) | 1284 |
| Race/ethnicity | | | | | | | |
| Mexican Americans | 03-04 | 1.10 (.786-1.55) | .877 (.612-1.40) | 2.93 (1.78-5.21) | 8.88 (5.50-15.4) | 19.0 (9.64-29.4) | 621 |
| Non-Hispanic blacks | 03-04 | 1.65 (1.19-2.30) | 1.53 (.901-2.45) | 5.81 (4.25-7.82) | 13.6 (9.76-27.9) | 32.9 (13.4-82.1) | 725 |
| Non-Hispanic whites | 03-04 | 1.44 (1.15-1.80) | 1.05 (.833-1.36) | 4.47 (2.73-6.83) | 14.3 (10.9-18.6) | 26.5 (18.6-32.0) | 1078 |

< LOD means less than the limit of detection for the urine levels not corrected for creatinine.
* Not calculated: proportion of results below limit of detection was too high to provide a valid result.

## Urinary Arsenocholine

Geometric mean and selected percentiles of urine concentrations (in µg/L) for the U.S. population from the National Health and Nutrition Examination Survey.

| | Survey years | Geometric mean (95% conf. interval) | Selected percentiles ( 95% confidence interval) | | | | Sample size |
|---|---|---|---|---|---|---|---|
| | | | 50th | 75th | 90th | 95th | |
| **Total** | 03-04 | * | < LOD | < LOD | < LOD | < LOD | 2568 |
| **Age group** | | | | | | | |
| 6-11 years | 03-04 | * | < LOD | < LOD | < LOD | < LOD | 292 |
| 12-19 years | 03-04 | * | < LOD | < LOD | < LOD | < LOD | 728 |
| 20 years and older | 03-04 | * | < LOD | < LOD | < LOD | < LOD | 1548 |
| **Gender** | | | | | | | |
| Males | 03-04 | * | < LOD | < LOD | < LOD | < LOD | 1284 |
| Females | 03-04 | * | < LOD | < LOD | < LOD | < LOD | 1284 |
| **Race/ethnicity** | | | | | | | |
| Mexican Americans | 03-04 | * | < LOD | < LOD | < LOD | < LOD | 621 |
| Non-Hispanic blacks | 03-04 | * | < LOD | < LOD | < LOD | < LOD | 725 |
| Non-Hispanic whites | 03-04 | * | < LOD | < LOD | < LOD | < LOD | 1078 |

Limit of detection (LOD, see Data Analysis section) for Survey year 03-04 is 0.6.
< LOD means less than the limit of detection, which may vary for some chemicals by year and by individual sample.
* Not calculated: proportion of results below limit of detection was too high to provide a valid result.

## Urinary Arsenocholine (creatinine corrected)

Geometric mean and selected percentiles of urine concentrations (in µg/g of creatinine) for the U.S. population from the National Health and Nutrition Examination Survey.

| | Survey years | Geometric mean (95% conf. interval) | Selected percentiles ( 95% confidence interval) | | | | Sample size |
|---|---|---|---|---|---|---|---|
| | | | 50th | 75th | 90th | 95th | |
| **Total** | 03-04 | * | < LOD | < LOD | < LOD | < LOD | 2568 |
| **Age group** | | | | | | | |
| 6-11 years | 03-04 | * | < LOD | < LOD | < LOD | < LOD | 292 |
| 12-19 years | 03-04 | * | < LOD | < LOD | < LOD | < LOD | 728 |
| 20 years and older | 03-04 | * | < LOD | < LOD | < LOD | < LOD | 1548 |
| **Gender** | | | | | | | |
| Males | 03-04 | * | < LOD | < LOD | < LOD | < LOD | 1284 |
| Females | 03-04 | * | < LOD | < LOD | < LOD | < LOD | 1284 |
| **Race/ethnicity** | | | | | | | |
| Mexican Americans | 03-04 | * | < LOD | < LOD | < LOD | < LOD | 621 |
| Non-Hispanic blacks | 03-04 | * | < LOD | < LOD | < LOD | < LOD | 725 |
| Non-Hispanic whites | 03-04 | * | < LOD | < LOD | < LOD | < LOD | 1078 |

< LOD means less than the limit of detection for the urine levels not corrected for creatinine.
* Not calculated: proportion of results below limit of detection was too high to provide a valid result.

## Urinary Arsenous (III) Acid

Geometric mean and selected percentiles of urine concentrations (in µg/L) for the U.S. population from the National Health and Nutrition Examination Survey.

| | Survey years | Geometric mean (95% conf. interval) | Selected percentiles ( 95% confidence interval) | | | | Sample size |
|---|---|---|---|---|---|---|---|
| | | | 50th | 75th | 90th | 95th | |
| Total | 03-04 | * | < LOD | < LOD | < LOD | < LOD | 2568 |
| **Age group** | | | | | | | |
| 6-11 years | 03-04 | * | < LOD | < LOD | < LOD | < LOD | 292 |
| 12-19 years | 03-04 | * | < LOD | < LOD | < LOD | 1.40 (<LOD-1.70) | 728 |
| 20 years and older | 03-04 | * | < LOD | < LOD | < LOD | < LOD | 1548 |
| **Gender** | | | | | | | |
| Males | 03-04 | * | < LOD | < LOD | < LOD | < LOD | 1284 |
| Females | 03-04 | * | < LOD | < LOD | < LOD | < LOD | 1284 |
| **Race/ethnicity** | | | | | | | |
| Mexican Americans | 03-04 | * | < LOD | < LOD | < LOD | 2.00 (<LOD-3.00) | 621 |
| Non-Hispanic blacks | 03-04 | * | < LOD | < LOD | < LOD | 1.20 (<LOD-1.80) | 725 |
| Non-Hispanic whites | 03-04 | * | < LOD | < LOD | < LOD | < LOD | 1078 |

Limit of detection (LOD, see Data Analysis section) for Survey year 03-04 is 1.2.
< LOD means less than the limit of detection, which may vary for some chemicals by year and by individual sample.
* Not calculated: proportion of results below limit of detection was too high to provide a valid result.

## Urinary Arsenous (III) Acid (creatinine corrected)

Geometric mean and selected percentiles of urine concentrations (in µg/g of creatinine) for the U.S. population from the National Health and Nutrition Examination Survey.

| | Survey years | Geometric mean (95% conf. interval) | Selected percentiles ( 95% confidence interval) | | | | Sample size |
|---|---|---|---|---|---|---|---|
| | | | 50th | 75th | 90th | 95th | |
| Total | 03-04 | * | < LOD | < LOD | < LOD | < LOD | 2568 |
| **Age group** | | | | | | | |
| 6-11 years | 03-04 | * | < LOD | < LOD | < LOD | < LOD | 292 |
| 12-19 years | 03-04 | * | < LOD | < LOD | < LOD | 1.95 (<LOD-2.76) | 728 |
| 20 years and older | 03-04 | * | < LOD | < LOD | < LOD | < LOD | 1548 |
| **Gender** | | | | | | | |
| Males | 03-04 | * | < LOD | < LOD | < LOD | < LOD | 1284 |
| Females | 03-04 | * | < LOD | < LOD | < LOD | < LOD | 1284 |
| **Race/ethnicity** | | | | | | | |
| Mexican Americans | 03-04 | * | < LOD | < LOD | < LOD | 3.08 (<LOD-4.44) | 621 |
| Non-Hispanic blacks | 03-04 | * | < LOD | < LOD | < LOD | 2.00 (<LOD-2.29) | 725 |
| Non-Hispanic whites | 03-04 | * | < LOD | < LOD | < LOD | < LOD | 1078 |

< LOD means less than the limit of detection for the urine levels not corrected for creatinine.
* Not calculated: proportion of results below limit of detection was too high to provide a valid result.

## Urinary Dimethylarsinic Acid

*Metabolite of Arsenic*

Geometric mean and selected percentiles of urine concentrations (in µg/L) for the U.S. population from the National Health and Nutrition Examination Survey.

| | Survey years | Geometric mean (95% conf. interval) | Selected percentiles ( 95% confidence interval) | | | | Sample size |
|---|---|---|---|---|---|---|---|
| | | | 50th | 75th | 90th | 95th | |
| **Total** | 03-04 | 3.71 (3.33-4.14) | 3.90 (3.00-4.00) | 6.00 (5.00-7.00) | 11.0 (9.20-12.0) | 16.0 (13.0-17.8) | 2568 |
| **Age group** | | | | | | | |
| 6-11 years | 03-04 | 3.73 (3.12-4.45) | 4.00 (3.00-4.00) | 6.00 (5.00-7.00) | 9.00 (7.00-12.0) | 12.0 (8.00-22.0) | 292 |
| 12-19 years | 03-04 | 3.85 (3.34-4.42) | 4.00 (3.00-4.00) | 6.00 (5.00-7.10) | 9.30 (7.70-12.0) | 13.0 (10.0-16.0) | 728 |
| 20 years and older | 03-04 | 3.69 (3.31-4.11) | 3.70 (3.00-4.00) | 6.00 (5.00-7.00) | 11.0 (10.0-12.0) | 16.0 (13.0-19.0) | 1548 |
| **Gender** | | | | | | | |
| Males | 03-04 | 4.12 (3.60-4.71) | 4.00 (3.70-4.30) | 6.00 (5.60-7.70) | 11.0 (9.00-15.0) | 17.0 (12.1-22.0) | 1284 |
| Females | 03-04 | 3.37 (3.00-3.78) | 3.00 (3.00-4.00) | 5.50 (4.80-6.20) | 10.0 (8.00-11.0) | 14.0 (11.0-17.7) | 1284 |
| **Race/ethnicity** | | | | | | | |
| Mexican Americans | 03-04 | 4.72 (4.27-5.22) | 4.80 (4.00-5.00) | 7.00 (6.00-9.00) | 12.0 (10.0-16.0) | 17.0 (12.0-25.0) | 621 |
| Non-Hispanic blacks | 03-04 | 4.27 (3.71-4.92) | 4.00 (3.50-5.00) | 7.00 (6.00-8.00) | 11.6 (9.00-15.0) | 16.0 (14.0-18.7) | 725 |
| Non-Hispanic whites | 03-04 | 3.27 (2.95-3.62) | 3.00 (3.00-3.80) | 5.00 (4.60-6.00) | 9.00 (7.00-10.0) | 12.0 (9.50-15.0) | 1078 |

Limit of detection (LOD  see Data Analysis section) for Survey year 03-04 is 1.7.

## Urinary Dimethylarsinic Acid (creatinine corrected)

*Metabolite of Arsenic*

Geometric mean and selected percentiles of urine concentrations (in µg/g of creatinine) for the U.S. population from the National Health and Nutrition Examination Survey.

| | Survey years | Geometric mean (95% conf. interval) | Selected percentiles ( 95% confidence interval) | | | | Sample size |
|---|---|---|---|---|---|---|---|
| | | | 50th | 75th | 90th | 95th | |
| **Total** | 03-04 | 3.69 (3 24-4.19) | 3.37 (2 94-3.91) | 5.71 (4.69-6.74) | 9.09 (7.61-11.5) | 13.0 (10.7-16.0) | 2568 |
| **Age group** | | | | | | | |
| 6-11 years | 03-04 | 4.34 (3 57-5.28) | 4.03 (3 20-4.80) | 6.32 (4.65-8.33) | 10.3 (7 00-13.9) | 13.9 (7 86-21.8) | 292 |
| 12-19 years | 03-04 | 2.74 (2 39-3.14) | 2.55 (2 27-2.94) | 3.77 (3.17-4.44) | 5.88 (4.65-6.67) | 7.18 (6.16-11.7) | 728 |
| 20 years and older | 03-04 | 3.79 (3 34-4.31) | 3.48 (3 00-4.00) | 5.95 (4 86-7.05) | 9.45 (8 00-12.0) | 13.5 (11.1-18.6) | 1548 |
| **Gender** | | | | | | | |
| Males | 03-04 | 3.48 (2 95-4.10) | 3.16 (2.70-3.82) | 5.46 (4.17-6.90) | 8.59 (6 92-12.0) | 12.3 (8 84-18.9) | 1284 |
| Females | 03-04 | 3.89 (3.49-4.34) | 3.57 (3.13-4.06) | 5.78 (4 95-6.67) | 9.32 (8 00-11.5) | 13.7 (10.6-18.6) | 1284 |
| **Race/ethnicity** | | | | | | | |
| Mexican Americans | 03-04 | 4.38 (3 80-5.05) | 4.11 (3 29-4.90) | 6.25 (4 84-8.15) | 10.3 (8 00-11.8) | 12.9 (11.1-15.2) | 621 |
| Non-Hispanic blacks | 03-04 | 3.08 (2.69-3.52) | 2.86 (2.60-3.24) | 4.34 (3 82-5.05) | 7.81 (5 82-9.45) | 10.4 (7.61-16.9) | 725 |
| Non-Hispanic whites | 03-04 | 3.44 (2 97-3.98) | 3.17 (2 80-3.73) | 5.16 (4 03-6.49) | 8.00 (6 32-10.9) | 11.1 (8 00-15.4) | 1078 |

## Urinary Monomethylarsonic Acid

*Metabolite of Arsenic*

Geometric mean and selected percentiles of urine concentrations (in µg/L) for the U.S. population from the National Health and Nutrition Examination Survey.

| | Survey years | Geometric mean (95% conf. interval) | Selected percentiles ( 95% confidence interval) | | | | Sample size |
|---|---|---|---|---|---|---|---|
| | | | 50th | 75th | 90th | 95th | |
| **Total** | 03-04 | * | < LOD | **1.20** (1.00-1.30) | **1.90** (1.60-2.10) | **2.40** (2.00-2.80) | 2567 |
| **Age group** | | | | | | | |
| 6-11 years | 03-04 | * | < LOD | **1.00** (<LOD-1.40) | **1.80** (1.30-2.60) | **2.30** (1.70-2.90) | 292 |
| 12-19 years | 03-04 | * | < LOD | **1.50** (1.10-1.80) | **2.20** (1.70-3.00) | **2.90** (2.20-3.60) | 728 |
| 20 years and older | 03-04 | * | < LOD | **1.20** (1.00-1.30) | **1.80** (1.50-2.10) | **2.30** (2.00-2.60) | 1547 |
| **Gender** | | | | | | | |
| Males | 03-04 | * | < LOD | **1.30** (1.10-1.60) | **2.00** (1.80-2.40) | **2.60** (2.10-3.00) | 1283 |
| Females | 03-04 | * | < LOD | **1.00** (<LOD-1.20) | **1.60** (1.30-1.90) | **2.10** (1.70-2.60) | 1284 |
| **Race/ethnicity** | | | | | | | |
| Mexican Americans | 03-04 | * | < LOD | **1.50** (1.20-1.90) | **2.20** (1.70-2.80) | **2.80** (2.00-4.40) | 621 |
| Non-Hispanic blacks | 03-04 | * | < LOD | **1.10** (<LOD-1.30) | **1.80** (1.40-2.00) | **2.20** (1.70-2.70) | 725 |
| Non-Hispanic whites | 03-04 | * | < LOD | **1.10** (.900-1.30) | **1.80** (1.40-2.00) | **2.10** (1.80-2.50) | 1077 |

Limit of detection (LOD, see Data Analysis section) for Survey year 03-04 is 0.9.
< LOD means less than the limit of detection, which may vary for some chemicals by year and by individual sample.
* Not calculated: proportion of results below limit of detection was too high to provide a valid result.

## Urinary Monomethylarsonic Acid (creatinine corrected)

*Metabolite of Arsenic*

Geometric mean and selected percentiles of urine concentrations (in µg/g of creatinine) for the U.S. population from the National Health and Nutrition Examination Survey.

| | Survey years | Geometric mean (95% conf. interval) | Selected percentiles ( 95% confidence interval) | | | | Sample size |
|---|---|---|---|---|---|---|---|
| | | | 50th | 75th | 90th | 95th | |
| **Total** | 03-04 | * | < LOD | **1.33** (1.18-1.54) | **2.22** (1.82-2.57) | **2.86** (2.40-3.53) | 2567 |
| **Age group** | | | | | | | |
| 6-11 years | 03-04 | * | < LOD | **1.63** (<LOD-1.81) | **2.31** (1.88-2.50) | **2.52** (2.31-3.07) | 292 |
| 12-19 years | 03-04 | * | < LOD | **1.10** (.853-1.23) | **1.53** (1.30-1.85) | **2.07** (1.71-2.22) | 728 |
| 20 years and older | 03-04 | * | < LOD | **1.36** (1.18-1.58) | **2.28** (1.82-2.79) | **3.00** (2.43-3.53) | 1547 |
| **Gender** | | | | | | | |
| Males | 03-04 | * | < LOD | **1.20** (1.05-1.36) | **1.88** (1.53-2.34) | **2.50** (2.07-3.45) | 1283 |
| Females | 03-04 | * | < LOD | **1.50** (<LOD-1.77) | **2.40** (1.96-2.86) | **3.00** (2.61-3.53) | 1284 |
| **Race/ethnicity** | | | | | | | |
| Mexican Americans | 03-04 | * | < LOD | **1.46** (1.11-1.93) | **2.30** (1.84-3.00) | **3.16** (2.40-3.85) | 621 |
| Non-Hispanic blacks | 03-04 | * | < LOD | **.816** (<LOD-.985) | **1.37** (1.14-1.61) | **1.88** (1.46-2.17) | 725 |
| Non-Hispanic whites | 03-04 | * | < LOD | **1.33** (1.15-1.62) | **2.28** (1.73-2.86) | **2.86** (2.35-3.75) | 1077 |

< LOD means less than the limit of detection for the urine levels not corrected for creatinine.
* Not calculated: proportion of results below limit of detection was too high to provide a valid result.

## Urinary Trimethylarsine oxide

Geometric mean and selected percentiles of urine concentrations (in µg/L) for the U.S. population from the National Health and Nutrition Examination Survey.

| | Survey years | Geometric mean (95% conf. interval) | 50th | Selected percentiles ( 95% confidence interval) 75th | 90th | 95th | Sample size |
|---|---|---|---|---|---|---|---|
| **Total** | 03-04 | * | < LOD | < LOD | < LOD | < LOD | 2568 |
| **Age group** | | | | | | | |
| 6-11 years | 03-04 | * | < LOD | < LOD | < LOD | < LOD | 292 |
| 12-19 years | 03-04 | * | < LOD | < LOD | < LOD | < LOD | 728 |
| 20 years and older | 03-04 | * | < LOD | < LOD | < LOD | < LOD | 1548 |
| **Gender** | | | | | | | |
| Males | 03-04 | * | < LOD | < LOD | < LOD | < LOD | 1284 |
| Females | 03-04 | * | < LOD | < LOD | < LOD | < LOD | 1284 |
| **Race/ethnicity** | | | | | | | |
| Mexican Americans | 03-04 | * | < LOD | < LOD | < LOD | < LOD | 621 |
| Non-Hispanic blacks | 03-04 | * | < LOD | < LOD | < LOD | < LOD | 725 |
| Non-Hispanic whites | 03-04 | * | < LOD | < LOD | < LOD | < LOD | 1078 |

Limit of detection (LOD, see Data Analysis section) for Survey year 03-04 is 1.0.
< LOD means less than the limit of detection, which may vary for some chemicals by year and by individual sample.
* Not calculated: proportion of results below limit of detection was too high to provide a valid result.

## Urinary Trimethylarsine oxide (creatinine corrected)

Geometric mean and selected percentiles of urine concentrations (in µg/g of creatinine) for the U.S. population from the National Health and Nutrition Examination Survey.

| | Survey years | Geometric mean (95% conf. interval) | 50th | Selected percentiles ( 95% confidence interval) 75th | 90th | 95th | Sample size |
|---|---|---|---|---|---|---|---|
| **Total** | 03-04 | * | < LOD | < LOD | < LOD | < LOD | 2568 |
| **Age group** | | | | | | | |
| 6-11 years | 03-04 | * | < LOD | < LOD | < LOD | < LOD | 292 |
| 12-19 years | 03-04 | * | < LOD | < LOD | < LOD | < LOD | 728 |
| 20 years and older | 03-04 | * | < LOD | < LOD | < LOD | < LOD | 1548 |
| **Gender** | | | | | | | |
| Males | 03-04 | * | < LOD | < LOD | < LOD | < LOD | 1284 |
| Females | 03-04 | * | < LOD | < LOD | < LOD | < LOD | 1284 |
| **Race/ethnicity** | | | | | | | |
| Mexican Americans | 03-04 | * | < LOD | < LOD | < LOD | < LOD | 621 |
| Non-Hispanic blacks | 03-04 | * | < LOD | < LOD | < LOD | < LOD | 725 |
| Non-Hispanic whites | 03-04 | * | < LOD | < LOD | < LOD | < LOD | 1078 |

< LOD means less than the limit of detection for the urine levels not corrected for creatinine.
* Not calculated: proportion of results below limit of detection was too high to provide a valid result.

# References

Agency for Toxic Substances and Disease Registry (ATSDR). Toxicological profile for arsenic. September 2005 [online]. Available at: http://www.atsdr.cdc.gov/toxpro2.html. 8/7/08

Ahsan H, Perrin M, Rahman A, Parvez F, Stute M, Zheng Y, et al. Associations between drinking water and urinary arsenic levels and skin lesions in Bangladesh. J Occup Environ Med 2000;42(12):1195-1201.

American Conference of Government Industrial Hygienists (ACGIH). Documentation of biological exposure indices. 7th edition. Cincinnati (OH): ACGIH Worldwide; 2001.

Aposhian HV, Gurzau ES, Le XC, Gurzau A, Healy SM, Lu X, et al. Occurrence of monomethylarsonous acid in urine of humans exposed to inorganic arsenic. Chem Res Toxicol 2000;13(8):693-697.

Blom S, Lagerkvist B, Linderholm H. Arsenic exposure to smelter workers. Clinical and neurophysiological studies. Scand J Work Environ Health 1985;11(4):265-269.

Bredfeldt TG, Jagadish B, Eblin KE, Mash EA, Gandolfi AJ. Monomethylarsonous acid induces transformation of human bladder cells. Toxicol Appl Pharmacol 2006;216(1):69-79.

Caceres DD, Pino P, Montesinos N, Atalah E, Amigo H, Loomis D. Exposure to inorganic arsenic in drinking water and total urinary arsenic concentration in a Chilean population. Environ Res 2005;98(2):151-159.

Calafat AM, Wong LY, Ye X, Reidy JA, Needham LL. Concentrations of the sunscreen agent benzophenone-3 in residents of the United States: National Health and Nutrition Examination Survey 2003-2004. Environ Health Perspect 2008;116(7):893-897.

Calderon RL, Hudgens E, Le XC, Schreinemachers D, Thomas DJ. Excretion of arsenic in urine as a function of exposure to arsenic in drinking water. Environ Health Perspect 1999;107(8):663-667. Chen CL, Hsu LI, Chiou HY, Hsueh YM, Chen SY, Wu MM, et al. Ingested arsenic, cigarette smoking, and lung cancer risk: a follow-up study in arseniasis-endemic areas in Taiwan. JAMA 2004;292(24):2984-2990.

Chen Y, Hall M, Graziano JH, Slavkovich V, van Geen A, Parvez F, et al. A prospective study of blood selenium levels and the risk of arsenic-related premalignant skin lesions. Cancer Epidemiol Biomarkers Prev 2007;16(2):207-213.

Chowdhury UK, Rahman MM, Sengupta MK, Lodh D, Chanda CR, Roy S, et al. Pattern of excretion of arsenic compounds [arsenite, arsenate, MMA(V), DMA(V)] in urine of children compared to adults from an arsenic exposed area in Bangladesh. J Environ Sci Health A Tox Hazard Subst Environ Eng 2003;38(1):87-113.

Christakopoulos A, Norin H, Sandstrom M, Thor H, Moldeus P, Ryhage R. Cellular metabolism of arsenocholine. J Appl Toxicol 1988;8(2):119-127.

Cohen SM, Arnold LL, Eldan M, Lewis AS, Beck BD. Methylated arsenicals: the implications of metabolism and carcinogenicity studies in rodents to human risk assessment. Crit Rev Toxicol 2006;36(2):99-133.

Gamble MV, Liu X, Ahsan H, Pilsner JR, Ilievski V, Slavkovich V, et al. Folate and arsenic metabolism: a double-blind, placebo-controlled folic acid-supplementation trial in Bangladesh. Am J Clin Nutr 2006;84(5):1093-1101.

Hopenhayn-Rich C, Biggs ML, Kalman DA, Moore LE, Smith AH. Arsenic methylation patterns before and after changing from high to lower concentrations of arsenic in drinking water. Environ Health Perspect 1996;104(11):1200-1207.

Hughes MF. Biomarkers of exposure: a case study with inorganic arsenic. Environ Health Perspect 2006;114(11):1790-1796.

Hysong TA, Burgess JL, Cebrian Garcia ME, O'Rourke MK. House dust and inorganic urinary arsenic in two Arizona mining towns. J Expo Anal Environ Epidemiol 2003;13(3):211-218.

International Agency for Research on Cancer (IARC). IARC Monographs on the Evaluation of Carcinogenic Risks to Humans. Volume 84. Some Drinking-water Disinfectants and Contaminants, including Arsenic. Summary of Data Reported and Evaluation. Updated September 2004 [online]. Available at URL: http://monographs.iarc.fr/ENG/Monographs/vol84/volume84.pdf. 8/7/07.

Jakubowski M, Trzcinka-Ochocka M, Razniewska G, Matczak W. Biological monitoring of occupational exposure to arsenic by determining urinary content of inorganic arsenic and its methylated metabolites. Int Arch Occup Environ Health 1998;71 Suppl:S29-32.

Josyula AB, McClellen H, Hysong TA, Kurzius-Spencer M, Poplin GS, Sturup S, et al. Reduction in urinary arsenic with bottled-water intervention. J Health Popul Nutr 2006;24(3):298-304.

Kalman DA, Hughes J, van Belle G, Burbacher T, Bolgiano D, Coble K, et al. The effect of variable environmental arsenic contamination on urinary concentrations of arsenic species. Environ Health Perspect 1990;89:145-151.

Kapaj S, Peterson H, Liber K, Bhattacharya P. Human health effects from chronic arsenic poisoning--a review. J Environ Sci Health A Tox Hazard Subst Environ Eng 2006;41(10):2399-2428.

Kumagai Y, Sumi D. Arsenic: signal transduction, transcription factor, and biotransformation involved in cellular response and toxicity. Annu Rev Pharmacol Toxicol 2007;47:243-262.

Kwon E, Zhang H, Wang Z, Jhangri GS, Lu X, Fok N, et al. Arsenic on the hands of children after playing in playgrounds. Environ Health Perspect 2004;112(14):1375-1380.

Lauwerys RR, Hoet P. Arsenic. In:Industrial Chemical Exposure. Guidelines for Biological Monitoring. 3rd Ed. Boca Raton (FL). Lewis Publishers. 2001. pp.36-37.

Meza MM, Kopplin MJ, Burgess JL, Gandolfi AJ. Arsenic drinking water exposure and urinary excretion among adults in the Yaqui Valley, Sonora, Mexico. Environ Res 2004;96(2):119-126.

Morton J, Mason H. Speciation of arsenic compounds in urine from occupationally unexposed and exposed persons in the U.K. using a routine LC-ICP-MS method. J Anal Toxicol 2006;30(5):293-301.

Naranmandura H, Ibata K, Suzuki KT. Toxicity of dimethylmonothioarsinic acid toward human epidermoid carcinoma A431 cells. Chem Res Toxicol 2007;20(8):1120-1125.

National Research Council (NRC). Arsenic in drinking water-2001 update. Washington (DC) National Academy Press; 2001.

Offergelt JA, Roels H, Buchet JP, Boeckx M, Lauwerys R. Relation between airborne arsenic trioxide and urinary excretion of inorganic arsenic and its methylated metabolites. Br J Ind Med 1992;49(6):387-393.

Pellizzari ED, Clayton CA. Assessing the measurement precision of various arsenic forms and arsenic exposure in the National Human Exposure Assessment Survey (NHEXAS). Environ Health Perspect 2006;114(2):220-227.

Raml R, Rumpler A, Goessler W, Vahter M, Li L, Ochi T, Francesconi KA. Thio-dimethylarsinate is a common metabolite in urine samples from arsenic-exposed women in Bangladesh. Toxicol Appl Pharmacol 2007;222(3):374-380.

Rubin CS, Holmes AK, Belson MG, Jones RL, Flanders WD, Kieszak SM, et al. Investigating childhood leukemia in Churchill County, Nevada. Environ Health Perspect 2007;115(1):151-157.

Schulz C, Conrad A, Becker K, Kolossa-Gehring M, Seiwert M, Seifert B. Twenty years of the German Environmental Survey (GerES): human biomonitoring--temporal and spatial (West Germany/East Germany) differences in population exposure. Int J Hyg Environ Health 2007;210(3-4):271-297.

Shalat SL, Solo-Gabriele HM, Fleming LE, Buckley BT, Black K, Jimenez M, et al. A pilot study of children's exposure to CCA-treated wood from playground equipment. Sci Total Environ 2006;367(1):80-88.

Smith AH, Marshall G, Yuan Y, Ferreccio C, Liaw J, von Ehrenstein

O, et al. Increased mortality from lung cancer and bronchiectasis in young adults after exposure to arsenic in utero and in early childhood. Environ Health Perspect 2006;114(8):1293-1296.

Steinmaus C, Moore LE, Shipp M, Kalman D, Rey OA, Biggs ML, et al. Genetic polymorphisms in MTHFR 677 and 1298, GSTM1 and T1, and metabolism of arsenic. J Toxicol Environ Health A 2007;70(2):159-170.

Sun G, Xu Y, Li X, Jin Y, Li B, Sun X. Urinary arsenic metabolites in children and adults exposed to arsenic in drinking water in Inner Mongolia, China. Environ Health Perspect 2007;115(4):648-652.

Tseng CH, Huang YK, Huang YL, Chung CJ, Yang MH, Chen CJ, et al. Arsenic exposure, urinary arsenic speciation, and peripheral vascular disease in blackfoot disease-hyperendemic villages in Taiwan. Toxicol Appl Pharmacol 2005;206(3):299-308. Erratum in: Toxicol Appl Pharmacol 2006;211(2):175.

Tseng CH. Arsenic methylation, urinary arsenic metabolites and human diseases: current perspective. J Environ Sci Health C Environ Carcinog Ecotoxicol Rev 2007;25(1):1-22.

U.S. Environmental Protection Agency (U.S. EPA). Arsenic in Drinking Water. Fact Sheet: Drinking Water Standard for Arsenic. EPA 815-F-00-015. January 2001 [online]. Available at URL: http://www.epa.gov/safewater/arsenic/regulations_factsheet.html. 8/7/07

U.S. Environmental Protection Agency (U.S. EPA). Integrated Risk Information System. Arsenic, inorganic. 1998 [online]. Available at URL: http://www.epa.gov/iris/subst/0278.htm. 8/7/07.

Vahter M, Friberg L, Rahnster B, Nygren A, Nolinder P. Airborne arsenic and urinary excretion of metabolites of inorganic arsenic among smelter workers. Int Arch Occup Environ Health 1986;57(2):79-91.

Valenzuela OL, Borja-Aburto VH, Garcia-Vargas GG, Cruz-Gonzalez MB, Garcia-Montalvo EA, Calderon-Aranda ES, et al. Urinary trivalent methylated arsenic species in a population chronically exposed to inorganic arsenic. Environ Health Perspect 2005;113(3):250-254.

World Health Organization (WHO). Arsenic and Arsenic Compounds. 2nd ed. Environmental Health Criteria 224. Geneva 2001. Available at URL: http://www.inchem.org/documents/ehc/ehc/ehc224.htm. 8/8/07

# Barium
CAS No. 7440-39-3

## General Information

Elemental barium is a silver-white metal which comprises approximately 0.05% of the earth's crust. In nature, it combines with other chemicals such as sulfur or carbon and oxygen. Some barium salts are freely soluble in water, whereas others are practically insoluble (e.g., barium sulfate and barium carbonate). Barium compounds are used by the oil and gas industries to make drilling muds. Barium compounds are also used commercially in paint, bricks, tiles, glass, rubber, depilatories, fireworks, and ceramics.

Medically, barium sulfate is used as a contrast medium for taking radiographs of the gastrointestinal tract. Barium salts have also been available as rodenticides.

The general population can be exposed to low amounts of barium in air, water, and food. Certain foods, such as brazil nuts, are high in barium (Genter, 2001). Small amounts of barium can be released into the air during mining and other industrial processes. Workers employed by industries that make or use barium compounds can be exposed to barium dust. In single dose animal studies, soluble forms of barium, such as barium chloride, were relatively well absorbed following inhalation (60-80% of a dose) or ingestion (11-32 % of a dose). Ingested soluble barium

## Urinary Barium

Geometric mean and selected percentiles of urine concentrations (in µg/L) for the U.S. population from the National Health and Nutrition Examination Survey.

| | Survey years | Geometric mean (95% conf. interval) | Selected percentiles ( 95% confidence interval) 50th | 75th | 90th | 95th | Sample size |
|---|---|---|---|---|---|---|---|
| **Total** | 99-00 | **1.50** (1.35-1.66) | **1.60** (1.50-1.90) | **3.10** (2.70-3.40) | **5.40** (4.60-6.10) | **6.90** (6.20-8.40) | 2180 |
| | 01-02 | **1.52** (1.41-1.65) | **1.63** (1.50-1.76) | **3.12** (2.77-3.51) | **5.24** (4.73-5.84) | **7.48** (6.54-8.12) | 2690 |
| | 03-04 | **1.49** (1.36-1.64) | **1.51** (1.35-1.72) | **2.91** (2.64-3.28) | **5.36** (4.86-5.71) | **7.54** (6.93-8.63) | 2558 |
| **Age group** | | | | | | | |
| 6-11 years | 99-00 | **2.15** (1.70-2.72) | **2.20** (1.90-2.50) | **4.00** (2.60-6.10) | **6.40** (5.20-8.30) | **8.30** (5.00-76.2) | 297 |
| | 01-02 | **1.80** (1.44-2.26) | **2.09** (1.74-2.49) | **3.63** (2.86-4.39) | **5.37** (4.26-7.38) | **6.88** (5.37-8.49) | 368 |
| | 03-04 | **2.21** (1.81-2.71) | **2.50** (1.81-2.75) | **4.76** (3.80-5.65) | **8.63** (5.59-11.8) | **11.8** (6.87-14.8) | 290 |
| 12-19 years | 99-00 | **1.97** (1.78-2.19) | **2.00** (1.70-2.30) | **3.50** (3.10-4.00) | **5.90** (4.80-7.00) | **9.70** (5.90-13.1) | 621 |
| | 01-02 | **2.03** (1.76-2.34) | **2.27** (1.96-2.53) | **4.11** (3.48-4.72) | **6.73** (5.55-7.87) | **9.02** (7.25-11.4) | 762 |
| | 03-04 | **2.16** (1.93-2.41) | **2.35** (2.06-2.63) | **4.11** (3.48-4.71) | **7.18** (6.00-8.29) | **9.63** (8.15-11.4) | 725 |
| 20 years and older | 99-00 | **1.36** (1.24-1.51) | **1.50** (1.30-1.70) | **2.80** (2.60-3.20) | **5.10** (4.30-5.50) | **6.40** (5.70-8.40) | 1262 |
| | 01-02 | **1.43** (1.32-1.54) | **1.50** (1.39-1.65) | **2.85** (2.55-3.27) | **4.86** (4.53-5.47) | **7.14** (6.08-8.12) | 1560 |
| | 03-04 | **1.34** (1.20-1.50) | **1.39** (1.19-1.56) | **2.54** (2.21-2.91) | **4.61** (3.99-5.30) | **6.61** (5.57-7.43) | 1543 |
| **Gender** | | | | | | | |
| Males | 99-00 | **1.70** (1.54-1.88) | **1.90** (1.80-2.00) | **3.20** (3.00-3.60) | **5.50** (4.20-6.70) | **7.50** (5.90-9.70) | 1083 |
| | 01-02 | **1.64** (1.47-1.82) | **1.80** (1.65-1.98) | **3.15** (2.76-3.73) | **5.52** (4.82-6.35) | **7.87** (6.49-9.32) | 1335 |
| | 03-04 | **1.62** (1.47-1.78) | **1.69** (1.49-1.85) | **3.09** (2.81-3.54) | **5.65** (5.14-6.16) | **8.56** (6.71-9.67) | 1281 |
| Females | 99-00 | **1.33** (1.15-1.53) | **1.50** (1.20-1.60) | **2.80** (2.30-3.30) | **5.20** (4.20-5.90) | **6.80** (5.60-10.4) | 1097 |
| | 01-02 | **1.43** (1.30-1.56) | **1.44** (1.29-1.63) | **3.11** (2.74-3.43) | **4.93** (4.44-5.88) | **7.15** (6.32-7.86) | 1355 |
| | 03-04 | **1.38** (1.24-1.54) | **1.39** (1.18-1.57) | **2.71** (2.41-3.15) | **4.95** (4.29-5.51) | **6.87** (5.65-8.10) | 1277 |
| **Race/ethnicity** | | | | | | | |
| Mexican Americans | 99-00 | **1.35** (1.25-1.46) | **1.40** (1.20-1.50) | **2.60** (2.30-2.90) | **4.50** (4.10-5.30) | **6.30** (5.50-6.80) | 692 |
| | 01-02 | **1.21** (1.06-1.37) | **1.25** (1.11-1.46) | **2.56** (2.04-2.91) | **4.35** (3.65-5.49) | **6.43** (5.21-8.22) | 683 |
| | 03-04 | **1.40** (1.15-1.70) | **1.45** (1.22-1.73) | **2.62** (1.78-3.38) | **4.07** (2.95-6.37) | **6.01** (4.01-7.88) | 618 |
| Non-Hispanic blacks | 99-00 | **1.34** (1.12-1.62) | **1.40** (1.20-1.60) | **2.50** (2.30-2.90) | **5.10** (3.70-6.60) | **7.40** (5.40-13.9) | 540 |
| | 01-02 | **1.30** (1.14-1.48) | **1.42** (1.22-1.62) | **2.61** (2.31-2.82) | **4.30** (3.70-5.18) | **5.99** (4.87-7.26) | 667 |
| | 03-04 | **1.27** (1.17-1.39) | **1.38** (1.26-1.48) | **2.34** (2.05-2.59) | **3.77** (3.35-4.36) | **5.86** (4.76-7.45) | 723 |
| Non-Hispanic whites | 99-00 | **1.56** (1.36-1.80) | **1.80** (1.60-2.00) | **3.30** (2.80-3.70) | **5.50** (4.50-6.30) | **7.50** (6.20-8.80) | 765 |
| | 01-02 | **1.61** (1.46-1.77) | **1.68** (1.54-1.85) | **3.31** (2.87-3.74) | **5.66** (4.94-6.30) | **7.73** (6.61-8.49) | 1132 |
| | 03-04 | **1.56** (1.37-1.78) | **1.61** (1.28-1.92) | **3.12** (2.75-3.70) | **5.57** (5.04-6.43) | **8.08** (6.87-9.53) | 1074 |

Limit of detection (LOD, see Data Analysis section) for Survey years 99-00, 01-02, and 03-04 are 0.12, 0.12, and 0.31, respectively.

was eliminated primarily in feces and to a lesser extent, in urine. Following intravenous injection in animals, about 75 % of a dose of soluble barium was eliminated within 3 days (Reeves, 1986). Insoluble barium salts, such as those used in medical radiographic procedures, are not absorbed when administered.

Human health effects from barium at low environmental doses or at biomonitored levels from low environmental exposures are unknown. The health effects of exposure to barium compounds depend on the dose, chemical form, water solubility, and route of exposure. Toxicity from soluble barium salts is rare, but can occur after intentional or accidental ingestion of barium carbonate in rodenticides

(Genter, 2001). Barium blocks cellular efflux of potassium resulting in profound hypokalemia. Symptoms following acute high dose include perioral paresthesias, vomiting, diarrhea, weakness, paralysis, hypertension, and cardiac dysrhythmias. Chronic accumulation of inhaled barium dust in the lung tissue may cause baritosis, a benign condition that may occur among barite ore miners. Chronic exposures to natural low levels of barium in drinking water have not produced general health effects or evidence of cardiovascular risk (Brenniman and Levy, 1984; Wones et al., 1990). Chronic high doses in animals resulted in kidney damage (McCauley et al., 1985; NTP, 1994; Perry et al., 1989). Barium is not rated for human carcinogenicity.

## Urinary Barium (creatinine corrected)

Geometric mean and selected percentiles of urine concentrations (in µg/g of creatinine) for the U.S. population from the National Health and Nutrition Examination Survey.

| | Survey years | Geometric mean (95% conf. interval) | 50th | 75th | 90th | 95th | Sample size |
|---|---|---|---|---|---|---|---|
| | | | Selected percentiles (95% confidence interval) | | | | |
| **Total** | 99-00 | 1.40 (1 26-1.56) | 1.41 (1 28-1.54) | 2.54 (2 20-2.91) | 4.68 (3 85-5.47) | 6.33 (5.47-8.09) | 2180 |
| | 01-02 | 1.44 (1 31-1.58) | 1.49 (1 35-1.63) | 2.76 (2 51-3.03) | 4.58 (4.15-4.96) | 6.24 (5 28-7.27) | 2689 |
| | 03-04 | 1.48 (1 37-1.60) | 1.41 (1 31-1.58) | 2.68 (2.44-2.89) | 4.92 (4 39-5.45) | 7.10 (6 29-7.77) | 2558 |
| **Age group** | | | | | | | |
| 6-11 years | 99-00 | 2.37 (1.68-3.32) | 2.38 (1 84-2.92) | 4.47 (2 55-6.46) | 10.2 (3.75-22.0) | 11.4 (5.46-22.0) | 297 |
| | 01-02 | 2.20 (1 91-2.52) | 2.41 (2.19-2.83) | 3.91 (3 29-4.51) | 5.01 (4 58-6.00) | 6.71 (5 20-8.47) | 368 |
| | 03-04 | 2.58 (2 22-2.99) | 3.00 (2 35-3.29) | 4.45 (3 57-5.54) | 6.69 (5 59-7.70) | 10.3 (6 53-21.0) | 290 |
| 12-19 years | 99-00 | 1.51 (1 34-1.70) | 1.40 (1 26-1.59) | 2.48 (1 97-3.06) | 4.36 (3 23-5.39) | 7.62 (4 24-11.4) | 621 |
| | 01-02 | 1.45 (1 33-1.59) | 1.56 (1 31-1.77) | 2.89 (2.68-3.12) | 4.52 (3 84-5.20) | 5.55 (4 81-6.10) | 762 |
| | 03-04 | 1.54 (1 36-1.75) | 1.59 (1 39-1.87) | 2.60 (2 24-3.48) | 4.97 (4 34-5.58) | 6.47 (5 38-7.77) | 725 |
| 20 years and older | 99-00 | 1.30 (1.19-1.42) | 1.33 (1 20-1.46) | 2.32 (2 08-2.62) | 4.29 (3.63-4.96) | 5.65 (5 28-6.33) | 1262 |
| | 01-02 | 1.37 (1 24-1.50) | 1.40 (1 24-1.52) | 2.53 (2 23-2.84) | 4.38 (4 02-5.00) | 6.55 (5 00-7.64) | 1559 |
| | 03-04 | 1.38 (1 26-1.50) | 1.32 (1 22-1.41) | 2.39 (2.13-2.70) | 4.39 (3.77-5.16) | 7.00 (5.45-8.50) | 1543 |
| **Gender** | | | | | | | |
| Males | 99-00 | 1.32 (1 22-1.42) | 1.36 (1 23-1.47) | 2.39 (2.11-2.57) | 4.24 (3.48-5.00) | 5.61 (4 39-10.2) | 1083 |
| | 01-02 | 1.30 (1.16-1.45) | 1.34 (1.19-1.50) | 2.46 (2.14-2.83) | 4.51 (3.73-4.96) | 5.42 (4 81-7.51) | 1334 |
| | 03-04 | 1.36 (1 26-1.47) | 1.31 (1.19-1.43) | 2.60 (2 37-2.75) | 4.36 (3 97-4.72) | 6.01 (5.45-6.96) | 1281 |
| Females | 99-00 | 1.49 (1 27-1.74) | 1.48 (1 29-1.68) | 2.65 (2.13-3.46) | 4.91 (3 96-6.38) | 7.36 (5 25-11.3) | 1097 |
| | 01-02 | 1.59 (1.45-1.75) | 1.64 (1.48-1.79) | 2.98 (2.75-3.30) | 4.76 (4 38-5.31) | 6.97 (5 86-7.52) | 1355 |
| | 03-04 | 1.60 (1.45-1.77) | 1.55 (1 35-1.73) | 2.78 (2 34-3.25) | 5.50 (4.43-6.86) | 7.88 (6 28-11.5) | 1277 |
| **Race/ethnicity** | | | | | | | |
| Mexican Americans | 99-00 | 1.21 (1.10-1.33) | 1.18 (1 05-1.38) | 2.39 (2.10-2.59) | 4.00 (3 33-4.80) | 5.31 (4 80-6.51) | 692 |
| | 01-02 | 1.18 (1 03-1.34) | 1.16 (1 00-1.38) | 2.33 (1 90-2.61) | 3.68 (3 29-4.10) | 4.96 (4 24-6.80) | 682 |
| | 03-04 | 1.29 (1 08-1.55) | 1.28 (1 03-1.53) | 2.25 (1.73-2.97) | 3.99 (2.79-5.03) | 4.99 (4 24-6.56) | 618 |
| Non-Hispanic blacks | 99-00 | .881 (.703-1.11) | .905 (.710-1.06) | 1.64 (1 36-2.00) | 3.27 (2 26-4.76) | 4.84 (3 57-10.8) | 540 |
| | 01-02 | .891 (.777-1.02) | .921 (.754-1.11) | 1.64 (1.44-2.03) | 2.86 (2.48-3.37) | 4.02 (3 52-4.68) | 667 |
| | 03-04 | .915 (.832-1.01) | .963 (.880-1.04) | 1.51 (1 39-1.75) | 2.62 (2 29-3.04) | 3.76 (3 22-4.72) | 723 |
| Non-Hispanic whites | 99-00 | 1.56 (1 38-1.77) | 1.55 (1 36-1.74) | 2.72 (2 27-3.24) | 5.00 (3 81-6.02) | 6.60 (5 52-10.2) | 765 |
| | 01-02 | 1.62 (1.49-1.76) | 1.66 (1.49-1.82) | 3.04 (2.76-3.32) | 4.96 (4 55-5.41) | 6.74 (5 57-7.64) | 1132 |
| | 03-04 | 1.64 (1.49-1.82) | 1.60 (1.40-1.76) | 2.88 (2 56-3.26) | 5.38 (4.67-6.28) | 7.57 (6.69-9.27) | 1074 |

Workplace standards for external air exposure to various barium salts have been established by OSHA, and a drinking water standard has been established by U.S. EPA. Information about external exposure (i.e., environmental levels) and health effects is available from ATSDR at: http://www.atsdr.cdc.gov/toxpro2.html.

**Biomonitoring Information**

Levels of urinary barium reflect recent exposure. Studies reporting urinary levels of barium in general populations have found values generally similar to those reported in NHANES 1999-2000, 2001-2002, and 2003-2004 (CDC, 2005; Minoia et al., 1990; Paschal et al., 1998). Barium levels determined in clinically submitted specimens were broadly comparable (Komaromy-Hiller et al., 2000) to levels in NHANES 1999-2000 and 2001-2002. Welders of barium-containing electrodes had median urinary levels of barium that were 60 times higher than the median levels in this *Report*; the welders had no obvious adverse clinical effects (Zschiesche et al., 1992). Urinary concentrations in acute poisonings are often hundreds to thousands of times higher than in this *Report*.

Finding a measurable amount of barium in urine does not mean that the level of barium causes an adverse health effect. Biomonitoring studies of levels of barium provide physicians and public health officials with reference values so that they can determine whether people have been exposed to higher levels of barium than are found in the general population. Biomonitoring data can also help scientists plan and conduct research on exposure and health effects.

**References**

Brenniman GR, Levy, PS. Epidemiological study of barium in Illinois drinking water supplies. In: Calabrese EJ, ed. Advances in modern toxicology. Princeton (NJ): Princeton Scientific Publications; 1984. p. 231-249.

Centers for Disease Control and Prevention (CDC). Third National Report on Human Exposure to Environmental Chemicals. Atlanta (GA). 2005.

Genter MB. Magnesium, calcium, strontium, barium, and radium In: Bingham A, Cohressen B, Powell C, eds. Patty's toxicology. 5th ed. New York: John Wiley & Sons, Inc.; 2001. p. 221-252

Komaromy-Hiller G, Ash KO, Costa R, Howerton K. Comparison of representative ranges based on U.S. patient population and literature reference intervals for urinary trace elements. Clin Chim Acta 2000;296(1-2):71-90.

McCauley PT, Douglas BH, Laurie RD, et al., Investigations into the effect of drinking water barium on rats. In: Inorganics in drinking water and cardiovascular disease. Calabrese EJ, ed. Princeton NJ: Princeton Scientific Publications, 1985; pp.197-210.

Minoia C, Sabbioni E, Apostoli P, Pietra R, Pozzoli L, Gallorini M, et al. Trace element reference values in tissues from inhabitants of the European community I. A study of 46 elements in urine, blood, and serum of Italian subjects. Sci Total Environ 1990;95:89-105.

National Toxicology Program (NTP). NTP, technical report on the toxicology and carcinogenesis studies of barium chloride dehydrate (CAS no. 10326-27-9) in F344/N rats and B6C3F1 mice (drinking water studies). 1994; [online]. Available at URL: http://ntp.niehs.nih.gov:8080/cs.html?charset=iso-8859-1&url=http%3A//ntp.niehs.nih.gov/ntp/htdocs/LT_rpts/tr432.pdf&qt=barium+chloride+dehydrate+1994&col=020rpt&n=3&la=en. 4/8/09

Paschal DC, Ting BG, Morrow JC, Pirkle JL, Jackson RJ, Sampson EJ, et al. Trace metals in urine of United States residents: reference range concentrations. Environ Res 1998;76(1):53-59.

Perry HM, Jr, Kopp SJ, Perry EF, et al., Hypertension and associated cardiovascular abnormalities induced by chronic barium feeding. J Toxicol Environ Health. 1989;28(3):373-388.

Reeves AL. Barium. In Friberg L, Nordberg GF, Vouk VB, eds. Handbook on the Toxicology of Metals, Vol 2: Specific Metals., 2nd Ed. New York: Elsevier; 1986. p. 84-94.

Wones RG, Stadler BL, Frohman, LA. Lack of effect of drinking water barium on cardiovascular risk factor. Environ Health Perspect 1990;85:355-359.

Zschiesche W, Schaller KH, Weltle D. Exposure to soluble barium compounds: an interventional study in arc welders. Int Arch Occup Environ Health 1992;64(1):13-23.

# Beryllium

CAS No. 7440-41-7

## General Information

Pure beryllium is a hard gray metal, the lightest of all metals, and can be found in mineral rocks, coal, soil, and volcanic dust. Beryllium compounds are commercially mined, and refined beryllium is used in mirrors and special metal alloys for the automobile, computer, nuclear, electrical, aircraft, and machine-parts industries. Beryllium is also used in the production of sports equipment such as golf clubs and bike frames. In medicine, beryllium is used in instruments, x-ray machines, and dental bridges. Burning coal and oil

can produce small amounts of beryllium dust that can be released into the air.

Exposure to beryllium occurs mostly in the workplace, near some hazardous waste sites, and from breathing tobacco smoke. Two types of minerals, bertrandite and beryl, are mined for commercial recovery of beryllium. Low-level beryllium exposure in the general population can occur through breathing air, eating food, or drinking water containing the metal. In studies of laboratory animals, inhaled insoluble beryllium sulfate was retained in the lungs and nearby lymph nodes; less than one percent of the inhaled dose was slowly absorbed into the blood and eventually incorporated into the skeleton. A half-life of 450

## Urinary Beryllium

Geometric mean and selected percentiles of urine concentrations (in µg/L) for the U.S. population from the National Health and Nutrition Examination Survey.

| | Survey years | Geometric mean (95% conf. interval) | 50th | 75th | 90th | 95th | Sample size |
|---|---|---|---|---|---|---|---|
| | | | \multicolumn{4}{c|}{Selected percentiles ( 95% confidence interval)} | |
| **Total** | 99-00 | * | < LOD | < LOD | < LOD | < LOD | 2465 |
| | 01-02 | * | < LOD | < LOD | < LOD | < LOD | 2690 |
| | 03-04 | * | < LOD | < LOD | < LOD | < LOD | 2558 |
| **Age group** | | | | | | | |
| 6-11 years | 99-00 | * | < LOD | < LOD | < LOD | < LOD | 340 |
| | 01-02 | * | < LOD | < LOD | < LOD | < LOD | 368 |
| | 03-04 | * | < LOD | < LOD | < LOD | < LOD | 290 |
| 12-19 years | 99-00 | * | < LOD | < LOD | < LOD | < LOD | 719 |
| | 01-02 | * | < LOD | < LOD | < LOD | .140 (<LOD-.170) | 762 |
| | 03-04 | * | < LOD | < LOD | < LOD | < LOD | 725 |
| 20 years and older | 99-00 | * | < LOD | < LOD | < LOD | < LOD | 1406 |
| | 01-02 | * | < LOD | < LOD | < LOD | < LOD | 1560 |
| | 03-04 | * | < LOD | < LOD | < LOD | < LOD | 1543 |
| **Gender** | | | | | | | |
| Males | 99-00 | * | < LOD | < LOD | < LOD | < LOD | 1227 |
| | 01-02 | * | < LOD | < LOD | < LOD | .130 (<LOD-.150) | 1335 |
| | 03-04 | * | < LOD | < LOD | < LOD | < LOD | 1281 |
| Females | 99-00 | * | < LOD | < LOD | < LOD | < LOD | 1238 |
| | 01-02 | * | < LOD | < LOD | < LOD | < LOD | 1355 |
| | 03-04 | * | < LOD | < LOD | < LOD | < LOD | 1277 |
| **Race/ethnicity** | | | | | | | |
| Mexican Americans | 99-00 | * | < LOD | < LOD | < LOD | < LOD | 884 |
| | 01-02 | * | < LOD | < LOD | < LOD | .130 (<LOD-.160) | 683 |
| | 03-04 | * | < LOD | < LOD | < LOD | < LOD | 618 |
| Non-Hispanic blacks | 99-00 | * | < LOD | < LOD | < LOD | < LOD | 568 |
| | 01-02 | * | < LOD | < LOD | < LOD | < LOD | 667 |
| | 03-04 | * | < LOD | < LOD | < LOD | < LOD | 723 |
| Non-Hispanic whites | 99-00 | * | < LOD | < LOD | < LOD | < LOD | 822 |
| | 01-02 | * | < LOD | < LOD | < LOD | < LOD | 1132 |
| | 03-04 | * | < LOD | < LOD | < LOD | < LOD | 1074 |

Limit of detection (LOD, see Data Analysis section) for Survey years 99-00, 01-02, and 03-04 are 0.13, 0.13, and 0.13, respectively.
< LOD means less than the limit of detection, which may vary for some chemicals by year and by individual sample.
* Not calculated: proportion of results below limit of detection was too high to provide a valid result.

days has been calculated for beryllium elimination from the human skeleton (IPCS, 1990).

Human health effects from beryllium at low environmental doses or at biomonitored levels from low environmental exposures are unknown. The effects of occupational exposure to beryllium depend on the concentration of beryllium in the inhaled air and the duration of air exposure. Air levels greater than 100 µg/m3 can result in erythema and edema of the lung mucosa, which produces pneumonitis. Chronic beryllium disease, or berylliosis, is a granulomatous interstitial lung disease that is caused by chronic beryllium inhalation and the resultant immunologic response. Genetic factors modify individual sensitivity

to beryllium and susceptibility to developing chronic beryllium disease (McCanlies et al., 2003; Maier, 2002). Skin exposure can result in delayed hypersensitivity reactions, including contact dermatitis and subcutaneous nodules.

Workplace air standards and guidelines for external exposure have been established by OSHA and ACGIH, respectively; and drinking water and environmental standards have been established by U. S. EPA. IARC has classified beryllium as a human carcinogen, based upon excess lung and central nervous system cancers in studies of workers. NTP considers beryllium to be a known human carcinogen. More information about external exposure

## Urinary Beryllium (creatinine corrected)

Geometric mean and selected percentiles of urine concentrations (in µg/g of creatinine) for the U.S. population from the National Health and Nutrition Examination Survey.

| | Survey years | Geometric mean (95% conf. interval) | Selected percentiles ( 95% confidence interval) | | | | Sample size |
|---|---|---|---|---|---|---|---|
| | | | 50th | 75th | 90th | 95th | |
| **Total** | 99-00 | * | < LOD | < LOD | < LOD | < LOD | 2465 |
| | 01-02 | * | < LOD | < LOD | < LOD | < LOD | 2689 |
| | 03-04 | * | < LOD | < LOD | < LOD | < LOD | 2558 |
| **Age group** | | | | | | | |
| 6-11 years | 99-00 | * | < LOD | < LOD | < LOD | < LOD | 340 |
| | 01-02 | * | < LOD | < LOD | < LOD | < LOD | 368 |
| | 03-04 | * | < LOD | < LOD | < LOD | < LOD | 290 |
| 12-19 years | 99-00 | * | < LOD | < LOD | < LOD | < LOD | 719 |
| | 01-02 | * | < LOD | < LOD | < LOD | **.231** (<LOD-.273) | 762 |
| | 03-04 | * | < LOD | < LOD | < LOD | < LOD | 725 |
| 20 years and older | 99-00 | * | < LOD | < LOD | < LOD | < LOD | 1406 |
| | 01-02 | * | < LOD | < LOD | < LOD | < LOD | 1559 |
| | 03-04 | * | < LOD | < LOD | < LOD | < LOD | 1543 |
| **Gender** | | | | | | | |
| Males | 99-00 | * | < LOD | < LOD | < LOD | < LOD | 1227 |
| | 01-02 | * | < LOD | < LOD | < LOD | **.281** (<LOD-.333) | 1334 |
| | 03-04 | * | < LOD | < LOD | < LOD | < LOD | 1281 |
| Females | 99-00 | * | < LOD | < LOD | < LOD | < LOD | 1238 |
| | 01-02 | * | < LOD | < LOD | < LOD | < LOD | 1355 |
| | 03-04 | * | < LOD | < LOD | < LOD | < LOD | 1277 |
| **Race/ethnicity** | | | | | | | |
| Mexican Americans | 99-00 | * | < LOD | < LOD | < LOD | < LOD | 884 |
| | 01-02 | * | < LOD | < LOD | < LOD | **.346** (<LOD-.391) | 682 |
| | 03-04 | * | < LOD | < LOD | < LOD | < LOD | 618 |
| Non-Hispanic blacks | 99-00 | * | < LOD | < LOD | < LOD | < LOD | 568 |
| | 01-02 | * | < LOD | < LOD | < LOD | < LOD | 667 |
| | 03-04 | * | < LOD | < LOD | < LOD | < LOD | 723 |
| Non-Hispanic whites | 99-00 | * | < LOD | < LOD | < LOD | < LOD | 822 |
| | 01-02 | * | < LOD | < LOD | < LOD | < LOD | 1132 |
| | 03-04 | * | < LOD | < LOD | < LOD | < LOD | 1074 |

< LOD means less than the limit of detection for the urine levels not corrected for creatinine.
* Not calculated: proportion of results below limit of detection was too high to provide a valid result.

(i.e., environmental levels) and health effects is available from ATSDR at: http://www.atsdr.cdc.gov/toxpro2.html.

## Biomonitoring Information

Urinary beryllium levels represent recent and accumulated exposure. Levels of beryllium in urine for the U.S. population were generally undetectable in NHANES 1999-2000, 2001-2002, and 2003-2004. In other studies, urinary levels for general populations have been either undetectable or had different detection limits than in this *Report* (Komaromy-Hiller et al., 2000; Minoia et al., 1990; Paschal et al., 1998). Hamilton et al. (1994) noted that analytical methods used in several general population studies appeared to have limits of detection that were insufficiently low (i.e., less than 0.1 µg/L). Apostoli and Schaller (2001) stated that detection limits in earlier studies were inadequate to estimate non-occupational exposures. They reported urinary beryllium levels ranging from 0.12 to 0.15 µg/L in workers exposed at the recommended threshold limit value (Apostoli and Schaller, 2001). Given these results, which approximate this *Report's* limit of detection, 0.13 µg/L, and the 95th percentile for males in NHANES 2001-2002, and the fact that most NHANES participant levels were undetectable, it is likely that urinary beryllium levels in the U.S. population are lower than levels in workers.

Finding a measurable amount of beryllium in urine does not mean that the level of beryllium causes an adverse health effect. Biomonitoring studies on levels of beryllium provide physicians and public health officials with reference values so that they can determine whether people have been exposed to higher levels of beryllium than are found in the general population. Biomonitoring data can also help scientists plan and conduct research on exposure and health effects.

## References

Apostoli P, Schaller KH. Urinary beryllium--a suitable tool for assessing occupational and environmental beryllium exposure. Int Arch Occup Environ Health 2001;74:162-166.

Centers for Disease Control and Prevention (CDC). Third National Report on Human Exposure to Environmental Chemicals. Atlanta (GA) 2005.

Hamilton EI, Sabbioni E, Van der Venne MT. Element reference values in tissues from inhabitants of the European community. VI. Review of elements in blood, plasma and urine and a critical evaluation of reference values for the United Kingdom population. Sci Total Environ 1994;158:165-190.

International Programme on Chemical Safety (IPCS).

Environmental Health Criteria. 106. Beryllium [online]. 1990. Available at URL: http://www.inchem.org/documents/ehc/ehc/ehc106 htm. 3/27/08

Komaromy-Hiller G, Ash KO, Costa R, Howerton K. Comparison of representative ranges based on U.S. patient population and literature reference intervals for urinary trace elements. Clin Chim Acta 2000;296(1-2):71-90.

Maier L. Genetic and exposure risks for chronic beryllium disease. Clin Chest Med 2002;23:827-839.

McCanlies EC, Kriess K, Andrew M, Weston A. HLA-DPB1 and chronic beryllium disease: a HuGE review. Am J Epidemiol 2003;157:388-398.

Minoia C, Sabbioni E, Apostoli P, Pietra R, Pozzoli L, Gallorini M, et al. Trace element reference values in tissues from inhabitants of the European community I. A study of 46 elements in urine, blood, and serum of Italian subjects. Sci Total Environ 1990;95:89-105.

Paschal DC, Ting BG, Morrow JC, Pirkle JL, Jackson RJ, Sampson EJ, et al. Trace metals in urine of United States residents: reference range concentrations. Environ Res 1998;76(1):53-59.

# Cadmium
CAS No. 7440-43-9

## General Information

Cadmium is a soft, malleable, bluish-white metal that is obtained chiefly as a by-product of processing zinc-containing ores (principally sphalerite, as zinc sulfide) and to a lesser extent, during refining of lead and copper from sulfide ore. The predominant commercial use of cadmium is in battery manufacturing. Other uses include pigment production, coatings and plating, plastic stabilizers, and nonferrous alloys. Since 2001, U.S. cadmium use has declined in response to environmental concerns (http://minerals.usgs.gov/minerals/pubs/commodity/cadmium). Important sources of airborne cadmium in the environment are burning fossil fuels such as coal or oil, and incineration of municipal waste materials. Cadmium also may be emitted into the air from zinc, lead, or copper smelters (U.S. EPA,

## Blood Cadmium

Geometric mean and selected percentiles of blood concentrations (in μg/L) for the U.S. population from the National Health and Nutrition Examination Survey.

| | Survey years | Geometric mean (95% conf. interval) | 50th | 75th | 90th | 95th | Sample size |
|---|---|---|---|---|---|---|---|
| **Total** | 99-00 | .412 (.378-.449) | .400 (.300-.400) | .600 (.500-.700) | 1.00 (1.00-1.10) | 1.40 (1.30-1.40) | 7970 |
| | 01-02 | * | .300 (.300-.400) | .500 (.500-.600) | 1.00 (.900-1.10) | 1.40 (1.20-1.70) | 8945 |
| | 03-04 | .304 (.289-.320) | .300 (.300-.300) | .500 (.500-.600) | 1.10 (1.00-1.20) | 1.60 (1.50-1.60) | 8372 |
| **Age group** | | | | | | | |
| 1-5 years | 99-00 | * | < LOD | .300 (<LOD-.400) | .400 (.300-.400) | .400 (.300-.700) | 723 |
| | 01-02 | * | < LOD | < LOD | < LOD | .300 (.300-.300) | 898 |
| | 03-04 | * | < LOD | < LOD | .200 (.200-.300) | .200 (.200-.400) | 910 |
| 6-11 years | 99-00 | * | < LOD | .300 (<LOD-.400) | .400 (.300-.500) | .500 (.400-.500) | 905 |
| | 01-02 | * | < LOD | < LOD | .300 (.300-.300) | .400 (.400-.400) | 1044 |
| | 03-04 | * | < LOD | .200 (<LOD-.200) | .300 (.200-.300) | .300 (.300-.300) | 856 |
| 12-19 years | 99-00 | .333 (.304-.366) | .300 (.300-.400) | .400 (.400-.500) | .800 (.600-1.00) | 1.10 (.900-1.20) | 2135 |
| | 01-02 | * | < LOD | .300 (.300-.400) | .500 (.400-.700) | .900 (.700-1.20) | 2231 |
| | 03-04 | * | .200 (<LOD-.200) | .300 (.300-.300) | .600 (.500-.700) | .900 (.800-1.10) | 2081 |
| 20 years and older | 99-00 | .468 (.426-.513) | .400 (.400-.500) | .700 (.600-.800) | 1.10 (1.00-1.20) | 1.50 (1.40-1.60) | 4207 |
| | 01-02 | .425 (.400-.452) | .400 (.400-.400) | .600 (.600-.700) | 1.10 (1.00-1.30) | 1.60 (1.40-1.90) | 4772 |
| | 03-04 | .378 (.359-.398) | .400 (.300-.400) | .600 (.600-.700) | 1.20 (1.20-1.30) | 1.80 (1.60-1.90) | 4525 |
| **Gender** | | | | | | | |
| Males | 99-00 | .403 (.368-.441) | .400 (.300-.400) | .600 (.500-.700) | 1.00 (.900-1.10) | 1.40 (1.30-1.50) | 3913 |
| | 01-02 | * | .300 (<LOD-.300) | .500 (.500-.600) | 1.00 (.900-1.10) | 1.50 (1.20-1.80) | 4339 |
| | 03-04 | .283 (.266-.300) | .300 (.200-.300) | .500 (.500-.500) | 1.10 (1.00-1.20) | 1.60 (1.50-1.60) | 4131 |
| Females | 99-00 | .421 (.386-.460) | .400 (.400-.400) | .600 (.500-.700) | 1.00 (1.00-1.10) | 1.30 (1.20-1.40) | 4057 |
| | 01-02 | .382 (.362-.403) | .400 (.300-.400) | .600 (.500-.600) | 1.00 (.900-1.10) | 1.40 (1.20-1.70) | 4606 |
| | 03-04 | .326 (.309-.344) | .300 (.300-.300) | .600 (.500-.600) | 1.10 (1.00-1.20) | 1.60 (1.50-1.70) | 4241 |
| **Race/ethnicity** | | | | | | | |
| Mexican Americans | 99-00 | .395 (.367-.424) | .400 (.400-.400) | .500 (.500-.600) | .800 (.700-1.00) | 1.20 (.900-1.30) | 2742 |
| | 01-02 | * | < LOD | .400 (.400-.500) | .600 (.500-.800) | 1.00 (.700-1.30) | 2268 |
| | 03-04 | .235 (.216-.255) | .200 (.200-.300) | .400 (.300-.400) | .600 (.500-.800) | 1.00 (.800-1.50) | 2085 |
| Non-Hispanic blacks | 99-00 | .393 (.361-.427) | .400 (.300-.400) | .600 (.500-.600) | 1.00 (.900-1.20) | 1.40 (1.20-1.60) | 1842 |
| | 01-02 | * | .300 (<LOD-.300) | .500 (.500-.600) | 1.00 (.900-1.10) | 1.40 (1.20-1.70) | 2219 |
| | 03-04 | .304 (.275-.337) | .300 (.300-.300) | .500 (.400-.600) | 1.00 (.900-1.20) | 1.50 (1.30-1.70) | 2292 |
| Non-Hispanic whites | 99-00 | .420 (.376-.470) | .400 (.300-.500) | .600 (.500-.700) | 1.10 (1.00-1.20) | 1.40 (1.30-1.50) | 2716 |
| | 01-02 | * | .300 (.300-.400) | .600 (.500-.600) | 1.00 (.900-1.20) | 1.50 (1.30-1.80) | 3806 |
| | 03-04 | .313 (.296-.331) | .300 (.300-.300) | .600 (.500-.600) | 1.10 (1.00-1.20) | 1.60 (1.50-1.70) | 3478 |

Limit of detection (LOD, see Data Analysis section) for Survey years 99-00, 01-02, and 03-04 are 0 3, 0.3, and 0.14, respectively.
< LOD means less than the limit of detection, which may vary for some chemicals by year and by individual sample.
* Not calculated: proportion of results below limit of detection was too high to provide a valid result.

2000). Cadmium in soil is absorbed by plants, including many food crops such as cereal grains, wheat, rice, potatoes, and various seeds. To a lesser extent, drinking water is a source for cadmium intake.

Cadmium is absorbed via inhalation and ingestion. Inhalation of cigarette smoke is a predominant source of exposure in smokers, whose body burdens of cadmium can be approximately twice that of nonsmokers. For nonsmokers who are not exposed to cadmium in the workplace, ingestion through food is the largest source of exposure. The gastrointestinal absorption of dietary cadmium is about 5% in adult men and 10% or higher in women (Diamond et al., 2003; Horiguchi et al., 2004a; Kikuchi et al., 2003), however, individual values vary and are affected by factors

such as dietary intake of essential nutrients (iron, calcium, zinc, copper) and protein. Cadmium absorption may be increased with iron deficiency (Berglund et al., 1994), a factor that may contribute to the higher absorption of cadmium by women (Diamond et al., 2003). With chronic exposure, cadmium accumulates in the liver and kidneys where it is bound to metallothionein, an inducible metal binding protein. About one-third to one half of the total body burden accumulates in the kidney tissues (Nordberg and Nordberg, 2001). The estimated half-life of cadmium in the kidney is from one to four decades (ATSDR, 1999; Diamond et al., 2003).

The kidney is a critical target and shows the earliest sign of cadmium toxicity. Renal tubular and glomerular damage,

## Urinary Cadmium

Geometric mean and selected percentiles of urine concentrations (in µg/L) for the U.S. population from the National Health and Nutrition Examination Survey.**

| | Survey years | Geometric mean (95% conf. interval) | Selected percentiles ( 95% confidence interval) 50th | 75th | 90th | 95th | Sample size |
|---|---|---|---|---|---|---|---|
| **Total** | 99-00 | .193 (.169-.220) | .232 ( 214-.249) | .475 (.436-.519) | .858 (.763-.980) | 1.20 (1.06-1.34) | 2257 |
| | 01-02 | .210 (.189-.235) | .230 ( 207-.255) | .458 (.423-.482) | .839 (.753-.919) | 1.20 (1.07-1.28) | 2690 |
| | 03-04 | .211 (.196-.226) | .210 ( 200-.230) | .450 (.400-.500) | .800 (.730-.880) | 1.15 ( 980-1.26) | 2543 |
| **Age group** | | | | | | | |
| 6-11 years | 99-00 | * | .078 ( 061-.101) | .141 (.115-.173) | .219 (.178-.233) | .279 ( 211-.507) | 310 |
| | 01-02 | .061 (<LOD-.081) | .077 ( 067-.092) | .140 (.112-.160) | .219 (.184-.262) | .282 ( 260-.326) | 368 |
| | 03-04 | .077 ( 065-.090) | .080 ( 060-.090) | .120 (.100-.160) | .180 (.160-.310) | .310 (.170-.610) | 287 |
| 12-19 years | 99-00 | .092 (.067-.126) | .128 (.107-.148) | .203 (.183-.232) | .329 ( 272-.372) | .426 ( 366-.596) | 648 |
| | 01-02 | .109 (.087-.136) | .135 (.114-.157) | .210 (.189-.247) | .327 ( 289-.366) | .452 ( 366-.480) | 762 |
| | 03-04 | .121 (.109-.134) | .130 (.110-.150) | .200 (.170-.210) | .300 ( 260-.360) | .390 ( 330-.490) | 724 |
| 20 years and older | 99-00 | .281 ( 253-.313) | .306 ( 261-.339) | .551 ( 510-.623) | .980 ( 836-1.13) | 1.32 (1.13-1.57) | 1299 |
| | 01-02 | .273 (.249-.299) | .280 ( 261-.308) | .545 (.493-.607) | .972 ( 855-1.06) | 1.28 (1.20-1.43) | 1560 |
| | 03-04 | .260 (.238-.284) | .270 ( 240-.300) | .530 (.470-.580) | .890 ( 800-.990) | 1.25 (1.09-1.46) | 1532 |
| **Gender** | | | | | | | |
| Males | 99-00 | .199 (.165-.241) | .227 (.193-.263) | .462 ( 381-.539) | .892 (.748-1.15) | 1.41 ( 980-1.83) | 1121 |
| | 01-02 | .201 (.177-.229) | .223 (.191-.257) | .445 ( 393-.481) | .875 (.741-1.03) | 1.22 (1.12-1.38) | 1335 |
| | 03-04 | .206 (.190-.222) | .210 (.190-.230) | .440 ( 390-.490) | .790 (.700-.870) | 1.01 ( 890-1.25) | 1277 |
| Females | 99-00 | .187 (.153-.229) | .239 ( 220-.255) | .492 (.456-.540) | .818 (.705-.980) | 1.10 (1.01-1.19) | 1136 |
| | 01-02 | .219 (.192-.251) | .234 ( 202-.265) | .466 (.433-.519) | .817 (.733-.886) | 1.17 ( 918-1.36) | 1355 |
| | 03-04 | .216 (.195-.238) | .210 ( 200-.240) | .450 (.400-.530) | .820 (.700-.960) | 1.20 (1.02-1.37) | 1266 |
| **Race/ethnicity** | | | | | | | |
| Mexican Americans | 99-00 | .191 (.157-.233) | .202 (.167-.221) | .447 ( 351-.551) | .813 ( 686-.977) | 1.12 ( 886-1.38) | 780 |
| | 01-02 | .160 (.135-.189) | .181 (.171-.198) | .322 ( 285-.362) | .559 (.430-.733) | .766 ( 633-1.15) | 683 |
| | 03-04 | .175 (.151-.203) | .170 (.150-.210) | .350 ( 290-.430) | .680 ( 520-.820) | 1.04 ( 820-1.20) | 614 |
| Non-Hispanic blacks | 99-00 | .283 ( 208-.387) | .316 ( 243-.412) | .633 (.498-.806) | 1.22 ( 892-1.38) | 1.48 (1.30-1.72) | 546 |
| | 01-02 | .277 ( 229-.336) | .302 ( 257-.354) | .589 (.476-.713) | 1.04 ( 843-1.38) | 1.51 (1.28-1.74) | 667 |
| | 03-04 | .265 ( 237-.295) | .270 ( 220-.320) | .550 (.440-.640) | .960 ( 810-1.17) | 1.52 (1.06-1.82) | 717 |
| Non-Hispanic whites | 99-00 | .175 (.148-.206) | .220 (.194-.246) | .455 ( 388-.510) | .848 (.714-1.01) | 1.17 ( 963-1.47) | 760 |
| | 01-02 | .204 (.179-.231) | .221 (.191-.255) | .445 ( 394-.479) | .817 (.717-.875) | 1.17 ( 989-1.24) | 1132 |
| | 03-04 | .209 (.192-.226) | .200 (.190-.220) | .440 ( 390-.500) | .790 (.700-.860) | 1.13 ( 940-1.26) | 1070 |

Limit of detection (LOD, see Data Analysis section) for Survey years 99-00, 01-02, and 03-04 are 0.06, 0.06, and 0.06, respectively.
* Not calculated: proportion of results below limit of detection was too high to provide a valid result.
**All results are corrected for molybdenum oxide interference in the ICP-MS method.

manifested by irreversible proteinuria and progressive reduction in glomerular filtration rate, can result from high dose chronic exposure, most often a result of occupational exposure (Roels et al., 1999). Most studies of relatively low level environmental exposure to cadmium have demonstrated associations between higher urine or blood cadmium levels and an increased prevalence of various biomarkers of renal tubular effects (Alfven et al., 2002; Jarup et al., 2000; Noonan et al., 2002; Olsson et al., 2002; Staessen et al., 1996, 1999). However, two studies in Japan did not find an association between cadmium in urine and renal biomarkers (Ezaki et al., 2003; Horiguchi et al., 2004b). Whether the markers of renal tubular effects found in populations with low environmental exposure are likely to progress or predict an increased risk for developing clinically evident renal dysfunction is unknown (Hotz et al., 1999).

During the 1950's and 1960's, a condition known as "itai-itai" ("ouch-ouch") affected postmenopausal women living in a cadmium-polluted region of Japan. This condition of painful osteomalacia or osteoporosis was associated with advanced renal tubular damage that led to increased urinary excretion of calcium and phosphorus and decreased hydroxylation of vitamin D metabolites. Kidney dysfunction that led to osteoporosis was associated with very high urine cadmium levels in residents of an area of China where extensive environmental cadmium pollution occurred (Jin et al., 2004). At lower environmental exposures, older adults and postmenopausal women with

## Urinary Cadmium (creatinine corrected)

Geometric mean and selected percentiles of urine concentrations (in µg/g of creatinine) for the U.S. population from the National Health and Nutrition Examination Survey.**

| | Survey years | Geometric mean (95% conf. interval) | Selected percentiles ( 95% confidence interval) | | | | Sample size |
|---|---|---|---|---|---|---|---|
| | | | 50th | 75th | 90th | 95th | |
| Total | 99-00 | .181 (.157-.209) | .219 (.199-.238) | .423 (.391-.446) | .712 (.645-.757) | .941 (.826-1 07) | 2257 |
| | 01-02 | .199 (.181-.218) | .212 (.194-.232) | .404 (.377-.440) | .690 (.630-.754) | .919 (.813-.998) | 2689 |
| | 03-04 | .210 (.201-.219) | .208 (.189-.226) | .412 (.381-.438) | .678 (.650-.716) | .940 (.833-1 04) | 2543 |
| **Age group** | | | | | | | |
| 6-11 years | 99-00 | * | .085 (.063-.107) | .148 (.123-.182) | .210 (.171-.316) | .316 (.184-.607) | 310 |
| | 01-02 | .075 (<LOD- 094) | .100 (.083-.112) | .166 (.136-.192) | .233 (.206-.281) | .318 (.221-.440) | 368 |
| | 03-04 | .090 (.078-.104) | .091 (.075-.104) | .126 (.111-.156) | .200 (.147-.350) | .308 (.178-.415) | 287 |
| 12-19 years | 99-00 | .071 (.051-.098) | .093 (.084-.106) | .147 (.130-.163) | .215 (.204-.240) | .283 (.222-.404) | 648 |
| | 01-02 | .078 (.067-.091) | .091 (.085-.101) | .137 (.123-.143) | .191 (.175-.234) | .280 (.234-.321) | 762 |
| | 03-04 | .086 (.077-.096) | .084 (.074-.097) | .122 (.113-.135) | .176 (.154-.198) | .234 (.187-.274) | 724 |
| 20 years and older | 99-00 | .267 (.247-.289) | .288 (.261-.304) | .484 (.433-.545) | .769 (.727-.818) | 1.07 (.927-1.17) | 1299 |
| | 01-02 | .261 (.236-.289) | .273 (.247-.303) | .481 (.426-.518) | .779 (.691-.850) | .979 (.874-1.12) | 1559 |
| | 03-04 | .268 (.255-.281) | .270 (.247-.292) | .490 (.444-.538) | .767 (.688-.830) | 1.02 (.909-1.14) | 1532 |
| **Gender** | | | | | | | |
| Males | 99-00 | .154 (.131-.182) | .176 (.158-.191) | .329 (.293-.382) | .617 (.537-.700) | .789 (.696-.929) | 1121 |
| | 01-02 | .159 (.143-.177) | .168 (.157-.182) | .335 (.304-.364) | .536 (.491-.653) | .757 (.690-.856) | 1334 |
| | 03-04 | .173 (.161-.187) | .162 (.143-.185) | .325 (.300-.352) | .591 (.560-.631) | .740 (.678-.795) | 1277 |
| Females | 99-00 | .211 (.170-.261) | .267 (.239-.308) | .473 (.423-.551) | .783 (.690-.917) | 1.09 (.813-1 38) | 1136 |
| | 01-02 | .245 (.216-.278) | .263 (.228-.297) | .479 (.414-.541) | .792 (.687-.884) | .985 (.876-1.16) | 1355 |
| | 03-04 | .252 (.238-.266) | .253 (.227-.288) | .487 (.438-.533) | .802 (.716-.906) | 1.06 (.940-1 21) | 1266 |
| **Race/ethnicity** | | | | | | | |
| Mexican Americans | 99-00 | .175 (.137-.223) | .181 (.144-.225) | .331 (.266-.418) | .622 (.441-.828) | .856 (.674-1.13) | 780 |
| | 01-02 | .156 (.136-.178) | .170 (.150-.184) | .282 (.263-.340) | .501 (.388-.614) | .693 (.507-.839) | 682 |
| | 03-04 | .163 (.147-.181) | .159 (.140-.183) | .296 (.256-.311) | .531 (.418-.667) | .718 (.562-.950) | 614 |
| Non-Hispanic blacks | 99-00 | .183 (.140-.240) | .202 (.168-.241) | .414 (.343-.472) | .663 (.516-.827) | .873 (.722-.962) | 546 |
| | 01-02 | .190 (.156-.232) | .196 (.174-.225) | .387 (.336-.449) | .686 (.559-.850) | .917 (.725-1 08) | 667 |
| | 03-04 | .190 (.173-.210) | .185 (.168-.207) | .338 (.288-.431) | .700 (.500-.818) | .865 (.708-1.10) | 717 |
| Non-Hispanic whites | 99-00 | .175 (.146-.209) | .219 (.191-.250) | .432 (.387-.470) | .729 (.666-.783) | 1.00 (.826-1.16) | 760 |
| | 01-02 | .205 (.184-.229) | .224 (.208-.242) | .421 (.382-.470) | .719 (.668-.784) | .931 (.806-1 05) | 1132 |
| | 03-04 | .220 (.207-.235) | .221 (.197-.253) | .434 (.398-.476) | .687 (.647-.767) | 1.00 (.830-1 08) | 1070 |

* Not calculated: proportion of results below limit of detection was too high to provide a valid result.
**All results are corrected for molybdenum oxide interference in the ICP-MS method.

greater urine cadmium levels may have an increased risk for bone fracture and diminished bone mineral density (Alfven et al., 2002; Staessen et al., 1999).

Acute and heavy exposure to airborne dusts and fumes, as may occur from welding cadmium-alloyed metals, has resulted in severe, potentially fatal pneumonitis (Fernandez et al., 1996). Chronic inhalation exposure to cadmium particulates was associated with changes in pulmonary function and chest radiographs that were consistent with emphysema (Davidson et al., 1988). Workplace exposure to airborne cadmium particulates was associated with decreases in olfactory function (Mascagni et al., 2003). Animal studies have demonstrated reproductive and teratogenic effects. Small epidemiologic studies have noted an inverse relationship between cadmium in cord blood, maternal blood or maternal urine and birth weight (Nishijo et al., 2002; Salpietro et al., 2002) and length at birth (Nishijo et al., 2004; Zhang et al., 2004).

Cadmium can produce lung, pituitary gland and kidney tumors in animals and has been associated with lung cancer in humans in occupational epidemiologic studies. Both IARC and NTP consider cadmium a human carcinogen. Waalkes (2003) provides an overview and summarizes potential mechanisms for carcinogenicity. Workplace standards and guidelines for air exposure to cadmium have been established by OSHA and ACGIH, respectively, and drinking water and environmental standards have been established by U.S. EPA. Information about external exposure (i.e., environmental levels) and health effects is available from ATSDR at: http://www.atsdr.cdc.gov/toxpro2.html.

**Biomonitoring Information**

Blood cadmium reflects both recent and cumulative exposures. In the typical environmental exposure, urinary cadmium reflects both cumulative exposure and the concentration of cadmium in the kidney.

Surveys of populations not known to have increased cadmium exposure have reported similar urine and blood levels (Becker et al., 2002; Becker et al., 2003; CDC, 2005; Friedman et al., 2006; Komaromy-Hiller et al., 2000; Wennberg et al., 2006; Wilhelm et al., 2006). Women had higher blood and urine cadmium levels compared to men of similar ages, with peak values observed in the fifth to sixth decades (CDC, 2005; Horiguchi et al., 2004b; Olsson et al., 2002; Wennberg et al., 2006). For NHANES 1999-2000, blood cadmium was also slightly higher in Mexican Americans and participants 20 years and older (CDC, 2005). Blood and urine cadmium levels are typically higher in cigarette smokers, intermediate in former smokers and lower in never-smokers (Becker et al., 2003; Becker et al., 2002; Mannino et al., 2004; Olsson et al., 2002). Blood cadmium levels are about twice as high in smokers compared to nonsmokers (Becker et al., 2003; Becker et al., 2002; Olsson et al., 2002). Several studies of populations residing in areas with higher cadmium soil concentrations or with frank cadmium pollution have reported mean blood and urine cadmium levels considerably higher (as much as 10 times higher) than control groups or representative U.S. data (CDC, 2005; Ezaki et al., 2003; Jarup et al., 2000; Jin et al., 2004; Staessen et al., 1999; Staessen et al., 1996; Suwazono et al., 2000). Creatinine-corrected urine cadmium values in U.S. study subjects living near a former zinc smelter were similar to those from an unexposed community and to those in this *Report* (Noonan et al., 2002).

People who are occupationally exposed may have blood and urine cadmium levels that are higher than those of the general population. The 95th percentiles for cadmium levels in this *Report* were less than the OSHA standards for both blood cadmium (5 µg/L) and urine cadmium (3 µg/gram of creatinine). Occupational standards are provided here for comparison only, not to imply a safety level for general population exposure.

Subtle increases in markers of renal tubular effects have been associated with urine cadmium levels as low as approximately 1 µg/gram of creatinine (Akesson et al., 2005; Ezaki et al., 2003; Jarup et al., 2000; Moriguchi et al., 2004; Noonan et al., 2002). However, two studies of women in Japan with lower exposures found no correlation between renal tubular effect markers and blood or urine cadmium levels (geometric means were 1.26 and 3.46 µg/gram of creatinine) (Ezaki et al., 2003; Horiguchi et al., 2004b). In postmenopausal women, decreased bone density was correlated with mean urinary cadmium levels of approximately 1 µg/gram of creatinine (Staessen et al., 1999). In adults aged 60 years and older, the risk of low bone mineral density increased by nearly three-fold when the blood cadmium exceeded 1.1 µg/L (Alfven et al., 2002). In this *Report* the urinary and blood cadmium levels at the 95th and 90th percentiles, respectively, approached these values associated with subclinical changes in renal function and bone mineral density. Further research is needed to address the public health consequences of such exposure in the United States.

Finding a measurable amount of cadmium in blood or urine does not mean that the levels of cadmium cause an adverse health effect. Biomonitoring studies on levels of cadmium provide physicians and public health officials with reference values so they can determine whether people have been exposed to higher levels of cadmium than are found in the general population. Biomonitoring data can also help scientists plan and conduct research on exposure and health effects.

## References

Akesson A, Lundh T, Vahter M, Bellerup P, Lidfeldt J, Nerbrand C, et al. Tubular and glomerular kidney effects in Swedish women with low environmental cadmium exposure. Environ Health Perspect 2005;13(11):1627-1631.

Agency for Toxic Substances and Disease Registry (ATSDR). Toxicological profile for cadmium update. 1999 [online]. Available at URL: http://www.atsdr.cdc.gov/toxprofiles/tp5.html. 4/8/09

Alfven T, Jarup L, Elinder CG. Cadmium and lead in blood in relation to low bone mineral density and tubular proteinuria. Environ Health Perspect 2002;110:699-702.

Becker K, Kaus S, Krause C, Lepom P, Schulz C, Seiwert M, et al. German Environmental Survey 1998 (GerES III): environmental pollutants in blood of the German population. Int J Hyg Environ Health 2002;205:297-308.

Becker K, Schulz C, Kaus S, Seiwert M, Seifert B. German environmental survey 1998 (GerES III): environmental pollutants in the urine of the German population. Int J Hyg Environ Health 2003; 206:15-24.

Berglund M, Akesson A, Nermell B, Vahter M. Intestinal absorption of dietary cadmium in women depends on body iron stores and fiber intake. Environ Health Perspect 1994; 102:1058-1066.

Centers for Disease Control and Prevention (CDC). Third National Report on Human Exposure to Environmental Chemicals. Atlanta (GA). 2005.

Davison AG, Fayers PM, Taylor AJ, Venables KM, Darbyshire J, Pickering CA, et al. Cadmium fume inhalation and emphysema. Lancet 1988;1(8587):663-667.

Diamond GL, Thayer WC, Choudhury H. Pharmacokinetic/ pharmacodynamics (PK/PD) modeling of risks of kidney toxicity from exposure to cadmium: estimates of dietary risks in the U.S. population. J Toxicol Environ Health 2003;66(Pt A):2141-2164.

Ezaki T, Tsukahara T, Moriguchi J, Furuki K, Fukui Y, Ukai H, et al. No clear-cut evidence for cadmium-induced renal tubular dysfunction among over 10,000 women in the Japanese general population: a nationwide large-scale survey. Int Arch Occup Environ Health 2003;76:186-196.

Fernandez MA, Sanz P, Palomar M, Serra J, Gadea E. Fatal chemical pneumonitis due to cadmium fumes. Occup Med 1996;46:372-374.

Friedman LS, Lukyanova EM, Kundiev YT, Shkiryak-Nizhnyk AZ, Chislovska NV, Mucha A, et al. Anthropometric, environmental, and dietary predictors of elevated blood cadmium levels in Ukranian children: Ukraine ELSPAC group. Environ Res 2006;102:83-89.

Horiguchi H, Oguma E, Sasaki S, Miyamoto K, Ikeda Y, Machida M, et al. Comprehensive study of the effects of age, iron deficiency, diabetes mellitus, and cadmium burden on dietary cadmium absorption in cadmium-exposed female Japanese farmers. Toxicol Appl Pharmacol 2004a; 196:114-123.

Horiguchi H, Oguma E, Sasaki S, Miyamoto K, Ikeda Y, Machida M, et al. Dietary exposure to cadmium at close to the current provisional tolerable weekly intake does not affect renal function among female Japanese farmers. Environ Res 2004b;95:20–31.

Hotz P, Buchet JP, Bernard A, Lison D, Lauwerys R. Renal effects of low-level environmental cadmium exposure: 5-year follow-up of a subcohort from the Cadmibel study. Lancet 1999;354:1508–1513.

Jarup L, Hellstrom L, Alfven T, Carlsson MD, Grubb A, Persson B, et al. Low level exposure to cadmium and early kidney damage: the OSCAR study [published erratum appears in Occup Environ Med 2002;59:497]. Occup Environ Med 2000;57:668-672.

Jin T, Nordberg G, Ye T, Bo M, Wang H, Zhu G, et al. Osteoporosis and renal dysfunction in a general population exposed to cadmium in China. Environ Res 2004;96:353-359.

Kikuchi Y, Nomiyama T, Kumagai N, Dekio F, Uemura T, Takebayashi T, et al. Uptake of cadmium in meals from the digestive tract of young non-smoking Japanese female volunteers. J Occup Health 2003;45:43-52.

Komaromy-Hiller G, Ash KO, Costa R, Howerton K. Comparison of representative ranges based on U.S. patient population and literature reference intervals for urinary trace elements. Clin Chim Acta 2000;296(1-2):71-90.

Mannino DM, Holguin F, Greves HM, Savage-Brown A, Stock AL, Jones RL. Urinary cadmium levels predict lower lung function in current and former smokers: data from the Third National Health and Nutrition Examination Survey. Thorax 2004;59:194-8.

Mascagni P, Consonni D, Bregante G, Chiappino G, Toffoletto F. Olfactory function in workers exposed to moderate airborne cadmium levels. Neurotoxicology 2003;24:717-724.

Moriguchi J, Ezaki T, Tsukahara T, Furuki K, Fukui Y, Okamoto S, et al. α1-Microglobulin as a promising marker of cadmium-induced tubular dysfunction, possibly better than β2-microglobulin. Toxicol Lett 2004;148(1-2):11-20.

Nishijo M, Nakagawa H, Honda R, Tanebe K, et al. Effects of maternal exposure to cadmium on pregnancy outcome and breast milk. Occup Environ Med 2002;59:394-397.

Nishijo M, Tawara K, Honda R, Nakagawa H, Tanebe K, Saito S. Relationship between newborn size and mother's blood cadmium levels, Toyama, Japan. Arch Environ Health. 2004;59(1):22-25.

Noonan CW, Sarasua SM, Campagna D, Kathman SJ, Lybarger JA, Mueller PW. Effects of exposure to low levels of environmental cadmium on renal biomarkers. Environ Health Perspect 2002;110:151-155.

Nordberg GF, Nordberg M. Biological monitoring of cadmium. In: Clarkson TW, Friberg L, Nordberg GF, Sager PR, eds. Biological monitoring of toxic metals. New York: Plenum Press; 2001. pp. 151-168.

Olsson IM, Bensryd I, Lundh T, Ottosson H, Skerfving S, Oskarsson A. Cadmium in blood and urine – impact of sex, age, dietary intake, iron status, and former smoking – association of renal effects. Environ Health Perspect 2002;110:1185-1190.

Roels HA, Hoet P, Lison D. Usefulness of biomarkers of exposure to inorganic mercury, lead, or cadmium in controlling occupational and environmental risks of nephrotoxicity. Ren Fail 1999;21(3-4):251-262.

Salpietro CD, Gangemi S, Minciullo PL, Bruiglia S, Merlino MV, Stelitano A, et al. Cadmium concentration in maternal and cord blood and infant birth weight: a study on healthy non-smoking women. J Perinat Med 2002;30(5):395-399.

Staessen JA, Buchet JP, Ginucchio G, Lauwerys R, Lijnen P, Roels H, et al. Public health implications of environmental exposure to cadmium and lead: an overview of epidemiological studies in Belgium. J Cardiovasc Risk 1996;3:26-41.

Staessen J, Roels HA, Emelianov D, Kuznetsova T, Thijs L, Vangronsveld J, et al. Environmental exposure to cadmium, forearm bone density, and risk of fractures: prospective population study. Lancet 1999;353:1140-1144.

Suwazono Y, Kobayashi E, Okubo Y, Nogawa K, Kido T, Nakagawa H. Renal effects of cadmium exposure in cadmium nonpolluted areas in Japan. Environ Res 2000;84 (Section A):44-55.

United States Environmental Protection Agency (U.S. EPA). 2000. Cadmium compounds. Hazard Summary, created 1992, Revised 2000 [online]. Available at URL: www.epa.gov/ttn/atw/hlthef/cadmium.html. 4/8/09

Waalkes MP. Cadmium carcinogenesis. Mutat Res 2003;533(1-2):107-120.

Wennberg M, Lundh T, Bergdahl IA, Gallmans G, Jansson J-H, Stegmayr B, et al. Time trends in burdens of cadmium, lead, and mercury in the population of northern Sweden. Environ Res 2006;100:330-338.

Wilhelm M, Schultz C, Schwenk M. Revised and new reference values for arsenic, cadmium, lead, and mercury in blood or urine of children: Basis for validation of human biomonitoring data in environmental medicine. Int J Hyg Environ Health 2006;209:301-305.

Zhang YL, Zhao YC, Wang JX, Zhu HD, Liu QF, Fan YG, et al. Effect of environmental exposure to cadmium on pregnancy outcome and fetal growth: a study on healthy pregnant women in China. J Environ Sci Health B 2004;39:2507-2515.

# Cesium

CAS No. 7440-46-2

## General Information

Cesium is a silver-white metal that is found naturally in rock, soil, and clay. Inorganic cesium compounds are used in photomultiplier and vacuum tubes, scintillation counters, infrared lamps, semiconductors, photographic emulsions, and high-power gas-ion devices, and as polymerization catalysts. Radioactive [137]Cs has been used medically to treat cancer.

Most human exposure to cesium occurs through the diet.

For absorbed cesium salts, the body half-life is estimated to be 70-109 days based on [137]Cs exposures. Little is known about the health effects of this metal, although cesium was generally of low toxicity when given to animals. However, cesium hydroxide is corrosive and irritating at high concentrations. Case investigations of ingestions of large doses of cesium chloride have reported decreased appetite, nausea, diarrhea, and cardiac arrhythmia (ATSDR, 2004). Human health effects from cesium at low environmental doses or at biomonitored levels from low environmental exposures are unknown. Workplace guidelines for cesium hydroxide are available from ACGIH and NIOSH. Whether cesium compounds are carcinogenic is unknown.

## Urinary Cesium

Geometric mean and selected percentiles of urine concentrations (in µg/L) for the U.S. population from the National Health and Nutrition Examination Survey.

| | Survey years | Geometric mean (95% conf. interval) | 50th | 75th | 90th | 95th | Sample size |
|---|---|---|---|---|---|---|---|
| **Total** | 99-00 | 4.35 (4.00-4.74) | 4.90 (4.40-5.40) | 7.10 (6.60-7.70) | 9.60 (8.80-10.3) | 11.5 (10.2-13.0) | 2464 |
| | 01-02 | 4.81 (4.40-5.26) | 5.49 (5.12-5.90) | 7.91 (7.47-8.39) | 10.4 (9.56-11.4) | 12.6 (11.1-13.8) | 2690 |
| | 03-04 | 4.67 (4.39-4.97) | 5.14 (4.84-5.49) | 7.68 (7.20-8.21) | 10.6 (9.55-11.4) | 12.7 (11.5-13.9) | 2558 |
| **Age group** | | | | | | | |
| 6-11 years | 99-00 | 4.87 (4.08-5.81) | 5.70 (4.60-6.70) | 7.30 (6.70-8.00) | 9.00 (7.90-10.1) | 9.70 (9.00-10.8) | 340 |
| | 01-02 | 4.87 (4.08-5.82) | 5.64 (4.69-6.56) | 7.96 (6.77-8.84) | 9.88 (8.64-10.6) | 11.1 (10.2-12.4) | 368 |
| | 03-04 | 5.21 (4.74-5.71) | 5.50 (4.76-6.37) | 8.08 (7.10-8.83) | 11.5 (8.86-12.9) | 12.9 (10.8-13.6) | 290 |
| 12-19 years | 99-00 | 4.55 (4.09-5.05) | 5.20 (4.40-5.60) | 6.90 (6.10-7.80) | 8.80 (8.10-9.50) | 10.7 (8.90-12.5) | 718 |
| | 01-02 | 5.22 (4.57-5.95) | 5.62 (5.16-6.12) | 7.55 (7.13-8.04) | 9.77 (9.12-11.1) | 12.0 (10.0-15.0) | 762 |
| | 03-04 | 5.04 (4.59-5.54) | 5.70 (5.16-6.07) | 7.53 (6.91-8.37) | 9.71 (8.80-10.4) | 11.6 (9.92-13.2) | 725 |
| 20 years and older | 99-00 | 4.26 (3.94-4.62) | 4.80 (4.40-5.30) | 7.10 (6.50-7.60) | 9.80 (8.90-10.7) | 11.7 (10.2-13.4) | 1406 |
| | 01-02 | 4.74 (4.32-5.20) | 5.43 (5.05-5.87) | 7.97 (7.43-8.52) | 10.6 (9.73-11.5) | 12.9 (11.2-14.2) | 1560 |
| | 03-04 | 4.56 (4.23-4.90) | 5.03 (4.60-5.42) | 7.66 (7.01-8.34) | 10.7 (9.40-11.5) | 12.9 (11.5-14.9) | 1543 |
| **Gender** | | | | | | | |
| Males | 99-00 | 4.84 (4.35-5.38) | 5.50 (4.60-6.00) | 7.50 (7.00-8.20) | 9.70 (8.80-11.3) | 11.7 (10.3-13.0) | 1226 |
| | 01-02 | 5.34 (4.89-5.84) | 6.13 (5.61-6.64) | 8.27 (7.84-9.08) | 10.8 (10.1-12.1) | 12.8 (11.3-15.0) | 1335 |
| | 03-04 | 5.03 (4.73-5.36) | 5.59 (5.17-6.00) | 7.98 (7.31-8.63) | 11.0 (9.53-11.8) | 12.9 (11.5-16.1) | 1281 |
| Females | 99-00 | 3.95 (3.63-4.29) | 4.50 (4.20-4.90) | 6.70 (6.20-7.30) | 9.10 (8.30-10.0) | 11.2 (9.90-12.9) | 1238 |
| | 01-02 | 4.36 (3.95-4.81) | 4.87 (4.45-5.25) | 7.33 (6.71-8.01) | 9.77 (9.07-11.0) | 12.4 (10.4-13.8) | 1355 |
| | 03-04 | 4.35 (4.03-4.70) | 4.79 (4.25-5.26) | 7.30 (6.87-7.81) | 10.2 (9.40-11.0) | 12.1 (11.2-13.6) | 1277 |
| **Race/ethnicity** | | | | | | | |
| Mexican Americans | 99-00 | 4.32 (3.82-4.89) | 4.80 (4.30-5.20) | 6.70 (6.40-7.20) | 9.10 (8.00-9.90) | 11.1 (9.60-12.7) | 884 |
| | 01-02 | 4.63 (4.10-5.24) | 5.29 (4.59-5.89) | 7.08 (6.42-7.99) | 9.13 (7.86-11.3) | 11.3 (8.81-14.9) | 683 |
| | 03-04 | 4.94 (4.64-5.27) | 5.62 (5.01-6.09) | 7.86 (7.15-8.46) | 10.3 (8.99-11.3) | 11.9 (10.7-14.7) | 618 |
| Non-Hispanic blacks | 99-00 | 4.94 (4.33-5.64) | 5.40 (4.80-6.40) | 7.50 (6.90-8.40) | 9.80 (8.80-10.8) | 11.6 (9.80-13.1) | 568 |
| | 01-02 | 4.93 (4.70-5.17) | 5.33 (5.05-5.64) | 7.36 (6.97-7.59) | 9.44 (8.71-9.68) | 10.7 (10.1-12.3) | 667 |
| | 03-04 | 4.71 (4.47-4.97) | 5.12 (4.71-5.49) | 7.17 (6.72-7.60) | 9.13 (8.52-9.99) | 10.7 (9.99-11.4) | 723 |
| Non-Hispanic whites | 99-00 | 4.25 (3.83-4.72) | 4.80 (4.20-5.50) | 7.20 (6.60-7.90) | 9.70 (8.90-10.7) | 11.8 (10.3-13.3) | 821 |
| | 01-02 | 4.77 (4.27-5.32) | 5.49 (4.99-6.05) | 7.98 (7.45-8.61) | 10.4 (9.54-11.4) | 12.6 (11.0-13.8) | 1132 |
| | 03-04 | 4.56 (4.22-4.94) | 5.02 (4.59-5.42) | 7.60 (7.00-8.23) | 10.7 (9.26-11.8) | 12.9 (11.5-14.7) | 1074 |

Limit of detection (LOD, see Data Analysis section) for Survey years 99-00, 01-02, and 03-04 are 0.14, 0.14, and 0.2, respectively.

## Biomonitoring Information

Urinary cesium levels reflect recent exposure. Two small studies of European populations reported urinary cesium levels similar to U.S. population results shown in this *Report* (Alimonti et al., 2005; Minoia et al., 1990). Using clinically submitted specimens, Komaromy-Hiller et al. (2000) found urinary cesium levels that were slightly lower than those reported for the U.S. population. Urinary cesium levels were similar in a group of forest fire fighters and residents living near the fire area (Wolfe et al., 2004), and were also roughly similar to those in this *Report*.

Finding a measurable amount of cesium in the urine does not mean that the levels of cesium cause an adverse health effect. Biomonitoring studies on levels of cesium can provide physicians and public health officials with reference values so that they can determine whether people have been exposed to higher levels of cesium than are found in the general population. Biomonitoring data can also help scientists plan and conduct research on exposure and health effects.

## Urinary Cesium (creatinine corrected)

Geometric mean and selected percentiles of urine concentrations (in µg/g of creatinine) for the U.S. population from the National Health and Nutrition Examination Survey.

| | Survey years | Geometric mean (95% conf. interval) | 50th | 75th | 90th | 95th | Sample size |
|---|---|---|---|---|---|---|---|
| **Total** | 99-00 | 4.10 (3 96-4.25) | 4.13 (3 97-4.27) | 5.41 (5 21-5.70) | 7.14 (6 83-7.50) | 8.64 (8 00-9.30) | 2464 |
| | 01-02 | 4.54 (4 30-4.79) | 4.44 (4 20-4.64) | 6.06 (5.66-6.47) | 8.18 (7.62-8.95) | 10.2 (8 84-11.7) | 2689 |
| | 03-04 | 4.64 (4.42-4.87) | 4.42 (4 21-4.74) | 6.11 (5.76-6.48) | 8.51 (7 99-9.15) | 10.6 (9.75-11.0) | 2558 |
| **Age group** | | | | | | | |
| 6-11 years | 99-00 | 5.34 (5 03-5.67) | 5.42 (5 03-6.04) | 6.63 (6.18-7.13) | 8.23 (7.13-9.41) | 9.90 (7 88-10.1) | 340 |
| | 01-02 | 5.95 (5.48-6.46) | 5.91 (5.43-6.53) | 7.77 (7 00-8.28) | 9.27 (8 35-11.9) | 11.9 (9 38-12.3) | 368 |
| | 03-04 | 6.07 (5.63-6.53) | 6.02 (5.45-6.49) | 8.30 (7.16-8.99) | 10.8 (9.15-11.8) | 11.9 (10.3-15.8) | 290 |
| 12-19 years | 99-00 | 3.43 (3 29-3.58) | 3.54 (3 29-3.68) | 4.35 (4.17-4.56) | 5.31 (4 97-5.79) | 6.67 (5 33-8.09) | 718 |
| | 01-02 | 3.73 (3.41-4.08) | 3.55 (3 36-3.74) | 4.74 (4.40-5.14) | 6.10 (5 35-7.63) | 8.08 (6.44-9.82) | 762 |
| | 03-04 | 3.60 (3 37-3.85) | 3.51 (3 33-3.72) | 4.53 (4 24-4.87) | 6.08 (5.14-6.94) | 7.27 (6.13-9.07) | 725 |
| 20 years and older | 99-00 | 4.08 (3 88-4.29) | 4.06 (3 85-4.29) | 5.39 (5 04-5.85) | 7.17 (6 84-7.58) | 8.61 (7 91-9.30) | 1406 |
| | 01-02 | 4.54 (4 30-4.78) | 4.43 (4 20-4.59) | 5.94 (5.64-6.40) | 8.15 (7.46-8.97) | 10.2 (8.74-11.7) | 1559 |
| | 03-04 | 4.68 (4.46-4.91) | 4.47 (4 27-4.80) | 6.11 (5 83-6.43) | 8.47 (7.76-9.17) | 10.5 (9.68-11.2) | 1543 |
| **Gender** | | | | | | | |
| Males | 99-00 | 3.78 (3.65-3.91) | 3.78 (3.61-3.96) | 4.96 (4.72-5.20) | 6.50 (6.18-6.70) | 7.71 (7 01-8.64) | 1226 |
| | 01-02 | 4.22 (3 96-4.51) | 4.10 (3 87-4.41) | 5.60 (5 27-6.03) | 7.67 (6 90-8.48) | 9.46 (8 22-11.5) | 1334 |
| | 03-04 | 4.24 (3 99-4.50) | 4.12 (3 89-4.37) | 5.66 (5.19-6.06) | 7.66 (6 90-8.40) | 9.00 (8 36-10.3) | 1281 |
| Females | 99-00 | 4.43 (4 20-4.68) | 4.45 (4.14-4.77) | 5.92 (5 36-6.47) | 7.70 (7.16-8.07) | 9.41 (8 00-10.4) | 1238 |
| | 01-02 | 4.86 (4 58-5.16) | 4.72 (4 50-5.06) | 6.54 (5 93-7.00) | 8.50 (7 84-9.79) | 10.3 (8 95-12.2) | 1355 |
| | 03-04 | 5.05 (4.77-5.35) | 4.77 (4.44-5.14) | 6.58 (6.14-7.22) | 9.43 (8 56-10.5) | 11.3 (10.7-12.3) | 1277 |
| **Race/ethnicity** | | | | | | | |
| Mexican Americans | 99-00 | 3.99 (3.73-4.25) | 3.95 (3.65-4.17) | 5.09 (4.79-5.39) | 6.65 (6 08-7.10) | 7.98 (7 20-8.95) | 884 |
| | 01-02 | 4.51 (4 00-5.08) | 4.51 (3 82-4.95) | 5.91 (5 31-6.64) | 7.77 (6.60-10.0) | 10.0 (7.60-20.5) | 682 |
| | 03-04 | 4.58 (4.16-5.05) | 4.51 (4.10-4.92) | 5.74 (5.42-6.09) | 7.53 (6 59-8.91) | 9.44 (8 24-10.6) | 618 |
| Non-Hispanic blacks | 99-00 | 3.21 (2 90-3.56) | 3.26 (3 05-3.44) | 4.30 (4 00-4.55) | 5.50 (5 00-5.98) | 6.33 (5 91-7.04) | 568 |
| | 01-02 | 3.38 (3.19-3.57) | 3.35 (3 05-3.60) | 4.41 (4.15-4.78) | 5.87 (5.63-6.29) | 6.75 (6.41-7.03) | 667 |
| | 03-04 | 3.38 (3 21-3.56) | 3.30 (3 08-3.50) | 4.31 (4 02-4.62) | 5.79 (5.12-6.47) | 6.98 (6 38-7.18) | 723 |
| Non-Hispanic whites | 99-00 | 4.26 (4 07-4.47) | 4.28 (4 05-4.50) | 5.66 (5 26-6.05) | 7.27 (6 84-7.83) | 8.75 (7 93-9.38) | 821 |
| | 01-02 | 4.81 (4 55-5.08) | 4.63 (4.42-4.96) | 6.33 (5 91-6.68) | 8.46 (7 84-9.39) | 10.3 (9 04-11.8) | 1132 |
| | 03-04 | 4.81 (4 52-5.12) | 4.56 (4 31-4.98) | 6.28 (5 95-6.71) | 8.63 (7 99-9.28) | 10.6 (9.43-11.0) | 1074 |

## References

Agency for Toxic Substances and Disease Registry (ATSDR). Toxicological profile for cesium.2004 [online]. Available at URL: http://www.atsdr.cdc.gov/toxprofiles/tp157.html. 4/8/09

Alimonti A, Forte G, Spezia S, Gatti A, Mincione G, Ronchi P, et al. Uncertainty of inductively coupled plasma mass spectrometry based measurements: An application to the analysis of urinary barium, cesium, antimony and tungsten. Rapid Commun Mass Spectrom 2005;19:3131-3138.

Centers for Disease Control and Prevention (CDC). Third National Report on Human Exposure to Environmental Chemicals. Atlanta (GA) 2005.

Komaromy-Hiller G, Ash KO, Costa R, Howerton K. Comparison of representative ranges based on U.S. patient population and literature reference intervals for urinary trace elements. Clin Chim Acta 2000;296(1-2):71-90.

Minoia C, Sabbioni E, Apostoli P, Pietra R, Pozzoli L, Gallorini M, et al. Trace element reference values in tissues from inhabitants of the European community I. A study of 46 elements in urine, blood, and serum of Italian subjects. Sci Total Environ 1990;95:89-105.

Wolfe MI, Mott JA, Voorhees RE, Sewell CM, Paschal D, Wood CM, et al. Assessment of urinary metals following exposure to a large vegetative fire, New Mexico, 2000. J Expo Anal Environ Epidemiol 2004;14:120-128.

# Cobalt

CAS No. 7440-48-4

## General Information

Cobalt is a magnetic element that occurs in nature either as a steel-gray, shiny, hard metal or in combination with other elements. The cobalt used in U.S. industry is imported or obtained by recycling scrap metal that contains cobalt. Among its many uses are manufacturing superalloys used in gas turbines in aircraft engines, hard metal (alloys of cobalt and tungsten carbide), blue-colored pigments, and fertilizers. Cobalt is used as a drying agent in paints, varnishes, and inks. It is also a component of

porcelain enamel applied to steel bathroom fixtures, large appliances, and kitchenware. Cobalt compounds are used as catalysts in producing oil and gas, and in synthesizing polyester and other materials. Cobalt compounds are also used in manufacturing battery electrodes, steel-belted radial tires, automobile airbags, diamond-polishing wheels, and magnetic recording media. Medical uses include joint and dental prostheses and radioactive cobalt in cancer chemotherapy.

Cobalt occurs naturally in airborne dust, seawater, and soil. It is emitted into the environment from burning coal and oil and car and truck exhaust. Usual human exposure is from food sources. Cobalt may be released into the systemic circulation of patients who receive joint prostheses that are

## Urinary Cobalt

Geometric mean and selected percentiles of urine concentrations (in µg/L) for the U.S. population from the National Health and Nutrition Examination Survey.

| | Survey years | Geometric mean (95% conf. interval) | Selected percentiles ( 95% confidence interval) | | | | Sample size |
|---|---|---|---|---|---|---|---|
| | | | 50th | 75th | 90th | 95th | |
| **Total** | 99-00 | .375 (.336-.419) | .410 (.370-.450) | .630 (.570-.680) | .950 (.890-1.03) | 1.32 (1.16-1.48) | 2465 |
| | 01-02 | .379 (.355-.404) | .410 (.380-.430) | .610 (.570-.660) | .940 (.870-1.00) | 1.28 (1.15-1.44) | 2690 |
| | 03-04 | .316 (.291-.343) | .330 (.300-.350) | .520 (.490-.550) | .820 (.750-.890) | 1.16 (1.08-1.26) | 2558 |
| **Age group** | | | | | | | |
| 6-11 years | 99-00 | .499 (.427-.583) | .530 (.450-.640) | .750 (.610-.900) | 1.03 (.880-1.12) | 1.22 (1.03-1.50) | 340 |
| | 01-02 | .452 (.377-.543) | .520 (.430-.610) | .710 (.670-.810) | 1.07 (.940-1.21) | 1.32 (1.17-1.53) | 368 |
| | 03-04 | .454 (.393-.523) | .460 (.410-.520) | .750 (.590-.900) | 1.24 (.910-1.47) | 1.68 (1.26-1.81) | 290 |
| 12-19 years | 99-00 | .519 (.463-.581) | .520 (.490-.570) | .820 (.670-.890) | 1.17 (1.01-1.47) | 1.52 (1.26-2.56) | 719 |
| | 01-02 | .515 (.469-.564) | .520 (.480-.570) | .750 (.690-.840) | 1.24 (1.07-1.32) | 1.59 (1.37-1.99) | 762 |
| | 03-04 | .461 (.428-.496) | .480 (.450-.520) | .740 (.650-.800) | 1.03 (.940-1.23) | 1.60 (1.14-1.92) | 725 |
| 20 years and older | 99-00 | .343 (.305-.386) | .370 (.330-.420) | .570 (.520-.640) | .880 (.810-.980) | 1.28 (1.07-1.39) | 1406 |
| | 01-02 | .352 (.333-.373) | .380 (.350-.410) | .560 (.520-.590) | .860 (.800-.930) | 1.15 (1.04-1.42) | 1560 |
| | 03-04 | .285 (.259-.313) | .300 (.270-.330) | .460 (.410-.510) | .690 (.660-.730) | 1.06 (.890-1.14) | 1543 |
| **Gender** | | | | | | | |
| Males | 99-00 | .371 (.331-.416) | .410 (.370-.450) | .580 (.540-.640) | .820 (.740-.900) | 1.01 (.900-1.12) | 1227 |
| | 01-02 | .367 (.338-.399) | .390 (.360-.420) | .550 (.520-.600) | .790 (.740-.850) | 1.05 (.960-1.14) | 1335 |
| | 03-04 | .294 (.270-.319) | .320 (.290-.340) | .480 (.440-.500) | .670 (.620-.710) | .870 (.790-.920) | 1281 |
| Females | 99-00 | .379 (.333-.431) | .410 (.340-.460) | .680 (.590-.790) | 1.17 (.930-1.36) | 1.50 (1.28-2.05) | 1238 |
| | 01-02 | .390 (.364-.417) | .430 (.400-.450) | .670 (.620-.700) | 1.06 (.980-1.16) | 1.46 (1.22-1.81) | 1355 |
| | 03-04 | .339 (.308-.372) | .340 (.310-.370) | .580 (.540-.610) | 1.04 (.900-1.13) | 1.47 (1.33-1.73) | 1277 |
| **Race/ethnicity** | | | | | | | |
| Mexican Americans | 99-00 | .418 (.348-.502) | .470 (.370-.530) | .670 (.630-.770) | 1.05 (.950-1.19) | 1.47 (1.25-1.67) | 884 |
| | 01-02 | .398 (.373-.424) | .430 (.410-.450) | .650 (.600-.710) | .950 (.850-1.03) | 1.20 (1.06-1.48) | 683 |
| | 03-04 | .374 (.350-.398) | .350 (.340-.390) | .580 (.530-.620) | 1.09 (.920-1.16) | 1.33 (1.16-1.73) | 618 |
| Non-Hispanic blacks | 99-00 | .434 (.405-.465) | .430 (.390-.470) | .680 (.620-.760) | 1.17 (1.04-1.26) | 1.45 (1.23-2.04) | 568 |
| | 01-02 | .435 (.388-.487) | .420 (.380-.460) | .650 (.540-.810) | 1.16 (.850-1.64) | 1.75 (1.32-2.22) | 667 |
| | 03-04 | .380 (.348-.414) | .380 (.360-.410) | .600 (.540-.680) | 1.01 (.890-1.09) | 1.28 (1.01-2.03) | 723 |
| Non-Hispanic whites | 99-00 | .369 (.316-.431) | .410 (.350-.460) | .630 (.550-.700) | .930 (.830-1.08) | 1.29 (1.02-1.65) | 822 |
| | 01-02 | .359 (.327-.394) | .390 (.360-.430) | .590 (.520-.660) | .870 (.800-.950) | 1.16 (1.04-1.32) | 1132 |
| | 03-04 | .301 (.270-.334) | .310 (.280-.340) | .500 (.460-.540) | .760 (.690-.850) | 1.09 (.950-1.26) | 1074 |

Limit of detection (LOD, see Data Analysis section) for Survey years 99-00, 01-02, and 03-04 are 0 07, 0.07, and 0.08, respectively.

fabricated from cobalt alloys (Lhotka et al., 2003). Cobalt constitutes 4% by weight of vitamin B-12 (cobalamin), an essential human nutrient. A nutritional requirement for cobalt other than that contained within dietary cobalamin has not been established. Exposure in the workplace may come from electroplating, refining or processing alloys, using hard metal cutting tools, or using diamond-polishing wheels that contain cobalt metal. Workplace standards and guidelines for external air exposure to cobalt and several of its compounds have been established by OSHA and ACGIH, respectively.

Cobalt is absorbed by oral and pulmonary routes. Human studies with $^{60}$Co administered as soluble cobalt chloride have reported oral absorption ranging from approximately 1 to 25 % (Smith et al., 1972). Once absorbed and distributed in the body, cobalt is excreted predominantly in the urine, and to a lesser extent, in the feces. Elimination reflects a multi-compartmental model dominated by compartments with half-lives on the order of several hours to a week, but with a minor fraction (10-15 %) exhibiting a half-life of several years (Mosconi et al., 1994; Smith et al., 1972). A portion of cobalt retained for long periods is concentrated in the liver. Lung retention of relatively insoluble cobalt compounds such as cobalt oxide may be prolonged, with pulmonary clearance half-lives of from one to two years (Hedge et al., 1979). Recent inhalation exposure to soluble cobalt compounds can be monitored by measuring cobalt in urine or blood (Lison et al., 1994).

## Urinary Cobalt (creatinine corrected)

Geometric mean and selected percentiles of urine concentrations (in µg/g of creatinine) for the U.S. population from the National Health and Nutrition Examination Survey.

| | Survey years | Geometric mean (95% conf. interval) | 50th | 75th | 90th | 95th | Sample size |
|---|---|---|---|---|---|---|---|
| **Total** | 99-00 | .353 (.319-.391) | .328 (.302-.365) | .515 (.457-.581) | .821 (.679-.963) | 1.16 (.938-1.50) | 2465 |
| | 01-02 | .358 (.333-.384) | .335 (.313-.360) | .523 (.487-.562) | .844 (.750-.955) | 1.16 (1.00-1.28) | 2689 |
| | 03-04 | .314 (.303-.325) | .290 (.278-.306) | .455 (.434-.481) | .737 (.703-.781) | 1.02 (.911-1.10) | 2558 |
| **Age group** | | | | | | | |
| 6-11 years | 99-00 | .547 (.467-.640) | .554 (.449-.647) | .774 (.626-.938) | 1.00 (.833-1.49) | 1.25 (.895-1.50) | 340 |
| | 01-02 | .552 (.508-.599) | .548 (.503-.609) | .756 (.660-.829) | 1.00 (.900-1.27) | 1.30 (1.03-1.73) | 368 |
| | 03-04 | .529 (.471-.593) | .500 (.463-.543) | .689 (.634-.750) | 1.04 (.760-1.29) | 1.29 (1.04-1.36) | 290 |
| 12-19 years | 99-00 | .391 (.353-.433) | .378 (.329-.407) | .537 (.469-.595) | .824 (.638-1.17) | 1.44 (.821-3.54) | 719 |
| | 01-02 | .368 (.343-.396) | .352 (.327-.372) | .534 (.471-.611) | .851 (.673-.949) | 1.06 (.932-1.24) | 762 |
| | 03-04 | .329 (.304-.355) | .316 (.277-.348) | .495 (.442-.561) | .738 (.630-.847) | .952 (.792-1.09) | 725 |
| 20 years and older | 99-00 | .328 (.297-.362) | .306 (.280-.328) | .471 (.428-.522) | .727 (.632-.905) | 1.12 (.861-1.36) | 1406 |
| | 01-02 | .337 (.313-.363) | .313 (.294-.337) | .475 (.435-.513) | .792 (.704-.955) | 1.15 (.963-1.33) | 1559 |
| | 03-04 | .293 (.282-.304) | .271 (.257-.286) | .400 (.380-.429) | .691 (.616-.744) | .976 (.829-1.10) | 1543 |
| **Gender** | | | | | | | |
| Males | 99-00 | .290 (.259-.324) | .279 (.248-.301) | .402 (.365-.449) | .608 (.534-.728) | .838 (.667-1.10) | 1227 |
| | 01-02 | .290 (.272-.310) | .278 (.256-.297) | .392 (.361-.425) | .644 (.574-.707) | .848 (.786-.929) | 1334 |
| | 03-04 | .247 (.237-.259) | .234 (.215-.250) | .333 (.313-.352) | .513 (.476-.585) | .700 (.630-.753) | 1281 |
| Females | 99-00 | .426 (.378-.479) | .407 (.362-.457) | .606 (.550-.694) | .960 (.781-1.29) | 1.50 (1.11-1.83) | 1238 |
| | 01-02 | .435 (.404-.468) | .408 (.382-.438) | .635 (.560-.708) | 1.00 (.879-1.19) | 1.29 (1.12-1.60) | 1355 |
| | 03-04 | .393 (.378-.409) | .361 (.342-.381) | .554 (.513-.615) | .937 (.850-1.00) | 1.29 (1.10-1.33) | 1277 |
| **Race/ethnicity** | | | | | | | |
| Mexican Americans | 99-00 | .386 (.339-.439) | .376 (.333-.419) | .598 (.500-.669) | .898 (.826-1.00) | 1.23 (1.11-1.35) | 884 |
| | 01-02 | .388 (.361-.417) | .361 (.333-.394) | .591 (.500-.662) | .872 (.777-.990) | 1.10 (.990-1.27) | 682 |
| | 03-04 | .346 (.326-.368) | .327 (.296-.349) | .542 (.487-.594) | .850 (.753-.963) | 1.14 (.963-1.35) | 618 |
| Non-Hispanic blacks | 99-00 | .282 (.275-.289) | .257 (.243-.279) | .417 (.378-.462) | .723 (.600-.785) | .975 (.757-1.60) | 568 |
| | 01-02 | .298 (.275-.323) | .268 (.251-.296) | .444 (.393-.505) | .728 (.582-.917) | 1.03 (.740-1.55) | 667 |
| | 03-04 | .273 (.248-.300) | .259 (.239-.281) | .388 (.344-.461) | .700 (.563-.842) | .964 (.733-1.15) | 723 |
| Non-Hispanic whites | 99-00 | .369 (.324-.421) | .352 (.313-.387) | .533 (.452-.611) | .861 (.667-1.16) | 1.25 (.895-1.57) | 822 |
| | 01-02 | .362 (.331-.396) | .343 (.313-.368) | .523 (.479-.562) | .830 (.736-.983) | 1.16 (.983-1.33) | 1132 |
| | 03-04 | .317 (.301-.334) | .291 (.274-.309) | .457 (.425-.488) | .738 (.683-.804) | 1.00 (.857-1.13) | 1074 |

Toxic effects of cobalt have been encountered in workplace settings. Cobalt compounds are a recognized cause of allergic contact dermatitis (Dickel et al., 2001; Lisi, 2003; Thomassen et al., 2001). Occupational exposure to cobalt-containing dusts has caused occupational asthma (Pisati and Zedda, 1994; Shirakawa et al., 1989). "Hard metal" disease, an interstitial lung disorder with findings that range from alveolitis to pulmonary fibrosis, has been associated with exposure to dusts that contain cobalt, usually in combination with tungsten carbide (Cugell et al., 1990). The extent to which cobalt exposure alone causes interstitial lung disease is unknown (Linna et al., 2003; Swennen et al., 1993).

Cobalt was once added as a foaming agent to beer, and this caused outbreaks of cardiomyopathy among heavy drinkers in the mid-1960's (Alexander et al., 1972). Case reports have also suggested a link between occupational cobalt exposure and cardiomyopathy (Jarvis et al., 1992). Cobalt compounds appear to stimulate erythropoietin production and were formerly used in the treatment of anemia (Goldberg et al., 1988). Pharmaceutical preparations of cobalt used in the past as hematinics were associated with the development of overt hypothyroidism (Kriss et al., 1955). A subclinical decrease in thyroid production was observed in a study of cobalt production workers (Swennen et al., 1993).

Cobalt compounds elicited numerous genotoxic effects in both *in vitro* and *in vivo* assays (De Boeck et al., 2003) and produced lung cancer in rats and mice after chronic inhalation (Bucher et al., 1999). An industry-wide study of hard metal workers in France observed an increased mortality from lung cancer (Moulin et al., 1998). IARC has classified cobalt metal with tungsten carbide and other soluble cobalt salts as possibly carcinogenic to humans. Information about external exposure (i.e., environmental levels) and health effects is available from ATSDR at: http://www.atsdr.cdc.gov/toxpro2.html.

## Biomonitoring Information

Urinary levels of cobalt decline rapidly within 24 hours after exposure ceases (Alexandersson et al., 1988). Urinary measurements mainly reflect recent exposure, although substantial occupational exposures have produced elevated urinary levels for many weeks. Smaller population surveys of European adults reported urinary cobalt levels that were roughly similar U.S. population results in this *Report* (Kristiansen et al., 1997; White and Sabbioni, 1998). Small studies of patients with hip replacements using metal alloy prostheses reported increased urinary cobalt concentrations, with mean levels that were about 15-20 times higher than in the general U.S. population (CDC, 2005; Daniel et al.,

2006; Dunstan et al., 2005; Iavicoli et al., 2006; MacDonald et al., 2003).

Persons with occupational exposure to cobalt often have urinary cobalt levels that are many times higher than those of the general population. The ACGIH biological exposure index (BEI) for inorganic forms of cobalt (except insoluble cobalt oxides) is 15 µg/L. Information about the BEI is provided here for comparison, not to imply that the BEI is a safe level for general population exposure. For workers exposed to cobalt in the air, a distinction is made between soluble and insoluble (oxides and metallic) cobalt (Christensen and Poulsen, 1994; Lison et al., 1994). Exposure to soluble cobalt salts will produce proportionately higher urinary levels because they are absorbed better. Correlations between air exposure levels and urinary cobalt levels in hard metal fabricators are well documented (Ichikawa et al., 1985; Krause et al., 2001; Lauwerys and Hoet, 2001; Linnainmaa and Kiilunen, 1997).

Finding a measurable amount of cobalt in the urine does not mean that the levels of cobalt cause an adverse health effect. Biomonitoring studies on levels of cobalt provide physicians and public health officials with reference values so that they can determine whether people have been exposed to higher levels of cobalt than are found in the general population. Biomonitoring data can also help scientists plan and conduct research on exposure and health effects.

## References

Alexander CS. Cobalt-beer cardiomyopathy. A clinical and pathological study of twenty-eight cases. Am J Med 1972;53:395-417.

Alexandersson R. Blood and urinary concentrations as estimators of cobalt exposure. Arch Environ Health 1988;43(4):299-303.

Bucher JR, Hailey JR, Roycroft JR, Haseman JK, Sills RC, Grumbein SL, et al., Inhalation toxicity and carcinogenicity studies of cobalt sulfate. Toxicol Sci 1999;49:56-67.

Centers for Disease Control and Prevention (CDC). Third National Report on Human Exposure to Environmental Chemicals. Atlanta (GA). 2005 [online]. Available at URL: http://www.cdc.gov/exposurereport/. 4/3/08

Christensen JM, Poulsen OM. A 1982-1992 surveillance programme on Danish pottery painters. biological levels and health effects following exposure to soluble or insoluble cobalt compounds in cobalt blue dyes. Sci Total Environ 1994;50(1-3):95-104.

Cugell DW, Morgan WKC, Perkins DG, Rubin A. The respiratory

effects of cobalt. Arch Intern Med 1990;150:177-183.

Daniel J, Ziaee H, Salama A, Pradhan C, McMinn DJ. The effect of the diameter of metal-on-metal bearings on systemic exposure to cobalt and chromium. J Bone Joint Surg Br 2006;88(4):443-448.

De Boeck M, Kirsch-Volders M, Lison D. Cobalt and antimony: genotoxicity and carcinogenicity. Mutat Res 2003;533:135-152.

Dickel H, Radulescu M, Weyher I, Diepgen TL. Occupationally-induced "isolated cobalt sensitization." Contact Dermatitis 2001;45:246-247.

Dunstan E, Sanghrajka AP, Tilley S, Unwin P, Blunn G, Cannon SR, et al. Metal ion levels after metal-on-metal proximal femoral replacements: a 30-year follow-up. J Bone Joint Surg Br 2005;87(5):628-631.

Goldberg MA, Dunning SP, Bunn HF. Regulation of the erythropoietin gene: evidence that the oxygen sensor is a heme protein. Science 1988;242:1412-1415.

Hedge AG, Thakker DM, Ghat IS. Long-term clearance of inhaled $^{60}$Co. Health Phys 1979;36:732-734.

Iavicoli I, Falcone G, Alessandrelli M, Cresti R, DeSantis V, Salvatori S, et al. The release of metals from metal-on-metal surface arthroplasty of the hip. J Trace Elem Med Biol 2006;20(1):25-31.

Ichikawa Y, Kuska Y, Goto S. Biological monitoring of cobalt exposure based on cobalt concentrations in blood and urine. Int Arch Occup Environ Health. 1985;55(4):269-276.

Jarvis JQ, Hammon E, Meier R, Robinson C. Cobalt cardiomyopathy. A report of two cases from mineral assay laboratories and a review of the literature. J Occup Med 1992;34:620-626.

Kraus T, Schramel P, Schaller KH, Zobelein P, Weber A, Angerer J. Exposure assessment in the hard metal manufacturing industry with special regard to tungsten and its compounds. Occup Environ Med 2001;58(10):631-634.

Kriss JP, Carnes WH, Gross RT. Hypothyroidism and thyroid hyperplasia in patients treated with cobalt JAMA 1955;157:117-121.

Kristiansen J, Christensen JM, Iversen BS, Sabbioni E. Toxic trace element reference levels in blood and urine: influence of gender and lifestyle factors. Sci Total Environ 1997;204:147-160.

Lauwerys RB, Hoet P. Industrial Chemical Exposure: Guidelines for Biological Monitoring. 3rd ed. Boca Raton (FL): Lewis Publishers, 2001.

Lhotka C, Szekeres T, Steffan I, Zhuber K, Zweymuller K.

Four-year study of cobalt and chromium blood levels in patients managed with two different metal-on-metal total hip replacements. J Orthop Res 2003;21(2):189-195.

Linna A, Oksa P, Palmroos P, Roto P, Laippala P, Uitti J. Respiratory health of cobalt production workers. Am J Ind Med 2003;44:124-132.

Linnainmaa M, Kiilunen M. Urinary cobalt as a measure of exposure in the wet sharpening of hard metal and satellite blades. Int Arch Occup Environ Health 1997;69(3):193-200.

Lisi P. Co-sensitivity between cobalt and other transition metals. Contact Dermatitis 2003;48:172-173.

Lison D, Buchet JP, Swennen B, Molders J, Lauwerys R. Biological monitoring of workers exposed to cobalt metal, salt, oxides, and hard metal dust. Occup Environ Med 1994;51(7):447-450.

MacDonald SJ, McCalden RW, Chess DG, Bourne RB, Rorabeck CH, Cleland D, et al. Metal-on-metal versus polyethylene in hip arthroplasty: a randomized clinical trial. Clin Orthop Relat Res 2003;406:282-296.

Mosconi G, Bacis M, Vitali MT, Leghissa P, Sabbioni E. Cobalt excretion in urine: results of a study on workers producing diamond grinding tools and on a control group. Sci Total Environ 1994;150;(1-3):133-139.

Moulin JJ, Wild P, Romazini S, Lasfargues G, Peltier A, Bozec C, et al. Lung cancer risk in hard-metal workers. Am J Epidemiol 1998;148:241-248.

Pisati G, Zedda S. Outcome of occupational asthma due to cobalt hypersensitivity. Sci Total Environ 1994;150(1-3):167-171.

Shirakawa T, Kusaka Y, Fujimura N, Goto S, Kato M, Heki S, et al. Occupational asthma from cobalt sensitivity in workers exposed to hard metal dust. Chest 1989;95:29-37.

Smith T, Edmonds CJ, Barnaby CF. Absorption and retention of cobalt in man by whole-body counting. Health Phys 1972;22:359-367.

Swennen B, Buchet JP, Stanescu D, Lison D, Lauwerys R. Epidemiological survey of workers exposed to cobalt oxides, cobalt salts, and cobalt metals. Br J Ind Med 1993;50(9):835-842.

Thomassen H, HoffmannB, Schank M, Hoher T, Thabe H. Meyer zum Buschenfelde K-H, et al. Cobalt-specific T lymphocytes in synovial tissue after an allergic reaction to cobalt alloy joint prosthesis. J Rheumatol 2001;28(5):1121-1128.

White MA, Sabbioni E. Trace element reference values in tissues from inhabitants of the European Union. X. a study of 13 elements in blood and urine of a United Kingdom population. Sci Total Environ 1998;216:253-270.

# Lead
CAS No. 7439-92-1

## General Information

Elemental lead is a soft, malleable, dense, blue-gray metal that occurs naturally in soils and rocks. Lead is most often mined from ores or recycled from scrap metal or batteries. Elemental lead can be combined with other elements to form inorganic and organic compounds, such as lead phosphate and tetraethyl lead. Lead has a variety of uses in manufacturing: storage batteries, solders, metal alloys (e.g. brass, bronze), plastics, leaded glass, ceramic glazes, ammunition, antique-molded or cast ornaments, and for radiation shielding. In the past, lead was added to gasoline and residential paints and used in soldering the seams of food cans. Lead was used in plumbing for centuries and may still be present.

Before the 1980's, the main source of lead exposure for the general U.S. population was aerosolized lead emitted from combustion engines that used leaded gasoline. Aerosolized lead is either inhaled or ingested after it is deposited on surfaces and food crops. Since lead has been eliminated from gasoline, adult lead exposures tend to be limited to

## Blood Lead

Geometric mean and selected percentiles of blood concentrations (in µg/dL) for the U.S. population from the National Health and Nutrition Examination Survey.

| | Survey years | Geometric mean (95% conf. interval) | Selected percentiles ( 95% confidence interval) | | | | Sample size |
|---|---|---|---|---|---|---|---|
| | | | 50th | 75th | 90th | 95th | |
| Total | 99-00 | 1.66 (1.60-1.72) | 1.60 (1.60-1.70) | 2.50 (2.40-2.60) | 3.80 (3.60-4.00) | 5.00 (4.70-5.50) | 7970 |
| | 01-02 | 1.45 (1.39-1.51) | 1.40 (1.40-1.50) | 2.20 (2.10-2.30) | 3.40 (3.20-3.60) | 4.50 (4.20-4.70) | 8945 |
| | 03-04 | 1.43 (1.36-1.50) | 1.40 (1.30-1.50) | 2.10 (2.10-2.20) | 3.20 (3.10-3.30) | 4.20 (3.90-4.40) | 8373 |
| **Age group** | | | | | | | |
| 1-5 years | 99-00 | 2.23 (1.96-2.53) | 2.20 (1.90-2.50) | 3.40 (2.80-3.90) | 4.90 (4.00-6.60) | 7.00 (6.10-8.30) | 723 |
| | 01-02 | 1.70 (1.55-1.87) | 1.60 (1.50-1.80) | 2.50 (2.20-2.90) | 4.20 (3.50-5.20) | 5.80 (4.70-6.90) | 898 |
| | 03-04 | 1.77 (1.60-1.95) | 1.70 (1.50-1.90) | 2.50 (2.30-2.80) | 3.90 (3.30-4.60) | 5.10 (4.10-6.60) | 911 |
| 6-11 years | 99-00 | 1.51 (1.36-1.66) | 1.40 (1.30-1.60) | 2.10 (1.80-2.50) | 3.30 (2.80-3.80) | 4.50 (3.40-6.20) | 905 |
| | 01-02 | 1.25 (1.14-1.36) | 1.20 (1.00-1.30) | 1.70 (1.60-2.00) | 2.80 (2.50-3.10) | 3.70 (3.00-4.70) | 1044 |
| | 03-04 | 1.25 (1.12-1.39) | 1.20 (1.10-1.40) | 1.80 (1.50-2.10) | 2.60 (2.10-3.10) | 3.30 (2.50-4.60) | 856 |
| 12-19 years | 99-00 | 1.10 (1.04-1.17) | 1.10 (1.00-1.20) | 1.50 (1.40-1.70) | 2.30 (2.10-2.40) | 2.90 (2.70-3.00) | 2135 |
| | 01-02 | .942 (.899-.986) | .900 (.900-1.00) | 1.30 (1.20-1.40) | 2.00 (1.90-2.10) | 2.70 (2.40-2.90) | 2231 |
| | 03-04 | .946 (.878-1.02) | .900 (.800-1.00) | 1.30 (1.20-1.40) | 1.90 (1.70-2.10) | 2.60 (2.20-3.00) | 2081 |
| 20 years and older | 99-00 | 1.75 (1.68-1.81) | 1.70 (1.60-1.80) | 2.60 (2.50-2.70) | 3.90 (3.70-4.10) | 5.20 (4.80-5.60) | 4207 |
| | 01-02 | 1.56 (1.49-1.62) | 1.60 (1.50-1.60) | 2.30 (2.30-2.40) | 3.60 (3.40-3.70) | 4.60 (4.30-5.00) | 4772 |
| | 03-04 | 1.52 (1.45-1.60) | 1.50 (1.40-1.60) | 2.30 (2.20-2.40) | 3.30 (3.20-3.50) | 4.30 (4.00-4.60) | 4525 |
| **Gender** | | | | | | | |
| Males | 99-00 | 2.01 (1.93-2.09) | 1.90 (1.90-2.00) | 2.90 (2.80-3.00) | 4.50 (4.10-4.80) | 6.00 (5.50-6.50) | 3913 |
| | 01-02 | 1.78 (1.71-1.86) | 1.80 (1.70-1.80) | 2.70 (2.50-2.80) | 3.90 (3.80-4.10) | 5.40 (5.00-5.50) | 4339 |
| | 03-04 | 1.69 (1.62-1.75) | 1.60 (1.50-1.70) | 2.50 (2.40-2.60) | 3.70 (3.40-3.90) | 4.80 (4.50-5.20) | 4132 |
| Females | 99-00 | 1.37 (1.32-1.43) | 1.30 (1.30-1.40) | 2.00 (1.90-2.10) | 3.10 (2.90-3.30) | 4.00 (3.80-4.20) | 4057 |
| | 01-02 | 1.19 (1.14-1.25) | 1.20 (1.10-1.20) | 1.80 (1.70-1.90) | 2.60 (2.50-2.80) | 3.60 (3.10-4.00) | 4606 |
| | 03-04 | 1.22 (1.14-1.31) | 1.20 (1.10-1.30) | 1.80 (1.70-2.00) | 2.70 (2.50-3.00) | 3.50 (3.10-3.80) | 4241 |
| **Race/ethnicity** | | | | | | | |
| Mexican Americans | 99-00 | 1.83 (1.75-1.91) | 1.80 (1.70-1.90) | 2.80 (2.60-2.90) | 4.20 (3.90-4.60) | 5.80 (5.10-6.60) | 2742 |
| | 01-02 | 1.46 (1.34-1.60) | 1.50 (1.30-1.60) | 2.30 (2.10-2.60) | 3.60 (3.40-4.20) | 5.40 (4.40-6.70) | 2268 |
| | 03-04 | 1.55 (1.43-1.69) | 1.50 (1.40-1.60) | 2.30 (2.10-2.50) | 3.50 (2.90-4.20) | 4.90 (3.90-6.40) | 2085 |
| Non-Hispanic blacks | 99-00 | 1.87 (1.75-2.00) | 1.80 (1.70-2.00) | 2.80 (2.60-3.00) | 4.30 (4.00-4.60) | 5.70 (5.20-6.10) | 1842 |
| | 01-02 | 1.65 (1.52-1.80) | 1.60 (1.40-1.70) | 2.60 (2.30-2.90) | 4.20 (3.80-4.70) | 5.80 (5.30-6.50) | 2219 |
| | 03-04 | 1.69 (1.52-1.89) | 1.60 (1.40-1.80) | 2.60 (2.20-3.00) | 4.10 (3.50-4.70) | 5.30 (4.60-6.60) | 2293 |
| Non-Hispanic whites | 99-00 | 1.62 (1.55-1.69) | 1.60 (1.50-1.70) | 2.40 (2.30-2.50) | 3.60 (3.40-3.90) | 5.00 (4.40-5.70) | 2716 |
| | 01-02 | 1.43 (1.37-1.48) | 1.40 (1.30-1.50) | 2.20 (2.10-2.20) | 3.20 (3.10-3.40) | 4.20 (3.90-4.50) | 3806 |
| | 03-04 | 1.37 (1.32-1.43) | 1.30 (1.30-1.40) | 2.10 (2.00-2.10) | 3.00 (2.80-3.20) | 3.90 (3.60-4.30) | 3478 |

Limit of detection (LOD, see Data Analysis section) for Survey years 99-00, 01-02, and 03-04 are 0 3, 0.3, and 0 28, respectively.

occupational (e.g., battery and radiator manufacturing) and recreational sources. However, the primary source of exposure in children is from deteriorated lead-based paint and the resulting dust and soil contamination (Manton et al., 2000). Children may also be exposed to lead brought into the home on the work clothes of adults whose work involves lead. Less common sources of incidental or unique lead exposure are numerous: lead-glazed ceramic pottery; stained glass framing; pewter utensils and drinking vessels; older plumbing systems with leaded pipes or lead soldered connections; lead-based painted surfaces undergoing renovation or demolition; imported children's trinkets and toys; lead-containing folk remedies and cosmetics; bullet fragments retained in human tissue; lead-contaminated

dust in indoor firing ranges; and contact with soil, dust, or water contaminated by mining or smelting operations. Small amounts of environmental lead also may result from burning fossil fuels (ATSDR, 2007; CDC, 1991).

Lead is absorbed into the body after fine lead particulates or fumes are inhaled, or after soluble lead compounds are ingested. Absorption of ingested lead can be as much as five times greater in children than adults and even greater when intakes of dietary minerals are deficient. In the blood, absorbed lead is bound to erythrocytes and then is distributed initially to multiple soft tissues and eventually into bone. Approximately half of the absorbed lead may be incorporated into bone, which is the site of approximately

## Urinary Lead

Geometric mean and selected percentiles of urine concentrations (in µg/L) for the U.S. population from the National Health and Nutrition Examination Survey.

| | Survey years | Geometric mean (95% conf. interval) | 50th | 75th | 90th | 95th | Sample size |
|---|---|---|---|---|---|---|---|
| | | | \multicolumn{4}{c}{Selected percentiles (95% confidence interval)} | |
| **Total** | 99-00 | .766 (.708-.828) | .800 (.800-.900) | 1.40 (1.30-1.50) | 2.20 (2.00-2.30) | 2.90 (2.60-3.30) | 2465 |
| | 01-02 | .677 (.637-.718) | .700 (.700-.800) | 1.20 (1.20-1.30) | 2.00 (1.90-2.20) | 2.70 (2.50-2.80) | 2690 |
| | 03-04 | .636 (.595-.680) | .640 (.580-.690) | 1.04 (.960-1.12) | 1.73 (1.52-1.86) | 2.29 (2.03-2.62) | 2558 |
| **Age group** | | | | | | | |
| 6-11 years | 99-00 | 1.07 (.955-1.20) | 1.10 (.900-1.30) | 1.50 (1.40-1.70) | 2.40 (1.80-3.10) | 3.40 (2.40-5.00) | 340 |
| | 01-02 | .753 (.661-.857) | .800 (.600-.900) | 1.20 (1.10-1.40) | 2.10 (1.60-2.40) | 2.60 (2.10-3.70) | 368 |
| | 03-04 | .795 (.671-.941) | .790 (.640-.900) | 1.35 (.970-1.86) | 2.27 (1.62-4.09) | 3.33 (2.23-4.41) | 290 |
| 12-19 years | 99-00 | .659 (.579-.749) | .700 (.600-.800) | 1.10 (.900-1.30) | 1.80 (1.40-2.20) | 2.20 (1.90-2.80) | 719 |
| | 01-02 | .564 (.526-.605) | .600 (.500-.600) | 1.00 (.800-1.10) | 1.60 (1.40-1.70) | 2.00 (1.80-2.40) | 762 |
| | 03-04 | .604 (.553-.660) | .630 (.570-.680) | .920 (.810-1.02) | 1.32 (1.14-1.80) | 1.86 (1.44-2.29) | 725 |
| 20 years and older | 99-00 | .752 (.691-.818) | .800 (.700-.900) | 1.40 (1.30-1.50) | 2.20 (2.00-2.40) | 2.90 (2.60-3.30) | 1406 |
| | 01-02 | .688 (.641-.738) | .700 (.700-.800) | 1.20 (1.20-1.30) | 2.00 (1.90-2.30) | 2.80 (2.50-2.90) | 1560 |
| | 03-04 | .625 (.579-.674) | .620 (.560-.700) | 1.04 (.960-1.11) | 1.70 (1.52-1.80) | 2.21 (2.04-2.49) | 1543 |
| **Gender** | | | | | | | |
| Males | 99-00 | .923 (.822-1.04) | .900 (.900-1.00) | 1.60 (1.40-1.80) | 2.50 (2.20-2.90) | 3.40 (2.90-3.80) | 1227 |
| | 01-02 | .808 (.757-.862) | .800 (.800-.900) | 1.40 (1.30-1.50) | 2.50 (2.20-2.70) | 3.20 (2.90-3.50) | 1335 |
| | 03-04 | .731 (.680-.785) | .730 (.680-.800) | 1.17 (1.07-1.27) | 2.03 (1.78-2.22) | 2.66 (2.33-2.91) | 1281 |
| Females | 99-00 | .642 (.589-.701) | .700 (.600-.800) | 1.20 (1.10-1.30) | 1.90 (1.60-2.20) | 2.40 (2.10-3.00) | 1238 |
| | 01-02 | .573 (.535-.613) | .600 (.600-.600) | 1.10 (1.00-1.10) | 1.60 (1.50-1.80) | 2.20 (1.90-2.40) | 1355 |
| | 03-04 | .558 (.506-.616) | .540 (.480-.620) | .920 (.820-1.04) | 1.49 (1.24-1.75) | 1.82 (1.59-2.30) | 1277 |
| **Race/ethnicity** | | | | | | | |
| Mexican Americans | 99-00 | 1.02 (.915-1.13) | 1.10 (.900-1.20) | 1.80 (1.60-1.90) | 2.90 (2.50-3.40) | 4.30 (3.10-5.40) | 884 |
| | 01-02 | .833 (.745-.931) | .900 (.700-1.00) | 1.50 (1.20-1.70) | 2.50 (2.00-2.90) | 3.30 (2.70-3.80) | 683 |
| | 03-04 | .815 (.710-.935) | .840 (.700-.990) | 1.31 (1.18-1.59) | 2.19 (1.86-2.50) | 2.66 (2.13-3.97) | 618 |
| Non-Hispanic blacks | 99-00 | 1.11 (1.00-1.23) | 1.10 (1.00-1.20) | 1.90 (1.50-2.10) | 3.00 (2.40-3.50) | 4.20 (3.30-5.70) | 568 |
| | 01-02 | .940 (.833-1.06) | .900 (.800-1.00) | 1.60 (1.30-1.80) | 2.70 (2.10-3.40) | 3.70 (2.90-4.80) | 667 |
| | 03-04 | .848 (.729-.986) | .850 (.710-1.00) | 1.40 (1.10-1.72) | 2.14 (1.78-2.64) | 2.82 (2.31-3.89) | 723 |
| Non-Hispanic whites | 99-00 | .695 (.625-.773) | .700 (.700-.900) | 1.30 (1.10-1.40) | 2.00 (1.80-2.40) | 2.70 (2.30-3.10) | 822 |
| | 01-02 | .610 (.572-.651) | .700 (.600-.700) | 1.10 (1.10-1.20) | 1.90 (1.70-2.00) | 2.40 (2.30-2.60) | 1132 |
| | 03-04 | .591 (.556-.628) | .590 (.540-.650) | .960 (.910-.990) | 1.52 (1.40-1.75) | 2.14 (1.78-2.51) | 1074 |

Limit of detection (LOD, see Data Analysis section) for Survey years 99-00, 01-02, and 03-04 are 0.1, 0.1, and 0.33, respectively.

90% of the body lead burden in most adults. The skeleton acts as a storage depot, and approximately 40 to 70% of lead in blood comes from the skeleton in environmentally exposed adults (Smith et al., 1996). Lead can cross the placenta and enter the developing fetal brain. Lead is cleared from the blood and soft tissues with a half-life of 1 to 2 months and more slowly from the skeleton, with a half-life of years to decades. Approximately 70% of lead excretion occurs via the urine, with lesser amounts eliminated via the feces; scant amounts are lost through sweat, hair, and nails (Leggett, 1993; O'Flaherty, 1993).

The toxic effects of lead result from its interference with the physiologic actions of calcium, zinc, and iron, through the inhibition of certain enzymes, and through binding to ion channels and regulatory proteins. Additional mechanisms include generating reactive oxygen species and altering gene expression (ATSDR, 2007). Large amounts of lead in the body can cause anemia, kidney injury, abdominal pain, seizures, encephalopathy, and paralysis. Equilibrated blood lead levels (BLLs) after chronic intake are associated with certain toxic effects. BLLs and associated toxic effects differ in children and adults. For instance, BLLs near 10 µg/dL can affect blood pressure in adults and neurodevelopment in children (Bellinger, 2004; CDC, 1991; Nash et al., 2003; Schwartz, 1995; Staessen et al., 1995). In 1991, based on prospective population studies, the Centers for Disease Control and Prevention (CDC) established a BLL of 10

## Urinary Lead (creatinine corrected)

Geometric mean and selected percentiles of urine concentrations (in µg/g of creatinine) for the U.S. population from the National Health and Nutrition Examination Survey.

| | Survey years | Geometric mean (95% conf. interval) | 50th | 75th | 90th | 95th | Sample size |
|---|---|---|---|---|---|---|---|
| | | | \[ Selected percentiles (95% confidence interval) \] | | | | |
| **Total** | 99-00 | .721 (.700-.742) | .701 (.677-.725) | 1.11 (1 05-1.15) | 1.70 (1.62-1.85) | 2.38 (2 22-2.79) | 2465 |
| | 01-02 | .639 (.603-.677) | .635 (.588-.676) | 1.03 (.963-1.08) | 1.52 (1.43-1.61) | 2.03 (1 89-2.22) | 2689 |
| | 03-04 | .632 (.603-.662) | .622 (.594-.655) | .979 (.920-1.03) | 1.49 (1 33-1.64) | 1.97 (1.73-2.26) | 2558 |
| **Age group** | | | | | | | |
| 6-11 years | 99-00 | 1.17 (.975-1.41) | 1.06 (.918-1.22) | 1.55 (1 22-1.97) | 2.71 (1.67-4.66) | 4.66 (1 97-18.0) | 340 |
| | 01-02 | .918 (.841-1.00) | .870 (.800-.933) | 1.27 (1.12-1.43) | 2.33 (1 59-3.64) | 3.64 (1 89-5.56) | 368 |
| | 03-04 | .926 (.812-1.06) | .914 (.781-1.03) | 1.45 (1.17-1.72) | 2.14 (1.62-3.47) | 3.47 (2.19-5.31) | 290 |
| 12-19 years | 99-00 | .496 (.460-.535) | .469 (.408-.508) | .709 (.655-.828) | 1.11 (.981-1.28) | 1.65 (1.15-2.79) | 719 |
| | 01-02 | .404 (.380-.428) | .375 (.342-.400) | .603 (.541-.702) | .990 (.882-1.18) | 1.41 (1 07-1.63) | 762 |
| | 03-04 | .432 (.404-.461) | .404 (.383-.436) | .623 (.551-.730) | .938 (.828-1.06) | 1.23 (1 09-1.35) | 725 |
| 20 years and older | 99-00 | .720 (.683-.758) | .712 (.667-.739) | 1.10 (1 02-1.18) | 1.69 (1 53-1.87) | 2.31 (2.15-2.62) | 1406 |
| | 01-02 | .658 (.617-.703) | .652 (.608-.702) | 1.05 (.992-1.11) | 1.51 (1.40-1.61) | 2.00 (1 85-2.19) | 1559 |
| | 03-04 | .641 (.606-.679) | .633 (.605-.670) | .988 (.917-1.04) | 1.47 (1 28-1.63) | 1.94 (1.72-2.12) | 1543 |
| **Gender** | | | | | | | |
| Males | 99-00 | .720 (.679-.763) | .693 (.645-.734) | 1.10 (.992-1.22) | 1.68 (1 50-2.09) | 2.43 (2.15-3.03) | 1227 |
| | 01-02 | .639 (.607-.673) | .638 (.586-.686) | 1.01 (.957-1.08) | 1.55 (1.41-1.61) | 2.06 (1 88-2.43) | 1334 |
| | 03-04 | .615 (.588-.644) | .593 (.561-.639) | .914 (.862-.977) | 1.44 (1 25-1.53) | 2.00 (1.71-2.28) | 1281 |
| Females | 99-00 | .722 (.681-.765) | .707 (.667-.746) | 1.11 (1 05-1.18) | 1.74 (1 50-2.02) | 2.38 (2 03-2.88) | 1238 |
| | 01-02 | .639 (.594-.688) | .625 (.571-.682) | 1.03 (.946-1.11) | 1.50 (1 39-1.61) | 1.98 (1 85-2.15) | 1355 |
| | 03-04 | .648 (.601-.698) | .649 (.604-.718) | 1.03 (.938-1.10) | 1.56 (1 34-1.73) | 1.96 (1.72-2.20) | 1277 |
| **Race/ethnicity** | | | | | | | |
| Mexican Americans | 99-00 | .940 (.876-1.01) | .887 (.796-1.03) | 1.43 (1 37-1.58) | 2.38 (2 08-2.77) | 3.46 (2.78-4.18) | 884 |
| | 01-02 | .810 (.731-.898) | .774 (.702-.893) | 1.29 (1 09-1.44) | 2.05 (1.75-2.50) | 2.78 (2 56-3.33) | 682 |
| | 03-04 | .755 (.681-.838) | .708 (.612-.851) | 1.18 (1 09-1.31) | 1.86 (1 50-2.26) | 2.31 (1 98-2.92) | 618 |
| Non-Hispanic blacks | 99-00 | .722 (.659-.790) | .671 (.583-.753) | 1.11 (.988-1.20) | 2.00 (1 56-2.51) | 2.83 (2 20-3.88) | 568 |
| | 01-02 | .644 (.559-.742) | .608 (.510-.710) | .962 (.853-1.20) | 1.79 (1 36-2.33) | 2.75 (2 04-3.98) | 667 |
| | 03-04 | .609 (.529-.701) | .569 (.492-.698) | .900 (.793-1.03) | 1.48 (1.11-1.97) | 2.24 (1.65-2.88) | 723 |
| Non-Hispanic whites | 99-00 | .696 (.668-.725) | .677 (.645-.718) | 1.07 (.997-1.14) | 1.66 (1 50-1.83) | 2.31 (1 94-2.82) | 822 |
| | 01-02 | .615 (.579-.654) | .621 (.571-.667) | 1.00 (.933-1.07) | 1.46 (1 37-1.52) | 1.88 (1.62-2.03) | 1132 |
| | 03-04 | .623 (.592-.655) | .618 (.587-.657) | .971 (.914-1.03) | 1.44 (1 25-1.61) | 1.85 (1.64-2.10) | 1074 |

µg/dL or higher as the level of concern in children. Recent studies have suggested that neurodevelopmental effects may occur at BLLs lower than 10 µg/dL (Canfield et al., 2003; Lanphear et al., 2000). Many animal studies have established the multiple neurotoxic effects of lead (ATSDR, 2007).

In occupationally exposed adults, subtle or nonspecific neurocognitive effects have been reported at BLLs as low as 20-30 µg/dL (Mantere et al., 1984; Schwartz et al., 2001), with overt encephalopathy, seizures, and peripheral neuropathy generally occurring at much higher levels (e.g., higher than 100-200 µg/dL). BLLs higher than 40 µg/dL can result in proximal tubular dysfunction and decreased glomerular filtration rate leading to interstitial and peritubular fibrosis when high body burdens persist. Low level environmental lead exposure may be associated with small decrements in renal function (Kim et al., 1996; Muntner et al., 2003; Payton et al., 1994). Results of studies of adults with either occupational or environmental lead exposure have shown consistent associations between increased BLLs and increased blood pressure (Nash et al., 2003; Schwartz, 1995; Staessen et al., 1995) and associations between increased bone lead concentrations and blood pressure (Hu et al., 1996; Korrick et al., 1999). High dose occupational lead exposure, usually with BLLs greater than 40 µg/dL, may alter sperm morphology, reduce sperm count, and decrease fertility (Alexander et al., 1996; Telisman et al., 2000). At low environmental exposures, lead in women may be associated with hypertension during pregnancy, premature delivery, and spontaneous abortion (Baghurst et al., 1987; Bellinger 2005; Borja-Aburto et al., 1999).

Workplace standards and guidelines for lead exposure and monitoring have been established by OSHA and ACGIH, respectively. Both drinking water and ambient air standards for lead have been established by the U.S. EPA. IARC considers inorganic lead compounds probable human carcinogens, and organic lead compounds not classifiable with respect to human carcinogenicity. NTP considers lead and its compounds reasonably anticipated to be human carcinogens. Information about external exposure (i.e., environmental levels) and health effects is available from ATSDR at: http://www.atsdr.cdc.gov/toxpro2.html.

**Biomonitoring Information**

Blood lead measurement is the preferred method of evaluating lead exposure and its human health effects. BLLs reflect both recent intake and equilibration with stored lead in other tissues, particularly in the skeleton. Urine levels may reflect recently absorbed lead, though there is greater individual variation in urine lead than in blood and greater potential for contamination.

The Adult Blood Lead Epidemiology and Surveillance program has tracked BLLs reported by states for mostly for occupational but also for non-occupational exposure in U.S. adult residents. Overall, the national prevalence rate for adults with BLLs 25 µg/dL or higher was 7.5 per 100,000 adults; the prevalence rate has declined annually since 1994 (CDC, 2006). A decrease in BLLs is evident also in adult NHANES results reported over past decades (CDC, 2005a). The U.S. adult population has similar or slightly lower BLLs than adults in other developed nations (CDC, 2005b). A general population survey of adults Germany in 1998 reported a geometric mean blood lead concentration of 3.07 µg/dL (Becker et al., 2002), almost double the geometric mean of 1.75 µg/dL in U.S. adults in the 1999-2000 NHANES sample. A general population survey of adults in Italy tested in 2000 found BLLs slightly more than double those reported for U.S. adults in the 1999-2000 NHANES sample (Apostoli et al., 2002a).

In NHANES 1999-2002 in children 1-5 years old, both the geometric mean (1.9 µg/dL) and percentage of children with BLLs greater than 10 µg/dL (1.6%) were lower than those from NHANES 1991-1994, when the geometric mean BLL was 2.7 µg/dL and 4.4% of children had BLLs of 10µg/dL or higher (CDC, 2005b; Pirkle et al., 1998). More recently, Jones et al (2009) showed that the prevalence of BLLs of 10 µg/dL or greater decreased from 8.6% in NHANES 1988-1991 to 1.4% in NHANES 1999-2004, which is an 84% decline. Temporal declines in children's BLLs have been found in other developed countries (Wilhelm et al., 2006). Surveillance data reported by U.S. state childhood lead programs also show a decline in the percentage of children younger than 6 years of age who had BLLs of 10 µg/dL or higher. Data submitted through state public health programs from 2006 showed that 1.21% of approximately 3.3 million children tested had BLLs of 10 µg/dL or higher (http://www.cdc.gov/nceh/lead/surv/database/State_Confirmed_byYear_1997_to_2006.xls). However, BLLs greater than 10 µg/dL continue to be more prevalent among children with known risk factors, including minority race or ethnicity; urban residence; residing in housing built before the 1950's; and low family income (CDC, 1991; CDC, 2002; Jones et al., 2009). For example, approximately 11,000 higher-risk children and adolescents who were tested from 2001 to 2002 at an urban medical center had higher BLLs than the NHANES sample; the geometric mean BLL was 3.2 µg/dL in males and 3.0 µg/dL in females (Soldin et al., 2003).

Biomonitoring studies on levels of lead provide physicians and public health officials with reference values so that they can determine whether people have been exposed to higher levels of lead than are found in the general population. Biomonitoring data can also help scientists plan and conduct research on exposure and health effects.

## References

Agency for Toxic Substances and Disease Registry (ATSDR). Toxicological profile for lead. Aug 2007 [online]. Available from URL: http://www.atsdr.cdc.gov/toxprofiles/tp13.html. 4/14/09

Alexander BH, Checkoway H, van Netten C, Muller CH, Ewers TG, Kaufman JD, et al. Semen quality of men employed at a lead smelter. Occup Environ Med 1996;53:411-416.

Apostoli P, Baj A, Bavazzano P, Ganzi A, Neri A, Ronchi L, et al. Blood lead reference values: the results of an Italian polycentric study. Sci Total Environ 2002;287:1-11.

Baghurst PA, Robertson EF, McMichael AJ, Vimpani FB, Wigg NR, Roberts RR. The Port Pirie cohort study: lead effects on pregnancy outcome and early childhood development. Neurotoxicol 1987;8(3):395-401.

Becker K, Kaus S, Krause C, Lepom P, Schulz C, Seiwert M, et al. German Environmental Survey 1998 (GerES III): environmental pollutants in blood of the German population. Int J Hyg Environ Health 2002;205:297-308.

Bellinger D. Lead. Pediatrics 2004;113(4):1016-1022.

Bellinger D. Teratogen update: lead and pregnancy. Birth Defects Research (Part A). 2005;73:409-420.

Borja-Aburto VH, Hertz-Picciotto I, Rojas LM, Farias P, Rios C, Blanco J. Blood lead levels measured prospectively and risk of spontaneous abortion. Am J Epidemiol 1999;150(6):590-597.

Canfield RL, Henderson CR, Cory-Slechta DA, Cox C, Jusko TA, Lanphear BP. Intellectual impairment in children with blood lead concentrations below 10 µg/dL. N Engl J Med 2003;348:1517-1526.

Centers for Disease Control and Prevention (CDC). Adult blood lead epidemiology and surveillance—United States, 2003-2004. MMWR Morb Mortal Wkly Rep 2006;55(32):876-879. Available at URL: http://www.cdc.gov/mmwr/preview/mmwrhtml/mm5532a2.htm. 4/14/09

Centers for Disease Control and Prevention (CDC). Blood lead levels—United States, 1999-2002. MMWR Morb Mortal Wkly Rep 2005a;54(20):513-516. Available at URL: http://www.cdc.gov/mmwr/preview/mmwrhtml/mm5420a5.htm. 4/14/09

Centers for Disease Control and Prevention (CDC). Managing Elevated Blood Lead Levels Among Young Children. Recommendations from the Advisory Committee on Childhood Lead Poisoning Prevention. Atlanta, Ga. CDC; 2002 [online]. Available at URL: http://www.cdc.gov/nceh/lead/CaseManagement/caseManage_main.htm. 4/14/09

Centers for Disease Control and Prevention (CDC). Preventing Lead Poisoning in Young Children. Atlanta (GA). 1991 [online]. Available at URL: http://www.cdc.gov/nceh/lead/publications/books/plpyc/contents.htm. 4/14/09

Centers for Disease Control and Prevention (CDC). Third National Report on Human Exposure to Environmental Chemicals. Atlanta (GA). 2005b.

Chiodo LM, Jacobson SW, Jacobson JL. Neurodevelopmental effects of postnatal lead exposure at very low levels. Neurotoxicol Teratol 2004;26:359-371.

Hu H, Aro A, Payton M, Korrick S, Sparrow D, Weiss ST, et al. The relationship of bone and blood lead to hypertension. JAMA 1996;275(15):1171-1176.

IARC Working Group on the Evaluation of Carcinogenic Risks to Humans. Inorganic and Organic Lead Compounds. IARC Monogr Eval Carcinog Risks Hum 2006;87:1-471.

Jones RL, Homa DM, Meyer PA, Brody DJ, Caldwell KL, Pirkle JL, et al. Trends in blood lead levels and blood lead testing among US children aged 1 to 5 yeas, 1988-2004. Pediatrics 2009;123:e376-e385. doi:10.1542/peds:2007-3608.

Kim R, Rotnitzky A, Sparrow D, Weiss ST, Wager C, Hu H. A longitudinal study of low-level lead exposure and impairment of renal function: the Normative Aging Study. JAMA 1996;275:1177-1181.

Korrick SA, Hunter DJ, Rotnitzky A, Hu H, Speizer FE. Lead and hypertension in a sample of middle-aged women. Am J Public Health 1999;89:330-335.

Lanphear BP, Dietrich K, Auinger P, Cox C. Cognitive deficits with blood lead concentrations < 10 µg/dL in US children and adolescents. Public Health Rep 2000;115:521-529.

Leggett RW. Age-specific kinetic model of lead metal in humans. Environ Health Perspect 1993;101(7):598-616.

Mantere P, Hänninen H, Hernberg S, Luukkonen R. A prospective follow-up study on psychological effects in workers exposed to low levels of lead. Scand J Work Environ Health 1984;10:43-50.

Manton WI, Angle CR, Stanek KL, Reese YR, Kuehnemann TJ. Acquisition and retention of lead by young children. Environ Res 2000;82:60-80.

Muntner P, Vupputyuri S, Coresh J, Batuman V. Blood lead and chronic kidney disease in the general United States population:

results from NHANES III. Kidney Int 2003;63:1044-1050.

Nash D, Magder L, Lustberg M, Sherwin R, Rubin R, Kaufmann R, et al. Blood lead, blood pressure, and hypertension in perimenopausal and postmenopausal women. JAMA 2003;289(12):1523-1531.

O'Flaherty EJ. Physiologically based models for bone-seeking elements. IV. Kinetics of lead disposition in humans. Toxicol Appl Pharmacol 1993;118:16-29.

Payton M, Hu H, Sparrow D, Weiss ST. Low-level lead exposure and renal function in the Normative Aging Study. Am J Epidemiol 1994;140:821-829.

Pirkle JL, Kaufmann RB, Brody DJ, Hickman T, Gunter EW, Paschal DC. Exposure of the U.S. population to lead: 1991-1994. Environ Health Perspect 1998;106:745-750.

Schwartz BS, Lee BK, Lee GS, Stewar WF, Lee SS, Hwang KY, et al. Association of blood lead, dimercaptosuccinic acid-chelatable lead, and tibia lead with neurobehavioral test scores in South Korean lead workers. Am J Epidemiol 2001;153(5):453-464.

Schwartz J. Lead, blood pressure and cardiovascular disease in men. Arch Environ Health 1995; 50:31-37.

Soldin OP, Hanak B, Soldin SJ. Blood lead concentrations in children: new ranges. Clin Chim Acta 2003;327:109-113.

Smith DR, Osterloh JD, Flegal AR. Use of endogenous, stable lead isotopes to determine release of lead from the skeleton. Environ Health Perspect 1996;104(1):60-66.

Staessen JA, Roels H, Lauwerys RR, Amery A. Low-level lead exposure and blood pressure. J Hum Hypertens 1995;9:303-327.

Telisman S, Cvitkovic P, Jurasovic J, Pizent A, Gavella M, Rocic B. Semen quality and reproductive endocrine function in relation to biomarkers of lead, cadmium, zinc, and copper in men. Environ Health Perspect 2000;108(1):45-53.

Wilhelm M, Schulz D, Schwenk M. Revised and new reference values for arsenic, cadmium, lead, and mercury in blood or urine of children: basis for validation of human biomonitoring data in environmental medicine. Int J Hyg Environ Health 2006;209:301-305.

# Mercury

CAS No. 7439-97-6

## General Information

Mercury is a naturally occurring metal that has elemental (metallic), inorganic, and organic forms. Elemental mercury is a shiny, silver-white liquid (quicksilver) obtained predominantly from the refining of mercuric sulfide in cinnabar ore. Elemental mercury is used to produce chlorine gas and caustic soda for industrial applications. Other major uses include electrical equipment (e.g., thermostats and switches), electrical lamps, thermometers, sphygmomanometers and barometers, and dental amalgam. Inhalation of elemental mercury volatilized from dental amalgam is a major source of mercury exposure in the general population (Halbach, 1994; Kingman et al., 1998; Woods et al., 2007). Accidental spills of elemental mercury, which create an episodic potential for volatization and inhalation of mercury vapor, have often required public health intervention (Zeitz et al., 2002). Also, elemental mercury is used in rituals practiced in some Latin American and Caribbean communities.

Elemental mercury is released into the air from the combustion of fossil fuels (primarily coal), solid-waste incineration, and mining and smelting. Atmospheric elemental mercury can be deposited on land and water. In addition, water can be contaminated by the direct release of elemental and inorganic mercury from industrial discharges. Metabolism of mercury by microorganisms in aquatic sediments creates methyl mercury, an organic form of mercury, which can bioaccumulate in aquatic and terrestrial food chains. The ingestion of methyl mercury, predominantly from fish and other seafood, constitutes the main source of dietary mercury exposure in the general population. Apart from methyl mercury, synthetic organomercury compounds were once used in pharmaceutical applications, and mercury compounds are still used as preservatives (e.g., thimerosal, phenylmercuric acetate) or topical antiseptics (e.g., merbromin).

Inorganic mercury exists in two oxidative states (mercurous and mercuric) that combine with other elements, such as chlorine (e.g., mercuric chloride), sulfur, or oxygen, to form inorganic mercury compounds or salts. Inorganic mercury compounds such as mercuric oxide are used in producing batteries and pigments and in synthesizing many organic chemicals. Some cosmetic skin creams from countries other than the U.S. may contain inorganic mercury. Imported folk and alternative medicines occasionally are contaminated with inorganic mercury.

The kinetics of the different forms of mercury vary considerably. Poorly absorbed from the gastrointestinal tract, elemental mercury is absorbed mainly by inhaling volatilized vapor, and is distributed to most tissues, with the highest concentrations occurring in the kidneys (Barregard et al., 1999 ; Hursh et al., 1980; IARC, 1993). After elemental mercury is absorbed, it is oxidized in

## Total Blood Mercury—2003-2004

Geometric mean and selected percentiles of blood concentrations (in µg/L) for the U.S. population from the National Health and Nutrition Examination Survey.

| | Survey years | Geometric mean (95% conf. interval) | Selected percentiles ( 95% confidence interval) | | | | Sample size |
|---|---|---|---|---|---|---|---|
| | | | 50th | 75th | 90th | 95th | |
| **Total** | 03-04 | .797 (.703-.903) | .800 (.700-.900) | 1.70 (1.50-1.90) | 3.30 (2.90-3.90) | 4.90 (4.30-5.50) | 8373 |
| **Age group** | | | | | | | |
| 1-5 years | 03-04 | .326 (.285-.372) | .300 (.300-.300) | .500 (.500-.700) | 1.00 (.800-1.60) | 1.80 (1.30-2.50) | 911 |
| 6-11 years | 03-04 | .419 (.363-.484) | .400 (.400-.500) | .700 (.700-.900) | 1.30 (1.00-1.60) | 1.90 (1.40-3.50) | 856 |
| 12-19 years | 03-04 | .490 (.418-.574) | .500 (.400-.600) | 1.00 (.800-1.20) | 1.80 (1.40-2.30) | 2.60 (2.10-3.30) | 2081 |
| 20 years and older | 03-04 | .979 (.860-1.12) | 1.00 (.800-1.10) | 2.00 (1.70-2.30) | 3.80 (3.20-4.40) | 5.40 (4.60-6.70) | 4525 |
| **Gender** | | | | | | | |
| Males | 03-04 | .814 (.714-.927) | .800 (.700-.900) | 1.80 (1.50-2.00) | 3.70 (3.20-4.30) | 5.40 (4.60-6.50) | 4132 |
| Females | 03-04 | .781 (.689-.886) | .800 (.700-.900) | 1.60 (1.40-1.80) | 3.00 (2.50-3.50) | 4.40 (3.60-5.30) | 4241 |
| **Race/ethnicity** | | | | | | | |
| Mexican Americans | 03-04 | .563 (.472-.672) | .600 (.500-.700) | 1.00 (.800-1.30) | 1.90 (1.60-2.40) | 3.00 (2.20-3.80) | 2085 |
| Non-Hispanic blacks | 03-04 | .877 (.753-1.02) | .900 (.800-1.00) | 1.60 (1.40-1.80) | 3.00 (2.30-4.00) | 4.40 (3.30-6.00) | 2293 |
| Non-Hispanic whites | 03-04 | .776 (.655-.919) | .800 (.700-.900) | 1.70 (1.40-2.00) | 3.20 (2.60-3.90) | 4.70 (4.00-5.60) | 3478 |

Limit of detection (LOD, see Data Analysis section) for Survey year 03-04 is 0.2.

the tissues to mercurous and mercuric inorganic forms. Blood concentrations decline initially with a rapid half-life of approximately 1-3 days followed by a slower half-life of approximately 1-3 weeks (Barregard et al., 1992; Sandborgh-Englund et al., 1998). The slow-phase half-life may be several weeks longer in persons with chronic occupational exposure (Sallsten et al., 1993). After exposure to elemental mercury, excretion of mercury occurs predominantly through the kidney (Sandborgh-Englund et al., 1998), and peak urine levels can lag behind peak blood levels by days to a few weeks (Barregard et al., 1992); thereafter, for both acute and chronic exposures, urinary mercury levels decline with a half-life of approximately 1-3 months (Roels et al., 1991; Jonsson et al., 1999).

Less than 15% of inorganic mercury is absorbed from the human gastrointestinal tract (Rahola et al., 1973). Lesser penetration of inorganic mercury occurs through the blood-brain barrier than occurs with either elemental or methyl mercury (Hattula and Rahola, 1975; Vahter et al., 1994). The half-life of inorganic mercury in blood is similar to the slow-phase half-life of mercury after inhalation of elemental mercury. Excretion occurs by renal and fecal routes.

The fraction of methyl mercury absorbed from the gastrointestinal tract is about 95% (Aberg et al., 1969; Miettinen et al., 1971). Methyl mercury enters the brain and other tissues (Vahter et al., 1994) and then undergoes slow dealkylation to inorganic mercury. Human pharmacokinetic studies indicate that methyl mercury declines in blood and the whole body with a half-life of approximately 50 days, with most elimination occurring through in the feces (Sherlock et al., 1984; Smith et al., 1994; Smith and Farris, 1996). Methyl mercury is incorporated into growing hair, a measure of accumulated dose (Cernichiari et al., 1995; Suzuki et al., 1993), and a useful marker of exposure in epidemiologic studies (Grandjean et al., 1992 and 1999; McDowell et al., 2004; Myers et al., 2003).

Transplacental transport of methyl mercury and elemental mercury has been demonstrated in animals (Kajiwara et al., 1996; Vimy et al., 1990). Mercury levels in the cord blood are higher than in the mother's blood (Stern and Smith, 2003), and the newborn's levels decline gradually over several weeks (Bjornberg et al., 2005). Inorganic mercury and methyl mercury are distributed into human breast milk in relatively low concentrations; the transfer

## Total Blood Mercury–1999-2002

Geometric mean and selected percentiles of blood concentrations (in µg/L) for males and females aged 1 to 5 years and females aged 16 to 49 years in the U.S. population, National Health and Nutrition Examination Survey, 1999-2002.

| | Survey years | Geometric mean (95% conf. interval) | Selected percentiles (95% confidence interval) | | | | Sample size |
|---|---|---|---|---|---|---|---|
| | | | 50th | 75th | 90th | 95th | |
| **Age Group** | | | | | | | |
| 1-5 years (females and males) | 99-00 | .343 (.297-.395) | .300 (.200-.300) | .500 (.500-.600) | 1.40 (1.00-2.30) | 2.30 (1.20-3.50) | 705 |
| | 01-02 | .318 (.268-.377) | .300 (.200-.300) | .700 (.500-.800) | 1.20 (.900-1.60) | 1.90 (1.40-2.90) | 872 |
| Females | 99-00 | .377 (.299-.475) | .200 (.200-.300) | .800 (.500-1.10) | 1.60 (1.00-2.80) | 2.70 (1.30-5.50) | 318 |
| | 01-02 | .329 (.265-.407) | .300 (.200-.300) | .700 (.500-.800) | 1.30 (1.00-2.10) | 2.60 (1.30-4.90) | 432 |
| Males | 99-00 | .317 (.269-.374) | .200 (.200-.300) | .500 (.500-.600) | 1.10 (.800-1.60) | 2.10 (1.10-3.50) | 387 |
| | 01-02 | .307 (.256-.369) | .300 (.200-.300) | .600 (.400-.700) | 1.30 (.900-1.70) | 1.70 (1.40-2.00) | 440 |
| 16-49 years (females only) | 99-00 | 1.02 (.825-1.27) | .900 (.800-1.20) | 2.00 (1.50-3.00) | 4.90 (3.70-6.30) | 7.10 (5.30-11.3) | 1709 |
| | 01-02 | .833 (.738-.940) | .700 (.700-.800) | 1.70 (1.40-1.90) | 3.00 (2.70-3.50) | 4.60 (3.70-5.90) | 1928 |
| **Race/ethnicity** (females, 16-49 years) | | | | | | | |
| Mexican Americans | 99-00 | .820 (.664-1.01) | .900 (.700-1.00) | 1.40 (1.20-2.00) | 2.60 (2.00-3.60) | 4.00 (2.70-5.50) | 579 |
| | 01-02 | .667 (.541-.824) | .700 (.500-.800) | 1.10 (1.00-1.40) | 2.10 (1.70-3.00) | 3.50 (2.30-4.40) | 527 |
| Non-hispanic blacks | 99-00 | 1.35 (1.06-1.73) | 1.30 (1.10-1.70) | 2.60 (1.80-3.40) | 4.80 (3.30-6.60) | 5.90 (4.20-11.7) | 370 |
| | 01-02 | 1.06 (.871-1.29) | 1.10 (.800-1.20) | 1.80 (1.50-2.20) | 3.20 (2.20-3.90) | 4.10 (3.30-6.00) | 436 |
| Non-hispanic whites | 99-00 | .944 (.726-1.23) | .900 (.700-1.10) | 1.90 (1.30-3.30) | 5.00 (3.00-6.90) | 6.90 (4.50-12.0) | 588 |
| | 01-02 | .800 (.697-.919) | .800 (.700-.800) | 1.50 (1.30-2.00) | 3.00 (2.20-3.70) | 4.60 (3.30-6.80) | 806 |

Limit of detection (LOD, see Data Analysis sec ion) for Survey years 99-00 and 01-02 are 0.14 and 0.14.

may be more efficient for inorganic mercury (Grandjean et al., 1995; Oskarsson et al., 1996). Mercury levels in breast milk also decline in the weeks after birth (Bjornberg et al., 2005; Drexler and Schaller, 1998; Sakamoto et al., 2002; Sakamoto et al., 2004).

The health effects of mercury are diverse and can depend on the form of the mercury to which a person is exposed and the dose and the duration of exposure. Acute, high-dose exposure to elemental mercury vapor may cause severe pneumonitis. At levels below those that cause acute lung injury, overt signs and symptoms of chronic inhalation may include tremor, gingivitis, and neurocognitive and behavioral disturbances, particularly irritability, depression, short-term memory loss, fatigue, anorexia, and sleep disturbance (Bidstrup et al., 1951; Smith et al., 1970; Smith et al., 1983). Low-level exposure from dental amalgams has not been associated with neurologic effects in children or adults (Bates et al., 2004; Bellinger et al., 2006; DeRouen et al., 2006; Factor-Litvak et al., 2003). Occupational exposure to elemental mercury vapor has been associated with subclinical effects on biomarkers of renal dysfunction (Cardenas et al., 1993).

Inorganic mercury exposure usually occurs by ingestion. Large amounts may cause irritant or corrosive effects on the gastrointestinal tract (Sanchez-Sicilia et al., 1963). Once absorbed, the most prominent effect is on the kidneys where mercury accumulates and may lead to renal tubular necrosis. Acrodynia is a sporadic and predominantly pediatric syndrome historically associated with calomel (mercuric oxide) in teething powders and occasionally other inorganic forms of mercury. The constellation of findings may include anorexia, insomnia, irritability, hypertension, maculopapular rash, pain in the extremities, and pinkish discoloration of the hands and feet (Tunnessen et al., 1987).

Overt poisoning from methyl mercury primarily affects the central nervous system, causing parasthesias, ataxia, dysarthria, hearing impairment, and progressive constriction of the visual fields, typically after a latent period of weeks to months. High-level prenatal exposure may result in a constellation of developmental deficits that includes mental retardation, cerebellar ataxia, dysarthria, limb deformities, altered physical growth, sensory impairments, and cerebral palsy (NRC, 2000). In recent epidemiologic studies, lower levels of prenatal exposure due to maternal seafood consumption have been associated with an increased risk for abnormal neurocognitive test results in children (NRC, 2000; Rice, 2004). Although recent investigations have suggested a possible link between chronic ingestion of methyl mercury and an increased risk for cardiovascular disease, the existence of a causal relation is unresolved (Chan and Egeland, 2004; Rissanen et al., 2000; Salonen et al., 1995; Stern 2005; Vupputuri et al., 2005).

Workplace standards for inorganic mercury exposure have been established by OSHA and ACGIH, and a drinking water

## Inorganic Blood Mercury

Geometric mean and selected percentiles of blood concentrations (in μg/L) for the U.S. population from the National Health and Nutrition Examination Survey.

| | Survey years | Geometric mean (95% conf. interval) | Selected percentiles (95% confidence interval) | | | | Sample size |
|---|---|---|---|---|---|---|---|
| | | | 50th | 75th | 90th | 95th | |
| **Total** | 03-04 | * | < LOD | < LOD | .600 ( 500-.600) | .700 (.700-.700) | 8147 |
| **Age group** | | | | | | | |
| 1-5 years | 03-04 | * | < LOD | < LOD | < LOD | .500 (<LOD-.600) | 792 |
| 6-11 years | 03-04 | * | < LOD | < LOD | < LOD | .600 ( 500-.600) | 842 |
| 12-19 years | 03-04 | * | < LOD | < LOD | .500 (<LOD-.500) | .600 ( 500-.600) | 2060 |
| 20 years and older | 03-04 | * | < LOD | < LOD | .600 ( 500-.600) | .700 (.700-.800) | 4453 |
| **Gender** | | | | | | | |
| Males | 03-04 | * | < LOD | < LOD | .500 ( 500-.600) | .600 ( 600-.700) | 4015 |
| Females | 03-04 | * | < LOD | < LOD | .600 ( 500-.600) | .700 (.700-.800) | 4132 |
| **Race/ethnicity** | | | | | | | |
| Mexican Americans | 03-04 | * | < LOD | < LOD | .500 ( 500-.600) | .700 ( 600-.800) | 2007 |
| Non-Hispanic blacks | 03-04 | * | < LOD | < LOD | .600 ( 500-.600) | .700 ( 600-.800) | 2240 |
| Non-Hispanic whites | 03-04 | * | < LOD | < LOD | .600 ( 500-.600) | .700 ( 600-.700) | 3406 |

Limit of detection (LOD, see Data Analysis section) for Survey year 03-04 is 0.42.
< LOD means less than the limit of detection, which may vary for some chemicals by year and by individual sample.
* Not calculated: proportion of results below limit of detection was too high to provide a valid result.

standard for inorganic mercury has been established by U.S. EPA. IARC considers methylmercury to be a possible human carcinogen and elemental and inorganic mercury to be unclassifiable with regard to human carcinogenicity. Information about external exposure (i.e., environmental levels) and health effects is available from the U.S. EPA at: http://www.epa.gov/mercury and from ATSDR at: http://www.atsdr.cdc.gov/toxprofiles.

## Biomonitoring Information

In the general population, the total blood mercury concentration is due mostly to the dietary intake of organic forms, particularly methyl mercury. Urinary mercury consists mostly of inorganic mercury (Cianciola et al., 1997; Kingman et al., 1998). These distinctions can help interpret mercury blood levels in people. Total blood mercury levels increase with greater fish consumption (Dewailly et al., 2001; Grandjean et al., 1995; Mahaffey et al., 2004; Sanzo et al., 2001; Schober et al., 2003). Urine mercury levels increase as more occlusal surfaces of teeth are filled with mercury-containing amalgams (Becker et al., 2003).

In Germany the geometric mean for blood mercury was 0.58 µg/L for 4645 adults, aged 18 to 69 years, who participated in a 1998 representative population survey (Becker et al., 2002). From 1996 through 1998, Benes et al. (2000) studied 1216 blood donors in the Czech Republic (896 men and 320 women, average age 33 years; 758 children, average age 9.9 years); the median concentration of blood mercury was

0.78 µg/L for adults and 0.46 µg/L for children. A cohort of 1127 U.S. military veterans (mean age 52.8 years, range 40 years to 78 years) had an average total blood mercury concentration of 2.55 µg/L. These men had no occupational exposure to mercury but previously had received dental amalgams at military facilities (Kingman et al., 1998).

Over the NHANES 1999-2006 survey periods, total blood mercury geometric mean levels in females aged 16-49 years did not change, although non-Hispanic black females had higher levels than non-Hispanic white or Mexican American females. Among the three racial/ethnic groups, total blood mercury increased with age, and the age-related changes differed across the groups (Caldwell et al., 2009). During the same survey periods, total blood mercury levels declined slightly in non-Hispanic black and Mexican American children, and increased slightly in non-Hispanic white children (Caldwell, et al., 2009). In NHANES 1999-2002, slightly higher total blood mercury levels were found in U.S. adult women in several ethnic subgroups (Hightower et al., 2006).

Clinically observable signs of ataxia and paresthesias may occur when blood mercury levels increase to approximately 100 µg/L after methyl mercury poisoning. However, the developing fetus may be the most susceptible to the effects of ongoing methyl mercury exposure (NRC, 2000). A cord blood mercury level of 85 µg/L (lower 95% confidence bound = 58 µg/L) is associated with a 5% increase in the prevalence of an abnormal Boston Naming Test (NRC,

## Urinary Mercury—2003-2004

Geometric mean and selected percentiles of urine concentrations (in µg/L) for the U.S. population from the National Health and Nutrition Examination Survey.

| | Survey years | Geometric mean (95% conf. interval) | 50th | 75th | 90th | 95th | Sample size |
|---|---|---|---|---|---|---|---|
| | | | \>\>\> Selected percentiles ( 95% confidence interval) | | | | |
| Total | 03-04 | .447 (.406-.492) | .420 (.360-.480) | 1.00 (.870-1.14) | 2.08 (1.78-2.42) | 3.19 (2.76-3.55) | 2538 |
| **Age group** | | | | | | | |
| 6-11 years | 03-04 | .254 (.213-.304) | .200 (.160-.250) | .440 (.330-.580) | 1.16 (.610-1.61) | 1.96 (1.13-2.97) | 287 |
| 12-19 years | 03-04 | .358 (.313-.408) | .330 (.290-.370) | .700 (.530-.840) | 1.60 (1.14-2.52) | 2.93 (1.88-3.66) | 722 |
| 20 years and older | 03-04 | .495 (.442-.555) | .480 (.410-.570) | 1.12 (.930-1.29) | 2.20 (1.85-2.65) | 3.33 (2.76-3.88) | 1529 |
| **Gender** | | | | | | | |
| Males | 03-04 | .433 (.405-.463) | .400 (.350-.460) | .940 (.840-1.05) | 1.88 (1.63-2.18) | 2.68 (2.34-3.05) | 1266 |
| Females | 03-04 | .460 (.396-.534) | .430 (.330-.530) | 1.07 (.870-1.28) | 2.26 (1.77-2.90) | 3.54 (2.76-4.31) | 1272 |
| **Race/ethnicity** | | | | | | | |
| Mexican Americans | 03-04 | .416 (.340-.509) | .360 (.280-.430) | .960 (.700-1.23) | 2.19 (1.39-3.24) | 3.16 (1.99-6.30) | 619 |
| Non-Hispanic blacks | 03-04 | .476 (.413-.549) | .430 (.360-.530) | .890 (.770-1.00) | 1.96 (1.60-2.31) | 3.09 (2.03-4.89) | 713 |
| Non-Hispanic whites | 03-04 | .441 (.382-.509) | .420 (.330-.520) | 1.01 (.840-1.23) | 2.08 (1.67-2.46) | 3.24 (2.67-3.60) | 1066 |

Limit of detection (LOD, see Data Analysis section) for Survey year 03-04 is 0.14.

2000). Levels in U.S. women of childbearing age have generally been much lower than these levels (CDC, 2005). ACGIH recommends that the blood levels due to inorganic mercury exposure in workers not exceed 15 µg/L. Blood mercury levels of women and children in NHANES 1999-2006 were also below levels established as occupational exposure guidelines (Caldwell, et al., 2009). Information about the biological exposure indices is provided here for comparison, not to imply a safety level for general population exposure.

Urinary mercury levels in recent German (Becker et al., 2003), Czech (Benes et al., 2002), and Italian (Apostoli et al., 2002) adult population surveys were similar to those in a U.S. representative sample of women aged 16-49 years reported in NHANES 1999-2006 (Caldwell, et al., 2009). In the study of U.S. military veterans with dental amalgams, mean urinary mercury was 3.1 µg/L. Urine mercury and the number of dental amalgams were correlated, and on average, the urine mercury increased by approximately 0.1 µg/L for each surface with a dental amalgam (Kingman et al., 1998). Recent studies in children with dental amalgams and urinary levels less than 5 µg/g of creatinine did not have changes in cognitive-behavioral testing when followed for 5-7 years (Bellinger et al., 2006; DeRouen et al., 2006). An expert-panel report recently prepared for the U.S. Department of Health and Human Services noted that several studies have observed a modest, reversible increase in urinary N-acetyl-glucosaminidase, a biomarker of perturbation in renal tubular function, among

workers with urinary mercury concentrations of 25-35 µg/L or greater (Barregard et al., 1988; Langworth et al., 1992). The ACGIH (2007) currently recommends that urinary inorganic mercury in workers not exceed 35 µg/g of creatinine.

Finding a measurable amount of mercury in blood or urine does not mean that the level of mercury causes an adverse health effect. Biomonitoring studies provide physicians and public health officials with reference ranges so that they can determine whether people have been exposed to higher levels of mercury than are found in the general population. Biomonitoring data will also help scientists plan and conduct research on exposure and health effects.

## Urinary Mercury (creatinine corrected)—2003-2004

Geometric mean and selected percentiles of urine concentrations (in µg/g of creatinine) for the U.S. population from the National Health and Nutrition Examination Survey.

| | Survey years | Geometric mean (95% conf. interval) | Selected percentiles ( 95% confidence interval) | | | | Sample size |
|---|---|---|---|---|---|---|---|
| | | | 50th | 75th | 90th | 95th | |
| **Total** | 03-04 | .443 (.404-.486) | .447 (.392-.498) | .909 (.785-1.00) | 1.65 (1.40-1.86) | 2.35 (1 88-2.85) | 2537 |
| **Age group** | | | | | | | |
| 6-11 years | 03-04 | .297 (.246-.358) | .276 (.208-.347) | .485 (.391-.630) | 1.25 (.667-1.79) | 1.79 (1.11-2.61) | 286 |
| 12-19 years | 03-04 | .255 (.225-.289) | .217 (.196-.275) | .464 (.376-.535) | 1.06 (.714-1.39) | 1.67 (1.13-2.03) | 722 |
| 20 years and older | 03-04 | .508 (.455-.566) | .525 (.447-.616) | 1.00 (.875-1.09) | 1.76 (1.46-2.11) | 2.54 (2 04-3.00) | 1529 |
| **Gender** | | | | | | | |
| Males | 03-04 | .365 (.333-.400) | .362 (.309-.417) | .696 (.620-.784) | 1.31 (1.18-1.44) | 1.87 (1 51-2.30) | 1266 |
| Females | 03-04 | .532 (.472-.599) | .545 (.455-.652) | 1.06 (.969-1.21) | 1.88 (1.64-2.30) | 2.77 (2.12-3.56) | 1271 |
| **Race/ethnicity** | | | | | | | |
| Mexican Americans | 03-04 | .384 (.307-.480) | .365 (.280-.455) | .768 (.619-.990) | 1.62 (1 23-2.16) | 2.32 (1.78-4.01) | 618 |
| Non-Hispanic blacks | 03-04 | .343 (.301-.391) | .306 (.265-.368) | .587 (.522-.687) | 1.28 (.964-1.63) | 2.13 (1.41-2.87) | 713 |
| Non-Hispanic whites | 03-04 | .463 (.400-.537) | .476 (.385-.588) | .970 (.800-1.07) | 1.67 (1 32-2.11) | 2.40 (1 88-2.90) | 1066 |

## Urinary Mercury—Females Aged 16-49 Years Old, 1999-2002

Geometric mean and selected percentiles of urine concentrations (in µg/L) for females aged 16 to 49 years in the U.S. population, National Health and Nutrition Examination Survey, 1999-2002.

| | Survey years | Geometric mean (95% conf. interval) | Selected percentiles (95% confidence interval) | | | | Sample size |
|---|---|---|---|---|---|---|---|
| | | | 50th | 75th | 90th | 95th | |
| **Age group** (females) | | | | | | | |
| 16-49 years | 99-00 | **.719** (.622-.831) | **.760** (.610-.910) | **1.62** (1.43-1.94) | **3.15** (2.55-3.92) | **5.00** (3.59-5.79) | 1748 |
| | 01-02 | **.606** (.553-.665) | **.580** (.500-.670) | **1.37** (1.23-1.55) | **2.91** (2.53-3.17) | **3.99** (3.50-4.63) | 1960 |
| **Race/ethnicity** (females, 16-49 years) | | | | | | | |
| Mexican Americans | 99-00 | **.724** (.656-.799) | **.650** (.560-.810) | **1.69** (1.45-2.07) | **3.68** (3.10-4.45) | **5.62** (4.91-7.38) | 595 |
| | 01-02 | **.592** (.502-.699) | **.560** (.420-.710) | **1.35** (1.09-1.76) | **2.84** (2.32-3.85) | **4.13** (2.81-6.24) | 531 |
| Non-Hispanic blacks | 99-00 | **1.06** (.832-1.35) | **1.03** (.850-1.51) | **2.30** (1.83-3.03) | **4.81** (3.41-6.18) | **6.98** (5.04-10.3) | 381 |
| | 01-02 | **.772** (.616-.966) | **.740** (.540-.930) | **1.76** (1.30-2.37) | **3.50** (2.57-4.97) | **5.18** (3.61-6.92) | 442 |
| Non-Hispanic whites | 99-00 | **.657** (.557-.774) | **.710** (.520-.870) | **1.50** (1.31-1.77) | **2.84** (2.39-3.32) | **4.05** (3.16-5.52) | 594 |
| | 01-02 | **.565** (.501-.637) | **.540** (.450-.650) | **1.31** (1.09-1.56) | **2.70** (2.22-3.16) | **3.62** (3.13-4.54) | 826 |

Limit of detection (LOD, see Data Analysis section) for Survey years 99-00 and 01-02 are 0.14 and 0.14.

## Urinary Mercury (creatinine corrected)—Females Aged 16-49 Years Old, 1999-2002

Geometric mean and selected percentiles of urine concentrations (in µg/g of creatinine) for females aged 16 to 49 years in the U.S. population, National Health and Nutrition Examination Survey, 1999-2002.

| | Survey years | Geometric mean (95% conf. interval) | Selected percentiles (95% confidence interval) | | | | Sample size |
|---|---|---|---|---|---|---|---|
| | | | 50th | 75th | 90th | 95th | |
| **Age group** (females) | | | | | | | |
| 16-49 years | 99-00 | **.710** (.624-.806) | **.723** (.636-.833) | **1.41** (1.24-1.65) | **2.48** (2.10-2.97) | **3.27** (2.85-3 92) | 1748 |
| | 01-02 | **.620** (.579-.664) | **.650** (.582-.709) | **1.27** (1.15-1.42) | **2.30** (2.07-2.45) | **3.00** (2.68-3 39) | 1960 |
| **Race/ethnicity** (females, 16-49 years) | | | | | | | |
| Mexican Americans | 99-00 | **.685** (.580-.809) | **.639** (.508-.790) | **1.45** (1.27-1.61) | **2.89** (2.21-3.42) | **4.51** (3.07-5.68) | 595 |
| | 01-02 | **.600** (.526-.686) | **.596** (.426-.709) | **1.32** (1.04-1.47) | **2.41** (2.14-2.77) | **3.21** (2.65-4.46) | 531 |
| Non-Hispanic blacks | 99-00 | **.658** (.520-.831) | **.615** (.475-.892) | **1.22** (.909-1.79) | **2.56** (1.69-3.99) | **3.99** (2.76-5.14) | 381 |
| | 01-02 | **.522** (.410-.665) | **.516** (.387-.664) | **1.03** (.742-1.47) | **1.97** (1.42-3.25) | **3.21** (1.87-4.44) | 442 |
| Non-Hispanic whites | 99-00 | **.706** (.605-.824) | **.721** (.631-.846) | **1.41** (1.23-1.72) | **2.46** (1.99-2.97) | **3.05** (2.46-4 00) | 594 |
| | 01-02 | **.632** (.578-.691) | **.655** (.569-.744) | **1.28** (1.14-1.45) | **2.30** (2.03-2.56) | **2.95** (2.45-3 53) | 826 |

## References

Aberg B, Ekman L, Falk R, Greitz U, Persson G, Snihs JO. Metabolism of methyl mercury ($^{203}$Hg) compounds in man. Arch Environ Health 1969;19:478-484.

ACGIH. 2007 TLVs and BEIs. Based on the Documentation of the Threshold Limit Values for Chemical Substances and Physical Agents and Biological Exposure Indices. Cincinnati (OH): Signature Publications.

Apostoli P, Cortesi I, Mangili A, Elia G, Drago I, Gagliardi T, et al. Assessment of reference values for mercury in urine: the results of an Italian polycentric study. Sci Total Environ 2002;289:13-24.

Barregard L, Hultberg B., Schuzt A, Sallsten G. Enzymuria in workers exposed to inorganic mercury. Int Arch Occup Environ Health 1988;61:65-69.

Barregard L, Sallsten G, Conradi N. Tissue levels of mercury determined in a deceased worker after occupational exposure. Int Arch Occup Environ Health 1999;72:169-173.

Barregard L, Sallsten G, Schutz A, Attewell R, Skerfving S, Jarvholm B. Kinetics of mercury in blood and urine after brief occupational exposure. Arch Environ Health 1992;7(3):176-184.

Bates MN, Fawcett J, Garrett N, Cutress T, Kjellstrom T. Health effects of dental amalgam exposure: a retrospective cohort study. Int J Epidemiol 2004;33:1-9.

Becker K, Kaus S, Krause C, Lepom P, Schulz C, Seiwert M, et al. German Environmental Survey 1998 (GerES III): environmental pollutants in blood of the German population. Int JHyg Environ Health 2002;205:297-308.

Becker K, Schulz C, Kaus S, Seiwert M, Seifert B. German environmental survey 1998 (GerES III): environmental pollutants in the urine of the German population. Int J Hyg Environ Health 2003; 206:15-24.

Bellinger DC, Trachtenberg F, Barregard L, Tavares M, Cernichiari E, Daniel D, McKinlay S. Neuropsychological and renal effects of dental amalgam in children: a randomized clinical trial. JAMA 2006;295(15):1775-1783.

Benes B, Spevackova V, Smid J, Cejchanova M, Cerna M, Subrt P, et al. The concentration levels of Cd, Pb, Hg, Cu, Zn, and Se in blood of the population in the Czech Republic. Cent Eur J Public Health 2000;8(2):117-119.

Bidstrup PL, Bonnell JA, Harvey DG, Locket S. Chronic mercury poisoning in men repairing direct-current meters. Lancet 1951;2:856-861.

Bjornberg KA, Vahter M, Berglund B, Niklasson B, Biennow M, Sandborgh-englund B. Transport of methylmercury and inorganic mercury to the fetus and breast-fed infant. Environ Health Perspect 2005;113(10):1381-1385.

Caldwell KL, Mortensen ME, Jones RL, Caudill SP, Osterloh JD. Total blood mercury concentrations in the U.S. population: 1999-2006. Int J Hyg Environ Health 2009;212:588-598.

Cardenas A, Roels H, Bernard AM, Barbon R, Buchet JP, Lauwerys RR, et al. Markers of early renal changes induced by industrial pollutants. I. Application to workers exposed to mercury vapour. Br J Ind Med 1993;50:17-27.

Cernichiari E, Brewer R, Myers GJ, Marsh DO, Lapham LW, Cox C, et al. Monitoring methylmercury during pregnancy: maternal hari predicts fetal brain exposure. Neurotoxicology 1995;16(4):705-710.

Centers for Disease Control and Prevention (CDC). Third National Report on Human Exposure to Environmental Chemicals. Atlanta (GA). 2005.

Chan JM, Egeland FM. Fish consumption, mercury exposure, and heart diseases. Nutr Rev 2004;62(2):68-72.

Cianciola ME, Echeverria D, Martin MD, Aposian HV, Woods JS. Epidemiologic assessment of measures used to indicate low-level exposure to mercury vapor (Hg°). J Toxicol Environ Health 1997; 52:19-33.

DeRouen TA, Martin MD, Leroux BG, Townes BD, Woods JS, Leitão J, Castro-Caldas A, Luis H, Bernardo M, Rosenbaum G, Martins IP. Neurobehavioral effects of dental amalgam in children: a randomized clinical trial. JAMA 2006;295(15):1784-1792.

Dewailly E, Ayotte P, Bruneau S, Lebel G, Levallois P, Weber JP. Exposure of the Inuit population of Nunavik (Arctic Quebec) to lead and mercury. Arch Environ Health 2001;56(4):350-357.

Drexler H, Schaller KH. The mercury concentration in breast milk resulting from amalgam fillings and dietary habits. Environ Res 1998;77(2):124-129.

Factor-Litvak P, Hasselgren G, Jacobs D, Begg M, Kline J, Geier J, et al. Mercury derived from dental amalgams and neuropsychologic function. Environ Health Perspect 2003;111:719-723.

Grandjean P, Budtz-Jorgensen E, White RF, Jorgensen PJ, Weihe P, Debes F, et al. Methylmercury exposure biomarkers as indicators of neurotoxicity in children aged 7 years. Am J Epidemiol 1999;149:301-305.

Grandjean P, Weihe P, Jorgensen PJ, Clarkson T, Cernichiari E, Videro T. Impact of maternal seafood diet on fetal exposure to mercury, selenium, and lead. Arch Environ Health 1992;47(3):185-195.

Grandjean P, Weihe P, Needham LL, Burse VW, Patterson DG Jr, Sampson EJ, et al. Relation of a seafood diet to mercury, selenium, arsenic, and polychlorinated biphenyl and other organochlorine concentrations in human milk. Environ Res 1995;71(1):29-38.

Halbach S. Amalgam tooth fillings and man's mercury burden. Hum Exp Toxicol 1994;13:496-501.

Hattula T, Rahola T. The distribution and biological half-time of [203]Hg in the human body according to a modified whole-body counting technique. Environ Physiol Biochem 1975;5:252-257.

Hightower JM, O'Hare A, Hernandez GT. Blood mercury reporting in NHANES: Identifying Asian, Pacific Islander, Native American, and multiracial groups. Environ Health Perspect 2006;114(2):173-175.

Hursh JB, Greenwood MR, Clarkson TW, Allen J, Demuth S. The effect of ethanol on the fate of mercury vapor inhaled by man. J Pharmacol Exp Ther 1980;214(3):520-527.

International Agency for Research on Cancer (IARC). IARC Monographs on the Evaluation of Risks to Humans. Volume 58. Beryllium, Cadmium, Mercury, and Exposures in the Glass Manufacturing industry. 1993. Available at URL: http://monographs.iarc.fr/ENG/Monographs/vol58/index.php. 7/15/09

Jonsson F, Sandborgh-Englund G, Johanson G. A compartmental model for the kinetics of mercury vapor in humans. Toxicol Appl Pharmacol 1999;155(2):161-168.

Kajiwara Y, Yasutake A, Adachi T, Hirayama K. methylmercury transport across the placenta via neutral amino acid carrier. Arch Toxicol 1996;70(5):310-314.

Kingman A, Albertini T, Brown LJ. Mercury concentrations in urine and whole blood associated with amalgam exposure in a US military population. J Dent Res 1998;77(3):461-467.

Langworth S, Elinder CG, Sundquist KG, Vesterberg O. Renal and immunological effects of occupational exposure to inorganic mercury. Br J Ind Med 1992;49(6):394-401.

McDowell MA, Dillon CF, Osterloh J, Bolger PM, Pellizzari E, Fernando R, et al. Hair mercury levels in U.S. children and women of childbearing age: reference range data from NHANES 1999-2000. Environ Health Perspect 2004;112(11):1165-1171.

Mehaffey KR, Clickner RP, Bodurow CC. Blood organic mercury and dietary intake: National Health and Nutrition Examination Survey, 1999 and 2000. Environ Health Perspect 2004;112(5):562-570.

Miettinen JK, Rahola T, Hattula T, Rissanen K, Tillander M. Elimination of [203]Hg-methyl mercury in man. Ann Clin Res 1971;3(2):116-122.

Myers GJ, Davidson PW, Cox C, Shamlaye CF, Palumbo D, Cernichari, et al. Prenatal methylmercury exposure from ocean fish consumption in the Seychelles child development study. Lancet 2003;361:1686-1692.

National Research Council (NRC). Toxicological effects of methylmercury. National Academy Press. Washington (DC). 2000.

Oskarsson A, Schultz A, Skerfving S, Hallen IP, Ohlin B, Lagerkvist BJ. Total and inorganic mercury in breast milk and blood in relation to fish consumption and amalgam fillings in lactating women. Arch Environ Health 1996;51(3):234-241.

Rahola T, Hattula T, Korolainen A, Miettinen JK. Elimination of free and protein-bound ionic mercury ([203]Hg[2+]) in man. Ann Clin Res 1973;5:214-219.

Rice DC. The US EPA reference dose for methyl mercury: sources of uncertainty. Environ Res 2004;95:406-13.

Rissanen T, Voutilainen S, Nyyssonen K, Lakka TA, Salonen JT. Fish oil-derived fatty acids, docosahexaenoic acid and docosapentaenoic acid, and the risk of acute coronary events—The Kuopio Ischaemic Heart Disease Risk Factor Study. Circulation 2000;103:2766-2679.

Roels HA, Boeckx M, Ceulemans E, Lauwerys RR. Urinary excretion of mercury after occupational exposure to mercury vapor and influence of the chelating agent meso-2,3-dimercaptosuccinic acid (DMSA). Br J Ind Med 1991;48:247-53.

Sakamoto M, Kubota M, Matsumoto S, Nakano A, Akagi H. Declining risk of methylmercury exposure to infants during lactation. Environ Res 2002;90:185-189.

Sakamoto M, Kubota M, Liu XJ, Murata K, Nakai K, Satoh H. Maternal and fetal mercury and n-3 polyunsaturated fatty acids as a risk and benefit of fish consumption to fetus. Environ Sci Technol 2004;38:3860-3863.

Salonen JT, Seppanen K, Nyyssonen K, Korpela H, Kauhanen J, Kantola M, et al. Intake of mercury from fish, lipid peroxidation, and the risk of myocardial infarction and coronary, cardiovascular, and any death in eastern Finnish men. Circulation 1995;91:645-655.

Sallsten G, Barregard L, Schutz A. Decrease in mercury concentration in blood after long term exposure: a kinetic study of chloralkali workers. Br J Ind Med 1993;50(9):814-821.

Sanchez-Sicilia L, Seto DS, Nakamoto S, Kolff WJ. Acute mercurial intoxication treated by hemodialysis. Ann Intern Med 1963;59(5):692-706.

Sandborgh-Englund G, Elinder CG, Langworth S, Schutz A, Ekstrand J. Mercury in biological fluids after amalgam removal. J Dent Res 1998;77(4):615-624.

Sanzo JM, Dorronsoro M, Amiano P, Amurrio A, Aguinagalde FX, Azpiri MA. Estimation and validation of mercury intake associated with fish consumption in an EPIC cohort of Spain. Public Health Nutr 2001;4(5):981-988.

Schober SE, Sinks TH, Jones RL, Bolger PM, McDowell M, Osterloh J, et al. Blood mercury levels in US children and women of childbearing age, 1999-2000. JAMA 2003;289(13):1667-1674.

Sherlock J, Hislop D, Newton G, Topping G, Whittle K. Elevation of mercury in human blood from controlled ingestion of methyl mercury in fish. Hum Toxicol 1984;2:117-131.

Smith JC, Allen PV, Turner MD, Most B, Fisher HL, Hall LL. The kinetics of intravenously administered methyl mercury in man. Toxicol Appl Pharmacol 1994;128(2):25125-25126.

Smith JC, Farris FF. Methyl mercury pharmacokinetics in man: a reevaluation. Toxicol Appl Pharmacol 1996;37:245-252.

Smith PJ, Langolf GD, Goldberg J. Effects of occupational exposure to elemental mercury on short term memory. Br J Ind Med 1983;40:413-419.

Smith RG, Vorwald AJ, Patil LS, Mooney TF. Effects of exposure to mercury in the manufacture of chlorine. Am Ind Hyg Assoc J 1970;31:687-700.

Stern AH. A review of the studies of the cardiovascular health effects of methylmercury with consideration of their suitability for risk assessment. Environ Res 2005;98(1):133-142.

Stern AH, Smith AE. An assessment of the cord blood: maternal blood methyl mercury ratio: implications for risk assessment. Environ Health Perspect 2003;111(12):1465-1470.

Suzuki T, Hongo T, Yoshinaga J, Imai H, Nakazawa M, Matsuo N, et al. The hair-organ relationship in mercury concentration in contemporary Japanese. Arch Environ Health 1993;48(4):221-229.

Tunnessen WW, McMahon KJ, Baser M. Acrodynia: exposure to mercury from fluorescent light bulbs. Pediatrics 1987;79:786-789.

Vahter M, Mottet NK, Friberg L, Lind B, Shen DD, Burbacher T. Speciation of mercury in the primate blood and brain following long-term exposure to methyl mercury. Toxicol Appl Pharmacol 1994;124:221-229.

Vimy MJ, Takahashi Y, Lorscheider FL. Maternal-fetal distribution of mercury (203Hg) released from dental amalgam fillings. Am J Physiol 1990;258(4 Pt 2):R939-945.

Vupputuri S, Longnecker MP, Daniels JL, Guo S, Sandler DP. Blood mercury level and blood pressure among US women: results from the National Health and Nutrition Examination Survey 1999-2000. Environ Res 2005;97(2):195-200.

Woods JS, Martin MD, Leroux BG, DeRouen TA, Leitao JG, Bernardo MF, et al. The contribution of dental amalgam to urinary mercury excretion in children. Environ Health Perspect 2007;115(10):1527-1531.

Zeitz P, Orr MF, Kaye WE. Public health consequences of mercury spills: hazardous substances emergency events surveillance system, 1993-1998. Environ Health Perspect 2002;110:129-132.

# Molybdenum
CAS No. 7439-98-7

### General Information

Elemental molybdenum is a silver-white, hard metal widely used to add strength and hardness and retard corrosion in metal alloys. Compounds of molybdenum are also used as corrosion inhibitors, hydrogenation catalysts, lubricants, chemical reagents in hospital laboratories, and in pigments for ceramics, inks, and paints. More recently, semiconductor and battery industries have begun to use molybdenum. Molybdenum occurs in natural waters and may be present in concentrations of several hundred micrograms per liter or higher in ground and surface water near mining operations or ore deposits.

Molybdenum is a nutritionally essential trace element that enters the body primarily from dietary sources. In humans, molybdenum is a cofactor for three enzyme classes—sulfite oxidase, aldehyde dehydrogenase, and xanthine oxidase (Kisker et al., 1997). The recommended dietary allowance for adult men and women is 45 µg/day (IOM, 2001), and the average dietary daily intake of molybdenum is approximately 100 µg/day (IOM, 2001; WHO, 1996). Gastrointestinal absorption of molybdenum averages 88-93% for dietary intakes of 22-1490 µg/day. Excretion occurs predominantly via the kidneys, which exert homeostatic regulation over molybdenum balance. At a daily oral molybdenum dose of 24 µg, urinary excretion over six days

### Urinary Molybdenum

Geometric mean and selected percentiles of urine concentrations (in µg/L) for the U.S. population from the National Health and Nutrition Examination survey.

| | Survey years | Geometric mean (95% conf. interval) | 50th | 75th | 90th | 95th | Sample size |
|---|---|---|---|---|---|---|---|
| **Total** | 99-00 | **45.9** (40.1-52.6) | **50.7** (44.6-58.4) | **84.9** (78.7-92.3) | **135** (125-146) | **180** (154-216) | 2257 |
| | 01-02 | **45.0** (42.1-48.0) | **52.4** (48.9-55.5) | **83.4** (79.1-88.7) | **124** (117-130) | **165** (145-176) | 2690 |
| | 03-04 | **39.7** (37.7-41.7) | **44.5** (41.6-46.7) | **78.5** (74.9-82.3) | **111** (105-118) | **138** (133-146) | 2558 |
| **Age group** | | | | | | | |
| 6-11 years | 99-00 | **78.2** (61.0-100) | **84.8** (67.7-105) | **126** (106-147) | **178** (147-259) | **267** (159-840) | 310 |
| | 01-02 | **63.3** (53.4-75.0) | **69.2** (63.0-77.6) | **109** (94.5-124) | **169** (138-197) | **197** (161-291) | 368 |
| | 03-04 | **62.2** (56.7-68.3) | **71.3** (55.7-84.1) | **108** (92.7-122) | **138** (127-152) | **181** (138-235) | 290 |
| 12-19 years | 99-00 | **54.3** (47.6-62.0) | **60.6** (52.2-70.3) | **93.3** (79.9-109) | **146** (112-171) | **188** (146-216) | 648 |
| | 01-02 | **60.6** (55.5-66.2) | **65.7** (58.7-73.1) | **97.1** (91.8-108) | **145** (129-159) | **179** (155-227) | 762 |
| | 03-04 | **52.5** (49.0-56.3) | **59.6** (55.5-65.1) | **87.3** (84.5-91.4) | **118** (105-125) | **143** (130-156) | 725 |
| 20 years and older | 99-00 | **41.7** (36.7-47.4) | **46.6** (40.5-52.5) | **76.7** (73.4-82.2) | **126** (114-134) | **168** (143-206) | 1299 |
| | 01-02 | **41.1** (38.3-44.1) | **47.6** (43.7-51.2) | **79.1** (71.9-83.6) | **114** (103-124) | **150** (130-166) | 1560 |
| | 03-04 | **35.9** (34.0-38.0) | **40.3** (37.6-42.1) | **71.5** (67.3-75.2) | **105** (98.6-111) | **133** (119-144) | 1543 |
| **Gender** | | | | | | | |
| Males | 99-00 | **52.7** (45.7-60.7) | **57.5** (48.5-68.4) | **93.2** (83.8-106) | **150** (128-187) | **215** (161-278) | 1121 |
| | 01-02 | **51.0** (46.6-55.7) | **56.9** (52.0-62.6) | **88.5** (81.6-96.5) | **130** (120-141) | **169** (145-194) | 1335 |
| | 03-04 | **45.5** (43.3-47.8) | **51.0** (48.1-55.4) | **85.8** (82.8-90.7) | **119** (112-130) | **148** (136-163) | 1281 |
| Females | 99-00 | **40.4** (34.8-46.8) | **45.6** (40.4-52.0) | **77.3** (71.0-85.7) | **119** (105-138) | **154** (132-180) | 1136 |
| | 01-02 | **39.9** (37.2-42.9) | **45.8** (42.8-49.3) | **78.4** (72.6-82.9) | **115** (104-128) | **158** (130-177) | 1355 |
| | 03-04 | **34.9** (32.2-37.7) | **37.9** (33.5-41.6) | **67.3** (64.6-72.2) | **101** (97.3-108) | **127** (114-139) | 1277 |
| **Race/ethnicity** | | | | | | | |
| Mexican Americans | 99-00 | **47.0** (42.1-52.4) | **53.2** (49.2-59.0) | **80.6** (73.7-91.7) | **121** (103-139) | **152** (120-217) | 780 |
| | 01-02 | **49.3** (46.5-52.3) | **55.7** (50.4-61.0) | **86.4** (80.8-94.1) | **133** (113-155) | **177** (142-207) | 683 |
| | 03-04 | **47.0** (43.1-51.1) | **54.4** (48.2-59.9) | **82.9** (73.2-91.0) | **121** (106-143) | **152** (141-169) | 618 |
| Non-Hispanic blacks | 99-00 | **57.7** (51.0-65.2) | **62.2** (55.0-71.5) | **97.8** (85.0-110) | **153** (126-188) | **206** (150-274) | 546 |
| | 01-02 | **53.2** (49.9-56.7) | **60.3** (55.1-63.8) | **90.0** (81.0-101) | **132** (121-147) | **166** (147-170) | 667 |
| | 03-04 | **46.0** (41.7-50.8) | **46.2** (40.9-55.2) | **82.3** (73.3-91.3) | **117** (109-129) | **156** (135-175) | 723 |
| Non-Hispanic whites | 99-00 | **44.5** (37.0-53.4) | **48.5** (41.1-59.8) | **85.0** (76.7-96.5) | **135** (119-154) | **187** (146-223) | 760 |
| | 01-02 | **42.2** (38.5-46.2) | **48.9** (44.2-53.2) | **80.7** (71.9-85.8) | **117** (108-129) | **152** (134-180) | 1132 |
| | 03-04 | **37.1** (34.7-39.6) | **41.3** (38.1-44.5) | **75.2** (69.2-79.6) | **107** (99.3-115) | **130** (119-142) | 1074 |

Limits of detection (LOD, see Data Analysis section) for survey years 99-00, 01-02, and 03-04 are 0.8, 0.8, and 1.5, respectively.

was 18% of the ingested dose; at daily oral doses of 95 µg and 428 µg, urinary excretion over six days rose to 50% and 67%, respectively, of the ingested dose (Turnlund et al., 1995). In industry, dust and other fine particles produced during refining or shaping of molybdenum or molybdenum-containing alloys are inhalational pathways of exposure.

Human health effects from molybdenum at low environmental doses or at biomonitored levels from low environmental exposures are unknown. Molybdenum is generally considered to be of low human toxicity, and clinical or epidemiologic evidence of adverse effects is limited. Chronic exposure to very high levels may result in higher serum uric acid levels and a gout-like illness (Koval'skiy et al., 1961; U.S. EPA, 1993). Based on studies finding adverse reproductive effects in rats and mice,

the Panel on Micronutrients of the Institute of Medicine identified a no observed adverse effect level (NOAEL) of 0.9 mg/kg/day and established a tolerable upper intake level of 0.03 mg/kg/day in humans (IOM, 2001). A long term inhalation bioassay of molybdenum trioxide in mice yielded "some evidence" of carcinogenicity (NTP, 1997). One case-control study suggested a possible link between occupational exposure to molybdenum and lung cancer (Droste et al., 1999), but available epidemiologic data are scant, and molybdenum has not been systematically evaluated for carcinogenicity by IARC.

**Biomonitoring Information**

Molybdenum is an essential element for health, and urinary levels reflect intake from all sources. Levels of molybdenum

## Urinary Molybdenum (creatinine corrected)

Geometric mean and selected percentiles of urine concentrations (in µg/g of creatinine) for the U.S. population from the National Health and Nutrition Examination survey.

| | Survey years | Geometric mean (95% conf. interval) | 50th | 75th | 90th | 95th | Sample size |
|---|---|---|---|---|---|---|---|
| | | | \ ( 95% confidence interval) | | | | |
| **Total** | 99-00 | 43.2 (40.0-46.6) | 41.6 (38.5-45.2) | 63.5 (59.3-68.8) | 108 (97.3-115) | 144 (125-171) | 2257 |
| | 01-02 | 42.5 (39.9-45.2) | 42.2 (40.1-45.2) | 62.0 (58.4-66.4) | 98.8 (90.1-109) | 130 (120-149) | 2689 |
| | 03-04 | 39.4 (37.6-41.3) | 39.2 (37.9-40.7) | 58.3 (55.6-61.5) | 89.0 (80.5-99.0) | 120 (107-135) | 2558 |
| **Age group** | | | | | | | |
| 6-11 years | 99-00 | 85.9 (73.7-100) | 79.3 (71.6-88.4) | 122 (107-133) | 173 (130-243) | 214 (154-1040) | 310 |
| | 01-02 | 77.2 (73.1-81.5) | 77.6 (71.8-84.5) | 109 (99.4-120) | 159 (129-170) | 185 (165-219) | 368 |
| | 03-04 | 72.5 (65.2-80.7) | 73.5 (65.1-79.9) | 101 (84.9-117) | 132 (107-158) | 160 (129-257) | 290 |
| 12-19 years | 99-00 | 41.9 (39.3-44.6) | 40.5 (37.7-44.4) | 57.3 (51.5-62.5) | 85.4 (67.4-107) | 112 (78.4-185) | 648 |
| | 01-02 | 43.4 (40.8-46.1) | 44.1 (40.8-47.2) | 60.8 (57.6-63.7) | 85.5 (79.7-93.8) | 106 (94.8-118) | 762 |
| | 03-04 | 37.5 (35.4-39.8) | 38.9 (36.9-41.8) | 53.2 (50.3-56.1) | 71.9 (64.6-76.9) | 81.0 (74.3-102) | 725 |
| 20 years and older | 99-00 | 39.6 (36.9-42.6) | 38.5 (36.1-41.0) | 56.4 (53.5-60.7) | 92.5 (83.1-100) | 122 (116-147) | 1299 |
| | 01-02 | 39.3 (36.8-42.0) | 39.6 (36.4-42.1) | 57.2 (52.9-61.0) | 86.7 (75.2-96.8) | 123 (109-139) | 1559 |
| | 03-04 | 36.9 (35.0-38.9) | 37.0 (35.7-38.4) | 53.5 (50.0-56.9) | 79.8 (75.9-87.5) | 118 (101-134) | 1543 |
| **Gender** | | | | | | | |
| Males | 99-00 | 40.8 (37.5-44.3) | 38.5 (37.2-40.4) | 62.4 (55.9-68.4) | 101 (83.9-118) | 131 (112-179) | 1121 |
| | 01-02 | 40.3 (37.1-43.8) | 40.2 (36.3-43.3) | 60.5 (54.8-66.3) | 91.3 (83.4-106) | 123 (107-155) | 1334 |
| | 03-04 | 38.3 (36.1-40.7) | 37.8 (36.1-39.3) | 56.3 (53.3-59.3) | 85.7 (77.2-96.7) | 118 (100-139) | 1281 |
| Females | 99-00 | 45.5 (41.5-50.0) | 44.1 (39.5-48.8) | 64.4 (59.5-70.5) | 112 (95.2-121) | 152 (122-181) | 1136 |
| | 01-02 | 44.6 (42.2-47.1) | 45.1 (42.2-46.9) | 63.6 (59.5-69.4) | 107 (92.5-119) | 136 (117-169) | 1355 |
| | 03-04 | 40.5 (38.1-43.0) | 41.1 (38.7-43.7) | 61.4 (56.8-65.1) | 90.1 (82.2-103) | 122 (115-142) | 1277 |
| **Race/ethnicity** | | | | | | | |
| Mexican Americans | 99-00 | 42.9 (40.6-45.4) | 43.2 (40.9-45.6) | 61.6 (57.2-65.5) | 89.5 (80.0-103) | 115 (93.7-137) | 780 |
| | 01-02 | 48.1 (44.3-52.2) | 48.4 (44.8-52.3) | 71.7 (66.4-76.0) | 103 (90.0-120) | 129 (109-155) | 682 |
| | 03-04 | 43.5 (40.5-46.8) | 43.5 (41.0-46.2) | 62.8 (56.8-67.2) | 85.9 (79.5-97.0) | 112 (97.0-133) | 618 |
| Non-Hispanic blacks | 99-00 | 37.2 (33.4-41.6) | 37.1 (33.0-41.2) | 55.9 (49.6-63.3) | 88.2 (69.1-112) | 119 (88.3-141) | 546 |
| | 01-02 | 36.5 (34.1-39.0) | 37.5 (35.1-38.9) | 57.1 (49.7-62.4) | 78.3 (71.5-92.0) | 109 (81.1-127) | 667 |
| | 03-04 | 33.1 (30.5-35.9) | 31.7 (30.1-34.7) | 47.2 (43.7-52.1) | 72.9 (64.6-78.4) | 90.5 (78.4-118) | 723 |
| Non-Hispanic whites | 99-00 | 44.5 (40.2-49.2) | 42.1 (38.8-47.3) | 65.3 (58.9-71.3) | 116 (101-126) | 172 (131-195) | 760 |
| | 01-02 | 42.5 (39.3-46.0) | 41.9 (39.3-45.6) | 61.2 (57.1-67.2) | 104 (88.7-120) | 138 (120-163) | 1132 |
| | 03-04 | 39.1 (37.2-41.1) | 39.3 (37.7-40.8) | 58.1 (54.6-61.4) | 87.4 (78.9-96.7) | 118 (106-134) | 1074 |

in urine for the U.S. population were well characterized in NHANES 1999-2000 and 2001-2002 (CDC, 2005); these levels were comparable to those reported for adults in smaller European population surveys (Iversen et al., 1998; Minoia et al., 2002; White and Sabbioni, 1998). Urinary molybdenum concentrations in infants may be slightly lower than those in other age groups (Sievers et al., 2001).

Finding a measurable amount of molybdenum in the urine does not mean that the level of molybdenum causes an adverse health effect. Biomonitoring studies on levels of molybdenum can provide physicians and public health officials with reference values so that they can determine whether people have been exposed to higher levels of molybdenum than are found in the general population. Biomonitoring data can also help scientists plan and conduct research on exposure and health effects.

## References

Centers for Disease Control and Prevention (CDC). Third National Report on Human Exposure to Environmental Chemicals. Atlanta (GA). 2005.

Droste JHJ, Weyler JJ, Van Meerbeeck JP, Vermeire PA, van Sprundel MP. Occupational risk factors of lung cancer: a hospital based case-control study. Occup Environ Med 1999; 56:322-327.

Institute of Medicine (IOM). Standing Committee on the Scientific Evaluation of Dietary Reference Intakes, Food and Nutrition Board. Dietary reference intakes for vitamin A, vitamin K, arsenic, boron, chromium, copper, iodine, iron, manganese, molybdenum, nickel, silicon, vanadium, and zinc: a report of the Panel on Micronutrients. Washington, (DC): National Academy Press; 2001. pp. 420-441. Available at URL: http://books nap. edu/openbook.php?record_id=10026&page=420. 4/14/09

Iversen BS, Menne C, White MA, Kristiansen J, Christensen JM, Sabbioni E. Inductively coupled plasma mass spectrometric determination of molybdenum in urine from a Danish population. Analyst 1998;123(1):81-85.

Kisker C, Schindelin H, Rees DC. Molybdenum-cofactor-containing enzymes: structure and mechanism. Ann Rev Biochem 1997;66:233-267.

Koval'skiy GA, Yarovaya GA, Shmavonyan DM. Changes of purine metabolism in man and animals under conditions of molybdenum biogeochemical provinces. Zhurnal Obshchey Biologii 1961;22(3):179-191.

Minoia C, Gatti A, Aprea C, Ronchi A, Sciarra G, Turci R, et al. Inductively coupled plasma mass spectrometric determination of molybdenum in urine. Rapid Comm Mass Spectrom 2002; 16:1313-1319.

National Toxicology Program (NTP). TR-462. Toxicology and carcinogenesis studies of molybdenum trioxide (CAS No. 1313-27-5) in F344 Rats and B6C3F1 Mice (inhalation studies) 1997 [online]. Available at URL: http://ntp niehs.nih.gov/index. cfm?objectid=070A72C6-E9C1-AE67-4BFAB97AD0F427E8. 4/14/09

Sievers E, Schleyerbach U, Schaub J. Molybdenum in infancy: methodical investigation of urinary excretion. J Trace Elem Med Biol 2001;15(2-3):149-154.

Turnlund JR, Keyes WR, Peiffer GL. Molybdenum absorption, excretion, and retention studied with stable isotopes in young men at five intakes of dietary molybdenum. Am J Clin Nutr 1995;62(4):790-796.

U.S. Environmental Protection Agency (U.S. EPA). Molybdenum 1993 [online]. Available at URL: http://www.epa.gov/iris/subst/0425 htm. 4/14/09

White MA, Sabbioni E. Trace element reference values in tissues from inhabitants of the European Union. X. A study of 13 elements in blood and urine of a United Kingdom population. Sci Total Environ 1998;216:253-270.

World Health Organization (WHO). Molybdenum. In: Trace elements in human nutrition and health. Geneva: WHO, 1996. pp. 144-154.

# Platinum
CAS No. 7440-06-4

## General Information

Platinum is a silver-gray, lustrous metal found naturally in extremely low amounts in the earth's crust and is typically associated with sulfide-ore bodies of nickel, copper, and iron. Important properties of platinum are resistance to corrosion, strength at high temperatures, and high catalytic activity. Platinum compounds are used in electrodes, jewelry, dental alloys, thick-film circuits printed on ceramic substrates, as oxidation catalysts in chemical manufacturing, and as drugs (e.g., cisplatin, carboplatin) in the treatment of cancer. Platinum-rhodium and platinum-palladium crystals are used as catalysts in petroleum refining and in vehicular catalytic converters to control exhaust emissions. Platinum-rhodium compounds are also used in glass and glass-fiber manufacture and in high-temperature thermocouples. Higher environmental soil concentrations of platinum from vehicular emissions have been found near roadways (Farago et al., 1998); however, the ambient air concentrations of platinum associated with its use in automotive engine catalytic converters are estimated to be thousands of times lower than occupational exposure limits.

Human health effects from platinum at low environmental

## Urinary Platinum

Geometric mean and selected percentiles of urine concentrations (in µg/L) for the U.S. population from the National Health and Nutrition Examination Survey.

| | Survey years | Geometric mean (95% conf. interval) | 50th | 75th | 90th | 95th | Sample size |
|---|---|---|---|---|---|---|---|
| | | | | | | | |
| **Total** | 99-00 | * | < LOD | < LOD | < LOD | < LOD | 2465 |
| | 01-02 | * | < LOD | < LOD | < LOD | < LOD | 2690 |
| | 03-04 | * | < LOD | < LOD | < LOD | < LOD | 2558 |
| **Age group** | | | | | | | |
| 6-11 years | 99-00 | * | < LOD | < LOD | < LOD | < LOD | 340 |
| | 01-02 | * | < LOD | < LOD | < LOD | < LOD | 368 |
| | 03-04 | * | < LOD | < LOD | < LOD | < LOD | 290 |
| 12-19 years | 99-00 | * | < LOD | < LOD | < LOD | < LOD | 719 |
| | 01-02 | * | < LOD | < LOD | < LOD | < LOD | 762 |
| | 03-04 | * | < LOD | < LOD | < LOD | < LOD | 725 |
| 20 years and older | 99-00 | * | < LOD | < LOD | < LOD | < LOD | 1406 |
| | 01-02 | * | < LOD | < LOD | < LOD | < LOD | 1560 |
| | 03-04 | * | < LOD | < LOD | < LOD | < LOD | 1543 |
| **Gender** | | | | | | | |
| Males | 99-00 | * | < LOD | < LOD | < LOD | < LOD | 1227 |
| | 01-02 | * | < LOD | < LOD | < LOD | < LOD | 1335 |
| | 03-04 | * | < LOD | < LOD | < LOD | < LOD | 1281 |
| Females | 99-00 | * | < LOD | < LOD | < LOD | < LOD | 1238 |
| | 01-02 | * | < LOD | < LOD | < LOD | < LOD | 1355 |
| | 03-04 | * | < LOD | < LOD | < LOD | < LOD | 1277 |
| **Race/ethnicity** | | | | | | | |
| Mexican Americans | 99-00 | * | < LOD | < LOD | < LOD | < LOD | 884 |
| | 01-02 | * | < LOD | < LOD | < LOD | < LOD | 683 |
| | 03-04 | * | < LOD | < LOD | < LOD | < LOD | 618 |
| Non-Hispanic blacks | 99-00 | * | < LOD | < LOD | < LOD | < LOD | 568 |
| | 01-02 | * | < LOD | < LOD | < LOD | < LOD | 667 |
| | 03-04 | * | < LOD | < LOD | < LOD | < LOD | 723 |
| Non-Hispanic whites | 99-00 | * | < LOD | < LOD | < LOD | < LOD | 822 |
| | 01-02 | * | < LOD | < LOD | < LOD | < LOD | 1132 |
| | 03-04 | * | < LOD | < LOD | < LOD | < LOD | 1074 |

Limit of detection (LOD, see Data Analysis section) for Survey years 99-00, 01-02, and 03-04 are 0 04, 0.04, and 0.07, respectively.
< LOD means less than the limit of detection, which may vary for some chemicals by year and by individual sample.
* Not calculated: proportion of results below limit of detection was too high to provide a valid result.

doses or at biomonitored levels from low environmental exposures are unknown. Toxicity is determined by the type of compound (e.g., metallic, inorganic salt, or organometallic), route of exposure (e.g., intravenous medicinal use, inhalational, cutaneous, oral), and duration of exposure. Platinum metal is biologically inert, whereas soluble platinum compounds (e.g., halogenated salts) encountered in occupational settings can cause platinum salt hypersensitivity with symptoms that include bronchitis and asthma after inhalational exposure and contact dermatitis after skin exposure. Animals exposed to cholorplatinate salts used in industry have demonstrated severe hypersensitivity with asthma-like symptoms and anaphylactic shock (Parrot et al., 1969; Saindelle et al., 1969). Platinum metal and

insoluble salts can produce eye irritation. When ingested or inhaled, platinum metal and insoluble salts are very poorly absorbed (<1% of a dose) and cleared from the body within a week after a single dose. Most absorbed platinum accumulates in the kidneys and is excreted in urine (Moore et al., 1975a, 1975b). The pharmaceutical cisplatin is an animal carcinogen and reasonably anticipated to be a human carcinogen as determined by NTP. The carcinogenicity of other platinum compounds remains uncertain. Workplace air standards for external exposure are established for soluble salts of platinum by OSHA and ACGIH, or recommended for the metal form by NIOSH (Czerczak and Gromiec, 2000). Information about external exposure (i.e., environmental levels) and health effects is available from

## Urinary Platinum (creatinine corrected)

Geometric mean and selected percentiles of urine concentrations (in µg/g of creatinine) for the U.S. population from the National Health and Nutrition Examination Survey.

| | Survey years | Geometric mean (95% conf. interval) | 50th | 75th | 90th | 95th | Sample size |
|---|---|---|---|---|---|---|---|
| **Total** | 99-00 | * | < LOD | < LOD | < LOD | < LOD | 2465 |
| | 01-02 | * | < LOD | < LOD | < LOD | < LOD | 2689 |
| | 03-04 | * | < LOD | < LOD | < LOD | < LOD | 2558 |
| **Age group** | | | | | | | |
| 6-11 years | 99-00 | * | < LOD | < LOD | < LOD | < LOD | 340 |
| | 01-02 | * | < LOD | < LOD | < LOD | < LOD | 368 |
| | 03-04 | * | < LOD | < LOD | < LOD | < LOD | 290 |
| 12-19 years | 99-00 | * | < LOD | < LOD | < LOD | < LOD | 719 |
| | 01-02 | * | < LOD | < LOD | < LOD | < LOD | 762 |
| | 03-04 | * | < LOD | < LOD | < LOD | < LOD | 725 |
| 20 years and older | 99-00 | * | < LOD | < LOD | < LOD | < LOD | 1406 |
| | 01-02 | * | < LOD | < LOD | < LOD | < LOD | 1559 |
| | 03-04 | * | < LOD | < LOD | < LOD | < LOD | 1543 |
| **Gender** | | | | | | | |
| Males | 99-00 | * | < LOD | < LOD | < LOD | < LOD | 1227 |
| | 01-02 | * | < LOD | < LOD | < LOD | < LOD | 1334 |
| | 03-04 | * | < LOD | < LOD | < LOD | < LOD | 1281 |
| Females | 99-00 | * | < LOD | < LOD | < LOD | < LOD | 1238 |
| | 01-02 | * | < LOD | < LOD | < LOD | < LOD | 1355 |
| | 03-04 | * | < LOD | < LOD | < LOD | < LOD | 1277 |
| **Race/ethnicity** | | | | | | | |
| Mexican Americans | 99-00 | * | < LOD | < LOD | < LOD | < LOD | 884 |
| | 01-02 | * | < LOD | < LOD | < LOD | < LOD | 682 |
| | 03-04 | * | < LOD | < LOD | < LOD | < LOD | 618 |
| Non-Hispanic blacks | 99-00 | * | < LOD | < LOD | < LOD | < LOD | 568 |
| | 01-02 | * | < LOD | < LOD | < LOD | < LOD | 667 |
| | 03-04 | * | < LOD | < LOD | < LOD | < LOD | 723 |
| Non-Hispanic whites | 99-00 | * | < LOD | < LOD | < LOD | < LOD | 822 |
| | 01-02 | * | < LOD | < LOD | < LOD | < LOD | 1132 |
| | 03-04 | * | < LOD | < LOD | < LOD | < LOD | 1074 |

< LOD means less than the limit of detection for the urine levels not corrected for creatinine.
* Not calculated: proportion of results below limit of detection was too high to provide a valid result.

the International Programme on Chemical Safety at http://www.inchem.org/documents/ehc/ehc/ehc125.htm.

## Biomonitoring Information

Urinary platinum levels reflect recent exposure. Levels of platinum in urine for the U.S. population were below the limit of detection (0.04 µg/L) in this *Report*. Several studies have shown that background concentrations in general populations were usually less than 0.005 µg/L (Iavicoli et al., 2004; Wilhelm et al., 2004) or less than 0.01 µg/L (Becker et al., 2003; Herr et al., 2003; Schierl et al., 1998).

One study found that traffic-control officers had no greater urinary platinum concentrations than office-based control subjects (Iavicoli et al., 2004). Gold-platinum dental restorations were correlated with increased urinary platinum concentrations, which elevate urinary platinum by five to twelve-fold (Begerow et al., 1999; Herr et al., 2003; Schierl, 2001). Platinum-industry and precious-metal workers had urinary concentrations about one-thousand times higher than general populations (Schierl et al., 1998). Modest (ten-fold or less) elevations in urinary platinum concentrations were associated with handling of cisplatin and carboplatin by pharmacy and other hospital personnel (Ensslin et al., 1997; Pethran et al., 2003).

Finding a measurable amount of platinum in the urine does not mean that the level of platinum causes an adverse health effect. Biomonitoring studies on levels of platinum provide physicians and public health officials with reference values so that they can determine whether people have been exposed to higher levels of platinum than are found in the general population. Biomonitoring data can also help scientists plan and conduct research on exposure and health effects.

## References

Becker K, Schulz C, Kaus S, Seiwert M, Seifert B. German environmental survey 1998 (GerES III): environmental pollutants in the urine of the German population. International Journal of Hygiene and Environmental Health 2003; 206:15-24.

Begerow J, Neuendorf J, Turfeld M, Raab W, Duneman L:Long-term urinary platinum, palladium, and gold excretion of patients after insertion of noble-metal dental alloys. Biomarkers 1999;4(1):27-36.

Czerczak S, Gromiec JP. Nickel, ruthenium, rhodium, palladium, osmium, and platinum. In: Bingham E, Cohrssen B, Powell CH, eds. Patty's Toxicology. 5th ed. New York: John Wiley & Sons; 2000. pp. 289-380.

Ensslin AS, Huber R, Pethran A, Rommelt H, Schierl R, Kulka U, et al. Biological monitoring of hospital pharmacy personnel occupationally exposed to cytostatic drugs: urinary excretion and cytogenetic studies. Int Arch Occup Environ Health 1997;70(3):205-208.

Farago ME, Kavanagh P, Blanks R, Kelly J, Kazantzis G, Thornton I, et al. Platinum concentrations in urban road dust and soil, and in blood and urine in the United Kingdom. Analyst 1998;123(3):451-454.

Herr CE, Jankofsky M, Angerer J, Kuster W, Stilianakis NI, Gieler U, et al. Influences on human internal exposure to environmental platinum. J Expo Anal Environ Epidemiol 2003;13(1):24-30.

Iavicoli I, Bocca B, Petrucci F, Senofonte O, Carelli G, Alimonti A, et al. Biomonitoring of traffic police officers exposed to airborne platinum. Occup Environ Med 2004;61(7):636-9.

International Programme on Chemical Safety (IPCS). Environmental Health Criteria 125. Platinum. 1991 [online]. Available at URL: http://www.inchem.org/documents/ehc/ehc/ehc125.htm. 3/31/08

Moore W Jr, Hysell D, Crocker W, Stara J: Biological fate of a single administration of 191Pt in rats following different routes of exposure. Environ Res 1975a;9:152-158.

Moore W Jr, Hysell D, Hall L, Campbell K, Stara J: Preliminary studies on the toxicity and metabolism of palladium and platinum. Environ Health Perspect 1975b;10:63-71.

Parrot JL, Hebert R, Saindelle A, Ruff F: Platinum and platinosis. Allergy and histamine release due to some platinum salts. Arch Environ Health:1969;19:685-691.

Pethran A, Schierl R, Hauff K, Grimm CH, Boos KS, Nowak D. Uptake of antineoplastic agents in pharmacy and hospital personnel. Part 1: monitoring of urinary concentrations. Int Arch Occup Environ Health 2003;76(1):5-10.

Saindelle A, Ruff F: Histamine release by sodium cholorplatinate. Br J Pharmacol 1969;35:313-321.

Schierl R. Urinary platinum levels associated with dental gold alloys. Arch Environ Health 2001;56(3):283-286.

Schierl R, Fries HG, van de Weyer C, Fruhmann G. Urinary excretion of platinum from platinum-industry workers. Occup Environ Med 1998;55(2):138-140.

Wilhelm M, Ewers U, Schulz C. Revised and new reference values for some trace elements in blood and urine for human biomonitoring in environmental medicine. Int J Hyg Environ Health 2004;207(1):69-73.

## Thallium

CAS No. 7440-28-0

### General Information

Elemental thallium is a blue-white metal found in small amounts in soil and in sulfide-based minerals. In the past, thallium was obtained as a by-product of smelting other metals; however, it has not been specifically mined or refined in the United States since 1984. It is still used in relatively small amounts in pharmaceutical and electronics manufacturing, the latter being the current major industrial consumer of thallium in this country. In the United States, thallium has been restricted from use in rodenticides and depilatory cosmetics.

Thallium exposure occurs primarily from industrial processes such as coal-burning and smelting. From these and other sources, thallium is produced in a fine particulate form that can be absorbed through inhalation or ingestion. Thallium disappears from the blood with a half-life of several days, representing distribution into other tissues. In addition, thallium readily crosses the placenta and also distributes into breast milk. Elimination from the body tissues occurs slowly through urine and feces (Blanchardon et al., 2005).

Human health effects from thallium at low environmental

### Urinary Thallium

Geometric mean and selected percentiles of urine concentrations (in µg/L) for the U.S. population from the National Health and Nutrition Examination Survey.

| | Survey years | Geometric mean (95% conf. interval) | Selected percentiles ( 95% confidence interval) | | | | Sample size |
|---|---|---|---|---|---|---|---|
| | | | 50th | 75th | 90th | 95th | |
| **Total** | 99-00 | .176 (.162-.192) | .200 (.180-.220) | .290 (.270-.330) | .400 (.370-.420) | .450 (.430-.480) | 2413 |
| | 01-02 | .165 (.154-.177) | .190 (.180-.200) | .280 (.260-.290) | .370 (.350-.390) | .440 (.410-.470) | 2653 |
| | 03-04 | .155 (.145-.165) | .170 (.160-.180) | .270 (.250-.290) | .370 (.340-.400) | .440 (.410-.490) | 2558 |
| **Age group** | | | | | | | |
| 6-11 years | 99-00 | .201 (.167-.243) | .210 (.150-.280) | .310 (.250-.350) | .410 (.330-.450) | .450 (.350-.590) | 336 |
| | 01-02 | .172 (.147-.202) | .200 (.160-.220) | .290 (.230-.330) | .350 (.340-.370) | .390 (.360-.430) | 362 |
| | 03-04 | .191 (.170-.215) | .190 (.170-.230) | .300 (.250-.370) | .430 (.360-.500) | .510 (.430-.690) | 290 |
| 12-19 years | 99-00 | .202 (.181-.225) | .220 (.200-.240) | .300 (.270-.340) | .410 (.390-.430) | .470 (.430-.510) | 697 |
| | 01-02 | .200 (.182-.220) | .220 (.190-.250) | .310 (.290-.320) | .370 (.350-.420) | .470 (.400-.500) | 746 |
| | 03-04 | .201 (.185-.218) | .220 (.210-.240) | .310 (.290-.320) | .410 (.360-.470) | .500 (.420-.560) | 725 |
| 20 years and older | 99-00 | .170 (.157-.183) | .190 (.180-.210) | .290 (.260-.320) | .400 (.370-.420) | .450 (.420-.480) | 1380 |
| | 01-02 | .159 (.147-.173) | .190 (.170-.200) | .270 (.250-.290) | .380 (.350-.400) | .440 (.410-.490) | 1545 |
| | 03-04 | .145 (.134-.156) | .160 (.150-.170) | .250 (.240-.270) | .360 (.330-.390) | .420 (.390-.460) | 1543 |
| **Gender** | | | | | | | |
| Males | 99-00 | .197 (.179-.217) | .220 (.200-.240) | .320 (.280-.350) | .400 (.370-.440) | .450 (.420-.520) | 1200 |
| | 01-02 | .184 (.173-.196) | .210 (.200-.230) | .290 (.280-.300) | .380 (.360-.400) | .430 (.400-.470) | 1313 |
| | 03-04 | .167 (.156-.178) | .190 (.180-.200) | .280 (.260-.300) | .370 (.340-.400) | .430 (.400-.480) | 1281 |
| Females | 99-00 | .159 (.145-.175) | .180 (.150-.200) | .270 (.250-.300) | .390 (.350-.420) | .460 (.410-.490) | 1213 |
| | 01-02 | .149 (.137-.163) | .160 (.150-.180) | .260 (.230-.290) | .370 (.330-.400) | .440 (.400-.500) | 1340 |
| | 03-04 | .144 (.133-.156) | .160 (.140-.170) | .250 (.230-.280) | .370 (.330-.410) | .450 (.410-.510) | 1277 |
| **Race/ethnicity** | | | | | | | |
| Mexican Americans | 99-00 | .172 (.150-.196) | .200 (.160-.230) | .270 (.250-.300) | .370 (.320-.420) | .450 (.370-.520) | 861 |
| | 01-02 | .160 (.148-.173) | .180 (.160-.200) | .260 (.240-.270) | .340 (.310-.360) | .400 (.350-.440) | 675 |
| | 03-04 | .171 (.160-.183) | .200 (.170-.220) | .280 (.260-.310) | .360 (.340-.420) | .450 (.390-.480) | 618 |
| Non-Hispanic blacks | 99-00 | .217 (.197-.239) | .230 (.220-.260) | .350 (.300-.390) | .450 (.400-.520) | .550 (.460-.630) | 561 |
| | 01-02 | .202 (.187-.218) | .220 (.200-.230) | .300 (.270-.340) | .410 (.380-.440) | .520 (.440-.590) | 657 |
| | 03-04 | .185 (.167-.206) | .190 (.170-.220) | .290 (.250-.330) | .410 (.330-.490) | .490 (.410-.640) | 723 |
| Non-Hispanic whites | 99-00 | .170 (.153-.188) | .200 (.170-.220) | .290 (.260-.330) | .400 (.360-.420) | .450 (.420-.480) | 801 |
| | 01-02 | .159 (.147-.172) | .180 (.170-.200) | .270 (.250-.290) | .360 (.330-.390) | .430 (.390-.460) | 1114 |
| | 03-04 | .146 (.135-.158) | .160 (.150-.170) | .260 (.240-.280) | .360 (.330-.380) | .410 (.380-.460) | 1074 |

Limit of detection (LOD, see Data Analysis section) for Survey years 99-00, 01-02, and 03-04 are 0.02, 0.02, and 0.02, respectively.

doses or at biomonitored levels from low environmental exposures are unknown. Thallium produces toxicity by replacing intracellular potassium in the body, although additional mechanisms of action are possible. Severe accidental thallium poisonings from ingesting of rat poisons that contained water-soluble thallium salt have occurred. Relatively high-dose intentional or accidental ingestion can result in gastrointestinal symptoms followed by multiorgan failure, neurologic injury, and death. Peripheral neuropathy and alopecia are well-documented effects of acute and chronic exposures. Chronic high-level exposures have been associated with weight loss, arthralgias, and polyneuropathy. (ATSDR, 1992)

Workplace air standards and guidelines for external exposure are established by OSHA and ACGIH, respectively, and a drinking water standard has been established by U.S. EPA. IARC and NTP consider the evidence for the carcinogenicity of thallium as inadequate or unclassifiable. Information about external exposure (i.e., environmental levels) and health effects is available from ATSDR at: http://www.atsdr.cdc.gov/toxpro2.html.

**Biomonitoring Information**

Urinary thallium levels reflect recent exposure. Levels of thallium in urine for the U.S. population have been well characterized in NHANES 1999-2000 and 2001-2002

## Urinary Thallium (creatinine corrected)

Geometric mean and selected percentiles of urine concentrations (in µg/g of creatinine) for the U.S. population from the National Health and Nutrition Examination Survey.

| | Survey years | Geometric mean (95% conf. interval) | 50th | 75th | 90th | 95th | Sample size |
|---|---|---|---|---|---|---|---|
| **Total** | 99-00 | .166 (.159-.173) | .168 (.162-.176) | .224 (.217-.233) | .297 (.273-.319) | .366 (.338-.387) | 2413 |
| | 01-02 | .156 (.151-.162) | .156 (.148-.164) | .215 (.208-.222) | .287 (.278-.300) | .349 (.337-.365) | 2652 |
| | 03-04 | .154 (.149-.158) | .153 (.146-.160) | .214 (.203-.222) | .286 (.274-.304) | .350 (.328-.369) | 2558 |
| **Age group** | | | | | | | |
| 6-11 years | 99-00 | .221 (.197-.248) | .222 (.196-.236) | .297 (.229-.356) | .375 (.318-.469) | .424 (.356-.600) | 336 |
| | 01-02 | .211 (.198-.226) | .207 (.198-.221) | .286 (.260-.321) | .370 (.333-.402) | .412 (.389-.456) | 362 |
| | 03-04 | .223 (.208-.238) | .216 (.198-.229) | .306 (.280-.346) | .412 (.346-.458) | .458 (.400-.532) | 290 |
| 12-19 years | 99-00 | .153 (.146-.160) | .154 (.146-.162) | .205 (.191-.219) | .258 (.231-.278) | .321 (.265-.364) | 697 |
| | 01-02 | .143 (.137-.150) | .145 (.135-.152) | .196 (.184-.207) | .272 (.250-.289) | .312 (.299-.333) | 746 |
| | 03-04 | .143 (.135-.152) | .146 (.131-.155) | .194 (.179-.208) | .254 (.234-.280) | .304 (.271-.327) | 725 |
| 20 years and older | 99-00 | .162 (.153-.171) | .167 (.155-.176) | .218 (.207-.230) | .286 (.271-.300) | .364 (.325-.389) | 1380 |
| | 01-02 | .153 (.147-.159) | .153 (.144-.161) | .210 (.200-.217) | .278 (.263-.293) | .343 (.313-.362) | 1544 |
| | 03-04 | .148 (.144-.153) | .149 (.141-.156) | .206 (.192-.215) | .273 (.258-.289) | .333 (.306-.353) | 1543 |
| **Gender** | | | | | | | |
| Males | 99-00 | .154 (.147-.161) | .156 (.149-.164) | .202 (.192-.214) | .269 (.254-.297) | .338 (.300-.364) | 1200 |
| | 01-02 | .146 (.140-.153) | .148 (.142-.157) | .192 (.184-.204) | .260 (.246-.278) | .307 (.291-.342) | 1312 |
| | 03-04 | .140 (.135-.146) | .142 (.134-.149) | .188 (.180-.198) | .264 (.235-.286) | .317 (.287-.350) | 1281 |
| Females | 99-00 | .178 (.167-.189) | .182 (.169-.197) | .244 (.226-.259) | .317 (.281-.366) | .380 (.333-.462) | 1213 |
| | 01-02 | .167 (.158-.176) | .167 (.153-.180) | .233 (.217-.250) | .313 (.282-.348) | .378 (.348-.402) | 1340 |
| | 03-04 | .167 (.162-.173) | .166 (.157-.177) | .235 (.222-.243) | .313 (.286-.333) | .368 (.340-.412) | 1277 |
| **Race/ethnicity** | | | | | | | |
| Mexican Americans | 99-00 | .158 (.147-.170) | .160 (.148-.176) | .213 (.200-.237) | .282 (.266-.304) | .343 (.306-.389) | 861 |
| | 01-02 | .156 (.145-.169) | .155 (.145-.167) | .204 (.191-.221) | .286 (.250-.317) | .361 (.301-.424) | 674 |
| | 03-04 | .159 (.148-.170) | .157 (.143-.172) | .211 (.187-.241) | .293 (.273-.324) | .369 (.326-.422) | 618 |
| Non-Hispanic blacks | 99-00 | .142 (.133-.152) | .140 (.129-.151) | .200 (.184-.214) | .278 (.244-.307) | .383 (.286-.462) | 561 |
| | 01-02 | .138 (.128-.150) | .136 (.125-.146) | .194 (.170-.212) | .256 (.238-.278) | .328 (.271-.387) | 657 |
| | 03-04 | .133 (.122-.145) | .128 (.119-.143) | .185 (.171-.200) | .255 (.237-.269) | .323 (.267-.377) | 723 |
| Non-Hispanic whites | 99-00 | .169 (.160-.179) | .173 (.167-.181) | .227 (.215-.240) | .300 (.272-.329) | .364 (.333-.377) | 801 |
| | 01-02 | .161 (.155-.167) | .161 (.153-.171) | .222 (.214-.231) | .292 (.278-.304) | .348 (.330-.383) | 1114 |
| | 03-04 | .154 (.148-.160) | .153 (.143-.162) | .214 (.200-.223) | .283 (.271-.304) | .333 (.313-.363) | 1074 |

(CDC, 2005) and are shown with results from NHANES 2003-2004 in this *Report*. These urine levels are generally comparable to levels observed in earlier studies of general populations (Brockhaus et al., 1981; Minoia et al., 1990; Paschal et al., 1998; Schaller et al., 1980; White and Sabbioni, 1998). Urinary concentrations of 100 µg/L in asymptomatic workers (500 times higher than median levels in the U.S. population) are thought to correspond to workplace exposures at the threshold limit value of 0.1 mg/m³ (Marcus, 1985). Brockhaus et al. (1981) studied 1,265 people living near a thallium-emitting cement plant in Germany. Nearby residents were exposed by eating garden plants that had been contaminated by the thallium. Seventy-eight percent of the urine specimens in that study contained greater than 1 µg/L, with concentrations ranging up to 76.5 µg/L. There was no increase in the prevalence of symptoms at levels less than 20 µg/L and only a slight increase in nonspecific symptoms greater than 20 µg/L.

Finding a measurable amount of thallium in urine does not mean that the level of thallium causes an adverse health effect. Biomonitoring studies on levels of thallium provide physicians and public health officials with reference values so that they can determine whether people have been exposed to higher levels of thallium than are found in the general population. Biomonitoring data can also help scientists plan and conduct research on exposure and health effects.

## References

Agency for Toxic Substances and Disease Registry (ATSDR). Toxicological profile for thallium. 1992 [online]. Available at URL: http://www.atsdr.cdc.gov/toxprofiles/tp54 html. 7/15/09

Blanchardon E, Challeton-de Vathaire C, Boisson P, Celier D, Martin J-C, Cassot G, et al. Long term retention and excretion of 201Tl in a patient after myocardial perfusion imaging. Radiat Prot Dosim. 2005;113(1):47-53.

Brockhaus A, Dolger R, Ewers U, Kramer U, Soddemann H, Wiegand H. Intake and health effects of thallium among a population living in the vicinity of a cement plant emitting thallium-containing dust. Int Arch Occup Environ Health 1981;48(4):375-389.

Centers for Disease Control and Prevention. Third National Report on Human Exposure to Environmental Chemicals. Atlanta (GA). 2005.

Marcus RL. Investigation of a working population exposed to thallium. J Soc Occup Med 1985;35(1):4-9.

Minoia C, Sabbioni E, Apostoli P, Pietra R, Pozzoli L, Gallorini

M, et al. Trace element reference values in tissues from inhabitants of the European community I. A study of 46 elements in urine, blood, and serum of Italian subjects. Sci Total Environ 1990;95:89-105.

Paschal DC, Ting BG, Morrow JC, Pirkle JL, Jackson RJ, Sampson EJ, et al. Trace metals in urine of United States residents: reference range concentrations. Environ Res 1998;76(1):53-59.

Schaller KH, Manke G, Raithel HJ, Buhlmeyer G, Schmidt M, Valentin H. Investigations of thallium-exposed workers in cement factories. Int Arch Occup Environ Health 1980;47(3):223-231.

White MA, Sabbioni E. Trace element reference values in tissues from inhabitants of the European Union. X. A study of 13 elements in blood and urine of a United Kingdom population. Sci Total Environ 1998;216:253-270.

# Tungsten
CAS No. 7440-33-7

## General Information

Tungsten is a steel-gray to tin-white metal that occurs naturally in the earth's crust, mainly as scheelite ($CaWO_4$). Tungsten is used mainly for producing hard metals, which are used in rock drills and metal-cutting tools, and for producing ferrotungsten, which is used in the steel industry. Tungsten compounds are used as lubricating agents, filaments for incandescent lamps, bronzes in pigments, and as catalysts in the petroleum industry.

Most background environmental exposures to tungsten are from the soluble forms such as tungstate salts that may occur in drinking water. Occupational exposure is from dusts released during grinding or drilling of hard metals. Human health effects from tungsten at low environmental doses or at biomonitored levels from low environmental exposures are unknown. Little information is available on the toxicity of tungsten. Although workers occupationally exposed to tungsten carbide may develop serious lung disease ("hard metal disease"), their illness may stem from exposure to cobalt mixed with tungsten carbide rather than to tungsten alone. Evidence is lacking for the carcinogenicity of tungsten, and it has not been classified with respect to its carcinogenicity by either IARC or NTP.

## Urinary Tungsten

Geometric mean and selected percentiles of urine concentrations (in µg/L) for the U.S. population from the National Health and Nutrition Examination Survey.

| | Survey years | Geometric mean (95% conf. interval) | 50th | 75th | 90th | 95th | Sample size |
|---|---|---|---|---|---|---|---|
| **Total** | 99-00 | .093 (.087-.100) | .090 (.080-.090) | .180 (.160-.190) | .320 (.280-.370) | .500 (.430-.550) | 2338 |
| | 01-02 | .082 (.073-.092) | .070 (.060-.090) | .160 (.140-.180) | .300 (.260-.350) | .460 (.370-.560) | 2652 |
| | 03-04 | .071 (.064-.078) | .070 (.060-.080) | .130 (.120-.140) | .270 (.230-.300) | .400 (.330-.480) | 2558 |
| **Age group** | | | | | | | |
| 6-11 years | 99-00 | .158 (.123-.204) | .160 (.120-.220) | .270 (.220-.350) | .510 (.380-.560) | .620 (.510-.950) | 320 |
| | 01-02 | .137 (.110-.170) | .140 (.110-.170) | .260 (.200-.350) | .460 (.360-.690) | .770 (.510-1.53) | 363 |
| | 03-04 | .130 (.111-.151) | .140 (.120-.150) | .240 (.190-.290) | .410 (.290-.500) | .500 (.370-.630) | 290 |
| 12-19 years | 99-00 | .113 (.097-.132) | .110 (.090-.130) | .210 (.180-.250) | .360 (.310-.440) | .530 (.380-.800) | 679 |
| | 01-02 | .113 (.095-.135) | .110 (.090-.130) | .210 (.180-.260) | .400 (.310-.520) | .570 (.430-.790) | 744 |
| | 03-04 | .105 (.090-.122) | .100 (.090-.120) | .190 (.160-.230) | .350 (.290-.460) | .530 (.350-1.00) | 725 |
| 20 years and older | 99-00 | .084 (.078-.091) | .080 (.070-.090) | .160 (.130-.180) | .280 (.260-.320) | .450 (.360-.520) | 1339 |
| | 01-02 | .073 (.065-.082) | .060 (.050-.070) | .140 (.110-.160) | .260 (.210-.310) | .380 (.310-.490) | 1545 |
| | 03-04 | .062 (.056-.068) | .060 (.050-.070) | .110 (.100-.120) | .210 (.180-.250) | .360 (.270-.430) | 1543 |
| **Gender** | | | | | | | |
| Males | 99-00 | .107 (.096-.120) | .100 (.090-.120) | .210 (.190-.230) | .390 (.310-.470) | .530 (.470-.650) | 1160 |
| | 01-02 | .088 (.074-.105) | .080 (.060-.100) | .170 (.140-.220) | .330 (.260-.390) | .490 (.380-.580) | 1307 |
| | 03-04 | .081 (.071-.093) | .080 (.070-.090) | .140 (.130-.170) | .300 (.250-.340) | .430 (.340-.560) | 1281 |
| Females | 99-00 | .082 (.077-.087) | .070 (.060-.080) | .150 (.130-.160) | .270 (.240-.300) | .400 (.320-.470) | 1178 |
| | 01-02 | .076 (.069-.084) | .060 (.060-.080) | .150 (.120-.170) | .280 (.230-.330) | .430 (.340-.560) | 1345 |
| | 03-04 | .062 (.056-.069) | .060 (.050-.070) | .110 (.100-.120) | .220 (.190-.250) | .370 (.270-.460) | 1277 |
| **Race/ethnicity** | | | | | | | |
| Mexican Americans | 99-00 | .113 (.095-.133) | .110 (.090-.130) | .200 (.160-.250) | .400 (.300-.520) | .550 (.420-.830) | 790 |
| | 01-02 | .101 (.093-.109) | .100 (.090-.110) | .190 (.170-.210) | .370 (.310-.430) | .570 (.450-.670) | 680 |
| | 03-04 | .086 (.073-.100) | .080 (.070-.100) | .170 (.120-.220) | .360 (.230-.620) | .640 (.410-.800) | 618 |
| Non-Hispanic blacks | 99-00 | .113 (.101-.126) | .100 (.090-.130) | .210 (.180-.250) | .370 (.290-.460) | .560 (.420-.810) | 562 |
| | 01-02 | .096 (.080-.116) | .090 (.070-.120) | .160 (.130-.250) | .310 (.270-.400) | .460 (.400-.590) | 649 |
| | 03-04 | .092 (.082-.104) | .090 (.080-.110) | .160 (.150-.180) | .300 (.250-.330) | .470 (.340-.550) | 723 |
| Non-Hispanic whites | 99-00 | .092 (.084-.100) | .080 (.070-.100) | .180 (.160-.200) | .320 (.270-.380) | .470 (.380-.550) | 802 |
| | 01-02 | .076 (.066-.088) | .060 (.050-.080) | .150 (.120-.180) | .290 (.230-.360) | .430 (.330-.620) | 1117 |
| | 03-04 | .065 (.058-.073) | .060 (.060-.070) | .120 (.100-.130) | .230 (.190-.290) | .380 (.320-.410) | 1074 |

Limit of detection (LOD, see Data Analysis section) for Survey years 99-00, 01-02, and 03-04 are 0 04, 0.04, and 0.04, respectively.

Workplace air standards for external exposure have been established by ACGIH and recommended by NIOSH.

## Biomonitoring Information

Levels of urinary tungsten reflect recent exposure. A nonrandom subsample from NHANES III demonstrated slightly higher values than those found in NHANES 1999-2000, 2001-2002, and 2003-2004 (Paschal et al., 1998), possibly due to methodologic, population, or exposure differences. A study of 14 unexposed adults yielded values similar to those in this *Report* (Schramel et al., 1997). In a Nevada community where tungsten was measured and found at increased levels in drinking water, the residents'

median urinary levels were as much as 15-fold higher than median levels in the U.S. population (CDC, 2003, 2005).

Workers involved in grinding operations that released tungsten metal into the air had elevated urinary levels that were more than 900 times higher than the overall geometric mean of the U.S. population in the NHANES 1999-2000 (Kraus et al., 2001). Using neutron activation analysis to measure urinary tungsten, Nicolaou et al. (1987) found that a control group of non-metal workers had mean levels that were similar to the 95th percentiles in this *Report*, whereas the tungsten-worker group had mean urine levels 35 times higher. Patients with medically-inserted tungsten embolization coils showed elevated tungsten levels in

## Urinary Tungsten (creatinine corrected)

Geometric mean and selected percentiles of urine concentrations (in µg/g of creatinine) for the U.S. population from the National Health and Nutrition Examination Survey.

| | Survey years | Geometric mean (95% conf. interval) | Selected percentiles (95% confidence interval) | | | | Sample size |
|---|---|---|---|---|---|---|---|
| | | | 50th | 75th | 90th | 95th | |
| **Total** | 99-00 | .087 (.080-.095) | .080 (.075-.086) | .146 (.136-.158) | .270 (.206-.333) | .383 (.302-.459) | 2338 |
| | 01-02 | .078 (.069-.087) | .074 (.064-.084) | .138 (.122-.154) | .255 (.216-.300) | .359 (.315-.436) | 2651 |
| | 03-04 | .070 (.063-.078) | .065 (.059-.074) | .117 (.107-.133) | .215 (.179-.253) | .333 (.255-.439) | 2558 |
| **Age group** | | | | | | | |
| 6-11 years | 99-00 | .174 (.150-.201) | .169 (.136-.198) | .293 (.216-.333) | .439 (.331-.667) | .667 (.452-.880) | 320 |
| | 01-02 | .168 (.144-.197) | .158 (.139-.190) | .275 (.231-.326) | .412 (.333-.554) | .634 (.436-1.28) | 363 |
| | 03-04 | .151 (.131-.174) | .144 (.119-.167) | .250 (.205-.283) | .333 (.278-.484) | .484 (.333-.739) | 290 |
| 12-19 years | 99-00 | .084 (.078-.091) | .079 (.074-.084) | .138 (.124-.158) | .231 (.180-.287) | .339 (.237-.465) | 679 |
| | 01-02 | .081 (.071-.092) | .081 (.072-.091) | .148 (.122-.167) | .250 (.208-.301) | .359 (.272-.431) | 744 |
| | 03-04 | .075 (.065-.086) | .071 (.061-.082) | .122 (.098-.148) | .197 (.167-.308) | .379 (.197-.582) | 725 |
| 20 years and older | 99-00 | .080 (.072-.089) | .075 (.067-.082) | .130 (.116-.146) | .218 (.179-.301) | .347 (.245-.426) | 1339 |
| | 01-02 | .070 (.063-.079) | .067 (.058-.075) | .119 (.099-.139) | .216 (.176-.267) | .333 (.253-.431) | 1544 |
| | 03-04 | .063 (.057-.071) | .059 (.053-.065) | .105 (.094-.117) | .181 (.155-.215) | .279 (.217-.370) | 1543 |
| **Gender** | | | | | | | |
| Males | 99-00 | .083 (.074-.094) | .073 (.063-.086) | .146 (.126-.165) | .279 (.198-.386) | .439 (.329-.605) | 1160 |
| | 01-02 | .071 (.060-.083) | .065 (.056-.077) | .125 (.098-.153) | .255 (.203-.306) | .364 (.300-.431) | 1306 |
| | 03-04 | .068 (.059-.079) | .062 (.054-.071) | .111 (.098-.133) | .216 (.170-.284) | .341 (.240-.500) | 1281 |
| Females | 99-00 | .091 (.085-.098) | .084 (.080-.091) | .145 (.136-.158) | .265 (.200-.301) | .339 (.300-.381) | 1178 |
| | 01-02 | .085 (.077-.094) | .083 (.075-.091) | .143 (.130-.161) | .258 (.216-.317) | .353 (.317-.538) | 1345 |
| | 03-04 | .072 (.065-.079) | .069 (.063-.078) | .121 (.108-.138) | .211 (.176-.237) | .333 (.261-.439) | 1277 |
| **Race/ethnicity** | | | | | | | |
| Mexican Americans | 99-00 | .106 (.093-.120) | .100 (.086-.116) | .184 (.152-.214) | .329 (.267-.392) | .497 (.354-.727) | 790 |
| | 01-02 | .098 (.090-.108) | .089 (.081-.100) | .164 (.143-.187) | .294 (.258-.375) | .555 (.410-.797) | 679 |
| | 03-04 | .079 (.065-.096) | .073 (.054-.093) | .136 (.103-.197) | .300 (.233-.426) | .482 (.344-.823) | 618 |
| Non-Hispanic blacks | 99-00 | .073 (.064-.083) | .071 (.061-.081) | .124 (.109-.154) | .201 (.188-.222) | .360 (.217-.465) | 562 |
| | 01-02 | .066 (.056-.077) | .060 (.049-.079) | .109 (.090-.125) | .199 (.153-.285) | .340 (.250-.414) | 649 |
| | 03-04 | .066 (.059-.074) | .067 (.055-.075) | .105 (.095-.120) | .186 (.150-.224) | .317 (.214-.358) | 723 |
| Non-Hispanic whites | 99-00 | .091 (.083-.100) | .082 (.077-.088) | .150 (.136-.169) | .279 (.200-.354) | .385 (.302-.462) | 802 |
| | 01-02 | .078 (.068-.088) | .073 (.061-.085) | .139 (.121-.157) | .253 (.209-.308) | .353 (.286-.453) | 1117 |
| | 03-04 | .069 (.060-.078) | .063 (.057-.071) | .116 (.104-.133) | .199 (.167-.237) | .299 (.222-.439) | 1074 |

blood, urine, and hair (Bachthaler et al., 2004). Urinary tungsten levels in many patients were hundreds-fold higher than observed in this *Report*.

Finding a measurable amount of tungsten in the urine does not mean that the level of tungsten causes an adverse health effect. Biomonitoring studies on levels of tungsten provide physicians and public health officials with reference values so that they can determine whether people have been exposed to higher levels of tungsten than are found in the general population. Biomonitoring data can also help scientists plan and conduct research on exposure and health effects.

## References

Bachthaler M, Lenhart M, Paetzel C, Feuerbach S, Link J, Manke C. Corrosion of tungsten coils after peripheral vascular embolization therapy: influence on outcome and tungsten load. Catheter Cardiovasc Interv 2004;62:380-384.

Centers for Disease Control and Prevention. National Center for Environmental Health. Cancer Clusters. Churchill County (Fallon). Nevada Exposure Asssessment. [online] 2003. Available at URL: http://www.cdc.gov/nceh/clusters/Fallon/study.htm. 4/15/09

Centers for Disease Control and Prevention. Third National Report on Human Exposure to Environmental Chemicals. Atlanta (GA). 2005.

Kraus T, Schramel P, Schaller KH, Zobelein P, Weber A, Angerer J. Exposure assessment in the hard metal manufacturing industry with special regard to tungsten and its compounds. Occup Environ Med 2001;58(10):631-634.

Nicolaou G, Pietra R, Sabioni E, Mosconi G, Cassina G, Seghizzi P. Multielement determination of metals in biological specimens of hard-metal workers: a study carried out by neutron activation analysis. J Trace Elem Electrolytes Health Dis 1987;(2):73-77.

Paschal DC, Ting BG, Morrow JC, Pirkle JL, Jackson RJ, Sampson EJ, et al. Trace metals in urine of United States residents: reference range concentrations. Environ Res 1998;76(1):53-59.

Schramel P, Wendler I, Angerer J. The determination of metals (antimony, bismuth, lead, cadmium, mercury, palladium, platinum, tellurium, thallium, tin and tungsten) in urine samples by inductively coupled plasma-mass spectrometry. Int Arch Occup Environ Health 1997;69(3):219-223.

# Uranium
CAS No. 7440-61-1

## General Information

Uranium is a silver-white metal that is extremely dense and weakly radioactive. It usually occurs as an oxide and is extracted from ores containing less than 1% natural uranium. Natural uranium is a mixture of three isotopes: $^{238}U$ (greater than 99%), $^{235}U$ (about 0.72%), and $^{234}U$. Uranium has many commercial uses, including nuclear weapons, nuclear fuel, in some ceramics, and as an aid in electron microscopy and photography. Depleted uranium (DU) refers to uranium in which the proportions of $^{235}U$

and $^{234}U$ isotopes have been reduced compared with the proportion in natural uranium. Since the 1990's, DU has been used by the military in armor-piercing ammunition and as a component of protective armor for tanks.

Variable concentrations of uranium occur naturally in drinking water sources. Thus, the primary exposure sources for nonoccupationally exposed persons are dietary (especially root vegetables) and drinking water. In workplaces that involve uranium mining, milling, or processing, human exposure occurs primarily by inhaling dust and other small particles. Exposure to DU may occur in military personnel from retention internal shrapnel that contains DU or exposure to dust generated from ammunition

## Urinary Uranium

Geometric mean and selected percentiles of urine concentrations (in µg/L) for the U.S. population from the National Health and Nutrition Examination Survey.

| | Survey years | Geometric mean (95% conf. interval) | 50th | 75th | 90th | 95th | Sample size |
|---|---|---|---|---|---|---|---|
| | | | | **Selected percentiles** ( 95% confidence interval) | | | |
| **Total** | 99-00 | .008 (.007-.009) | .007 (.006-.008) | .013 (.010-.017) | .027 (.021-.038) | .046 (.037-.056) | 2464 |
| | 01-02 | .009 (.007-.010) | .008 (.007-.009) | .014 (.012-.018) | .030 (.023-.039) | .046 (.034-.062) | 2690 |
| | 03-04 | .008 (.007-.008) | .007 (.006-.007) | .011 (.010-.013) | .021 (.017-.026) | .031 (.026-.037) | 2557 |
| **Age group** | | | | | | | |
| **6-11 years** | 99-00 | .009 (.007-.011) | .007 (.006-.009) | .013 (.009-.022) | .032 (.019-.048) | .048 (.033-.066) | 340 |
| | 01-02 | .008 (.007-.010) | .008 (.006-.010) | .014 (.010-.020) | .026 (.020-.036) | .040 (.025-.049) | 368 |
| | 03-04 | .008 (.007-.009) | .007 (.006-.009) | .012 (.009-.016) | .020 (.016-.026) | .028 (.020-.039) | 289 |
| **12-19 years** | 99-00 | .009 (.008-.011) | .009 (.008-.010) | .015 (.012-.018) | .026 (.020-.043) | .044 (.028-.072) | 719 |
| | 01-02 | .010 (.008-.012) | .010 (.008-.012) | .017 (.013-.023) | .030 (.022-.042) | .042 (.027-.088) | 762 |
| | 03-04 | .010 (.009-.011) | .009 (.008-.010) | .015 (.012-.018) | .028 (.023-.036) | .038 (.036-.053) | 725 |
| **20 years and older** | 99-00 | .008 (.006-.009) | .007 (.005-.008) | .013 (.010-.017) | .027 (.021-.040) | .046 (.036-.056) | 1405 |
| | 01-02 | .009 (.007-.010) | .008 (.007-.009) | .014 (.012-.017) | .031 (.022-.040) | .046 (.034-.065) | 1560 |
| | 03-04 | * | .006 (.005-.007) | .011 (.009-.012) | .019 (.016-.026) | .029 (.024-.038) | 1543 |
| **Gender** | | | | | | | |
| **Males** | 99-00 | .009 (.008-.011) | .008 (.007-.010) | .015 (.012-.021) | .036 (.024-.046) | .053 (.040-.067) | 1227 |
| | 01-02 | .009 (.008-.011) | .009 (.007-.010) | .015 (.013-.021) | .033 (.024-.045) | .047 (.035-.065) | 1335 |
| | 03-04 | .008 (.007-.009) | .007 (.006-.008) | .013 (.011-.016) | .023 (.019-.027) | .031 (.027-.035) | 1280 |
| **Females** | 99-00 | .007 (.006-.008) | .006 (.005-.007) | .012 (.009-.015) | .023 (.016-.033) | .036 (.026-.050) | 1237 |
| | 01-02 | .008 (.007-.010) | .008 (.006-.009) | .014 (.011-.017) | .027 (.019-.037) | .041 (.029-.063) | 1355 |
| | 03-04 | * | .006 (.005-.007) | .010 (.009-.011) | .018 (.013-.027) | .031 (.022-.039) | 1277 |
| **Race/ethnicity** | | | | | | | |
| **Mexican Americans** | 99-00 | .017 (.012-.023) | .016 (.011-.021) | .033 (.020-.054) | .060 (.040-.127) | .114 (.054-.279) | 883 |
| | 01-02 | .013 (.010-.016) | .012 (.009-.016) | .022 (.017-.030) | .040 (.031-.054) | .055 (.046-.069) | 683 |
| | 03-04 | .014 (.011-.017) | .013 (.009-.018) | .024 (.017-.034) | .041 (.028-.073) | .064 (.039-.158) | 618 |
| **Non-Hispanic blacks** | 99-00 | .009 (.007-.011) | .008 (.006-.010) | .014 (.010-.020) | .028 (.018-.049) | .052 (.030-.067) | 568 |
| | 01-02 | .008 (.007-.009) | .008 (.007-.009) | .012 (.011-.015) | .021 (.017-.027) | .030 (.023-.037) | 667 |
| | 03-04 | .008 (.008-.009) | .007 (.007-.008) | .012 (.011-.013) | .021 (.017-.027) | .031 (.023-.045) | 722 |
| **Non-Hispanic whites** | 99-00 | .007 (.006-.009) | .007 (.006-.007) | .012 (.009-.016) | .023 (.017-.037) | .043 (.027-.051) | 822 |
| | 01-02 | .008 (.007-.009) | .007 (.006-.009) | .013 (.011-.016) | .026 (.019-.035) | .037 (.029-.050) | 1132 |
| | 03-04 | * | .006 (.005-.007) | .010 (.009-.012) | .018 (.015-.023) | .027 (.020-.036) | 1074 |

Limit of detection (LOD, see Data Analysis section) for Survey years 99-00, 01-02, and 03-04 are 0.004, 0 004, and 0 005, respectively.
* Not calculated: proportion of results below limit of detection was too high to provide a valid result.

impact.

Soluble forms of uranium salts are poorly absorbed in the gastrointestinal tract. Depending upon the specific compound and solubility, 0.1%-6% of an ingested dose may be absorbed. Inhaled uranium-containing particles are retained in the lungs, where limited absorption occurs (less than 5%). In cases of retained DU shrapnel, the shrapnel acts as a source of chronic, low level exposure. After long term or repeated exposure, kidneys, liver, and bones can accumulate uranium with the largest amounts being stored in bones (Li et al., 2005). Uranium is eliminated in feces and urine; about 50% of the absorbed dose is eliminated in the urine within the first 24 hours. After exposure to soluble

uranium salts, the initial half-life of uranium is about 15 days (Bhattacharyya et al., 1992), which represents distribution and excretion, with much slower elimination from bone. After inhalation, the half-life of insoluble uranium in the lungs is several years (Durakovic et al., 2003).

Human health effects from uranium at low environmental doses or at biomonitored levels from low environmental exposures are unknown. Radiation risks from exposure to natural uranium are very low. Health effects from uranium exposure result from chemical toxicity to the kidney, which can occur occasionally from high occupational exposure. Studies of persons with chronic exposure to soluble uranium salts in drinking water have not shown kidney

## Urinary Uranium (creatinine corrected)

Geometric mean and selected percentiles of urine concentrations (in µg/g of creatinine) for the U.S. population from the National Health and Nutrition Examination Survey.

| | Survey years | Geometric mean (95% conf. interval) | 50th | 75th | 90th | 95th | Sample size |
|---|---|---|---|---|---|---|---|
| | | | \<-- Selected percentiles ( 95% confidence interval) --\> | | | | |
| **Total** | 99-00 | .007 (.006-.009) | .007 (.006-.009) | .013 (.010-.016) | .024 (.019-.030) | .034 (.027-.053) | 2464 |
| | 01-02 | .008 (.007-.010) | .007 (.006-.009) | .014 (.011-.018) | .026 (.020-.034) | .040 (.028-.058) | 2689 |
| | 03-04 | .008 (.007-.008) | .007 (.006-.008) | .012 (.010-.014) | .021 (.017-.025) | .029 (.023-.039) | 2557 |
| **Age group** | | | | | | | |
| 6-11 years | 99-00 | .009 (.007-.012) | .008 (.006-.011) | .015 (.010-.024) | .030 (.016-.044) | .037 (.030-.077) | 340 |
| | 01-02 | .010 (.008-.011) | .010 (.008-.012) | .015 (.013-.019) | .027 (.018-.032) | .033 (.027-.048) | 368 |
| | 03-04 | .009 (.008-.010) | .008 (.007-.010) | .013 (.011-.017) | .024 (.016-.039) | .033 (.022-.050) | 289 |
| 12-19 years | 99-00 | .007 (.006-.008) | .006 (.005-.008) | .010 (.009-.014) | .020 (.014-.030) | .030 (.019-.074) | 719 |
| | 01-02 | .007 (.006-.008) | .007 (.006-.008) | .012 (.009-.016) | .020 (.015-.026) | .026 (.020-.042) | 762 |
| | 03-04 | .007 (.006-.008) | .006 (.005-.007) | .010 (.008-.013) | .019 (.015-.027) | .034 (.022-.041) | 725 |
| 20 years and older | 99-00 | .007 (.006-.009) | .007 (.006-.009) | .013 (.010-.016) | .024 (.019-.029) | .034 (.025-.051) | 1405 |
| | 01-02 | .008 (.007-.010) | .007 (.006-.009) | .014 (.011-.019) | .027 (.020-.039) | .043 (.030-.063) | 1559 |
| | 03-04 | * | .007 (.006-.008) | .012 (.010-.014) | .020 (.017-.024) | .028 (.022-.038) | 1543 |
| **Gender** | | | | | | | |
| Males | 99-00 | .007 (.006-.009) | .006 (.005-.008) | .011 (.009-.015) | .021 (.017-.028) | .035 (.024-.056) | 1227 |
| | 01-02 | .007 (.006-.008) | .007 (.006-.008) | .012 (.010-.015) | .022 (.018-.028) | .033 (.025-.047) | 1334 |
| | 03-04 | .007 (.006-.008) | .006 (.006-.007) | .010 (.009-.012) | .019 (.015-.024) | .026 (.019-.039) | 1280 |
| Females | 99-00 | .008 (.007-.010) | .007 (.006-.010) | .013 (.010-.017) | .025 (.019-.033) | .034 (.027-.054) | 1237 |
| | 01-02 | .009 (.008-.011) | .009 (.007-.011) | .016 (.012-.021) | .029 (.021-.042) | .045 (.031-.067) | 1355 |
| | 03-04 | * | .008 (.007-.009) | .013 (.011-.016) | .022 (.018-.028) | .031 (.025-.041) | 1277 |
| **Race/ethnicity** | | | | | | | |
| Mexican Americans | 99-00 | .015 (.011-.022) | .015 (.011-.020) | .029 (.016-.058) | .059 (.027-.146) | .100 (.042-.270) | 883 |
| | 01-02 | .012 (.010-.016) | .012 (.009-.016) | .021 (.015-.028) | .033 (.024-.053) | .050 (.034-.080) | 682 |
| | 03-04 | .013 (.010-.016) | .013 (.009-.017) | .022 (.016-.029) | .035 (.026-.051) | .051 (.034-.061) | 618 |
| Non-Hispanic blacks | 99-00 | .006 (.004-.007) | .005 (.004-.006) | .008 (.006-.013) | .017 (.011-.029) | .028 (.018-.048) | 568 |
| | 01-02 | .005 (.005-.006) | .005 (.005-.006) | .008 (.007-.010) | .013 (.011-.014) | .017 (.014-.029) | 667 |
| | 03-04 | .006 (.005-.006) | .005 (.005-.006) | .009 (.008-.009) | .013 (.012-.015) | .018 (.014-.024) | 722 |
| Non-Hispanic whites | 99-00 | .007 (.006-.009) | .007 (.006-.009) | .012 (.010-.015) | .021 (.017-.027) | .030 (.024-.050) | 822 |
| | 01-02 | .008 (.007-.009) | .007 (.006-.009) | .013 (.011-.016) | .025 (.018-.032) | .034 (.025-.051) | 1132 |
| | 03-04 | * | .007 (.006-.008) | .011 (.010-.013) | .019 (.015-.024) | .027 (.020-.040) | 1074 |

* Not calculated: proportion of results below limit of detection was too high to provide a valid result.

injury associated with elevated urinary uranium levels (Kurttio et al., 2006; McDiarmid et al., 2006). IARC and NTP have no ratings for uranium human carcinogenicity.

Workplace air standards and guidelines for external exposure to soluble and insoluble uranium compounds have been established by OSHA and ACGIH, respectively. Drinking water and other environmental standards have been established by U.S. EPA. Information about external exposure (i.e., environmental levels) and health effects is available from ATSDR at: http://www.atsdr.cdc.gov/toxpro2.html.

**Biomonitoring Information**

Levels of urinary uranium reflect recent and accumulated exposure. A previous nonrandom subsample from NHANES III (n = 499) (Ting et al., 1999) and other small populations have shown urinary concentrations that are similar to those in NHANES 1999-2000, 2001-2002, and 2003-2004 (Dang et al.,1992; Galletti, 2003; Karpas et al.,1996; Tolmachev et al., 2006). Older studies have demonstrated urinary uranium concentrations that are consistent with levels in the U.S. population, in that the levels were below their respective detection limits (Byrne et al., 1991; Hamilton et al., 1994; Komaromy-Hiller et al., 2000). In a study of 105 persons exposed to natural uranium in well water, urinary levels of uranium were as high as 9.55 µg/L (median 0.162 µg/L) (Orloff et al., 2004). Eighty-five percent of those levels were above the 95th percentile of the NHANES 1999-2000 population. In two studies of a Finnish population with high natural uranium concentrations in their drinking water, the median urinary concentration was 0.078 µg/L (ranging up to 5.65 µg/L), and no consistent effects on multiple endpoints of kidney function were found. (Kurttio et al., 2002, 2006).

The U.S. Nuclear Regulatory Commission (NRC) has set an action level of 15 µg/L urinary uranium to protect people who are occupationally exposed (U.S. NRC, 1978). Recent studies of veterans have been conducted to examine concerns about DU exposure during military conflicts. A cohort of 46 U.S. soldiers evaluated before, during, and after deployment had geometric mean urinary uranium concentrations that were less than the NHANES 1999-2000 and 2001-2002 geometric means at all three time periods, although slightly increased during and after deployment, (May et al., 2004). In 17 U.S. soldiers who had been injured and had embedded DU shrapnel for as long as eight years, the median urinary uranium concentration was 2.61 µg/g creatinine. In the same study, 28 soldiers who may have been exposed to DU by inhalation, ingestion, or wound contamination, but in whom no shrapnel was embedded, had a mean urinary uranium concentration of 0.066 µg/g

creatinine (Gwiazda et al., 2004). In a much larger study of 446 Gulf War veterans who were concerned about past exposure to DU, the geometric mean urinary uranium concentration was 0.011 µg/L (McDiarmid et al., 2004). Follow up of 32 veterans with embedded shrapnel showed that increased urinary uranium levels persisted more than 12 years after the first exposure (McDiarmid et al., 2006). Six workers in a depleted uranium program showed concentrations of 0.110 to 45 µg/L (Ejnik et al., 2000). Urinary uranium measurements in 103 Canadian military personnel showed mean urinary levels slightly less than geometric mean in this *Report* (Ough et al., 2002).

Finding a measurable amount of uranium in urine does not mean that the level of uranium causes an adverse health effect. Biomonitoring studies on levels of uranium provide physicians and public health officials with reference values so that they can determine whether people have been exposed to higher levels of uranium than are found in the general population. Biomonitoring data can also help scientists plan and conduct research on exposure and health effects.

**References**

Bhattacharyya MH, Breitenstein BD, Metivier H, Muggenburg BA, Stradling GN, Volf V. Guidebook for the treatment of accidental internal radionuclide contamination of workers. In: Gerber GB, Thomas RG, eds. Radiation protection dosimetry. Vol. 41 (1). Kent (England): Nuclear Technology Publishing; 1992. pp. 1-49.

Byrne AR, Benedik L. Uranium content of blood, urine and hair of exposed and non-exposed persons determined by radiochemical neutron activation analysis, with emphasis on quality control. Sci Total Environ 1991;107:143-157.

Centers for Disease Control and Prevention (CDC). Third National Report on Human Exposure to Environmental Chemicals. Atlanta (GA). 2005.

Dang HS, Pullat VR, Pillai KC. Determining the normal concentration of uranium in urine and application of the data to its biokinetics. Health Phys 1992;62:562-566.

Durakovic A, Horan P, Dietz LA, Zimmerman I. Estimate of the time zero lung burden of depleted uranium in Persian Gulf War veterans by the 24-hour urinary excretion and exponential decay analysis. Mil Med 2003;168(8):600-605.

Ejnik JW, Carmichael AJ, Hamilton MM, McDiarmid M, Squibb K, Boyd P, et al. Determination of the isotopic composition of uranium in urine by inductively coupled plasma mass spectrometry. Health Phys 2000;78:143-146.

Galletti M, D'Annibale L, Pinto V, Cremisini C. Uranium daily intake and urinary excretion: a preliminary study in Italy. Health Phys 2003;85:228-235.

Gwiazda RH, Squibb K, McDiarmid M, Smith D. Detection of depleted uranium in urine of veterans from the 1991 Gulf War. Health Phys 2004;86:12-18.

Hamilton EI, Sabbioni E, Van der Venne MT. Element reference values in tissues from inhabitants of the European community. VI. Review of elements in blood, plasma and urine and a critical evaluation of reference values for the United Kingdom population. Sci Total Environ 1994;158:165-190.

Karpas Z, Halicz L, Roiz J, Marko R, Katorza E, Lorber A, et al. Inductively coupled plasma mass spectrometry as a simple, rapid, and inexpensive method for determination of uranium in urine and fresh water: comparison with LIF. Health Phys 1996;71(6):879-85.

Komaromy-Hiller G, Ash KO, Costa R, Howerton K. Comparison of representative ranges based on U.S. patient population and literature reference intervals for urinary trace elements. Clin Chim Acta 2000;296(1-2):71-90.

Kurttio P, Auvinen A, Salonen L, Saha H, Pekkanen J, Makelainen I, et al. Renal effects of uranium in drinking water. Environ Health Perspect 2002;110(4):337-342.

Kurttio P, Harmionen A, Saha H, Salonen L, Karpas Z, Komulainen H, Auvinen A. Kidney toxicity of ingested uranium from drinking water. Am J Kidney Dis 2006;47(6):972-982.

Li WB, Roth P, Wahl W, Oeh U, Hollriegl V, Paretzke HG. Biokinetic modeling of uranium in man after injection and ingestion. Radiat Environ Biophys 2005;44:29-40.

May LM, Heller J, Kalinsky V, Ejnik J, Cordero S, Oberbroekling KJ, et al. Military deployment human exposure assessment: urine total and isotopic uranium sampling results. J Toxicol Environ Health A 2004;67(8-10):697-714.

McDiarmid MA, Squibb K, Engelhardt SM. Biologic monitoring for urinary uranium in Gulf War I veterans. Health Phys 2004;87:51-56.

McDiarmid MA, Englehardt SA, Oliver M, Gucer P, Wilson PD, Kane R, et al. Biological monitoring and surveillance results of Gulf War I veterans exposed to depleted uranium. Int Arch Occup Environ Health 2006;79(1):11-21.

Orloff KG, Mistry K, Charp P, Metcalf S, Marino R, Shelly T, et al. Human exposure to uranium in groundwater. Environ Res 2004;94:319-326.

Ough EA, Lewis BM, Andrews WS, Bennett LG, Hancock RG, Scott K. An examination of uranium levels in Canadian forces personnel who served in the Gulf War and Kosovo. Health Phys 2002;82(4): 527-532.

Ting BG, Paschal DC, Jarrett JM, Pirkle JL, Jackson RJ, Sampson EJ, et al. Uranium and thorium in urine of United States residents: reference range concentrations. Environ Res 1999;81:45-51.

Tolmachev S, Kuwabara J, Noguchi H. concentration and daily excretion of uranium in urine of Japanese. Health Phys 2006;91(2):144-153.

U.S. Nuclear Regulatory Commission (U.S. NRC). U.S. Nuclear Regulatory Commission (NRC) Guide 8.22–Bioassay at uranium mills. Washington (DC): NRC; July 1978.

# Perchlorate
CAS No. 7601-90-3

## General Information

Perchlorate is an inorganic chemical containing one chlorine and four oxygen atoms. It is normally found and produced as the anion of a sodium, potassium, or ammonium salt. Perchlorate is stable under most environmental and physiological conditions, but has strong oxidant properties in the presence of concentrated acids, certain catalytic metals, and reducing agents. The ammonium salt of the perchlorate ion has been manufactured in the military defense and aerospace industries primarily for use as an oxidizer in solid propellant systems for rockets and missiles. Other manufactured uses include fireworks, matches, and limited applications in pharmaceutics, laboratory analysis, leather tanning, fabric dyeing, and electroplating. In addition, small amounts of perchlorate can form naturally in the atmosphere (Dasgupta et al., 2006) and accumulate in nitrate-rich mineral deposits mined for use in fertilizers

(Urbansky, 2002).

Perchlorate was added to the U.S. EPA's Contaminant Candidate List (CCL) for drinking water in 1998 following discoveries of its presence in drinking water supplies throughout the southwestern United States (U.S.EPA, 1998). Perchlorate has been characterized as a mobile and persistent ground and surface water contaminant. Drinking water, milk, and certain plants with high water content (e.g., lettuce) can be the main sources of intake for humans (FDA, 2007). Perchlorate is excreted unchanged from the human body with an estimated elimination half-life of about 7.5 hours and has a small estimated volume of distribution (Crump and Gibbs, 2005).

Animal and human studies have shown that perchlorate can inhibit thyroid hormone production (NAS, 2005). Large doses of perchlorate have been used as a medicine to treat hyperthyroidism and to diagnose disorders related to thyroid or iodine metabolism. Inhibition of iodine uptake by competition for the sodium/iodide symporter in the thyroid can be estimated in humans by measuring radioiodine uptake

## Urinary Perchlorate

Geometric mean and selected percentiles of urine concentrations (in µg/L) for the U.S. population from the National Health and Nutrition Examination Survey.

| | Survey years | Geometric mean (95% conf. interval) | 50th | 75th | 90th | 95th | Sample size |
|---|---|---|---|---|---|---|---|
| **Total** | 01-02 | 3.54 (3.29-3.81) | 3.70 (3.50-4.00) | 6.30 (5.80-6.90) | 10.0 (9.10-11.0) | 14.0 (11.0-17.0) | 2820 |
| | 03-04 | 3.22 (2.93-3.55) | 3.30 (2.90-3.80) | 5.50 (5.00-6.40) | 9.50 (8.40-11.0) | 13.0 (12.0-15.0) | 2522 |
| **Age group** | | | | | | | |
| 6-11 years | 01-02 | 4.93 (4.22-5.76) | 5.20 (4.40-6.40) | 8.10 (6.90-9.80) | 12.0 (9.30-19.0) | 19.0 (12.0-23.0) | 374 |
| | 03-04 | 4.32 (3.67-5.09) | 4.60 (4.00-5.20) | 7.90 (5.70-9.50) | 13.0 (8.81-16.0) | 16.0 (11.0-29.0) | 314 |
| 12-19 years | 01-02 | 3.80 (3.44-4.20) | 4.40 (3.80-4.80) | 6.80 (6.30-7.30) | 10.0 (8.90-11.0) | 13.0 (11.0-17.0) | 828 |
| | 03-04 | 3.62 (3.19-4.12) | 3.80 (3.20-4.40) | 6.40 (5.50-7.10) | 9.80 (7.90-12.0) | 13.0 (10.0-18.0) | 721 |
| 20 years and older | 01-02 | 3.35 (3.08-3.65) | 3.50 (3.20-3.70) | 5.90 (5.30-6.60) | 10.0 (8.70-11.0) | 13.0 (11.0-17.0) | 1618 |
| | 03-04 | 3.05 (2.75-3.38) | 3.20 (2.70-3.60) | 5.20 (4.70-6.10) | 9.10 (7.90-10.0) | 12.0 (11.0-14.0) | 1487 |
| **Gender** | | | | | | | |
| Males | 01-02 | 4.19 (3.93-4.46) | 4.40 (4.20-4.60) | 7.10 (6.40-7.90) | 11.0 (9.70-12.0) | 14.0 (11.0-19.0) | 1335 |
| | 03-04 | 3.75 (3.39-4.16) | 3.90 (3.40-4.40) | 6.40 (5.60-7.50) | 11.0 (9.20-12.0) | 14.0 (13.0-17.0) | 1229 |
| Females | 01-02 | 3.01 (2.74-3.31) | 3.10 (2.70-3.40) | 5.40 (5.00-6.00) | 9.20 (8.20-11.0) | 13.0 (11.0-17.0) | 1485 |
| | 03-04 | 2.79 (2.49-3.11) | 2.90 (2.50-3.20) | 4.90 (4.40-5.50) | 8.20 (6.90-9.84) | 11.0 (8.80-15.0) | 1293 |
| **Race/ethnicity** | | | | | | | |
| Mexican Americans | 01-02 | 4.02 (3.47-4.66) | 4.40 (3.70-5.00) | 7.10 (5.80-8.40) | 12.0 (9.40-13.0) | 14.0 (12.0-18.0) | 708 |
| | 03-04 | 3.76 (3.45-4.11) | 3.96 (3.50-4.40) | 6.20 (5.30-7.50) | 11.0 (9.10-12.0) | 15.0 (12.0-17.0) | 617 |
| Non-Hispanic blacks | 01-02 | 3.51 (3.07-4.03) | 3.70 (3.10-4.10) | 5.90 (5.10-7.00) | 9.20 (7.80-12.0) | 15.0 (11.0-20.0) | 681 |
| | 03-04 | 3.21 (2.90-3.56) | 3.20 (2.87-3.50) | 5.40 (4.60-6.30) | 8.60 (7.50-11.0) | 13.0 (9.30-17.0) | 652 |
| Non-Hispanic whites | 01-02 | 3.51 (3.18-3.88) | 3.70 (3.40-4.10) | 6.30 (5.70-7.10) | 10.0 (8.90-11.0) | 14.0 (11.0-18.0) | 1228 |
| | 03-04 | 3.26 (2.89-3.68) | 3.30 (2.80-4.00) | 5.60 (4.90-6.80) | 9.40 (8.10-11.0) | 13.0 (11.0-15.0) | 1092 |

Limit of detection (LOD, see Data Analysis section) for Survey years 01-02 and 03-04 are 0.05 and 0.05.
2001-2002 performed on surplus samples (variable unavailable of NHANES website)

inhibition (RUI). Short term human studies of the effect of perchlorate on RUI have been used for risk estimation (Greer et al., 2002; Lawrence et al. 2001, 2002; NAS, 2005; U.S.EPA, 2005). In these small short-term experimental studies on males and studies of male perchlorate workers with doses or estimated exposures thousands-fold higher than known environmental exposures, up to 68% RUI has been demonstrated, but without effects on serum levels of thyroid stimulating hormone or thyroxine (Braverman et al., 2005; Greer et al., 2002). However, in a representative sample of U.S. women with urinary levels of iodine less than 100 micrograms per day, urinary perchlorate at environmental exposure levels were inversely associated with thyroxine levels and positively associated with levels of thyroid stimulating hormone (Blount et al., 2006; Steinmaus et al., 2007).

During gestation and infancy, it is known that maternal and congenital hypothyroidism adversely effects neurological development and decreases learning capability. In the U.S., congenital hypothyroidism is a condition for which nearly all newborn blood is screened. Ecologic studies from screening programs with elevated perchlorate in the regional drinking water have indicated no increased prevalence of abnormal neonatal screening tests for this disorder in these regions (Kelsh et al., 2003; Lamm and Doemland, 1999; Li et al., 2000). Also, altered thyroid function was not found in Chilean pregnant women or their newborns with mean urinary perchlorate levels about 40-fold higher than average U.S. levels, although iodine intake was higher than U.S. levels and sufficient in most participants (Tellez et al., 2005). Many factors may be important in consideration of perchlorate action on the thyroid: dose; dietary iodine intake; gender; age; menopausal status; chronicity of exposure; and the presence of other substances known to affect thyroid function (e.g., nitrate, thiocyanate, medications).

Though it produces follicular cell thyroid tumors in animal studies at goitrogenic doses, perchlorate is negative in most genotoxic assays (U.S.EPA, 2005), suggesting its tumorgenic effect is a result of a chronic increase in thyroid stimulating hormone indirectly resulting from iodine uptake inhibition. Follicular cell thyroid tumors would

## Urinary Perchlorate (creatinine corrected)

Geometric mean and selected percentiles of urine concentrations (in µg/g of creatinine) for the U.S. population from the National Health and Nutrition Examination Survey.

| | Survey years | Geometric mean (95% conf. interval) | 50th | 75th | 90th | 95th | Sample size |
|---|---|---|---|---|---|---|---|
| | | | \<\-\-\-\-\-\- Selected percentiles (95% confidence interval) \-\-\-\-\-\-\> | | | | |
| **Total** | 01-02 | 3.56 (3 34-3.80) | 3.39 (3.18-3.66) | 5.61 (5 29-6.00) | 9.36 (8.19-10.3) | 12.7 (11.0-14.3) | 2818 |
| | 03-04 | 3.14 (2 89-3.41) | 3.00 (2 80-3.30) | 4.90 (4 50-5.30) | 8.40 (7 20-9.50) | 12.0 (11.0-14.0) | 2504 |
| **Age group** | | | | | | | |
| 6-11 years | 01-02 | 5.71 (5 22-6.25) | 5.83 (5.19-6.25) | 8.33 (7.41-9.74) | 13.1 (11.1-16.0) | 17.5 (13.1-22.6) | 374 |
| | 03-04 | 5.24 (4.61-5.96) | 5.10 (4.70-5.50) | 7.20 (6.40-10.0) | 13.0 (8 90-20.0) | 20.0 (11.0-44.0) | 313 |
| 12-19 years | 01-02 | 2.95 (2.64-3.29) | 2.89 (2 56-3.39) | 4.50 (3 97-5.26) | 7.12 (6.60-8.10) | 9.87 (7.46-13.4) | 827 |
| | 03-04 | 2.70 (2.45-2.98) | 2.70 (2 50-3.00) | 4.20 (3.70-4.50) | 6.30 (5.10-7.50) | 8.00 (6 90-11.0) | 715 |
| 20 years and older | 01-02 | 3.46 (3 20-3.73) | 3.26 (3 04-3.58) | 5.37 (4 93-5.91) | 9.09 (7.61-10.2) | 12.3 (10.1-14.3) | 1617 |
| | 03-04 | 3.03 (2.76-3.32) | 2.90 (2.60-3.20) | 4.70 (4 30-5.10) | 8.10 (6 90-9.40) | 11.0 (9.60-15.0) | 1476 |
| **Gender** | | | | | | | |
| Males | 01-02 | 3.40 (3 20-3.60) | 3.25 (3 04-3.47) | 5.35 (4 93-5.86) | 8.80 (7 52-9.87) | 11.4 (10.1-13.0) | 1335 |
| | 03-04 | 3.07 (2 81-3.35) | 2.90 (2.70-3.20) | 4.80 (4 30-5.30) | 7.30 (6 50-9.70) | 12.0 (9.70-15.0) | 1220 |
| Females | 01-02 | 3.72 (3 39-4.09) | 3.60 (3 20-4.10) | 5.99 (5 33-6.67) | 10.0 (8.15-12.1) | 13.4 (11.4-16.0) | 1483 |
| | 03-04 | 3.21 (2 87-3.59) | 3.10 (2 80-3.40) | 5.00 (4.60-5.60) | 8.90 (7 00-11.0) | 12.0 (9 90-15.0) | 1284 |
| **Race/ethnicity** | | | | | | | |
| Mexican Americans | 01-02 | 3.77 (3 22-4.40) | 3.51 (3 02-4.44) | 6.05 (4 93-7.64) | 10.4 (8 37-13.0) | 14.4 (11.6-17.4) | 708 |
| | 03-04 | 3.42 (3.16-3.70) | 3.30 (3 00-3.50) | 5.40 (4.60-6.10) | 9.20 (7.60-11.0) | 13.0 (11.0-19.0) | 616 |
| Non-Hispanic blacks | 01-02 | 2.53 (2 24-2.87) | 2.54 (2.12-2.84) | 4.08 (3 51-4.93) | 6.87 (5 93-8.43) | 10.1 (8 33-12.2) | 680 |
| | 03-04 | 2.22 (2 00-2.45) | 2.10 (1 90-2.30) | 3.40 (3.10-3.90) | 6.20 (4.60-8.00) | 8.50 (6.60-11.0) | 648 |
| Non-Hispanic whites | 01-02 | 3.76 (3.46-4.08) | 3.54 (3 22-4.02) | 5.82 (5.44-6.25) | 9.52 (8 30-10.5) | 12.8 (11.3-14.6) | 1227 |
| | 03-04 | 3.35 (2 99-3.75) | 3.20 (2 90-3.50) | 5.10 (4.60-5.60) | 8.80 (7 20-10.0) | 12.0 (10.0-17.0) | 1080 |

2001-2002 performed on surplus samples (variable unavailable of NHANES website)

be unlikely to occur without overt perturbation of thyroid homeostasis. Additional information about exposure and health effects is available from the U.S.EPA at: http://www.epa.gov/safewater/ccl/perchlorate/perchlorate.html and from ATSDR at: http://www.atsdr.cdc.gov/toxpro2.html.

## Biomonitoring Information

Urinary perchlorate levels reflect recent exposure. Blount et al. (2007) analyzed a subsample of NHANES 2001-2002 which demonstrated detectable perchlorate in all urinary samples and showed slightly higher levels in children as compared to adults. When these NHANES 2001-2002 urinary levels of perchlorate are used to calculate daily oral intakes for the U.S. population, most of the population is considered to be below the U.S. EPA reference dose (Blount et al., 2007). The levels seen in NHANES 2003-2004 show a similar pattern to NHANES 2001-2002. Compared to a previous study of pregnant women in three Chilean communities with varying perchlorate levels in the drinking water, the women in the community with the highest drinking water levels had mean urinary perchlorate levels about 40 times greater than the geometric mean for participants in NHANES 2001-2002 aged 20 years and older (Tellez et al., 2005). Also, the 95th percentile of NHANES 2001-2002 participants aged 20 years and older have urinary perchlorate levels that are several thousand times less than urinary levels measured during occupational exposure of perchlorate workers (Braverman et al., 2005).

Finding a measurable amount of perchlorate in urine does not mean that the level of perchlorate causes an adverse health effect. Biomonitoring studies of urinary perchlorate provide physicians and public health officials with reference values so that they can determine whether or not people have been exposed to higher levels of perchlorate than levels found in the general population. Biomonitoring data can also help scientists plan and conduct research on exposure and health effects.

## References

Blount BC, Pirkle JL, Osterloh JD, Valentin-Blasini L, Caldwell KL. Urinary perchlorate and thyroid hormone levels in adolescent and adult men and women living in the United States. Environ Health Perspect 2006;114(12):1865-1871.

Blount BC, Valentin-Blasini L, Osterloh JD, Mauldin JP, Pirkle JL. Perchlorate Exposure of the US Population, 2001-2002. J Expo Sci Environ Epidemiol 2007;17(4):400-407.

Braverman LE, He X, Pino S, Cross M, Magnani B, Lamm SH, et al. The effect of perchlorate, thiocyanate, and nitrate on thyroid function in workers exposed to perchlorate long-term. J Clin Endocrinol Metab 2005;90(2):700-706.

Crump KS, Gibbs JP. Benchmark calculations for perchlorate from three human cohorts. Environ Health Perspect 2005;113(8):1001-1008.

Dasgupta PK, Dyke JV, Kirk AB, Jackson WA. Perchlorate in the United States. Analysis of relative source contributions to the food chain. Environ Sci Technol 2006;40(21):6608-6614.

Food and Drug Administration (FDA). CFSAN/Office of Plant & Dairy Foods. Preliminary Estimation of Perchlorate Dietary Exposure Based on FDA 2004/2005 Exploratory Data. May 2007. Available at URL: http://www.fda.gov/Food/FoodSafety/FoodContaminantsAdulteration/ChemicalContaminants/Perchlorate/ucm077653.htm. Page Last Updated: 05/28/2009. 6/2/09

Greer MA, Goodman G, Pleus RC, Greer SE. Health effects assessment for environmental perchlorate contamination: the dose response for inhibition of thyroidal radioiodine uptake in humans. Environ Health Perspect 2002;110(9):927-937. Erratum in: Environ Health Perspect 2005;113(11):A732.

Kelsh MA, Buffler PA, Daaboul JJ, Rutherford GW, Lau EC, Barnard JC, et al. Primary congenital hypothyroidism, newborn thyroid function, and environmental perchlorate exposure among residents of a Southern California community. J Occup Environ Med 2003;45(10):1116-1127. Erratum in: J Occup Environ Med 2004;46(5):509.

Lamm SH, Doemland M. Has perchlorate in drinking water increased the rate of congenital hypothyroidism? J Occup Environ Med 1999;41(5):409-411.

Lawrence J, Lamm S, Braverman LE. Low dose perchlorate (3 mg daily) and thyroid function. Thyroid 2001;11(3):295.

Lawrence JE, Lamm SH, Pino S, Richman K, Braverman LE. The effect of short-term low-dose perchlorate on various aspects of thyroid function. Thyroid 2000;10(8):659-663.

Li Z, Li FX, Byrd D, Deyhle GM, Sesser DE, Skeels MR, et al. Neonatal thyroxine level and perchlorate in drinking water. J Occup Environ Med 2000;42(2):200-205.

National Academy of Sciences (NAS). Health Implications of Perchlorate Ingestion. National Research Council of the National Academies. Washington (DC): National Academy Press; 2005.

Steinmaus C, Miller MD, Howd R. Impact of smoking and thiocyanate on perchlorate and thyroid hormone associations in the 2001-2002 national health and nutrition examination survey. Environ Health Perspect 2007;115(9):1333-1338.

Tellez RT, Chacon PM, Abarca CR, Blount BC, Landingham CB, Crump KS, et al. Long-term environmental exposure to perchlorate through drinking water and thyroid function during pregnancy and the neonatal period. Thyroid 2005;15(9):963-975.

U.S. Environmental Protection Agency (U.S. EPA). Perchlorate. Integrated Risk Information System (IRIS). Revised 2/11/05. Available from URL: http://cfpub.epa.gov/iris/quickview. cfm?substance_nmbr=1007.1/15/06

U.S. Environmental Protection Agency (U.S. EPA). Drinking Water Contaminant Candidate List. Doc. No. EPA/600/F-98/002 Washington (DC). 1988.

Urbansky TF. Perchlorate as an environmental contaminant. Environ Sci Pollut Res Int 2002;9(3):187-192.

# Perfluorochemicals

## General Information

The perfluorochemicals (PFCs) are molecules in which all bonds of the alkyl chain are carbon-fluorine bonds except for the terminal functional group. Discussed here are perfluoroalkyl acids, amides, and alcohols which are by-products, end products, or processing aids used in the synthesis of fluoropolymers. Fluoropolymers have applications in waterproofing and protective coatings of clothes, furniture, and other products; and also as constituents of floor polish, adhesives, fire retardant foam, and insulation of electrical wire. A major application of one important fluoropolymer, polytetrafluoroethylene, has been the heat-resistant non-stick coatings used on cooking ware and other protected surfaces. Because of their properties, fluoropolymer products are used in a wide range of industries including aerospace, automotive, building/construction, chemical processing, electrical and electronics, semiconductor, and textiles. There are many other fluorocarbon type chemicals which are not addressed here, such as perfluorochemical telomers, finalized perfluorochemical polymer products, chlorofluorocarbons and investigational blood substitutes.

Perfluorooctanoic acid (PFOA) has been manufactured since the 1950s, primarily as its ammonium salt, as a solubilization aid in the synthesis of polytetrafluoroethylene. PFOA is usually not a residual contaminant in non-stick surfaces made of polytetrafluoroethylene. Worldwide annual production of PFOA was estimated to be 260 metric tons in 1999 (Prevedouros et al., 2006). Production rates and emission rates have fallen since 2002 after conversion to a new synthesis process. Other perfluoroalkyl carboxylates of various chain lengths were also formed in the process used prior to 2002. However, current manufacturing practices reduce the formation of these by exclusively using fluorotelomers (Prevedouros et al., 2006).

Perfluorooctanesulfonyl fluoride (POSF) was synthesized as a polymerization starting material. POSF-based polymers have been used in a wide variety of products such as waterproofing, textiles, and fire protection. Other PFCs (including small amounts of PFOA) can also form as side-reaction by-products in the synthesis of POSF (e.g., perfluorooctane sulfonamide, PFOSA), or form as degradation products during its reaction to create the intermediate reacting monomers, N-methylperfluorooctanesulfonamidoethanol (MeFOSE) and N-ethylperfluorooctanesulfonamidoethanol (EtFOSE), or form in the final product (e.g., perfluorooctane sulfonate, PFOS) (Hekster et al., 2003; Olsen et al., 2005; U.S. EPA, 2003). MeFOSE and EtFOSE have been used in food packaging and textile treatments, and their oxidation products, N-methylperfluorooctane-sulfonamidoacetic acid (Me-PFOSA-AcOH) and N-ethylperfluorooctanesulfonamidoacetic acid (Et-PFOSA-AcOH), respectively, may be markers of food or consumer exposures. In addition, several pathways (during manufacturing) can lead to formation of PFOS or other sulfonyl-containing PFCs as residual contaminants in the final polymer products. Perfluorohexane sulfonate (PFHxS) has also been used to synthesize the fluoropolymers used in firefighting foams and some carpet treatments. U.S. manufacture of POSF-based products began ending in about 2000. Global production that year for POSF materials was 3700 metric tons (Prevedouros et al., 2006). Perfluorononanoic acid (PFNA) was an impurity in the process that produces PFOS.

The PFCs have limited water solubility, low volatility (as salts or ionized) and can remain in the environment and bioconcentrate in animals (e.g., some fish bioconcentrate

## Perfluorinated Chemicals in this *Report*

| Perfluorinated Compounds | CAS number | Abbreviation |
|---|---|---|
| Serum Perfluorobutane Sulfonic Acid | | PFBuS |
| Serum Perfluorodecanoic Acid | 335-76-2 | PFDeA |
| Serum Perfluorododecanoic Acid | 307-55-1 | PFDoA |
| Serum Perfluoroheptanoic Acid | 375-85-9 | PFHpA |
| Serum Perfluorohexane Sulfonic Acid | 355-46-4 | PFHxS |
| Serum Perfluorononanoic Acid | 375-95-1 | PFNA |
| Serum Perfluorooctanoic Acid | 335-67-1 | PFOA |
| Serum Perfluorooctane Sulfonic Acid | 1763-23-1 | PFOS |
| Serum Perfluorooctane Sulfonamide | 754-91-6 | PFOSA |
| Serum 2-(*N*-Ethyl-Perfluorooctane sulfonamido) Acetic Acid | | Et-PFOSA-AcOH |
| Serum 2-(*N*-Methyl-perfluorooctane sulfonamido) Acetic Acid | | Me-PFOSA-AcOH |
| Serum Perfluoroundecanoic Acid | 2058-94-8 | PFUA |

PFOS greater than 2000-fold over aquatic levels). PFOS and PFOA levels in archived bird eggs from Sweden have increased thirtyfold from 1968 to 2003 (Holmstrom et al., 2005). PFCs have been identified in surface coastal and ocean waters (Yamashita et al., 2005), in a wide variety of marine and land animals (Kannan et al., 2005; Keller et al., 2005; Taniyasu et al., 2003), and in human blood and semen (Calafat et al., 2006a; Guruge et al., 2005; Kannan et al., 2004; Olsen et al., 2003a and 2004a). In some cases, environmental breakdown products of the telomers used to make fluoropolymers or the metabolic products of fluorochemicals in the body can produce PFCs that are measured human blood. For instance, the 8-2 telomer, heptadecafluoro-1-decanol, may metabolize or degrade to PFOA (Dinglasan et al., 2004). It is unclear if environmentally degraded telomer products are a major source of other PFCs.

All sources of human exposure are uncertain, but probably include dietary sources (Kannan et al., 2004; Prevedouros et al., 2006; Tittlemier et al., 2007). PFOA (and probably other perfluoroalkyl acids) exist in the anionic state at physiologic and environmental pHs and their distribution in the body is determined, in part, by high protein binding in plasma and other proteins. Unlike many organohalogen contaminant chemicals, the perfluoroalkyl acids (PFOA and PFOS) do not tend to accumulate in fat tissue, but still can have long residence times in the body. PFOA is mostly excreted in the urine in animal studies, but limited observations in humans suggest that only one-fifth of the total body clearance is renal (Harada et al., 2005). The elimination half-life of

PFOA in humans is roughly estimated to be 3.5 years and for PFOS, approximately 4.8 years (Olsen et al., 2007a). Excepting PFOS and PFOA, there is limited information on the sources, environmental fate, human toxicokinetics, or effects of other PFCs. The PFCs often measured in human serum are listed in the table.

Human health effects from PFCs at low environmental doses or at biomonitored levels from low environmental exposures are unknown. The ammonium salt of PFOA has been tested at high doses in mammalian animal studies and produced altered weights of the liver, kidney, thymus and spleen; hepatotoxicity; endocrine and immune effects; and in offspring, growth retardation and delayed sexual maturation (Kennedy et al., 2004; Lau et al., 2004; U.S. EPA, 2003). Both PFOA and perfluorodecanoic acid have been shown to reduce androgen levels in laboratory animal studies (Biegel et al., 1995; Bookstaff et al., 1990). PFOA preparations used in many studies may also contain a small percentage of other chain length perfluoroalkyl acids (i.e., C5, C6, C7). The liver toxicity of several PFCs is evident by vacuolization and lipid accumulation in both rodent and monkey livers (Seacat et al., 2002; Lau et al., 2004) and may be attributable to the ability of PFCs to affect intracellular lipid binding proteins, peroxisomal proliferation, and β-oxidation of lipids (Kudo et al., 2000, 2003; Vanden Heuvel et al., 1993). Some of the effects in animals may be mediated through peroxisomal proliferation, including immunologic effects and tumor induction, but the relevance of peroxisomal pathways in humans is unclear (Kennedy et al., 2004). PFOA has been reported to cause liver, pancreas,

## Serum Perfluorobutane sulfonic acid (PFBuS)

Geometric mean and selected percentiles of serum concentrations (in µg/L) for the U.S. population from the National Health and Nutrition Examination Survey.

| | Survey years | Geometric mean (95% conf. interval) | Selected percentiles (95% confidence interval) | | | | Sample size |
|---|---|---|---|---|---|---|---|
| | | | 50th | 75th | 90th | 95th | |
| Total | 03-04 | * | < LOD | < LOD | < LOD | < LOD | 2094 |
| **Age group** | | | | | | | |
| 12-19 years | 03-04 | * | < LOD | < LOD | < LOD | < LOD | 640 |
| 20 years and older | 03-04 | * | < LOD | < LOD | < LOD | < LOD | 1454 |
| **Gender** | | | | | | | |
| Males | 03-04 | * | < LOD | < LOD | < LOD | < LOD | 1053 |
| Females | 03-04 | * | < LOD | < LOD | < LOD | < LOD | 1041 |
| **Race/ethnicity** | | | | | | | |
| Mexican Americans | 03-04 | * | < LOD | < LOD | < LOD | < LOD | 485 |
| Non-Hispanic blacks | 03-04 | * | < LOD | < LOD | < LOD | < LOD | 538 |
| Non-Hispanic whites | 03-04 | * | < LOD | < LOD | < LOD | < LOD | 962 |

Limit of detection (LOD, see Data Analysis section) for Survey year 03-04 is 0.4.
< LOD means less than the limit of detection, which may vary for some chemicals by year and by individual sample.
* Not calculated: proportion of results below limit of detection was too high to provide a valid result.

and testicular tumors in high dose animal testing (Biegel et al., 2001; Cook et al., 1992; Kennedy et al., 2004). Effects on serum liver enzymes in limited observational studies of human occupational exposures are unclear. Two recent cross-sectional human studies observed a negative correlation of birth weight with serum levels of PFOA (Apelberg et al., 2007; Fei et al., 2007).

Due to marked intergender differences in the elimination of PFOA in rats and substantial differences in the half-life of PFOA in rats, monkeys, and humans, the potential to estimate risks to humans from animal doses is uncertain. However, animal and human serum PFOA levels have been compared: serum levels associated with toxic effects in animals are 66-11,108 times higher than background serum levels in humans (Butenoff et al., 2004; U.S. EPA, 2003). A study of workers chronically exposed to primarily PFOA showed no biochemical evidence of hepatotoxicity or hormonal changes (adrenal, reproductive, thyroidal), and there was no clear evidence of excess all-cause or disease-specific mortality, or increased cancer rates (Alexander et al., 2003; Olsen et al., 1999; U.S. EPA, 2003).

Serum PFOS levels associated with toxicity in test animals were 310-1550 fold higher than 95 percent of the levels found in a study of adults (Olsen et al., 2003a, 2005). Animal studies of PFOS have demonstrated weight loss, hepatotoxicity, and changes in thyroid hormone concentrations (Grasty et al., 2003; Thibodeaux et al., 2003; Lau et al., 2004). At doses causing maternal toxicity, developmental and teratogenic effects were demonstrated in offspring. At high but non-toxic maternal doses of PFOS, development in offspring was stunted and hypothyroxinemia was observed. Late gestational exposure to PFOS in animal studies has also demonstrated early neonatal lethality, possibly related to lung immaturity (Lau et al., 2003). PFOA, PFOS, and other PFCs have not been classified as to human carcinogenicity by IARC or NTP.

**Biomonitoring Information**

Serum levels of PFCs (particularly PFOA and PFOS) tend to reflect cumulative exposure over several years. Twelve different PFCs were measured in the sera of NHANES 2003-2004 participants. Roughly similar levels of PFCs in serum have also been measured previously in other samples of the U.S. population. In such studies, PFOS, PFOA, perfluorohexanesulfonate (PFHxS), and perfluorononanoic acid (PFNA) are detectable in a high percentage of the participants and PFOS levels are generally 3-10 times higher than PFOA levels (Calafat et al., 2007a, 2007b; Olsen et al., 2003a, 2005). Analysis of the NHANES 2003-2004 subsample demonstrated higher levels of PFOA and PFOS in males and a slight increase in levels of PFOS with age (Calafat et al., 2007b). Slightly higher levels of PFOS and PFOA in males than females have been noted in several other studies (Calafat et al., 2007a; Harada et al., 2004; Olsen et al., 2003a). In comparing three separate reports on adults, elderly and children, the median PFCs values tend to be roughly similar in these age categories (Olsen et al., 2003a, 2004a, 2004b), and no substantial age trends were seen within adults ages 20-69 (Olsen et al., 2003a).

### Serum Perfluorodecanoic acid (PFDeA)

Geometric mean and selected percentiles of serum concentrations (in µg/L) for the U.S. population from the National Health and Nutrition Examination Survey.

| | Survey years | Geometric mean (95% conf. interval) | 50th | 75th | 90th | 95th | Sample size |
|---|---|---|---|---|---|---|---|
| Total | 03-04 | * | < LOD | .300 (<LOD- 500) | .600 (.400-1.10) | .900 (.500-1 80) | 2094 |
| **Age group** | | | | | | | |
| 12-19 years | 03-04 | * | < LOD | < LOD | .500 (<LOD-1.00) | .800 (.300-1 20) | 640 |
| 20 years and older | 03-04 | * | < LOD | .400 (<LOD- 500) | .700 (.400-1 00) | .900 (.500-1 80) | 1454 |
| **Gender** | | | | | | | |
| Males | 03-04 | * | < LOD | .400 (<LOD- 500) | .800 (.400-1.40) | 1.10 (.600-2.10) | 1053 |
| Females | 03-04 | * | < LOD | .300 (<LOD-.400) | .500 (.400-.800) | .800 (.500-1 20) | 1041 |
| **Race/ethnicity** | | | | | | | |
| Mexican Americans | 03-04 | * | < LOD | < LOD | .500 (.400-.500) | .600 (.500-.800) | 485 |
| Non-Hispanic blacks | 03-04 | * | < LOD | .400 (<LOD-.700) | .800 (.400-1 50) | 1.00 (.500-3.10) | 538 |
| Non-Hispanic whites | 03-04 | * | < LOD | .300 (<LOD- 500) | .600 (.400-1 00) | .900 (.500-1 80) | 962 |

Limit of detection (LOD, see Data Analysis section) for Survey year 03-04 is 0 3.
< LOD means less than the limit of detection, which may vary for some chemicals by year and by individual sample.
* Not calculated: proportion of results below limit of detection was too high to provide a valid result.

In a study of 598 blood donors aged 20-69 (Olsen et al., 2003*a*), surprisingly little variance in across five widely-dispersed U.S. cities was seen in median PFC levels. PFOS and PFOA were shown to be highly correlated in that study and also in NHANES 2003-2004 (Calafat et al., 2007*b*), possibly due to PFOA being a by-product in POSF-related production. The median levels of various PFCs in Olsen et al. (2003*a*) were similar to those of pooled samples (1990 through 2002) of the U.S. population (Calafat et al., 2006*a*). Olsen et al (2005) also showed that PFCs serum concentrations increased from 1974 to 1989 in 58 paired samples: 25% for PFOS, 162% for PFOA, and 204% for Et-PFOSA-AcOH. Recently, Olsen et al. (2007*b*) reported reductions in PFOS and PFOA concentrations for a group of Red Cross blood donors in the United States from 2000 to 2005.

Serum levels of PFCs, particularly PFOS, appear to be higher in the U.S. than in some other countries: about two to threefold higher than in Columbia, Brazil, Poland, Belgium, Malaysia, Korea and Japan; and about eight to sixteenfold higher than in Italy and India (Kannan et al., 2004); and more than thirtyfold higher than in Peru (Calafat et al., 2006*b*). Notably, the sample sizes were small in these studies. In Japan, PFOS levels tended to vary within regions of the country ranging from U.S. median levels to about fivefold lower levels (Harada et al., 2004). PFC levels for the U.S. population, representing environmental exposures, are much lower than those reported for occupational exposure. In monitored workers employed at a POSF production facility with no biochemical or clinically observable effects, median levels of PFOS and PFOA were over 40 to 300-fold higher, respectively (Olsen et al., 2003*b*).

Finding a measurable amount of PFCs in serum does not mean that the levels of PFCs cause an adverse health effect. Biomonitoring studies of serum PFCs can provide physicians and public health officials with reference values so that they can determine whether or not people have been exposed to higher levels of PFCs than are found in the general population. Biomonitoring data can also help scientists plan and conduct research on exposure and health effects.

## Serum Perfluorododecanoic acid (PFDoA)

Geometric mean and selected percentiles of serum concentrations (in µg/L) for the U.S. population from the National Health and Nutrition Examination Survey.

| | Survey years | Geometric mean (95% conf. interval) | Selected percentiles ( 95% confidence interval) | | | | Sample size |
|---|---|---|---|---|---|---|---|
| | | | 50th | 75th | 90th | 95th | |
| Total | 03-04 | * | < LOD | < LOD | < LOD | < LOD | 2094 |
| **Age group** | | | | | | | |
| 12-19 years | 03-04 | * | < LOD | < LOD | < LOD | < LOD | 640 |
| 20 years and older | 03-04 | * | < LOD | < LOD | < LOD | < LOD | 1454 |
| **Gender** | | | | | | | |
| Males | 03-04 | * | < LOD | < LOD | < LOD | < LOD | 1053 |
| Females | 03-04 | * | < LOD | < LOD | < LOD | < LOD | 1041 |
| **Race/ethnicity** | | | | | | | |
| Mexican Americans | 03-04 | * | < LOD | < LOD | < LOD | < LOD | 485 |
| Non-Hispanic blacks | 03-04 | * | < LOD | < LOD | < LOD | < LOD | 538 |
| Non-Hispanic whites | 03-04 | * | < LOD | < LOD | < LOD | < LOD | 962 |

Limit of detection (LOD, see Data Analysis section) for Survey year 03-04 is 1 0.
< LOD means less than the limit of detection, which may vary for some chemicals by year and by individual sample.
* Not calculated: proportion of results below limit of detection was too high to provide a valid result.


## Serum Perfluoroheptanoic acid (PFHpA)

Geometric mean and selected percentiles of serum concentrations (in µg/L) for the U.S. population from the National Health and Nutrition Examination Survey.

| | Survey years | Geometric mean (95% conf. interval) | Selected percentiles ( 95% confidence interval) | | | | Sample size |
|---|---|---|---|---|---|---|---|
| | | | 50th | 75th | 90th | 95th | |
| Total | 03-04 | * | < LOD | < LOD | < LOD | .400 (<LOD- 500) | 2094 |
| **Age group** | | | | | | | |
| 12-19 years | 03-04 | * | < LOD | < LOD | .400 (<LOD- 600) | .600 (.500-.900) | 640 |
| 20 years and older | 03-04 | * | < LOD | < LOD | < LOD | < LOD | 1454 |
| **Gender** | | | | | | | |
| Males | 03-04 | * | < LOD | < LOD | < LOD | .300 (<LOD-.400) | 1053 |
| Females | 03-04 | * | < LOD | < LOD | < LOD | .400 (.300-.600) | 1041 |
| **Race/ethnicity** | | | | | | | |
| Mexican Americans | 03-04 | * | < LOD | < LOD | < LOD | .500 (<LOD- 900) | 485 |
| Non-Hispanic blacks | 03-04 | * | < LOD | < LOD | < LOD | < LOD | 538 |
| Non-Hispanic whites | 03-04 | * | < LOD | < LOD | < LOD | .300 (<LOD- 500) | 962 |

Limit of detection (LOD, see Data Analysis section) for Survey year 03-04 is 0 3.
< LOD means less than the limit of detection, which may vary for some chemicals by year and by individual sample.
* Not calculated: proportion of results below limit of detection was too high to provide a valid result.

## Serum Perfluorohexane sulfonic acid (PFHxS)

Geometric mean and selected percentiles of serum concentrations (in µg/L) for the U.S. population from the National Health and Nutrition Examination Survey.

| | Survey years | Geometric mean (95% conf. interval) | Selected percentiles (95% confidence interval) | | | | Sample size |
|---|---|---|---|---|---|---|---|
| | | | 50th | 75th | 90th | 95th | |
| Total | 03-04 | 1.93 (1.73-2.16) | 1.90 (1.70-2.10) | 3.30 (2.80-3.90) | 5.90 (4.80-7.20) | 8.30 (7.10-9.70) | 2094 |
| Age group | | | | | | | |
| 12-19 years | 03-04 | 2.44 (2.05-2.90) | 2.40 (1.80-3.20) | 4.90 (4.00-6.30) | 9.50 (6.80-12 5) | 13.3 (9.90-19 6) | 640 |
| 20 years and older | 03-04 | 1.86 (1.67-2.08) | 1.80 (1.60-2.10) | 3.00 (2.60-3.60) | 5.50 (4.50-6.70) | 7.60 (6.30-9.40) | 1454 |
| Gender | | | | | | | |
| Males | 03-04 | 2.17 (1.87-2.51) | 2.10 (1.80-2.40) | 3.40 (2.80-4.50) | 6.10 (4.60-8.10) | 8.50 (6.50-10 5) | 1053 |
| Females | 03-04 | 1.72 (1.56-1.91) | 1.60 (1.40-1.80) | 2.90 (2.50-3.50) | 5.80 (4.60-7.10) | 8.20 (6.70-10 0) | 1041 |
| Race/ethnicity | | | | | | | |
| Mexican Americans | 03-04 | 1.42 (1.17-1.72) | 1.50 (1.20-1.70) | 2.30 (1.90-2.90) | 4.30 (3.10-5.10) | 5.50 (4.00-8.90) | 485 |
| Non-Hispanic blacks | 03-04 | 1.92 (1.62-2.26) | 1.90 (1.60-2.20) | 3.50 (2.80-4.60) | 6.00 (5.00-7.10) | 8.30 (6.30-12 0) | 538 |
| Non-Hispanic whites | 03-04 | 2.01 (1.77-2.27) | 1.90 (1.70-2.20) | 3.30 (2.80-4.10) | 6.10 (4.70-7.80) | 8.20 (6.90-10.1) | 962 |

Limit of detection (LOD, see Data Analysis section) for Survey year 03-04 is 0.3.

## Serum Perfluorononanoic acid (PFNA)

Geometric mean and selected percentiles of serum concentrations (in µg/L) for the U.S. population from the National Health and Nutrition Examination Survey.

| | Survey years | Geometric mean (95% conf. interval) | Selected percentiles (95% confidence interval) | | | | Sample size |
|---|---|---|---|---|---|---|---|
| | | | 50th | 75th | 90th | 95th | |
| Total | 03-04 | .966 ( 816-1.14) | 1.00 ( 900-1.10) | 1.50 (1.20-1.80) | 2.30 (1.60-4.30) | 3.20 (1.80-7.70) | 2094 |
| Age group | | | | | | | |
| 12-19 years | 03-04 | .852 ( 697-1.04) | .800 (.700-1.00) | 1.20 (1.00-1.60) | 1.90 (1.20-3.70) | 2.80 (1.30-6.30) | 640 |
| 20 years and older | 03-04 | .984 ( 835-1.16) | 1.00 ( 900-1.10) | 1.50 (1.20-1.80) | 2.40 (1.60-4.40) | 3.40 (1.80-8.40) | 1454 |
| Gender | | | | | | | |
| Males | 03-04 | 1.09 ( 912-1.30) | 1.10 ( 900-1.20) | 1.60 (1.40-1.90) | 2.40 (1.70-5.00) | 4.00 (1.80-8.70) | 1053 |
| Females | 03-04 | .861 (.721-1.03) | .900 ( 800-1.00) | 1.30 (1.00-1.70) | 2.20 (1.40-3.40) | 3.00 (1.70-6.10) | 1041 |
| Race/ethnicity | | | | | | | |
| Mexican Americans | 03-04 | .689 ( 586-.809) | .700 ( 600-.900) | 1.10 ( 900-1.40) | 1.60 (1.30-2.00) | 2.00 (1.60-2.80) | 485 |
| Non-Hispanic blacks | 03-04 | 1.14 ( 834-1.54) | 1.10 ( 900-1.40) | 1.70 (1.20-2.90) | 3.20 (1.50-6.50) | 4.70 (2.10-9.30) | 538 |
| Non-Hispanic whites | 03-04 | .963 ( 826-1.12) | .900 ( 900-1.10) | 1.50 (1.20-1.70) | 2.30 (1.60-3.60) | 3.00 (1.80-6.20) | 962 |

Limit of detection (LOD, see Data Analysis section) for Survey year 03-04 is 0.1.

## Serum Perfluorooctanoic acid (PFOA)

Geometric mean and selected percentiles of serum concentrations (in µg/L) for the U.S. population from the National Health and Nutrition Examination Survey.

| | Survey years | Geometric mean (95% conf. interval) | Selected percentiles ( 95% confidence interval) | | | | Sample size |
|---|---|---|---|---|---|---|---|
| | | | 50th | 75th | 90th | 95th | |
| Total | 03-04 | 3.95 (3.65-4 27) | 4.10 (3.80-4.40) | 5.80 (5.30-6.40) | 7.80 (6.70-9 60) | 9.80 (7.40-14.1) | 2094 |
| **Age group** | | | | | | | |
| 12-19 years | 03-04 | 3.89 (3.47-4 35) | 4.00 (3.50-4 50) | 5.40 (4.60-6.10) | 7.00 (5.60-9 20) | 8.60 (5.90-12.6) | 640 |
| 20 years and older | 03-04 | 3.96 (3.67-4 27) | 4.10 (3.90-4.40) | 5.90 (5.40-6 50) | 7.80 (6.80-9 60) | 9.90 (7.60-14.2) | 1454 |
| **Gender** | | | | | | | |
| Males | 03-04 | 4.47 (4.07-4 91) | 4.60 (4.30-5 00) | 6.30 (5.70-7 20) | 8.40 (6.80-12.5) | 10.7 (7.40-17.5) | 1053 |
| Females | 03-04 | 3.50 (3.21-3 82) | 3.60 (3.30-3 90) | 5.20 (4.70-5 80) | 7.10 (6.30-8 20) | 8.60 (7.40-10.6) | 1041 |
| **Race/ethnicity** | | | | | | | |
| Mexican Americans | 03-04 | 3.11 (2.84-3.40) | 3.30 (3.10-3.70) | 4.50 (4.20-5 20) | 6.70 (5.70-7 30) | 7.60 (6.70-10.5) | 485 |
| Non-Hispanic blacks | 03-04 | 3.37 (2.99-3.79) | 3.70 (3.20-4 20) | 5.20 (4.40-6 30) | 7.70 (5.30-11.6) | 9.60 (6.50-13.9) | 538 |
| Non-Hispanic whites | 03-04 | 4.18 (3.85-4 53) | 4.30 (3.90-4.70) | 6.00 (5.50-6.70) | 7.90 (7.20-9 20) | 9.90 (7.60-13.3) | 962 |

Limit of detection (LOD, see Data Analysis section) for Survey year 03-04 is 0.1.

## Serum Perfluorooctane sulfonic acid (PFOS)

Geometric mean and selected percentiles of serum concentrations (in µg/L) for the U.S. population from the National Health and Nutrition Examination Survey.

| | Survey years | Geometric mean (95% conf. interval) | Selected percentiles ( 95% confidence interval) | | | | Sample size |
|---|---|---|---|---|---|---|---|
| | | | 50th | 75th | 90th | 95th | |
| Total | 03-04 | 20.7 (19.2-22.3) | 21.2 (19.8-22.4) | 30.0 (27.5-33.0) | 41.3 (35.6-50.0) | 54.6 (44.0-66.5) | 2094 |
| **Age group** | | | | | | | |
| 12-19 years | 03-04 | 19.3 (17.5-21.4) | 19.9 (17.8-22.0) | 27.1 (23.7-30.2) | 36.5 (28.6-45.6) | 42.6 (35.1-52.1) | 640 |
| 20 years and older | 03-04 | 20.9 (19.3-22.5) | 21.4 (19.8-22.8) | 30.4 (28.1-33.0) | 42.7 (35.7-53.3) | 57.8 (45.7-69.4) | 1454 |
| **Gender** | | | | | | | |
| Males | 03-04 | 23.2 (21.1-25.6) | 23.9 (22.4-25.5) | 32.2 (28.8-35.9) | 45.3 (35.5-62.7) | 62.7 (43.8-81.8) | 1053 |
| Females | 03-04 | 18.4 (17.0-20.0) | 18.2 (16.9-19.8) | 27.4 (23.8-30.2) | 39.8 (34.4-42.6) | 46.6 (42.3-61.5) | 1041 |
| **Race/ethnicity** | | | | | | | |
| Mexican Americans | 03-04 | 14.7 (13.0-16.6) | 15.9 (13.4-17.9) | 21.2 (18.7-23.5) | 28.1 (24.1-35.0) | 35.5 (28.9-38.5) | 485 |
| Non-Hispanic blacks | 03-04 | 21.6 (19.1-24.4) | 22.1 (19.6-24.9) | 32.3 (28.1-36.2) | 43.8 (37.2-57.3) | 57.7 (43.8-78.4) | 538 |
| Non-Hispanic whites | 03-04 | 21.4 (19.9-23.1) | 22.0 (20.5-23.0) | 30.2 (27.7-33.3) | 41.7 (35.7-49.6) | 56.3 (44.0-70.0) | 962 |

Limit of detection (LOD, see Data Analysis section) for Survey year 03-04 is 0.4.

## Serum Perfluorooctane sulfonamide (PFOSA)

Geometric mean and selected percentiles of serum concentrations (in µg/L) for the U.S. population from the National Health and Nutrition Examination Survey.

| | Survey years | Geometric mean (95% conf. interval) | Selected percentiles ( 95% confidence interval) | | | | Sample size |
|---|---|---|---|---|---|---|---|
| | | | 50th | 75th | 90th | 95th | |
| **Total** | 03-04 | * | < LOD | < LOD | .300 ( 200-.300) | .300 ( 300-.400) | 2094 |
| **Age group** | | | | | | | |
| 12-19 years | 03-04 | * | < LOD | < LOD | .300 ( 200-.300) | .300 ( 200-.500) | 640 |
| 20 years and older | 03-04 | * | < LOD | < LOD | .300 ( 200-.300) | .300 ( 300-.400) | 1454 |
| **Gender** | | | | | | | |
| Males | 03-04 | * | < LOD | < LOD | .300 ( 200-.300) | .300 ( 200-.500) | 1053 |
| Females | 03-04 | * | < LOD | < LOD | .300 ( 200-.300) | .300 ( 300-.500) | 1041 |
| **Race/ethnicity** | | | | | | | |
| Mexican Americans | 03-04 | * | < LOD | < LOD | < LOD | .200 (<LOD-.300) | 485 |
| Non-Hispanic blacks | 03-04 | * | < LOD | < LOD | .300 ( 200-.300) | .300 ( 200-.500) | 538 |
| Non-Hispanic whites | 03-04 | * | < LOD | < LOD | .300 ( 200-.300) | .300 ( 300-.500) | 962 |

Limit of detection (LOD, see Data Analysis section) for Survey year 03-04 is 0.2.
< LOD means less than the limit of detection, which may vary for some chemicals by year and by individual sample.
* Not calculated: proportion of results below limit of detection was too high to provide a valid result.

## Serum 2-(N-Ethyl-perfluorooctane sulfonamido) acetic acid (Et-PFOSA-AcOH)

Geometric mean and selected percentiles of serum concentrations (in µg/L) for the U.S. population from the National Health and Nutrition Examination Survey.

| | Survey years | Geometric mean (95% conf. interval) | Selected percentiles ( 95% confidence interval) | | | | Sample size |
|---|---|---|---|---|---|---|---|
| | | | 50th | 75th | 90th | 95th | |
| **Total** | 03-04 | * | < LOD | < LOD | < LOD | < LOD | 2094 |
| **Age group** | | | | | | | |
| 12-19 years | 03-04 | * | < LOD | < LOD | < LOD | < LOD | 640 |
| 20 years and older | 03-04 | * | < LOD | < LOD | < LOD | < LOD | 1454 |
| **Gender** | | | | | | | |
| Males | 03-04 | * | < LOD | < LOD | < LOD | < LOD | 1053 |
| Females | 03-04 | * | < LOD | < LOD | < LOD | < LOD | 1041 |
| **Race/ethnicity** | | | | | | | |
| Mexican Americans | 03-04 | * | < LOD | < LOD | < LOD | < LOD | 485 |
| Non-Hispanic blacks | 03-04 | * | < LOD | < LOD | < LOD | .400 (<LOD-.500) | 538 |
| Non-Hispanic whites | 03-04 | * | < LOD | < LOD | < LOD | < LOD | 962 |

Limit of detection (LOD, see Data Analysis section) for Survey year 03-04 is 0.4.
< LOD means less than the limit of detection, which may vary for some chemicals by year and by individual sample.
* Not calculated: proportion of results below limit of detection was too high to provide a valid result.

## Serum 2-(N-Methyl-perfluorooctane sulfonamido) acetic acid (Me-PFOSA-AcOH)

Geometric mean and selected percentiles of serum concentrations (in µg/L) for the U.S. population from the National Health and Nutrition Examination Survey.

| | Survey years | Geometric mean (95% conf. interval) | Selected percentiles ( 95% confidence interval) | | | | Sample size |
|---|---|---|---|---|---|---|---|
| | | | 50th | 75th | 90th | 95th | |
| Total | 03-04 | * | < LOD | .700 (<LOD-.700) | 1.00 (.900-1.10) | 1.30 (1.10-1 50) | 2094 |
| **Age group** | | | | | | | |
| 12-19 years | 03-04 | * | < LOD | .700 (<LOD- 800) | 1.10 (.900-1 30) | 1.50 (1.20-1 80) | 640 |
| 20 years and older | 03-04 | * | < LOD | .700 (<LOD-.700) | 1.00 (.900-1.10) | 1.20 (1.10-1 60) | 1454 |
| **Gender** | | | | | | | |
| Males | 03-04 | * | < LOD | .700 (<LOD-.700) | 1.10 (.900-1 20) | 1.30 (1.10-1.70) | 1053 |
| Females | 03-04 | * | < LOD | .600 (<LOD-.700) | 1.00 (.900-1.10) | 1.10 (1.00-1 80) | 1041 |
| **Race/ethnicity** | | | | | | | |
| Mexican Americans | 03-04 | * | < LOD | < LOD | .700 (<LOD- 900) | .900 (<LOD-1.30) | 485 |
| Non-Hispanic blacks | 03-04 | * | < LOD | .800 (<LOD- 900) | 1.10 (.900-1.40) | 1.50 (1.10-1 80) | 538 |
| Non-Hispanic whites | 03-04 | * | < LOD | .700 (<LOD- 800) | 1.00 (.900-1.10) | 1.30 (1.10-1 60) | 962 |

Limit of detection (LOD, see Data Analysis section) for Survey year 03-04 is 0 6.
< LOD means less than the limit of detection, which may vary for some chemicals by year and by individual sample.
* Not calculated: proportion of results below limit of detection was too high to provide a valid result.

## Serum Perfluoroundecanoic acid (PFUA)

Geometric mean and selected percentiles of serum concentrations (in µg/L) for the U.S. population from the National Health and Nutrition Examination Survey.

| | Survey years | Geometric mean (95% conf. interval) | Selected percentiles ( 95% confidence interval) | | | | Sample size |
|---|---|---|---|---|---|---|---|
| | | | 50th | 75th | 90th | 95th | |
| Total | 03-04 | * | < LOD | < LOD | < LOD | .600 (<LOD-1.30) | 2094 |
| **Age group** | | | | | | | |
| 12-19 years | 03-04 | * | < LOD | < LOD | < LOD | .300 (<LOD-1.10) | 640 |
| 20 years and older | 03-04 | * | < LOD | < LOD | .300 (<LOD- 600) | .600 (<LOD-1.40) | 1454 |
| **Gender** | | | | | | | |
| Males | 03-04 | * | < LOD | < LOD | .400 (<LOD-1.00) | .700 (<LOD-2.30) | 1053 |
| Females | 03-04 | * | < LOD | < LOD | < LOD | .400 (<LOD-.700) | 1041 |
| **Race/ethnicity** | | | | | | | |
| Mexican Americans | 03-04 | * | < LOD | < LOD | < LOD | < LOD | 485 |
| Non-Hispanic blacks | 03-04 | * | < LOD | < LOD | .600 (<LOD-1.40) | .900 (.300-2 90) | 538 |
| Non-Hispanic whites | 03-04 | * | < LOD | < LOD | < LOD | .500 (<LOD- 900) | 962 |

Limit of detection (LOD, see Data Analysis section) for Survey year 03-04 is 0 3.
< LOD means less than the limit of detection, which may vary for some chemicals by year and by individual sample.
* Not calculated: proportion of results below limit of detection was too high to provide a valid result.

## References

Alexander BH, Olsen GW, Burris JM, Mandel JH, Mandel JS. Mortality of employees of a perfluorooctanesulphonyl fluoride manufacturing facility. Occup Environ Med 2003;60(10):722-729.

Apelberg BJ, Witter FR, Herbstman JB, Calafat AM, Halden RU, et al. Cord serum concentrations of perfluorooctane sulfonate and perfluorooctanoate in relation to weight and size at birth. Environ Health Perspect 2007;115(11):1670-1676.

Biegel LB, Hurtt ME, Frame SR, O'Connor JC, Cook JC. Mechanisms of extrahepatic tumor induction by peroxisome proliferators in male CD rats. Toxicol Sci 2001;60(1):44-55.

Biegel LB, Liu RC, Hurtt ME, Cook JC. Effects of ammonium perfluorooctanoate on Leydig cell function: in vitro, in vivo, and ex vivo studies. Toxicol Appl Pharmacol 1995;134(1):18-25.

Bookstaff RC, Moore RW, Ingall GB, Peterson RE. Androgenic deficiency in male rats treated with perfluorodecanoic acid. Toxicol Appl Pharmacol 1990;104(2):322-333.

Butenhoff JL, Gaylor DW, Moore JA, Olsen GW, Rodricks J, Mandel JH, et al. Characterization of risk for general population exposure to perfluorooctanoate. Regul Toxicol Pharmacol 2004;39(3):363-380.

Calafat AM, Kuklenyik Z, Caudill SP, Reidy JA, Needham LL. Perfluorochemicals in pooled serum samples from United States residents in 2001 and 2002. Environ Sci Technol 2006a;40:2128-2134.

Calafat AM, Needham LL, Kuklenyik Z, Reidy JA, Tully JS, Aguilar-Villalobos M, et al. Perfluorinated chemicals in selected residents of the American continent. Chemosphere 2006b;63:490-496.

Calafat AM, Kuklenyik Z, Reidy JA, Caudill SP, Tully JS, Needham LL. Serum concentrations of 11 polyfluoroalkyl compounds in the U.S. population: Data from the National Health and Nutrition Examination Survey (NHANES) 1999–2000. Environ Sci Technol 2007a;41:2237-2242.

Calafat AM, Wong LY, Kuklenyik Z, Reidy JA, Needham LL. Polyfluoroalkyl chemicals in the U.S. population: data from the National Health and Nutrition Examination Survey (NHANES) 2003-2004 and comparisons with NHANES 1999-2000. Environ Health Perspect. 2007b;115(11):1596-1602.

Cook JC, Murray SM, Frame SR, Hurtt ME. Induction of Leydig cell adenomas by ammonium perfluorooctanoate: a possible endocrine-related mechanism. Toxicol Appl Pharmacol 1992;113(2):209-217.

Dinglasan MJ, Ye Y, Edwards EA, Mabury SA. Fluorotelomer alcohol biodegradation yields poly- and perfluorinated acids. Environ Sci Technol 2004;38(10):2857-2864.

Fei C, McLaughlin JK, Tarone RE, Olsen J. Perfluorinated chemicals and fetal growth: A study within the Danish National Birth cohort. Environ Health Perspect 2007;115(11):1677-1682.

Grasty RC, Grey BE, Lau CS, Rogers JM. Prenatal window of susceptibility to perfluorooctane sulfonate-induced neonatal mortality in the Sprague-Dawley rat. Birth Defects Res B Dev Reprod Toxicol 2003;68(6):465-471.

Guruge KS, Taniyasu S, Yamashita N, Wijeratna S, Mohotti KM, Seneviratne HR, et al. Perfluorinated organic compounds in human blood serum and seminal plasma: a study of urban and rural tea worker populations in Sri Lanka. J Environ Monit 2005;7(4):371-377.

Harada K, Inoue K, Morikawa A, Yoshinaga T, Saito N, Koizumi A. Renal clearance of perfluorooctane sulfonate and perfluorooctanoate in humans and their species-specific excretion. Environ Res 2005;99(2):253-261.

Harada K, Saito N, Inoue K, Yoshinaga T, Watanabe T, Sasaki S, Kamiyama S,Koizumi A. The influence of time, sex and geographic factors on levels of perfluorooctanesulfonate and perfluorooctanoate in human serum over the last 25 years. J Occup Health 2004;46(2):141-147.

Hekster FM, Laane RW, de Voogt P. Environmental and toxicity effects of perfluoroalkylated substances. Rev Environ Contam Toxicol 2003;179:99-121.

Holmstrom KE, Jarnberg U, Bignert A. Temporal trends of PFOS and PFOA in guillemot eggs from the Baltic Sea,1968--2003. Environ Sci Technol 2005;39(1):80-84.

Kannan K, Corsolini S, Falandysz J, Fillmann G, Kumar KS, Loganathan BG, et al. Perfluorooctanesulfonate and related fluorochemicals in human blood from several countries. Environ Sci Technol 2004;38(17):4489-4495.

Kannan K, Yun SH, Evans TJ. Chlorinated, brominated, and perfluorinated contaminants in livers of polar bears from Alaska. Environ Sci Technol 2005;39(23):9057-9063.

Keller JM, Kannan K, Taniyasu S, Yamashita N, Day RD, Arendt MD, et al. Perfluorinated compounds in the plasma of loggerhead and Kemp's ridley sea turtles from the southeastern coast of the United States. Environ Sci Technol 2005;39(23):9101-9108.

Kennedy GL Jr, Butenhoff JL, Olsen GW, O'Connor JC, Seacat AM, Perkins RG, et al. The toxicology of perfluorooctanoate. Crit Rev Toxicol 2004;34(4):351-384.

Kudo N, Bandai N, Suzuki E, Katakura M, Kawashima Y. Induction by perfluorinated fatty acids with different carbon chain length of peroxisomal beta-oxidation in the liver of rats. Chem Biol Interact 2000;124(2):119-132.

Kudo N, Kawashima Y. Induction of triglyceride accumulation in the liver of rats by perfluorinated fatty acids with different carbon chain lengths: comparison with induction of peroxisomal beta-oxidation. Biol Pharm Bull 2003;26(1):47-51.

Lau C, Butenhoff JL, Rogers JM. The developmental toxicity of perfluoroalkyl acids and their derivatives. Toxicol Appl Pharmacol 2004;198(2):231-241.

Lau C, Thibodeaux JR, Hanson RG, Rogers JM, Grey BE, Stanton ME, et al. Exposure to perfluorooctane sulfonate during pregnancy in rat and mouse. II: postnatal evaluation. Toxicol Sci 2003;74(2):382-392.

Olsen GW, Burris JM, Mandel JH, Zobel LR. Serum perfluorooctane sulfonate and hepatic and lipid clinical chemistry tests in fluorochemical production employees. J Occup Environ Med 1999;41(9):799-806.

Olsen GW, Church TR, Miller JP, Burris JM, Hansen KJ, Lundberg JK, et al. Perfluorooctanesulfonate and other fluorochemicals in the serum of American Red Cross adult blood donors. Environ Health Perspect 2003a;111(16):1892-1901. (Erratum in: Environ Health Perspect. 2003a;111(16):1900)

Olsen GW, Burris JM, Burlew MM, Mandel JH. Epidemiologic assessment of worker serum perfluorooctanesulfonate (PFOS) and perfluorooctanoate (PFOA) concentrations and medical surveillance examinations. J Occup Environ Med 2003b;45(3):260-270.

Olsen GW, Church TR, Larson EB, van Belle G, Lundberg JK, Hansen KJ, et al. Serum concentrations of perfluorooctanesulfonate and other fluorochemicals in an elderly population from Seattle, Washington. Chemosphere 2004a;54(11):1599-1611.

Olsen GW, Church TR, Hansen KJ, Burris JM, Butenhoff JL, Mandel JH. Quantitative evaluation of perfluorooctanesulfonate (PFOS) and other fluorochemicals in the serum of children. J Children's Health 2004b;2(1):53-76.

Olsen GW, Huang HY, Helzlsouer KJ, Hansen KJ, Butenhoff JL, Mandel JH. Historical comparison of perfluorooctanesulfonate, perfluorooctanoate andother fluorochemicals in human blood. Environ Health Perspect 2005;113(5):539-545.

Olsen GW, Burris JM, Ehresman DJ, Froehlich JW, Seacat AM, Butenhoff JL, et al. Half-life of serum elimination of perfluoroo ctanesulfonate,perfluorohexanesulfonate, and perfluorooctanoate in retired fluorochemical production workers. Environ Health Perspect. 2007a;115(9):1298-1305.

Olsen GW, Mair DC, Reagen WK, Ellefson ME, Ehresman DJ, Butenhoff JL, et al.. Preliminary evidence of a decline in perfluorooctanesulfonate (PFOS) and perfluorooctanoate (PFOA) concentrations in American Red Cross blood donors. Chemosphere 2007b;68:105–111.

Prevedouros K, Cousins IT, Buck RC, Korzeniowski SH. Sources, fate and transport of perfluorocarboxylates. Environ Sci Technol 2006;40(1):32-44.

Seacat AM, Thomford PJ, Hansen KJ, Olsen GW, Case MT, Butenhoff JL. Subchronic toxicity studies on perfluorooctanesulfonate potassium salt in cynomolgus monkeys. Toxicol Sci 2002;68(1):249-264.

Taniyasu S, Kannan K, Horii Y, Hanari N, Yamashita N. A survey of perfluorooctane sulfonate and related perfluorinated organic compounds in water, fish, birds, and humans from Japan. Environ Sci Technol 2003;37(12):2634-2639.

Thibodeaux JR, Hanson RG, Rogers JM, Grey BE, Barbee BD, Richards JH, et al. Exposure to perfluorooctane sulfonate during pregnancy in rat and mouse. I: maternal and prenatal evaluations. Toxicol Sci 2003;74(2):369-381. (Erratum in: Toxicol Sci 2004;82(1):359.)

Tittlemier SA, Pepper K, Seymour C, Moisey J, Bronson R, Cao XL et al. Dietary exposure of Canadians to perfluorinated carboxylates and perfluorooctane sulfonate via consumption of meat, fish, fast foods, and food items prepared in their packaging. J Ag Food Chem 2007;55:3203-3210.

U.S. Environmental Protection Agency (U.S. EPA). Preliminary Risk Assessment of the Developmental Toxicity Associated with Exposure to Perfluorooctanoic Acid and its Salts. 2003. Available from URL: http://www.epa.gov/opptintr/pfoa/pfoara.htm. 1/15/06

Vanden Heuvel JP, Sterchele PF, Nesbit DJ, Peterson RE. Coordinate induction of acyl-CoA binding protein, fatty acid binding protein and peroxisomal beta-oxidation by peroxisome proliferators. Biochim Biophys Acta 1993;1177(2):183-190.

Yamashita N, Kannan K, Taniyasu S, Horii Y, Petrick G, Gamo T. A global survey of perfluorinated acids in oceans. Mar Pollut Bull 2005;51(8-12):658-668.

# Phthalates

## General Information

Phthalates are industrial chemicals that are added to plastics to impart flexibility and resilience and are often referred to as *plasticizers*. Phthalates are also used as solubilizing and stabilizing agents in other applications. There are numerous products that contain phthalates: adhesives; automotive plastics; detergents; lubricating oils; some medical devices and pharmaceuticals; plastic raincoats; solvents; vinyl tiles and flooring; and personal-care products, such as soap, shampoo, deodorants, lotions, fragrances, hair spray, and nail polish. Phthalates are often used in polyvinyl chloride type plastics, such as plastic bags, garden hoses, inflatable recreational toys, blood product storage bags, intravenous medical tubing, and toys (ATSDR, 2001, 2002). Because they are not chemically bound to the plastics to which they are added, phthalates can be released into the environment during use or disposal of the product. Various phthalate esters have been measured in specific foods, indoor and ambient air, indoor dust, water sources, and sediments (Clark et al., 2003).

People are exposed through ingestion, inhalation, and, to a lesser extent, dermal contact with products that contain phthalates. For the general population, dietary sources have been considered as the major exposure route, followed by inhaling indoor air. Infants may have relatively greater exposures from ingesting indoor dust containing some phthalates (Clark et al., 2003). Human milk can be a source of phthalate exposure for nursing infants (Calafat et al., 2004; Mortensen et al., 2005). The intravenous or parenteral exposure route can be important in patients undergoing medical procedures involving devices or materials containing phthalates. In settings where workers may be exposed to higher air phthalate concentrations than the general population, urinary metabolite and air phthalate concentrations are roughly correlated (Liss et al., 1985; Nielsen et al., 1985; Pan et al., 2006).

Phthalates are metabolized and excreted quickly and do not accumulate in the body (Anderson et al., 2001). Ingested phthalate diesters are initially hydrolyzed in the intestine to the corresponding monoesters, which are then absorbed (Albro et al., 1982; Albro and Lavenhar, 1989). Absorbed monoester metabolites are usually oxidized in the body and, in humans, excreted in urine largely as glucuronide conjugates (Albro et al., 1982; Dirven et al., 1993). The table shows the phthalate diesters, corresponding monoester metabolites, and other oxidized metabolites included in this *Report*.

Human health effects from phthalates at low environmental doses or at biomonitored levels from low environmental exposures are unknown. Phthalates have low acute animal toxicity. In chronic rodent studies, several of the phthalates produced testicular injury, liver injury, liver cancer, and teratogenicity, but these effects either have not been demonstrated when tested in non-human primates or are yet to be studied. *In vitro* studies showed that certain phthalates can bind to estrogen receptors and may have weak estrogenic or anti-estrogenic activity (Coldham et al., 1997; Harris et al., 1997; Jobling et al., 1995), but *in vivo* studies did not support phthalates having estrogenic effects (Milligan et al., 1998; Okubo et al., 2003; Parks et al., 2000; Zacharewski et al., 1998); however, not all phthalates

## Phthalates and Urinary Metabolites in this *Report*

| Phthalate name (CAS number) | Abbreviation | Urinary metabolite (CAS number) | Abbreviation |
|---|---|---|---|
| Benzylbutyl phthalate (85-68-7) | BzBP | Mono-benzyl phthalate (2528-16-7) (some mono-n-butyl phthalate) | MBzP |
| Dibutyl phthalates (84-74-2) | DBP | Mono-isobutyl phthalate | MiBP |
| | | Mono-n-butyl phthalate (131-70-4) | MnBP |
| Dicyclohexyl phthalate (84-61-7) | DCHP | Mono-cyclohexyl phthalate (7517-36-4) | MCHP |
| Diethyl phthalate (84-66-2) | DEP | Mono-ethyl phthalate (2306-33-4) | MEP |
| Di-2-ethylhexyl phthalate (117-81-7) | DEHP | Mono-2-ethylhexyl phthalate (4376-20-9) | MEHP |
| | | Mono-(2-ethyl-5-hydroxyhexyl) phthalate | MEHHP |
| | | Mono-(2-ethyl-5-oxohexyl) phthalate | MEOHP |
| | | Mono-(2-ethyl-5-carboxypentyl) phthalate (40809-41-4) | MECPP |
| Di-isononyl phthalate (28553-12-0) | DiNP | Mono-isononyl phthalate | MiNP |
| Dimethyl phthalate (131-11-3) | DMP | Mono-methyl phthalate (4376-18-5) | MMP |
| Di-n-octyl phthalate (117-84-0) | DOP | Mono-(3-carboxypropyl) phthalate | MCPP |
| | | Mono-n-octyl phthalate (5393-19-1) | MOP |

and metabolites have been tested. In animals, phthalates produced anti-androgenic effects by reducing testosterone production and, at very high levels, reducing estrogen production, effects that may be mediated by inhibiting testicular and ovarian steroidogenesis. High doses of di-2-ethylhexyl phthalate (DEHP), dibutyl phthalate (DBP), and benzylbutyl phthalate (BzBP) during the fetal period produced lowered testosterone levels, testicular atrophy, and Sertoli cell abnormalities in the male animals and, at higher doses, ovarian abnormalities in the female animals (Jarfelt et al., 2005; Lovekamp-Swan and Davis, 2003; McKee et al., 2004; NTP-CERHR, 2000a, 2000b, 2000c, 2006). Phthalate urinary metabolite levels in men evaluated at an infertility clinic were associated with several measures of sperm function and morphology (Duty et al., 2004; Hauser et al., 2007), but similar findings were not present in young Swedish men with comparable or higher median levels of urinary metabolites (Jonsson et al., 2005).

The monoester metabolites are thought to mediate toxic effects for some of the phthalates, but there are known species-related differences in the hydrolysis of diester phthalates, efficiency of intestinal absorption, and extent of metabolite conjugation to glucuronide (Albro et al., 1982; Kessler et al., 2004; Rhodes et al., 1986). These differences may contribute to species-specific differences in toxicity (ATSDR, 2001, 2002). Also, phthalates have been shown to induce peroxisomal proliferation in rodents, which may be a pathway to the development of liver toxicity and cancers in these animals. However, peroxisomal proliferation may not be a relevant pathway in humans (Rusyn et al., 2006).

The National Toxicology Program's Center for the Evaluation of Risks to Human Reproduction (NTP-CERHR) has reviewed the developmental and reproductive effects of specific phthalates (http://cerhr.niehs.nih.gov/reports/index.html). Information about external exposure (i.e., environmental levels) and health effects is also available for some phthalates from ATSDR at: http://www.atsdr.cdc.gov/toxpro2.html.

## Biomonitoring Information

Urinary levels of phthalate metabolites reflect recent exposure to the parent phthalate diester. The proportions of each metabolite for a given phthalate may vary by differing routes of exposure (Liss et al., 1985; Peck and Albro, 1982). Variation occurs from person to person in the proportions or amounts of a metabolite excreted after similar doses (Anderson et al., 2001); variation also occurs in the same person during repetitive monitoring (Fromme et al., 2007; Hauser et al., 2004; Hoppin et al., 2002). Population estimates of concentrations of specific phthalate

metabolites may differ by age, gender, and race/ethnicity (Silva et al., 2004).

Finding a measurable amount of one or more phthalate metabolites in urine does not mean that the levels of the metabolites or the parent phthalate cause an adverse health effect. Biomonitoring studies on levels of phthalate metabolites provide physicians and public health officials with reference values so that they can determine whether people have been exposed to higher levels of phthalates than are found in the general population. Biomonitoring data can also help scientists plan and conduct research on exposure and health effects.

## References

Agency for Toxic Substances and Disease Registry (ATSDR). Toxicological profile for di-n-butyl phthalate update [online]. 2001. Available at URL: http://www.atsdr.cdc.gov/toxprofiles/tp135.html. 4/20/09

Agency for Toxic Substances and Disease Registry (ATSDR). Toxicological profile for di(2-ethylhexyl)phthalate update [online]. 2002. Available at URL: http://www.atsdr.cdc.gov/toxprofiles/tp9 html. 4/20/09

Albro PW, Corbett JT, Schroeder JL, Jordan S, Matthews HB. Pharmacokinetics, interactions with macromolecules and species differences in metabolism of DEHP. Environ Health Perspect 1982;45:19-25.

Albro PW and Lavenhar SR. Metabolism of di(2-ethylhexyl) phthalate. Drug Metab Rev 1989;21:13-34.

Anderson WA, Castle L, Scotter MJ, Massey RC, Springall C. A biomarker approach to measuring human dietary exposure to certain phthalate diesters. Food Addit Contam 2001;18(12):1068-1074.

Calafat AM, Slakman AR, Silva MJ, Herbert AR, Needham LL. Automated solid phase extraction and quantitative analysis of human milk for 13 phthalate metabolites. J Chromatogr B 2004;805:49-56.

Clark K, Cousins IT, Mackay D. Assessment of critical exposure pathways. In Staples CA (ed), The Handbook of Environmental Chemistry, Vol.3, Part Q: Phthalate Esters. 2003;New York, Springer, pp. 227-262.

Coldham NG, Dave M, Silvapathasundaram S, McDonnell DP, Connor C, Sauer MJ. Evaluation of a recombinant yeast cell estrogen screening assay. Environ Health Perspect 1997; 105:734-742.

Dirven HA, van der Broek PH, Jongeneelen FJ. Determination of four metabolites of the plasticizer di (2-ethylhexyl) phthalate in human urine samples. Int Arch Occup Environ Health 1993;64(8):555-560.

Duty SM, Calafat AM, Silva MJ, Brock JW, Ryan L, Chen Z, et al. The relationship between environmental exposure to phthalates and computer-aided sperm analysis motion parameters. J Androl 2004;25(2):293-302.

Fromme H, Bolte G, Koch HM, Angerer J, Boehmer S, Drexler H, et al. Occurrence and daily variation of phthalate metabolites in the urine of an adult population. Int J Hyg Environ Health 2007;210:21-33.

Harris CA, Henttu P, Park MG, Sumpter JP. The estrogenic activity of phthalate esters in vitro. Environ Health Perspect 1997;105:802-811.

Hauser R, Meeker JD, Park S, Silva MJ, Calafat AM. Temporal variability of urinary phthalate metabolite levels in men of reproductive age [published erratum appears in Environ Health Perspect 2004;112(17):1740]. Environ Health Perspect 2004;112(17):1734-1740.

Hauser R, Meeker JD, Singh NP, Silva MJ, Ryan L, Duty S, et al. DNA damage in human sperm is related to urinary levels of phthalate monoester and oxidative metabolites. Hum Reprod 2007;22(3):688-695.

Hoppin JA, Brock JW, Davis BJ, Baird DD. Reproducibility of urinary phthalate metabolites in first morning urine samples. Environ Health Perspect 2002;110(5):515-518.

Jarfelt K, Dalgaard M, Hass U, Borch J, Jacobsen H, Ladefoged O. Antiandrogenic effects in male rats perinatally exposed to a mixture of di(2-ethylhexyl) phthalate and di(2-ethylhexyl) adipate. Reprod Toxicol 2005;19(4):505-515.

Jobling S, Reynolds T, White R, Parker MG, Sumpter JP. A variety of environmentally persistent chemicals including some phthalate plasticizers are weakly estrogenic. Environ Health Perspect 1995;103:582-587.

Jonsson BAG, Richthoff J, Rylander L, Giwercman A, Hagmar L. Urinary phthalate metabolites and biomarkers of reproductive function in young men. Epidemiol 2005;16(4):487-493.

Kessler W, Numtip W, Grote K, Csanády G, Chahoud I, Filser J. Blood burden of di(2-ethylhexylphthalate (DEHP) and its primary metabolite mono(2-ethylhexyl) phthalate (MEHP) in pregnant and non-pregnant rats and marmosets. Toxicol Appl Pharmacol 2004;195:142-153.

Liss GM, Albro PW, Hartle RW, Stringer WT. Urine phthalate determinations as an index of occupational exposure to phthalic anhydride and di (2-ethylhexyl) phthalate. Scand J Work Environ Health 1985;11(5):381-387.

Lovekamp-Swan T, Davis BJ. Mechanisms of phthalate ester

toxicity in the female reproductive system. Environ Health Perspect 2003;111(2):139-145.

McKee RH, Butala JH, David RM, Gans G. NTP center for the evaluation of risks to human reproduction reports on phthalates: addressing the data gaps [review]. Reprod Toxicol 2004;18(1):1-22.

Milligan SR, Balasubramanian AV, Kalita JC. Relative potency of xenobiotic estrogens in an acute in vivo mammalian assay. Environ Health Perspect 1998;106(1):23-26.

Mortensen GK, Main KM, Andersson A-M, Leffers H, Skakkebaek NE. Determination of phthalate monoesters in human milk, consumer milk, and infant formula by tandem mass spectrometry (LC-MS-MS). Anal Bioanal Chem 2005;382:1084-1092.

Nielsen J, Akesson B, Skerfving S. Phthalate ester exposure—air levels and health of workers processing polyvinylchloride. Am Ind Hyg Assoc J 1985;46(11):643-647.

NTP-CERHR. National Toxicology Program-Center for the Evaluation of Risks to Human Reproduction. Monograph on the Potential Human Reproductive and Developmental Effects of Butyl Benzyl Phthalate (BBP). Research Triangle Park (NC). 2000a [online]. Available at URL: http://cerhr niehs.nih.gov/ chemicals/phthalates/bb-phthalate/bbp-eval html. 6/2/09

NTP-CERHR. National Toxicology Program-Center for the Evaluation of Risks to Human Reproduction. Monograph on the Potential Human Reproductive and Developmental Effects of Di-n-Butyl Phthalate (DBP). Research Triangle Park (NC). 2000b [online]. Available at URL: http://cerhr.niehs nih.gov/chemicals/ phthalates/dbp/dbp-eval.html. 6/2/09

NTP-CERHR. National Toxicology Program-Center for the Evaluation of Risks to Human Reproduction. Monograph on the Potential Human Reproductive and Developmental Effects of Di(2-ethylhexyl) Phthalate (DEHP). Research Triangle Park (NC). 2000c [online]. Available at URL: http://cerhr niehs.nih. gov/chemicals/dehp/dehp-eval.html. 6/2/09

NTP-CERHR. National Toxicology Program-Center for the Evaluation of Risks to Human Reproduction. Draft Update Monograph on the Potential Human Reproductive and Developmental Effects of Di(2-ethylhexyl) Phthalate (DEHP). Research Triangle Park (NC). 2006 [online]. Available at URL: http://cerhr niehs.nih.gov/chemicals/dehp/dehp-eval.html. 6/2/09

Okubo T, Suzuki T, Yokoyama Y, Kano K, Kano I. Estimation of estrogenic and anti-estrogenic activities of some phthalate diesters and monoesters by MCF-7 cell proliferation assay in vitro. Biol Pharm Bull 2003;26(8):1219-24.

Pan G, Hanaoka T, Yoshimura M, Zhang S, Wang P, Tsukino H, et al. Decreased serum free testosterone in workers exposed to high levels of di-n-butyl phthalate (DBP) and di-2-ethylhexyl phthalate (DEHP): a cross-sectional study in China. Environ Health Perspect 2006;114(11):1643-1648.

Parks LG, Ostby JS, Lambright CR, Abbott BD, Klinefelter GR, Barlow NJ, et al. The plasticizer diethylhexyl phthalate induces malformations by decreasing fetal testosterone synthesis during sexual differentiation in the male rat. Toxicol Sci 2000;58:339-349.

Peck CC, Albro PW. Toxic potential of the plasticizer di (2-ethylhexyl) phthalate in the context of its disposition and metabolism in primates and man. Environ Health Perspect 1982;45:11-17.

Rhodes C, Orton TC, Pratt IA, Batten PL, Bratt H, Jackson SJ, et al. Comparative pharmacokinetics and subacute toxicity of di(2-ethylhexyl)phthalate (DEHP) in rats and marmosets: Extrapolation of effects in rodents to man. Environ Health Perspect 1986;65:299-308.

Rusyn I, Peters JM, Cunningham ML. Modes of action and species-specific effects of di-(2-ethylhexyl)phthalate in the liver. Crit Rev Toxicol 2006;36:459-479.

Silva MJ, Barr DB, Reidy JA, Malek NA, Hodge CC, Caudill SP, et al. Urinary levels of seven phthalate metabolites in the U.S. population from the National Health and Nutrition Examination Survey (NHANES) 1999-2000 [published erratum appears in Environ Health Perspect 2004; 112(5):A270]. Environ Health Perspect 2004;112(3):331-338.

Zacharewski TR, Meek MD, Clemons JH, Wu ZF, Fielden MR, Matthews JB. Examination of the in vitro and in vivo estrogenic activities of eight commercial phthalate esters. Toxicol Sci 1998;46:282-293.

# Benzylbutyl Phthalate

CAS No. 85-68-7

## General Information

Benzylbutyl phthalate (BzBP) is a solvent and additive used in products such as adhesives, vinyl tile, sealants, car care products, and to a lesser extent, some personal care products. BzBP can be released into the environment during its production and, because it is not bound to products in which it is incorporated, it can be released into the ambient air during use or disposal of the products. Food crops take up BzBP, and diet is the major source for general population exposure. People exposed to BzBP will excrete mono-benzyl phthalate (MBzP) and small amounts of mono-n-butyl phthalate in their urine. High dose BzBP and its monoester metabolites, including MBzP, can produce developmental and reproductive toxicity in rodents, particularly male animals (McKee et al., 2004; NTP-CERHR, 2000). IARC considers BzBP not classifiable with respect to human carcinogenicity.

## Biomonitoring Information

The median levels of MBzP in NHANES subsamples from 1999-2000, 2001-2002, and 2003-2004 were generally similar those reported in U.S. residents (Blount et al., 2000), in a small sample of pregnant women in New

## Urinary Mono-benzyl phthalate (MBzP)
*Metabolite of Benzylbutyl phthalate (BzBP)*
Geometric mean and selected percentiles of urine concentrations (in µg/L) for the U.S. population from the National Health and Nutrition Examination Survey.

| | Survey years | Geometric mean (95% conf. interval) | Selected percentiles ( 95% confidence interval) | | | | Sample size |
|---|---|---|---|---|---|---|---|
| | | | 50th | 75th | 90th | 95th | |
| **Total** | 99-00 | 15.3 (13.7-17.1) | 17.0 (15.3-18.9) | 35.4 (32.6-39.7) | 67.1 (55.3-82.4) | 103 (94.6-116) | 2541 |
| | 01-02 | 15.1 (13.9-16.3) | 15.8 (14.8-17.4) | 38.0 (34.5-41.2) | 80.8 (71.3-88.2) | 122 (102-142) | 2782 |
| | 03-04 | 13.7 (12.7-14.9) | 14.3 (12.8-16.4) | 32.3 (30.1-35.0) | 66.5 (57.3-75.6) | 101 (85.3-125) | 2605 |
| **Age group** | | | | | | | |
| 6-11 years | 99-00 | 39.4 (32.9-47.2) | 40.3 (33.8-48.6) | 82.0 (55.8-98.1) | 129 (98.1-214) | 214 (108-399) | 328 |
| | 01-02 | 33.4 (29.1-38.4) | 37.0 (26.6-43.4) | 68.5 (61.6-92.8) | 166 (116-191) | 235 (183-330) | 393 |
| | 03-04 | 33.9 (28.2-40.6) | 35.0 (30.1-39.8) | 63.8 (50.4-92.4) | 145 (110-213) | 255 (146-365) | 342 |
| 12-19 years | 99-00 | 25.6 (21.9-30.0) | 28.3 (22.3-34.8) | 51.2 (43.7-58.5) | 88.5 (67.2-115) | 125 (93.7-170) | 752 |
| | 01-02 | 23.2 (19.9-27.2) | 24.9 (21.2-31.0) | 55.5 (47.4-62.9) | 113 (91.8-133) | 169 (134-198) | 742 |
| | 03-04 | 22.1 (19.4-25.1) | 24.9 (22.3-27.2) | 49.9 (39.8-64.6) | 89.8 (71.1-120) | 152 (99.9-190) | 729 |
| 20 years and older | 99-00 | 12.4 (10.9-14.2) | 13.8 (12.1-15.6) | 29.2 (25.2-33.1) | 52.0 (43.9-62.5) | 86.3 (54.7-119) | 1461 |
| | 01-02 | 12.7 (11.7-13.9) | 13.9 (12.8-14.9) | 31.8 (28.5-33.5) | 65.4 (53.8-76.3) | 99.7 (82.8-121) | 1647 |
| | 03-04 | 11.4 (10.3-12.7) | 12.1 (10.8-13.5) | 27.0 (23.6-29.4) | 54.2 (47.1-61.5) | 79.5 (66.5-94.8) | 1534 |
| **Gender** | | | | | | | |
| Males | 99-00 | 16.2 (14.1-18.6) | 17.7 (15.2-20.0) | 35.4 (31.5-40.3) | 69.4 (59.9-87.2) | 108 (96.3-130) | 1215 |
| | 01-02 | 15.6 (13.6-17.9) | 16.0 (14.6-18.5) | 37.0 (33.1-43.0) | 78.4 (63.5-97.4) | 122 (88.2-183) | 1371 |
| | 03-04 | 14.6 (13.2-16.2) | 15.1 (13.2-17.5) | 32.3 (29.5-35.6) | 65.6 (53.6-79.6) | 101 (78.6-132) | 1250 |
| Females | 99-00 | 14.6 (12.7-16.6) | 16.1 (14.2-19.2) | 35.8 (30.8-41.4) | 63.7 (53.7-82.4) | 103 (84.2-116) | 1326 |
| | 01-02 | 14.6 (13.1-16.3) | 15.4 (13.8-17.9) | 38.1 (32.3-43.8) | 81.4 (68.3-91.6) | 122 (102-143) | 1411 |
| | 03-04 | 13.0 (11.8-14.2) | 13.3 (12.1-15.6) | 33.3 (29.5-36.2) | 67.1 (58.8-72.4) | 101 (84.4-120) | 1355 |
| **Race/ethnicity** | | | | | | | |
| Mexican Americans | 99-00 | 13.9 (12.1-16.1) | 15.7 (13.4-16.9) | 33.0 (27.5-36.1) | 67.5 (55.5-84.0) | 98.8 (80.6-150) | 814 |
| | 01-02 | 13.2 (10.8-16.2) | 14.8 (10.8-18.5) | 29.5 (26.2-38.1) | 70.4 (53.0-85.4) | 94.7 (70.3-161) | 677 |
| | 03-04 | 14.9 (13.2-16.7) | 15.5 (13.5-18.3) | 32.4 (27.7-35.4) | 71.4 (48.6-92.3) | 99.8 (86.5-145) | 652 |
| Non-Hispanic blacks | 99-00 | 23.0 (20.7-25.5) | 23.1 (20.5-25.6) | 49.3 (44.0-55.6) | 94.7 (80.0-130) | 138 (106-241) | 603 |
| | 01-02 | 23.8 (21.0-26.9) | 24.2 (19.9-28.0) | 50.6 (41.5-62.9) | 101 (86.4-127) | 143 (127-179) | 703 |
| | 03-04 | 18.9 (16.3-21.8) | 20.0 (15.4-24.6) | 43.8 (38.9-49.0) | 80.9 (70.0-106) | 120 (99.7-172) | 699 |
| Non-Hispanic whites | 99-00 | 14.3 (12.7-16.1) | 16.1 (14.3-18.6) | 34.0 (30.6-38.4) | 58.7 (51.3-74.1) | 103 (74.1-116) | 912 |
| | 01-02 | 14.0 (12.7-15.4) | 14.6 (13.4-15.6) | 35.6 (32.2-39.5) | 76.6 (66.1-90.3) | 122 (93.2-155) | 1216 |
| | 03-04 | 12.9 (11.5-14.3) | 13.2 (11.7-16.0) | 30.5 (27.8-35.1) | 63.8 (53.6-72.4) | 91.5 (76.3-122) | 1088 |

Limit of detection (LOD, see Data Analysis section) for Survey years 99-00, 01-02, and 03-04 are 0 8, 0.3, and 0.1, respectively.

York City (Adibi et al., 2003), in men attending a Boston infertility clinic (Duty et al., 2004; Hauser et al., 2007), in young Swedish men (Jonsson et al., 2005), and in a small sample of German residents (Koch et al., 2003). In an annual sample of German university students, median urine levels of MBzP were about one-half the median levels in NHANES subsamples from 1999-2002 (Wittassek et al., 2007). A small study of African-American women in Washington, DC reported median urinary MBzP levels that were about twice the levels of adults and females reported in NHANES 1999-2002 (CDC, 2005; Hoppin et al., 2002). Limited studies in children younger than 2 years old have found median and geometric mean urine MBzP that were similar to children aged 6-11 years in the NHANES subsamples (Brock et al., 2002; Weuve et al., 2006). In

NHANES 1999-2000, the adjusted geometric mean levels of urinary MBzP were significantly higher in several subgroups: children compared to adolescents and adults; adolescents compared with adults; and females compared to males (Silva et al., 2004).

Finding a measurable amount of MBzP in the urine does not mean that the levels of MBzP or the parent compound cause an adverse health effect. Biomonitoring studies on levels of urinary MBzP provide physicians and public health officials with reference values so that they can determine whether people have been exposed to higher levels of BzBP than are found in the general population. Biomonitoring data can also help scientists plan and conduct research on exposure and health effects.

## Urinary Mono-benzyl phthalate (MBzP) (creatinine corrected)
*Metabolite of Benzylbutyl phthalate (BzBP)*
Geometric mean and selected percentiles of urine concentrations (in µg/g of creatinine) for the U.S. population from the National Health and Nutrition Examination Survey.

| | Survey years | Geometric mean (95% conf. interval) | 50th | 75th | 90th | 95th | Sample size |
|---|---|---|---|---|---|---|---|
| | | | **Selected percentiles** ( 95% confidence interval) | | | | |
| **Total** | 99-00 | **14.0** (13.0-15.0) | **13.3** (12.8-14.3) | **25.1** (23.4-27.2) | **50.1** (41.5-58.8) | **77.4** (69.6-86.3) | 2541 |
| | 01-02 | **14.1** (13.2-15.1) | **13.5** (12.7-14.4) | **26.6** (24.7-29.1) | **54.8** (49.1-58.5) | **90.4** (74.4-102) | 2782 |
| | 03-04 | **12.9** (12.2-13.7) | **12.6** (11.2-13.6) | **24.6** (22.2-26.4) | **46.0** (41.0-51.5) | **70.0** (62.4-79.9) | 2605 |
| **Age group** | | | | | | | |
| 6-11 years | 99-00 | **40.0** (33.6-47.6) | **38.6** (30.2-51.3) | **73.5** (56.6-99.2) | **104** (89.4-142) | **142** (99.8-173) | 328 |
| | 01-02 | **38.1** (34.4-42.1) | **37.4** (33.8-42.2) | **67.9** (55.8-80.4) | **134** (116-176) | **195** (121-305) | 393 |
| | 03-04 | **35.8** (30.5-42.1) | **32.2** (27.9-40.5) | **60.8** (50.1-79.4) | **136** (85.5-213) | **229** (99.7-397) | 342 |
| 12-19 years | 99-00 | **17.3** (15.4-19.4) | **17.1** (14.6-20.3) | **28.3** (24.3-34.8) | **49.7** (38.8-69.3) | **70.0** (49.6-81.9) | 752 |
| | 01-02 | **17.9** (15.7-20.5) | **18.1** (15.7-20.8) | **33.9** (29.3-38.6) | **67.7** (55.8-85.9) | **100** (80.7-123) | 742 |
| | 03-04 | **16.6** (15.4-17.8) | **16.9** (15.4-18.2) | **30.1** (25.1-35.5) | **52.2** (40.7-61.8) | **77.7** (54.9-115) | 729 |
| 20 years and older | 99-00 | **11.8** (10.7-12.9) | **12.1** (11.1-12.9) | **20.1** (18.4-23.3) | **34.6** (30.6-40.9) | **57.2** (41.3-73.9) | 1461 |
| | 01-02 | **12.0** (11.2-12.9) | **11.8** (11.1-12.5) | **21.6** (19.9-23.7) | **42.3** (35.8-48.3) | **64.9** (54.2-78.3) | 1647 |
| | 03-04 | **11.0** (10.3-11.7) | **10.5** (9.69-11.6) | **19.7** (18.2-21.4) | **36.6** (34.8-39.1) | **55.8** (46.9-62.4) | 1534 |
| **Gender** | | | | | | | |
| Males | 99-00 | **12.7** (11.8-13.6) | **12.4** (11.6-13.0) | **23.7** (21.5-26.1) | **44.5** (35.5-57.0) | **73.5** (48.5-99.8) | 1215 |
| | 01-02 | **12.7** (11.4-14.2) | **11.9** (10.9-13.2) | **24.1** (21.0-26.4) | **49.1** (43.7-56.1) | **80.3** (60.9-104) | 1371 |
| | 03-04 | **11.5** (10.6-12.4) | **11.1** (9.73-12.5) | **21.1** (19.5-23.6) | **39.4** (34.2-49.7) | **62.9** (51.9-83.1) | 1250 |
| Females | 99-00 | **15.3** (13.8-16.8) | **14.7** (13.3-16.0) | **25.9** (24.1-29.3) | **56.4** (46.8-60.6) | **80.4** (60.2-117) | 1326 |
| | 01-02 | **15.6** (14.2-17.3) | **15.1** (13.9-16.5) | **29.4** (25.8-34.1) | **58.5** (49.9-69.4) | **95.8** (69.4-116) | 1411 |
| | 03-04 | **14.4** (13.4-15.6) | **13.9** (12.8-15.1) | **27.9** (24.7-31.4) | **51.9** (43.4-60.3) | **73.4** (63.7-90.2) | 1355 |
| **Race/ethnicity** | | | | | | | |
| Mexican Americans | 99-00 | **12.6** (11.4-14.0) | **11.9** (10.9-13.2) | **24.1** (21.5-26.5) | **46.5** (42.0-53.8) | **68.2** (56.4-93.8) | 814 |
| | 01-02 | **12.4** (10.7-14.4) | **11.9** (9.95-14.9) | **23.7** (19.5-29.0) | **46.6** (36.5-61.6) | **71.6** (51.1-120) | 677 |
| | 03-04 | **13.4** (11.7-15.4) | **12.5** (11.5-13.4) | **24.1** (21.0-27.8) | **53.0** (38.3-64.8) | **77.8** (57.1-125) | 652 |
| Non-Hispanic blacks | 99-00 | **14.8** (13.5-16.3) | **13.7** (12.2-15.2) | **26.9** (22.5-31.8) | **56.3** (39.5-76.0) | **86.8** (64.4-99.8) | 603 |
| | 01-02 | **16.7** (14.7-19.0) | **15.7** (13.7-19.3) | **33.4** (26.5-38.0) | **60.1** (53.7-69.4) | **108** (75.6-116) | 703 |
| | 03-04 | **13.4** (11.8-15.3) | **13.6** (11.6-15.6) | **24.1** (21.9-28.7) | **50.0** (41.2-57.8) | **74.7** (59.0-90.5) | 699 |
| Non-Hispanic whites | 99-00 | **14.0** (12.7-15.3) | **13.4** (12.9-14.8) | **25.3** (23.1-27.4) | **53.3** (38.8-64.8) | **78.0** (67.4-90.3) | 912 |
| | 01-02 | **13.8** (12.8-14.9) | **13.0** (12.1-14.3) | **25.7** (23.8-27.9) | **53.1** (46.5-58.5) | **89.2** (69.0-109) | 1216 |
| | 03-04 | **12.7** (11.8-13.7) | **12.5** (10.8-13.8) | **24.4** (21.6-26.7) | **41.9** (39.0-48.8) | **65.6** (57.5-79.5) | 1088 |

## References

Adibi JJ, Perera FP, Jedrychowski W, Camann DE, Barr D, Jacek R, et al. Prenatal exposures to phthalates among women in New York City and Krakow, Poland. Environ Health Perspect 2003;111(14):1719-1722.

Blount BC, Silva MJ, Caudill SP, Needham LL, Pirkle JL, Sampson EJ, et al. Levels of seven urinary phthalate metabolites in a human reference population. Environ Health Perspect 2000;108(10):979-982.

Brock JW, Caudill SP, Silva MJ, Needham LL, Hilborn ED. Phthalate monoesters levels in the urine of young children. Bull Environ Contam Toxicol 2002;68:309-314.

Centers for Disease Control and Prevention (CDC). Third National Report on Human Exposure to Environmental Chemicals. Atlanta (GA). 2005.

Duty SM, Calafat AM, Silva MJ, Brock JW, Ryan L, Chen Z, et al. The relationship between environmental exposure to phthalates and computer-aided sperm analysis motion parameters. J Androl 2004;25(2):293-302.

Hauser R, Meeker JD, Singh NP, Silva MJ, Ryan L, Duty S, et al. DNA damage in human sperm is related to urinary levels of phthalate monoester and oxidative metabolites. Hum Reprod 2007;22(3):688-695.

Hoppin JA, Brock JW, Davis BJ, Baird DD. Reproducibility of urinary phthalate metabolites in first morning urine samples. Environ Health Perspect 2002;110(5):515-518.

Jonsson BAG, Richthoff J, Rylander L, Giwercman A, Hagmar L. Urinary phthalate metabolites and biomarkers of reproductive function in young men. Epidemiol 2005;16(4):487-493.

Koch HM, Rossbach B, Drexler H, Angerer J. Internal exposure of the general population to DEHP and other phthalates - determination of secondary and primary phthalate monoester metabolites in urine. Environ Res 2003;93:177-185.

McKee RH, Butala JH, David RM, Gans G. NTP center for the evaluation of risks to human reproduction reports on phthalates: addressing the data gaps [review]. Reprod Toxicol 2004;18(1):1-22.

NTP-CERHR. National Toxicology Program-Center for the Evaluation of Risks to Human Reproduction. Monograph on the Potential Human Reproductive and Developmental Effects of Butyl Benzyl Phthalate (BBP). Research Triangle Park (NC). 2000 [online]. Available at URL: http://cerhr.niehs.nih.gov/chemicals/phthalates/bb-phthalate/bbp-eval.html. 4/20/09

Silva MJ, Barr DB, Reidy JA, Malek NA, Hodge CC, Caudill SP, et al. Urinary levels of seven phthalate metabolites in the U.S. population from the National Health and Nutrition Examination Survey (NHANES) 1999-2000 [published erratum appears in Environ Health Perspect 2004; 112(5):A270]. Environ Health Perspect 2004;112(3):331-338.

Weuve J, Sanchez GN, Calafat AM, Schettler T, Green RA, Hu H, et al. Exposure to phthalates in neonatal intensive care unit infants: urinary concentrations of monoesters and oxidative metabolites. Environ Health Perspect 2006;114(9):1424-1431.

Wittassek M, Wiesmuller GA, Koch HM, Eckard R, Dobler L, Helm D, et al. Internal phthalate exposure over the last two decades—a retrospective human biomonitoring study. Int J Hyg Environ Health 2007;210(3-4):319-333.

# Di-n-butyl Phthalate
CAS No. 84-74-2

# Di-isobutyl Phthalate
CAS No. 84-69-5

## General Information

Dibutyl phthalates (both di-n-butyl and di-isobutyl phthalates, referred to as DBP) are industrial solvents or additives used in many personal care products such as nail polish and cosmetics, and also in some printing inks, pharmaceutical coatings, and insecticides. People exposed to dibutyl phthalates will excrete mono-n-butyl phthalate (MnBP) and mono-isobutyl phthalate (MiBP) in their urine. When total DBP metabolites have been measured, they have been referred to as monobutyl phthalate (MBP). Small amounts of mono-3-carboxypropyl phthalate are also produced from di-n-butyl phthalate. In addition, exposure to benzylbutyl phthalate (BzBP) will also result in small amounts of mono-n-butyl phthalate appearing in the urine. Following oral administration of DBP to humans, about 65% to 80% of a dose is eliminated in urine within 24 hours,

mostly as MnBP (Anderson et al., 2001). DBP can produce reproductive toxicity in male rodents (McKee et al., 2004; NTP-CERHR, 2000). OSHA has established a workplace air standard for external exposure to DBP; NIOSH and ACGIH have established guidelines for workplace air exposure to di-n-butyl phthalate. Neither IARC nor NTP has evaluated dibutyl phthalates with respect to human carcinogenicity.

## Biomonitoring Information

Median concentrations reported in the NHANES 1999-2000, 2001-2002 and 2003-2004 subsamples were similar to MBP levels reported in U.S. residents (Blount et al., 2000; CDC, 2005), in men attending a Boston infertility clinic (Duty et al., 2004; Hauser et al., 2007), in a small sample of pregnant women in New York City (Adibi et al., 2003), and in a small sample of Japanese adults (Itoh et al., 2005). Median MBP levels in two European studies were about two to six times higher than median levels in this *Report* (Jonsson et al., 2005; Koch et al., 2003). Studies of children found age-related differences in urine MBP levels. Compared with the median for 6 to 11 year olds in NHANES 1999-2004 (CDC, 2005), the median

## Urinary Mono-isobutyl phthalate (MiBP)
*Metabolite of Di-isobutyl phthalate (DBP)*
Geometric mean and selected percentiles of urine concentrations (in µg/L) for the U.S. population from the National Health and Nutrition Examination Survey.

| | Survey years | Geometric mean (95% conf. interval) | Selected percentiles ( 95% confidence interval) | | | | Sample size |
|---|---|---|---|---|---|---|---|
| | | | 50th | 75th | 90th | 95th | |
| Total | 01-02 | 2.71 (2.49-2 94) | 2.70 (2.40-3 00) | 5.70 (5.30-6.10) | 12.0 (11.4-12.7) | 17.9 (16.3-19.8) | 2782 |
| | 03-04 | 3.80 (3.40-4 25) | 4.20 (3.70-4 80) | 8.40 (7.40-9 50) | 15.0 (13.1-17.3) | 21.3 (18.6-26.0) | 2605 |
| **Age group** | | | | | | | |
| 6-11 years | 01-02 | 4.22 (3.28-5.43) | 4.40 (3.20-6 20) | 10.7 (7.30-13.4) | 18.6 (14.2-22.0) | 23.4 (20.4-27.8) | 393 |
| | 03-04 | 6.56 (5.24-8 22) | 7.00 (5.10-9.10) | 12.8 (9.40-17.7) | 24.3 (19.6-34.5) | 40.6 (29.3-48.5) | 342 |
| 12-19 years | 01-02 | 3.48 (2.90-4.17) | 3.80 (2.90-4.40) | 7.40 (6.00-9 00) | 14.5 (11.7-18.6) | 22.3 (16.2-33.4) | 742 |
| | 03-04 | 4.55 (3.73-5 55) | 5.60 (4.50-6 30) | 10.1 (8.00-11.4) | 17.1 (13.3-20.9) | 22.7 (18.5-29.1) | 729 |
| 20 years and older | 01-02 | 2.46 (2.30-2 63) | 2.40 (2.20-2.70) | 5.10 (4.80-5 50) | 10.6 (9.40-12.0) | 16.3 (13.6-18.5) | 1647 |
| | 03-04 | 3.46 (3.11-3 84) | 3.90 (3.40-4 30) | 7.50 (6.70-8 50) | 13.3 (11.5-16.5) | 19.9 (16.0-25.0) | 1534 |
| **Gender** | | | | | | | |
| Males | 01-02 | 2.73 (2.50-2 97) | 2.80 (2.40-3 20) | 5.60 (5.00-6.10) | 11.6 (10.1-12.6) | 16.6 (13.6-20.1) | 1371 |
| | 03-04 | 4.07 (3.56-4 66) | 4.30 (3.80-5.10) | 9.20 (7.50-10.2) | 16.0 (13.3-18.5) | 22.7 (17.3-30.3) | 1250 |
| Females | 01-02 | 2.68 (2.44-2 96) | 2.60 (2.30-3 00) | 5.80 (5.30-6 50) | 12.6 (11.0-14.7) | 18.7 (16.3-24.0) | 1411 |
| | 03-04 | 3.56 (3.19-3 97) | 4.10 (3.50-4 50) | 8.00 (7.10-9.10) | 14.2 (12.5-16.6) | 20.5 (17.9-23.0) | 1355 |
| **Race/ethnicity** | | | | | | | |
| Mexican Americans | 01-02 | 3.26 (2.72-3 91) | 3.40 (2.70-4 30) | 7.20 (6.20-9 30) | 12.2 (11.2-14.7) | 18.4 (14.1-25.6) | 677 |
| | 03-04 | 4.81 (3.85-6 02) | 5.10 (4.00-6.70) | 10.2 (8.20-12.6) | 18.3 (13.5-24.5) | 26.0 (19.0-38.5) | 652 |
| Non-Hispanic blacks | 01-02 | 4.90 (4.46-5 37) | 5.30 (4.60-6 00) | 10.7 (9.20-12.0) | 18.3 (16.1-20.1) | 25.5 (20.7-31.3) | 703 |
| | 03-04 | 6.67 (5.97-7.46) | 6.90 (6.30-7 50) | 12.6 (10.9-14.7) | 25.7 (17.7-31.0) | 33.5 (27.3-43.9) | 699 |
| Non-Hispanic whites | 01-02 | 2.33 (2.10-2 59) | 2.30 (1.90-2 60) | 4.90 (4.40-5 30) | 9.60 (8.30-11.6) | 15.6 (13.0-18.6) | 1216 |
| | 03-04 | 3.17 (2.82-3 56) | 3.50 (3.00-4 00) | 6.80 (5.90-7 90) | 12.5 (10.6-14.5) | 17.6 (14.7-20.8) | 1088 |

Limit of detection (LOD, see Data Analysis section) for Survey years 01-02 and 03-04 are 1 0 and 0.3.

for neonates was lower (by about half) and the median for toddlers was higher (by about sixfold) (Brock et al., 2002; Weuve et al., 2006). In an analysis of NHANES 1999-2000, the adjusted geometric mean levels of urinary MBP were significantly higher in children aged 6 to 11 years than in either adolescents or adults (Silva et al., 2004). Differences in urinary MBP population estimates by gender have also been shown (Silva et al., 2004). An analysis of NHANES 2001-2002 showed similar age- and gender- related differences in the adjusted geometric mean levels of urinary MiBP and MnBP (CDC, 2005).

Studies measuring urinary MnBP have reported variable median values compared to the NHANES 2001-2002 and 2003-2004 subsamples, ranging from more than one-tenth the NHANES median (Itoh et al., 2005), to about two to fourfold higher (Fromme et al., 2007). Between 1998 and 2003, samples from German university students had consistently higher median urine levels of MnBP and MiBP, up to four and 13 fold, respectively, than adults in NHANES subsamples during the same time period. Over this time, the students' median values for MiBP levels remained relatively unchanged, while MnBP declined (Wittassek et al., 2007).

Finding a measurable amount of MnBP or MiBP in urine does not mean that these levels or the parent compound cause an adverse health effect. Biomonitoring studies on levels of MnBP and MiBP provide physicians and public health officials with reference values so that they can determine whether people have been exposed to higher levels of dibutyl phthalates than are found in the general population. Biomonitoring data can also help scientists plan and conduct research on exposure and health effects.

## Urinary Mono-isobutyl phthalate (MiBP) (creatinine corrected)
*Metabolite of Di-isobutyl phthalate (DBP)*
Geometric mean and selected percentiles of urine concentrations (in µg/g of creatinine) for the U.S. population from the National Health and Nutrition Examination Survey.

| | Survey years | Geometric mean (95% conf. interval) | Selected percentiles ( 95% confidence interval) | | | | Sample size |
|---|---|---|---|---|---|---|---|
| | | | 50th | 75th | 90th | 95th | |
| Total | 01-02 | 2.54 (2.36-2.73) | 2.46 (2.26-2.68) | 4.54 (4.20-4.86) | 8.02 (7.78-8.66) | 12.0 (10.8-13 5) | 2782 |
| | 03-04 | 3.57 (3.18-4.00) | 3.57 (3.15-4.08) | 6.21 (5.36-7.17) | 10.9 (9.47-12.7) | 15.4 (12.8-18 6) | 2605 |
| **Age group** | | | | | | | |
| 6-11 years | 01-02 | 4.81 (3.89-5.94) | 5.18 (4.13-6.32) | 9.20 (7.03-11.7) | 15.2 (11.1-24 3) | 24.3 (13.9-40 3) | 393 |
| | 03-04 | 6.94 (5.79-8.31) | 7.03 (5.29-8.95) | 11.8 (9.56-15.1) | 18.6 (15.1-25.1) | 28.7 (21.8-36 9) | 342 |
| 12-19 years | 01-02 | 2.68 (2.29-3.15) | 2.83 (2.39-3.33) | 4.79 (4.04-5.51) | 7.62 (6.18-10 2) | 12.8 (8.76-15 6) | 742 |
| | 03-04 | 3.41 (2.86-4.05) | 3.69 (2.99-4.31) | 5.75 (4.69-7.04) | 9.32 (7.17-12 0) | 13.5 (9.52-20.1) | 729 |
| 20 years and older | 01-02 | 2.33 (2.20-2.46) | 2.26 (2.08-2.43) | 3.89 (3.65-4.25) | 7.31 (7.00-7.78) | 10.6 (9.46-11 3) | 1647 |
| | 03-04 | 3.32 (3.00-3.68) | 3.33 (3.00-3.81) | 5.59 (4.93-6.51) | 9.84 (8.65-11 2) | 13.5 (11.4-16 0) | 1534 |
| **Gender** | | | | | | | |
| Males | 01-02 | 2.22 (2.09-2.35) | 2.18 (1.97-2.37) | 3.76 (3.58-4.11) | 7.38 (6.64-7.95) | 11.1 (10.1-12 5) | 1371 |
| | 03-04 | 3.20 (2.80-3.66) | 3.19 (2.74-3.56) | 5.84 (4.79-6.56) | 10.0 (8.27-12 2) | 13.9 (11.5-19.1) | 1250 |
| Females | 01-02 | 2.88 (2.61-3.18) | 2.85 (2.52-3.18) | 5.14 (4.67-5.89) | 8.66 (8.02-10.1) | 13.7 (11.1-15 0) | 1411 |
| | 03-04 | 3.96 (3.56-4.42) | 4.00 (3.57-4.45) | 6.73 (5.64-7.80) | 11.6 (10.2-13 0) | 15.7 (13.0-18.7) | 1355 |
| **Race/ethnicity** | | | | | | | |
| Mexican Americans | 01-02 | 3.07 (2.58-3.66) | 2.98 (2.53-3.82) | 5.82 (4.91-6.99) | 10.6 (8.28-13 3) | 16.0 (12.6-19.4) | 677 |
| | 03-04 | 4.34 (3.47-5.43) | 4.47 (3.53-5.24) | 7.75 (6.33-9.69) | 13.1 (11.9-16 8) | 23.3 (17.9-26.1) | 652 |
| Non-Hispanic blacks | 01-02 | 3.44 (3.20-3.69) | 3.52 (2.95-3.81) | 6.11 (5.03-7.04) | 10.6 (8.94-12.4) | 15.6 (12.6-19.7) | 703 |
| | 03-04 | 4.74 (4.07-5.51) | 4.65 (4.10-5.30) | 7.81 (6.38-10 0) | 15.2 (10.8-18.4) | 19.9 (15.7-28.7) | 699 |
| Non-Hispanic whites | 01-02 | 2.31 (2.11-2.52) | 2.20 (2.01-2.43) | 3.80 (3.53-4.39) | 7.30 (6.72-7.78) | 10.7 (9.62-12 6) | 1216 |
| | 03-04 | 3.13 (2.76-3.54) | 3.17 (2.76-3.72) | 5.28 (4.55-6.21) | 8.92 (7.64-10 3) | 11.8 (10.2-15.1) | 1088 |

# Urinary Mono-n-butyl phthalate (MnBP)
*Metabolite of Dibutyl phthalate (DBP) and Benzylbutyl phthalate (BzBP)*

Geometric mean and selected percentiles of urine concentrations (in µg/L) for the U.S. population from the National Health and Nutrition Examination Survey.

| | Survey years | Geometric mean (95% conf. interval) | Selected percentiles ( 95% confidence interval) | | | | Sample size |
|---|---|---|---|---|---|---|---|
| | | | 50th | 75th | 90th | 95th | |
| **Total** | 99-00* | 24.6 (22.1-27.4) | 26.0 (23.6-29.2) | 51.6 (44.5-60.3) | 98.6 (90.2-114) | 150 (121-169) | 2541 |
| | 01-02 | 18.9 (17.4-20.6) | 20.4 (19.2-21.8) | 40.4 (36.5-44.2) | 73.6 (65.3-85.6) | 108 (94.1-122) | 2782 |
| | 03-04 | 21.1 (19.8-22.5) | 23.2 (21.2-24.8) | 42.7 (38.5-47.2) | 80.7 (70.2-93.9) | 122 (104-137) | 2605 |
| **Age group** | | | | | | | |
| 6-11 years | 99-00* | 41.4 (35.6-48.0) | 40.0 (36.2-49.2) | 75.5 (59.1-92.8) | 124 (98.4-159) | 166 (127-279) | 328 |
| | 01-02 | 31.1 (26.6-36.5) | 32.4 (25.6-37.1) | 62.1 (51.3-76.9) | 107 (84.3-136) | 159 (110-290) | 393 |
| | 03-04 | 36.3 (30.7-42.9) | 36.7 (28.5-47.5) | 71.3 (56.9-87.2) | 137 (107-162) | 191 (150-243) | 342 |
| 12-19 years | 99-00* | 36.0 (30.8-42.1) | 36.3 (30.6-44.9) | 68.6 (55.9-79.7) | 119 (90.2-159) | 165 (121-227) | 752 |
| | 01-02 | 25.1 (21.6-29.2) | 26.7 (22.0-32.7) | 52.6 (48.4-60.4) | 92.4 (72.7-121) | 148 (106-185) | 742 |
| | 03-04 | 26.7 (24.1-29.5) | 28.2 (25.2-33.1) | 52.0 (45.3-60.9) | 97.5 (74.7-116) | 134 (110-158) | 729 |
| 20 years and older | 99-00* | 21.6 (19.0-24.5) | 23.1 (19.7-26.1) | 46.3 (36.9-53.6) | 95.0 (78.7-111) | 143 (117-161) | 1461 |
| | 01-02 | 17.0 (15.4-18.8) | 19.1 (17.1-20.4) | 35.1 (31.6-40.2) | 64.8 (57.3-79.7) | 95.4 (84.6-113) | 1647 |
| | 03-04 | 19.0 (17.7-20.5) | 20.7 (18.9-22.9) | 38.4 (35.7-42.7) | 74.7 (64.1-82.6) | 108 (90.7-127) | 1534 |
| **Gender** | | | | | | | |
| Males | 99-00* | 22.0 (20.1-24.1) | 23.2 (20.4-26.3) | 43.1 (36.6-49.5) | 84.4 (71.3-96.2) | 116 (97.8-132) | 1215 |
| | 01-02 | 17.7 (16.0-19.6) | 19.3 (17.3-21.0) | 34.5 (30.3-40.6) | 62.1 (54.1-75.5) | 95.2 (75.5-117) | 1371 |
| | 03-04 | 20.0 (18.1-22.0) | 21.1 (19.0-24.0) | 39.4 (35.5-43.4) | 65.5 (59.0-73.0) | 95.9 (79.8-111) | 1250 |
| Females | 99-00* | 27.3 (23.6-31.5) | 30.0 (25.9-33.3) | 59.7 (51.6-69.6) | 120 (98.3-145) | 167 (143-223) | 1326 |
| | 01-02 | 20.2 (18.2-22.4) | 21.7 (19.7-24.3) | 46.7 (43.1-51.1) | 85.0 (72.7-92.5) | 121 (106-136) | 1411 |
| | 03-04 | 22.2 (21.2-23.3) | 24.4 (23.4-25.8) | 47.3 (42.7-53.0) | 95.9 (79.9-114) | 137 (122-156) | 1355 |
| **Race/ethnicity** | | | | | | | |
| Mexican Americans | 99-00* | 23.4 (21.8-25.1) | 26.3 (23.9-28.1) | 48.1 (41.2-56.7) | 92.2 (78.9-101) | 117 (104-131) | 814 |
| | 01-02 | 20.1 (16.6-24.5) | 23.1 (18.0-26.5) | 42.1 (34.0-51.5) | 77.1 (62.9-92.5) | 112 (84.6-143) | 677 |
| | 03-04 | 24.1 (19.8-29.5) | 26.9 (20.2-32.0) | 47.4 (38.0-58.5) | 85.6 (61.7-117) | 127 (99.8-165) | 652 |
| Non-Hispanic blacks | 99-00* | 37.0 (31.9-42.9) | 38.7 (33.4-44.5) | 78.2 (58.7-91.8) | 118 (108-143) | 167 (143-197) | 603 |
| | 01-02 | 29.6 (26.6-33.1) | 31.5 (28.7-34.1) | 58.3 (51.2-63.4) | 93.2 (79.5-121) | 138 (110-184) | 703 |
| | 03-04 | 30.1 (28.4-31.9) | 31.5 (29.7-34.1) | 64.1 (58.3-67.1) | 106 (94.8-119) | 144 (115-168) | 699 |
| Non-Hispanic whites | 99-00* | 21.8 (19.3-24.6) | 23.2 (19.5-27.5) | 46.3 (37.5-53.3) | 90.2 (74.7-106) | 142 (111-161) | 912 |
| | 01-02 | 17.6 (16.0-19.3) | 19.2 (17.0-21.0) | 36.6 (32.4-42.6) | 69.2 (59.2-87.6) | 107 (89.8-123) | 1216 |
| | 03-04 | 18.9 (17.6-20.3) | 20.7 (18.9-22.8) | 38.4 (35.5-42.7) | 71.3 (60.1-80.0) | 101 (90.7-124) | 1088 |

Limits of detection (LOD, see Data Analysis section) for survey years 99-00, 01-02, and 03-04 are 0.9, 1.1, and 0.4, respectively.

*In the 1999-2000 survey period, concentrations of mono-isobutyl phthalate and mono-n-butyl phthalate were measured together and expressed as a combined value, referred to as monobutyl phthalate (MBP).

## Urinary Mono-n-butyl phthalate (MnBP) (creatinine corrected)
*Metabolite of Dibutyl phthalate (DBP) and Benzylbutyl phthalate (BzBP)*

Geometric mean and selected percentiles of urine concentrations (in µg/g of creatinine) for the U.S. population from the National Health and Nutrition Examination Survey.

| | Survey years | Geometric mean (95% conf. interval) | Selected percentiles ( 95% confidence interval) | | | | Sample size |
|---|---|---|---|---|---|---|---|
| | | | 50th | 75th | 90th | 95th | |
| **Total** | 99-00* | 22.4 (20.6-24.4) | 21.9 (19.8-24 3) | 38.9 (35.0-41 8) | 68.3 (60.3-78 3) | 97.7 (81.4-131) | 2541 |
| | 01-02 | 17.8 (16.7-19 0) | 17.4 (16.3-18.4) | 30.3 (28.1-32 3) | 52.4 (47.4-61 0) | 81.3 (71.0-92 5) | 2782 |
| | 03-04 | 19.8 (18.5-21 2) | 19.3 (17.7-20 8) | 33.9 (30.9-38 5) | 59.0 (52.9-68.1) | 91.6 (74.1-115) | 2605 |
| **Age group** | | | | | | | |
| 6-11 years | 99-00* | 41.9 (37.4-47.1) | 39.1 (34.3-49 0) | 65.9 (56.7-80 0) | 108 (71.2-179) | 159 (102-263) | 328 |
| | 01-02 | 35.4 (31.7-39 6) | 35.1 (29.3-38 9) | 55.4 (50.1-62 3) | 84.0 (69.0-113) | 147 (93.8-235) | 393 |
| | 03-04 | 38.4 (33.8-43 6) | 39.0 (34.7-42 6) | 59.3 (52.9-68.1) | 104 (83.6-119) | 137 (108-198) | 342 |
| 12-19 years | 99-00* | 24.3 (21.2-27 8) | 23.7 (20.6-27.4) | 37.6 (31.6-43 8) | 63.3 (52.4-76.4) | 88.1 (61.5-142) | 752 |
| | 01-02 | 19.4 (17.3-21.7) | 20.3 (17.5-22 3) | 34.9 (30.5-37 9) | 53.4 (45.2-73 9) | 89.7 (60.3-106) | 742 |
| | 03-04 | 20.0 (18.7-21 3) | 19.8 (18.2-21.7) | 30.7 (27.9-34 8) | 52.7 (43.4-65.4) | 74.4 (56.0-90 9) | 729 |
| 20 years and older | 99-00* | 20.4 (18.6-22.4) | 19.5 (18.1-21.4) | 34.9 (30.3-40 0) | 62.4 (53.4-72.1) | 91.0 (70.4-135) | 1461 |
| | 01-02 | 16.1 (15.0-17 3) | 15.5 (14.2-16 5) | 26.3 (24.2-28 6) | 44.2 (38.7-51.1) | 71.6 (61.2-85 6) | 1647 |
| | 03-04 | 18.3 (17.0-19 6) | 17.7 (16.6-19 2) | 31.0 (27.4-34 0) | 53.3 (46.5-64 2) | 83.8 (65.3-114) | 1534 |
| **Gender** | | | | | | | |
| Males | 99-00* | 17.3 (16.1-18 6) | 17.0 (15.5-18 8) | 28.6 (25.8-32.1) | 49.3 (42.6-53 5) | 64.7 (57.3-71 5) | 1215 |
| | 01-02 | 14.4 (13.5-15.4) | 13.7 (12.9-14 9) | 22.9 (20.8-24 6) | 39.9 (35.6-44 0) | 60.0 (50.5-76 2) | 1371 |
| | 03-04 | 15.7 (14.5-16 9) | 14.8 (13.6-16 0) | 25.4 (23.6-28.1) | 41.4 (37.0-47 5) | 59.4 (50.3-81 5) | 1250 |
| Females | 99-00* | 28.6 (25.3-32 3) | 28.8 (25.5-30 5) | 50.6 (41.9-56 3) | 84.3 (69.2-106) | 134 (93.6-155) | 1326 |
| | 01-02 | 21.7 (19.6-23 9) | 21.6 (19.7-23 6) | 35.8 (33.0-38.7) | 64.9 (58.9-70 2) | 91.5 (81.4-103) | 1411 |
| | 03-04 | 24.8 (22.9-26 8) | 24.1 (21.6-26 8) | 42.9 (39.2-48 9) | 74.9 (64.2-86 6) | 117 (83.6-139) | 1355 |
| **Race/ethnicity** | | | | | | | |
| Mexican Americans | 99-00* | 21.2 (19.3-23 3) | 20.0 (18.2-22 9) | 40.1 (32.6-44 3) | 63.6 (57.5-70.1) | 82.9 (73.9-100) | 814 |
| | 01-02 | 19.0 (16.2-22 2) | 19.2 (16.3-21 9) | 33.7 (28.3-39 6) | 61.0 (43.9-84 0) | 86.7 (60.6-128) | 677 |
| | 03-04 | 21.8 (17.7-26 8) | 20.4 (17.4-24 0) | 37.6 (29.6-50.1) | 75.3 (55.6-92 0) | 96.3 (76.4-164) | 652 |
| Non-Hispanic blacks | 99-00* | 23.9 (21.3-26 8) | 25.0 (20.7-28.1) | 42.2 (35.9-49 6) | 70.0 (61.1-83 9) | 96.2 (83.9-105) | 603 |
| | 01-02 | 20.8 (18.8-23.1) | 20.2 (19.2-22 8) | 34.5 (30.9-36 8) | 62.8 (50.6-74 6) | 85.6 (72.1-99 0) | 703 |
| | 03-04 | 21.4 (19.5-23.4) | 22.0 (19.6-24 8) | 35.4 (31.6-42.7) | 65.7 (54.0-75 3) | 94.0 (71.1-128) | 699 |
| Non-Hispanic whites | 99-00* | 21.3 (19.1-23 8) | 20.5 (18.6-23 2) | 36.4 (31.5-41 0) | 67.1 (56.7-78.4) | 97.7 (73.5-142) | 912 |
| | 01-02 | 17.4 (16.2-18 6) | 16.5 (15.3-17 8) | 29.0 (26.6-32 2) | 51.1 (46.0-60 0) | 81.4 (68.1-99 0) | 1216 |
| | 03-04 | 18.6 (17.3-20.1) | 17.9 (16.7-19 8) | 31.6 (27.7-37 8) | 53.3 (48.2-61 5) | 81.5 (64.2-108) | 1088 |

*In the 1999-2000 survey period, concentrations of mono-isobutyl phthalate and mono-n-butyl phthalate were measured together and expressed as a combined value.

## References

Adibi JJ, Perera FP, Jedrychowski W, Camann DE, Barr D, Jacek R, et al. Prenatal exposures to phthalates among women in New York City and Krakow, Poland. Environ Health Perspect 2003;111(14):1719-1722.

Anderson WA, Castle L, Scotter MJ, Massey RC, Springall C. A biomarker approach to measuring human dietary exposure to certain phthalate diesters. Food Addit Contam 2001;18(12):1068-1074.

Blount BC, Silva MJ, Caudill SP, Needham LL, Pirkle JL, Sampson EJ, et al. Levels of seven urinary phthalate metabolites in a human reference population. Environ Health Perspect 2000;108(10)979-982.

Brock JW, Caudill SP, Silva MJ, Needham LL, Hilborn ED. Phthalate monoesters levels in the urine of young children. Bull Environ Contam Toxicol 2002;68:309-314.

Centers for Disease Control and Prevention (CDC). Third National Report on Human Exposure to Environmental Chemicals. Atlanta (GA). 2005.

Duty SM, Calafat AM, Silva MJ, Brock JW, Ryan L, Chen Z, et al. The relationship between environmental exposure to phthalates and computer-aided sperm analysis motion parameters. J Androl 2004;25(2):293-302.

Fromme H, Bolte G, Koch HM, Angerer J, Boehmer S, Drexler H, et al. Occurrence and daily variation of phthalate metabolites in the urine of an adult population. Int J Hyg Environ Health 2007;210:21-33.

Hauser R, Meeker JD, Singh NP, Silva MJ, Ryan L, Duty S, et al. DNA damage in human sperm is related to urinary levels of phthalate monoester and oxidative metabolites. Hum Reprod 2007;22(3):688-695.

Itoh H, Yoshida K, Masunaga S. Evaluation of the effect of a governmental control of human exposure to two phthalates in Japan using a urinary biomarker approach. Int J Hyg Environ Health 2005;208:237-245.

Jonsson BAG, Richthoff J, Rylander L, Giwercman A, Hagmar L. Urinary phthalate metabolites and biomarkers of reproductive function in young men. Epidemiol 2005;16(4):487-493.

Koch HM, Rossbach B, Drexler H, Angerer J. Internal exposure of the general population to DEHP and other phthalates - determination of secondary and primary phthalate monoester metabolites in urine. Environ Res 2003;93:177-185.

McKee RH, Butala JH, David RM, Gans G. NTP center for the evaluation of risks to human reproduction reports on phthalates: addressing the data gaps [review]. Reprod Toxicol 2004;18(1):1-22.

NTP-CERHR. National Toxicology Program-Center for the Evaluation of Risks to Human Reproduction. Monograph on the Potential Human Reproductive and Developmental Effects of Di-n-Butyl Phthalate (DBP). Research Triangle Park (NC). 2000 [online]. Available at URL: http://cerhr.niehs.nih.gov/chemicals/phthalates/dbp/dbp-eval.html. 4/20/09

Silva MJ, Barr DB, Reidy JA, Malek NA, Hodge CC, Caudill SP, et al. Urinary levels of seven phthalate metabolites in the U.S. population from the National Health and Nutrition Examination Survey (NHANES) 1999-2000 [published erratum appears in Environ Health Perspect 2004; 112(5):A270]. Environ Health Perspect 2004;112(3):331-338.

Weuve J, Sanchez GN, Calafat AM, Schettler T, Green RA, Hu H, et al. Exposure to phthalates in neonatal intensive care unit infants: urinary concentrations of monoesters and oxidative metabolites. Environ Health Perspect 2006;114(9):1424-1431.

Wittassek M, Wiesmuller GA, Koch HM, Eckard R, Dobler L, Helm D, et al. Internal phthalate exposure over the last two decades—a retrospective human biomonitoring study. Int J Hyg Environ Health 2007;210(3-4):319-33.

# Dicyclohexyl Phthalate
CAS No. 84-61-7

## General Information

Dicyclohexyl phthalate (DCHP) is used to stabilize some rubbers, resins, and polymers, including nitrocellulose, polyvinyl acetate, and polyvinyl chloride. People exposed to DCHP will excrete mono-cyclohexyl phthalate (MCHP) in their urine. Neither IARC nor NTP has evaluated DCHP with respect to human carcinogenicity.

## Biomonitoring Information

Urinary levels of MCHP are infrequently measured and the

limited population-based surveys available to date have reported most levels below the limit of detection. In this *Report,* only levels at or above the 90th percentile could be characterized.

Finding a measurable amount of MCHP in urine does not mean that the levels of MCHP or the parent compound cause an adverse health effect. Biomonitoring studies on levels of urinary MCHP provide physicians and public health officials with reference values so that they can determine whether people have been exposed to higher levels of DHCP than are found in the general population. Biomonitoring data can also help scientists plan and conduct research on exposure and health effects.

### Urinary Mono-cyclohexyl phthalate (MCHP)
*Metabolite of Dicyclohexyl phthalate (DCHP)*

Geometric mean and selected percentiles of urine concentrations (in µg/L) for the U.S. population from the National Health and Nutrition Examination Survey.

| | Survey years | Geometric mean (95% conf. interval) | Selected percentiles (95% confidence interval) | | | | Sample size |
|---|---|---|---|---|---|---|---|
| | | | 50th | 75th | 90th | 95th | |
| **Total** | 99-00 | * | < LOD | < LOD | < LOD | 1.10 (<LOD-1.70) | 2541 |
| | 01-02 | * | < LOD | < LOD | .400 ( 300-.500) | .500 (.400-.600) | 2782 |
| | 03-04 | * | < LOD | < LOD | < LOD | .300 ( 200-.400) | 2605 |
| **Age group** | | | | | | | |
| 6-11 years | 99-00 | * | < LOD | < LOD | 1.00 (<LOD-1.10) | 1.70 (1.00-3.80) | 328 |
| | 01-02 | * | < LOD | < LOD | .400 ( 300-.500) | .600 ( 500-.700) | 393 |
| | 03-04 | * | < LOD | < LOD | .300 (<LOD-.400) | .500 ( 300-.500) | 342 |
| 12-19 years | 99-00 | * | < LOD | < LOD | 1.00 (<LOD-1.50) | 1.70 (1.00-2.50) | 752 |
| | 01-02 | * | < LOD | < LOD | .400 ( 300-.500) | .500 (.400-.600) | 742 |
| | 03-04 | * | < LOD | < LOD | .200 (<LOD-.300) | .400 ( 300-.600) | 729 |
| 20 years and older | 99-00 | * | < LOD | < LOD | < LOD | < LOD | 1461 |
| | 01-02 | * | < LOD | < LOD | .400 (<LOD-.500) | .500 (.400-.600) | 1647 |
| | 03-04 | * | < LOD | < LOD | < LOD | .300 ( 200-.300) | 1534 |
| **Gender** | | | | | | | |
| Males | 99-00 | * | < LOD | < LOD | < LOD | 1.10 (<LOD-2.00) | 1215 |
| | 01-02 | * | < LOD | < LOD | .400 ( 300-.500) | .500 (.400-.600) | 1371 |
| | 03-04 | * | < LOD | < LOD | < LOD | .300 ( 300-.400) | 1250 |
| Females | 99-00 | * | < LOD | < LOD | < LOD | 1.10 (<LOD-1.90) | 1326 |
| | 01-02 | * | < LOD | < LOD | .400 (<LOD-.400) | .500 (.400-.500) | 1411 |
| | 03-04 | * | < LOD | < LOD | < LOD | .300 ( 200-.500) | 1355 |
| **Race/ethnicity** | | | | | | | |
| Mexican Americans | 99-00 | * | < LOD | < LOD | < LOD | < LOD | 814 |
| | 01-02 | * | < LOD | < LOD | .400 (<LOD-.500) | .500 ( 300-.700) | 677 |
| | 03-04 | * | < LOD | < LOD | < LOD | .300 ( 200-.500) | 652 |
| Non-Hispanic blacks | 99-00 | * | < LOD | < LOD | < LOD | 1.10 ( 900-1.20) | 603 |
| | 01-02 | * | < LOD | < LOD | .400 ( 300-.500) | .500 (.400-.700) | 703 |
| | 03-04 | * | < LOD | < LOD | .300 ( 200-.300) | .400 ( 300-.500) | 699 |
| Non-Hispanic whites | 99-00 | * | < LOD | < LOD | < LOD | 1.00 (<LOD-1.70) | 912 |
| | 01-02 | * | < LOD | < LOD | .400 (<LOD-.400) | .500 (.400-.600) | 1216 |
| | 03-04 | * | < LOD | < LOD | < LOD | .300 ( 200-.400) | 1088 |

Limit of detection (LOD, see Data Analysis section) for Survey years 99-00, 01-02, and 03-04 are 0.9, 0.3, and 0.2, respectively.
< LOD means less than the limit of detection, which may vary for some chemicals by year and by individual sample.
* Not calculated: proportion of results below limit of detection was too high to provide a valid result.

## Urinary Mono-cyclohexyl phthalate (MCHP) (creatinine corrected)
*Metabolite of Dicyclohexyl phthalate (DCHP)*

Geometric mean and selected percentiles of urine concentrations (in µg/g of creatinine) for the U.S. population from the National Health and Nutrition Examination Survey.

| | Survey years | Geometric mean (95% conf. interval) | Selected percentiles ( 95% confidence interval) | | | | Sample size |
|---|---|---|---|---|---|---|---|
| | | | 50th | 75th | 90th | 95th | |
| **Total** | 99-00 | * | < LOD | < LOD | < LOD | 3.00 (<LOD-3.33) | 2541 |
| | 01-02 | * | < LOD | < LOD | .610 (.530-.690) | .910 (.770-1 00) | 2782 |
| | 03-04 | * | < LOD | < LOD | < LOD | .450 (.400-.500) | 2605 |
| **Age group** | | | | | | | |
| 6-11 years | 99-00 | * | < LOD | < LOD | 1.54 (<LOD-2.34) | 2.82 (1.54-6.44) | 328 |
| | 01-02 | * | < LOD | < LOD | .690 (.510-.740) | .940 (.690-1.17) | 393 |
| | 03-04 | * | < LOD | < LOD | .370 (<LOD-530) | .530 (.350-.830) | 342 |
| 12-19 years | 99-00 | * | < LOD | < LOD | 1.22 (<LOD-1.54) | 1.67 (1.36-1 82) | 752 |
| | 01-02 | * | < LOD | < LOD | .470 (.380-.660) | .770 (.530-1.18) | 742 |
| | 03-04 | * | < LOD | < LOD | .220 (<LOD- 270) | .380 (.240-.620) | 729 |
| 20 years and older | 99-00 | * | < LOD | < LOD | < LOD | < LOD | 1461 |
| | 01-02 | * | < LOD | < LOD | .630 (<LOD- 690) | .910 (.770-1 05) | 1647 |
| | 03-04 | * | < LOD | < LOD | < LOD | .450 (.400-.500) | 1534 |
| **Gender** | | | | | | | |
| Males | 99-00 | * | < LOD | < LOD | < LOD | 2.14 (<LOD-3.16) | 1215 |
| | 01-02 | * | < LOD | < LOD | .510 (.420-.660) | .880 (.670-1 06) | 1371 |
| | 03-04 | * | < LOD | < LOD | < LOD | .330 (.290-.500) | 1250 |
| Females | 99-00 | * | < LOD | < LOD | < LOD | 3.33 (<LOD-3.53) | 1326 |
| | 01-02 | * | < LOD | < LOD | .670 (<LOD-.770) | .910 (.800-1.10) | 1411 |
| | 03-04 | * | < LOD | < LOD | < LOD | .500 (.420-.590) | 1355 |
| **Race/ethnicity** | | | | | | | |
| Mexican Americans | 99-00 | * | < LOD | < LOD | < LOD | < LOD | 814 |
| | 01-02 | * | < LOD | < LOD | .590 (<LOD- 690) | .950 (.790-1.11) | 677 |
| | 03-04 | * | < LOD | < LOD | < LOD | .390 (.310-.560) | 652 |
| Non-Hispanic blacks | 99-00 | * | < LOD | < LOD | < LOD | 1.43 (1.12-1.74) | 603 |
| | 01-02 | * | < LOD | < LOD | .410 (.360-.490) | .590 (.500-.710) | 703 |
| | 03-04 | * | < LOD | < LOD | .250 (.170-.310) | .330 (.260-.470) | 699 |
| Non-Hispanic whites | 99-00 | * | < LOD | < LOD | < LOD | 3.16 (<LOD-3.53) | 912 |
| | 01-02 | * | < LOD | < LOD | .630 (<LOD-.740) | .910 (.770-1 06) | 1216 |
| | 03-04 | * | < LOD | < LOD | < LOD | .480 (.420-.530) | 1088 |

< LOD means less than the limit of detection for the urine levels not corrected for creatinine.
* Not calculated: proportion of results below limit of detection was too high to provide a valid result.

# Diethyl Phthalate
CAS No. 84-66-2

## General Information

Diethyl phthalate (DEP) is a solvent used in many consumer products, particularly those containing fragrances. Products that may contain DEP include perfumes, colognes, deodorants, soaps, shampoos, and hand lotions. People exposed to DEP eliminate mono-ethyl phthalate (MEP) in their urine. Workplace air guidelines for external exposure to DEP have been established by ACGIH and NIOSH. Neither IARC nor NTP has evaluated DEP with respect to human carcinogenicity.

## Biomonitoring Information

MEP levels in the NHANES 1999-2000, 2001-2002, and 2003-2004 subsamples were similar to median or geometric mean levels in small samples of pregnant women in New York City (Adibi et al., 2003) and African-American women in Washington, DC (Hoppin et al., 2002), and also in men attending a Boston infertility clinic (Hauser et al., 2007). In contrast, a sample of young Swedish males entering the military had median urinary MEP levels that were somewhat higher than males in the NHANES subsamples. A small study of children less than 2 years old reported mean urine MEP levels that were about twice as high as levels in children (aged 6-11 years) in NHANES 2001-

## Urinary Mono-ethyl phthalate (MEP)
*Metabolite of Diethyl phthalate (DEP)*

Geometric mean and selected percentiles of urine concentrations (in µg/L) for the U.S. population from the National Health and Nutrition Examination Survey.

| | Survey years | Geometric mean (95% conf. interval) | Selected percentiles ( 95% confidence interval) 50th | 75th | 90th | 95th | Sample size |
|---|---|---|---|---|---|---|---|
| **Total** | 99-00 | 179 (156-204) | 164 (136-201) | 454 (370-538) | 1260 (1010-1480) | 2840 (2150-3770) | 2536 |
| | 01-02 | 178 (159-199) | 169 (141-194) | 465 (415-527) | 1230 (1040-1440) | 2500 (1860-3220) | 2782 |
| | 03-04 | 193 (169-220) | 174 (151-208) | 502 (457-555) | 1380 (1170-1750) | 2700 (2160-3310) | 2605 |
| **Age group** | | | | | | | |
| 6-11 years | 99-00 | 91.3 (74.8-111) | 75.4 (62.1-93.7) | 197 (129-249) | 378 (290-730) | 756 (379-1070) | 328 |
| | 01-02 | 85.1 (71.2-102) | 71.9 (61.9-92.5) | 183 (142-217) | 451 (315-636) | 808 (572-1090) | 393 |
| | 03-04 | 95.3 (82.3-110) | 81.7 (70.3-103) | 196 (170-241) | 521 (295-571) | 827 (542-1440) | 342 |
| 12-19 years | 99-00 | 211 (160-278) | 193 (141-256) | 564 (419-818) | 1510 (1050-2150) | 3260 (1550-4420) | 752 |
| | 01-02 | 197 (159-243) | 184 (148-227) | 479 (387-651) | 1260 (983-1480) | 2070 (1470-3050) | 742 |
| | 03-04 | 225 (187-270) | 221 (165-294) | 557 (432-695) | 1250 (973-1560) | 2310 (1360-3310) | 729 |
| 20 years and older | 99-00 | 190 (164-219) | 180 (140-221) | 482 (390-590) | 1340 (1010-1660) | 3480 (2230-4640) | 1456 |
| | 01-02 | 191 (171-214) | 181 (152-212) | 498 (441-567) | 1350 (1060-1660) | 2720 (2160-3670) | 1647 |
| | 03-04 | 205 (176-238) | 188 (158-219) | 533 (471-629) | 1590 (1220-2070) | 2980 (2250-3800) | 1534 |
| **Gender** | | | | | | | |
| Males | 99-00 | 179 (149-215) | 154 (119-197) | 523 (372-650) | 1440 (1020-2280) | 3500 (2130-4560) | 1214 |
| | 01-02 | 182 (157-211) | 171 (139-199) | 502 (419-603) | 1450 (1060-2110) | 3100 (2110-4390) | 1371 |
| | 03-04 | 197 (173-224) | 171 (148-201) | 536 (449-654) | 1520 (1210-2070) | 2910 (2210-3480) | 1250 |
| Females | 99-00 | 178 (154-206) | 174 (138-210) | 425 (350-508) | 988 (880-1230) | 2230 (1370-3880) | 1322 |
| | 01-02 | 174 (153-198) | 167 (139-194) | 427 (387-498) | 1050 (879-1310) | 1860 (1490-2500) | 1411 |
| | 03-04 | 189 (160-225) | 182 (138-219) | 478 (392-564) | 1260 (969-1640) | 2590 (1800-3420) | 1355 |
| **Race/ethnicity** | | | | | | | |
| Mexican Americans | 99-00 | 181 (157-209) | 174 (146-210) | 441 (390-541) | 1280 (851-1510) | 1720 (1460-2130) | 813 |
| | 01-02 | 226 (195-262) | 220 (190-264) | 530 (444-660) | 1490 (1050-2110) | 2630 (1540-4460) | 677 |
| | 03-04 | 267 (239-298) | 249 (212-307) | 597 (523-688) | 1640 (1320-2180) | 3050 (2230-4300) | 652 |
| Non-Hispanic blacks | 99-00 | 322 (275-377) | 306 (256-350) | 789 (635-949) | 1890 (1410-2270) | 3610 (2130-4640) | 603 |
| | 01-02 | 352 (324-384) | 357 (290-407) | 853 (709-1090) | 2160 (1620-2470) | 3540 (2810-5070) | 703 |
| | 03-04 | 357 (310-412) | 306 (253-414) | 948 (769-1150) | 2500 (1840-2980) | 4370 (2780-5910) | 699 |
| Non-Hispanic whites | 99-00 | 152 (133-175) | 134 (108-157) | 367 (287-482) | 986 (798-1340) | 2470 (1590-3880) | 908 |
| | 01-02 | 158 (141-178) | 147 (119-177) | 413 (366-451) | 1020 (905-1230) | 2320 (1560-2720) | 1216 |
| | 03-04 | 167 (145-193) | 148 (125-175) | 418 (366-477) | 1210 (954-1480) | 2250 (1590-3290) | 1088 |

Limit of detection (LOD, see Data Analysis section) for Survey years 99-00, 01-02, and 03-04 are 1 2, 0.9, and 0.4, respectively.

2002 (Brock et al., 2002). Median MEP levels found in a small sample of German residents (Koch et al., 2003) were slightly lower than levels found in NHANES 2001-2002.

In an analysis of NHANES 1999-2000, the adjusted geometric mean levels of urinary MEP were lower in the group aged 6-11 years than in either of the other age groups. This age-related trend is opposite the direction seen for other phthalates. Other population estimates also differed by sex and race ethnicity (Silva et al., 2004). Analysis of NHANES 2001-2002 showed similar findings, with adjusted geometric mean levels of urinary MEP that increased with age (CDC, 2005).

Finding a measurable amount of MEP in urine does not mean that the levels of MEP or the parent compound cause an adverse health effect. Biomonitoring studies on levels of MEP provide physicians and public health officials with reference values so that they can determine whether people have been exposed to higher levels of DEP than are found in the general population. Biomonitoring data can also help scientists plan and conduct research on exposure and health effects.

## Urinary Mono-ethyl phthalate (MEP) (creatinine corrected)
*Metabolite of Diethyl phthalate (DEP)*
Geometric mean and selected percentiles of urine concentrations (in µg/g of creatinine) for the U.S. population from the National Health and Nutrition Examination Survey.

| | Survey years | Geometric mean (95% conf. interval) | 50th | 75th | 90th | 95th | Sample size |
|---|---|---|---|---|---|---|---|
| **Total** | 99-00 | 163 (149-178) | 141 (129-157) | 360 (307-422) | 905 (753-1180) | 1950 (1670-2310) | 2536 |
| | 01-02 | 167 (150-185) | 148 (133-162) | 388 (330-435) | 969 (805-1180) | 1840 (1450-2200) | 2782 |
| | 03-04 | 181 (163-202) | 153 (137-177) | 452 (386-504) | 1110 (889-1290) | 2040 (1640-2540) | 2605 |
| **Age group** | | | | | | | |
| 6-11 years | 99-00 | 92.6 (77.9-110) | 79.6 (65.7-110) | 165 (127-208) | 341 (219-554) | 625 (400-784) | 328 |
| | 01-02 | 96.9 (82.5-114) | 81.2 (66.3-105) | 177 (135-224) | 512 (290-802) | 843 (512-1320) | 393 |
| | 03-04 | 101 (87.0-117) | 87.0 (66.5-113) | 180 (145-203) | 470 (310-596) | 719 (470-1330) | 342 |
| 12-19 years | 99-00 | 142 (119-169) | 122 (93.0-156) | 364 (275-495) | 879 (676-1260) | 1760 (1000-2000) | 752 |
| | 01-02 | 152 (126-184) | 140 (111-180) | 330 (249-409) | 808 (590-1100) | 1330 (868-1840) | 742 |
| | 03-04 | 168 (141-201) | 150 (123-184) | 363 (292-485) | 791 (589-1080) | 1470 (987-2220) | 729 |
| 20 years and older | 99-00 | 179 (161-199) | 154 (136-177) | 390 (336-452) | 1010 (803-1460) | 2170 (1790-3350) | 1456 |
| | 01-02 | 181 (164-200) | 160 (146-182) | 419 (363-486) | 1060 (884-1320) | 2120 (1520-2790) | 1647 |
| | 03-04 | 197 (174-223) | 177 (147-202) | 512 (423-632) | 1230 (989-1610) | 2290 (1770-3200) | 1534 |
| **Gender** | | | | | | | |
| Males | 99-00 | 141 (124-159) | 120 (107-134) | 324 (249-415) | 1000 (693-1480) | 1950 (1460-2900) | 1214 |
| | 01-02 | 148 (130-168) | 126 (110-147) | 352 (282-425) | 1100 (839-1480) | 2120 (1490-3030) | 1371 |
| | 03-04 | 154 (139-171) | 127 (108-150) | 390 (341-465) | 1070 (852-1360) | 2000 (1610-2410) | 1250 |
| Females | 99-00 | 187 (165-211) | 158 (142-179) | 377 (307-495) | 822 (697-1170) | 1930 (1170-3410) | 1322 |
| | 01-02 | 187 (166-210) | 171 (148-188) | 407 (355-473) | 860 (712-1100) | 1430 (1190-2010) | 1411 |
| | 03-04 | 211 (180-248) | 181 (148-217) | 508 (379-634) | 1120 (889-1400) | 2250 (1440-3330) | 1355 |
| **Race/ethnicity** | | | | | | | |
| Mexican Americans | 99-00 | 164 (142-190) | 154 (136-174) | 382 (314-472) | 814 (673-974) | 1330 (974-1920) | 813 |
| | 01-02 | 213 (182-249) | 199 (164-242) | 461 (396-572) | 1080 (860-1650) | 1940 (1410-2630) | 677 |
| | 03-04 | 241 (213-271) | 233 (202-270) | 533 (417-665) | 1230 (956-1610) | 2270 (1810-3140) | 652 |
| Non-Hispanic blacks | 99-00 | 208 (183-236) | 196 (166-228) | 443 (390-505) | 1030 (762-1700) | 1920 (1230-2590) | 603 |
| | 01-02 | 247 (226-271) | 227 (185-270) | 557 (478-618) | 1240 (961-1480) | 2090 (1550-2800) | 703 |
| | 03-04 | 254 (225-287) | 212 (188-246) | 619 (476-791) | 1530 (1200-1970) | 2590 (2160-3500) | 699 |
| Non-Hispanic whites | 99-00 | 149 (135-165) | 128 (111-142) | 313 (239-387) | 856 (655-1390) | 1950 (1480-2740) | 908 |
| | 01-02 | 157 (142-173) | 136 (124-150) | 338 (288-402) | 919 (712-1160) | 1590 (1320-2170) | 1216 |
| | 03-04 | 165 (144-189) | 135 (120-158) | 386 (338-485) | 989 (831-1330) | 1920 (1400-2780) | 1088 |

## References

Adibi JJ, Perera FP, Jedrychowski W, Camann DE, Barr D, Jacek R, et al. Prenatal exposures to phthalates among women in New York City and Krakow, Poland. Environ Health Perspect 2003;111(14):1719-1722.

Brock JW, Caudill SP, Silva MJ, Needham LL, Hilborn ED. Phthalate monoesters levels in the urine of young children. Bull Environ Contam Toxicol 2002;68:309-314.

Centers for Disease Control and Prevention (CDC). Third National Report on Human Exposure to Environmental Chemicals. Atlanta (GA). 2005.

Hauser R, Meeker JD, Singh NP, Silva MJ, Ryan L, Duty S, et al. DNA damage in human sperm is related to urinary levels of phthalate monoester and oxidative metabolites. Hum Reprod 2007;22(3):688-695.

Hoppin JA, Brock JW, Davis BJ, Baird DD. Reproducibility of urinary phthalate metabolites in first morning urine samples. Environ Health Perspect 2002;110(5):515-518.

Koch HM, Rossbach B, Drexler H, Angerer J. Internal exposure of the general population to DEHP and other phthalates - determination of secondary and primary phthalate monoester metabolites in urine. Environ Res 2003;93:177-185.

Silva MJ, Barr DB, Reidy JA, Malek NA, Hodge CC, Caudill SP, et al. Urinary levels of seven phthalate metabolites in the U.S. population from the National Health and Nutrition Examination Survey (NHANES) 1999-2000 [published erratum appears in Environ Health Perspect 2004; 112(5):A270]. Environ Health Perspect 2004;112(3):331-338.

# Di-2-ethylhexyl Phthalate
CAS No. 117-81-7

## General Information

Di-2-ethylhexyl phthalate (DEHP) is primarily used to produce flexibility in plastics, mainly polyvinyl chloride, which is used for many consumer products, toys, packaging film, and blood product storage and intravenous delivery systems. Concentrations in plastic materials may reach 40% by weight. DEHP has been removed from or replaced in most toys and food packaging in the United States.

Following ingestion, DEHP is metabolized to more than 30 metabolites which are rapidly eliminated in urine, and in humans, as glucuronide conjugates (Albro et al., 1982; Albro and Lavenhar, 1989; ATSDR, 2002; Peck and Albro,1982). Four metabolites were measured in this *Report*: mono-(2-ethyl-5-hexyl) phthalate (MEHP), mono-(2-ethyl-5-oxohexyl) phthalate (MEOHP), mono-(2-ethyl-5-hydroxyhexyl) phthalate (MEHHP) and mono-(2-ethyl-5-carboxypentyl) phthalate (MECPP).

MEHP is primarily formed by the hydrolysis of DEHP in the gastrointestinal tract and then absorbed. DEHP present in medical devices and parenteral delivery systems results in the diester rather than the monoester form being directly introduced into the blood. After parenteral administration,

## Urinary Mono-2-ethylhexyl phthalate (MEHP)
*Metabolite of Di-2-ethylhexyl phthalate (DEHP)*
Geometric mean and selected percentiles of urine concentrations (in µg/L) for the U.S. population from the National Health and Nutrition Examination Survey.

| | Survey years | Geometric mean (95% conf. interval) | 50th | 75th | 90th | 95th | Sample size |
|---|---|---|---|---|---|---|---|
| Total | 99-00 | 3.43 (3.19-3.69) | 3.20 (3.00-3.60) | 7.60 (6.80-8.40) | 14.9 (13.5-17.4) | 23.8 (19.2-28.6) | 2541 |
| | 01-02 | 4.27 (3.80-4.79) | 4.20 (3.70-4.90) | 9.80 (8.40-11.6) | 23.0 (19.1-27.9) | 39.2 (31.8-50.0) | 2782 |
| | 03-04 | 2.34 (2.10-2.62) | 1.90 (1.70-2.40) | 5.30 (4.50-6.60) | 15.1 (11.4-20.6) | 31.0 (21.4-42.0) | 2605 |
| **Age group** | | | | | | | |
| 6-11 years | 99-00 | 5.12 (4.42-5.92) | 4.90 (3.70-6.40) | 11.1 (8.30-13.6) | 19.0 (13.8-36.1) | 35.3 (15.6-130) | 328 |
| | 01-02 | 4.41 (3.90-5.00) | 4.40 (4.10-5.30) | 9.30 (7.90-11.7) | 19.7 (14.6-25.9) | 31.4 (21.8-47.9) | 393 |
| | 03-04 | 2.84 (2.10-3.84) | 2.70 (1.80-4.10) | 6.40 (4.40-9.60) | 13.9 (7.80-27.6) | 27.6 (11.3-64.7) | 342 |
| 12-19 years | 99-00 | 3.75 (3.24-4.35) | 3.70 (2.90-4.60) | 8.10 (6.40-9.40) | 15.3 (11.4-20.5) | 22.8 (19.1-29.2) | 752 |
| | 01-02 | 4.57 (3.96-5.27) | 4.50 (3.70-5.10) | 11.0 (9.50-14.4) | 23.0 (17.7-32.7) | 42.5 (25.9-57.5) | 742 |
| | 03-04 | 2.77 (2.25-3.41) | 2.50 (2.00-3.00) | 6.40 (4.50-8.60) | 18.6 (10.2-35.6) | 40.6 (20.7-58.4) | 729 |
| 20 years and older | 99-00 | 3.21 (2.94-3.51) | 3.00 (2.70-3.40) | 7.30 (6.40-8.00) | 14.5 (12.1-17.0) | 22.7 (17.5-27.0) | 1461 |
| | 01-02 | 4.20 (3.63-4.86) | 4.10 (3.50-5.00) | 9.50 (8.10-11.9) | 23.5 (18.0-29.8) | 39.5 (30.3-57.1) | 1647 |
| | 03-04 | 2.23 (2.03-2.44) | 1.70 (1.50-2.00) | 5.10 (4.50-6.00) | 15.1 (10.9-19.7) | 29.5 (20.4-40.0) | 1534 |
| **Gender** | | | | | | | |
| Males | 99-00 | 3.68 (3.31-4.10) | 3.40 (2.90-3.90) | 8.00 (7.40-8.80) | 16.0 (14.0-19.0) | 25.3 (19.5-36.7) | 1215 |
| | 01-02 | 4.31 (3.84-4.83) | 4.30 (3.70-5.10) | 9.70 (8.30-11.2) | 23.0 (16.9-29.8) | 37.9 (29.9-48.4) | 1371 |
| | 03-04 | 2.56 (2.26-2.90) | 2.20 (1.70-2.60) | 6.00 (4.60-7.70) | 17.2 (11.3-26.3) | 33.3 (24.9-55.5) | 1250 |
| Females | 99-00 | 3.21 (2.91-3.54) | 3.10 (2.80-3.50) | 7.10 (5.90-8.50) | 13.6 (12.1-17.2) | 21.9 (15.6-28.5) | 1326 |
| | 01-02 | 4.23 (3.67-4.86) | 4.10 (3.50-5.00) | 9.80 (8.40-12.2) | 23.0 (19.5-28.4) | 43.5 (31.4-53.7) | 1411 |
| | 03-04 | 2.15 (1.92-2.42) | 1.80 (1.50-2.10) | 4.90 (4.10-5.70) | 13.2 (10.0-18.1) | 27.8 (17.5-40.7) | 1355 |
| **Race/ethnicity** | | | | | | | |
| Mexican Americans | 99-00 | 3.49 (3.16-3.85) | 3.50 (3.10-3.90) | 7.00 (5.70-8.60) | 13.3 (10.7-18.7) | 23.9 (17.4-27.3) | 814 |
| | 01-02 | 4.32 (3.75-4.98) | 4.70 (3.80-5.70) | 10.1 (8.50-11.4) | 19.6 (16.6-23.0) | 28.5 (24.2-39.9) | 677 |
| | 03-04 | 2.35 (1.87-2.96) | 2.20 (1.50-3.00) | 5.10 (4.30-6.60) | 11.2 (7.50-16.5) | 18.5 (11.6-38.2) | 652 |
| Non-Hispanic blacks | 99-00 | 4.82 (3.92-5.93) | 5.20 (4.10-5.80) | 9.50 (7.60-11.4) | 19.5 (12.9-26.5) | 29.5 (18.6-60.3) | 603 |
| | 01-02 | 6.60 (5.57-7.82) | 6.70 (5.40-8.10) | 15.4 (13.0-18.7) | 32.9 (26.5-41.4) | 52.6 (41.0-84.0) | 703 |
| | 03-04 | 3.61 (3.07-4.23) | 3.50 (3.00-4.00) | 8.50 (7.10-11.4) | 22.9 (16.5-28.6) | 35.2 (29.3-49.1) | 699 |
| Non-Hispanic whites | 99-00 | 3.16 (2.89-3.46) | 2.80 (2.50-3.10) | 7.40 (6.30-8.40) | 14.5 (12.2-17.4) | 22.4 (16.9-28.5) | 912 |
| | 01-02 | 3.85 (3.37-4.40) | 3.70 (3.10-4.40) | 8.70 (7.80-9.90) | 20.9 (17.3-25.9) | 37.9 (29.9-49.5) | 1216 |
| | 03-04 | 2.14 (1.92-2.39) | 1.70 (1.40-1.90) | 4.80 (4.00-5.80) | 13.6 (9.50-20.0) | 31.0 (18.1-48.9) | 1088 |

Limit of detection (LOD, see Data Analysis section) for Survey years 99-00, 01-02, and 03-04 are 1.2, 1.0, and 0 9, respectively.

hydrolysis of DEHP most likely also occurs in the blood, and subsequent metabolism is similar to that following ingestion (Koch et al., 2005a, 2005b, 2005c). MEOHP, MEHHP, and MECPP are produced by the oxidative metabolism of MEHP and are present at roughly three- to five-fold higher concentrations than MEHP in urine (Barr et al., 2003; Fromme et al., 2007; Koch et al., 2003).

MEHP is the putative toxic metabolite of DEHP. Liver toxicity, decreased testicular weight, and testicular atrophy have been observed in rodents fed high doses over a short term or with chronic dosing (McKee et al., 2004; NTP-CERHR, 2000c, 2006). In contrast, marmoset monkeys fed high dose DEHP for longer than a year did

not demonstrate testicular or liver toxicity (NTP-CERHR, 2006). Very high doses of DEHP have suppressed estradiol production in female rats (Lovecamp-Swan and Davis, 2003). The Food and Drug Administration determined that in adults, the amounts of DEHP or MEHP received from intravenous delivery systems or blood transfusions (DEHP is hydrolyzed to MEHP in stored blood) would result in short-term elevations similar to background levels (FDA, 2001). However, critically ill neonates and infants receiving selected or multiple intensive procedures, such as exchange transfusions, extracorporeal membrane oxygenation, and parenteral nutrition, could receive higher exposures than the general population (Calafat et al., 2004; FDA, 2001; Loff et al., 2000; Weuve et al., 2006).

## Urinary Mono-2-ethylhexyl phthalate (MEHP) (creatinine corrected)
*Metabolite of Di-2-ethylhexyl phthalate (DEHP)*
Geometric mean and selected percentiles of urine concentrations (in µg/g of creatinine) for the U.S. population from the National Health and Nutrition Examination Survey.

| | Survey years | Geometric mean (95% conf. interval) | 50th | 75th | 90th | 95th | Sample size |
|---|---|---|---|---|---|---|---|
| **Total** | 99-00 | 3.12 (2 95-3.31) | 3.08 (2 82-3.27) | 5.88 (5 38-6.25) | 10.8 (9.62-12.5) | 18.9 (15.0-21.8) | 2541 |
| | 01-02 | 4.00 (3 58-4.48) | 3.90 (3.44-4.47) | 7.94 (7 22-9.02) | 18.0 (15.3-21.5) | 32.8 (25.2-42.9) | 2782 |
| | 03-04 | 2.20 (2 01-2.41) | 1.89 (1.68-2.19) | 4.31 (3 84-4.74) | 10.8 (8.72-13.8) | 25.4 (16.7-34.7) | 2605 |
| **Age group** | | | | | | | |
| 6-11 years | 99-00 | 5.19 (4 55-5.93) | 5.37 (4 52-5.95) | 9.11 (8 06-11.4) | 21.6 (11.5-41.9) | 41.9 (13.5-86.2) | 328 |
| | 01-02 | 5.03 (4.47-5.65) | 5.38 (4 51-6.21) | 9.90 (7 87-11.5) | 21.1 (13.8-28.8) | 31.4 (24.3-40.7) | 393 |
| | 03-04 | 3.00 (2 30-3.93) | 2.80 (1 93-4.09) | 5.86 (4.69-7.70) | 14.3 (8 54-24.4) | 28.7 (14.1-45.3) | 342 |
| 12-19 years | 99-00 | 2.53 (2.14-2.99) | 2.35 (2 05-2.76) | 5.83 (4 38-6.29) | 9.66 (7.41-11.5) | 12.1 (10.5-17.3) | 752 |
| | 01-02 | 3.53 (3 09-4.03) | 3.67 (2 89-4.48) | 7.47 (6 51-8.67) | 15.2 (11.7-21.9) | 25.2 (17.7-32.8) | 742 |
| | 03-04 | 2.07 (1.74-2.48) | 1.88 (1.60-2.23) | 4.25 (3.19-5.62) | 11.6 (6 83-23.2) | 24.8 (11.6-37.9) | 729 |
| 20 years and older | 99-00 | 3.03 (2 83-3.25) | 2.98 (2.73-3.23) | 5.55 (4 90-6.06) | 10.0 (8.60-12.9) | 17.5 (13.8-22.1) | 1461 |
| | 01-02 | 3.97 (3.49-4.52) | 3.82 (3 26-4.38) | 7.79 (7 00-9.00) | 18.3 (15.3-21.8) | 34.5 (23.1-47.9) | 1647 |
| | 03-04 | 2.14 (1 98-2.31) | 1.84 (1.63-2.08) | 4.14 (3.78-4.40) | 10.5 (8 38-12.9) | 25.6 (15.9-36.3) | 1534 |
| **Gender** | | | | | | | |
| Males | 99-00 | 2.89 (2.60-3.22) | 2.76 (2 52-2.96) | 5.58 (4.71-6.08) | 10.3 (9 35-12.4) | 21.6 (14.1-27.7) | 1215 |
| | 01-02 | 3.50 (3 08-3.99) | 3.33 (2 83-3.90) | 7.00 (6.49-7.77) | 16.2 (12.8-20.9) | 31.6 (20.5-49.4) | 1371 |
| | 03-04 | 2.01 (1 82-2.21) | 1.71 (1.46-1.89) | 4.14 (3.49-4.81) | 10.4 (7.68-16.2) | 23.3 (15.1-41.1) | 1250 |
| Females | 99-00 | 3.36 (3.11-3.63) | 3.33 (2 91-3.80) | 6.15 (5 55-6.77) | 11.1 (9.11-14.0) | 17.3 (12.4-24.6) | 1326 |
| | 01-02 | 4.54 (4 02-5.13) | 4.47 (3 85-5.14) | 9.28 (7 94-10.3) | 20.3 (16.6-24.4) | 34.7 (27.1-42.0) | 1411 |
| | 03-04 | 2.40 (2.15-2.69) | 2.16 (1 84-2.40) | 4.40 (3 97-4.89) | 10.9 (8 27-16.0) | 27.0 (17.5-34.6) | 1355 |
| **Race/ethnicity** | | | | | | | |
| Mexican Americans | 99-00 | 3.16 (2.72-3.68) | 3.15 (2 52-3.81) | 5.88 (4 86-7.24) | 11.6 (9.63-13.1) | 15.7 (12.6-23.1) | 814 |
| | 01-02 | 4.07 (3.60-4.61) | 4.18 (3 82-4.90) | 7.80 (6.64-9.49) | 16.4 (13.6-18.9) | 24.9 (19.8-28.7) | 677 |
| | 03-04 | 2.12 (1.74-2.59) | 1.94 (1 50-2.42) | 4.06 (3 29-4.93) | 9.38 (5.72-15.4) | 16.8 (9 86-38.6) | 652 |
| Non-Hispanic blacks | 99-00 | 3.11 (2 59-3.73) | 3.13 (2 50-3.61) | 5.84 (4.43-7.32) | 10.2 (8 05-15.6) | 18.4 (11.6-35.2) | 603 |
| | 01-02 | 4.63 (3 96-5.42) | 4.59 (3 97-5.02) | 9.93 (7 95-12.4) | 21.2 (16.0-33.2) | 39.9 (27.7-48.1) | 703 |
| | 03-04 | 2.56 (2 24-2.92) | 2.28 (2 02-2.78) | 5.17 (4.48-6.83) | 13.2 (10.5-16.2) | 27.5 (18.4-36.0) | 699 |
| Non-Hispanic whites | 99-00 | 3.09 (2 84-3.36) | 3.08 (2.73-3.47) | 5.87 (5.11-6.67) | 10.6 (8 95-13.5) | 20.0 (14.0-24.6) | 912 |
| | 01-02 | 3.81 (3 34-4.35) | 3.67 (3.11-4.33) | 7.78 (6.74-9.35) | 17.0 (14.1-21.8) | 32.8 (21.5-46.9) | 1216 |
| | 03-04 | 2.12 (1 91-2.35) | 1.82 (1.60-2.13) | 4.11 (3.49-4.42) | 10.7 (7.42-15.1) | 27.0 (15.1-37.4) | 1088 |

OSHA has established a workplace air standard for external exposure to DEHP; NIOSH and ACGIH have established guidelines for workplace air exposure to DEHP. IARC considers DEHP to be unclassifiable with respect to human carcinogenicity. NTP determined that DEHP is reasonably anticipated to be a human carcinogen.

**Biomonitoring Information**

The levels of MEHP reported in NHANES 1999-2000, 2001-2002, and 2003-2004 appear roughly comparable to those reported previously in several small U.S. studies involving adults (Blount et al., 2000), pregnant women in New York City (Adibi et al., 2003), and low income African-American women in Washington, DC (Hoppin et al., 2002). In contrast, a sample of South Korean women had higher urine MEHP levels: the geometric mean was about ten times higher than for females in each of the NHANES survey periods (Koo and Lee, 2005; CDC, 2005). Median urine MEHP levels in a small group of Japanese adults, in a group of Swedish male military recruits, and in samples of men attending an infertility clinic were similar to median values for adults and males, respectively, in NHANES 1999-2000 and 2001-2002 subsamples (Duty et al., 2004,

2005; Itoh et al., 2005).

In another sample of men attending an infertility clinic, the median and 95th percentile values of urinary MEHP were similar, but MEHHP and MEOHP were about three to five times higher than comparable values found in males in two NHANES survey periods (1999-2000, 2001-2002) (CDC, 2005; Hauser et al., 2007). Compared with the U.S. population in this *Report,* urinary MEHP, MEOHP, and MEHHP levels were similar or up to twofold higher in a sample of German residents (Koch et al., 2003; Preuss et al., 2005) and German children (Becker et al., 2004; Koch et al., 2004). During 2001-2003, median levels of urinary MEOHP and MEHHP appeared to be similar in samples of German university students and the adults in this *Report* (Wittasek et al., 2007).

In separate analyses of NHANES 1999-2000 and NHANES 2001-2002, the adjusted geometric mean levels of urinary MEHP were significantly higher in children compared with adolescents and adults, and in females compared with males (CDC, 2005; Silva et al., 2004). South Korean children had geometric mean urine MEHP levels that were about three times higher than the U.S. children in this *Report* (Koo and

### Urinary Mono-(2-ethyl-5-hydroxyhexyl) phthalate (MEHHP)

*Metabolite of Di-2-ethylhexyl phthalate (DEHP)*

Geometric mean and selected percentiles of urine concentrations (in µg/L) for the U.S. population from the National Health and Nutrition Examination Survey.

| | Survey years | Geometric mean (95% conf. interval) | 50th | 75th | 90th | 95th | Sample size |
|---|---|---|---|---|---|---|---|
| **Total** | 01-02 | 20.0 (17.8-22.5) | 20.1 (17.8-22.4) | 43.6 (38.0-49.7) | 92.3 (77.0-108) | 192 (131-256) | 2782 |
| | 03-04 | 21.7 (19.3-24.4) | 21.2 (18.7-24.1) | 49.1 (40.5-56.9) | 121 (91.3-164) | 266 (165-383) | 2605 |
| **Age group** | | | | | | | |
| 6-11 years | 01-02 | 33.6 (29.7-37.9) | 32.9 (26.9-39.1) | 66.9 (49.7-74.0) | 127 (103-148) | 216 (137-280) | 393 |
| | 03-04 | 36.9 (28.4-47.9) | 36.5 (26.5-47.0) | 77.4 (49.1-103) | 164 (79.9-350) | 318 (164-400) | 342 |
| 12-19 years | 01-02 | 24.9 (21.3-29.1) | 25.3 (22.9-31.3) | 50.6 (40.7-64.5) | 107 (78.5-148) | 216 (117-330) | 742 |
| | 03-04 | 28.3 (23.0-34.8) | 29.8 (25.9-33.9) | 56.9 (45.4-73.7) | 157 (84.1-299) | 317 (176-553) | 729 |
| 20 years and older | 01-02 | 18.1 (15.7-20.9) | 17.8 (14.7-20.7) | 39.8 (32.7-48.0) | 86.2 (65.7-107) | 175 (110-279) | 1647 |
| | 03-04 | 19.5 (17.7-21.5) | 18.4 (16.6-21.0) | 41.9 (36.9-51.2) | 107 (88.2-136) | 225 (148-384) | 1534 |
| **Gender** | | | | | | | |
| Males | 01-02 | 22.0 (19.5-24.7) | 21.2 (19.4-24.2) | 48.0 (41.4-54.4) | 94.2 (80.8-110) | 212 (130-256) | 1371 |
| | 03-04 | 24.1 (20.9-27.9) | 22.9 (19.2-27.9) | 51.0 (40.5-59.8) | 133 (94.8-220) | 317 (162-470) | 1250 |
| Females | 01-02 | 18.3 (15.7-21.4) | 18.2 (14.9-22.1) | 39.8 (34.3-46.0) | 86.0 (69.4-115) | 170 (119-273) | 1411 |
| | 03-04 | 19.7 (17.4-22.2) | 19.4 (16.7-22.8) | 46.4 (37.5-54.4) | 103 (84.1-148) | 214 (140-318) | 1355 |
| **Race/ethnicity** | | | | | | | |
| Mexican Americans | 01-02 | 18.5 (16.2-21.1) | 19.1 (16.3-21.6) | 36.3 (31.6-44.0) | 79.9 (66.4-93.9) | 123 (100-161) | 677 |
| | 03-04 | 18.9 (15.4-23.4) | 19.8 (17.6-22.3) | 37.5 (30.0-45.6) | 72.2 (52.4-115) | 116 (71.6-327) | 652 |
| Non-Hispanic blacks | 01-02 | 29.8 (26.1-34.1) | 30.9 (27.2-34.3) | 61.9 (52.6-69.4) | 126 (108-157) | 276 (157-339) | 703 |
| | 03-04 | 30.8 (26.8-35.5) | 29.1 (25.3-32.3) | 65.6 (53.7-76.3) | 154 (113-178) | 275 (174-401) | 699 |
| Non-Hispanic whites | 01-02 | 19.1 (16.7-21.9) | 19.2 (16.9-21.4) | 41.7 (35.3-50.7) | 91.1 (75.6-110) | 212 (130-275) | 1216 |
| | 03-04 | 20.8 (18.6-23.3) | 19.7 (17.2-22.5) | 47.5 (39.4-56.1) | 120 (91.3-165) | 270 (155-403) | 1088 |

Limit of detection (LOD, see Data Analysis section) for Survey years 01-02 and 03-04 are 1 0 and 0.3.

Lee, 2005). Younger children eliminate higher proportions of urinary MEHHP and MEOHP relative to MEHP, with the difference increasing as age decreases; this may be the result of differences in metabolism and/or excretion (NTP-CERHR, 2006). Studies of hospitalized neonates have reported urinary geometric mean levels of MEHP, MEOHP, and MEHHP that were two to five times higher, or more (depending on the intensity of DEHP-product exposure), than the geometric means of children in the NHANES subsamples for all three survey periods (Calafat et al., 2004; Weuve et al., 2006). Small studies of plasma and platelet donors have reported very high levels of MEHP, MEOHP, MEHHP and MECPP in urine collected shortly after these procedures (Koch et al., 2005b, 2005c).

Finding a measurable amount of one or more DEHP metabolites in urine does not mean that the levels of the metabolites or the parent compound cause an adverse health effect. Biomonitoring studies on levels of urinary DEHP metabolites provide physicians and public health officials with reference values so that they can determine whether people have been exposed to higher levels of DEHP than are found in the general population. Biomonitoring data can also help scientists plan and conduct research on exposure and health effects.

### Urinary Mono-(2-ethyl-5-hydroxyhexyl) phthalate (MEHHP) (creatinine corrected)
*Metabolite of Di-2-ethylhexyl phthalate (DEHP)*

Geometric mean and selected percentiles of urine concentrations (in µg/g of creatinine) for the U.S. population from the National Health and Nutrition Examination Survey.

| | Survey years | Geometric mean (95% conf. interval) | Selected percentiles ( 95% confidence interval) | | | | Sample size |
|---|---|---|---|---|---|---|---|
| | | | 50th | 75th | 90th | 95th | |
| **Total** | 01-02 | 18.8 (17.0-20.7) | 16.6 (14.9-18 5) | 32.2 (27.8-37.1) | 71.1 (58.7-88 3) | 143 (101-200) | 2782 |
| | 03-04 | 20.4 (18.7-22 3) | 17.7 (16.3-19 6) | 35.8 (30.5-43 3) | 93.5 (74.0-128) | 182 (134-262) | 2605 |
| **Age group** | | | | | | | |
| 6-11 years | 01-02 | 38.2 (34.3-42 6) | 34.3 (29.9-38 9) | 60.6 (51.9-76.4) | 107 (96.3-147) | 211 (122-313) | 393 |
| | 03-04 | 39.0 (31.1-48 9) | 36.6 (25.3-49 3) | 65.6 (49.8-91 3) | 129 (77.1-253) | 211 (123-708) | 342 |
| 12-19 years | 01-02 | 19.2 (17.0-21 8) | 17.8 (15.6-20 0) | 34.9 (29.2-42.7) | 73.4 (58.4-80.7) | 102 (86.6-160) | 742 |
| | 03-04 | 21.2 (18.1-24.7) | 18.6 (16.9-21.7) | 38.7 (29.7-53.4) | 103 (62.7-209) | 212 (100-358) | 729 |
| 20 years and older | 01-02 | 17.1 (15.2-19 3) | 15.0 (13.3-16.7) | 27.7 (23.2-34 0) | 63.7 (48.3-86 9) | 137 (84.4-203) | 1647 |
| | 03-04 | 18.8 (17.5-20 2) | 16.3 (15.4-17 5) | 31.6 (28.1-35 3) | 83.8 (67.2-106) | 171 (129-246) | 1534 |
| **Gender** | | | | | | | |
| Males | 01-02 | 17.9 (16.2-19.7) | 15.4 (13.8-17 9) | 32.2 (27.8-36 8) | 73.4 (55.3-91 8) | 137 (97.7-224) | 1371 |
| | 03-04 | 18.9 (17.1-20 9) | 17.1 (15.2-18 6) | 32.7 (26.6-41 6) | 93.4 (68.8-123) | 193 (108-291) | 1250 |
| Females | 01-02 | 19.7 (17.3-22.4) | 17.6 (15.4-19 5) | 32.1 (26.8-38 6) | 70.5 (57.8-93.7) | 156 (93.7-201) | 1411 |
| | 03-04 | 21.9 (19.7-24 5) | 18.7 (16.8-20 9) | 39.3 (33.8-46 9) | 94.3 (72.8-136) | 171 (146-261) | 1355 |
| **Race/ethnicity** | | | | | | | |
| Mexican Americans | 01-02 | 17.4 (15.9-19.1) | 15.7 (14.4-17 5) | 30.6 (26.0-34.7) | 65.9 (50.6-83 9) | 103 (75.5-128) | 677 |
| | 03-04 | 17.1 (14.3-20.4) | 15.4 (13.2-17.7) | 29.3 (23.8-36 8) | 57.3 (45.7-97 6) | 105 (70.1-195) | 652 |
| Non-Hispanic blacks | 01-02 | 20.9 (18.8-23 3) | 19.7 (17.5-21 8) | 38.3 (32.1-46 0) | 93.5 (69.2-123) | 164 (130-183) | 703 |
| | 03-04 | 21.9 (20.1-23 8) | 19.5 (17.3-22 6) | 40.1 (35.8-45 3) | 102 (75.5-122) | 164 (133-269) | 699 |
| Non-Hispanic whites | 01-02 | 18.9 (17.0-21 0) | 16.3 (14.8-18.4) | 32.1 (27.3-37 3) | 70.8 (56.9-93.7) | 177 (98.0-242) | 1216 |
| | 03-04 | 20.5 (18.5-22 8) | 17.8 (16.2-19.7) | 35.3 (29.7-44 9) | 96.2 (75.8-136) | 211 (136-283) | 1088 |

## Urinary Mono-(2-ethyl-5-oxohexyl) phthalate (MEOHP)
*Metabolite of Di-2-ethylhexyl phthalate (DEHP)*

Geometric mean and selected percentiles of urine concentrations (in µg/L) for the U.S. population from the National Health and Nutrition Examination Survey.

| | Survey years | Geometric mean (95% conf. interval) | Selected percentiles ( 95% confidence interval) | | | | Sample size |
|---|---|---|---|---|---|---|---|
| | | | 50th | 75th | 90th | 95th | |
| Total | 01-02 | 13.5 (12.0-15.0) | 14.0 (12.5-15.1) | 29.6 (25.2-34.0) | 59.9 (50.4-70.9) | 120 (87.2-156) | 2782 |
| | 03-04 | 14.5 (13.0-16.1) | 14.4 (12.4-16.7) | 31.4 (27.4-36.6) | 76.7 (59.4-102) | 157 (106-232) | 2605 |
| **Age group** | | | | | | | |
| 6-11 years | 01-02 | 23.3 (20.9-26.1) | 22.9 (18.5-28.1) | 46.5 (38.1-52.0) | 81.6 (64.7-109) | 142 (93.9-178) | 393 |
| | 03-04 | 25.1 (19.6-32.3) | 25.8 (19.3-31.4) | 51.1 (32.1-76.5) | 97.9 (58.8-197) | 197 (97.6-261) | 342 |
| 12-19 years | 01-02 | 17.5 (15.1-20.3) | 18.6 (16.2-20.7) | 35.0 (27.7-42.1) | 70.7 (52.2-104) | 118 (74.0-174) | 742 |
| | 03-04 | 19.5 (16.0-23.7) | 20.3 (18.4-23.5) | 37.8 (32.6-44.6) | 110 (54.6-168) | 212 (103-326) | 729 |
| 20 years and older | 01-02 | 12.0 (10.5-13.9) | 12.3 (10.4-14.1) | 26.0 (21.6-32.1) | 52.3 (41.8-68.3) | 116 (74.9-160) | 1647 |
| | 03-04 | 12.9 (11.8-14.1) | 12.4 (10.9-14.5) | 27.0 (25.0-30.9) | 68.9 (55.0-86.5) | 139 (92.7-216) | 1534 |
| **Gender** | | | | | | | |
| Males | 01-02 | 14.5 (13.0-16.2) | 14.6 (13.1-16.2) | 31.6 (25.6-34.7) | 60.4 (52.3-71.4) | 129 (84.4-167) | 1371 |
| | 03-04 | 15.6 (13.6-17.9) | 14.7 (12.7-18.1) | 31.8 (27.2-39.5) | 83.8 (59.4-134) | 185 (96.2-277) | 1250 |
| Females | 01-02 | 12.5 (10.8-14.6) | 13.1 (11.2-15.0) | 28.1 (23.7-33.5) | 57.5 (45.8-72.7) | 115 (81.8-147) | 1411 |
| | 03-04 | 13.4 (11.9-15.1) | 13.7 (11.4-16.4) | 29.5 (26.1-36.6) | 68.6 (53.7-88.1) | 143 (88.2-210) | 1355 |
| **Race/ethnicity** | | | | | | | |
| Mexican Americans | 01-02 | 13.1 (11.6-14.9) | 13.4 (11.6-15.0) | 25.5 (21.6-30.8) | 56.6 (40.6-70.3) | 77.3 (70.5-101) | 677 |
| | 03-04 | 12.8 (10.5-15.5) | 13.6 (11.4-15.6) | 25.3 (20.4-29.9) | 46.6 (32.3-70.8) | 76.0 (51.6-153) | 652 |
| Non-Hispanic blacks | 01-02 | 19.6 (17.1-22.5) | 20.1 (17.9-22.4) | 39.0 (34.8-44.2) | 80.5 (71.4-97.4) | 153 (102-228) | 703 |
| | 03-04 | 20.2 (17.7-23.0) | 20.1 (17.0-22.5) | 40.0 (33.9-46.9) | 92.6 (68.8-130) | 173 (104-247) | 699 |
| Non-Hispanic whites | 01-02 | 12.8 (11.2-14.6) | 13.2 (11.6-14.6) | 28.5 (23.6-34.0) | 58.6 (48.8-70.9) | 126 (83.7-172) | 1216 |
| | 03-04 | 13.8 (12.4-15.4) | 13.4 (11.3-16.3) | 31.0 (27.0-36.3) | 77.6 (59.4-102) | 161 (98.7-241) | 1088 |

Limit of detection (LOD, see Data Analysis section) for Survey years 01-02 and 03-04 are 1.1 and 0.5.

## Urinary Mono-(2-ethyl-5-oxohexyl) phthalate (MEOHP) (creatinine corrected)
*Metabolite of Di-2-ethylhexyl phthalate (DEHP)*
Geometric mean and selected percentiles of urine concentrations (in µg/g of creatinine) for the U.S. population from the National Health and Nutrition Examination Survey.

| | Survey years | Geometric mean (95% conf. interval) | Selected percentiles ( 95% confidence interval) | | | | Sample size |
|---|---|---|---|---|---|---|---|
| | | | 50th | 75th | 90th | 95th | |
| Total | 01-02 | 12.6 (11.5-13 9) | 11.2 (10.2-12 3) | 21.3 (18.3-23 8) | 45.2 (37.1-58.1) | 87.0 (68.0-124) | 2782 |
| | 03-04 | 13.6 (12.4-14 8) | 12.1 (11.0-12 9) | 24.3 (20.9-27 8) | 63.0 (47.8-75 8) | 118 (94.1-153) | 2605 |
| **Age group** | | | | | | | |
| 6-11 years | 01-02 | 26.6 (24.0-29.4) | 22.8 (20.3-25 0) | 43.3 (33.6-47.1) | 74.7 (69.0-91 9) | 131 (83.0-183) | 393 |
| | 03-04 | 26.6 (21.4-33 0) | 25.3 (17.8-32.4) | 43.6 (34.2-63 2) | 77.1 (63.0-118) | 121 (76.3-435) | 342 |
| 12-19 years | 01-02 | 13.5 (12.0-15 2) | 12.0 (10.8-14 3) | 23.4 (20.0-28 5) | 48.4 (39.2-54 9) | 70.5 (55.0-97 2) | 742 |
| | 03-04 | 14.6 (12.6-16 9) | 12.7 (11.6-14.4) | 25.5 (20.7-33 8) | 67.9 (42.3-143) | 153 (61.8-209) | 729 |
| 20 years and older | 01-02 | 11.4 (10.2-12 8) | 10.1 (8.89-11.4) | 17.5 (15.2-21 8) | 38.4 (30.5-52 5) | 84.3 (53.3-128) | 1647 |
| | 03-04 | 12.4 (11.5-13 3) | 11.0 (10.0-12 0) | 20.9 (18.6-22 8) | 53.9 (40.7-70 2) | 109 (88.6-130) | 1534 |
| **Gender** | | | | | | | |
| Males | 01-02 | 11.8 (10.7-13 0) | 10.2 (8.93-11.7) | 21.2 (18.5-23 3) | 46.1 (35.3-58.7) | 84.2 (69.6-104) | 1371 |
| | 03-04 | 12.3 (11.1-13 5) | 11.1 (10.0-12 0) | 21.6 (17.6-26 9) | 59.1 (45.4-72 0) | 120 (72.0-162) | 1250 |
| Females | 01-02 | 13.5 (11.9-15 2) | 12.0 (10.8-13.7) | 21.5 (18.0-25 6) | 44.8 (36.8-61 6) | 92.3 (61.0-139) | 1411 |
| | 03-04 | 14.9 (13.4-16.7) | 12.7 (11.4-14 2) | 26.6 (21.8-30 6) | 65.6 (48.0-90.1) | 118 (97.0-157) | 1355 |
| **Race/ethnicity** | | | | | | | |
| Mexican Americans | 01-02 | 12.4 (11.4-13 5) | 11.0 (10.5-12 3) | 20.9 (18.5-24.4) | 44.6 (33.4-56 2) | 65.9 (53.1-83.1) | 677 |
| | 03-04 | 11.5 (9.81-13 6) | 10.7 (9.04-12 3) | 18.8 (15.6-24 6) | 39.1 (31.8-53 9) | 63.0 (47.2-121) | 652 |
| Non-Hispanic blacks | 01-02 | 13.8 (12.3-15.4) | 13.1 (12.0-14 2) | 23.9 (20.0-29 3) | 58.3 (45.3-79.7) | 101 (81.3-124) | 703 |
| | 03-04 | 14.3 (13.1-15 6) | 13.3 (11.3-15 5) | 24.8 (21.7-27.7) | 61.2 (46.8-76 6) | 105 (79.7-152) | 699 |
| Non-Hispanic whites | 01-02 | 12.7 (11.4-14 0) | 11.1 (9.90-12 3) | 20.8 (18.0-23 9) | 45.7 (35.9-64 9) | 96.0 (68.5-161) | 1216 |
| | 03-04 | 13.7 (12.2-15 3) | 12.0 (10.5-12 9) | 24.9 (20.7-28 6) | 69.5 (51.4-95 3) | 124 (90.3-182) | 1088 |

## Urinary Mono-(2-ethyl-5-carboxypentyl) phthalate (MECPP)
*Metabolite of Di-2-ethylhexyl phthalate (DEHP)*

Geometric mean and selected percentiles of urine concentrations (in µg/L) for the U.S. population from the National Health and Nutrition Examination Survey.

| | Survey years | Geometric mean (95% conf. interval) | 50th | 75th | 90th | 95th | Sample size |
|---|---|---|---|---|---|---|---|
| | | | Selected percentiles ( 95% confidence interval) | | | | |
| Total | 03-04 | 34.7 (31.0-38.9) | 33.0 (29.1-37.4) | 71.8 (61.7-84.8) | 168 (133-240) | 339 (235-506) | 2605 |
| **Age group** | | | | | | | |
| 6-11 years | 03-04 | 58.2 (44.7-75.6) | 51.6 (39.2-67.6) | 112 (71.4-182) | 314 (124-524) | 391 (238-781) | 342 |
| 12-19 years | 03-04 | 44.6 (36.8-54.0) | 42.7 (38.4-47.6) | 86.5 (67.3-108) | 220 (120-397) | 448 (235-808) | 729 |
| 20 years and older | 03-04 | 31.3 (28.6-34.4) | 29.2 (26.2-33.0) | 63.5 (56.5-73.9) | 157 (130-187) | 312 (199-457) | 1534 |
| **Gender** | | | | | | | |
| Males | 03-04 | 37.9 (33.1-43.5) | 34.7 (30.0-39.5) | 73.7 (60.8-91.9) | 187 (133-300) | 388 (222-660) | 1250 |
| Females | 03-04 | 31.9 (28.1-36.2) | 31.3 (27.5-35.8) | 69.3 (58.9-81.9) | 154 (128-199) | 312 (182-441) | 1355 |
| **Race/ethnicity** | | | | | | | |
| Mexican Americans | 03-04 | 31.9 (27.1-37.6) | 31.5 (26.8-37.4) | 57.4 (45.9-71.8) | 116 (86.0-162) | 175 (133-355) | 652 |
| Non-Hispanic blacks | 03-04 | 42.6 (37.0-49.2) | 38.3 (33.8-46.9) | 82.5 (68.7-103) | 191 (146-246) | 339 (244-468) | 699 |
| Non-Hispanic whites | 03-04 | 33.8 (30.1-37.9) | 32.1 (27.6-37.5) | 72.4 (62.0-87.7) | 167 (133-240) | 354 (220-560) | 1088 |

Limit of detection (LOD, see Data Analysis section) for Survey year 03-04 is 0 3.

## Urinary Mono-(2-ethyl-5-carboxypentyl) phthalate (MECPP) (creatinine corrected)
*Metabolite of Di-2-ethylhexyl phthalate (DEHP)*

Geometric mean and selected percentiles of urine concentrations (in µg/g of creatinine) for the U.S. population from the National Health and Nutrition Examination Survey.

| | Survey years | Geometric mean (95% conf. interval) | 50th | 75th | 90th | 95th | Sample size |
|---|---|---|---|---|---|---|---|
| | | | Selected percentiles ( 95% confidence interval) | | | | |
| Total | 03-04 | 32.6 (29.6-36.0) | 27.0 (24.3-30.6) | 54.6 (48.0-63.5) | 139 (109-186) | 251 (192-356) | 2605 |
| **Age group** | | | | | | | |
| 6-11 years | 03-04 | 61.5 (49.0-77.2) | 52.2 (41.6-73.8) | 104 (74.2-140) | 210 (111-500) | 372 (192-988) | 342 |
| 12-19 years | 03-04 | 33.4 (28.7-38.7) | 27.1 (23.9-32.0) | 55.0 (43.8-83.8) | 168 (92.5-289) | 294 (159-387) | 729 |
| 20 years and older | 03-04 | 30.1 (27.7-32.7) | 25.1 (22.9-27.6) | 49.1 (44.1-55.2) | 126 (101-154) | 237 (191-315) | 1534 |
| **Gender** | | | | | | | |
| Males | 03-04 | 29.8 (26.8-33.1) | 23.5 (21.4-27.1) | 50.7 (42.2-61.7) | 132 (98.0-191) | 248 (159-422) | 1250 |
| Females | 03-04 | 35.5 (31.6-40.0) | 30.6 (26.4-35.5) | 58.3 (48.8-71.8) | 144 (108-192) | 251 (192-349) | 1355 |
| **Race/ethnicity** | | | | | | | |
| Mexican Americans | 03-04 | 28.8 (25.4-32.6) | 24.7 (22.4-26.3) | 46.7 (39.0-56.3) | 94.7 (73.2-137) | 152 (118-238) | 652 |
| Non-Hispanic blacks | 03-04 | 30.3 (27.7-33.2) | 27.0 (23.2-30.7) | 51.1 (41.6-64.0) | 135 (100-161) | 212 (173-252) | 699 |
| Non-Hispanic whites | 03-04 | 33.4 (29.5-37.7) | 27.0 (23.5-31.6) | 56.8 (48.6-69.4) | 145 (109-198) | 294 (193-385) | 1088 |

# References

Adibi JJ, Perera FP, Jedrychowski W, Camann DE, Barr D, Jacek R, et al. Prenatal exposures to phthalates among women in New York City and Krakow, Poland. Environ Health Perspect 2003;111(14):1719-1722.

Agency for Toxic Substances and Disease Registry (ATSDR). Toxicological profile for di(2-ethylhexyl)phthalate update [online]. 2002. Available at URL: http://www.atsdr.cdc.gov/toxprofiles/tp9 html. 4/20/09

Albro PW, Corbett JT, Schroeder JL, Jordan S, Matthews HB. Pharmacokinetics, interactions with macromolecules and species differences in metabolism of DEHP. Environ Health Perspect 1982;45:19-25.

Albro PW and Lavenhar SR. Metabolism of di(2-ethylhexyl) phthalate. Drug Metab Rev 1989;21:13-34.

Barr DB, Silva MJ, Kato K, Reidy JA, Malek NA, Hurtz D, et al. Assessing human exposure to phthalates using monoesters and their oxidized metabolites as biomarkers. Environ Health Perspect 2003;111(9):1148-1151.

Becker K, Seiwert M, Angerer J, Heger W, Koch HM, Nagorka R, et al. DEHP metabolites in urine of children and DEHP in house dust. Int J Hyg Environ Health 2004;207(5):409-417.

Blount BC, Silva MJ, Caudill SP, Needham LL, Pirkle JL, Sampson EJ, et al. Levels of seven urinary phthalate metabolites in a human reference population. Environ Health Perspect 2000;108(10)979-982.

Calafat AM, Needham LL, Silva MJ, Lambert G. Exposure to di-(2-ethylhexyl) phthalate among premature neonates in a neonatal intensive care unit. Pediatrics 2004;113:e429-e434.

Centers for Disease Control and Prevention (CDC). Third National Report on Human Exposure to Environmental Chemicals. Atlanta (GA). 2005.

Duty SM, Calafat AM, Silva MJ, Brock JW, Ryan L, Chen Z, et al. The relationship between environmental exposure to phthalates and computer-aided sperm analysis motion parameters. J Androl 2004;25(2):293-302.

Duty SM, Calafat AM, Silva MJ, Ryan L, Hauser R. Phthalate exposure and reproductive hormones in adult men. Hum Reprod 2005;20(3):604-610.

Food and Drug Administration (FDA). Safety assessment of di(2-ethylhexyl)phthalate (DEHP) released form PCV medical devices. 2001 [online]. Available at URL: http://www.fda.gov/cdrh/ost/dehp-pvc.pdf. 4/20/09

Fromme H, Bolte G, Koch HM, Angerer J, Boehmer S, Drexler H, et al. Occurrence and daily variation of phthalate metabolites in the urine of an adult population. Int J Hyg Environ Health 2007;210:21-33.

Hauser R, Meeker JD, Singh NP, Silva MJ, Ryan L, Duty S, et al. DNA damage in human sperm is related to urinary levels of phthalate monoester and oxidative metabolites. Hum Reprod 2007;22(3):688-695.

Hoppin JA, Brock JW, Davis BJ, Baird DD. Reproducibility of urinary phthalate metabolites in first morning urine samples. Environ Health Perspect 2002;110(5):515-518.

Itoh H, Yoshida K, Masunaga S. Evaluation of the effect of a governmental control of human exposure to two phthalates in Japan using a urinary biomarker approach. Int J Hyg Environ Health 2005;208:237-245.

Koch HM, Angerer J, Drexler H, Eckstein R, Weisbach V. Di(2-ethylhexyl)phthalate (DEHP) exposure of voluntary plasma and platelet donors. Int J Hyg Environ Health 2005c;208:489-498.

Koch HM, Bolt HM, Preuss R, Angerer J. New metabolites of di(2-ethylhexyl)phthalate (DEHP) in human urine and serum after single oral doses of deuterium-labelled DEHP. Arch Toxicol 2005a;79:367-376.

Koch HM, Bolt HM, Preuss R, Eckstein R, Weisback V, Angerer J. Intravenous exposure to di(2-ethylhexyl)phthalate (DEHP) : metabolites of DEHP in urine after a voluntary platelet donation. Arch Toxicol 2005b;79:689-693.

Koch HM, Drexler H, Angerer J. Internal exposure of nursery-school children and their parents and teachers to di(2-ethylhexyl) phthalate (DEHP). Int J Hyg Environ Health. 2004;207:15-22.

Koch HM, Rossbach B, Drexler H, Angerer J. Internal exposure of the general population to DEHP and other phthalates - determination of secondary and primary phthalate monoester metabolites in urine. Environ Res 2003;93:177-185.

Koo HJ, Lee BM. Human monitoring of phthalates and risk assessment. J Toxicol Environ Health Part A 2005;68:1379-1392.

Loff S, Kabs F, Witt K, Sartoris J, Mandl B, Niessen KH, et al. Polyvinylchloride infusion lines expose infants to large amounts of toxic plasticizers. J Pediatr Surg 2000;35(12):1775-1781.

Lovekamp-Swan T, Davis BJ. Mechanisms of phthalate ester toxicity in the female reproductive system. Environ Health Perspect 2003;111(2):139-145.

McKee RH, Butala JH, David RM, Gans G. NTP center for the evaluation of risks to human reproduction reports on phthalates: addressing the data gaps [review]. Reprod Toxicol 2004;18(1):1-22.

NTP-CERHR. National Toxicology Program-Center for the Evaluation of Risks to Human Reproduction. Monograph on the Potential Human Reproductive and Developmental Effects of Di(2-ethylhexyl) Phthalate (DEHP). Research Triangle Park (NC). 2000c [online]. Available at URL: http://cerhr.niehs.nih.gov/chemicals/dehp/dehp-eval.html. 6/2/09

NTP-CERHR. National Toxicology Program-Center for the Evaluation of Risks to Human Reproduction. Draft Update Monograph on the Potential Human Reproductive and Developmental Effects of Di(2-ethylhexyl) Phthalate (DEHP). Research Triangle Park (NC). 2006 [online]. Available at URL: http://cerhr.niehs.nih.gov/chemicals/dehp/dehp-eval.html. 6/2/09

Peck CC, Albro PW. Toxic potential of the plasticizer di (2-ethylhexyl) phthalate in the context of its disposition and metabolism in primates and man. Environ Health Perspect 1982;45:11-17.

Silva MJ, Barr DB, Reidy JA, Malek NA, Hodge CC, Caudill SP, et al. Urinary levels of seven phthalate metabolites in the U.S. population from the National Health and Nutrition Examination Survey (NHANES) 1999-2000 [published erratum appears in Environ Health Perspect 2004; 112(5):A270]. Environ Health Perspect 2004;112(3):331-338.

Weuve J, Sanchez GN, Calafat AM, Schettler T, Green RA, Hu H, et al. Exposure to phthalates in neonatal intensive care unit infants: urinary concentrations of monoesters and oxidative metabolites. Environ Health Perspect 2006;114(9):1424-1431.

Wittassek M, Wiesmuller GA, Koch HM, Eckard R, Dobler L, Helm D, et al. Internal phthalate exposure over the last two decades—a retrospective human biomonitoring study. Int J Hyg Environ Health 2007;210(3-4):319-333.

# Di-isononyl Phthalate

CAS No. 28553-12-0

## General Information

Di-isononyl phthalate (DiNP) is a mixture of phthalates with branched alkyl side chains of varying length (C8, C9, and C10). DiNP is primarily used to produce flexible plastics and has replaced di-2-ethylhexyl phthalate (DEHP) in some plastics, though not in medical products. DiNP is widely used in such products as toys, flooring, gloves, drinking straws, garden hoses, and in sealants used for food packaging. People exposed to DiNP will excrete small amounts of mono-isononyl phthalate (MiNP) and other secondary oxidative metabolites. Urinary MiNP represents only about 2% of a dose (Koch and Angerer, 2007; Silva et al., 2006a, 2006b). Because DiNP is a complex mixture, MiNP may not reflect exposure to all the chemical components.

DiNP administered to rodents produced liver and kidney toxicity, and may cause liver tumors by a mechanism involving peroxisomal proliferation. High dose DiNP was a developmental toxicant in rodents (NTP-CERHR, 2000). Although DiNP is considered an animal carcinogen, neither IARC nor NTP has evaluated DiNP with respect to human carcinogenicity.

## Urinary Mono-isononyl phthalate (MiNP)
*Metabolite of Di-isononyl phthalate (DiNP)*

Geometric mean and selected percentiles of urine concentrations (in μg/L) for the U.S. population from the National Health and Nutrition Examination Survey.

| | Survey years | Geometric mean (95% conf. interval) | 50th | 75th | 90th | 95th | Sample size |
|---|---|---|---|---|---|---|---|
| **Total** | 99-00 | * | < LOD | < LOD | < LOD | 3.50 (<LOD-13.8) | 2541 |
| | 01-02 | * | < LOD | < LOD | < LOD | < LOD | 2782 |
| | 03-04 | * | < LOD | < LOD | < LOD | 1.00 (<LOD-1.30) | 2605 |
| **Age group** | | | | | | | |
| 6-11 years | 99-00 | * | < LOD | < LOD | < LOD | 6.20 (<LOD-22.5) | 328 |
| | 01-02 | * | < LOD | < LOD | < LOD | < LOD | 393 |
| | 03-04 | * | < LOD | < LOD | 1.00 (<LOD-1.50) | 1.70 (1.20-3.10) | 342 |
| 12-19 years | 99-00 | * | < LOD | < LOD | < LOD | 2.30 (<LOD-20.3) | 752 |
| | 01-02 | * | < LOD | < LOD | < LOD | .900 (<LOD-1.10) | 742 |
| | 03-04 | * | < LOD | < LOD | < LOD | 1.40 (<LOD-1.80) | 729 |
| 20 years and older | 99-00 | * | < LOD | < LOD | < LOD | 3.10 (<LOD-13.2) | 1461 |
| | 01-02 | * | < LOD | < LOD | < LOD | < LOD | 1647 |
| | 03-04 | * | < LOD | < LOD | < LOD | < LOD | 1534 |
| **Gender** | | | | | | | |
| Males | 99-00 | * | < LOD | < LOD | .800 (<LOD-5.40) | 4.90 (<LOD-18.9) | 1215 |
| | 01-02 | * | < LOD | < LOD | < LOD | < LOD | 1371 |
| | 03-04 | * | < LOD | < LOD | < LOD | 1.00 (<LOD-1.80) | 1250 |
| Females | 99-00 | * | < LOD | < LOD | < LOD | 2.50 (<LOD-6.80) | 1326 |
| | 01-02 | * | < LOD | < LOD | < LOD | .900 (<LOD-1.10) | 1411 |
| | 03-04 | * | < LOD | < LOD | < LOD | < LOD | 1355 |
| **Race/ethnicity** | | | | | | | |
| Mexican Americans | 99-00 | * | < LOD | < LOD | < LOD | 1.50 (<LOD-2.80) | 814 |
| | 01-02 | * | < LOD | < LOD | < LOD | 1.00 (<LOD-1.40) | 677 |
| | 03-04 | * | < LOD | < LOD | < LOD | < LOD | 652 |
| Non-Hispanic blacks | 99-00 | * | < LOD | < LOD | 2.30 (<LOD-13.8) | 6.80 (<LOD-30.2) | 603 |
| | 01-02 | * | < LOD | < LOD | < LOD | 1.00 (<LOD-1.70) | 703 |
| | 03-04 | * | < LOD | < LOD | < LOD | 1.30 (1.00-2.00) | 699 |
| Non-Hispanic whites | 99-00 | * | < LOD | < LOD | < LOD | 3.50 (<LOD-16.0) | 912 |
| | 01-02 | * | < LOD | < LOD | < LOD | < LOD | 1216 |
| | 03-04 | * | < LOD | < LOD | < LOD | < LOD | 1088 |

Limit of detection (LOD, see Data Analysis section) for Survey years 99-00, 01-02, and 03-04 are 0.8, 0.8, and 1.0, respectively.
< LOD means less than the limit of detection, which may vary for some chemicals by year and by individual sample.
* Not calculated: proportion of results below limit of detection was too high to provide a valid result.

## Biomonitoring Information

MiNP was detected mainly at the 95th percentiles in this *Report*. A low detection rate was also reported in a small sample of African-American women in Washington, DC (Hoppin et al., 2002).

Finding a measurable amount of MiNP in urine does not mean that the levels of MiNP or the parent compound cause an adverse health effect. Biomonitoring studies on levels of MiNP provide physicians and public health officials with reference values so that they can determine whether people have been exposed to higher levels of DiNP than are found in the general population. Biomonitoring data can also help

scientists plan and conduct research on exposure and health effects.

## Urinary Mono-isononyl phthalate (MiNP) (creatinine corrected)

*Metabolite of Di-isononyl phthalate (DiNP)*

Geometric mean and selected percentiles of urine concentrations (in μg/g of creatinine) for the U.S. population from the National Health and Nutrition Examination Survey.

| | Survey years | Geometric mean (95% conf. interval) | Selected percentiles ( 95% confidence interval) | | | | Sample size |
|---|---|---|---|---|---|---|---|
| | | | 50th | 75th | 90th | 95th | |
| **Total** | 99-00 | * | < LOD | < LOD | < LOD | 4.29 (<LOD-8.31) | 2541 |
| | 01-02 | * | < LOD | < LOD | < LOD | < LOD | 2782 |
| | 03-04 | * | < LOD | < LOD | < LOD | 2.92 (<LOD-3.18) | 2605 |
| **Age group** | | | | | | | |
| 6-11 years | 99-00 | * | < LOD | < LOD | < LOD | 6.00 (<LOD-14.2) | 328 |
| | 01-02 | * | < LOD | < LOD | < LOD | < LOD | 393 |
| | 03-04 | * | < LOD | < LOD | 2.41 (<LOD-3.13) | 3.27 (2.41-4 67) | 342 |
| 12-19 years | 99-00 | * | < LOD | < LOD | < LOD | 2.00 (<LOD-7.65) | 752 |
| | 01-02 | * | < LOD | < LOD | < LOD | 2.07 (<LOD-3.33) | 742 |
| | 03-04 | * | < LOD | < LOD | < LOD | 1.97 (<LOD-2.59) | 729 |
| 20 years and older | 99-00 | * | < LOD | < LOD | < LOD | 4.62 (<LOD-8.07) | 1461 |
| | 01-02 | * | < LOD | < LOD | < LOD | < LOD | 1647 |
| | 03-04 | * | < LOD | < LOD | < LOD | < LOD | 1534 |
| **Gender** | | | | | | | |
| Males | 99-00 | * | < LOD | < LOD | 2.00 (<LOD-3.71) | 4.24 (<LOD-10.2) | 1215 |
| | 01-02 | * | < LOD | < LOD | < LOD | < LOD | 1371 |
| | 03-04 | * | < LOD | < LOD | < LOD | 2.31 (<LOD-2.95) | 1250 |
| Females | 99-00 | * | < LOD | < LOD | < LOD | 4.29 (<LOD-7.65) | 1326 |
| | 01-02 | * | < LOD | < LOD | < LOD | 2.73 (<LOD-2.86) | 1411 |
| | 03-04 | * | < LOD | < LOD | < LOD | < LOD | 1355 |
| **Race/ethnicity** | | | | | | | |
| Mexican Americans | 99-00 | * | < LOD | < LOD | < LOD | 3.53 (<LOD-5.00) | 814 |
| | 01-02 | * | < LOD | < LOD | < LOD | 2.40 (<LOD-2.73) | 677 |
| | 03-04 | * | < LOD | < LOD | < LOD | < LOD | 652 |
| Non-Hispanic blacks | 99-00 | * | < LOD | < LOD | 2.03 (<LOD-5.31) | 4.29 (<LOD-14.3) | 603 |
| | 01-02 | * | < LOD | < LOD | < LOD | 1.76 (<LOD-2.14) | 703 |
| | 03-04 | * | < LOD | < LOD | < LOD | 2.19 (1.67-2 50) | 699 |
| Non-Hispanic whites | 99-00 | * | < LOD | < LOD | < LOD | 5.45 (<LOD-10.0) | 912 |
| | 01-02 | * | < LOD | < LOD | < LOD | < LOD | 1216 |
| | 03-04 | * | < LOD | < LOD | < LOD | < LOD | 1088 |

< LOD means less than the limit of detection for the urine levels not corrected for creatinine.
* Not calculated: proportion of results below limit of detection was too high to provide a valid result.

## References

Hoppin JA, Brock JW, Davis BJ, Baird DD. Reproducibility of urinary phthalate metabolites in first morning urine samples. Environ Health Perspect 2002;110(5):515-518.

Koch HM, Angerer J. Di-iso-nonylphthalate (DINP) metabolites in human urine after a single oral dose of deuterium-labelled DINP. Int J Hyg Environ Health 2007;79:210:9-19.

NTP-CERHR. National Toxicology Program-Center for the Evaluation of Risks to Human Reproduction. Monograph on the Potential Human Reproductive and Developmental Effects of Di-n-octyl Phthalate (DnOP). Research Triangle Park (NC). 2000 [online]. Available at URL: http://cerhr.niehs.nih.gov/chemicals/phthalates/dnop/dnop-eval.html. 6/2/09

Silva MJ, Kato K, Wolf C, Samandar El, Silva SS, Gray EL, et al. Urinary biomarkers of di-isononyl phthalate in rats. Toxicol 2006a;223:101-112.

Silva MJ, Reidy JA, Preu Jr JL, Needham LL, Calafat AM. Oxidative metabolites of diisononyl phthalate as biomarkers for human exposure assessment. Environ Health Perspect 2006b;114(8):1158-1161.

# Dimethyl Phthalate
CAS No.131-11-3

## General Information

Dimethyl phthalate (DMP) is used in manufacturing solid rocket propellant and consumer products such as insect repellents and plastics. People exposed to DMP will excrete mono-methyl phthalate (MMP) in their urine. A workplace air standard for external exposure to DMP has been established by OSHA, and guidelines established by ACGIH and NIOSH. Neither IARC nor NTP has evaluated DBP with respect to human carcinogenicity.

## Biomonitoring Information

In NHANES 2001-2002 and 2003-2004, the urinary levels of MMP were similar. Among men attending a Boston infertility clinic, at least 75% had detectable urine MMP levels, and the median value was similar to the median urine MMP levels for both males and adults in this *Report* (Hauser et al., 2007). Analysis of the NHANES 2001-

2002 levels showed that adjusted geometric mean levels of urinary MMP were higher in children aged 6-11 years than either groups aged 12-19 years or 20 years and older. Females had higher levels than males (CDC, 2005).

Finding a measurable amount of MMP in urine does not mean that the levels of MMP or the parent compound cause an adverse health effect. Biomonitoring studies on levels of urinary MMP provide physicians and public health officials with reference values so that they can determine whether people have been exposed to higher levels of DMP than are found in the general population. Biomonitoring data can also help scientists plan and conduct research on exposure and health effects.

## Urinary Mono-methyl phthalate (MMP)
*Metabolite of Dimethyl phthalate (DMP)*

Geometric mean and selected percentiles of urine concentrations (in µg/L) for the U.S. population from the National Health and Nutrition Examination Survey.

| | Survey years | Geometric mean (95% conf. interval) | Selected percentiles ( 95% confidence interval) | | | | Sample size |
|---|---|---|---|---|---|---|---|
| | | | 50th | 75th | 90th | 95th | |
| Total | 01-02 | 1.15 (.985-1 34) | 1.50 (1.30-1 80) | 3.30 (2.90-3.70) | 6.00 (5.10-7 50) | 9.80 (8.00-12.5) | 2782 |
| | 03-04 | * | 1.30 (<LOD-1.70) | 3.90 (3.00-4 90) | 9.70 (7.70-12.2) | 16.3 (12.0-20.4) | 2605 |
| **Age group** | | | | | | | |
| 6-11 years | 01-02 | 1.45 (1.13-1 87) | 1.90 (1.40-2 80) | 4.00 (3.40-4 90) | 7.20 (6.00-8 00) | 11.8 (7.60-20.8) | 393 |
| | 03-04 | 2.10 (1.67-2 63) | 1.70 (1.20-2.40) | 4.30 (2.80-6.40) | 9.50 (6.40-18.8) | 18.8 (9.40-33.4) | 342 |
| 12-19 years | 01-02 | 1.59 (1.28-1 96) | 2.10 (1.80-2 50) | 3.90 (3.30-4.70) | 8.50 (5.30-10.5) | 13.0 (9.60-17.8) | 742 |
| | 03-04 | * | 1.50 (1.00-2 20) | 4.40 (3.00-7 00) | 13.3 (7.40-20.9) | 21.8 (17.8-31.5) | 729 |
| 20 years and older | 01-02 | 1.06 (.904-1 25) | 1.40 (1.10-1 60) | 3.10 (2.50-3 50) | 5.60 (4.60-7.10) | 9.20 (7.40-12.3) | 1647 |
| | 03-04 | * | 1.20 (<LOD-1.50) | 3.80 (2.80-4 90) | 9.30 (7.10-11.8) | 14.3 (10.8-19.9) | 1534 |
| **Gender** | | | | | | | |
| Males | 01-02 | 1.17 (.962-1.43) | 1.50 (1.30-1 90) | 3.30 (2.90-4 00) | 5.90 (4.80-7 90) | 9.20 (7.10-13.5) | 1371 |
| | 03-04 | * | 1.30 (1.00-1 80) | 4.00 (3.20-5 20) | 10.0 (7.30-13.5) | 17.7 (11.8-20.4) | 1250 |
| Females | 01-02 | 1.13 (.973-1 31) | 1.40 (1.10-1.70) | 3.30 (2.80-3.70) | 6.40 (5.00-7 80) | 10.3 (8.20-16.2) | 1411 |
| | 03-04 | * | 1.20 (<LOD-1.60) | 3.60 (2.80-4.70) | 9.50 (7.70-12.2) | 15.3 (11.7-22.9) | 1355 |
| **Race/ethnicity** | | | | | | | |
| Mexican Americans | 01-02 | 1.21 (1.02-1.45) | 1.60 (1.30-1.70) | 3.30 (2.70-4 00) | 5.60 (4.70-7 30) | 8.60 (6.40-15.2) | 677 |
| | 03-04 | * | 1.40 (1.10-1 80) | 4.00 (2.50-6 30) | 9.60 (7.30-13.4) | 15.0 (11.4-18.8) | 652 |
| Non-Hispanic blacks | 01-02 | 1.64 (1.37-1 98) | 2.10 (1.70-2.70) | 4.40 (3.60-5.10) | 8.30 (6.20-10.1) | 11.0 (9.50-13.4) | 703 |
| | 03-04 | 2.16 (1.64-2 84) | 1.70 (1.00-2 80) | 5.10 (3.70-7 00) | 11.4 (7.30-17.3) | 17.8 (10.2-39.4) | 699 |
| Non-Hispanic whites | 01-02 | 1.08 (.906-1 29) | 1.40 (1.10-1.70) | 3.20 (2.50-3 60) | 5.60 (4.70-6.70) | 9.70 (7.10-14.0) | 1216 |
| | 03-04 | * | 1.20 (<LOD-1.60) | 3.60 (2.80-4 80) | 9.70 (7.50-12.2) | 16.5 (12.0-20.4) | 1088 |

Limit of detection (LOD, see Data Analysis section) for Survey years 01-02 and 03-04 are 0 2 and 1.0.
< LOD means less than the limit of detection, which may vary for some chemicals by year and by individual sample.
* Not calculated: proportion of results below limit of detection was too high to provide a valid result.

# Urinary Mono-methyl phthalate (MMP) (creatinine corrected)
*Metabolite of Dimethyl phthalate (DMP)*

Geometric mean and selected percentiles of urine concentrations (in µg/g of creatinine) for the U.S. population from the National Health and Nutrition Examination Survey.

| | Survey years | Geometric mean (95% conf. interval) | Selected percentiles ( 95% confidence interval) | | | | Sample size |
|---|---|---|---|---|---|---|---|
| | | | 50th | 75th | 90th | 95th | |
| Total | 01-02 | 1.08 ( 936-1.25) | 1.33 (1.13-1.55) | 2.62 (2.36-2.97) | 5.00 (3.97-6.02) | 8.00 (6.07-11 0) | 2782 |
| | 03-04 | * | 1.53 (<LOD-1.79) | 3.45 (2.76-4.37) | 7.95 (5.83-11 8) | 13.5 (11.3-18.1) | 2605 |
| **Age group** | | | | | | | |
| 6-11 years | 01-02 | 1.65 (1.28-2.14) | 2.32 (1.72-2.86) | 3.97 (3.27-4.71) | 7.20 (5.99-9.41) | 13.2 (7.60-22 5) | 393 |
| | 03-04 | 2.22 (1.75-2.81) | 1.88 (1.49-2.60) | 4.96 (2.81-6.49) | 9.67 (6.15-14 6) | 16.2 (12.1-34 5) | 342 |
| 12-19 years | 01-02 | 1.23 (1.01-1.48) | 1.51 (1.32-1.82) | 2.84 (2.52-3.33) | 5.36 (3.68-6.39) | 7.27 (5.64-11.4) | 742 |
| | 03-04 | * | 1.34 (1.12-1.73) | 3.19 (2.26-4.43) | 7.84 (4.95-12.1) | 13.3 (9.49-19.1) | 729 |
| 20 years and older | 01-02 | 1.00 ( 868-1.16) | 1.21 (1.05-1.40) | 2.44 (2.14-2.68) | 4.53 (3.49-6.02) | 7.72 (5.52-11.4) | 1647 |
| | 03-04 | * | 1.52 (<LOD-1.79) | 3.39 (2.69-4.31) | 7.69 (5.40-11 8) | 13.3 (10.1-18 9) | 1534 |
| **Gender** | | | | | | | |
| Males | 01-02 | .954 (.794-1.15) | 1.17 (1.02-1.40) | 2.37 (2.03-2.75) | 4.18 (3.45-5.64) | 6.42 (4.94-9.59) | 1371 |
| | 03-04 | * | 1.35 (1.15-1.52) | 2.95 (2.26-4.09) | 7.11 (5.00-10 2) | 11.8 (9.05-13 3) | 1250 |
| Females | 01-02 | 1.21 (1.06-1.38) | 1.45 (1.23-1.82) | 2.87 (2.58-3.06) | 5.56 (4.55-7.14) | 10.0 (7.20-15 3) | 1411 |
| | 03-04 | * | 1.83 (<LOD-2.10) | 3.87 (3.04-4.96) | 9.41 (6.41-13 6) | 16.5 (12.5-23 5) | 1355 |
| **Race/ethnicity** | | | | | | | |
| Mexican Americans | 01-02 | 1.14 ( 975-1.34) | 1.48 (1.30-1.63) | 2.50 (2.20-2.94) | 4.19 (3.77-5.76) | 8.47 (5.58-12 5) | 677 |
| | 03-04 | * | 1.36 (1.15-1.71) | 3.56 (2.45-4.90) | 7.53 (5.62-9.64) | 12.5 (9.44-16 9) | 652 |
| Non-Hispanic blacks | 01-02 | 1.15 ( 949-1.40) | 1.39 (1.29-1.67) | 2.70 (2.36-2.95) | 4.87 (4.21-5.93) | 8.09 (5.86-11 0) | 703 |
| | 03-04 | 1.53 (1.21-1.94) | 1.40 (1.07-1.75) | 3.14 (2.26-4.37) | 7.50 (4.29-14 6) | 13.7 (7.70-20.7) | 699 |
| Non-Hispanic whites | 01-02 | 1.07 ( 914-1.26) | 1.30 (1.05-1.58) | 2.62 (2.32-2.99) | 5.22 (3.68-6.82) | 8.26 (6.07-12 6) | 1216 |
| | 03-04 | * | 1.56 (<LOD-1.89) | 3.50 (2.71-4.67) | 8.10 (6.00-11 9) | 13.6 (11.3-18 9) | 1088 |

< LOD means less than the limit of detection for the urine levels not corrected for creatinine.
* Not calculated: proportion of results below limit of detection was too high to provide a valid result.

## References

Centers for Disease Control and Prevention (CDC). Third National Report on Human Exposure to Environmental Chemicals. Atlanta (GA). 2005.

Hauser R, Meeker JD, Singh NP, Silva MJ, Ryan L, Duty S, et al. DNA damage in human sperm is related to urinary levels of phthalate monoester and oxidative metabolites. Hum Reprod 2007;22(3):688-695.

## Di-n-octyl Phthalate
CAS No. 117-84-0

### General Information

Di-n-octyl phthalate (DOP) is added to polyvinyl chloride resins used in diverse products including floorings, carpet tiles, vinyl gloves, garden hoses, wire and cable insulation, and adhesives. In addition, DOP may be added to polyvinyl chloride with food applications, such as package sealants and bottle cap liners. People exposed to DOP will excrete primarily mono-3-carboxypropyl phthalate (MCPP) and smaller amounts of mono-n-octyl phthalate (MOP) and other oxidative metabolites in their urine. In rodent studies, oral DOP produces liver and thyroid toxicity (NTP-CERHR, 2000). Neither IARC nor NTP has evaluated DOP with respect to human carcinogenicity.

### Biomonitoring Information

In NHANES 1999-2000, MOP was only detectable at the 90th and 95th percentiles, and less frequently detected in the 2001-2002 and 2003-2004 survey periods. A low

detection rate was reported in small samples of German residents (Koch et al., 2003) and of African-American women in Washington, DC (Hoppin et al., 2002). MCPP levels measured in NHANES 2001-2002 and 2003-2004 subsamples had overall median values that were roughly similar to a smaller sample of U.S. adults (Calafat et al., 2006).

Finding a measurable amount of MCPP or MOP in urine does not mean that the levels of MCPP or MOP or the parent compound cause an adverse health effect. Biomonitoring studies on levels of MCPP and MOP provide physicians and public health officials with reference values so that they can determine whether people have been exposed to higher levels of DOP than are found in the general population. Biomonitoring data can also help scientists plan and conduct research on exposure and health effects.

### Urinary Mono-(3-carboxypropyl) phthalate (MCPP)
*Metabolite of Di-n-octyl phthalate (DOP)*

Geometric mean and selected percentiles of urine concentrations (in µg/L) for the U.S. population from the National Health and Nutrition Examination Survey.

| | Survey years | Geometric mean (95% conf. interval) | 50th | 75th | 90th | 95th | Sample size |
|---|---|---|---|---|---|---|---|
| **Total** | 01-02 | 2.75 (2.49-3.04) | 3.10 (2.80-3.30) | 5.70 (5.10-6.40) | 10.0 (8.90-11 3) | 14.6 (12.7-17 5) | 2782 |
| | 03-04 | 2.91 (2.79-3.04) | 3.10 (3.00-3.30) | 5.70 (5.20-6.10) | 10.2 (9.20-11 8) | 15.3 (13.8-16 2) | 2605 |
| **Age group** | | | | | | | |
| 6-11 years | 01-02 | 6.11 (5.46-6.84) | 6.70 (5.40-7.50) | 11.8 (10.2-13 3) | 20.1 (17.8-23.1) | 24.7 (22.2-31 6) | 393 |
| | 03-04 | 6.86 (5.80-8.11) | 7.10 (6.00-8.90) | 12.7 (10.4-16.4) | 22.0 (17.2-27.7) | 29.2 (22.3-36 6) | 342 |
| 12-19 years | 01-02 | 3.71 (3.18-4.33) | 4.00 (3.40-4.70) | 7.10 (6.10-8.10) | 11.5 (9.50-12.7) | 14.1 (11.8-19 0) | 742 |
| | 03-04 | 3.72 (3.33-4.15) | 4.10 (3.50-4.60) | 7.20 (5.80-8.40) | 11.0 (9.50-13 6) | 15.4 (13.4-17 9) | 729 |
| 20 years and older | 01-02 | 2.37 (2.11-2.66) | 2.60 (2.20-3.00) | 4.80 (4.30-5.40) | 8.10 (7.20-9.50) | 12.0 (10.1-14 2) | 1647 |
| | 03-04 | 2.53 (2.41-2.66) | 2.80 (2.60-2.90) | 4.90 (4.50-5.20) | 8.10 (7.50-8.90) | 13.2 (10.8-14 3) | 1534 |
| **Gender** | | | | | | | |
| Males | 01-02 | 2.89 (2.64-3.17) | 3.10 (2.80-3.40) | 5.70 (5.00-6.80) | 9.90 (8.70-120) | 14.2 (12.4-18.1) | 1371 |
| | 03-04 | 3.25 (3.01-3.52) | 3.30 (3.00-3.60) | 6.00 (5.60-6.80) | 11.8 (10.1-13 6) | 16.0 (14.2-20 0) | 1250 |
| Females | 01-02 | 2.62 (2.29-2.99) | 3.00 (2.50-3.30) | 5.70 (5.00-6.30) | 10.0 (8.50-11 5) | 14.7 (11.2-20 3) | 1411 |
| | 03-04 | 2.63 (2.44-2.83) | 3.00 (2.60-3.20) | 5.20 (4.70-5.80) | 9.20 (8.20-10 3) | 13.4 (11.0-16 2) | 1355 |
| **Race/ethnicity** | | | | | | | |
| Mexican Americans | 01-02 | 2.67 (2.26-3.16) | 3.00 (2.30-3.50) | 5.30 (4.40-5.90) | 9.20 (7.30-12.4) | 13.6 (10.4-18.7) | 677 |
| | 03-04 | 3.08 (2.86-3.32) | 3.10 (2.80-3.40) | 5.50 (4.80-6.10) | 9.90 (7.90-12 6) | 13.7 (11.5-19 8) | 652 |
| Non-Hispanic blacks | 01-02 | 3.09 (2.81-3.40) | 3.30 (2.90-3.60) | 6.30 (5.50-6.50) | 10.9 (9.10-13 0) | 15.1 (13.5-22.4) | 703 |
| | 03-04 | 3.30 (3.01-3.62) | 3.20 (2.90-3.60) | 6.10 (5.50-6.90) | 11.6 (9.30-13.4) | 20.1 (13.6-25 5) | 699 |
| Non-Hispanic whites | 01-02 | 2.72 (2.40-3.08) | 3.00 (2.60-3.30) | 5.80 (4.80-6.80) | 10.3 (8.90-11 9) | 15.8 (12.6-19 5) | 1216 |
| | 03-04 | 2.87 (2.73-3.02) | 3.10 (2.90-3.30) | 5.60 (5.00-6.00) | 10.1 (9.10-12 0) | 15.2 (13.4-16.1) | 1088 |

Limit of detection (LOD, see Data Analysis section) for Survey years 01-02 and 03-04 are 0.4 and 0 2.

## Urinary Mono-(3-carboxypropyl) phthalate (MCPP) (creatinine corrected)

*Metabolite of Di-n-octyl phthalate (DOP)*

Geometric mean and selected percentiles of urine concentrations (in µg/g of creatinine) for the U.S. population from the National Health and Nutrition Examination Survey.

| | Survey years | Geometric mean (95% conf. interval) | Selected percentiles ( 95% confidence interval) | | | | Sample size |
|---|---|---|---|---|---|---|---|
| | | | 50th | 75th | 90th | 95th | |
| Total | 01-02 | 2.58 (2.35-2 83) | 2.47 (2.25-2.76) | 4.08 (3.87-4.48) | 7.24 (6.58-8 00) | 11.4 (10.0-12.5) | 2782 |
| | 03-04 | 2.74 (2.56-2 93) | 2.60 (2.42-2.79) | 4.39 (3.94-4 86) | 7.70 (6.65-8 60) | 10.7 (9.53-11.9) | 2605 |
| **Age group** | | | | | | | |
| 6-11 years | 01-02 | 6.96 (6.29-7.70) | 7.08 (5.83-7 87) | 11.2 (9.15-14.0) | 20.7 (15.5-22.3) | 26.4 (20.7-27.0) | 393 |
| | 03-04 | 7.25 (6.43-8.18) | 7.06 (5.93-7 59) | 11.2 (9.38-12.4) | 19.1 (14.4-25.6) | 26.9 (19.3-29.0) | 342 |
| 12-19 years | 01-02 | 2.86 (2.52-3 25) | 2.94 (2.50-3 36) | 4.59 (4.03-5 23) | 6.69 (6.30-7 25) | 9.55 (8.03-10.7) | 742 |
| | 03-04 | 2.78 (2.54-3 05) | 2.75 (2.53-2 99) | 4.55 (4.05-5.15) | 6.61 (6.15-7 20) | 8.24 (7.00-10.2) | 729 |
| 20 years and older | 01-02 | 2.24 (2.03-2.47) | 2.20 (2.00-2.40) | 3.51 (3.11-3 95) | 5.39 (4.82-6.18) | 7.71 (6.71-9 28) | 1647 |
| | 03-04 | 2.43 (2.27-2 61) | 2.38 (2.19-2 56) | 3.70 (3.33-4 08) | 6.09 (5.38-7 06) | 8.79 (7.84-9 56) | 1534 |
| **Gender** | | | | | | | |
| Males | 01-02 | 2.35 (2.17-2 56) | 2.20 (2.02-2.42) | 3.76 (3.45-4 20) | 7.17 (6.27-8 06) | 11.5 (9.28-15.1) | 1371 |
| | 03-04 | 2.55 (2.39-2.72) | 2.36 (2.22-2.47) | 4.14 (3.52-4 86) | 7.84 (6.80-8.79) | 11.6 (10.2-13.5) | 1250 |
| Females | 01-02 | 2.81 (2.48-3.18) | 2.76 (2.46-3 02) | 4.39 (3.97-4 92) | 7.66 (6.17-8 69) | 11.0 (8.62-15.9) | 1411 |
| | 03-04 | 2.93 (2.68-3 20) | 2.89 (2.58-3 23) | 4.53 (4.09-5 00) | 7.58 (6.44-8 57) | 10.0 (8.60-11.6) | 1355 |
| **Race/ethnicity** | | | | | | | |
| Mexican Americans | 01-02 | 2.52 (2.21-2 88) | 2.37 (2.07-2.73) | 4.29 (3.73-5 00) | 7.36 (5.58-10.3) | 11.4 (8.36-14.5) | 677 |
| | 03-04 | 2.78 (2.56-3 02) | 2.63 (2.30-2 96) | 4.32 (3.66-4 96) | 8.14 (6.72-10.3) | 12.8 (9.37-17.1) | 652 |
| Non-Hispanic blacks | 01-02 | 2.17 (2.02-2 33) | 2.07 (1.88-2 28) | 3.68 (3.25-4 07) | 6.73 (5.46-7.70) | 10.0 (8.27-13.1) | 703 |
| | 03-04 | 2.34 (2.13-2 58) | 2.17 (1.99-2.45) | 3.96 (3.33-4.43) | 6.93 (6.03-8 80) | 13.4 (9.32-15.9) | 699 |
| Non-Hispanic whites | 01-02 | 2.69 (2.42-3 00) | 2.57 (2.25-2 94) | 4.19 (3.87-4.79) | 7.63 (6.58-8.45) | 11.8 (10.0-14.7) | 1216 |
| | 03-04 | 2.83 (2.60-3 09) | 2.65 (2.43-2 96) | 4.55 (3.90-5.16) | 7.79 (6.59-8.79) | 10.6 (9.43-11.3) | 1088 |

## Urinary Mono-n-octyl phthalate (MOP)
*Metabolite of Di-n-octyl phthalate (DOP)*

Geometric mean and selected percentiles of urine concentrations (in µg/L) for the U.S. population from the National Health and Nutrition Examination Survey.

| | Survey years | Geometric mean (95% conf. interval) | Selected percentiles ( 95% confidence interval) | | | | Sample size |
|---|---|---|---|---|---|---|---|
| | | | 50th | 75th | 90th | 95th | |
| **Total** | 99-00 | * | < LOD | < LOD | 1.60 (1.20-2.00) | 2.90 (2.30-3.40) | 2541 |
| | 01-02 | * | < LOD | < LOD | < LOD | < LOD | 2782 |
| | 03-04 | * | < LOD | < LOD | < LOD | < LOD | 2605 |
| **Age group** | | | | | | | |
| 6-11 years | 99-00 | * | < LOD | < LOD | 2.20 ( 900-3.50) | 3.20 (1.70-5.00) | 328 |
| | 01-02 | * | < LOD | < LOD | < LOD | < LOD | 393 |
| | 03-04 | * | < LOD | < LOD | < LOD | < LOD | 342 |
| 12-19 years | 99-00 | * | < LOD | < LOD | 1.70 ( 900-2.50) | 2.80 (2.00-4.20) | 752 |
| | 01-02 | * | < LOD | < LOD | < LOD | < LOD | 742 |
| | 03-04 | * | < LOD | < LOD | < LOD | < LOD | 729 |
| 20 years and older | 99-00 | * | < LOD | < LOD | 1.50 (1.10-1.90) | 2.90 (2.10-3.50) | 1461 |
| | 01-02 | * | < LOD | < LOD | < LOD | < LOD | 1647 |
| | 03-04 | * | < LOD | < LOD | < LOD | < LOD | 1534 |
| **Gender** | | | | | | | |
| Males | 99-00 | * | < LOD | < LOD | 1.60 (1.10-2.20) | 2.80 (2.00-3.50) | 1215 |
| | 01-02 | * | < LOD | < LOD | < LOD | < LOD | 1371 |
| | 03-04 | * | < LOD | < LOD | < LOD | < LOD | 1250 |
| Females | 99-00 | * | < LOD | < LOD | 1.50 (1.20-2.10) | 3.10 (2.20-3.80) | 1326 |
| | 01-02 | * | < LOD | < LOD | < LOD | < LOD | 1411 |
| | 03-04 | * | < LOD | < LOD | < LOD | < LOD | 1355 |
| **Race/ethnicity** | | | | | | | |
| Mexican Americans | 99-00 | * | < LOD | < LOD | 1.10 (<LOD-1.40) | 1.60 (1.40-2.60) | 814 |
| | 01-02 | * | < LOD | < LOD | < LOD | < LOD | 677 |
| | 03-04 | * | < LOD | < LOD | < LOD | < LOD | 652 |
| Non-Hispanic blacks | 99-00 | * | < LOD | < LOD | 1.90 (<LOD-3.00) | 3.00 (2.20-4.10) | 603 |
| | 01-02 | * | < LOD | < LOD | < LOD | < LOD | 703 |
| | 03-04 | * | < LOD | < LOD | < LOD | < LOD | 699 |
| Non-Hispanic whites | 99-00 | * | < LOD | < LOD | 1.60 (1.20-2.10) | 3.00 (2.30-3.50) | 912 |
| | 01-02 | * | < LOD | < LOD | < LOD | < LOD | 1216 |
| | 03-04 | * | < LOD | < LOD | < LOD | < LOD | 1088 |

Limit of detection (LOD, see Data Analysis section) for Survey years 99-00, 01-02, and 03-04 are 0.9, 1.0, and 1.0, respectively.
< LOD means less than the limit of detection, which may vary for some chemicals by year and by individual sample.
* Not calculated: proportion of results below limit of detection was too high to provide a valid result.

# Urinary Mono-n-octyl phthalate (MOP) (creatinine corrected)
*Metabolite of Di-n-octyl phthalate (DOP)*

Geometric mean and selected percentiles of urine concentrations (in µg/g of creatinine) for the U.S. population from the National Health and Nutrition Examination Survey.

| | Survey years | Geometric mean (95% conf. interval) | 50th | 75th | 90th | 95th | Sample size |
|---|---|---|---|---|---|---|---|
| **Total** | 99-00 | * | < LOD | < LOD | 2.40 (2.07-2 61) | 3.53 (2.95-4 29) | 2541 |
| | 01-02 | * | < LOD | < LOD | < LOD | < LOD | 2782 |
| | 03-04 | * | < LOD | < LOD | < LOD | < LOD | 2605 |
| **Age group** | | | | | | | |
| 6-11 years | 99-00 | * | < LOD | < LOD | 2.22 (1.60-3.75) | 3.75 (1.97-10.3) | 328 |
| | 01-02 | * | < LOD | < LOD | < LOD | < LOD | 393 |
| | 03-04 | * | < LOD | < LOD | < LOD | < LOD | 342 |
| 12-19 years | 99-00 | * | < LOD | < LOD | 1.49 (1.29-1.71) | 1.88 (1.54-3 33) | 752 |
| | 01-02 | * | < LOD | < LOD | < LOD | < LOD | 742 |
| | 03-04 | * | < LOD | < LOD | < LOD | < LOD | 729 |
| 20 years and older | 99-00 | * | < LOD | < LOD | 2.60 (2.07-2 91) | 3.53 (3.00-4 62) | 1461 |
| | 01-02 | * | < LOD | < LOD | < LOD | < LOD | 1647 |
| | 03-04 | * | < LOD | < LOD | < LOD | < LOD | 1534 |
| **Gender** | | | | | | | |
| Males | 99-00 | * | < LOD | < LOD | 1.82 (1.54-2 07) | 2.56 (1.94-3.45) | 1215 |
| | 01-02 | * | < LOD | < LOD | < LOD | < LOD | 1371 |
| | 03-04 | * | < LOD | < LOD | < LOD | < LOD | 1250 |
| Females | 99-00 | * | < LOD | < LOD | 3.00 (2.50-3 55) | 4.29 (3.33-6 23) | 1326 |
| | 01-02 | * | < LOD | < LOD | < LOD | < LOD | 1411 |
| | 03-04 | * | < LOD | < LOD | < LOD | < LOD | 1355 |
| **Race/ethnicity** | | | | | | | |
| Mexican Americans | 99-00 | * | < LOD | < LOD | 1.82 (<LOD-2.80) | 3.33 (2.60-4 00) | 814 |
| | 01-02 | * | < LOD | < LOD | < LOD | < LOD | 677 |
| | 03-04 | * | < LOD | < LOD | < LOD | < LOD | 652 |
| Non-Hispanic blacks | 99-00 | * | < LOD | < LOD | 1.36 (<LOD-1.94) | 2.22 (1.50-3 27) | 603 |
| | 01-02 | * | < LOD | < LOD | < LOD | < LOD | 703 |
| | 03-04 | * | < LOD | < LOD | < LOD | < LOD | 699 |
| Non-Hispanic whites | 99-00 | * | < LOD | < LOD | 2.61 (2.14-3 08) | 3.64 (3.15-5 00) | 912 |
| | 01-02 | * | < LOD | < LOD | < LOD | < LOD | 1216 |
| | 03-04 | * | < LOD | < LOD | < LOD | < LOD | 1088 |

< LOD means less than the limit of detection for the urine levels not corrected for creatinine.
* Not calculated: proportion of results below limit of detection was too high to provide a valid result.

## References

Calafat AM, Silva MJ, Reidy JA, Gray LE, Samander E, Preau Jr JL, et al. Mono-(3-carboxypropyl)phthalate, a metabolite of di-n-octyl phthalate. J Toxicol Environ Health Part A 2006;69:215-227.

Hoppin JA, Brock JW, Davis BJ, Baird DD. Reproducibility of urinary phthalate metabolites in first morning urine samples. Environ Health Perspect 2002;110(5):515-518.

Koch HM, Rossbach B, Drexler H, Angerer J. Internal exposure of the general population to DEHP and other phthalates - determination of secondary and primary phthalate monoester metabolites in urine. Environ Res 2003;93:177-185.

NTP-CERHR. National Toxicology Program-Center for the Evaluation of Risks to Human Reproduction. Monograph on the Potential Human Reproductive and Developmental Effects of Di-isononyl Phthalate (DiOP). Research Triangle Park (NC). 2000 [online]. Available at URL: http://cerhr.niehs.nih.gov/chemicals/phthalates/dinp/dinp-eval.html. 6/2/09

# Phytoestrogens

## General Informatgraceion

Phytoestrogens are naturally occurring polycyclic phenols found in certain plants. These are chemicals that may have weak estrogenic effects when they are ingested and metabolized. Two important groups of phytoestrogens are isoflavones and lignans. The table shows the phytoestrogen classes, examples, and some human urinary metabolites.

The isoflavones considered here include formononetin, daidzein, biochanin A, genistein, O-desmethylangolensin, and equol. Plant sources of isoflavones include legumes, with the largest contribution coming from soy-based foods. Because soy flour and soy protein isolates may be added to processed meats, meat substitutes, breads, and protein food bars, these items can be a major source of isoflavones (Grace et al., 2004; Lampe et al., 1999). However, the isoflavone content of soy protein preparations can vary widely and is affected by production techniques (Erdman et al., 2004). Daidzein and genistein are the main soy isoflavones. Kudzu root, used in some dietary supplements, also contains appreciable amounts of daidzein. Naringenin, a precursor to genistein, is found in some citrus fruits. Formononetin and biochanin A are methylated isoflavones found in clovers, which may be used in red clover dietary supplements; these isoflavones are metabolized in the body to daidzein and genistein, respectively.

Ingested daidzein is further metabolized to O-desmethylangolensin and to equol by intestinal bacteria. Equol, but not O-desmethylangolensin, has estrogenic activity. About 30% of adults can be characterized as equol producers and demonstrate higher serum equol levels after daidzein consumption (Cassidy et al., 2006; Setchell et al., 2003). This ability to produce equol may be related to an individual's intestinal microflora and influenced by dietary

habits (Rowland et al., 2000). The relevance of equol-producer status to potential health related effects is unclear (Vafeiadou et al., 2006).

Lignans include matairesinol and secoisolariciresinol, which are transformed by intestinal bacteria into the estrogenic compounds enterolactone and enterodiol, respectively (Cornwell et al., 2004; Rowland et al., 2003). Enterodiol may also interconvert with enterolactone. Lignans are found in flax seeds, whole wheat flour, tea, some fruits, and other cereal grains. Other phytoestrogens of interest are resveratrol and trans-resveratrol, found in grape skins, wine, and peanuts.

Diet is the source of human exposure to phytoestrogens. The absorption and metabolism of phytoestrogens demonstrate large interindividual variability, which may relate to differences in both human pharmacokinetics and metabolism by intestinal bacteria. Phytoestrogens are ingested in their naturally occurring beta-glycosidic forms. The beta-glycosidic forms are hydrolyzed to their aglycones in the intestine, absorbed, and then glucuronidated in the intestinal wall and liver (Doerge et al., 2000; Rowland et al., 2003). The glucuronidated metabolites of isoflavones predominate in blood and urine (Rozman et al., 2006a; Setchell et al., 2001).

The isoflavones are excreted from the body about 24 hours after ingestion, mainly in urine and, to a lesser extent, in feces. Urinary concentrations of daidzein and genistein did not correlate well with the ingested doses, possibly due to limited absorption of these isoflavones at higher doses (Setchell et al., 2003a). In contrast, plasma and urine lignan concentrations after flax seed consumption increased in a dose-dependent manner (Nesbitt et al., 1999). Equol excretion may depend on diet, the type of intestinal bacteria present, and individual genetic factors (Rowland et al., 2000; Setchell et al., 2002; Setchell and Cassidy, 1999).

## Phytoestrogens and Urinary Metabolites in this *Report*

| Phytoestrogen Class | Phytoestrogen or Metabolite (CAS number) |
|---|---|
| Isoflavones | Daidzein (486-66-8)<br>O-Desmethylangolensin (21255-69-6)<br>Equol (531-95-3)<br>Genistein (466-72-0) |
| Lignans | Enterolactone (78473-71-9)<br>Enterodiol (80226-00-2) |

After hydrolysis to the aglycone forms, phytoestrogens can weakly bind to estrogen-beta receptors (ER-beta) which are expressed in arteries and smooth muscle. Individual phytoestrogens may be either estrogen agonists or antagonists. Equol has more potent estrogenic activity than its precursor, daidzein. Equol also has been shown to have antiandrogenic activity in animals (Lund et al., 2004; Magee and Rowland, 2004). Genistein binds ER-beta with greater affinity than equol (Doerge and Sheehan, 2002). Although far less potent, phytoestrogens can be present in concentrations 100 to 1000 times greater than the endogenously produced estrogens. Soy-based infant formula can result in plasma concentrations of isoflavones in infants that are 13,000-22,000 times higher than endogenous estrogen concentrations in infants (Setchell et al., 1997). Phytoestrogens may also act through pathways other than the interaction with estrogen receptors. These actions include inhibiting the transformation of estrone to estradiol, inhibiting enzymes important for steroid biosynthesis and cell growth, and having antioxidant and anti-angiogenesis activities. (Adlercreutz et al., 1995a; Dixon and Ferreira, 2002; Sirtori et al., 2005). Numerous studies of either dietary soy or phytoestrogens and health outcomes have demonstrated inconsistent or inconclusive results. Consensus reviews of these studies suggest that no evidence clearly shows that dietary phytoestrogens significantly reduce cardiovascular disease risk, reduce postmenopausal vasomotor symptoms, improve bone

## Urinary Daidzein

Geometric mean and selected percentiles of urine concentrations (in µg/L) for the U.S. population from the National Health and Nutrition Examination Survey.

| | Survey years | Geometric mean (95% conf. interval) | Selected percentiles (95% confidence interval) | | | | Sample size |
|---|---|---|---|---|---|---|---|
| | | | 50th | 75th | 90th | 95th | |
| **Total** | 99-00 | 75.1 (61.9-91.1) | 69.8 (57.8-82.6) | 229 (184-298) | 538 (471-702) | 1320 (1020-1540) | 2553 |
| | 01-02 | 51.7 (46.6-57.5) | 52.3 (48.9-57.4) | 192 (151-226) | 577 (447-725) | 1250 (863-1640) | 2794 |
| | 03-04 | 66.7 (60.4-73.7) | 62.0 (54.1-69.7) | 195 (171-219) | 590 (500-675) | 1070 (893-1330) | 2594 |
| **Age group** | | | | | | | |
| 6-11 years | 99-00 | 90.5 (75.1-109) | 101 (70.3-138) | 257 (172-430) | 510 (437-840) | 1130 (657-1740) | 330 |
| | 01-02 | 84.9 (71.6-101) | 72.7 (56.3-97.0) | 261 (155-385) | 605 (437-989) | 1060 (645-1500) | 396 |
| | 03-04 | 84.9 (71.6-101) | 66.8 (55.4-92.8) | 229 (151-314) | 574 (371-654) | 818 (625-1060) | 341 |
| 12-19 years | 99-00 | 123 (91.4-166) | 124 (85.6-168) | 326 (227-454) | 833 (445-1490) | 1460 (861-2410) | 753 |
| | 01-02 | 69.3 (52.6-91.3) | 70.2 (52.5-87.5) | 255 (185-344) | 774 (573-984) | 1360 (922-1950) | 744 |
| | 03-04 | 89.0 (75.2-105) | 78.0 (59.0-104) | 248 (197-332) | 808 (500-968) | 1200 (900-1790) | 729 |
| 20 years and older | 99-00 | 67.6 (55.4-82.4) | 60.9 (49.3-74.1) | 215 (167-239) | 518 (459-573) | 1320 (978-1540) | 1470 |
| | 01-02 | 46.4 (41.4-52.0) | 49.1 (40.8-53.4) | 176 (133-216) | 520 (396-703) | 1210 (771-1900) | 1654 |
| | 03-04 | 61.9 (55.2-69.4) | 57.9 (48.7-68.5) | 180 (150-214) | 554 (416-695) | 1110 (857-1360) | 1524 |
| **Gender** | | | | | | | |
| Males | 99-00 | 88.9 (71.4-111) | 80.6 (66.6-112) | 262 (198-355) | 587 (501-989) | 1540 (989-2080) | 1220 |
| | 01-02 | 49.8 (42.8-57.9) | 50.8 (46.0-55.0) | 190 (137-240) | 498 (386-694) | 920 (717-1380) | 1375 |
| | 03-04 | 73.8 (63.4-85.9) | 65.2 (56.1-76.4) | 214 (156-311) | 709 (535-900) | 1200 (969-1380) | 1244 |
| Females | 99-00 | 64.1 (52.9-77.6) | 57.8 (45.0-73.2) | 199 (150-244) | 476 (389-722) | 1220 (566-1700) | 1333 |
| | 01-02 | 53.6 (48.1-59.8) | 55.7 (49.8-62.7) | 199 (149-234) | 642 (511-816) | 1470 (1170-1980) | 1419 |
| | 03-04 | 60.7 (53.6-68.8) | 57.4 (49.1-67.6) | 175 (159-201) | 466 (381-622) | 884 (654-1380) | 1350 |
| **Race/ethnicity** | | | | | | | |
| Mexican Americans | 99-00 | 78.9 (59.8-104) | 66.2 (48.4-87.1) | 254 (170-402) | 806 (534-1020) | 1360 (968-2780) | 816 |
| | 01-02 | 39.2 (28.5-54.0) | 39.9 (28.8-59.9) | 169 (100-291) | 515 (388-669) | 896 (613-1480) | 679 |
| | 03-04 | 57.4 (50.2-65.7) | 45.5 (35.2-53.3) | 178 (130-236) | 686 (487-934) | 1390 (934-1650) | 653 |
| Non-Hispanic blacks | 99-00 | 91.9 (71.9-118) | 103 (81.6-133) | 286 (243-377) | 553 (459-824) | 1190 (640-1900) | 607 |
| | 01-02 | 66.1 (48.2-90.7) | 72.9 (52.8-97.3) | 255 (182-393) | 757 (448-1400) | 1410 (757-2480) | 706 |
| | 03-04 | 75.0 (56.1-100) | 66.0 (50.7-86.6) | 241 (151-340) | 622 (408-875) | 1190 (660-2300) | 699 |
| Non-Hispanic whites | 99-00 | 74.4 (61.5-89.9) | 66.9 (56.2-78.2) | 216 (157-298) | 512 (438-745) | 1360 (989-1710) | 917 |
| | 01-02 | 48.6 (43.8-54.0) | 49.8 (42.8-54.2) | 171 (137-204) | 504 (389-658) | 1140 (774-1620) | 1222 |
| | 03-04 | 65.8 (58.6-74.0) | 62.0 (52.8-71.9) | 191 (165-215) | 572 (416-722) | 1070 (823-1330) | 1079 |

Limit of detection (LOD, see Data Analysis section) for Survey years 99-00, 01-02, and 03-04 are 0 5, 1.6, and 1 6, respectively.

mineral density, or reduce cancer risk (Cornwell et al., 2004; Messina et al., 2006; NAMS, 2000; Nedrow et al., 2006; Sacks et al., 2006; Sirtori et al., 2005).

Adverse effects on fertility have been observed in animals that graze on red clover. Results of chronic feeding studies in pregnant animals suggest that high doses of phytoestrogens alter the fetal hormonal environment (Cornwell et al., 2004). Studies of children who had been fed soy-based formula as infants and who were followed through adolescence (Klein, 1998) and young adulthood (Strom et al., 2001) found no adverse reproductive or endocrine effects. *In vitro* and animal studies suggest that soy isoflavones may have immunologic and thyroid effects (Doerge and Sheehan,

2002; Sirtori et al., 2005). The Center for the Evaluation of Risks to Human Reproduction (CERHR) of the National Toxicology Program reviewed developmental and reproductive toxicity of both soy formula and genistein and concluded that available data were inadequate to determine whether soy formula has developmental or reproductive toxicity (Rozman et al., 2006*a*). The expert review panel expressed negligible concern for adverse effects in the general population consuming dietary sources of genistein (Rozman et al., 2006*b*).

## Biomonitoring Information

The concentrations of urinary phytoestrogens observed

### Urinary Daidzein (creatinine corrected)

Geometric mean and selected percentiles of urine concentrations (in µg/g of creatinine) for the U.S. population from the National Health and Nutrition Examination Survey.

| | Survey years | Geometric mean (95% conf. interval) | Selected percentiles ( 95% confidence interval) | | | | Sample size |
|---|---|---|---|---|---|---|---|
| | | | 50th | 75th | 90th | 95th | |
| Total | 99-00 | 68.5 (55.9-83.9) | 65.1 (52.8-80.8) | 204 (156-249) | 560 (471-629) | 944 (836-1150) | 2553 |
| | 01-02 | 48.5 (43.7-54.0) | 48.3 (43.1-56.5) | 166 (140-196) | 500 (391-608) | 957 (801-1180) | 2794 |
| | 03-04 | 62.5 (58.3-67.0) | 56.1 (50.0-63.6) | 164 (144-187) | 502 (429-591) | 1060 (825-1150) | 2594 |
| **Age group** | | | | | | | |
| 6-11 years | 99-00 | 92.6 (76.3-112) | 93.1 (71.2-114) | 251 (157-324) | 552 (363-838) | 1070 (781-2150) | 330 |
| | 01-02 | 96.4 (79.0-118) | 85.9 (60.3-127) | 275 (159-395) | 655 (452-733) | 938 (683-1140) | 396 |
| | 03-04 | 90.4 (77.2-106) | 72.8 (58.2-99.5) | 201 (152-240) | 454 (329-638) | 702 (526-1200) | 341 |
| 12-19 years | 99-00 | 83.1 (58.4-118) | 85.6 (53.8-126) | 207 (138-386) | 628 (295-1060) | 1000 (628-2380) | 753 |
| | 01-02 | 53.4 (40.8-70.0) | 50.9 (38.3-77.6) | 181 (142-248) | 549 (385-718) | 1030 (622-1360) | 744 |
| | 03-04 | 66.6 (55.7-79.6) | 56.4 (43.9-74.6) | 179 (151-217) | 517 (370-753) | 877 (617-1240) | 729 |
| 20 years and older | 99-00 | 63.8 (51.5-79.1) | 59.3 (48.7-75.0) | 194 (151-234) | 554 (471-624) | 908 (783-1180) | 1470 |
| | 01-02 | 43.9 (39.4-48.9) | 43.8 (37.4-53.3) | 153 (125-186) | 428 (348-590) | 946 (728-1220) | 1654 |
| | 03-04 | 59.2 (54.3-64.5) | 51.7 (46.4-62.6) | 155 (131-185) | 501 (404-658) | 1090 (808-1240) | 1524 |
| **Gender** | | | | | | | |
| Males | 99-00 | 69.7 (54.7-88.8) | 70.2 (51.3-84.3) | 198 (147-276) | 623 (494-836) | 1050 (884-1290) | 1220 |
| | 01-02 | 40.5 (34.8-47.1) | 41.7 (34.5-47.9) | 139 (107-179) | 348 (260-553) | 788 (585-947) | 1375 |
| | 03-04 | 57.7 (49.4-67.3) | 48.9 (41.6-58.3) | 160 (126-205) | 467 (368-600) | 919 (665-1200) | 1244 |
| Females | 99-00 | 67.4 (54.8-82.9) | 62.6 (51.1-80.9) | 207 (152-250) | 509 (356-624) | 850 (610-1410) | 1333 |
| | 01-02 | 57.6 (50.8-65.2) | 59.5 (48.1-73.4) | 191 (159-227) | 615 (536-722) | 1180 (924-1430) | 1419 |
| | 03-04 | 67.4 (60.8-74.9) | 65.1 (54.6-73.4) | 165 (143-191) | 564 (409-699) | 1090 (757-1370) | 1350 |
| **Race/ethnicity** | | | | | | | |
| Mexican Americans | 99-00 | 72.5 (59.1-88.9) | 64.2 (47.1-91.1) | 243 (176-310) | 677 (468-1080) | 1380 (753-2690) | 816 |
| | 01-02 | 36.9 (27.8-49.0) | 37.1 (24.8-57.9) | 146 (101-225) | 441 (307-596) | 722 (565-1160) | 679 |
| | 03-04 | 51.8 (45.0-59.6) | 47.7 (35.9-58.3) | 159 (117-209) | 502 (354-686) | 1130 (779-1390) | 653 |
| Non-Hispanic blacks | 99-00 | 59.1 (46.5-75.1) | 67.6 (52.1-87.1) | 172 (134-207) | 381 (316-533) | 802 (562-1010) | 607 |
| | 01-02 | 46.4 (33.7-63.8) | 49.8 (35.5-69.7) | 169 (104-249) | 504 (263-773) | 939 (542-1530) | 706 |
| | 03-04 | 53.1 (42.5-66.4) | 44.7 (28.6-72.1) | 147 (121-191) | 415 (275-538) | 727 (538-1040) | 699 |
| Non-Hispanic whites | 99-00 | 72.8 (60.3-88.0) | 67.5 (55.3-81.5) | 207 (160-249) | 560 (442-659) | 908 (742-1350) | 917 |
| | 01-02 | 48.1 (43.4-53.3) | 47.0 (42.1-56.0) | 163 (137-191) | 463 (375-627) | 957 (805-1220) | 1222 |
| | 03-04 | 64.9 (59.8-70.3) | 58.2 (50.4-66.3) | 165 (138-204) | 516 (385-667) | 1090 (786-1250) | 1079 |

in the NHANES 1999-2000, 2000-2001, and 2003-2004 subsamples generally reflect a diet consumed in the U.S. that is lower in isoflavones than in lignans. This is consistent with a Western diet in which whole grains and cereals, rather than soybean products, contribute the bulk of phytoestrogens (CDC, 2005). Enterolactone levels were highest, followed by daidzein, enterodiol, genistein, equol, and O-desmethylangolensin. Isoflavone levels at the higher percentiles may reflect dietary supplementation with soy products. The relationship between the dose and urinary excretion is linear for many phytoestrogens, except for equol (Karr et al., 1997; Slavin et al., 1998). Because excretory half-lives are reported to be in the range of 3-10 hours (Lu et al., 1995; Setchell et al., 2001), urinary concentrations reflect recent consumption.

Levels of lignans (enterolactone, enterodiol) in the NHANES 1999-2000, 2001-2002, and 2003-2004 subsamples appeared broadly similar to levels found in studies of postmenopausal women in the United Kingdom (Grace et al., 2004); men and women in the U. S. (Valentin-Blasini et al., 2003); men and women in Minnesota (Lampe et al., 1999); postmenopausal Dutch women (den Tonkelaar et al., 2001); young African-American, Latina, and Japanese women in the San Francisco Bay Area (Horn-Ross et al., 1997); Japanese men and women (Adlercreutz et al., 1991; Uehara et al., 2000a); premenopausal omnivorous women in Boston (Adlercreutz et al., 1986); and healthy

## Urinary O-Desmethylangolensin

Geometric mean and selected percentiles of urine concentrations (in µg/L) for the U.S. population from the National Health and Nutrition Examination Survey.

| | Survey years | Geometric mean (95% conf. interval) | Selected percentiles ( 95% confidence interval) | | | | Sample size |
|---|---|---|---|---|---|---|---|
| | | | 50th | 75th | 90th | 95th | |
| **Total** | 99-00 | 4.39 (3.37-5.73) | 4.98 (3.65-6.77) | 22.7 (18.7-30.1) | 100 (74.8-141) | 222 (182-250) | 2271 |
| | 01-02 | 4.08 (3.53-4.73) | 3.30 (2.70-4.20) | 19.8 (16.7-24.6) | 96.0 (70.1-135) | 260 (161-437) | 2794 |
| | 03-04 | 4.91 (4.34-5.55) | 4.60 (4.00-5.20) | 23.6 (18.6-27.2) | 95.9 (70.7-122) | 230 (185-342) | 2581 |
| **Age group** | | | | | | | |
| 6-11 years | 99-00 | 5.60 (3.85-8.15) | 7.52 (3.43-15.2) | 36.2 (20.3-45.0) | 78.7 (43.4-191) | 176 (74.8-264) | 287 |
| | 01-02 | 6.19 (4.51-8.49) | 5.90 (3.80-9.30) | 26.9 (15.7-52.1) | 122 (61.5-215) | 281 (161-466) | 396 |
| | 03-04 | 6.33 (4.30-9.30) | 6.10 (3.50-10.6) | 24.0 (17.0-33.8) | 70.8 (51.4-122) | 138 (80.9-256) | 341 |
| 12-19 years | 99-00 | 6.04 (3.76-9.70) | 7.60 (5.13-13.5) | 36.6 (22.0-57.3) | 107 (63.4-165) | 194 (107-238) | 667 |
| | 01-02 | 5.92 (4.46-7.87) | 5.20 (3.70-7.60) | 33.6 (18.0-56.8) | 125 (91.2-172) | 299 (172-435) | 744 |
| | 03-04 | 6.37 (4.95-8.18) | 5.30 (3.80-8.10) | 33.9 (18.2-50.5) | 110 (82.2-198) | 257 (175-415) | 729 |
| 20 years and older | 99-00 | 4.05 (3.12-5.26) | 4.46 (3.31-5.64) | 19.8 (16.0-26.5) | 101 (80.8-150) | 228 (179-259) | 1317 |
| | 01-02 | 3.65 (3.08-4.32) | 2.80 (2.30-3.70) | 17.0 (13.9-22.4) | 81.5 (63.0-128) | 260 (135-526) | 1654 |
| | 03-04 | 4.56 (4.02-5.17) | 4.40 (3.60-4.90) | 22.0 (17.8-25.6) | 94.0 (67.6-131) | 230 (187-398) | 1511 |
| **Gender** | | | | | | | |
| Males | 99-00 | 4.97 (3.71-6.66) | 5.62 (4.12-8.73) | 29.1 (19.8-42.9) | 121 (74.1-190) | 235 (177-332) | 1087 |
| | 01-02 | 3.81 (3.08-4.71) | 3.30 (2.60-4.50) | 17.4 (13.2-24.6) | 82.8 (58.4-116) | 194 (123-324) | 1375 |
| | 03-04 | 4.90 (3.93-6.12) | 4.60 (3.40-5.50) | 23.0 (16.6-30.1) | 92.9 (70.7-129) | 222 (159-332) | 1240 |
| Females | 99-00 | 3.92 (2.97-5.16) | 4.22 (3.18-5.51) | 19.4 (14.1-26.1) | 83.8 (61.1-114) | 192 (123-250) | 1184 |
| | 01-02 | 4.36 (3.64-5.23) | 3.40 (2.50-4.60) | 21.3 (16.8-29.2) | 107 (70.6-199) | 394 (230-746) | 1419 |
| | 03-04 | 4.91 (4.26-5.66) | 4.60 (3.90-5.50) | 23.9 (18.1-27.4) | 99.3 (63.5-155) | 283 (160-433) | 1341 |
| **Race/ethnicity** | | | | | | | |
| Mexican Americans | 99-00 | 2.41 (1.55-3.73) | 2.14 (1.31-3.37) | 21.0 (10.6-30.5) | 97.6 (59.7-140) | 191 (122-320) | 721 |
| | 01-02 | 2.44 (1.51-3.94) | 1.40 (.500-3.40) | 13.1 (5.80-27.6) | 66.4 (33.5-102) | 152 (75.8-265) | 679 |
| | 03-04 | 2.54 (1.86-3.48) | 1.90 (1.00-3.40) | 14.4 (9.00-18.1) | 62.3 (40.3-99.5) | 146 (99.5-254) | 652 |
| Non-Hispanic blacks | 99-00 | 5.74 (4.55-7.24) | 8.71 (5.82-10.9) | 33.5 (22.1-52.4) | 108 (78.3-156) | 192 (149-255) | 538 |
| | 01-02 | 5.35 (4.00-7.14) | 5.30 (2.90-7.30) | 32.7 (22.0-52.4) | 128 (75.9-216) | 308 (150-436) | 706 |
| | 03-04 | 5.49 (4.05-7.46) | 4.20 (3.30-6.10) | 26.1 (13.4-49.0) | 117 (86.2-166) | 221 (177-354) | 698 |
| Non-Hispanic whites | 99-00 | 4.50 (3.26-6.22) | 4.99 (3.43-7.10) | 22.5 (17.1-34.4) | 103 (72.0-152) | 228 (177-259) | 826 |
| | 01-02 | 4.13 (3.43-4.96) | 3.40 (2.60-4.40) | 17.9 (15.5-23.8) | 98.7 (67.4-153) | 260 (153-526) | 1222 |
| | 03-04 | 5.27 (4.63-5.99) | 5.30 (4.40-6.00) | 24.2 (18.8-28.5) | 99.5 (67.6-149) | 246 (183-409) | 1070 |

Limit of detection (LOD, see Data Analysis section) for Survey years 99-00, 01-02, and 03-04 are 0 2, 0.4, and 0.4, respectively.

postmenopausal Finnish women who were omnivores and vegetarians (Uehara et al., 2000*a,b*). Vegetarian women in Boston and Helsinki (Adlercreutz et al., 1986), men and women consuming an experimental cruciferous diet (Kirkman et al., 1995), and Boston women consuming a macrobiotic diet excreted significantly higher urinary levels of these lignans (Hutchins, 1995a). Urinary enterolactone and enterodiol levels have been reported to vary by age, gender, race/ethnicity, and income (Valentin-Blasini et al., 2003). Men were shown to have higher urinary mean levels of the isoflavones and higher levels of total phytoestrogens when compared with women (Lampe et al., 1999).

Levels of isoflavones (daidzein, genistein, equol, and O-desmethylangolensin) in the NHANES 1999-2004 subsamples appeared broadly similar to those seen in young Caucasian, African-American, Latino, and Japanese women in the San Francisco Bay area (CDC, 2005; Horn-Ross et al., 1997); men and women in the United States (Valentin-Blasini et al., 2003; Lampe et al., 1999); Caucasian and Filipino women living in Hawaii (Maskarinec et al., 1998); postmenopausal women from Holland (den Tonkelaar et al., 2001) and the United Kingdom (Grace et al., 2004); omnivorous and vegetarian Helsinki women (Uehara et al., 2000 *a,b*); and premenopausal omnivorous Boston women (Hutchins, 1995*a,b*).

Isoflavone levels seen in the NHANES 1999-2004

## Urinary O-Desmethylangolensin (creatinine corrected)

Geometric mean and selected percentiles of urine concentrations (in μg/g of creatinine) for the U.S. population from the National Health and Nutrition Examination Survey.

| | Survey years | Geometric mean (95% conf. interval) | Selected percentiles (95% confidence interval) | | | | Sample size |
|---|---|---|---|---|---|---|---|
| | | | 50th | 75th | 90th | 95th | |
| **Total** | 99-00 | 4.03 (2.97-5.45) | 4.44 (3.10-6.34) | 21.8 (15.3-31.6) | 90.4 (62.9-122) | 167 (140-218) | 2271 |
| | 01-02 | 3.83 (3.32-4.43) | 3.24 (2.55-4.12) | 18.9 (16.1-23.3) | 85.2 (65.1-117) | 281 (149-412) | 2794 |
| | 03-04 | 4.58 (4.20-5.01) | 4.09 (3.53-4.59) | 19.6 (17.4-22.6) | 92.9 (76.5-120) | 201 (183-261) | 2581 |
| **Age group** | | | | | | | |
| 6-11 years | 99-00 | 6.00 (4.04-8.91) | 7.15 (3.94-16.6) | 28.8 (14.3-45.0) | 83.3 (45.0-167) | 179 (88.2-262) | 287 |
| | 01-02 | 7.03 (5.05-9.77) | 6.49 (4.24-11.6) | 29.9 (16.3-54.1) | 101 (75.3-199) | 305 (134-464) | 396 |
| | 03-04 | 6.73 (4.55-9.97) | 5.97 (4.09-8.28) | 27.7 (15.6-42.3) | 86.1 (45.2-135) | 149 (84.3-189) | 341 |
| 12-19 years | 99-00 | 4.13 (2.33-7.35) | 5.71 (2.82-11.5) | 26.0 (14.7-44.4) | 71.4 (40.8-122) | 122 (75.2-262) | 667 |
| | 01-02 | 4.57 (3.44-6.07) | 3.88 (2.82-5.32) | 26.0 (18.0-35.9) | 95.0 (61.4-129) | 259 (129-331) | 744 |
| | 03-04 | 4.76 (3.71-6.11) | 4.26 (3.13-5.97) | 22.9 (14.3-39.2) | 86.4 (49.0-149) | 185 (101-261) | 729 |
| 20 years and older | 99-00 | 3.82 (2.84-5.13) | 3.90 (2.69-5.73) | 20.2 (12.9-29.2) | 96.5 (61.8-133) | 172 (140-252) | 1317 |
| | 01-02 | 3.46 (2.95-4.04) | 2.74 (2.03-3.64) | 16.8 (13.7-20.3) | 78.9 (58.2-124) | 281 (143-467) | 1654 |
| | 03-04 | 4.35 (3.96-4.78) | 3.75 (3.23-4.35) | 18.7 (15.7-22.6) | 95.2 (76.5-131) | 228 (192-284) | 1511 |
| **Gender** | | | | | | | |
| Males | 99-00 | 3.95 (2.79-5.58) | 4.50 (2.88-6.50) | 24.5 (13.8-40.5) | 96.5 (62.4-122) | 210 (125-265) | 1087 |
| | 01-02 | 3.10 (2.48-3.86) | 2.87 (2.00-3.96) | 15.0 (10.4-19.7) | 60.7 (41.5-90.2) | 154 (96.4-301) | 1375 |
| | 03-04 | 3.83 (3.10-4.73) | 3.33 (2.41-4.35) | 15.6 (13.9-19.0) | 76.2 (51.1-99.5) | 193 (124-255) | 1240 |
| Females | 99-00 | 4.10 (3.00-5.61) | 4.17 (2.91-6.34) | 20.4 (14.4-27.2) | 86.0 (49.1-145) | 155 (100-205) | 1184 |
| | 01-02 | 4.68 (3.87-5.68) | 3.74 (2.77-4.88) | 26.8 (18.7-34.0) | 111 (70.3-205) | 399 (175-739) | 1419 |
| | 03-04 | 5.45 (4.71-6.30) | 4.81 (4.09-5.92) | 24.3 (19.6-28.9) | 106 (78.5-163) | 255 (193-343) | 1341 |
| **Race/ethnicity** | | | | | | | |
| Mexican Americans | 99-00 | 2.19 (1.49-3.24) | 1.88 (1.15-3.10) | 16.6 (11.3-25.8) | 71.2 (52.3-113) | 136 (90.5-251) | 721 |
| | 01-02 | 2.30 (1.48-3.57) | 1.45 (.770-3.37) | 11.8 (4.91-23.6) | 46.7 (31.4-87.8) | 108 (54.7-218) | 679 |
| | 03-04 | 2.30 (1.68-3.15) | 1.65 (.850-3.06) | 13.2 (6.63-21.2) | 51.6 (36.9-75.4) | 125 (84.1-165) | 652 |
| Non-Hispanic blacks | 99-00 | 3.65 (2.90-4.60) | 5.22 (3.58-6.75) | 23.8 (17.6-32.1) | 67.1 (52.1-79.7) | 116 (81.9-239) | 538 |
| | 01-02 | 3.75 (2.76-5.10) | 3.56 (2.14-5.48) | 22.8 (14.5-30.4) | 78.5 (46.5-175) | 218 (98.5-339) | 706 |
| | 03-04 | 3.89 (3.03-4.99) | 3.12 (1.96-4.96) | 17.0 (11.3-26.7) | 80.0 (58.6-104) | 159 (120-255) | 698 |
| Non-Hispanic whites | 99-00 | 4.42 (3.12-6.27) | 4.68 (3.05-7.23) | 22.3 (15.3-37.9) | 102 (57.6-148) | 177 (140-215) | 826 |
| | 01-02 | 4.08 (3.41-4.89) | 3.51 (2.45-4.57) | 21.2 (16.3-27.4) | 96.4 (69.8-126) | 300 (153-464) | 1222 |
| | 03-04 | 5.18 (4.70-5.70) | 4.58 (3.89-5.39) | 21.6 (17.4-27.7) | 103 (77.7-149) | 225 (185-272) | 1070 |

subsamples were 4 to 50 times lower than levels observed in Japanese men and women (Adlercreutz et al., 1991; CDC, 2005; Uehara et al., 2000a); Japanese women (Arai et al., 2000); postmenopausal Chinese women (Zheng et al., 1999); Singaporean women (Chen et al., 1999; Seow et al., 1998); and Japanese women living in Hawaii (Maskarinec et al., 1998). Genistein and daidzein levels in NHANES 1999-2004 subsamples were twice as high as levels reported in people consuming a carotenoid diet, but lower than levels found in people consuming a cruciferous diet; O-desmethylangolensin levels were seven times lower (Kirkman et al., 1995). Levels of genistein, daidzein, and O-desmethylangolensin in urine of people consuming a soy diet were 6 to 100 times higher than levels

found in NHANES 1999-2004 subsamples (CDC, 2005). Supplementing an omnivorous U.S. diet over a three month period with 60 grams of soy powder for female subjects increased isoflavone levels by more than thirteen-fold. (Albertazzi et al., 1999). Among U.S. adults, non-Hispanic whites were reported to have higher urinary isoflavone levels than non-Hispanic blacks or Hispanics (Valentin-Blasini et al., 2003).

Finding a measurable amount of one or more phytoestrogen metabolites in urine does not mean that the levels of the metabolites or the parent phytoestrogen cause an adverse health effect. Biomonitoring studies on the levels of phytoestrogen metabolites provide physicians and public

## Urinary Enterodiol

Geometric mean and selected percentiles of urine concentrations (in µg/L) for the U.S. population from the National Health and Nutrition Examination Survey.

| | Survey years | Geometric mean (95% conf. interval) | Selected percentiles ( 95% confidence interval) | | | | Sample size |
|---|---|---|---|---|---|---|---|
| | | | 50th | 75th | 90th | 95th | |
| Total | 99-00 | 26.6 (21.9-32.3) | 34.0 (29.4-38.7) | 78.8 (62.6-95.5) | 165 (135-215) | 266 (215-335) | 2527 |
| | 01-02 | 35.7 (32.5-39.3) | 39.4 (36.3-43.4) | 89.2 (80.7-96.9) | 181 (162-205) | 253 (223-308) | 2794 |
| | 03-04 | 39.5 (36.1-43.3) | 44.9 (40.6-50.3) | 106 (97.2-115) | 242 (212-264) | 367 (311-423) | 2594 |
| **Age group** | | | | | | | |
| 6-11 years | 99-00 | 26.5 (17.1-41.0) | 29.4 (21.2-44.2) | 78.7 (44.2-109) | 215 (91.1-279) | 276 (131-458) | 327 |
| | 01-02 | 33.6 (29.8-37.8) | 35.5 (29.4-43.7) | 78.1 (63.8-87.0) | 152 (113-171) | 203 (167-327) | 396 |
| | 03-04 | 42.0 (34.5-51.1) | 42.1 (34.4-49.2) | 91.4 (74.4-110) | 199 (126-289) | 312 (217-525) | 341 |
| 12-19 years | 99-00 | 29.8 (23.8-37.2) | 34.0 (27.4-42.0) | 84.4 (59.1-101) | 166 (112-234) | 253 (182-337) | 744 |
| | 01-02 | 35.3 (30.5-40.9) | 37.7 (34.8-43.4) | 84.2 (72.1-96.9) | 165 (128-206) | 238 (169-343) | 744 |
| | 03-04 | 45.1 (39.4-51.6) | 46.3 (38.7-56.9) | 99.5 (84.9-109) | 191 (161-269) | 325 (275-415) | 729 |
| 20 years and older | 99-00 | 26.1 (21.8-31.3) | 34.3 (29.8-38.7) | 78.3 (63.5-94.8) | 160 (132-196) | 263 (189-335) | 1456 |
| | 01-02 | 36.1 (31.8-41.0) | 40.4 (36.0-45.7) | 91.2 (79.3-105) | 190 (161-220) | 256 (224-312) | 1654 |
| | 03-04 | 38.4 (34.2-43.0) | 44.9 (40.1-51.9) | 112 (98.8-125) | 255 (215-274) | 398 (320-448) | 1524 |
| **Gender** | | | | | | | |
| Males | 99-00 | 25.3 (19.5-32.7) | 33.0 (28.0-38.0) | 72.6 (54.7-94.3) | 149 (109-219) | 258 (169-286) | 1206 |
| | 01-02 | 35.2 (31.8-39.1) | 40.5 (36.8-44.8) | 90.6 (82.3-103) | 184 (158-198) | 263 (223-338) | 1375 |
| | 03-04 | 39.7 (36.2-43.6) | 45.1 (40.5-51.1) | 102 (92.9-115) | 231 (186-266) | 361 (268-460) | 1244 |
| Females | 99-00 | 27.9 (23.4-33.3) | 36.0 (29.9-40.3) | 84.4 (71.8-97.9) | 177 (146-219) | 280 (219-375) | 1321 |
| | 01-02 | 36.2 (32.2-40.7) | 38.5 (35.3-43.4) | 87.0 (75.6-98.5) | 175 (152-212) | 248 (220-283) | 1419 |
| | 03-04 | 39.3 (33.8-45.5) | 44.9 (38.3-53.0) | 110 (97.3-124) | 250 (203-294) | 398 (309-464) | 1350 |
| **Race/ethnicity** | | | | | | | |
| Mexican Americans | 99-00 | 21.7 (19.5-24.1) | 28.0 (24.7-34.7) | 70.4 (60.8-78.8) | 143 (117-169) | 213 (169-256) | 791 |
| | 01-02 | 30.5 (25.7-36.3) | 34.0 (29.0-39.2) | 75.9 (58.8-89.7) | 159 (119-202) | 244 (192-298) | 679 |
| | 03-04 | 33.1 (26.4-41.6) | 38.7 (31.2-47.6) | 95.2 (78.1-115) | 198 (125-307) | 307 (186-480) | 653 |
| Non-Hispanic blacks | 99-00 | 25.8 (21.7-30.7) | 31.2 (24.4-35.9) | 66.0 (50.2-86.7) | 157 (122-193) | 260 (185-336) | 608 |
| | 01-02 | 35.0 (28.9-42.3) | 38.7 (33.2-49.2) | 83.7 (70.0-103) | 169 (132-191) | 225 (175-339) | 706 |
| | 03-04 | 40.4 (34.9-46.7) | 47.1 (40.4-53.7) | 100 (81.3-123) | 212 (157-254) | 293 (232-417) | 699 |
| Non-Hispanic whites | 99-00 | 29.2 (24.0-35.4) | 37.6 (31.3-43.8) | 85.8 (68.3-99.4) | 171 (138-228) | 270 (187-375) | 915 |
| | 01-02 | 35.6 (31.8-40.0) | 40.4 (36.1-44.7) | 89.6 (78.5-101) | 175 (153-198) | 254 (214-337) | 1222 |
| | 03-04 | 39.8 (35.5-44.7) | 45.8 (38.9-54.9) | 109 (95.8-126) | 255 (206-267) | 365 (294-424) | 1079 |

Limit of detection (LOD, see Data Analysis section) for Survey years 99-00, 01-02, and 03-04 are 0 8, 1.5, and 1 5, respectively.

health officials with reference values so that they can determine whether people have been exposed to higher levels of phytoestrogens than those found in the general population. Biomonitoring data can also help scientists plan and conduct research on exposure and health effects.

## Urinary Enterodiol (creatinine corrected)

Geometric mean and selected percentiles of urine concentrations (in µg/g of creatinine) for the U.S. population from the National Health and Nutrition Examination Survey.

| | Survey years | Geometric mean (95% conf. interval) | 50th | 75th | 90th | 95th | Sample size |
|---|---|---|---|---|---|---|---|
| | | | \* Selected percentiles (95% confidence interval) | | | | |
| **Total** | 99-00 | 24.2 (20.3-28.9) | 29.9 (25.0-34.7) | 70.5 (59.6-82.1) | 146 (124-177) | 240 (199-320) | 2527 |
| | 01-02 | 33.5 (30.7-36.7) | 37.6 (33.0-42.1) | 79.2 (72.6-87.3) | 149 (136-164) | 224 (197-250) | 2794 |
| | 03-04 | 37.0 (33.6-40.7) | 41.7 (37.9-45.4) | 95.9 (85.6-106) | 194 (171-213) | 294 (247-368) | 2594 |
| **Age group** | | | | | | | |
| 6-11 years | 99-00 | 27.0 (18.6-39.3) | 33.7 (21.8-43.7) | 62.7 (43.0-108) | 168 (81.6-290) | 290 (150-411) | 327 |
| | 01-02 | 38.1 (32.5-44.7) | 39.3 (30.8-53.1) | 78.3 (66.6-103) | 188 (147-244) | 304 (242-389) | 396 |
| | 03-04 | 44.7 (37.4-53.5) | 46.6 (38.5-58.3) | 93.3 (73.9-125) | 177 (128-205) | 215 (181-413) | 341 |
| 12-19 years | 99-00 | 20.1 (16.7-24.2) | 24.1 (19.6-30.1) | 55.1 (42.6-71.7) | 99.5 (91.5-116) | 158 (121-177) | 744 |
| | 01-02 | 27.2 (23.3-31.8) | 28.7 (24.9-34.9) | 62.7 (54.9-71.0) | 104 (84.2-139) | 152 (111-225) | 744 |
| | 03-04 | 33.8 (30.3-37.7) | 34.8 (33.2-38.8) | 67.6 (64.1-73.9) | 130 (107-164) | 221 (138-324) | 729 |
| 20 years and older | 99-00 | 24.7 (20.6-29.5) | 30.6 (26.0-34.8) | 73.0 (62.5-84.5) | 157 (129-184) | 242 (199-344) | 1456 |
| | 01-02 | 34.2 (30.3-38.5) | 39.6 (32.5-45.3) | 84.1 (73.8-93.3) | 152 (136-169) | 224 (193-250) | 1654 |
| | 03-04 | 36.7 (32.5-41.4) | 42.0 (37.1-47.8) | 103 (91.8-111) | 205 (173-239) | 327 (256-431) | 1524 |
| **Gender** | | | | | | | |
| Males | 99-00 | 19.8 (15.4-25.4) | 25.4 (20.0-31.4) | 55.1 (46.4-64.2) | 122 (94.6-168) | 199 (145-282) | 1206 |
| | 01-02 | 28.7 (26.0-31.7) | 31.4 (27.0-36.8) | 71.3 (64.2-78.0) | 136 (114-160) | 212 (179-259) | 1375 |
| | 03-04 | 31.1 (27.5-35.0) | 34.8 (32.3-38.5) | 78.0 (68.8-92.7) | 165 (128-211) | 249 (187-361) | 1244 |
| Females | 99-00 | 29.3 (25.0-34.4) | 35.4 (29.5-41.6) | 85.2 (74.5-92.3) | 165 (141-201) | 321 (226-370) | 1321 |
| | 01-02 | 38.9 (34.9-43.3) | 43.9 (39.3-48.7) | 88.3 (74.7-102) | 157 (139-174) | 235 (180-304) | 1419 |
| | 03-04 | 43.6 (38.3-49.7) | 49.0 (43.4-57.7) | 109 (98.8-123) | 215 (178-270) | 377 (278-443) | 1350 |
| **Race/ethnicity** | | | | | | | |
| Mexican Americans | 99-00 | 19.6 (17.3-22.2) | 23.5 (19.7-28.7) | 60.6 (49.8-77.7) | 134 (114-154) | 193 (154-227) | 791 |
| | 01-02 | 28.7 (24.5-33.7) | 31.0 (27.0-37.3) | 64.1 (55.0-77.5) | 133 (94.4-183) | 223 (143-337) | 679 |
| | 03-04 | 29.9 (23.8-37.4) | 34.0 (26.5-42.8) | 74.1 (62.0-101) | 176 (118-234) | 241 (189-364) | 653 |
| Non-Hispanic blacks | 99-00 | 16.6 (13.9-19.7) | 18.8 (14.4-22.9) | 47.3 (37.7-55.8) | 113 (85.9-145) | 169 (131-272) | 608 |
| | 01-02 | 24.5 (19.7-30.6) | 27.0 (22.6-33.4) | 57.5 (48.2-73.2) | 117 (92.2-143) | 157 (118-246) | 706 |
| | 03-04 | 28.6 (24.5-33.4) | 30.4 (26.1-36.1) | 68.3 (53.4-87.5) | 126 (96.3-191) | 203 (153-227) | 699 |
| Non-Hispanic whites | 99-00 | 28.6 (24.3-33.6) | 34.4 (28.9-39.3) | 75.8 (65.3-87.2) | 163 (130-197) | 252 (203-363) | 915 |
| | 01-02 | 35.3 (31.6-39.4) | 40.9 (34.3-46.8) | 83.3 (74.7-90.3) | 152 (136-173) | 225 (189-275) | 1222 |
| | 03-04 | 39.3 (34.4-44.8) | 45.5 (38.4-53.0) | 105 (90.2-116) | 202 (168-234) | 299 (244-374) | 1079 |

## Urinary Enterolactone

Geometric mean and selected percentiles of urine concentrations (in µg/L) for the U.S. population from the National Health and Nutrition Examination Survey.

| | Survey years | Geometric mean (95% conf. interval) | Selected percentiles ( 95% confidence interval) | | | | Sample size |
|---|---|---|---|---|---|---|---|
| | | | 50th | 75th | 90th | 95th | |
| **Total** | 99-00 | **239** (200-286) | **315** (245-381) | **726** (595-879) | **1970** (1440-2370) | **2800** (2500-3140) | 2548 |
| | 01-02 | **259** (233-287) | **350** (314-389) | **807** (739-873) | **1590** (1440-1820) | **2720** (1870-3430) | 2794 |
| | 03-04 | **298** (265-334) | **395** (331-464) | **900** (819-969) | **1790** (1560-2040) | **2620** (2360-2880) | 2594 |
| **Age group** | | | | | | | |
| 6-11 years | 99-00 | **308** (219-432) | **356** (243-474) | **721** (520-1320) | **1730** (973-2840) | **2840** (1700-3590) | 331 |
| | 01-02 | **288** (245-339) | **329** (271-412) | **680** (566-794) | **1380** (929-1620) | **2200** (1420-2550) | 396 |
| | 03-04 | **384** (287-513) | **414** (299-567) | **926** (589-1190) | **1660** (1140-2280) | **2360** (1700-3440) | 341 |
| 12-19 years | 99-00 | **250** (191-327) | **317** (242-410) | **672** (454-888) | **1760** (973-2480) | **2920** (1950-4330) | 746 |
| | 01-02 | **267** (231-308) | **321** (255-399) | **729** (617-856) | **1480** (1230-1800) | **2180** (1560-3440) | 744 |
| | 03-04 | **314** (267-369) | **400** (333-468) | **866** (736-1050) | **1690** (1410-2080) | **2620** (2000-2890) | 729 |
| 20 years and older | 99-00 | **230** (193-274) | **310** (242-375) | **734** (599-888) | **2000** (1490-2390) | **2790** (2510-3540) | 1471 |
| | 01-02 | **254** (223-289) | **357** (314-397) | **835** (760-914) | **1660** (1460-1890) | **2840** (1890-3610) | 1654 |
| | 03-04 | **286** (253-324) | **394** (311-465) | **900** (824-960) | **1820** (1560-2060) | **2630** (2350-3100) | 1524 |
| **Gender** | | | | | | | |
| Males | 99-00 | **254** (212-304) | **351** (266-418) | **778** (579-1050) | **2000** (1580-2400) | **2730** (2430-3350) | 1219 |
| | 01-02 | **262** (233-295) | **340** (314-387) | **873** (769-957) | **1810** (1490-2470) | **3050** (1990-4070) | 1375 |
| | 03-04 | **314** (280-351) | **425** (376-477) | **938** (840-1060) | **1760** (1540-2050) | **2620** (2060-3230) | 1244 |
| Females | 99-00 | **226** (180-284) | **287** (236-339) | **684** (560-799) | **1890** (1200-2460) | **2830** (2100-4330) | 1329 |
| | 01-02 | **255** (226-288) | **357** (298-397) | **759** (680-840) | **1450** (1190-1700) | **2200** (1710-2950) | 1419 |
| | 03-04 | **283** (233-343) | **371** (278-465) | **859** (706-984) | **1810** (1440-2170) | **2630** (2210-3440) | 1350 |
| **Race/ethnicity** | | | | | | | |
| Mexican Americans | 99-00 | **212** (169-265) | **281** (230-335) | **631** (539-732) | **1650** (950-2210) | **2690** (2380-3350) | 813 |
| | 01-02 | **275** (221-342) | **347** (312-395) | **778** (671-913) | **1520** (1090-1920) | **2340** (1610-2990) | 679 |
| | 03-04 | **275** (239-316) | **376** (316-435) | **849** (744-958) | **1560** (1320-1860) | **2240** (1860-3100) | 653 |
| Non-Hispanic blacks | 99-00 | **262** (196-349) | **363** (293-440) | **759** (629-925) | **1730** (1000-2420) | **2500** (1870-3280) | 605 |
| | 01-02 | **278** (226-342) | **418** (341-479) | **769** (686-853) | **1450** (1160-1840) | **2000** (1540-2420) | 706 |
| | 03-04 | **328** (285-378) | **437** (362-526) | **942** (768-1110) | **1580** (1360-1820) | **2280** (1880-2640) | 699 |
| Non-Hispanic whites | 99-00 | **247** (196-311) | **317** (240-403) | **752** (616-955) | **2040** (1600-2450) | **3000** (2460-3880) | 917 |
| | 01-02 | **267** (235-303) | **357** (307-397) | **834** (750-923) | **1630** (1420-1890) | **2780** (1820-3740) | 1222 |
| | 03-04 | **299** (254-352) | **396** (299-488) | **900** (789-996) | **1810** (1510-2140) | **2680** (2310-3230) | 1079 |

Limit of detection (LOD  see Data Analysis section) for Survey years 99-00  01-02  and 03-04 are 0 6  1.9  and 1 9  respectively.

# Urinary Enterolactone (creatinine corrected)

Geometric mean and selected percentiles of urine concentrations (in µg/g of creatinine) for the U.S. population from the National Health and Nutrition Examination Survey.

| | Survey years | Geometric mean (95% conf. interval) | 50th | 75th | 90th | 95th | Sample size |
|---|---|---|---|---|---|---|---|
| **Total** | 99-00 | 218 (184-260) | 284 (247-336) | 733 (613-869) | 1580 (1290-1830) | 2250 (1860-2830) | 2548 |
| | 01-02 | 243 (220-268) | 324 (293-360) | 756 (668-858) | 1430 (1250-1580) | 2120 (1720-2450) | 2794 |
| | 03-04 | 279 (245-317) | 371 (324-430) | 810 (697-911) | 1590 (1350-1910) | 2400 (2000-2890) | 2594 |
| **Age group** | | | | | | | |
| 6-11 years | 99-00 | 315 (238-416) | 384 (266-435) | 704 (495-1110) | 1580 (1110-2010) | 2100 (1580-3040) | 331 |
| | 01-02 | 327 (274-391) | 349 (263-478) | 738 (603-994) | 1420 (1140-1800) | 2020 (1420-2940) | 396 |
| | 03-04 | 409 (310-540) | 470 (354-632) | 904 (669-1150) | 1480 (1090-2420) | 2300 (1480-2690) | 341 |
| 12-19 years | 99-00 | 169 (133-214) | 210 (172-264) | 486 (371-615) | 1150 (742-1540) | 1850 (1310-2350) | 746 |
| | 01-02 | 206 (178-239) | 255 (223-293) | 619 (466-753) | 1110 (869-1480) | 1500 (1140-2080) | 744 |
| | 03-04 | 235 (202-273) | 285 (255-307) | 631 (533-744) | 1230 (993-1350) | 1510 (1240-2230) | 729 |
| 20 years and older | 99-00 | 217 (181-261) | 288 (249-350) | 785 (653-923) | 1640 (1330-1890) | 2310 (1890-3110) | 1471 |
| | 01-02 | 240 (213-271) | 331 (300-375) | 786 (672-915) | 1460 (1300-1630) | 2180 (1890-2470) | 1654 |
| | 03-04 | 274 (236-318) | 377 (316-448) | 823 (697-937) | 1700 (1430-1980) | 2480 (2040-3100) | 1524 |
| **Gender** | | | | | | | |
| Males | 99-00 | 199 (170-234) | 263 (228-309) | 664 (490-828) | 1380 (1200-1710) | 2030 (1780-2480) | 1219 |
| | 01-02 | 213 (191-238) | 287 (255-316) | 682 (601-764) | 1350 (1090-1580) | 1980 (1570-2550) | 1375 |
| | 03-04 | 245 (215-280) | 330 (288-372) | 729 (676-808) | 1330 (1160-1580) | 2040 (1590-2380) | 1244 |
| Females | 99-00 | 238 (191-297) | 303 (260-379) | 819 (662-968) | 1720 (1390-2010) | 2550 (1940-3390) | 1329 |
| | 01-02 | 274 (241-312) | 356 (313-407) | 833 (710-1000) | 1490 (1320-1670) | 2150 (1890-2410) | 1419 |
| | 03-04 | 314 (257-385) | 414 (327-510) | 866 (704-1090) | 1840 (1460-2280) | 2840 (2220-3910) | 1350 |
| **Race/ethnicity** | | | | | | | |
| Mexican Americans | 99-00 | 194 (165-228) | 254 (225-282) | 605 (519-695) | 1340 (969-1740) | 2100 (1620-2790) | 813 |
| | 01-02 | 259 (213-314) | 362 (296-409) | 730 (586-905) | 1240 (1010-1490) | 1630 (1240-2540) | 679 |
| | 03-04 | 248 (217-282) | 350 (310-403) | 724 (657-826) | 1320 (1020-1560) | 1820 (1460-2170) | 653 |
| Non-Hispanic blacks | 99-00 | 168 (125-226) | 214 (173-274) | 546 (411-732) | 1130 (874-1450) | 1590 (1120-2560) | 605 |
| | 01-02 | 195 (155-245) | 302 (257-331) | 562 (470-629) | 985 (821-1130) | 1490 (1080-1730) | 706 |
| | 03-04 | 233 (197-274) | 303 (276-347) | 621 (512-707) | 1050 (917-1350) | 1550 (1170-2220) | 699 |
| Non-Hispanic whites | 99-00 | 241 (194-300) | 323 (279-388) | 828 (674-997) | 1780 (1390-2020) | 2490 (1930-3340) | 917 |
| | 01-02 | 264 (232-301) | 339 (299-393) | 833 (719-944) | 1530 (1340-1880) | 2410 (1940-2800) | 1222 |
| | 03-04 | 294 (246-353) | 399 (326-488) | 836 (707-980) | 1660 (1330-2040) | 2500 (1990-3350) | 1079 |

## Urinary Equol

Geometric mean and selected percentiles of urine concentrations (in µg/L) for the U.S. population from the National Health and Nutrition Examination Survey.

| | Survey years | Geometric mean (95% conf. interval) | Selected percentiles ( 95% confidence interval) | | | | Sample size |
|---|---|---|---|---|---|---|---|
| | | | 50th | 75th | 90th | 95th | |
| Total | 99-00 | 8.37 (7.21-9.72) | 8.02 (6.27-9.90) | 17.2 (15.2-19.8) | 35.0 (28.9-41.6) | 53.7 (40.1-74.2) | 2182 |
| | 01-02 | 9.17 (7.76-10.8) | 9.00 (7.40-10.5) | 19.6 (16.6-23.5) | 42.1 (34.3-51.5) | 73.5 (53.6-89.2) | 2794 |
| | 03-04 | 8.02 (7.07-9.10) | 8.00 (6.80-9.40) | 18.2 (15.2-20.8) | 36.6 (31.3-40.0) | 64.9 (45.4-97.9) | 2590 |
| **Age group** | | | | | | | |
| 6-11 years | 99-00 | 10.5 (7.65-14.3) | 11.7 (5.43-18.6) | 24.9 (17.5-29.5) | 34.4 (29.5-53.3) | 56.1 (30.1-149) | 272 |
| | 01-02 | 12.2 (10.2-14.6) | 13.7 (11.1-16.2) | 26.2 (17.9-37.9) | 50.4 (35.0-84.3) | 85.4 (50.4-159) | 396 |
| | 03-04 | 12.4 (9.71-15.8) | 12.1 (8.40-17.8) | 24.4 (20.1-31.2) | 46.7 (33.5-82.3) | 85.8 (44.9-118) | 341 |
| 12-19 years | 99-00 | 10.9 (8.64-13.8) | 10.8 (8.52-13.4) | 22.3 (16.0-34.9) | 42.9 (34.1-71.3) | 71.6 (48.1-210) | 657 |
| | 01-02 | 10.2 (8.50-12.1) | 10.5 (8.20-12.5) | 20.5 (16.8-24.8) | 43.1 (30.1-56.1) | 70.0 (46.3-99.2) | 744 |
| | 03-04 | 10.6 (8.97-12.4) | 10.5 (8.70-12.2) | 22.6 (19.3-26.4) | 39.9 (34.8-45.1) | 61.9 (45.1-113) | 729 |
| 20 years and older | 99-00 | 7.79 (6.79-8.94) | 7.43 (5.71-8.85) | 16.0 (13.6-18.1) | 33.1 (24.4-39.7) | 52.2 (36.3-93.9) | 1253 |
| | 01-02 | 8.70 (7.29-10.4) | 8.00 (6.20-10.2) | 18.6 (15.0-22.3) | 41.3 (34.1-47.4) | 73.5 (53.9-89.0) | 1654 |
| | 03-04 | 7.28 (6.37-8.33) | 7.20 (6.00-8.70) | 16.0 (14.2-19.2) | 33.9 (28.2-38.9) | 63.0 (41.3-121) | 1520 |
| **Gender** | | | | | | | |
| Males | 99-00 | 9.15 (7.37-11.4) | 8.44 (6.36-11.2) | 19.0 (15.9-24.0) | 35.6 (29.2-54.8) | 71.3 (39.7-166) | 1042 |
| | 01-02 | 9.41 (7.99-11.1) | 9.20 (7.70-10.8) | 20.1 (16.7-26.1) | 43.1 (32.4-53.1) | 61.7 (51.8-81.5) | 1375 |
| | 03-04 | 8.56 (7.54-9.72) | 8.70 (7.20-10.2) | 19.0 (15.9-21.6) | 38.0 (31.9-44.2) | 72.6 (45.4-100) | 1240 |
| Females | 99-00 | 7.70 (6.79-8.75) | 7.57 (5.79-9.04) | 15.6 (12.7-18.9) | 33.6 (26.7-37.7) | 48.2 (37.1-62.9) | 1140 |
| | 01-02 | 8.94 (7.38-10.8) | 8.60 (6.70-10.7) | 19.0 (15.6-22.9) | 41.6 (33.3-51.5) | 79.8 (56.6-122) | 1419 |
| | 03-04 | 7.55 (6.44-8.84) | 7.30 (6.20-9.00) | 16.9 (14.7-19.8) | 33.8 (28.3-40.0) | 60.3 (42.5-116) | 1350 |
| **Race/ethnicity** | | | | | | | |
| Mexican Americans | 99-00 | 5.24 (4.77-5.76) | 4.51 (3.65-5.18) | 9.48 (7.96-10.3) | 18.5 (14.5-22.6) | 30.9 (21.6-48.4) | 726 |
| | 01-02 | 7.22 (6.04-8.62) | 6.50 (4.40-9.10) | 14.2 (11.3-20.1) | 31.4 (21.1-41.0) | 42.4 (38.1-60.2) | 679 |
| | 03-04 | 6.08 (5.08-7.28) | 5.70 (4.70-6.80) | 12.5 (9.80-15.4) | 26.1 (18.1-39.7) | 43.6 (34.3-88.2) | 653 |
| Non-Hispanic blacks | 99-00 | 6.73 (5.20-8.71) | 6.24 (3.86-10.0) | 15.1 (12.7-17.6) | 27.6 (19.4-35.6) | 36.4 (28.9-49.4) | 514 |
| | 01-02 | 7.15 (6.06-8.43) | 6.10 (4.70-7.60) | 14.7 (12.0-18.7) | 30.9 (22.8-41.9) | 45.7 (36.1-90.5) | 706 |
| | 03-04 | 7.35 (6.16-8.79) | 7.90 (6.00-9.60) | 16.5 (14.2-18.3) | 32.0 (25.1-37.5) | 47.0 (37.8-68.2) | 696 |
| Non-Hispanic whites | 99-00 | 9.26 (7.80-11.0) | 8.98 (6.73-11.9) | 19.0 (16.1-22.8) | 36.2 (30.1-45.4) | 56.1 (42.1-89.4) | 758 |
| | 01-02 | 9.91 (7.95-12.4) | 10.0 (7.30-12.6) | 22.0 (17.4-27.4) | 44.4 (35.1-57.5) | 74.4 (55.1-107) | 1222 |
| | 03-04 | 8.52 (7.26-10.0) | 8.80 (7.10-10.3) | 19.3 (15.4-23.0) | 37.7 (31.7-44.2) | 73.1 (46.7-120) | 1078 |

Limit of detection (LOD  see Data Analysis section) for Survey years 99-00  01-02  and 03-04 are 3 0  3.3  and 3 3  respectively.

## Urinary Equol (creatinine corrected)

Geometric mean and selected percentiles of urine concentrations (in μg/g of creatinine) for the U.S. population from the National Health and Nutrition Examination Survey.

| | Survey years | Geometric mean (95% conf. interval) | 50th | 75th | 90th | 95th | Sample size |
|---|---|---|---|---|---|---|---|
| **Total** | 99-00 | 7.70 (6.82-8.70) | 7.96 (6.87-9.35) | 16.2 (13.2-18.6) | 30.6 (26.9-35.1) | 50.3 (41.8-67.3) | 2182 |
| | 01-02 | 8.60 (7.26-10.2) | 7.98 (6.62-9.76) | 17.6 (14.8-21.8) | 37.8 (30.3-46.3) | 62.6 (50.0-85.0) | 2794 |
| | 03-04 | 7.52 (6.83-8.29) | 7.29 (6.56-8.18) | 14.6 (13.3-15.7) | 27.8 (24.7-31.9) | 50.6 (39.9-75.1) | 2590 |
| **Age group** | | | | | | | |
| 6-11 years | 99-00 | 10.3 (7.83-13.5) | 11.4 (7.46-16.3) | 22.6 (14.7-27.2) | 32.7 (25.5-46.0) | 47.8 (32.7-150) | 272 |
| | 01-02 | 13.9 (11.2-17.2) | 14.0 (10.6-17.0) | 28.8 (19.6-39.8) | 54.4 (34.9-99.8) | 88.2 (56.8-186) | 396 |
| | 03-04 | 13.2 (10.9-15.9) | 13.2 (9.19-17.5) | 24.2 (20.6-28.0) | 41.6 (35.2-64.1) | 93.5 (45.4-117) | 341 |
| 12-19 years | 99-00 | 7.61 (6.17-9.39) | 8.02 (6.72-9.29) | 14.0 (11.4-20.4) | 27.5 (20.8-38.3) | 47.4 (27.5-149) | 657 |
| | 01-02 | 7.83 (6.68-9.17) | 7.77 (6.29-9.13) | 17.4 (14.9-19.2) | 31.9 (25.3-41.7) | 54.3 (33.0-76.7) | 744 |
| | 03-04 | 7.91 (6.59-9.49) | 8.11 (6.80-9.09) | 14.5 (11.8-17.5) | 30.1 (21.0-38.2) | 40.6 (32.6-66.9) | 729 |
| 20 years and older | 99-00 | 7.45 (6.60-8.41) | 7.63 (6.34-9.22) | 15.3 (12.7-17.7) | 30.8 (25.0-37.2) | 53.2 (41.2-71.8) | 1253 |
| | 01-02 | 8.23 (6.93-9.79) | 7.52 (5.97-9.56) | 16.6 (14.0-20.8) | 36.4 (29.3-42.9) | 58.7 (47.9-85.0) | 1654 |
| | 03-04 | 6.98 (6.30-7.73) | 6.76 (6.05-7.65) | 13.6 (12.5-14.9) | 24.6 (21.9-29.4) | 42.8 (35.7-81.6) | 1520 |
| **Gender** | | | | | | | |
| Males | 99-00 | 7.01 (5.93-8.29) | 7.31 (5.63-8.78) | 13.8 (11.7-17.6) | 29.3 (21.4-41.8) | 54.1 (35.8-81.0) | 1042 |
| | 01-02 | 7.66 (6.39-9.18) | 7.43 (5.81-9.16) | 16.2 (14.0-19.4) | 32.9 (27.9-40.4) | 54.3 (37.8-67.1) | 1375 |
| | 03-04 | 6.71 (6.02-7.47) | 6.63 (5.78-7.29) | 13.3 (11.9-15.5) | 25.7 (23.1-30.3) | 51.1 (37.1-76.7) | 1240 |
| Females | 99-00 | 8.41 (7.33-9.66) | 8.71 (7.33-10.1) | 17.7 (15.1-20.0) | 31.6 (27.5-37.2) | 46.3 (41.0-56.5) | 1140 |
| | 01-02 | 9.60 (7.99-11.5) | 8.66 (6.97-10.6) | 19.2 (15.7-23.7) | 41.7 (32.3-55.9) | 85.0 (61.7-115) | 1419 |
| | 03-04 | 8.38 (7.39-9.51) | 8.29 (7.03-9.28) | 15.1 (14.0-16.6) | 30.6 (25.0-32.5) | 45.4 (38.7-102) | 1350 |
| **Race/ethnicity** | | | | | | | |
| Mexican Americans | 99-00 | 4.89 (4.36-5.47) | 4.73 (3.90-5.27) | 8.85 (8.18-9.91) | 22.3 (16.5-26.8) | 37.1 (25.3-57.6) | 726 |
| | 01-02 | 6.79 (5.82-7.92) | 6.81 (5.55-8.04) | 14.9 (11.7-17.8) | 29.1 (22.9-36.0) | 41.3 (31.4-47.1) | 679 |
| | 03-04 | 5.48 (4.60-6.54) | 4.72 (3.95-5.78) | 10.1 (7.76-13.4) | 24.4 (17.2-30.9) | 35.6 (27.6-102) | 653 |
| Non-Hispanic blacks | 99-00 | 4.36 (3.41-5.57) | 4.57 (2.94-6.23) | 10.2 (7.96-12.0) | 17.1 (14.8-19.8) | 26.0 (19.6-32.0) | 514 |
| | 01-02 | 5.01 (4.26-5.89) | 4.48 (3.80-5.42) | 11.0 (8.80-13.0) | 22.7 (16.5-29.3) | 35.4 (24.8-46.7) | 706 |
| | 03-04 | 5.23 (4.44-6.16) | 5.28 (4.67-6.09) | 10.3 (8.61-12.3) | 20.2 (17.1-23.9) | 29.4 (23.9-42.3) | 696 |
| Non-Hispanic whites | 99-00 | 9.13 (7.85-10.6) | 9.51 (7.63-11.2) | 18.0 (15.2-21.6) | 35.4 (29.5-41.3) | 56.5 (46.0-73.0) | 758 |
| | 01-02 | 9.81 (7.93-12.1) | 9.17 (7.06-12.2) | 19.8 (15.4-25.6) | 41.3 (30.7-55.9) | 66.4 (56.8-85.0) | 1222 |
| | 03-04 | 8.40 (7.50-9.41) | 8.17 (7.13-9.19) | 15.6 (14.1-17.1) | 30.6 (25.0-32.8) | 56.8 (38.0-107) | 1078 |

## Urinary Genistein

Geometric mean and selected percentiles of urine concentrations (in µg/L) for the U.S. population from the National Health and Nutrition Examination Survey.

| | Survey years | Geometric mean (95% conf. interval) | Selected percentiles ( 95% confidence interval) | | | | Sample size |
|---|---|---|---|---|---|---|---|
| | | | 50th | 75th | 90th | 95th | |
| **Total** | 99-00 | **24.4** (19.7-30.3) | **27.0** (22.5-32.8) | **93.6** (75.8-118) | **284** (244-331) | **563** (413-709) | 2557 |
| | 01-02 | **33.0** (30.1-36.2) | **29.0** (26.8-31.8) | **92.5** (77.9-109) | **306** (240-372) | **619** (523-719) | 2794 |
| | 03-04 | **31.1** (29.0-33.3) | **26.2** (23.9-29.7) | **87.8** (78.8-102) | **286** (239-313) | **528** (402-610) | 2594 |
| **Age group** | | | | | | | |
| 6-11 years | 99-00 | **27.6** (21.1-36.1) | **31.9** (18.1-42.6) | **104** (67.6-151) | **220** (151-315) | **376** (272-725) | 331 |
| | 01-02 | **39.2** (33.4-46.0) | **31.7** (25.8-39.6) | **94.1** (62.3-158) | **258** (190-426) | **502** (258-830) | 396 |
| | 03-04 | **33.6** (27.8-40.6) | **29.3** (23.1-37.8) | **79.4** (56.7-111) | **193** (146-274) | **351** (207-376) | 341 |
| 12-19 years | 99-00 | **43.7** (34.2-55.7) | **45.4** (34.3-60.5) | **138** (93.7-179) | **319** (245-464) | **547** (321-777) | 754 |
| | 01-02 | **34.1** (27.2-42.8) | **29.0** (26.1-32.9) | **90.6** (71.5-113) | **278** (216-363) | **470** (360-687) | 744 |
| | 03-04 | **34.7** (29.3-41.0) | **29.0** (23.4-37.6) | **111** (69.3-141) | **304** (206-376) | **530** (358-671) | 729 |
| 20 years and older | 99-00 | **21.9** (17.6-27.2) | **24.0** (21.7-28.4) | **86.2** (67.5-108) | **293** (235-343) | **566** (412-744) | 1472 |
| | 01-02 | **32.1** (28.8-35.8) | **28.8** (25.4-33.4) | **93.4** (77.3-110) | **312** (235-389) | **627** (537-790) | 1654 |
| | 03-04 | **30.2** (27.8-32.8) | **25.9** (22.3-29.8) | **87.8** (77.9-103) | **296** (239-321) | **557** (412-653) | 1524 |
| **Gender** | | | | | | | |
| Males | 99-00 | **29.8** (22.2-40.0) | **31.9** (26.3-37.2) | **108** (79.1-151) | **335** (257-440) | **709** (437-981) | 1222 |
| | 01-02 | **32.2** (27.9-37.2) | **29.5** (25.4-33.7) | **91.2** (73.4-103) | **239** (190-331) | **474** (335-719) | 1375 |
| | 03-04 | **33.7** (29.6-38.4) | **27.3** (23.4-33.0) | **92.6** (68.6-124) | **310** (228-351) | **562** (443-653) | 1244 |
| Females | 99-00 | **20.3** (17.0-24.2) | **23.1** (20.1-26.3) | **84.7** (59.6-105) | **242** (203-288) | **446** (339-619) | 1335 |
| | 01-02 | **33.7** (30.9-36.8) | **28.7** (26.0-32.3) | **97.0** (79.9-118) | **387** (253-500) | **666** (598-807) | 1419 |
| | 03-04 | **28.7** (25.5-32.4) | **25.0** (22.4-28.4) | **85.0** (71.2-106) | **256** (218-308) | **467** (356-620) | 1350 |
| **Race/ethnicity** | | | | | | | |
| Mexican Americans | 99-00 | **31.1** (25.1-38.5) | **30.0** (25.1-37.3) | **117** (83.9-179) | **328** (248-479) | **573** (419-1180) | 819 |
| | 01-02 | **28.3** (22.0-36.4) | **25.6** (19.6-32.5) | **74.8** (48.8-111) | **225** (174-314) | **424** (323-523) | 679 |
| | 03-04 | **31.1** (27.5-35.2) | **25.2** (19.1-32.6) | **83.2** (63.6-120) | **319** (252-537) | **653** (537-851) | 653 |
| Non-Hispanic blacks | 99-00 | **26.7** (19.2-37.0) | **32.9** (24.4-41.5) | **103** (84.8-137) | **257** (213-367) | **495** (329-926) | 608 |
| | 01-02 | **37.6** (27.4-51.6) | **35.3** (23.6-49.5) | **95.5** (71.1-142) | **378** (192-530) | **598** (375-1120) | 706 |
| | 03-04 | **32.3** (24.0-43.4) | **27.4** (18.8-44.9) | **84.8** (60.5-113) | **279** (163-412) | **514** (323-852) | 699 |
| Non-Hispanic whites | 99-00 | **23.6** (19.1-29.3) | **25.6** (21.7-32.0) | **91.4** (68.0-122) | **288** (227-353) | **566** (395-734) | 917 |
| | 01-02 | **30.9** (27.8-34.4) | **27.6** (24.6-30.8) | **89.7** (71.1-105) | **278** (226-365) | **626** (485-755) | 1222 |
| | 03-04 | **30.8** (28.2-33.6) | **26.2** (22.6-31.0) | **93.6** (78.8-112) | **279** (225-313) | **504** (376-610) | 1079 |

Limit of detection (LOD  see Data Analysis section) for Survey years 99-00  01-02  and 03-04 are 0 3  0.8  and 0 8  respectively.

## Urinary Genistein (creatinine corrected)

Geometric mean and selected percentiles of urine concentrations (in µg/g of creatinine) for the U.S. population from the National Health and Nutrition Examination Survey.

| | Survey years | Geometric mean (95% conf. interval) | 50th | 75th | 90th | 95th | Sample size |
|---|---|---|---|---|---|---|---|
| **Total** | 99-00 | **22.3** (17.7-28.1) | **23.8** (18.8-28.9) | **84.7** (67.2-105) | **222** (182-279) | **381** (334-497) | 2557 |
| | 01-02 | **30.9** (28.5-33.6) | **25.9** (23.4-29.2) | **83.3** (72.2-96.3) | **256** (211-296) | **427** (375-490) | 2794 |
| | 03-04 | **29.1** (27.3-31.0) | **24.6** (21.3-27.5) | **77.7** (67.3-90.9) | **231** (203-279) | **510** (388-619) | 2594 |
| **Age group** | | | | | | | |
| 6-11 years | 99-00 | **28.3** (21.1-37.9) | **27.8** (15.8-41.3) | **94.3** (60.5-145) | **209** (148-317) | **490** (279-895) | 331 |
| | 01-02 | **44.5** (37.0-53.5) | **37.9** (29.7-49.0) | **112** (76.5-146) | **252** (173-371) | **504** (252-713) | 396 |
| | 03-04 | **35.8** (29.7-43.0) | **35.4** (24.9-43.2) | **78.6** (60.9-119) | **172** (130-243) | **297** (168-618) | 341 |
| 12-19 years | 99-00 | **29.4** (22.3-38.8) | **32.0** (23.8-41.6) | **83.2** (64.1-104) | **184** (130-295) | **336** (184-816) | 754 |
| | 01-02 | **26.3** (21.3-32.5) | **21.0** (17.8-26.5) | **66.2** (47.9-91.5) | **200** (149-298) | **321** (261-435) | 744 |
| | 03-04 | **25.9** (21.8-30.9) | **21.8** (17.0-29.1) | **65.6** (51.0-83.1) | **201** (145-313) | **366** (297-455) | 729 |
| 20 years and older | 99-00 | **20.6** (16.3-26.2) | **21.6** (17.7-26.2) | **83.1** (64.9-107) | **234** (190-287) | **381** (325-562) | 1472 |
| | 01-02 | **30.4** (27.6-33.4) | **24.8** (21.9-30.0) | **83.2** (68.5-99.0) | **269** (208-328) | **435** (374-518) | 1654 |
| | 03-04 | **28.9** (26.7-31.3) | **24.0** (20.1-27.5) | **78.5** (66.1-92.9) | **253** (209-302) | **542** (399-673) | 1524 |
| **Gender** | | | | | | | |
| Males | 99-00 | **23.3** (16.8-32.3) | **23.8** (17.5-32.2) | **86.2** (64.7-115) | **236** (178-330) | **523** (323-889) | 1222 |
| | 01-02 | **26.2** (23.1-29.8) | **22.1** (19.4-26.0) | **67.6** (57.4-78.1) | **186** (144-237) | **350** (278-418) | 1375 |
| | 03-04 | **26.4** (22.8-30.5) | **21.5** (17.3-26.2) | **70.1** (51.1-90.5) | **203** (159-235) | **415** (346-600) | 1244 |
| Females | 99-00 | **21.3** (17.5-26.0) | **23.2** (17.5-29.3) | **83.1** (57.2-106) | **211** (154-283) | **357** (283-398) | 1335 |
| | 01-02 | **36.2** (32.8-39.9) | **29.6** (25.2-34.3) | **107** (88.4-129) | **321** (269-355) | **547** (427-729) | 1419 |
| | 03-04 | **31.9** (28.7-35.5) | **27.1** (23.6-31.6) | **87.1** (71.1-102) | **278** (209-324) | **548** (363-763) | 1350 |
| **Race/ethnicity** | | | | | | | |
| Mexican Americans | 99-00 | **28.4** (23.3-34.7) | **27.9** (22.5-35.0) | **109** (91.5-137) | **257** (209-380) | **562** (257-981) | 819 |
| | 01-02 | **26.6** (21.6-32.9) | **21.0** (16.1-28.9) | **61.6** (50.6-76.8) | **205** (147-270) | **372** (271-479) | 679 |
| | 03-04 | **28.0** (24.8-31.8) | **23.5** (18.5-28.1) | **69.2** (52.3-92.8) | **254** (187-390) | **608** (417-764) | 653 |
| Non-Hispanic blacks | 99-00 | **17.1** (12.4-23.7) | **19.5** (15.7-26.1) | **59.5** (43.1-93.7) | **179** (132-245) | **299** (222-446) | 608 |
| | 01-02 | **26.4** (19.3-36.1) | **22.7** (16.4-33.6) | **69.4** (42.2-115) | **217** (139-317) | **384** (217-747) | 706 |
| | 03-04 | **22.8** (18.1-28.8) | **19.6** (14.3-27.1) | **55.0** (39.6-78.1) | **182** (107-240) | **311** (210-514) | 699 |
| Non-Hispanic whites | 99-00 | **23.2** (18.5-29.0) | **24.9** (19.0-31.7) | **86.1** (68.4-105) | **232** (178-295) | **381** (325-523) | 917 |
| | 01-02 | **30.6** (28.2-33.2) | **25.4** (22.7-29.5) | **82.0** (68.3-96.3) | **248** (207-320) | **427** (365-518) | 1222 |
| | 03-04 | **30.4** (27.9-33.0) | **26.2** (21.5-31.4) | **79.6** (69.1-99.6) | **238** (195-321) | **534** (352-688) | 1079 |

# References

Adlercreutz CH, Goldin BR, Gorbach SL, Hockerstedt KA, Watanabe S, Hamalainen EK, et al. Soybean phytoestrogens intake and cancer risk. J Nutr 1995*a*;125(3 Suppl):757S-770S.

Adlercreutz H, Fotsis T, Bannwart C, Wahala K, Makela T, Brunow G, et al. Determination of urinary lignans and phytoestrogen metabolites, potential antiestrogens and anticarcinogens in urine of women on various habitual diets. J Steroid Biochem 1986;25:791-797.

Adlercreutz H, Honjo H, Higashi A, Fotsis T, Hamalainen E, Hasegawa T, et al. Urinary excretion of lignans and isoflavone phytoestrogens in Japanese men and women consuming a traditional Japanese diet. Am J Clin Nutr 1991;54:1093-1100.

Albertazzi P, Pansini F, Bottazi M, Bonaccorsi G, De Aloysio D, Morton MS. Dietary soy supplementation and phytoestrogen levels. Obstet Gynecol 1999;94(2):229-231.

Arai Y, Uehara M, Sato Y, Kimura M, Eboshida A, Adlercreutz H, et al. Comparison of isoflavones among dietary intake, plasma concentration and urinary excretion for accurate estimation of phytoestrogen intake. J Epidemiol 2000;10:127-135.

Cassidy A, Brown JE, Hawdon A, Faughnan MA, King LJ, Millward J, et al. Factors affecting the bioavailability of soy isoflavones in humans after ingestion of physiologically relevant levels from different soy foods. J. Nutr 2006;136:45-51.

Centers for Disease Control and Prevention (CDC). Third National Report on Human Exposure to Environmental Chemicals. Atlanta (GA). 2005

Chen Z, Zheng W, Custer LJ, Dai Q, Shu X, Jin F, et al. Usual dietary consumption of soy foods and its correlation with the excretion rate of isoflavonoids in overnight urine samples among Chinese women in Shanghai. Nutr Cancer 1999;33:82-87.

Cornwell T, Cohick W, Raskin I. Dietary phytoestrogens and health. Phytochemistry 2004;65(8):995-1016.

den Tonkelaar I, Keinan-Boker L, Van't Veer P, Arts CJM, Adlercreutz H, Thijssen JHH, et al. Urinary phytoestrogens and postmenopausal breast cancer risk. Cancer Epidemiol Biomarkers and Prev 2001;10:223-228.

Dixon RA, Ferreira D. Genistein. Phytochemistry 2002;60(3):205-211.

Doerge DR, Sheehan DM. Goitrogenic and estrogenic activity of soy isoflavones. Environ Health Perspect 2002;110 (Suppl 3):349-353.

Doerge DR, Chang HC, Churchwell MI, Holder CL. Analysis of soy isoflavone conjugation in vitro and in human blood using liquid chromatography-mass spectrometry. Drug Metab Disp 2000;283:298-307.

Erdman JW Jr, Badger TM, Lampe JW, Setchell KDR, Messina M. Not all soy products are created equal: Caution needed in interpretation of research results. J Nutr 2004;134:1229S-1233S.

Grace PB, Taylor JI, Low Y, Luben RN, Mulligan AA, Botting NP, et al. Phytoestrogen concentrations in serum and spot urine as biomarkers for dietary phytoestrogen intake and their relation to breast cancer risk in European prospective investigation of cancer and nutrition—Norfolk. Cancer Epidemiol Biomarkers and Prev 2004;13:698-708.

Horn-Ross PL, Barnes S, Kirk M, Coward L, Parsonnet J, Hiatt RA. Urinary phytoestrogen levels in young women from a multiethnic population. Cancer Epidemiol Biomarkers Prev 1997;6:339-345.

Hutchins AM, Lampe JW, Martini MC, Campbell DR, Slavin JL. Vegetables, fruits and legumes: effect on isoflavonoid phytoestrogen and lignan excretion J Am Diet Assoc 1995*a*;95:769-774.

Hutchins AM, Slavin JL, Lampe JW. Urinary isoflavonoid phytoestrogen and lignan excretion after consumption of fermented and unfermented soy products. J Am Diet Assoc 1995*b*;95(5):545-551.

Karr SC, Lampe JW, Hutchins AM, Slavin JL. Urinary isoflavonoid excretion in humans is dose dependent at low to moderate levels of soy-protein consumption. Am J Clin Nutr 1997;66:46-51.

Kirkman LM, Lampe JW, Campbell D, Martini M, Slavin J. Urinary lignan and isoflavonoid excretion in men and women consuming vegetable and soy diets. Nutr Cancer 1995;24:1-12.

Klein KO. Isoflavones, soy-based infant formulas, and relevance to endocrine function. Nutr Rev 1998;56:193-204.

Lampe JW, Gustafson DR, Hutchins AM, Martini MG, Li S, Wahala K, et al. Urinary isoflavonoid and lignan excretion on a western diet: relation to soy, vegetable and fruit intake. Cancer Epidemiol Biomarkers and Prev 1999;8:699-707.

Lu LJ, Grady JJ, Marshall MV, Ramanujam VM, Anderson KE. Altered time course of urinary daidzein and genistein excretion during chronic soya diet in healthy male subjects. Nutr Cancer 1995;24:311-323.

Lund TD, Munson DJ, Haldy ME, Setchell KDR, Lephart ED, Handa RJ. Equol is a novel anti-androgen that inhibits prostate growth and hormone feedback. Biol Reprod 2004;70:1188-1195.

Magee PJ and Rowland IR. Phyto-oestrogens, their mechanism of action: current evidence for a role in breast and prostate cancer. Br J Nutr 2004;91:513-531.

Maskarinec G, Singh S, Meng L, Franke AA. Dietary soy intake and urinary isoflavone excretion among women from a multiethnic population. Cancer Epidemiol Biomarkers and Prev 1998;7:613-619.

Messina M, McCaskill-Stevens W, Lampe JW. Addressing the soy and breast cancer relationship: Review, commentary, and workshop proceedings. J Natl Cancer Inst 2006;98(18):1275-1284.

The North American Menopause Society (NAMS). The role of isoflavones in menopausal health. Concensus opinion of The North American Menopause Society. Menopause 2000;7(4):215-229.

Nedrow A, Miller J, Walker M, Nygren P, Huffman LH, Nelson HD. Comlementary and alternative therapies for the management of menopause-related symptoms. A systematic evidence review. Arch Intern Med 2006;166:1453-1465.

Nesbitt PD, Lam Y, Thompson LU. Human metabolism of mammalian lignan precursors in raw and processed flaxseed. Am J Clin Nutr 1999;69(3):549-555.

Rowland I, Faughnan M, Hoey L, Wahala K, Williamson G, Cassidy A. Bioavailability of phyto-estrogens Br J Nutr 2003;89 (Suppl 1):S45-S58.

Rowland IR, Wiseman H, Sanders TAB, Adlercreutz H, Bowey Ea. Interindividual variation in metabolism of soy isoflavones and lignans: Influence of habitual diet on equol production by the gut microflora. Nutr Cancer 2000;36:27-32.

Rozman KK, Bhatia J, Calafat AM, Chambers C, Culty M, Etzel RA, et al. NTP-CERHR expert panel report on the reproductive and developmental toxicity of soy formula. Birth Defects Res (Part B) 2006a;77:280-397.

Rozman KK, Bhatia J, Calafat AM, Chambers C, Culty M, Etzel RA, et al. NTP-CERHR expert panel report on the reproductive and developmental toxicity of genistein. Birth Defects Res (Part B) 2006b;77:485-638.

Sacks FM, Lichtenstein A, Van Horn L, Harris W, Kris-Etherton P, Winston M. Soy protein, isoflavones, and cardiovascular health. An American Heart Association Science Advisory for Professionals from the Nutrition Committee. Circulation 2006;113:1034-1044.

Seow A, Shi CY, Franke AA, Hankin JH, Lee H, Yu MC. Isoflavonoid levels in spot urine are associated with frequency of dietary soy intake in a population-based sample of middle-aged and older Chinese in Singapore. Cancer Epidemiol Biomarkers Prev 1998;7:135-140.

Setchell KD, Brown NM, Desai P, Zimmer-Nechemias L, Wolfe BE, Brashear WT, et al. Bioavailability of pure isoflavones in healthy humans and analysis of commercial soy isoflavone supplements. J Nutr 2001;131(4 Suppl):1362S-1375S.

Setchell KDR, Brown NM, Desai PB, Zimmer-Nechimias L, Wolfe B, Jakate AS, et al. Bioavailability, disposition, and dose-response effects of soy isoflavones when consumed by healthy women at physiologically typical dietary intakes. J Nutr. 2003b; 133:1027-1035.

Setchell KDR, Brown NM, Lydeking-Olsen E. The clinical importance of the metabolite equol—a clue to the effectiveness of soy and its isoflavones. J Nutr 2002;132(12):3577-3584.

Setchell KDR, Cassidy A. Dietary isoflavones: biological effects and relevance to human health. J Nutr 1999;129(3):758S-767S.

Setchell KDR, Faughnan MS, Acades T, Zimmer-Nechemias L, Brown NM, Wolfe BE, et al. Comparing the pharmacokinetics of daidzein and genistein with the use of 13C-labeled tracers in premenopausal women. Am J Clin Nutr 2003a;77:411-419.

Setchell KDR, Zimmer-Nechemias L, Cai J, Heubi JE. Exposure of infants to phyto-oestrogens from soy-based infant formula. Lancet 1997;350(9070):23-27.

Sirtori CR, Arnold A, Johnson SK. Phytoestrogens: End of a tale? Ann Med 2005;37:423-438.

Slavin JL, Karr SC, Hutchins AM, Lampe JW. Influence of soybean processing, habitual diet, and soy dose on urinary isoflavonoid excretion. Am J Clin Nutr 1998;68(6 Suppl):1492S-1495S.

Strom BL, Schinnar R, Ziegler EE, Barnhart KT, Sammel MD, Macones GA, et al. Exposure to soy-based formula in infancy and endocrinological and reproductive outcomes in young adulthood. JAMA 2001;286:807-814.

Uehara M, Arai Y, Watanabe S, Adlercreutz H. Comparison of plasma and urinary phytoestrogens in Japanese and Finnish women by time-resolved fluoroimmunoassay. Biofactors 2000a;12:217-225.

Uehara M, Lapcik O, Hampl R, Al-maharik N, Makela T, Wahala K, et al. Rapid analysis of phytoestrogens in human by time-resolved fluoroimmunoassay. J Steroid Biochem Mol Biol (Oxford) 2000b;72:273-282.

Vafeiadou K, Hall WL, Williams CM. Does genotype and equol-production status affect response to isoflavones? Data from a pan-European study on the effects of isoflavones on cardiovascular risk markers in post-menopausal women. Proc Nutr Soc 2006;65:106-115.

Valentin-Blasini L, Blount B, Caudill S, ,Needham L. Urinary and serum concentrations of seven phytoestrogens in a human reference population subset. J Expos Anal Environ Epidemiol 2003;13:276-282.

Zheng W, Dai Q, Custer LJ, Shu XO, Wen WQ, Jin F, et, al. Urinary excretion of isoflavonoids and the risk of breast cancer. Cancer Epidemiol Biomarkers Prev 1999;8(1):35-40.

# Polybrominated Diphenyl Ethers and 2,2',4,4',5,5'-Hexabromobiphenyl (BB-153)

## General Information

Polybrominated diphenyl ethers (PBDEs) are a class of synthetic chemicals first produced commercially in the 1970s. They are added to products such as foam padding, textiles, or plastics to retard combustion. 2,2',4,4',5,5'-hexabromobiphenyl (BB-153) is a brominated biphenyl that was used as a flame retardant in the U.S. until the 1970s. Its use was phased out following an accidental contamination of cattle feed in the state of Michigan with the contamination extending to other animals, the environment, and into humans (Fries, 1985).

Three major commercial mixtures of PBDEs have been produced and used. These are named for the average number of bromines attached to the diphenyl ether structure, e.g., pentaBDE. The pentaBDE technical mixture contains 50-60% of PBDE congeners with five bromines, 24-38% with four bromines (tetraBDEs) and 4-8% with six bromines (hexaBDE), though reports on mixtures vary (Alaee et al., 2003; Birnbaum and Staskal, 2004; OECD, 1994). Commercial pentaBDEs are often added to polyurethane foams used in mattresses, upholstered furniture, and carpet padding. OctaBDE technical mixtures contain 10-12% of PBDE congeners with six bromines, 43-44% with seven bromines, 31-35% with eight bromines and 10-11% with nine bromines. OctaBDE mixtures are added to acrylonitrile-butadiene-styrene used in computer and appliance casings, and also to some polyolefins and nylon. DecaBDE is the most widely used PBDE globally and greater than 97% of its content includes PBDEs with ten bromines. It is added to polystyrene, polybutylene, nylon, polypropylene, and other thermoelastic polymers used in adhesives, wire insulation, casings for televisions and computers, and in some non-clothing textiles (OECD, 1994; Sjödin et al., 2003; WSDH, 2004). PBDEs are often combined with antimony trioxide to enhance the fire protection offered by the PBDEs. For example, protected polypropylene can contain 23% decaBDE and 8% antimony trioxide by weight. PBDE content in protected products varies from 3-33% (Gill et al., 2004).

PBDE production makes up about 25% of all fire retardant production. In 2000, global production was 67,000 metric tons annually with about 80% of the total being decaBDE (Birnbaum and Staskal, 2004; WSDH, 2004). Most of the pentaBDE produced has been used within the U.S. About 40% and 44% of the global production of octaBDE and decaBDE were also used in the U.S. Since PBDEs are not chemically bound to the flame-retarded material, they can enter the environment from volatilization, leaching, or degradation of PBDE-containing products (Gill et al., 2004). Also, PBDEs can enter the environment from manufacturer-related releases. When thermally decomposed, PBDEs can produce polybrominated dibenzo-*p*-dioxins and dibenzofurans (Watanabe and Sakai, 2003). Manufacturers of pentaBDE and octaBDE in the U.S. were to have phased out production of these chemicals by 2004 and U.S. EPA issued a rule to prevent new production (U.S. EPA, 2005). PBDEs are generally persistent in the environment and have been measured in aquatic sediments and aquatic and terrestrial animals, especially in fish where PBDEs are known to bioconcentrate. Several studies of stored biologic specimens have shown dramatic increases in PBDE concentrations over the last several decades, for example, in archived bird eggs (Norstrom et al., 2002).

Human exposure to PBDEs is thought to result from

## Polybrominated Diphenyl Ethers in this *Report*

| Polybrominated Diphenyl Ether (IUPAC number) | CAS Number |
|---|---|
| Serum 2,2',4-Tribromodiphenyl ether (BDE 17) | 147217-75-2 |
| Serum 2,4,4'-Tribromodiphenyl ether (BDE 28) | 41318-75-6 |
| Serum 2,2',4,4'-Tetrabromodiphenyl ether (BDE 47) | 5436-43-1 |
| Serum 2,3',4,4'-Tetrabromodiphenyl ether (BDE 66) | 189084-61-5 |
| Serum 2,2',3,4,4'-Pentabromodiphenyl ether (BDE 85) | 182346-21-0 |
| Serum 2,2',4,4',5-Pentabromodiphenyl ether (BDE 99) | 60328-60-9 |
| Serum 2,2',4,4',6-Pentabromodiphenyl ether (BDE 100) | 189084-64-8 |
| Serum 2,2',4,4',5,5'-Hexabromodiphenyl ether (BDE 153) | 68631-49-2 |
| Serum 2,2',4,4',5,6'-Hexabromodiphenyl ether (BDE 154) | 207122-15-4 |
| Serum 2,2',3,4,4',5',6-Heptabromodiphenyl ether (BDE 183) | 207122-16-5 |

dietary sources, including fish, fatty foods, and mother's milk. However, oral ingestion from dust and leachates may be a larger source (Sjödin et al, 2004b), particularly for children (Jones-Otazo et al., 2005; Stapleton et al., 2005). Once absorbed, PBDEs distribute into body fat. The metabolism and elimination of PBDEs in humans are not well characterized. One occupational study indicated that decaBDE has an elimination half-life of 11-18 days and the octaBDEs have half-lives ranging between 37-91 days (Thuresson et al., 2006). In animals, PBDE elimination occurs primarily through fecal excretion with decaBDE being more rapidly eliminated than the other less brominated PBDEs (Gill et al., 2004; Hardy, 2002). Some PBDEs measured in human serum are listed in the table.

Human health effects from PBDEs at low environmental doses or at biomonitored levels from low environmental exposures are unknown. In animal studies, PBDEs have low acute toxicity, but have demonstrated effects on thyroid function, neurodevelopment, hepatic enzyme induction and hepatic injury in subchronic or chronic dosing studies (Birnbaum and Staskal, 2004; Branchi et al., 2002; Gill et al., 2004; Hallgren and Darnerud, 2002; Viberg et al., 2003 and 2004; Zhou et al., 2002). Some developmental and behavioral effects may be mediated by the aforementioned effect on the thyroid, by alteration in cholinergic function (Branchi et al., 2003; Dufault et al., 2005), or by altered intracellular signaling within brain cells (Kodavanti et al., 2005). The lesser brominated PBDEs have been reported to have fetotoxic and reproductive effects, to alter expression of estrogen-regulated genes and receptors, and to have anti-

androgenic effects (Ceccatelli et al., 2006; Gill et al., 2004; Kuriyama et al., 2005; Stoker et al., 2005; Talsness et al., 2005; WSDH, 2004). PentaBDE is considered more toxic than decaBDE and the most sensitive effects of pentaBDE in animal studies are neurodevelopmental and reproductive. In a study of electronics dismantlers, serum levels of PBDEs were not generally higher than in nonexposed workers and were not associated with changes in thyroid function (Julander et al., 2005). PBDEs are not considered genotoxic and are not classified by IARC and NTP with respect to human carcinogenicity. Additional information about external exposure (i.e., environmental levels) and health effects is available from ATSDR at: http://www. atsdr.cdc.gov/toxpro2.html.

**Biomonitoring Information**

Levels of PBDEs in serum reflect cumulative exposure over the recent months to years of exposure. The PBDE congeners measured for biomonitoring often include those containing three bromines (BDE-17, BDE-28), four bromines (BDE-47, BDE-66), five bromines (BDE-85, BDE-99, BDE-100), six bromines (BDE-153, BDE-154) and seven bromines (BDE-183). Analysis of the NHANES 2003-2004 subsample showed detection of BDE-47 (a tetraBDE present in commercial pentaBDEs) in nearly all participants and detection of BDE-28, BDE-99, BDE-100, and BDE-153 in greater than 60 percent of participants (Sjödin et al., 2008). Levels of these PBDEs tended to be well-correlated with each other. Serum levels of BDE-47, BDE-99, and BDE-153 were found to decrease with

## Serum 2,2',4-Tribromodiphenyl ether (BDE 17) (lipid adjusted)

Geometric mean and selected percentiles of serum concentrations (in ng/g of lipid or parts per billion on a lipid-weight basis) for the U.S. population from the National Health and Nutrition Examination Survey.

| | Survey years | Geometric mean (95% conf. interval) | Selected percentiles ( 95% confidence interval) | | | | Sample size |
|---|---|---|---|---|---|---|---|
| | | | 50th | 75th | 90th | 95th | |
| Total | 03-04 | * | < LOD | < LOD | < LOD | < LOD | 1992 |
| **Age group** | | | | | | | |
| 12-19 years | 03-04 | * | < LOD | < LOD | < LOD | < LOD | 607 |
| 20 years and older | 03-04 | * | < LOD | < LOD | < LOD | < LOD | 1385 |
| **Gender** | | | | | | | |
| Males | 03-04 | * | < LOD | < LOD | < LOD | < LOD | 964 |
| Females | 03-04 | * | < LOD | < LOD | < LOD | < LOD | 1028 |
| **Race/ethnicity** | | | | | | | |
| Mexican Americans | 03-04 | * | < LOD | < LOD | < LOD | < LOD | 482 |
| Non-Hispanic blacks | 03-04 | * | < LOD | < LOD | < LOD | < LOD | 491 |
| Non-Hispanic whites | 03-04 | * | < LOD | < LOD | < LOD | < LOD | 892 |

Limit of detection (LOD, see Data Analysis section) for Survey year 03-04 is 1.0.
< LOD means less than the limit of detection, which may vary for some chemicals by year and by individual sample.
* Not calculated: proportion of results below limit of detection was too high to provide a valid result.

increasing age from 12-19 to 20-39 to 40-59 years, and then increase slightly in the 60 years and older age group. Slight differences by gender and race/ethnicity were also observed for several PBDEs (Sjödin et al., 2008).

From the 1970s to the late 1990s, levels of BDE-47 had increased in samples of breast milk and sera in Sweden and Norway, respectively (Meironyté et al., 1999; Thomsen et al., 2002). Also, in small samplings of residents in Japan and U.S., serum levels have been shown to increase by more than fivefold to twentyfold over the past two decades (Koizumi et al., 2005; Schecter et al., 2005; Sjödin et al., 2004a). Several small studies of U.S. residents have shown increasing levels of BDE-47 during recent decades that were 3-10 times higher than contemporary European residents (Petreas et al., 2003; Sjödin et al., 2003). Serum levels of PBDEs in the NHANES 2003-2004 subsample (Sjödin et al., 2008) also appeared generally higher than those reported for Japan, Sweden, and Norway (Koizumi et al., 2005; Thomsen et al., 2002; Thuresson et al., 2006). In most studies, BDE-47 demonstrates the highest levels of all the measured PBDEs.

Detection of BB-153 was also prevalent in the NHANES 2003-2004 subsample and increased with age (Sjödin et al., 2008). This age trend may be due to the longer time that BB-153 stays in the body or due to greater past exposures in older people. Mexican Americans and NHANES participants born in foreign countries had lower serum concentrations of BB-153 (Sjödin et al, 2008). Levels of BB-153 in NHANES 2003-2004 were about one-fourth to

one-fortieth of the levels of BDE-47, depending on the age group. In human sera from Sweden, BB-153 was generally not detected as compared to detectable levels a small regional sample of U.S. residents (Sjödin et al., 2001).

Finding measurable amounts of PBDEs or BB-153 in serum does not mean that the levels of these chemicals cause an adverse health effect. Biomonitoring studies of serum PBDEs and BB-153 can provide physicians and public health officials with reference values so that they can determine whether people have been exposed to higher levels of PBDEs or BB-153 than levels found in the general population. Biomonitoring data can also help scientists plan and conduct research on exposure and health effects.

## Serum 2,4,4'-Tribromodiphenyl ether (BDE 28) (lipid adjusted)

Geometric mean and selected percentiles of serum concentrations (in ng/g of lipid or parts per billion on a lipid-weight basis) for the U.S. population from the National Health and Nutrition Examination Survey.

| | Survey years | Geometric mean (95% conf. interval) | Selected percentiles ( 95% confidence interval) | | | | Sample size |
|---|---|---|---|---|---|---|---|
| | | | 50th | 75th | 90th | 95th | |
| Total | 03-04 | 1.19 (1.03-1.37) | 1.10 (1.00-1.30) | 2.20 (1.90-2.60) | 4.80 (3.30-6.70) | 8.00 (5.40-11.3) | 1987 |
| Age group | | | | | | | |
| 12-19 years | 03-04 | 1.30 (1.15-1.46) | 1.20 (1.10-1.50) | 2.40 (2.00-2.60) | 4.00 (2.90-5.60) | 6.10 (4.00-9.40) | 598 |
| 20 years and older | 03-04 | 1.17 (1.01-1.37) | 1.10 (.900-1.30) | 2.20 (1.90-2.70) | 5.00 (3.30-7.20) | 8.20 (6.00-10.9) | 1389 |
| Gender | | | | | | | |
| Males | 03-04 | 1.21 (1.05-1.39) | 1.10 (1.00-1.30) | 2.30 (2.00-2.70) | 5.10 (3.50-7.30) | 8.20 (6.00-11.3) | 964 |
| Females | 03-04 | 1.17 (.990-1.38) | 1.10 (.900-1.40) | 2.10 (1.80-2.60) | 4.60 (3.00-6.90) | 7.80 (4.70-11.8) | 1023 |
| Race/ethnicity | | | | | | | |
| Mexican Americans | 03-04 | 1.43 (1.29-1.59) | 1.40 (1.20-1.50) | 2.40 (2.00-2.90) | 4.70 (3.70-5.50) | 7.30 (5.60-8.30) | 488 |
| Non-Hispanic blacks | 03-04 | 1.21 (1.03-1.42) | 1.10 (.900-1.30) | 2.20 (1.80-2.50) | 5.30 (3.50-6.70) | 8.40 (5.40-12.3) | 470 |
| Non-Hispanic whites | 03-04 | 1.17 (.968-1.42) | 1.10 (.900-1.30) | 2.20 (1.80-2.70) | 4.90 (3.00-8.00) | 8.00 (4.50-13.6) | 905 |

Limit of detection (LOD, see Data Analysis section) for Survey year 03-04 is 0.8.

## Serum 2,2',4,4'-Tetrabromodiphenyl ether (BDE 47) (lipid adjusted)

Geometric mean and selected percentiles of serum concentrations (in ng/g of lipid or parts per billion on a lipid-weight basis) for the U.S. population from the National Health and Nutrition Examination Survey.

| | Survey years | Geometric mean (95% conf. interval) | Selected percentiles ( 95% confidence interval) | | | | Sample size |
|---|---|---|---|---|---|---|---|
| | | | 50th | 75th | 90th | 95th | |
| Total | 03-04 | 20.5 (17.6-23.9) | 19.2 (15.7-22.3) | 41.1 (35.6-49.2) | 85.1 (66.8-127) | 163 (108-240) | 2016 |
| Age group | | | | | | | |
| 12-19 years | 03-04 | 28.2 (24.6-32.3) | 27.2 (22.1-33.6) | 53.6 (44.9-63.6) | 104 (82.4-145) | 174 (115-211) | 615 |
| 20 years and older | 03-04 | 19.5 (16.5-23.1) | 18.0 (14.6-21.6) | 39.1 (32.8-47.0) | 83.3 (63.0-127) | 163 (102-240) | 1401 |
| Gender | | | | | | | |
| Males | 03-04 | 21.4 (18.1-25.3) | 19.2 (15.8-24.0) | 45.2 (37.3-54.9) | 94.3 (66.8-148) | 168 (112-382) | 981 |
| Females | 03-04 | 19.6 (16.4-23.5) | 19.1 (14.1-23.2) | 38.4 (31.8-46.4) | 79.5 (60.7-121) | 155 (102-239) | 1035 |
| Race/ethnicity | | | | | | | |
| Mexican Americans | 03-04 | 25.5 (23.0-28.1) | 23.6 (21.2-25.5) | 47.1 (38.2-56.5) | 87.2 (72.0-105) | 151 (105-195) | 478 |
| Non-Hispanic blacks | 03-04 | 24.3 (20.9-28.2) | 21.4 (18.2-25.6) | 47.5 (40.7-53.2) | 116 (81.8-149) | 242 (136-481) | 499 |
| Non-Hispanic whites | 03-04 | 19.5 (16.1-23.7) | 17.4 (14.4-22.2) | 40.2 (33.1-51.9) | 85.1 (60.3-142) | 163 (90.2-283) | 912 |

Limit of detection (LOD, see Data Analysis section) for Survey year 03-04 is 4.2.

## Serum 2,3',4,4'-Tetrabromodiphenyl ether (BDE 66) (lipid adjusted)

Geometric mean and selected percentiles of serum concentrations (in ng/g of lipid or parts per billion on a lipid-weight basis) for the U.S. population from the National Health and Nutrition Examination Survey.

| | Survey years | Geometric mean (95% conf. interval) | Selected percentiles ( 95% confidence interval) | | | | Sample size |
|---|---|---|---|---|---|---|---|
| | | | 50th | 75th | 90th | 95th | |
| Total | 03-04 | * | < LOD | < LOD | < LOD | 1.30 (1.00-2.10) | 1999 |
| Age group | | | | | | | |
| 12-19 years | 03-04 | * | < LOD | < LOD | < LOD | 1.30 (<LOD-1.90) | 606 |
| 20 years and older | 03-04 | * | < LOD | < LOD | < LOD | 1.30 (1.00-2.20) | 1393 |
| Gender | | | | | | | |
| Males | 03-04 | * | < LOD | < LOD | < LOD | 1.40 (1.00-2.60) | 970 |
| Females | 03-04 | * | < LOD | < LOD | < LOD | 1.10 (<LOD-2.20) | 1029 |
| Race/ethnicity | | | | | | | |
| Mexican Americans | 03-04 | * | < LOD | < LOD | < LOD | 1.20 (<LOD-1.60) | 461 |
| Non-Hispanic blacks | 03-04 | * | < LOD | < LOD | 1.00 (<LOD-2.00) | 2.40 (1.40-5.10) | 496 |
| Non-Hispanic whites | 03-04 | * | < LOD | < LOD | < LOD | 1.20 (<LOD-2.50) | 914 |

Limit of detection (LOD, see Data Analysis section) for Survey year 03-04 is 1.0.
< LOD means less than the limit of detection, which may vary for some chemicals by year and by individual sample.
* Not calculated: proportion of results below limit of detection was too high to provide a valid result.

## Serum 2,2',3,4,4'-Pentabromodiphenyl ether (BDE 85) (lipid adjusted)

Geometric mean and selected percentiles of serum concentrations (in ng/g of lipid or parts per billion on a lipid-weight basis) for the U.S. population from the National Health and Nutrition Examination Survey.

| | Survey years | Geometric mean (95% conf. interval) | Selected percentiles ( 95% confidence interval) | | | | Sample size |
|---|---|---|---|---|---|---|---|
| | | | 50th | 75th | 90th | 95th | |
| Total | 03-04 | * | < LOD | < LOD | < LOD | 4.10 (2.80-6.30) | 2000 |
| **Age group** | | | | | | | |
| 12-19 years | 03-04 | * | < LOD | < LOD | 2.80 (<LOD-3.50) | 4.00 (3.50-6.30) | 610 |
| 20 years and older | 03-04 | * | < LOD | < LOD | < LOD | 4.10 (2.50-6.70) | 1390 |
| **Gender** | | | | | | | |
| Males | 03-04 | * | < LOD | < LOD | 2.40 (<LOD-3.30) | 4.80 (3.10-8.40) | 967 |
| Females | 03-04 | * | < LOD | < LOD | < LOD | 3.60 (<LOD-5.20) | 1033 |
| **Race/ethnicity** | | | | | | | |
| Mexican Americans | 03-04 | * | < LOD | < LOD | < LOD | 3.70 (2.80-4.80) | 484 |
| Non-Hispanic blacks | 03-04 | * | < LOD | < LOD | 3.50 (2.50-4.40) | 6.90 (3.10-18.0) | 493 |
| Non-Hispanic whites | 03-04 | * | < LOD | < LOD | < LOD | 3.90 (<LOD-7.50) | 895 |

Limit of detection (LOD, see Data Analysis section) for Survey year 03-04 is 2.4.
< LOD means less than the limit of detection, which may vary for some chemicals by year and by individual sample.
* Not calculated: proportion of results below limit of detection was too high to provide a valid result.

## Serum 2,2',4,4',5-Pentabromodiphenyl ether (BDE 99) (lipid adjusted)

Geometric mean and selected percentiles of serum concentrations (in ng/g of lipid or parts per billion on a lipid-weight basis) for the U.S. population from the National Health and Nutrition Examination Survey.

| | Survey years | Geometric mean (95% conf. interval) | Selected percentiles ( 95% confidence interval) | | | | Sample size |
|---|---|---|---|---|---|---|---|
| | | | 50th | 75th | 90th | 95th | |
| Total | 03-04 | * | < LOD | 9.20 (7.50-11.1) | 21.7 (17.0-29.1) | 42.2 (33.3-54.8) | 1985 |
| **Age group** | | | | | | | |
| 12-19 years | 03-04 | 6.88 (6.14-7.72) | 5.70 (<LOD-7.70) | 12.9 (11.4-15.7) | 27.9 (19.6-37.9) | 45.2 (35.9-56.8) | 602 |
| 20 years and older | 03-04 | * | < LOD | 8.50 (7.10-10.5) | 20.6 (15.5-28.8) | 41.6 (30.8-57.3) | 1383 |
| **Gender** | | | | | | | |
| Males | 03-04 | 5.28 (<LOD-6.14) | < LOD | 10.0 (8.40-11.6) | 24.5 (18.0-37.3) | 45.5 (33.8-57.3) | 964 |
| Females | 03-04 | * | < LOD | 8.70 (6.60-10.6) | 18.3 (14.7-28.8) | 41.2 (22.9-60.3) | 1021 |
| **Race/ethnicity** | | | | | | | |
| Mexican Americans | 03-04 | 5.90 (5.45-6.39) | 5.50 (<LOD-5.80) | 10.8 (9.30-12.6) | 20.0 (17.0-23.5) | 30.8 (24.5-41.7) | 478 |
| Non-Hispanic blacks | 03-04 | 6.22 (5.42-7.12) | 5.00 (<LOD-5.70) | 11.5 (9.60-13.1) | 30.2 (21.5-42.2) | 74.7 (30.2-155) | 479 |
| Non-Hispanic whites | 03-04 | * | < LOD | 8.90 (6.80-11.3) | 21.7 (15.3-34.0) | 43.6 (30.7-71.4) | 903 |

Limit of detection (LOD, see Data Analysis section) for Survey year 03-04 is 5.0.
* Not calculated: proportion of results below limit of detection was too high to provide a valid result.

## Serum 2,2',4,4',6-Pentabromodiphenyl ether (BDE 100) (lipid adjusted)

Geometric mean and selected percentiles of serum concentrations (in ng/g of lipid or parts per billion on a lipid-weight basis) for the U.S. population from the National Health and Nutrition Examination Survey.

| | Survey years | Geometric mean (95% conf. interval) | Selected percentiles ( 95% confidence interval) | | | | Sample size |
|---|---|---|---|---|---|---|---|
| | | | 50th | 75th | 90th | 95th | |
| Total | 03-04 | 3.93 (3.42-4.51) | 3.60 (3.10-4.10) | 7.80 (6.80-9.00) | 18.4 (15.4-22.0) | 36.5 (24.6-54.0) | 2040 |
| Age group | | | | | | | |
| 12-19 years | 03-04 | 5.17 (4.46-6.00) | 4.90 (3.80-6.10) | 9.50 (7.90-12.8) | 19.3 (14.4-26.2) | 34.3 (25.2-45.0) | 622 |
| 20 years and older | 03-04 | 3.77 (3.24-4.38) | 3.30 (2.90-4.00) | 7.40 (6.20-9.00) | 18.3 (15.0-22.2) | 36.6 (23.2-59.2) | 1418 |
| Gender | | | | | | | |
| Males | 03-04 | 4.16 (3.55-4.86) | 3.80 (3.10-4.50) | 8.50 (7.50-9.90) | 18.5 (14.9-25.1) | 44.1 (21.9-61.5) | 994 |
| Females | 03-04 | 3.72 (3.15-4.40) | 3.30 (2.80-4.10) | 7.10 (6.00-8.00) | 18.4 (14.4-23.1) | 33.3 (23.3-46.0) | 1046 |
| Race/ethnicity | | | | | | | |
| Mexican Americans | 03-04 | 4.58 (4.03-5.22) | 4.30 (3.80-5.20) | 8.10 (6.80-9.10) | 14.9 (11.4-20.3) | 26.7 (20.3-36.2) | 488 |
| Non-Hispanic blacks | 03-04 | 4.72 (4.01-5.55) | 4.30 (3.30-5.20) | 9.50 (7.80-10.9) | 24.1 (16.6-34.3) | 41.3 (26.0-79.2) | 503 |
| Non-Hispanic whites | 03-04 | 3.78 (3.17-4.51) | 3.30 (2.90-4.10) | 7.70 (6.20-9.70) | 18.6 (14.5-23.3) | 40.5 (22.6-59.2) | 921 |

Limit of detection (LOD, see Data Analysis section) for Survey year 03-04 is 1.4.

## Serum 2,2',4,4',5,5'-Hexabromodiphenyl ether (BDE 153) (lipid adjusted)

Geometric mean and selected percentiles of serum concentrations (in ng/g of lipid or parts per billion on a lipid-weight basis) for the U.S. population from the National Health and Nutrition Examination Survey.

| | Survey years | Geometric mean (95% conf. interval) | Selected percentiles ( 95% confidence interval) | | | | Sample size |
|---|---|---|---|---|---|---|---|
| | | | 50th | 75th | 90th | 95th | |
| Total | 03-04 | 5.69 (5.11-6.34) | 4.80 (4.20-5.30) | 11.3 (9.90-12.8) | 32.6 (27.9-40.3) | 65.7 (54.9-88.4) | 2039 |
| Age group | | | | | | | |
| 12-19 years | 03-04 | 8.05 (6.68-9.70) | 7.50 (6.10-9.90) | 15.3 (11.7-19.4) | 31.0 (22.9-44.2) | 52.9 (35.9-68.5) | 621 |
| 20 years and older | 03-04 | 5.41 (4.83-6.05) | 4.40 (3.80-5.10) | 10.6 (9.00-12.3) | 32.8 (26.5-45.9) | 73.3 (58.2-90.4) | 1418 |
| Gender | | | | | | | |
| Males | 03-04 | 6.85 (5.99-7.84) | 5.50 (4.80-6.70) | 12.7 (11.2-16.5) | 49.3 (31.0-62.9) | 88.4 (63.4-115) | 994 |
| Females | 03-04 | 4.78 (4.20-5.43) | 4.10 (3.40-5.00) | 9.70 (7.40-11.9) | 26.0 (20.2-31.6) | 54.5 (34.6-62.9) | 1045 |
| Race/ethnicity | | | | | | | |
| Mexican Americans | 03-04 | 5.11 (4.32-6.06) | 4.80 (4.20-5.40) | 8.70 (6.50-11.0) | 17.2 (13.0-25.3) | 34.0 (18.3-55.1) | 487 |
| Non-Hispanic blacks | 03-04 | 6.05 (5.35-6.83) | 5.50 (4.80-6.20) | 12.9 (9.90-17.5) | 30.0 (21.0-44.2) | 53.1 (36.8-63.3) | 503 |
| Non-Hispanic whites | 03-04 | 5.85 (5.03-6.81) | 4.90 (3.90-5.70) | 11.9 (9.90-15.2) | 39.0 (28.5-54.9) | 75.9 (58.0-93.2) | 921 |

Limit of detection (LOD, see Data Analysis section) for Survey year 03-04 is 2.2.

## Serum 2,2',4,4',5,6'-Hexabromodiphenyl ether (BDE 154) (lipid adjusted)

Geometric mean and selected percentiles of serum concentrations (in ng/g of lipid or parts per billion on a lipid-weight basis) for the U.S. population from the National Health and Nutrition Examination Survey.

| | Survey years | Geometric mean (95% conf. interval) | Selected percentiles ( 95% confidence interval) | | | | Sample size |
|---|---|---|---|---|---|---|---|
| | | | 50th | 75th | 90th | 95th | |
| Total | 03-04 | * | < LOD | .900 (.800-1.10) | 2.10 (1.70-2.70) | 4.20 (2.80-5.40) | 2014 |
| Age group | | | | | | | |
| 12-19 years | 03-04 | * | < LOD | 1.20 (1.00-1.40) | 2.70 (2.00-3.00) | 4.00 (3.00-4.80) | 614 |
| 20 years and older | 03-04 | * | < LOD | .900 (.800-1.10) | 2.00 (1.60-2.60) | 4.20 (2.70-5.70) | 1400 |
| Gender | | | | | | | |
| Males | 03-04 | * | < LOD | 1.00 (.800-1.20) | 2.30 (1.80-3.00) | 4.30 (3.20-6.50) | 976 |
| Females | 03-04 | * | < LOD | .900 (.800-1.00) | 1.80 (1.40-2.80) | 4.20 (2.50-5.70) | 1038 |
| Race/ethnicity | | | | | | | |
| Mexican Americans | 03-04 | * | < LOD | 1.00 (.900-1.10) | 1.80 (1.40-2.30) | 3.90 (2.30-4.50) | 477 |
| Non-Hispanic blacks | 03-04 | * | < LOD | 1.20 (.900-1.40) | 2.70 (2.30-4.40) | 5.30 (3.10-8.70) | 498 |
| Non-Hispanic whites | 03-04 | * | < LOD | .900 (.800-1.10) | 2.00 (1.50-2.80) | 4.20 (2.50-6.70) | 913 |

Limit of detection (LOD, see Data Analysis section) for Survey year 03-04 is 0.8.
* Not calculated: proportion of results below limit of detection was too high to provide a valid result.

## Serum 2,2',3,4,4',5',6-Heptabromodiphenyl ether (BDE 183) (lipid adjusted)

Geometric mean and selected percentiles of serum concentrations (in ng/g of lipid or parts per billion on a lipid-weight basis) for the U.S. population from the National Health and Nutrition Examination Survey.

| | Survey years | Geometric mean (95% conf. interval) | Selected percentiles ( 95% confidence interval) | | | | Sample size |
|---|---|---|---|---|---|---|---|
| | | | 50th | 75th | 90th | 95th | |
| Total | 03-04 | * | < LOD | < LOD | < LOD | < LOD | 1993 |
| Age group | | | | | | | |
| 12-19 years | 03-04 | * | < LOD | < LOD | < LOD | < LOD | 604 |
| 20 years and older | 03-04 | * | < LOD | < LOD | < LOD | < LOD | 1389 |
| Gender | | | | | | | |
| Males | 03-04 | * | < LOD | < LOD | < LOD | 1.70 (<LOD-2.60) | 962 |
| Females | 03-04 | * | < LOD | < LOD | < LOD | < LOD | 1031 |
| Race/ethnicity | | | | | | | |
| Mexican Americans | 03-04 | * | < LOD | < LOD | < LOD | < LOD | 484 |
| Non-Hispanic blacks | 03-04 | * | < LOD | < LOD | < LOD | 1.80 (<LOD-2.70) | 482 |
| Non-Hispanic whites | 03-04 | * | < LOD | < LOD | < LOD | < LOD | 901 |

Limit of detection (LOD, see Data Analysis section) for Survey year 03-04 is 1.7.
< LOD means less than the limit of detection, which may vary for some chemicals by year and by individual sample.
* Not calculated: proportion of results below limit of detection was too high to provide a valid result.

## Serum 2,2',4,4',5,5'-Hexabromobiphenyl (BB 153) (lipid adjusted)

Geometric mean and selected percentiles of serum concentrations (in ng/g of lipid or parts per billion on a lipid-weight basis) for the U.S. population from the National Health and Nutrition Examination Survey.

| | Survey years | Geometric mean (95% conf. interval) | Selected percentiles ( 95% confidence interval) | | | | Sample size |
|---|---|---|---|---|---|---|---|
| | | | 50th | 75th | 90th | 95th | |
| Total | 03-04 | 2.29 (1.82-2.87) | 2.20 (2.00-2.60) | 4.40 (3.40-6.30) | 12.8 (6.60-25.5) | 27.2 (11.7-60.9) | 2032 |
| Age group | | | | | | | |
| 12-19 years | 03-04 | * | < LOD | 1.10 (.900-1.60) | 2.70 (2.00-3.00) | 4.10 (2.90-4.70) | 616 |
| 20 years and older | 03-04 | 2.72 (2.14-3.47) | 2.50 (2.20-2.80) | 4.90 (3.60-7.90) | 13.6 (7.20-34.6) | 34.6 (12.8-66.8) | 1416 |
| Gender | | | | | | | |
| Males | 03-04 | 2.76 (2.21-3.45) | 2.70 (2.30-3.20) | 5.40 (3.90-8.50) | 15.8 (9.30-27.8) | 35.4 (13.5-70.3) | 987 |
| Females | 03-04 | 1.92 (1.50-2.46) | 2.00 (1.60-2.30) | 3.60 (2.80-4.90) | 9.70 (4.60-27.5) | 23.9 (7.40-56.6) | 1045 |
| Race/ethnicity | | | | | | | |
| Mexican Americans | 03-04 | 1.11 (.917-1.33) | 1.10 (<LOD-1.30) | 2.60 (2.00-3.00) | 6.00 (3.50-8.60) | 10.0 (6.50-15.2) | 484 |
| Non-Hispanic blacks | 03-04 | 2.35 (1.64-3.37) | 2.10 (1.70-2.80) | 4.80 (3.00-12.1) | 13.9 (7.00-38.2) | 29.7 (12.1-70.2) | 503 |
| Non-Hispanic whites | 03-04 | 2.66 (2.06-3.42) | 2.50 (2.20-2.80) | 4.90 (3.40-7.80) | 13.5 (6.60-36.4) | 34.6 (11.6-70.3) | 917 |

Limit of detection (LOD, see Data Analysis section) for Survey year 03-04 is 0.8.
* Not calculated: proportion of results below limit of detection was too high to provide a valid result.

# References

Alaeea M, Arias P, Sjödin A, Bergmand A. An overview of commercially used brominated flame retardants, their applications, their use patterns in different countries/regions and possible modes of release. Environ Int 2003;29:683– 689.

Birnbaum LS, Staskal DF. Brominated flame retardants: cause for concern? Environ Health Perspect 2004;112:9–17.

Branchi I, Alleva E, Costa LG. Effects of perinatal exposure to a polybrominated diphenyl ether (PBDE 99) on mouse neurobehavioural development. Neurotoxicology 2002;23(3):375-384.

Branchi I, Capone F, Alleva E, Costa LG. Polybrominated diphenyl ethers: neurobehavioral effects following developmental exposure. Neurotoxicology 2003;24(3):449-462.

Ceccatelli R, Faass O, Schlumpf M, Lichtensteiger W. Gene expression and estrogen sensitivity in rat uterus after developmental exposure to the polybrominated diphenylether PBDE 99 and PCB. Toxicology 2006;220(2-3):104-116.

Dufault C, Poles G, Driscoll LL. Brief postnatal PBDE exposure alters learning and the cholinergic modulation of attention in rats. Toxicol Sci 2005;88(1):172-180.

Fries GF. The PBB episode in Michigan: an overall appraisal. Crit Rev Toxicol 1985;16(2):105-156.

Gill U, Chu I, Ryan JJ, Feeley M. Polybrominated diphenyl ethers: human tissue levels and toxicology. Rev Environ Contam Toxicol 2004;183:55-97.

Hallgren S, Darnerud PO. Polybrominated diphenyl ethers (PBDEs), polychlorinated biphenyls (PCBs) and chlorinated paraffins (CPs) in rats-testing interactions and mechanisms for thyroid hormone effects. Toxicology 2002;177(2-3):227-243.

Hardy ML. The toxicology of the three commercial polybrominated diphenyl oxide (ether) flame retardants. Chemosphere 2002;46(5):757-777.

Jones-Otazo HA, Clarke JP, Diamond ML, Archbold JA, Ferguson G, Harner et al. Is house dust the missing exposure pathway for PBDEs? An analysis of the urban fate and human exposure to PBDEs. Environ Sci Technol 2005;39(14):5121-5130.

Julander A, Karlsson M, Hagstrom K, Ohlson CG, Engwall M, Bryngelsson IL, et al. Polybrominated diphenyl ethers--plasma levels and thyroid status of workers at an electronic recycling facility. Int Arch Occup Environ Health 2005;78(7):584-592.

Kodavanti PR, Ward TR, Ludewig G, Robertson LW, Birnbaum LS. Polybrominated diphenyl ether (PBDE) effects in rat neuronal cultures: 14C-PBDE accumulation, biological effects, and structure-activity relationships. Toxicol Sci 2005;88(1):181-192.

Koizumi A, Yoshinaga T, Harada K, Inoue K, Morikawa A, Muroi J, et al. Assessment of human exposure to polychlorinated biphenyls and polybrominated diphenyl ethers in Japan using archived samples from the early 1980s and mid-1990s. Environ Res 2005;99(1):31-39.

Kuriyama SN, Talsness CE, Grote K, Chahoud I. Developmental exposure to low dose PBDE 99: effects on male fertility and neurobehavior in rat offspring. Environ Health Perspect 2005;113(2):149-154.

Meironyte D, Noren K, Bergman A. Analysis of polybrominated diphenyl ethers in Swedish human milk. A time-related trend study, 1972-1997. J Toxicol Environ Health A 1999;58(6):329-341.

Norstrom RJ, Simon M, Moisey J, Wakeford B, Weseloh DV. Geographical distribution (2000) and temporal trends (1981-2000) of brominated diphenyl ethers in Great Lakes hewing gull eggs. Environ Sci Technol 2002;36(22):4783-4789.

Organization for Economic Co-operation and Development (OECD). OECE Environment Monograph Series No. 102. Risk Reduction Monograph No. 3: Selected Brominated Flame Retardants – Background and National Experience with Reducing Risk.1994. Paris, France.

Petreas M, She J, Brown FR, Winkler J, Windham G, Rogers E, et al. High body burdens of 2,2',4,4'-tetrabromodiphenyl ether (BDE-47) in California women. Environ Health Perspect 2003;111(9):1175-1179.

Schecter A, Papke O, Tung KC, Joseph J, Harris TR, Dahlgren J. Polybrominated diphenyl ether flame retardants in the U.S. population: current levels, temporal trends, and comparison with dioxins, dibenzofurans, and polychlorinated biphenyls. J Occup Environ Med 2005;47(3):199-211.

Sjödin A, Patterson DG Jr, Bergman A. Brominated flame retardants in serum from U.S. blood donors. Environ Sci Technol. 2001;35(19):3830-3833.

Sjödin A, Patterson DG Jr, Bergman A. A review on human exposure to brominated flame retardants—particularly polybrominated diphenyl ethers. Environ Int 2003;29(6):829-839.

Sjödin A, Jones RS, Focant JF, Lapeza C, Wang RY, McGahee EE 3rd, et al. Retrospective time-trend study of polybrominated diphenyl ether and polybrominated and polychlorinated biphenyl levels in human serum from the United States. Environ Health Perspect. 2004a;112(6):654-658.

Sjödin A, PäpkeO, McGahee E, Jones R, Focant JF, Pless-Mulloli T, et al. Concentration of polybrominated diphenyl ethers

(PBDEs) in household dust from various countries - inhalation a potential route of human exposure. Organohalogen Compounds 2004*b*;66:3817-3822.

Sjödin A, Wong LY, Jones RS, Park A, Zhang Y, Hodge C, et al. Serum concentrations of polybrominated diphenyl ethers (PBDEs) and polybrominated biphenyl (PBB) in the United States population: 2003-2004. Environ Sci Technol. 2008;42(4):1377-1384.

Stapleton HM, Dodder NG, Offenberg JH, Schantz MM, Wise SA. Polybrominated diphenyl ethers in house dust and clothes dryer lint. Environ Sci Technol 2005;39(4):925-931.

Stoker TE, Cooper RL, Lambright CS, Wilson VS, Furr J, Gray LE. In vivo and in vitro anti-androgenic effects of DE-71, a commercial polybrominated diphenyl ether (PBDE) mixture. Toxicol Appl Pharmacol 2005;207(1):78-88.

Talsness CE, Shakibaei M, Kuriyama SN, Grande SW, Sterner-Kock A, Schnitker P, et al. Ultrastructural changes observed in rat ovaries following in utero and lactational exposure to low doses of a polybrominated flame retardant. Toxicol Lett 2005;157(3):189-202.

Thomsen C, Lundanes E, Becher G. Brominated flame retardants in archived serum samples from Norway: a study on temporal trends and the role of age. Environ Sci Technol. 2002;36(7):1414-1418.

Thuresson K, Hoglund P, Hagmar L, Sjödin A, Bergman A, Jakobsson K. Apparent half-lives of hepta- to decabrominated diphenyl ethers in human serum as determined in occupationally exposed workers. Environ Health Perspect 2006;114(2):176-181.

U.S. Environmental Protection Agency (U.S. EPA). Polybrominated diphenylethers (PBDEs) Significant New Use Rule (SNUR) Questions and Answers. 2005. Revised 1/12/06. Available from URL: http://www.epa.gov/oppt/pbde/pubs/qanda.htm, 1/30/06

Viberg H, Fredriksson A, Eriksson P. Investigations of strain and/or gender differences in developmental neurotoxic effects of polybrominated diphenyl ethers in mice. Toxicol Sci 2004;81(2):344-353.

Viberg H, Fredriksson A, Eriksson P. Neonatal exposure to polybrominated diphenyl ether (PBDE 153) disrupts spontaneous behaviour, impairs learning and memory, and decreases hippocampal cholinergic receptors in adult mice. Toxicol Appl Pharmacol 2003;192(2):95-106.

Washington State Department of Health (WSDH). Washington State polybrominated diphenyl ether (PBDE) Chemical Action Plan: Interim Plan. December 31, 2004. Department of Ecology Publication No. 04-03-056. Also available URL: http://www.ecy.wa.gov/biblio/0403056.html. 1/30/06

Watanabe I, Sakai S. Environmental release and behavior of brominated flame retardants. Environ Int 2003;29(6):665-682.

Zhou T, Taylor MM, DeVito MJ, Crofton KM. Developmental exposure to brominated diphenyl ethers results in thyroid hormone disruption. Toxicol Sci 2002;66(1):105-116.

# Non-Dioxin-Like Polychlorinated Biphenyls

*(The coplanar and mono-ortho-substituted PCBs are discussed in the section titled "Dioxin-Like Chemicals: Polychlorinated Dibenzo-p-dioxins, Polychlorinated Dibenzofurans, and Coplanar and Mono-ortho-substituted Polychlorinated Biphenyls.")*

## General Information

Polychlorinated biphenyls (PCBs) are a class of chlorinated aromatic hydrocarbon chemicals that once were used as heat-exchanger, transformer, and hydraulic fluids, and as additives to paints, oils, joint caulking, and floor tiles. Peak production occurred in the early 1970s, and production was banned in the United States after 1979. More than 1.5 billion pounds of PCBs were manufactured in the United States prior to 1977. The continued concern about these chemicals is because of their persistence in the environment and accumulation in wildlife and the animal food chain.

Food is the main source of exposure for the general population. PCBs enter the food chain by a variety of routes, including migration into food from external sources, contamination of animal feeds, and accumulation in the fatty tissues of animals. PCBs are found at higher concentrations in fatty foods (e.g., dairy products and fish). The transfer of PCBs from mother to infant via breast milk is another important source of exposure. The lesser-chlorinated PCBs are more volatile and indoor inhalational exposure from buildings containing caulking made with these PCBs prior to 1979 can increase background serum levels (Johansson et al., 2003; Kohler et al., 2005). Other sources of exposure in the general population include the release of these chemicals from PCB-containing waste sites and from fires involving transformers and capacitors. Additionally, the heat from fires can result in the production of polychlorinated dibenzofurans from PCBs. In certain

## Non-Dioxin-like Polychlorinated Biphenyls in this *Report*

| Non-dioxin-like polychlorinated biphenyls (IUPAC number) | CAS number |
|---|---|
| Polychlorinated biphenyls (general class) | 1336-36-3 |
| 2,4,4'-Trichlorobiphenyl (PCB 28) | 7012-37-5 |
| 2,2',3,5'-Tetrachlorobiphenyl (PCB 44) | 41464-39-5 |
| 2,2',4,5'-Tetrachlorobiphenyl (PCB 49) | 41464-40-8 |
| 2,2',5,5'-Tetrachlorobiphenyl (PCB 52) | 35693-99-3 |
| 2,3',4,4'-Tetrachlorobiphenyl (PCB 66) | 32598-10-0 |
| 2,4,4',5-Tetrachlorobiphenyl (PCB 74) | 32690-93-0 |
| 2,2',3,4,5'-Pentachlorobiphenyl (PCB 87) | 38380-02-8 |
| 2,2',4,4',5-Pentachlorobiphenyl (PCB 99) | 38380-01-7 |
| 2,2',4,5,5'-Pentachlorobiphenyl (PCB 101) | 37680-73-2 |
| 2,3,3',4',6-Pentachlorobiphenyl (PCB 110) | 38380-03-9 |
| 2,2',3,3',4,4'-Hexachlorobiphenyl (PCB 128) | 38380-07-3 |
| 2,2',3,4,4',5'-Hexachlorobiphenyl (PCB 138) | 35065-28-2 |
| 2,3,3',4,4',6-Hexachlorobiphenyl (PCB 158) | 74472-42-7 |
| 2,2',3,4,5,5'-Hexachlorobiphenyl (PCB 146) | 51908-16-8 |
| 2,2',3,4,5',6-Hexachlorobiphenyl (PCB 149) | 38380-04-0 |
| 2,2',3,5,5',6-Hexachlorobiphenyl (PCB 151) | 52663-63-5 |
| 2,2',4,4',5,5'-Hexachlorobiphenyl (PCB 153) | 35065-27-1 |
| 2,2',3,3',4,4',5-Heptachlorobiphenyl (PCB 170) | 35065-30-6 |
| 2,2',3,3',4,5,5'-Heptachlorobiphenyl (PCB 172) | 52663-74-8 |
| 2,2',3,3',4,5',6-Heptachlorobiphenyl (PCB 177) | 52663-70-4 |
| 2,2',3,3',5,5',6-Heptachlorobiphenyl (PCB 178) | 52663-67-9 |
| 2,2',3,4,4',5,5'-Heptachlorobiphenyl (PCB 180) | 35065-29-3 |
| 2,2',3,4,4',5',6-Heptachlorobiphenyl (PCB 183) | 52663-69-1 |
| 2,2',3,4,5,5',6-Heptachlorobiphenyl (PCB 187) | 52663-68-0 |
| 2,2',3,3',4,4',5,5'-Octachlorobiphenyl (PCB 194) | 35694-08-7 |
| 2,2',3,3',4,4',5,6-Octachlorobiphenyl (PCB 195) | 52663-78-2 |
| 2,2',3,3',4,4',5,6'-Octachlorobiphenyl (PCB 196) | 42740-50-1 |
| 2,2',3,3',4,5,5',6'-Octachlorobiphenyl (PCB 199) | 52663-75-9 |
| 2,2',3,4,4',5,5',6-Octachlorobiphenyl (PCB 203) | 52663-76-0 |
| 2,2',3,3',4,4',5,5',6-Nonachlorobiphenyl (PCB 206) | 40186-72-9 |
| 2,2'3,3'4,4'5,5'6,6'-Decachlorobiphenyl (PCB 209) | 2051-24-3 |

occupational settings, workers can be exposed to PCBs such as when repairing or manufacturing transformers, capacitors, and hydraulic systems, and when remediating hazardous-waste sites. Both U.S. FDA and OSHA have developed criteria on the allowable levels of these chemicals in foods and the workplace. The U.S. EPA has also set criteria for allowable levels in water and waste materials. The international Stockholm Convention on Persistent Organic Pollutants of 2001 establishes the most stringent guidelines to date regarding elimination, restriction and unintentional production of PCBs and selected organochlorine chemicals (Porta and Zumeta, 2002).

Exposure to these chemicals nearly always occurs as mixtures rather than from individual PCBs. The different types of PCB chemicals are known as congeners, which are compounds that are distinguished by the number of chlorine atoms and their location on the biphenyl structure. PCB congeners can be divided into the coplanar, the mono-*ortho*-substituted PCBs, and other non-dioxin-like PCBs. The significance of this designation is that the coplanar and some of the mono-*ortho*-substituted PCBs have dioxin-like toxicologic effects. Structural nomenclature is available at: http://www.epa.gov/oswer/riskassessment/pdf/1340-erasc-003.pdf. The non-dioxin-like PCBs and

their metabolites do not interact substantially with the aryl hydrocarbon receptor (AhR) and may act through different pathways than the dioxin-like chemicals, so their effects are not represented in the use of toxic equivalency factors (TEFs) (Carpenter, 2006). The non-dioxin-like PCBs measured in this *Report* are listed in the table.

Human health effects that have been reported after investigations of occupational and accidental exposures to high levels of PCBs include elevations of serum hepatic enzymes, dermal changes, inconsistent associations with serum lipid levels, and some types of cancer (e.g., liver, biliary) (ATSDR, 2000; Carpenter, 2006; Charles et al., 2001; Negri et al., 2003). Animal studies have demonstrated varied effects of PCBs including neurotoxicity, immune suppression, altered thyroid and reproductive function, and liver cancer (Carpenter, 2006; U.S.EPA, 2008). Effects of PCBs in humans are difficult to study due to coexposures to the dioxin-like chemicals and other organochlorine chemicals. (Also see the section titled: "Dioxin-Like Chemicals: Polychlorinated Dibenzo-*p*-dioxins, Polychlorinated Dibenzofurans, and the Coplanar and Mono-*ortho*-substituted Polychlorinated Biphenyls").

Transplacental transfer of PCBs after maternal

## Serum 2,4,4'-Trichlorobiphenyl (PCB 28) (lipid adjusted)

Geometric mean and selected percentiles of serum concentrations (in ng/g of lipid or parts per billion on a lipid-weight basis) for the U.S. population from the National Health and Nutrition Examination Survey.

| | Survey years# | Geometric mean (95% conf. interval) | Selected percentiles ( 95% confidence interval) | | | | Sample size |
|---|---|---|---|---|---|---|---|
| | | | 50th | 75th | 90th | 95th | |
| **Total** | 99-00 | * | < LOD | < LOD | < LOD | < LOD | 1849 |
| | 03-04 | 4.90 (4.60-5.22) | 4.96 (4 65-5.26) | 6.79 (6.40-7.31) | 9.39 (8.70-10.1) | 11.3 (10.7-11.8) | 1866 |
| **Age group** | | | | | | | |
| 12-19 years | 99-00 | * | < LOD | < LOD | < LOD | < LOD | 647 |
| | 03-04 | 5.02 (4.48-5.63) | 4.88 (4 26-5.48) | 7.20 (5.90-8.60) | 10.2 (8.40-11.5) | 11.7 (10.7-13.3) | 590 |
| 20 years and older | 99-00 | * | < LOD | < LOD | < LOD | < LOD | 1202 |
| | 03-04 | 4.88 (4.61-5.17) | 4.98 (4 67-5.26) | 6.78 (6.40-7.25) | 9.10 (8.70-9 87) | 11.1 (10 6-11.8) | 1276 |
| **Gender** | | | | | | | |
| Males | 99-00 | * | < LOD | < LOD | < LOD | < LOD | 886 |
| | 03-04 | 4.81 (4.47-5.16) | 4.86 (4.45-5.20) | 6.70 (6.07-7.50) | 9.39 (8.34-10.4) | 10.8 (10 5-11.4) | 926 |
| Females | 99-00 | * | < LOD | < LOD | < LOD | < LOD | 963 |
| | 03-04 | 4.99 (4.66-5.35) | 5.07 (4.73-5.37) | 6.90 (6.49-7.40) | 9.37 (8.72-10.1) | 11.6 (10.7-13.1) | 940 |
| **Race/ethnicity** | | | | | | | |
| Mexican Americans | 99-00 | * | < LOD | < LOD | < LOD | < LOD | 618 |
| | 03-04 | 4.95 (4.55-5.38) | 4.90 (4.40-5.70) | 6.70 (6.07-7.90) | 8.94 (8.17-9.70) | 10.5 (9.02-14.7) | 413 |
| Non-Hispanic blacks | 99-00 | * | < LOD | < LOD | < LOD | < LOD | 392 |
| | 03-04 | 4.95 (4.20-5.84) | 6.03 (4.10-5.60) | 7.20 (5.62-8.80) | 10.2 (8.51-12.4) | 13.1 (10 8-15.3) | 459 |
| Non-Hispanic whites | 99-00 | * | < LOD | < LOD | < LOD | < LOD | 687 |
| | 03-04 | 4.89 (4.58-5.22) | 4.90 (4 61-5.26) | 6.76 (6.33-7.32) | 9.40 (8.70-10.3) | 11.1 (10 6-11.8) | 876 |

Limit of detection (LOD, see Data Analysis section) for Survey years 99-00 and 03-04 are 32.4 and 1.7.
< LOD means less than the limit of detection, which may vary for some chemicals by year and by individual sample.
* Not calculated: proportion of results below limit of detection was too high to provide a valid result.
# Data not available for Survey years 2001-2002.

environmental exposure has been reported to be associated with altered psychomotor development in children and lower birth weight and size in newborns ( Hertz-Picciotto et al., 2005; Jacobson and Jacobson, 1996; Koopman-Essenboom et al., 1996; Longnecker et al., 2003; Lundqvist et al., 2006; Sagiv et al., 2007; Sala et al., 2001), although other studies have either not confirmed these findings or found that such effects do not persist into toddler and school aged children (Gladen and Rogan, 1991; Gray et al., 2005; Hertz-Picciotto et al., 2005; Koopman-Essenboom et al., 1996; Wolff et al., 2007). Many animal studies demonstrate that high dose PCB impairs neurodevelopment or their hydroxylated metabolites may interfere with thyroid hormone-dependent neurodevelopment (Kimura-Kuroda et al., 2007; Nguon et al., 2005; Purkey et al., 2004; Roegge et al., 2006).

The non-dioxin-like PCBs weakly interact with estrogen and thyroid receptors and with transport proteins, and the hydroxylated metabolites of PCBs may be more potent mediators of these actions (Azulmozhiraja et al., 2005; DeCastro et al., 2006; Langer et al., 2005; Purkey et al., 2004; Kitamura etal., 2005; You et al., 2006). Variations in thyroid hormone levels have been associated with PCB exposures in human populations (Langer et al., 2007a; Meeker et al., 2007; Otake et al., 2007; Wang et al.,

2005). Though only limited investigation of estrogenic or reproductive effects has occurred in women, inconsistent associations of PCB levels with altered spermatogenesis and reproductive hormone levels have been reported in environmentally exposed men (Giwercman et al., 2006; Rignell-Hydbom et al., 2005; Toft et al., 2006).

PCBs are not considered directly genotoxic. They are classified as probable human carcinogens by IARC and are classified by NTP as reasonably anticipated to be carcinogens. Early studies associated workplace PCB exposures with increased deaths from cancer of the liver, gallbladder, biliary tract, gastrointestinal tract, brain and malignant melanoma (Knerr and Schrenk, 2006). Follow up studies of these earlier investigations have shown no increase in deaths or cancers, with the exception of liver cancer (Kimbrough et al., 2003; Prince et al., 2006; Ross, 2004), though the contributions of dioxin-like chemicals or other organochlorines were unclear. Recent studies have associated PCB exposures with other cancers (De Roos et al., 2005; Engel et al., 2007; Prince et al., 2006). Information about external exposure (i.e., environmental levels) and health effects is available from ATSDR at: http://www.atsdr.cdc.gov/toxpro2.html and from the U.S. EPA at: http://www.epa.gov/iris.

## Serum 2,4,4'-Trichlorobiphenyl (PCB 28) (whole weight)

Geometric mean and selected percentiles of serum concentrations (in ng/g of serum or parts per billion) for the U.S. population from the National Health and Nutrition Examination Survey.

| | Survey years# | Geometric mean (95% conf. interval) | Selected percentiles ( 95% confidence interval) 50th | 75th | 90th | 95th | Sample size |
|---|---|---|---|---|---|---|---|
| **Total** | 99-00 | * | < LOD | < LOD | < LOD | < LOD | 1849 |
| | 03-04 | .030 (.028-.032) | .030 (.028-.032) | .041 ( 039-.043) | .057 (.055-.060) | .067 (.063-071) | 1866 |
| **Age group** | | | | | | | |
| 12-19 years | 99-00 | * | < LOD | < LOD | < LOD | < LOD | 647 |
| | 03-04 | .025 (.023-.028) | .025 (.021-.028) | .035 ( 030-.042) | .051 (.042-.061) | .061 (.051- 070) | 590 |
| 20 years and older | 99-00 | * | < LOD | < LOD | < LOD | < LOD | 1202 |
| | 03-04 | .031 (.029-.033) | .031 (.029-.032) | .042 ( 040-.043) | .058 (.055-.061) | .067 (.063- 071) | 1276 |
| **Gender** | | | | | | | |
| Males | 99-00 | * | < LOD | < LOD | < LOD | < LOD | 886 |
| | 03-04 | .030 (.028-.032) | .030 (.027-.032) | .041 ( 037-.044) | .056 (.051-.061) | .065 (.061- 070) | 926 |
| Females | 99-00 | * | < LOD | < LOD | < LOD | < LOD | 963 |
| | 03-04 | .030 (.028-.032) | .030 (.028-.032) | .042 ( 039-.044) | .058 (.055-.061) | .070 (.064- 075) | 940 |
| **Race/ethnicity** | | | | | | | |
| Mexican Americans | 99-00 | * | < LOD | < LOD | < LOD | < LOD | 618 |
| | 03-04 | .030 (.028-.033) | .031 (.027-.035) | .041 ( 036-.044) | .053 (.048-.059) | .063 (.054- 070) | 413 |
| Non-Hispanic blacks | 99-00 | * | < LOD | < LOD | < LOD | < LOD | 392 |
| | 03-04 | .028 (.024-.033) | .029 (.024-.033) | .039 ( 034-.047) | .059 (.047-.070) | .070 (.064- 082) | 459 |
| Non-Hispanic whites | 99-00 | * | < LOD | < LOD | < LOD | < LOD | 687 |
| | 03-04 | .030 (.028-.032) | .030 (.028-.032) | .041 ( 039-.043) | .058 (.055-.061) | .068 (.062- 075) | 876 |

< LOD means less than the limit of detection for the lipid adjusted serum level, which may vary for some chemicals by year and by individual sample.
* Not calculated: proportion of results below limit of detection was too high to provide a valid result.
# Data not available for Survey years 2001-2002.

## Biomonitoring Information

Measurement of serum PCBs generally reflect cumulative past exposure. Levels of non-dioxin-like PCBs in NHANES 2003-2004 are observed to be roughly similar to the previous two NHANES survey periods. Many PCBs can remain in the body for years after exposure, though some of the PCBs with fewer chlorine atoms have short residence times. The levels of individual PCB congeners in the body may vary by exposure source and by differences in pharmacokinetics, i.e., those with longer half-lives accumulate to higher levels. Adult age-related accumulations in the non-dioxin-like PCBs have been observed in many studies (Apostoli et al., 2005; Park et al., 2007; Patterson et al., 1994). Breastfeeding is a major source of PCBs, with serum levels increasing after birth in breastfed infants and then decreasing in early adolescence due to dilution as body mass increases (Barr et al., 2006). Fish consumption from the Great Lakes region contributed a twofold to tenfold increase in the mean concentrations of non-dioxin-like PCBs over referent populations (Patterson et al., 1994; Turyk et al., 2006). Arctic native Alaskans who consumed locally-caught fish, meat, and eggs had mean serum levels of total PCB that were nearly three times higher than the adult NHANES 1999-2000 subsample (Carpenter et al., 2005; CDC, 2005; Needham et al., 2005). Much higher levels due to contaminated fish intake have also been noted also in eastern Europe (Langer et al., 2007b).

The concentrations of the di-*ortho*-substituted PCBs are usually higher than the mono-*ortho*-substituted PCBs, which in turn are higher than the coplanar PCBs (CDC, 2005; Glynn et al., 2000; Longnecker et al., 2000; Patterson et al., 1994). The most frequently detected di-*ortho*-chlorine-substituted PCBs in population studies are 138, 153, and 180 (CDC, 2005; Heudorf et al., 2002; Patterson et al., 1994 and 2009; Turyk et al., 2006). These three congeners contributed a substantial portion of the total PCB concentration observed in pooled specimens representative of a New Zealand population (Bates et al., 2004); in a small population of Swedish men (Glynn et al., 2000), and in blood bank specimens from Canada (Longnecker et al., 2000). In the U.S representative subsample from NHANES 1999-2000, non-dioxin-like PCBs 138, 153, and 180 accounted for 65% of the measured total sum of PCBs (Needham et al., 2005) and for 78% of the total in a referent population of 311 Italian residents in 2001-2003 (Apostoli et al., 2005). Non-dioxin-like PCBs with five, six, and seven chlorines attached comprised about 80% of the total PCBs in human serum, or alternatively, PCBs 138, 153, 180, 187 and 118 composed 57% of the total PCB concentration in a small sample of South Korean

residents and incineration workers (Park et al., 2007). In the sera of Yucheng victims analyzed 15 years after the rice oil contamination event (See the section "Dioxin-Like Chemicals" for further discussion.),73% of the total PCB concentration was contributed by PCBs 99, 138, 153, 156, 170, 179, and 180 (Hsu et al., 2005).

As has been shown for other organochlorines, median serum lipid-adjusted levels of PCB 153 declined by 38% from 1991 to 2001 in a small sample of Swedish men (Hagmar et al., 2006). In four biannual surveys covering the years 1996-2003, about 400 German fourth grade children were sampled each period and demonstrated a decrease of more than one-half in mean whole blood levels of PCBs 138, 153, and 180 (Link et al., 2005). Lipid adjusted levels of the non-dioxin-like PCBs seen in the U.S representative subsample from NHANES 2001-2002 are generally lower than levels in selected populations during the 1980s to 1990s (CDC, 2005; Glynn et al., 2000; Longnecker et al., 2000; Patterson et al., 1994).

In a convenience sample of 624 urban Germans aged 0-65 years conducted during 1998 (Heudorf et al., 2002), 95th percentile levels for PCBs 138, 153, and 180 were similar or up to two-fold higher than 95th percentile levels in the U.S. NHANES 1999-2000 subsample (CDC, 2005). In contrast, a representative pooled sampling of New Zealand residents in 1996-1997 demonstrated slightly lower levels than for NHANES 1999-2000 (Bates et al., 2004). In two separate Italian studies of a regional reference population and a convenience sample in 2001-2003, median serum levels of PCBs 138, 153, and 180, as well as the sum of measurable PCBs, were about fivefold higher than NHANES 1999-2000 (Apostoli et al., 2005; CDC, 2005; Needham et al., 2005; Turci et al., 2006). Mean levels of PCBs 153 and 180 in 753 adult native Americans were approximately similar to the 95th percentile for the overall adult NHANES 2001-2002 population (CDC, 2005; DeCaprio et al., 2005). In some other countries, comparable population levels are ten or more times higher than those reported for NHANES subsamples from 1999-2000 and 2001-2002 (CDC, 2005; Jursa et al.,2006; Petrik et al., 2006). In the sera of Yucheng victims analyzed at 15 years following the rice oil contamination event, mean serum lipid adjusted levels of PCBs 99, 153, 170, and 180 were several to eightfold higher than the 95th percentiles of NHANES 1999-2000 (Hsu et al., 2005).

Finding a measurable amount of one or more PCBs in serum does not mean that the levels of the PCBs cause an adverse health effect. Biomonitoring studies of serum PCBs can provide physicians and public health officials with reference values so that they can determine whether or not people have been exposed to higher levels of PCBs than levels found in the general population. Biomonitoring data can also help scientists plan and conduct research on exposure and health effects.

## Serum 2,2'3,5'-Tetrachlorobiphenyl (PCB 44) (lipid adjusted)

Geometric mean and selected percentiles of serum concentrations (in ng/g of lipid or parts per billion on a lipid-weight basis) for the U.S. population from the National Health and Nutrition Examination Survey.

| | Survey years | Geometric mean (95% conf. interval) | Selected percentiles ( 95% confidence interval) | | | | Sample size |
|---|---|---|---|---|---|---|---|
| | | | 50th | 75th | 90th | 95th | |
| **Total** | 03-04 | 2.06 (1.93-2.19) | 2.05 (1 90-2.20) | 3.03 (2.90-3.20) | 4.40 (4.10-4 86) | 5.70 (5.40-6.10) | 1890 |
| **Age group** | | | | | | | |
| 12-19 years | 03-04 | 2.45 (2.22-2.70) | 2.44 (2.10-2.70) | 3.68 (3.19-4.37) | 5.78 (5.13-6 30) | 7.99 (6.20-9.10) | 597 |
| 20 years and older | 03-04 | 2.00 (1.88-2.13) | 2.00 (1 90-2.11) | 2.97 (2.80-3.20) | 4.27 (3.85-4.70) | 5.44 (5.00-5.89) | 1293 |
| **Gender** | | | | | | | |
| Males | 03-04 | 2.12 (2.01-2.25) | 2.12 (2 00-2.30) | 3.11 (2.97-3.31) | 4.52 (4.10-5 20) | 5.89 (5.38-6.80) | 942 |
| Females | 03-04 | 1.99 (1.82-2.18) | 1.98 (1 80-2.20) | 2.94 (2.72-3.21) | 4.30 (3.77-5 05) | 5.60 (5.00-6.20) | 948 |
| **Race/ethnicity** | | | | | | | |
| Mexican Americans | 03-04 | 2.09 (1.88-2.31) | 2.10 (1 90-2.39) | 3.10 (2.52-3.73) | 4.20 (3.30-6.10) | 5.69 (3.80-7.40) | 427 |
| Non-Hispanic blacks | 03-04 | 2.21 (1.94-2.52) | 2.12 (1 80-2.56) | 3.18 (2.72-3.94) | 4.90 (3.90-6 32) | 6.32 (5.01-9.62) | 464 |
| Non-Hispanic whites | 03-04 | 2.03 (1.87-2.19) | 2.01 (1 90-2.20) | 3.07 (2.90-3.29) | 4.40 (4.01-4 95) | 5.70 (5.25-6.35) | 877 |

Limit of detection (LOD, see Data Analysis section) for Survey year 03-04 is 0.4.

## Serum 2,2'3,5'-Tetrachlorobiphenyl (PCB 44) (whole weight)

Geometric mean and selected percentiles of serum concentrations (in ng/g of serum or parts per billion) for the U.S. population from the National Health and Nutrition Examination Survey.

| | Survey years | Geometric mean (95% conf. interval) | Selected percentiles ( 95% confidence interval) | | | | Sample size |
|---|---|---|---|---|---|---|---|
| | | | 50th | 75th | 90th | 95th | |
| **Total** | 03-04 | .013 (.012- 013) | .013 (.012-.014) | .018 (.017-.020) | .026 (.024-.028) | .032 ( 030-.034) | 1890 |
| **Age group** | | | | | | | |
| 12-19 years | 03-04 | .012 (.011- 014) | .013 (.011-.014) | .019 (.016-.021) | .029 (.024-.031) | .037 ( 030-.042) | 597 |
| 20 years and older | 03-04 | .013 (.012- 013) | .013 (.012-.014) | .018 (.017-.020) | .025 (.023-.027) | .031 ( 029-.034) | 1293 |
| **Gender** | | | | | | | |
| Males | 03-04 | .013 (.012- 014) | .013 (.012-.014) | .018 (.017-.020) | .026 (.024-.028) | .034 ( 030-.038) | 942 |
| Females | 03-04 | .012 (.011- 013) | .012 (.011-.013) | .018 (.016-.020) | .025 (.023-.028) | .030 ( 028-.032) | 948 |
| **Race/ethnicity** | | | | | | | |
| Mexican Americans | 03-04 | .013 (.011- 014) | .013 (.011-.014) | .017 (.015-.020) | .023 (.018-.031) | .027 ( 021-.049) | 427 |
| Non-Hispanic blacks | 03-04 | .013 (.011- 014) | .012 (.010-.014) | .018 (.015-.022) | .026 (.021-.034) | .035 ( 026-.040) | 464 |
| Non-Hispanic whites | 03-04 | .012 (.012- 014) | .012 (.011-.014) | .019 (.017-.020) | .026 (.024-.028) | .032 ( 029-.035) | 877 |

## Serum 2,2',4,5'-Tetrachlorobiphenyl (PCB 49) (lipid adjusted)

Geometric mean and selected percentiles of serum concentrations (in ng/g of lipid or parts per billion on a lipid-weight basis) for the U.S. population from the National Health and Nutrition Examination Survey.

| | Survey years | Geometric mean (95% conf. interval) | Selected percentiles ( 95% confidence interval) | | | | Sample size |
|---|---|---|---|---|---|---|---|
| | | | 50th | 75th | 90th | 95th | |
| Total | 03-04 | 1.29 (1.20-1.39) | 1.35 (1.24-1.45) | 1.90 (1.80-2.10) | 2.80 (2.60-3.08) | 3.53 (3.33-3.80) | 1876 |
| Age group | | | | | | | |
| 12-19 years | 03-04 | 1.54 (1.37-1.72) | 1.59 (1.33-1.80) | 2.30 (2.00-2.84) | 3.60 (3.10-4.13) | 4.66 (3.80-5.73) | 590 |
| 20 years and older | 03-04 | 1.26 (1.17-1.35) | 1.33 (1.22-1.40) | 1.90 (1.78-2.03) | 2.69 (2.50-2.80) | 3.36 (3.15-3.63) | 1286 |
| Gender | | | | | | | |
| Males | 03-04 | 1.36 (1.27-1.45) | 1.40 (1.30-1.50) | 2.00 (1.90-2.20) | 3.00 (2.60-3.23) | 3.79 (3.36-4.10) | 932 |
| Females | 03-04 | 1.23 (1.12-1.35) | 1.30 (1.13-1.40) | 1.80 (1.70-2.04) | 2.66 (2.38-3.01) | 3.39 (3.02-3.73) | 944 |
| Race/ethnicity | | | | | | | |
| Mexican Americans | 03-04 | 1.33 (1.20-1.48) | 1.46 (1.20-1.57) | 2.00 (1.67-2.30) | 2.70 (2.17-3.80) | 3.56 (2.63-4.20) | 426 |
| Non-Hispanic blacks | 03-04 | 1.40 (1.23-1.59) | 1.40 (1.20-1.64) | 2.06 (1.70-2.80) | 3.23 (2.80-3.70) | 3.88 (3.33-5.53) | 453 |
| Non-Hispanic whites | 03-04 | 1.26 (1.15-1.38) | 1.32 (1.20-1.40) | 1.90 (1.78-2.11) | 2.77 (2.50-3.10) | 3.45 (3.20-3.90) | 876 |

Limit of detection (LOD, see Data Analysis section) for Survey year 03-04 is 0.4.

## Serum 2,2',4,5'-Tetrachlorobiphenyl (PCB 49) (whole weight)

Geometric mean and selected percentiles of serum concentrations (in ng/g of serum or parts per billion) for the U.S. population from the National Health and Nutrition Examination Survey.

| | Survey years | Geometric mean (95% conf. interval) | Selected percentiles ( 95% confidence interval) | | | | Sample size |
|---|---|---|---|---|---|---|---|
| | | | 50th | 75th | 90th | 95th | |
| Total | 03-04 | .008 (.007-.008) | .008 (.007-.009) | .012 ( 011-.012) | .016 (.015-.017) | .019 (.018-021) | 1876 |
| Age group | | | | | | | |
| 12-19 years | 03-04 | .008 (.007-.009) | .008 (.007-.009) | .012 ( 010-.013) | .018 (.015-.019) | .022 (.018-025) | 590 |
| 20 years and older | 03-04 | .008 (.007-.008) | .008 (.007-.009) | .012 ( 011-.013) | .015 (.015-.017) | .019 (.018-021) | 1286 |
| Gender | | | | | | | |
| Males | 03-04 | .008 (.008-.009) | .008 (.008-.009) | .012 ( 011-.013) | .017 (.015-.018) | .021 (.019-022) | 932 |
| Females | 03-04 | .007 (.007-.008) | .008 (.007-.008) | .011 ( 010-.012) | .015 (.014-.017) | .018 (.017-019) | 944 |
| Race/ethnicity | | | | | | | |
| Mexican Americans | 03-04 | .008 (.007-.009) | .008 (.007-.009) | .011 ( 010-.014) | .015 (.012-.018) | .018 (.015-023) | 426 |
| Non-Hispanic blacks | 03-04 | .008 (.007-.009) | .008 (.007-.009) | .012 ( 010-.014) | .017 (.015-.020) | .021 (.017-026) | 453 |
| Non-Hispanic whites | 03-04 | .008 (.007-.009) | .008 (.007-.009) | .012 ( 011-.013) | .016 (.015-.017) | .019 (.018-021) | 876 |

## Serum 2,2',5,5'-Tetrachlorobiphenyl (PCB 52) (lipid adjusted)

Geometric mean and selected percentiles of serum concentrations (in ng/g of lipid or parts per billion on a lipid-weight basis) for the U.S. population from the National Health and Nutrition Examination Survey.

| | Survey years | Geometric mean (95% conf. interval) | Selected percentiles ( 95% confidence interval) | | | | Sample size |
|---|---|---|---|---|---|---|---|
| | | | 50th | 75th | 90th | 95th | |
| **Total** | 99-00 | * | < LOD | < LOD | < LOD | < LOD | 1912 |
| | 01-02 | * | < LOD | < LOD | < LOD | 16.5 (14 3-17.2) | 1537 |
| | 03-04 | 2.66 (2.43-2.91) | 2.74 (2 50-3.00) | 4.17 (3.72-4.60) | 5.91 (5.40-6 67) | 7.60 (7.01-8.00) | 1897 |
| **Age group** | | | | | | | |
| 12-19 years | 99-00 | * | < LOD | < LOD | < LOD | < LOD | 664 |
| | 01-02 | * | < LOD | < LOD | 16.2 (<LOD-23 8) | 22.9 (16 9-32.3) | 291 |
| | 03-04 | 3.16 (2.81-3.56) | 3.22 (2 60-3.96) | 5.15 (4.46-5.79) | 7.60 (6.55-8 33) | 9.20 (7.80-12.5) | 597 |
| 20 years and older | 99-00 | * | < LOD | < LOD | < LOD | < LOD | 1248 |
| | 01-02 | * | < LOD | < LOD | < LOD | 16.0 (13 5-16.9) | 1246 |
| | 03-04 | 2.59 (2.36-2.84) | 2.70 (2.46-2.92) | 4.06 (3.60-4.43) | 5.70 (5.16-6.49) | 7.15 (6.62-7.80) | 1300 |
| **Gender** | | | | | | | |
| Males | 99-00 | * | < LOD | < LOD | < LOD | < LOD | 908 |
| | 01-02 | * | < LOD | < LOD | < LOD | 16.0 (<LOD-17.5) | 716 |
| | 03-04 | 2.75 (2.54-2.98) | 2.80 (2 55-3.20) | 4.36 (3.90-4.88) | 5.94 (5.51-6 80) | 7.80 (7.29-8.49) | 946 |
| Females | 99-00 | * | < LOD | < LOD | < LOD | < LOD | 1004 |
| | 01-02 | * | < LOD | < LOD | < LOD | 16.6 (14 0-18.2) | 821 |
| | 03-04 | 2.57 (2.30-2.87) | 2.70 (2.40-2.96) | 3.96 (3.52-4.30) | 5.86 (4.96-6 67) | 7.15 (6.57-8.10) | 951 |
| **Race/ethnicity** | | | | | | | |
| Mexican Americans | 99-00 | * | < LOD | < LOD | < LOD | < LOD | 631 |
| | 01-02 | * | < LOD | < LOD | < LOD | 16.9 (<LOD-20.6) | 366 |
| | 03-04 | 2.88 (2.56-3.24) | 3.00 (2.70-3.30) | 4.41 (3.60-5.30) | 6.00 (4.71-8.11) | 7.83 (5.70-12.0) | 426 |
| Non-Hispanic blacks | 99-00 | * | < LOD | < LOD | < LOD | < LOD | 408 |
| | 01-02 | * | < LOD | < LOD | < LOD | 16.6 (<LOD-20.9) | 282 |
| | 03-04 | 2.74 (2.35-3.19) | 2.58 (2 08-3.40) | 4.11 (3.30-5.60) | 6.92 (5.10-8.70) | 8.70 (7.10-10.2) | 464 |
| Non-Hispanic whites | 99-00 | * | < LOD | < LOD | < LOD | < LOD | 716 |
| | 01-02 | * | < LOD | < LOD | < LOD | 16.6 (14.7-17.5) | 773 |
| | 03-04 | 2.60 (2.35-2.88) | 2.70 (2.40-2.98) | 4.17 (3.70-4.60) | 5.79 (5.20-6.75) | 7.37 (6.80-7.87) | 885 |

Limit of detection (LOD, see Data Analysis section) for Survey years 99-00, 01-02, and 03-04 are 12.5, 12.4, and 0.8, respectively.
< LOD means less than the limit of detection, which may vary for some chemicals by year and by individual sample.
* Not calculated: proportion of results below limit of detection was too high to provide a valid result.

## Serum 2,2',5,5'-Tetrachlorobiphenyl (PCB 52) (whole weight)

Geometric mean and selected percentiles of serum concentrations (in ng/g of serum or parts per billion) for the U.S. population from the National Health and Nutrition Examination Survey.

| | Survey years | Geometric mean (95% conf. interval) | 50th | 75th | 90th | 95th | Sample size |
|---|---|---|---|---|---|---|---|
| **Total** | 99-00 | * | < LOD | < LOD | < LOD | < LOD | 1912 |
| | 01-02 | * | < LOD | < LOD | < LOD | .090 (.080-.100) | 1537 |
| | 03-04 | .016 (.015-.018) | .017 (.015-.019) | .024 ( 022-.028) | .035 (.032-.037) | .043 (.039- 046) | 1897 |
| **Age group** | | | | | | | |
| 12-19 years | 99-00 | * | < LOD | < LOD | < LOD | < LOD | 664 |
| | 01-02 | * | < LOD | < LOD | .080 (<LOD-.100) | .100 (.080-.140) | 291 |
| | 03-04 | .016 (.014-.018) | .017 (.014-.019) | .026 ( 022-.029) | .037 (.032-.041) | .042 (.037- 056) | 597 |
| 20 years and older | 99-00 | * | < LOD | < LOD | < LOD | < LOD | 1248 |
| | 01-02 | * | < LOD | < LOD | < LOD | .090 (.080- 090) | 1246 |
| | 03-04 | .016 (.015-.018) | .017 (.015-.019) | .024 ( 022-.028) | .034 (.031-.036) | .043 (.038- 045) | 1300 |
| **Gender** | | | | | | | |
| Males | 99-00 | * | < LOD | < LOD | < LOD | < LOD | 908 |
| | 01-02 | * | < LOD | < LOD | < LOD | .090 (<LOD-.110) | 716 |
| | 03-04 | .017 (.016-.018) | .018 (.016-.020) | .025 ( 023-.029) | .036 (.032-.039) | .044 (.040- 048) | 946 |
| Females | 99-00 | * | < LOD | < LOD | < LOD | < LOD | 1004 |
| | 01-02 | * | < LOD | < LOD | < LOD | .090 (.080-.100) | 821 |
| | 03-04 | .016 (.014-.017) | .016 (.014-018) | .024 ( 021-.028) | .033 (.030-036) | .042 (.036- 046) | 951 |
| **Race/ethnicity** | | | | | | | |
| Mexican Americans | 99-00 | * | < LOD | < LOD | < LOD | < LOD | 631 |
| | 01-02 | * | < LOD | < LOD | < LOD | .090 (<LOD-.110) | 366 |
| | 03-04 | .018 (.016-.020) | .018 (.016-.021) | .025 ( 022-.030) | .035 (.028-.044) | .044 (.032- 064) | 426 |
| Non-Hispanic blacks | 99-00 | * | < LOD | < LOD | < LOD | < LOD | 408 |
| | 01-02 | * | < LOD | < LOD | < LOD | .090 (<LOD-.110) | 282 |
| | 03-04 | .016 (.014-.018) | .015 (.012-.019) | .022 ( 019-.031) | .035 (.029-.043) | .043 (.035- 049) | 464 |
| Non-Hispanic whites | 99-00 | * | < LOD | < LOD | < LOD | < LOD | 716 |
| | 01-02 | * | < LOD | < LOD | < LOD | .090 (.080-.100) | 773 |
| | 03-04 | .016 (.014-.018) | .017 (.014-.019) | .024 ( 022-.028) | .035 (.032-.037) | .043 (.038- 047) | 885 |

< LOD means less than the limit of detection for the lipid adjusted serum level, which may vary for some chemicals by year and by individual sample.
* Not calculated: proportion of results below limit of detection was too high to provide a valid result.

## Serum 2,3',4,4'-Tetrachlorobiphenyl (PCB 66) (lipid adjusted)

Geometric mean and selected percentiles of serum concentrations (in ng/g of lipid or parts per billion on a lipid-weight basis) for the U.S. population from the National Health and Nutrition Examination Survey.

| | Survey years | Geometric mean (95% conf. interval) | Selected percentiles ( 95% confidence interval) | | | | Sample size |
|---|---|---|---|---|---|---|---|
| | | | 50th | 75th | 90th | 95th | |
| **Total** | 99-00 | * | < LOD | < LOD | < LOD | < LOD | 1931 |
| | 01-02 | * | < LOD | < LOD | < LOD | < LOD | 2250 |
| | 03-04 | 1.39 (1.32-1.47) | 1.37 (1 30-1.40) | 1.97 (1.90-2.10) | 3.10 (2.94-3 26) | 4.10 (3.90-4.55) | 1898 |
| **Age group** | | | | | | | |
| 12-19 years | 99-00 | * | < LOD | < LOD | < LOD | < LOD | 671 |
| | 01-02 | * | < LOD | < LOD | < LOD | < LOD | 724 |
| | 03-04 | 1.24 (1.14-1.34) | 1.20 (1.10-1.26) | 1.76 (1.62-2.00) | 2.40 (2.30-2.70) | 3.25 (2.70-4.10) | 598 |
| 20 years and older | 99-00 | * | < LOD | < LOD | < LOD | < LOD | 1260 |
| | 01-02 | * | < LOD | < LOD | < LOD | < LOD | 1526 |
| | 03-04 | 1.42 (1.34-1.49) | 1.40 (1 30-1.43) | 2.00 (1.90-2.12) | 3.10 (2.97-3.40) | 4.20 (3.90-4.71) | 1300 |
| **Gender** | | | | | | | |
| Males | 99-00 | * | < LOD | < LOD | < LOD | < LOD | 919 |
| | 01-02 | * | < LOD | < LOD | < LOD | < LOD | 1047 |
| | 03-04 | 1.29 (1.20-1.39) | 1.30 (1 20-1.38) | 1.87 (1.72-2.01) | 2.70 (2.50-3 00) | 3.30 (2.96-3.82) | 947 |
| Females | 99-00 | * | < LOD | < LOD | < LOD | < LOD | 1012 |
| | 01-02 | * | < LOD | < LOD | < LOD | < LOD | 1203 |
| | 03-04 | 1.50 (1.42-1.58) | 1.41 (1 38-1.50) | 2.10 (1.92-2.30) | 3.70 (3.20-4 00) | 5.08 (4.10-5.46) | 951 |
| **Race/ethnicity** | | | | | | | |
| Mexican Americans | 99-00 | * | < LOD | < LOD | < LOD | < LOD | 636 |
| | 01-02 | * | < LOD | < LOD | < LOD | < LOD | 548 |
| | 03-04 | 1.19 (1.09-1.30) | 1.14 (1 00-1.30) | 1.60 (1.48-1.73) | 2.23 (1.80-3 20) | 3.20 (2.46-3.60) | 427 |
| Non-Hispanic blacks | 99-00 | * | < LOD | < LOD | < LOD | < LOD | 414 |
| | 01-02 | * | < LOD | < LOD | < LOD | < LOD | 495 |
| | 03-04 | 1.50 (1.34-1.68) | 1.38 (1 21-1.50) | 2.31 (1.80-2.80) | 3.80 (3.10-4 80) | 5.46 (4.30-8.60) | 464 |
| Non-Hispanic whites | 99-00 | * | < LOD | < LOD | < LOD | < LOD | 723 |
| | 01-02 | * | < LOD | < LOD | < LOD | < LOD | 1047 |
| | 03-04 | 1.39 (1.31-1.47) | 1.39 (1 30-1.45) | 1.96 (1.90-2.10) | 3.01 (2.71-3 28) | 4.09 (3.70-4.33) | 885 |

Limit of detection (LOD, see Data Analysis section) for Survey years 99-00, 01-02, and 03-04 are 12.4, 12.4, and 0.8, respectively.
< LOD means less than the limit of detection, which may vary for some chemicals by year and by individual sample.
* Not calculated: proportion of results below limit of detection was too high to provide a valid result.

## Serum 2,3',4,4'-Tetrachlorobiphenyl (PCB 66) (whole weight)

Geometric mean and selected percentiles of serum concentrations (in ng/g of serum or parts per billion) for the U.S. population from the National Health and Nutrition Examination Survey.

| | Survey years | Geometric mean (95% conf. interval) | Selected percentiles ( 95% confidence interval) | | | | Sample size |
|---|---|---|---|---|---|---|---|
| | | | 50th | 75th | 90th | 95th | |
| **Total** | 99-00 | * | < LOD | < LOD | < LOD | < LOD | 1931 |
| | 01-02 | * | < LOD | < LOD | < LOD | < LOD | 2250 |
| | 03-04 | .008 (.008-.009) | .008 (.008-.009) | .012 ( 012-.013) | .019 (.018-.021) | .025 (.024-.030) | 1898 |
| **Age group** | | | | | | | |
| 12-19 years | 99-00 | * | < LOD | < LOD | < LOD | < LOD | 671 |
| | 01-02 | * | < LOD | < LOD | < LOD | < LOD | 724 |
| | 03-04 | .006 (.006-.007) | .006 (.005-.007) | .009 ( 008-.010) | .013 (.012-.014) | .017 (.013-.019) | 598 |
| 20 years and older | 99-00 | * | < LOD | < LOD | < LOD | < LOD | 1260 |
| | 01-02 | * | < LOD | < LOD | < LOD | < LOD | 1526 |
| | 03-04 | .009 (.008-.009) | .008 (.008-.009) | .013 ( 012-.013) | .020 (.019-.022) | .026 (.024-.032) | 1300 |
| **Gender** | | | | | | | |
| Males | 99-00 | * | < LOD | < LOD | < LOD | < LOD | 919 |
| | 01-02 | * | < LOD | < LOD | < LOD | < LOD | 1047 |
| | 03-04 | .008 (.007-.009) | .008 (.007-.008) | .011 ( 010-.013) | .017 (.016-.019) | .020 (.019-.022) | 947 |
| Females | 99-00 | * | < LOD | < LOD | < LOD | < LOD | 1012 |
| | 01-02 | * | < LOD | < LOD | < LOD | < LOD | 1203 |
| | 03-04 | .009 (.009-.010) | .009 (.008-.009) | .013 ( 012-.014) | .022 (.021-.024) | .032 (.026-.034) | 951 |
| **Race/ethnicity** | | | | | | | |
| Mexican Americans | 99-00 | * | < LOD | < LOD | < LOD | < LOD | 636 |
| | 01-02 | * | < LOD | < LOD | < LOD | < LOD | 548 |
| | 03-04 | .007 (.007-.008) | .007 (.006-.008) | .010 ( 009-.011) | .015 (.011-.018) | .018 (.014-.020) | 427 |
| Non-Hispanic blacks | 99-00 | * | < LOD | < LOD | < LOD | < LOD | 414 |
| | 01-02 | * | < LOD | < LOD | < LOD | < LOD | 495 |
| | 03-04 | .009 (.008-.009) | .008 (.007-.009) | .013 ( 011-.015) | .022 (.019-.030) | .036 (.024-.070) | 464 |
| Non-Hispanic whites | 99-00 | * | < LOD | < LOD | < LOD | < LOD | 723 |
| | 01-02 | * | < LOD | < LOD | < LOD | < LOD | 1047 |
| | 03-04 | .009 (.008-.009) | .008 (.008-.009) | .012 ( 012-.013) | .019 (.018-.022) | .025 (.023-.030) | 885 |

< LOD means less than the limit of detection for the lipid adjusted serum level, which may vary for some chemicals by year and by individual sample.
* Not calculated: proportion of results below limit of detection was too high to provide a valid result.

## Serum 2,4,4',5-Tetrachlorobiphenyl (PCB 74) (lipid adjusted)

Geometric mean and selected percentiles of serum concentrations (in ng/g of lipid or parts per billion on a lipid-weight basis) for the U.S. population from the National Health and Nutrition Examination Survey.

| | Survey years | Geometric mean (95% conf. interval) | 50th | 75th | 90th | 95th | Sample size |
|---|---|---|---|---|---|---|---|
| **Total** | 99-00 | * | < LOD | < LOD | 20.8 (17.9-23.4) | 29.0 (24 5-32.3) | 1924 |
| | 01-02 | * | < LOD | 13.2 (11.0-15.7) | 23.5 (20.2-27.7) | 33.0 (26 9-38.7) | 2307 |
| | 03-04 | 4.81 (4.63-4.99) | 4.36 (3 90-4.88) | 8.72 (8.30-9.28) | 15.8 (14.7-17.7) | 22.3 (19.7-25.5) | 1898 |
| **Age group** | | | | | | | |
| 12-19 years | 99-00 | * | < LOD | < LOD | < LOD | < LOD | 671 |
| | 01-02 | * | < LOD | < LOD | < LOD | < LOD | 758 |
| | 03-04 | 2.20 (2.02-2.39) | 2.20 (2 03-2.33) | 2.98 (2.80-3.30) | 4.19 (3.60-4.73) | 5.32 (4.20-6.90) | 598 |
| 20 years and older | 99-00 | * | < LOD | 12.6 (<LOD-14.4) | 22.4 (19.5-25.6) | 30.0 (26 2-35.8) | 1253 |
| | 01-02 | * | < LOD | 14.7 (12.4-17.1) | 25.2 (21.4-28.9) | 34.8 (28 8-41.4) | 1549 |
| | 03-04 | 5.38 (5.16-5.62) | 5.00 (4 60-5.50) | 9.60 (8.90-10.6) | 17.1 (15.7-18.5) | 24.1 (20 8-27.7) | 1300 |
| **Gender** | | | | | | | |
| Males | 99-00 | * | < LOD | < LOD | 15.4 (13.0-17.8) | 21.6 (18 3-24.4) | 915 |
| | 01-02 | * | < LOD | 10.6 (<LOD-12 3) | 20.2 (15.4-24.9) | 28.8 (20 8-38.2) | 1075 |
| | 03-04 | 4.06 (3.82-4.31) | 3.62 (3 30-4.00) | 6.71 (6.20-7.77) | 12.4 (10.8-13.1) | 15.8 (14 6-18.5) | 947 |
| Females | 99-00 | * | < LOD | 13.9 (<LOD-16.4) | 24.6 (21.9-28.5) | 31.9 (28 8-40.3) | 1009 |
| | 01-02 | * | < LOD | 15.8 (13.5-18.7) | 26.1 (23.2-29.3) | 35.9 (31.4-41.4) | 1232 |
| | 03-04 | 5.65 (5.33-5.98) | 5.38 (4 84-5.95) | 10.9 (9.30-12.1) | 19.1 (17.4-21.1) | 27.4 (22 9-29.6) | 951 |
| **Race/ethnicity** | | | | | | | |
| Mexican Americans | 99-00 | * | < LOD | < LOD | < LOD | 15.8 (12 8-18.2) | 636 |
| | 01-02 | * | < LOD | < LOD | 13.3 (<LOD-18.1) | 19.6 (16 2-23.0) | 567 |
| | 03-04 | 2.43 (2.10-2.80) | 2.12 (1 90-2.40) | 3.34 (2.90-4.16) | 6.10 (5.25-7.40) | 10.4 (6.61-12.2) | 427 |
| Non-Hispanic blacks | 99-00 | * | < LOD | < LOD | 29.0 (18.6-38.4) | 43.8 (35.4-64.0) | 411 |
| | 01-02 | * | < LOD | 12.0 (<LOD-14 2) | 21.7 (16.4-26.9) | 31.9 (24 5-41.0) | 515 |
| | 03-04 | 4.96 (4.21-5.83) | 4.00 (3.45-4.65) | 9.17 (6.80-12.4) | 23.0 (14.6-35.1) | 40.2 (23 0-68.2) | 464 |
| Non-Hispanic whites | 99-00 | * | < LOD | < LOD | 21.6 (18.9-24.0) | 29.0 (24 3-32.3) | 719 |
| | 01-02 | * | < LOD | 14.7 (12.2-17.3) | 25.8 (21.3-30.1) | 35.9 (29 0-42.5) | 1061 |
| | 03-04 | 5.23 (4.98-5.50) | 4.91 (4 38-5.65) | 9.30 (8.60-10.4) | 16.1 (15.1-18.2) | 21.9 (19 2-25.2) | 885 |

Limit of detection (LOD, see Data Analysis section) for Survey years 99-00, 01-02, and 03-04 are 12.4, 10 5, and 0.8, respectively.
< LOD means less than the limit of detection, which may vary for some chemicals by year and by individual sample.
* Not calculated: proportion of results below limit of detection was too high to provide a valid result.

## Serum 2,4,4',5-Tetrachlorobiphenyl (PCB 74) (whole weight)

Geometric mean and selected percentiles of serum concentrations (in ng/g of serum or parts per billion) for the U.S. population from the National Health and Nutrition Examination Survey.

| | Survey years | Geometric mean (95% conf. interval) | Selected percentiles ( 95% confidence interval) | | | | Sample size |
|---|---|---|---|---|---|---|---|
| | | | 50th | 75th | 90th | 95th | |
| **Total** | 99-00 | * | < LOD | < LOD | .140 (.120-.150) | .180 (.160- 220) | 1924 |
| | 01-02 | * | < LOD | .090 ( 070-.100) | .150 (.140-.180) | .210 (.180- 270) | 2307 |
| | 03-04 | .029 (.028-.031) | .027 (.024-.029) | .058 ( 053-.062) | .104 (.093-.121) | .153 (.135-.171) | 1898 |
| **Age group** | | | | | | | |
| 12-19 years | 99-00 | * | < LOD | < LOD | < LOD | < LOD | 671 |
| | 01-02 | * | < LOD | < LOD | < LOD | < LOD | 758 |
| | 03-04 | .011 (.010-.012) | .011 (.010-.012) | .015 ( 014-.018) | .021 (.019-.025) | .026 (.021- 033) | 598 |
| 20 years and older | 99-00 | * | < LOD | .080 (<LOD-.100) | .150 (.140-.160) | .200 (.170- 230) | 1253 |
| | 01-02 | * | < LOD | .100 ( 080-.110) | .170 (.140-.190) | .230 (.200- 280) | 1549 |
| | 03-04 | .034 (.032-.035) | .031 (.028-.033) | .064 ( 059-.068) | .115 (.103-.128) | .167 (.143-.186) | 1300 |
| **Gender** | | | | | | | |
| Males | 99-00 | * | < LOD | < LOD | .100 (.090-.120) | .150 (.130-.170) | 915 |
| | 01-02 | * | < LOD | .070 (<LOD-.080) | .130 (.100-.170) | .190 (.140- 250) | 1075 |
| | 03-04 | .025 (.023-.027) | .023 (.021-.027) | .043 ( 040-.050) | .077 (.067-.087) | .103 (.092-.118) | 947 |
| Females | 99-00 | * | < LOD | .100 (<LOD-.110) | .160 (.140-.180) | .220 (.190- 250) | 1009 |
| | 01-02 | * | < LOD | .100 ( 090-.110) | .170 (.150-.190) | .240 (.210- 290) | 1232 |
| | 03-04 | .034 (.032- 037) | .031 (.027-.036) | .071 ( 062-.085) | .130 (.120-.143) | .186 (.154- 216) | 951 |
| **Race/ethnicity** | | | | | | | |
| Mexican Americans | 99-00 | * | < LOD | < LOD | < LOD | .110 (.080-.130) | 636 |
| | 01-02 | * | < LOD | < LOD | .090 (<LOD-.120) | .140 (.110-.160) | 567 |
| | 03-04 | .015 (.013-.017) | .013 (.011-.016) | .022 ( 019-.026) | .042 (.032-.054) | .071 (.049- 097) | 427 |
| Non-Hispanic blacks | 99-00 | * | < LOD | < LOD | .170 (.110-.250) | .280 (.220-.420) | 411 |
| | 01-02 | * | < LOD | .070 (<LOD-.080) | .130 (.100-.170) | .200 (.150- 250) | 515 |
| | 03-04 | .028 (.024-.033) | .022 (.019-.025) | .055 ( 038-.077) | .153 (.090-.215) | .236 (.143- 337) | 464 |
| Non-Hispanic whites | 99-00 | * | < LOD | < LOD | .150 (.130-.160) | .190 (.160- 210) | 719 |
| | 01-02 | * | < LOD | .100 ( 080-.110) | .170 (.140-.200) | .230 (.190- 280) | 1061 |
| | 03-04 | .032 (.030-.034) | .030 (.027-.033) | .064 ( 058-.067) | .113 (.096-.123) | .153 (.131-.176) | 885 |

< LOD means less than the limit of detection for the lipid adjusted serum level, which may vary for some chemicals by year and by individual sample.
* Not calculated: proportion of results below limit of detection was too high to provide a valid result.

## Serum 2,2',3,4,5'-Pentachlorobiphenyl (PCB 87) (lipid adjusted)

Geometric mean and selected percentiles of serum concentrations (in ng/g of lipid or parts per billion on a lipid-weight basis) for the U.S. population from the National Health and Nutrition Examination Survey.

| | Survey years | Geometric mean (95% conf. interval) | Selected percentiles ( 95% confidence interval) | | | | Sample size |
|---|---|---|---|---|---|---|---|
| | | | 50th | 75th | 90th | 95th | |
| **Total** | 01-02 | * | < LOD | < LOD | < LOD | < LOD | 2298 |
| | 03-04 | .656 (.579-.744) | .900 (.800-.980) | 1.32 (1.24-1.46) | 2.02 (1.90-2.17) | 2.70 (2.40-3.03) | 1892 |
| **Age group** | | | | | | | |
| 12-19 years | 01-02 | * | < LOD | < LOD | < LOD | < LOD | 758 |
| | 03-04 | .706 (.629-.792) | .860 (.800-1.00) | 1.56 (1.32-1.69) | 2.25 (2.05-2 60) | 3.44 (2.27-3.98) | 596 |
| 20 years and older | 01-02 | * | < LOD | < LOD | < LOD | < LOD | 1540 |
| | 03-04 | .650 (.568-.742) | .900 (.800-.970) | 1.30 (1.22-1.40) | 2.00 (1.85-2.17) | 2.60 (2.35-2.91) | 1296 |
| **Gender** | | | | | | | |
| Males | 01-02 | * | < LOD | < LOD | < LOD | < LOD | 1069 |
| | 03-04 | .665 (.606-.730) | .900 (.800-.970) | 1.40 (1.30-1.50) | 2.05 (1.90-2 27) | 2.70 (2.33-3.08) | 945 |
| Females | 01-02 | * | < LOD | < LOD | < LOD | < LOD | 1229 |
| | 03-04 | .648 (.545-.771) | .870 (.780-1.00) | 1.30 (1.20-1.41) | 2.00 (1.84-2 23) | 2.60 (2.35-3.08) | 947 |
| **Race/ethnicity** | | | | | | | |
| Mexican Americans | 01-02 | * | < LOD | < LOD | < LOD | < LOD | 564 |
| | 03-04 | .693 (.569- 843) | .840 (.700-1.00) | 1.49 (1.14-1.70) | 2.00 (1.64-2.40) | 2.30 (2.00-3.10) | 427 |
| Non-Hispanic blacks | 01-02 | * | < LOD | < LOD | < LOD | < LOD | 515 |
| | 03-04 | .824 (.723- 939) | 1.05 (.950-1.10) | 1.70 (1.32-2.10) | 2.81 (2.48-3 09) | 3.42 (3.00-4.14) | 462 |
| Non-Hispanic whites | 01-02 | * | < LOD | < LOD | < LOD | < LOD | 1056 |
| | 03-04 | .625 (.531-.735) | .830 (.780-.940) | 1.30 (1.20-1.40) | 1.97 (1.85-2.17) | 2.49 (2.30-2.80) | 882 |

Limit of detection (LOD, see Data Analysis section) for Survey years 01-02 and 03-04 are 10.5 and 0.4.
< LOD means less than the limit of detection, which may vary for some chemicals by year and by individual sample.
* Not calculated: proportion of results below limit of detection was too high to provide a valid result.

## Serum 2,2',3,4,5'-Pentachlorobiphenyl (PCB 87) (whole weight)

Geometric mean and selected percentiles of serum concentrations (in ng/g of serum or parts per billion) for the U.S. population from the National Health and Nutrition Examination Survey.

| | Survey years | Geometric mean (95% conf. interval) | Selected percentiles ( 95% confidence interval) | | | | Sample size |
|---|---|---|---|---|---|---|---|
| | | | 50th | 75th | 90th | 95th | |
| **Total** | 01-02 | * | < LOD | < LOD | < LOD | < LOD | 2298 |
| | 03-04 | .004 (.004-.005) | .005 (.005-.006) | .008 ( 008-.009) | .012 (.012-.013) | .017 (.015- 017) | 1892 |
| **Age group** | | | | | | | |
| 12-19 years | 01-02 | * | < LOD | < LOD | < LOD | < LOD | 758 |
| | 03-04 | .004 (.003-.004) | .005 (.004-.005) | .008 ( 007-.008) | .011 (.010-.013) | .016 (.011- 021) | 596 |
| 20 years and older | 01-02 | * | < LOD | < LOD | < LOD | < LOD | 1540 |
| | 03-04 | .004 (.004-.005) | .006 (.005-.006) | .008 ( 008-.009) | .012 (.011-.014) | .017 (.014- 018) | 1296 |
| **Gender** | | | | | | | |
| Males | 01-02 | * | < LOD | < LOD | < LOD | < LOD | 1069 |
| | 03-04 | .004 (.004-.005) | .006 (.005-.006) | .009 ( 008-.009) | .013 (.012-.014) | .017 (.015- 018) | 945 |
| Females | 01-02 | * | < LOD | < LOD | < LOD | < LOD | 1229 |
| | 03-04 | .004 (.003-.005) | .005 (.005-.006) | .008 ( 007-.009) | .012 (.011-.013) | .016 (.014- 017) | 947 |
| **Race/ethnicity** | | | | | | | |
| Mexican Americans | 01-02 | * | < LOD | < LOD | < LOD | < LOD | 564 |
| | 03-04 | .004 (.003-.005) | .005 (.004-.006) | .008 ( 007-.010) | .011 (.009-.014) | .014 (.011- 022) | 427 |
| Non-Hispanic blacks | 01-02 | * | < LOD | < LOD | < LOD | < LOD | 515 |
| | 03-04 | .005 (.004-.005) | .006 (.006-.006) | .009 ( 008-.012) | .015 (.014-.017) | .020 (.017- 027) | 462 |
| Non-Hispanic whites | 01-02 | * | < LOD | < LOD | < LOD | < LOD | 1056 |
| | 03-04 | .004 (.003-.005) | .005 (.005-.006) | .008 ( 007-.009) | .012 (.011-.013) | .016 (.014- 017) | 882 |

< LOD means less than the limit of detection for the lipid adjusted serum level, which may vary for some chemicals by year and by individual sample.
* Not calculated: proportion of results below limit of detection was too high to provide a valid result.

## Serum 2,2',4,4',5-Pentachlorobiphenyl (PCB 99) (lipid adjusted)

Geometric mean and selected percentiles of serum concentrations (in ng/g of lipid or parts per billion on a lipid-weight basis) for the U.S. population from the National Health and Nutrition Examination Survey.

| | Survey years | Geometric mean (95% conf. interval) | 50th | 75th | 90th | 95th | Sample size |
|---|---|---|---|---|---|---|---|
| **Total** | 99-00 | * | < LOD | < LOD | 13.1 (<LOD-14.7) | 19.1 (16 2-20.6) | 1897 |
| | 01-02 | * | < LOD | < LOD | 17.6 (15.3-21.0) | 26.3 (22.1-30.5) | 2281 |
| | 03-04 | 4.16 (3.82-4.54) | 3.79 (3.43-4.10) | 6.53 (5.76-7.56) | 13.0 (10.5-16.1) | 18.0 (16.7-19.4) | 1877 |
| **Age group** | | | | | | | |
| 12-19 years | 99-00 | * | < LOD | < LOD | < LOD | < LOD | 654 |
| | 01-02 | * | < LOD | < LOD | < LOD | < LOD | 758 |
| | 03-04 | 2.34 (2.08-2.64) | 2.30 (2 05-2.60) | 3.20 (2.80-3.86) | 5.16 (3.80-6.12) | 6.00 (4.77-10.0) | 587 |
| 20 years and older | 99-00 | * | < LOD | < LOD | 13.9 (<LOD-16 0) | 20.0 (17 2-21.6) | 1243 |
| | 01-02 | * | < LOD | 10.8 (<LOD-12 3) | 19.4 (16.7-22.3) | 29.0 (23 5-32.1) | 1523 |
| | 03-04 | 4.52 (4.14-4.94) | 4.08 (3.75-4.45) | 7.10 (6.08-8.53) | 14.7 (10.9-17.0) | 18.6 (17.1-21.3) | 1290 |
| **Gender** | | | | | | | |
| Males | 99-00 | * | < LOD | < LOD | < LOD | 16.7 (13 8-20.5) | 905 |
| | 01-02 | * | < LOD | < LOD | 17.0 (13.8-21.0) | 24.9 (19 8-30.1) | 1061 |
| | 03-04 | 3.97 (3.64-4.33) | 3.69 (3 31-4.00) | 6.11 (5.44-7.00) | 11.1 (9.40-14.3) | 16.8 (12 9-19.0) | 936 |
| Females | 99-00 | * | < LOD | < LOD | 13.9 (<LOD-16 2) | 20.3 (17 3-23.5) | 992 |
| | 01-02 | * | < LOD | < LOD | 18.0 (15.8-22.2) | 28.5 (22 5-33.2) | 1220 |
| | 03-04 | 4.35 (3.94-4.81) | 3.90 (3.43-4.70) | 7.05 (6.00-8.46) | 15.3 (11.5-17.3) | 18.9 (17 5-22.8) | 941 |
| **Race/ethnicity** | | | | | | | |
| Mexican Americans | 99-00 | * | < LOD | < LOD | < LOD | < LOD | 624 |
| | 01-02 | * | < LOD | < LOD | < LOD | 13.8 (10.7-17.4) | 562 |
| | 03-04 | 2.33 (2.08-2.62) | 2.20 (1 90-2.47) | 3.35 (2.80-4.02) | 5.21 (4.50-6.10) | 6.35 (5.53-7.55) | 426 |
| Non-Hispanic blacks | 99-00 | * | < LOD | < LOD | 21.1 (17.0-31.1) | 32.0 (22 9-57.4) | 400 |
| | 01-02 | * | < LOD | 11.7 (10.6-13.1) | 22.5 (18.8-25.8) | 29.0 (23 0-37.2) | 510 |
| | 03-04 | 5.54 (4.53-6.77) | 4.81 (3 80-5.80) | 10.4 (7.20-15.3) | 23.1 (16.7-29.7) | 31.7 (24 2-49.1) | 447 |
| Non-Hispanic whites | 99-00 | * | < LOD | < LOD | 12.5 (<LOD-14 5) | 18.2 (14 3-20.8) | 715 |
| | 01-02 | * | < LOD | < LOD | 18.5 (15.3-22.3) | 28.5 (22.1-32.4) | 1046 |
| | 03-04 | 4.23 (3.80-4.72) | 3.90 (3.40-4.44) | 6.70 (5.70-8.00) | 12.6 (9.73-15.8) | 17.3 (15 5-18.1) | 883 |

Limit of detection (LOD, see Data Analysis section) for Survey years 99-00, 01-02, and 03-04 are 12.5, 10 5, and 0.6, respectively.
< LOD means less than the limit of detection, which may vary for some chemicals by year and by individual sample.
* Not calculated: proportion of results below limit of detection was too high to provide a valid result.

## Serum 2,2',4,4',5-Pentachlorobiphenyl (PCB 99) (whole weight)

Geometric mean and selected percentiles of serum concentrations (in ng/g of serum or parts per billion) for the U.S. population from the National Health and Nutrition Examination Survey.

| | Survey years | Geometric mean (95% conf. interval) | Selected percentiles ( 95% confidence interval) | | | | Sample size |
|---|---|---|---|---|---|---|---|
| | | | 50th | 75th | 90th | 95th | |
| **Total** | 99-00 | * | < LOD | < LOD | .090 (<LOD-.100) | .120 (.100-.150) | 1897 |
| | 01-02 | * | < LOD | < LOD | .120 (.100-.140) | .180 (.150- 210) | 2281 |
| | 03-04 | .025 (.023-.028) | .024 (.021-.026) | .042 ( 038-.049) | .082 (.067-.102) | .119 (.102-.140) | 1877 |
| **Age group** | | | | | | | |
| 12-19 years | 99-00 | * | < LOD | < LOD | < LOD | < LOD | 654 |
| | 01-02 | * | < LOD | < LOD | < LOD | < LOD | 758 |
| | 03-04 | .012 (.011-.013) | .012 (.010-.013) | .017 ( 015-.019) | .025 (.019-.032) | .032 (.025- 045) | 587 |
| 20 years and older | 99-00 | * | < LOD | < LOD | .090 (<LOD-.100) | .130 (.110-.150) | 1243 |
| | 01-02 | * | < LOD | .070 (<LOD-.080) | .130 (.110-.160) | .190 (.160- 210) | 1523 |
| | 03-04 | .028 (.026-.031) | .026 (.024-.028) | .046 ( 041-.054) | .093 (.073-.110) | .127 (.110-.153) | 1290 |
| **Gender** | | | | | | | |
| Males | 99-00 | * | < LOD | < LOD | < LOD | .110 (.090-.130) | 905 |
| | 01-02 | * | < LOD | < LOD | .110 (.090-.140) | .160 (.120- 200) | 1061 |
| | 03-04 | .025 (.022-.027) | .023 (.021-.025) | .040 ( 036-.045) | .070 (.059-.090) | .110 (.078-.132) | 936 |
| Females | 99-00 | * | < LOD | < LOD | .100 (<LOD-.110) | .130 (.100-.170) | 992 |
| | 01-02 | * | < LOD | < LOD | .130 (.110-.160) | .200 (.160- 210) | 1220 |
| | 03-04 | .026 (.024-.029) | .024 (.020-.028) | .045 ( 040-.053) | .095 (.078-.111) | .130 (.110-.158) | 941 |
| **Race/ethnicity** | | | | | | | |
| Mexican Americans | 99-00 | * | < LOD | < LOD | < LOD | < LOD | 624 |
| | 01-02 | * | < LOD | < LOD | < LOD | .100 (.070-.120) | 562 |
| | 03-04 | .014 (.012-.016) | .013 (.011-.016) | .022 ( 019-.026) | .036 (.030-.040) | .046 (.036- 058) | 426 |
| Non-Hispanic blacks | 99-00 | * | < LOD | < LOD | .140 (.110-.180) | .210 (.150-.400) | 400 |
| | 01-02 | * | < LOD | .070 ( 060-.090) | .140 (.110-.150) | .190 (.140- 230) | 510 |
| | 03-04 | .032 (.026-.039) | .027 (.023-.033) | .060 ( 042-.086) | .149 (.112-.172) | .211 (.150- 306) | 447 |
| Non-Hispanic whites | 99-00 | * | < LOD | < LOD | .090 (<LOD-.100) | .110 (.090-.150) | 715 |
| | 01-02 | * | < LOD | < LOD | .120 (.100-.160) | .190 (.160- 210) | 1046 |
| | 03-04 | .026 (.023-.029) | .025 (.022-.027) | .043 ( 038-.051) | .081 (.065-.102) | .112 (.098-.127) | 883 |

< LOD means less than the limit of detection for the lipid adjusted serum level, which may vary for some chemicals by year and by individual sample.
* Not calculated: proportion of results below limit of detection was too high to provide a valid result.

## Serum 2,2',4,5,5'-Pentachlorobiphenyl (PCB 101) (lipid adjusted)

Geometric mean and selected percentiles of serum concentrations (in ng/g of lipid or parts per billion on a lipid-weight basis) for the U.S. population from the National Health and Nutrition Examination Survey.

| | Survey years | Geometric mean (95% conf. interval) | Selected percentiles ( 95% confidence interval) | | | | Sample size |
|---|---|---|---|---|---|---|---|
| | | | 50th | 75th | 90th | 95th | |
| **Total** | 99-00 | * | < LOD | < LOD | < LOD | < LOD | 1929 |
| | 01-02 | * | < LOD | < LOD | < LOD | < LOD | 2307 |
| | 03-04 | 1.65 (1.51-1.81) | 1.70 (1 50-1.80) | 2.70 (2.50-2.94) | 4.40 (3.97-4 82) | 5.83 (5.29-6.66) | 1897 |
| **Age group** | | | | | | | |
| 12-19 years | 99-00 | * | < LOD | < LOD | < LOD | < LOD | 669 |
| | 01-02 | * | < LOD | < LOD | < LOD | < LOD | 758 |
| | 03-04 | 1.93 (1.76-2.11) | 1.73 (1 51-2.10) | 3.20 (3.00-3.60) | 5.05 (4.23-5 87) | 7.25 (5.10-8.30) | 598 |
| 20 years and older | 99-00 | * | < LOD | < LOD | < LOD | < LOD | 1260 |
| | 01-02 | * | < LOD | < LOD | < LOD | < LOD | 1549 |
| | 03-04 | 1.62 (1.46-1.78) | 1.67 (1 50-1.80) | 2.64 (2.40-2.90) | 4.40 (3.88-4.75) | 5.51 (5.00-6.60) | 1299 |
| **Gender** | | | | | | | |
| Males | 99-00 | * | < LOD | < LOD | < LOD | < LOD | 918 |
| | 01-02 | * | < LOD | < LOD | < LOD | < LOD | 1075 |
| | 03-04 | 1.71 (1.59-1.84) | 1.75 (1 60-1.90) | 2.80 (2.60-3.10) | 4.50 (3.97-5 06) | 6.00 (5.35-6.75) | 947 |
| Females | 99-00 | * | < LOD | < LOD | < LOD | < LOD | 1011 |
| | 01-02 | * | < LOD | < LOD | < LOD | < LOD | 1232 |
| | 03-04 | 1.60 (1.41-1.81) | 1.61 (1.41-1.82) | 2.57 (2.30-2.98) | 4.40 (3.71-4 94) | 5.60 (4.88-7.25) | 950 |
| **Race/ethnicity** | | | | | | | |
| Mexican Americans | 99-00 | * | < LOD | < LOD | < LOD | < LOD | 634 |
| | 01-02 | * | < LOD | < LOD | < LOD | < LOD | 567 |
| | 03-04 | 1.72 (1.55-1.92) | 1.70 (1 50-1.96) | 3.00 (2.30-3.80) | 4.40 (3.56-5 38) | 5.38 (4.10-6.60) | 427 |
| Non-Hispanic blacks | 99-00 | * | < LOD | < LOD | < LOD | < LOD | 413 |
| | 01-02 | * | < LOD | < LOD | < LOD | < LOD | 515 |
| | 03-04 | 1.69 (1.38-2.07) | 1.70 (1 50-2.16) | 3.00 (2.57-3.80) | 5.88 (3.88-7 39) | 7.68 (6.60-11.9) | 464 |
| Non-Hispanic whites | 99-00 | * | < LOD | < LOD | < LOD | < LOD | 724 |
| | 01-02 | * | < LOD | < LOD | < LOD | < LOD | 1061 |
| | 03-04 | 1.61 (1.46-1.79) | 1.61 (1.41-1.80) | 2.60 (2.37-2.90) | 4.40 (3.75-4 61) | 5.50 (5.00-6.15) | 885 |

Limit of detection (LOD, see Data Analysis section) for Survey years 99-00, 01-02, and 03-04 are 25.7, 10 5, and 0.6, respectively.
< LOD means less than the limit of detection, which may vary for some chemicals by year and by individual sample.
* Not calculated: proportion of results below limit of detection was too high to provide a valid result.

## Serum 2,2',4,5,5'-Pentachlorobiphenyl (PCB 101) (whole weight)

Geometric mean and selected percentiles of serum concentrations (in ng/g of serum or parts per billion) for the U.S. population from the National Health and Nutrition Examination Survey.

| | Survey years | Geometric mean (95% conf. interval) | Selected percentiles ( 95% confidence interval) | | | | Sample size |
|---|---|---|---|---|---|---|---|
| | | | 50th | 75th | 90th | 95th | |
| **Total** | 99-00 | * | < LOD | < LOD | < LOD | < LOD | 1929 |
| | 01-02 | * | < LOD | < LOD | < LOD | < LOD | 2307 |
| | 03-04 | .010 (.009-.011) | .010 (.009-.012) | .016 ( 015-.018) | .027 (.024-.028) | .033 (.031-037) | 1897 |
| **Age group** | | | | | | | |
| 12-19 years | 99-00 | * | < LOD | < LOD | < LOD | < LOD | 669 |
| | 01-02 | * | < LOD | < LOD | < LOD | < LOD | 758 |
| | 03-04 | .010 (.009-.011) | .009 (.008-.011) | .016 ( 014-.018) | .024 (.021-.028) | .030 (.025-044) | 598 |
| 20 years and older | 99-00 | * | < LOD | < LOD | < LOD | < LOD | 1260 |
| | 01-02 | * | < LOD | < LOD | < LOD | < LOD | 1549 |
| | 03-04 | .010 (.009-.011) | .011 (.009-.012) | .016 ( 015-.018) | .027 (.024-.029) | .034 (.031-037) | 1299 |
| **Gender** | | | | | | | |
| Males | 99-00 | * | < LOD | < LOD | < LOD | < LOD | 918 |
| | 01-02 | * | < LOD | < LOD | < LOD | < LOD | 1075 |
| | 03-04 | .011 (.010-.011) | .011 (.010-.012) | .017 ( 016-.019) | .025 (.024-.029) | .037 (.031-041) | 947 |
| Females | 99-00 | * | < LOD | < LOD | < LOD | < LOD | 1011 |
| | 01-02 | * | < LOD | < LOD | < LOD | < LOD | 1232 |
| | 03-04 | .010 (.009-.011) | .010 (.009-.011) | .015 ( 014-.018) | .027 (.022-.029) | .032 (.030-036) | 950 |
| **Race/ethnicity** | | | | | | | |
| Mexican Americans | 99-00 | * | < LOD | < LOD | < LOD | < LOD | 634 |
| | 01-02 | * | < LOD | < LOD | < LOD | < LOD | 567 |
| | 03-04 | .011 (.009-.012) | .011 (.009-.012) | .018 ( 014-.021) | .024 (.020-.030) | .029 (.022-052) | 427 |
| Non-Hispanic blacks | 99-00 | * | < LOD | < LOD | < LOD | < LOD | 413 |
| | 01-02 | * | < LOD | < LOD | < LOD | < LOD | 515 |
| | 03-04 | .010 (.008-.012) | .011 (.008-.013) | .016 ( 013-.022) | .032 (.023-.041) | .045 (.032-059) | 464 |
| Non-Hispanic whites | 99-00 | * | < LOD | < LOD | < LOD | < LOD | 724 |
| | 01-02 | * | < LOD | < LOD | < LOD | < LOD | 1061 |
| | 03-04 | .010 (.009-.011) | .010 (.009-.011) | .016 ( 014-.018) | .025 (.024-.027) | .031 (.029-037) | 885 |

< LOD means less than the limit of detection for the lipid adjusted serum level, which may vary for some chemicals by year and by individual sample.
* Not calculated: proportion of results below limit of detection was too high to provide a valid result.

## Serum 2,3,3',4',6-Pentachlorobiphenyl (PCB 110) (lipid adjusted)

Geometric mean and selected percentiles of serum concentrations (in ng/g of lipid or parts per billion on a lipid-weight basis) for the U.S. population from the National Health and Nutrition Examination Survey.

| | Survey years | Geometric mean (95% conf. interval) | Selected percentiles ( 95% confidence interval) | | | | Sample size |
|---|---|---|---|---|---|---|---|
| | | | 50th | 75th | 90th | 95th | |
| **Total** | 01-02 | * | < LOD | < LOD | < LOD | < LOD | 2298 |
| | 03-04 | 1.22 (1.11-1.33) | 1.20 (1.10-1.36) | 1.96 (1.80-2.20) | 3.40 (3.10-3 57) | 4.42 (3.88-4.95) | 1882 |
| **Age group** | | | | | | | |
| 12-19 years | 01-02 | * | < LOD | < LOD | < LOD | < LOD | 758 |
| | 03-04 | 1.44 (1.30-1.59) | 1.30 (1 20-1.50) | 2.50 (2.19-2.91) | 4.13 (3.40-4 90) | 5.40 (4.30-7.68) | 593 |
| 20 years and older | 01-02 | * | < LOD | < LOD | < LOD | < LOD | 1540 |
| | 03-04 | 1.19 (1.08-1.30) | 1.20 (1 09-1.33) | 1.88 (1.71-2.11) | 3.30 (2.95-3 50) | 4.18 (3.66-4.94) | 1289 |
| **Gender** | | | | | | | |
| Males | 01-02 | * | < LOD | < LOD | < LOD | < LOD | 1069 |
| | 03-04 | 1.26 (1.18-1.35) | 1.30 (1.19-1.40) | 2.05 (1.80-2.30) | 3.42 (3.07-3.70) | 4.61 (3.80-5.00) | 939 |
| Females | 01-02 | * | < LOD | < LOD | < LOD | < LOD | 1229 |
| | 03-04 | 1.17 (1.04-1.32) | 1.20 (1 00-1.36) | 1.82 (1.70-2.20) | 3.40 (2.77-3 57) | 4.40 (3.57-5.54) | 943 |
| **Race/ethnicity** | | | | | | | |
| Mexican Americans | 01-02 | * | < LOD | < LOD | < LOD | < LOD | 564 |
| | 03-04 | 1.33 (1.18-1.51) | 1.29 (1.13-1.50) | 2.30 (1.80-2.95) | 3.40 (2.70-4 30) | 4.10 (3.30-5.50) | 420 |
| Non-Hispanic blacks | 01-02 | * | < LOD | < LOD | < LOD | < LOD | 515 |
| | 03-04 | 1.36 (1.20-1.53) | 1.30 (1.14-1.50) | 2.10 (1.72-3.00) | 4.19 (2.91-5.10) | 5.32 (4.40-6.89) | 464 |
| Non-Hispanic whites | 01-02 | * | < LOD | < LOD | < LOD | < LOD | 1056 |
| | 03-04 | 1.17 (1.05-1.31) | 1.20 (1 00-1.33) | 1.86 (1.70-2.16) | 3.40 (2.93-3 57) | 4.19 (3.69-4.95) | 877 |

Limit of detection (LOD, see Data Analysis section) for Survey years 01-02 and 03-04 are 10.5 and 0.8.
< LOD means less than the limit of detection, which may vary for some chemicals by year and by individual sample.
* Not calculated: proportion of results below limit of detection was too high to provide a valid result.

## Serum 2,3,3',4',6-Pentachlorobiphenyl (PCB 110) (whole weight)

Geometric mean and selected percentiles of serum concentrations (in ng/g of serum or parts per billion) for the U.S. population from the National Health and Nutrition Examination Survey.

| | Survey years | Geometric mean (95% conf. interval) | Selected percentiles ( 95% confidence interval) | | | | Sample size |
|---|---|---|---|---|---|---|---|
| | | | 50th | 75th | 90th | 95th | |
| **Total** | 01-02 | * | < LOD | < LOD | < LOD | < LOD | 2298 |
| | 03-04 | .007 (.007-.008) | .007 (.007-.008) | .012 ( 011-.013) | .019 (.018-.021) | .026 (.023- 028) | 1882 |
| **Age group** | | | | | | | |
| 12-19 years | 01-02 | * | < LOD | < LOD | < LOD | < LOD | 758 |
| | 03-04 | .007 (.007-.008) | .007 (.006-.008) | .013 ( 010-.015) | .020 (.017-.022) | .026 (.019- 037) | 593 |
| 20 years and older | 01-02 | * | < LOD | < LOD | < LOD | < LOD | 1540 |
| | 03-04 | .007 (.007-.008) | .007 (.007-.008) | .012 ( 011-.013) | .019 (.017-.021) | .025 (.023- 028) | 1289 |
| **Gender** | | | | | | | |
| Males | 01-02 | * | < LOD | < LOD | < LOD | < LOD | 1069 |
| | 03-04 | .008 (.007-.008) | .008 (.007-.009) | .013 ( 011-.014) | .019 (.018-.021) | .028 (.022- 031) | 939 |
| Females | 01-02 | * | < LOD | < LOD | < LOD | < LOD | 1229 |
| | 03-04 | .007 (.006-.008) | .007 (.006-.008) | .011 ( 010-.013) | .019 (.016-.022) | .024 (.021- 027) | 943 |
| **Race/ethnicity** | | | | | | | |
| Mexican Americans | 01-02 | * | < LOD | < LOD | < LOD | < LOD | 564 |
| | 03-04 | .008 (.007-.009) | .008 (.007-.010) | .014 ( 011-.016) | .019 (.016-.022) | .022 (.017- 043) | 420 |
| Non-Hispanic blacks | 01-02 | * | < LOD | < LOD | < LOD | < LOD | 515 |
| | 03-04 | .008 (.007-.009) | .008 (.006-.009) | .012 ( 010-.016) | .023 (.017-.028) | .028 (.023- 032) | 464 |
| Non-Hispanic whites | 01-02 | * | < LOD | < LOD | < LOD | < LOD | 1056 |
| | 03-04 | .007 (.006-.008) | .007 (.006-.008) | .012 ( 010-.013) | .019 (.017-.021) | .026 (.022- 029) | 877 |

< LOD means less than the limit of detection for the lipid adjusted serum level, which may vary for some chemicals by year and by individual sample.
* Not calculated: proportion of results below limit of detection was too high to provide a valid result.

## Serum 2,2',3,3',4,4'-Hexachlorobiphenyl (PCB 128) (lipid adjusted)

Geometric mean and selected percentiles of serum concentrations (in ng/g of lipid or parts per billion on a lipid-weight basis) for the U.S. population from the National Health and Nutrition Examination Survey.

| | Survey years | Geometric mean (95% conf. interval) | Selected percentiles ( 95% confidence interval) | | | | Sample size |
|---|---|---|---|---|---|---|---|
| | | | 50th | 75th | 90th | 95th | |
| **Total** | 99-00 | * | < LOD | < LOD | < LOD | < LOD | 1927 |
| | 01-02 | * | < LOD | < LOD | < LOD | < LOD | 2298 |
| | 03-04 | * | < LOD | < LOD | < LOD | .600 ( 500-.700) | 1877 |
| **Age group** | | | | | | | |
| 12-19 years | 99-00 | * | < LOD | < LOD | < LOD | < LOD | 668 |
| | 01-02 | * | < LOD | < LOD | < LOD | < LOD | 758 |
| | 03-04 | * | < LOD | < LOD | < LOD | .510 (<LOD-.700) | 589 |
| 20 years and older | 99-00 | * | < LOD | < LOD | < LOD | < LOD | 1259 |
| | 01-02 | * | < LOD | < LOD | < LOD | < LOD | 1540 |
| | 03-04 | * | < LOD | < LOD | < LOD | .620 (.490-.800) | 1288 |
| **Gender** | | | | | | | |
| Males | 99-00 | * | < LOD | < LOD | < LOD | < LOD | 917 |
| | 01-02 | * | < LOD | < LOD | < LOD | < LOD | 1069 |
| | 03-04 | * | < LOD | < LOD | < LOD | .600 (.420-.770) | 937 |
| Females | 99-00 | * | < LOD | < LOD | < LOD | < LOD | 1010 |
| | 01-02 | * | < LOD | < LOD | < LOD | < LOD | 1229 |
| | 03-04 | * | < LOD | < LOD | < LOD | .630 ( 500-.800) | 940 |
| **Race/ethnicity** | | | | | | | |
| Mexican Americans | 99-00 | * | < LOD | < LOD | < LOD | < LOD | 636 |
| | 01-02 | * | < LOD | < LOD | < LOD | < LOD | 564 |
| | 03-04 | * | < LOD | < LOD | < LOD | < LOD | 424 |
| Non-Hispanic blacks | 99-00 | * | < LOD | < LOD | < LOD | < LOD | 409 |
| | 01-02 | * | < LOD | < LOD | < LOD | < LOD | 515 |
| | 03-04 | * | < LOD | < LOD | .670 (.500-.800) | 1.00 (.770-2.10) | 455 |
| Non-Hispanic whites | 99-00 | * | < LOD | < LOD | < LOD | < LOD | 725 |
| | 01-02 | * | < LOD | < LOD | < LOD | < LOD | 1056 |
| | 03-04 | * | < LOD | < LOD | < LOD | .500 (.420-.600) | 878 |

Limit of detection (LOD, see Data Analysis section) for Survey years 99-00, 01-02, and 03-04 are 12.4, 10 5, and 0.4, respectively.
< LOD means less than the limit of detection, which may vary for some chemicals by year and by individual sample.
* Not calculated: proportion of results below limit of detection was too high to provide a valid result.

## Serum 2,2',3,3',4,4'-Hexachlorobiphenyl (PCB 128) (whole weight)

Geometric mean and selected percentiles of serum concentrations (in ng/g of serum or parts per billion) for the U.S. population from the National Health and Nutrition Examination Survey.

| | Survey years | Geometric mean (95% conf. interval) | Selected percentiles ( 95% confidence interval) | | | | Sample size |
|---|---|---|---|---|---|---|---|
| | | | 50th | 75th | 90th | 95th | |
| **Total** | 99-00 | * | < LOD | < LOD | < LOD | < LOD | 1927 |
| | 01-02 | * | < LOD | < LOD | < LOD | < LOD | 2298 |
| | 03-04 | * | < LOD | < LOD | < LOD | .004 (.003-.004) | 1877 |
| **Age group** | | | | | | | |
| 12-19 years | 99-00 | * | < LOD | < LOD | < LOD | < LOD | 668 |
| | 01-02 | * | < LOD | < LOD | < LOD | < LOD | 758 |
| | 03-04 | * | < LOD | < LOD | < LOD | .003 (<LOD-.004) | 589 |
| 20 years and older | 99-00 | * | < LOD | < LOD | < LOD | < LOD | 1259 |
| | 01-02 | * | < LOD | < LOD | < LOD | < LOD | 1540 |
| | 03-04 | * | < LOD | < LOD | < LOD | .004 (.004-.005) | 1288 |
| **Gender** | | | | | | | |
| Males | 99-00 | * | < LOD | < LOD | < LOD | < LOD | 917 |
| | 01-02 | * | < LOD | < LOD | < LOD | < LOD | 1069 |
| | 03-04 | * | < LOD | < LOD | < LOD | .004 (.003-.005) | 937 |
| Females | 99-00 | * | < LOD | < LOD | < LOD | < LOD | 1010 |
| | 01-02 | * | < LOD | < LOD | < LOD | < LOD | 1229 |
| | 03-04 | * | < LOD | < LOD | < LOD | .004 (.003-.005) | 940 |
| **Race/ethnicity** | | | | | | | |
| Mexican Americans | 99-00 | * | < LOD | < LOD | < LOD | < LOD | 636 |
| | 01-02 | * | < LOD | < LOD | < LOD | < LOD | 564 |
| | 03-04 | * | < LOD | < LOD | < LOD | < LOD | 424 |
| Non-Hispanic blacks | 99-00 | * | < LOD | < LOD | < LOD | < LOD | 409 |
| | 01-02 | * | < LOD | < LOD | < LOD | < LOD | 515 |
| | 03-04 | * | < LOD | < LOD | .004 (.003-.005) | .006 (.005-.013) | 455 |
| Non-Hispanic whites | 99-00 | * | < LOD | < LOD | < LOD | < LOD | 725 |
| | 01-02 | * | < LOD | < LOD | < LOD | < LOD | 1056 |
| | 03-04 | * | < LOD | < LOD | < LOD | .003 (.002-.004) | 878 |

< LOD means less than the limit of detection for the lipid adjusted serum level, which may vary for some chemicals by year and by individual sample.
* Not calculated: proportion of results below limit of detection was too high to provide a valid result.

## Serum 2,2',3,4,4',5' and 2,3,3',4,4',6-Hexachlorobiphenyl (PCB 138 & 158) (lipid adjusted)

Geometric mean and selected percentiles of serum concentrations (in ng/g of lipid or parts per billion on a lipid-weight basis) for the U.S. population from the National Health and Nutrition Examination Survey.

| | Survey years | Geometric mean (95% conf. interval) | Selected percentiles ( 95% confidence interval) | | | | Sample size |
|---|---|---|---|---|---|---|---|
| | | | 50th | 75th | 90th | 95th | |
| **Total** | 99-00 | * | < LOD | < LOD | 49.3 (42.9-55.8) | 71.2 (59 8-82.7) | 1930 |
| | 01-02 | 19.9 (18.0-22 0) | 20.2 (18.2-23.1) | 40.4 (35.3-45.1) | 70.1 (61.8-78.8) | 94.6 (82 5-107) | 2293 |
| | 03-04 | 15.1 (14.1-16.1) | 15.1 (13.6-16 6) | 30.5 (28.1-34.0) | 55.4 (47.3-63.3) | 75.3 (69 0-81.8) | 1896 |
| **Age group** | | | | | | | |
| 12-19 years | 99-00 | * | < LOD | < LOD | < LOD | < LOD | 669 |
| | 01-02 | * | < LOD | < LOD | 17.0 (13.7-20.2) | 23.1 (17.7-41.2) | 748 |
| | 03-04 | 4.97 (4.45-5.55) | 4.57 (4.10-5.02) | 7.39 (6.35-8.63) | 12.7 (10.4-14.5) | 15.2 (13.1-21.3) | 598 |
| 20 years and older | 99-00 | * | < LOD | < LOD | 54.7 (47.4-60.8) | 72.8 (66 0-88.9) | 1261 |
| | 01-02 | 23.3 (21.1-25 8) | 24.0 (21.4-26 8) | 44.6 (40.4-49.2) | 73.9 (66.2-83.0) | 100 (88 8-109) | 1545 |
| | 03-04 | 17.7 (16.5-19 0) | 17.6 (15.5-20.4) | 34.3 (30.0-38.8) | 59.6 (50.6-66.9) | 77.4 (72 3-87.7) | 1298 |
| **Gender** | | | | | | | |
| Males | 99-00 | * | < LOD | < LOD | 47.2 (<LOD-55.7) | 68.2 (55.7-83.8) | 918 |
| | 01-02 | 20.1 (17.9-22 6) | 20.5 (17.6-23 5) | 39.2 (32.2-46.0) | 69.2 (58.1-82.5) | 94.6 (77 8-109) | 1066 |
| | 03-04 | 14.9 (13.8-15 9) | 14.4 (12.9-15 8) | 29.6 (26.6-33.8) | 56.3 (45.3-62.3) | 75.8 (63 3-87.7) | 947 |
| Females | 99-00 | * | < LOD | < LOD | 53.7 (44.7-61.2) | 72.1 (61 2-88.9) | 1012 |
| | 01-02 | 19.7 (17.8-21.7) | 20.2 (18.2-23.1) | 41.8 (37.5-45.9) | 70.1 (63.4-78.5) | 93.9 (80 2-109) | 1227 |
| | 03-04 | 15.3 (14.0-16 8) | 15.8 (14.2-17 8) | 31.8 (28.3-36.6) | 54.6 (47.3-64.4) | 72.5 (68.4-80.9) | 949 |
| **Race/ethnicity** | | | | | | | |
| Mexican Americans | 99-00 | * | < LOD | < LOD | < LOD | < LOD | 636 |
| | 01-02 | * | < LOD | 18.6 (13.6-23.4) | 33.3 (26.5-44.2) | 51.8 (42 3-57.6) | 559 |
| | 03-04 | 7.06 (6.02-8.28) | 6.52 (5 20-7.60) | 12.3 (8.91-16.0) | 23.6 (18.9-28.3) | 29.2 (24.7-36.1) | 427 |
| Non-Hispanic blacks | 99-00 | * | < LOD | < LOD | 72.6 (61.7-89.4) | 122 (86 5-185) | 412 |
| | 01-02 | 22.3 (19.3-25 6) | 22.0 (18.4-27.1) | 46.5 (38.0-55.6) | 91.5 (70.1-112) | 122 (91 5-169) | 513 |
| | 03-04 | 17.8 (14.9-21 3) | 15.9 (12.5-21 0) | 41.2 (30.6-57.3) | 86.5 (69.4-110) | 153 (94 6-191) | 464 |
| Non-Hispanic whites | 99-00 | * | < LOD | < LOD | 49.3 (41.4-55.8) | 70.1 (55.7-85.2) | 727 |
| | 01-02 | 21.5 (19.2-24 0) | 22.1 (19.6-24 9) | 43.0 (37.7-48.0) | 70.7 (62.3-79.7) | 96.1 (79.1-110) | 1057 |
| | 03-04 | 16.0 (14.5-17.7) | 15.8 (14.6-18.4) | 31.4 (28.2-36.6) | 55.1 (47.2-62.3) | 71.6 (64 0-75.8) | 883 |

Limit of detection (LOD, see Data Analysis section) for Survey years 99-00, 01-02, and 03-04 are 41.1, 10 5, and 0.4, respectively.
< LOD means less than the limit of detection, which may vary for some chemicals by year and by individual sample.
* Not calculated: proportion of results below limit of detection was too high to provide a valid result.

## Serum 2,2',3,4,4',5' and 2,3,3',4,4',6-Hexachlorobiphenyl (PCB 138 & 158) (whole weight)

Geometric mean and selected percentiles of serum concentrations (in ng/g of serum or parts per billion) for the U.S. population from the National Health and Nutrition Examination Survey.

| | Survey years | Geometric mean (95% conf. interval) | Selected percentiles ( 95% confidence interval) | | | | Sample size |
|---|---|---|---|---|---|---|---|
| | | | 50th | 75th | 90th | 95th | |
| **Total** | 99-00 | * | < LOD | < LOD | .340 (.300-.370) | .460 (.390- 530) | 1930 |
| | 01-02 | .122 (.110-.135) | .120 (.110-.140) | .270 ( 230-.290) | .460 (.410-.510) | .650 (.560-.700) | 2293 |
| | 03-04 | .092 (.086-.099) | .095 (.082-.105) | .206 (.180-.231) | .359 (.326-.392) | .477 (.450- 528) | 1896 |
| **Age group** | | | | | | | |
| 12-19 years | 99-00 | * | < LOD | < LOD | < LOD | < LOD | 669 |
| | 01-02 | * | < LOD | < LOD | .090 (.060-.110) | .110 (.090- 210) | 748 |
| | 03-04 | .025 (.023-.028) | .023 (.020-.027) | .037 ( 030-.047) | .062 (.049-.074) | .079 (.067-.103) | 598 |
| 20 years and older | 99-00 | * | < LOD | < LOD | .360 (.320-.390) | .490 (.400- 560) | 1261 |
| | 01-02 | .148 (.133-.163) | .150 (.140-.170) | .290 ( 270-.320) | .510 (.450-.550) | .680 (.610-.720) | 1545 |
| | 03-04 | .111 (.103-.120) | .114 (.099-.128) | .232 ( 204-.256) | .383 (.354-.416) | .506 (.467- 594) | 1298 |
| **Gender** | | | | | | | |
| Males | 99-00 | * | < LOD | < LOD | .320 (<LOD-.370) | .420 (.370- 530) | 918 |
| | 01-02 | .125 (.112-.140) | .130 (.110-.140) | .260 ( 230-.290) | .460 (.370-.540) | .630 (.510-.710) | 1066 |
| | 03-04 | .092 (.085-.099) | .091 (.079-.103) | .198 (.172-.229) | .354 (.316-.379) | .474 (.389- 562) | 947 |
| Females | 99-00 | * | < LOD | < LOD | .340 (.300-.370) | .490 (.390- 540) | 1012 |
| | 01-02 | .119 (.107-.132) | .120 (.110-.150) | .270 ( 230-.300) | .460 (.420-.500) | .660 (.590-.700) | 1227 |
| | 03-04 | .093 (.084-.102) | .098 (.085-.115) | .212 (.178-.244) | .373 (.325-.417) | .482 (.450- 568) | 949 |
| **Race/ethnicity** | | | | | | | |
| Mexican Americans | 99-00 | * | < LOD | < LOD | < LOD | < LOD | 636 |
| | 01-02 | * | < LOD | .110 ( 090-.150) | .240 (.170-.330) | .350 (.270-.430) | 559 |
| | 03-04 | .043 (.036-.051) | .040 (.032-.049) | .080 ( 068-.100) | .148 (.122-.203) | .239 (.147- 346) | 427 |
| Non-Hispanic blacks | 99-00 | * | < LOD | < LOD | .470 (.360-.670) | .830 (.530-1.22) | 412 |
| | 01-02 | .125 (.108-.146) | .130 (.090-.160) | .290 ( 230-.350) | .560 (.420-.680) | .770 (.560-1.06) | 513 |
| | 03-04 | .101 (.084-.122) | .087 (.068-.113) | .239 (.186-.326) | .568 (.424-.811) | .965 (.698-1.09) | 464 |
| Non-Hispanic whites | 99-00 | * | < LOD | < LOD | .340 (.300-.370) | .440 (.370- 530) | 727 |
| | 01-02 | .133 (.119-.149) | .140 (.120-.160) | .280 ( 250-.300) | .460 (.420-.530) | .650 (.550-.720) | 1057 |
| | 03-04 | .099 (.089-.109) | .104 (.091-.121) | .216 (.179-.252) | .355 (.320-.390) | .467 (.410- 520) | 883 |

< LOD means less than the limit of detection for the lipid adjusted serum level, which may vary for some chemicals by year and by individual sample.
* Not calculated: proportion of results below limit of detection was too high to provide a valid result.

## Serum 2,2',3,4',5,5'-Hexachlorobiphenyl (PCB 146) (lipid adjusted)

Geometric mean and selected percentiles of serum concentrations (in ng/g of lipid or parts per billion on a lipid-weight basis) for the U.S. population from the National Health and Nutrition Examination Survey.

| | Survey years | Geometric mean (95% conf. interval) | Selected percentiles ( 95% confidence interval) | | | | Sample size |
|---|---|---|---|---|---|---|---|
| | | | 50th | 75th | 90th | 95th | |
| **Total** | 99-00 | * | < LOD | < LOD | < LOD | 13.3 (<LOD-16.1) | 1923 |
| | 01-02 | * | < LOD | < LOD | 11.0 (<LOD-12 5) | 15.4 (13 6-16.9) | 2299 |
| | 03-04 | 2.17 (2.02-2.32) | 2.21 (2 03-2.54) | 4.80 (4.38-5.21) | 8.27 (7.10-9 50) | 11.7 (10 2-13.3) | 1894 |
| **Age group** | | | | | | | |
| 12-19 years | 99-00 | * | < LOD | < LOD | < LOD | < LOD | 667 |
| | 01-02 | * | < LOD | < LOD | < LOD | < LOD | 758 |
| | 03-04 | .620 (.562- 685) | .600 (.520-.690) | 1.02 (.870-1.20) | 1.67 (1.50-1 80) | 2.30 (1.79-2.97) | 594 |
| 20 years and older | 99-00 | * | < LOD | < LOD | < LOD | 14.3 (<LOD-17.1) | 1256 |
| | 01-02 | * | < LOD | < LOD | 11.8 (10.7-13.5) | 16.5 (14 6-18.1) | 1541 |
| | 03-04 | 2.60 (2.41-2.79) | 2.60 (2.40-2.90) | 5.27 (4.82-5.88) | 8.81 (8.00-9 80) | 12.7 (10.7-15.2) | 1300 |
| **Gender** | | | | | | | |
| Males | 99-00 | * | < LOD | < LOD | < LOD | 13.1 (<LOD-17.1) | 915 |
| | 01-02 | * | < LOD | < LOD | 11.0 (<LOD-13 0) | 15.4 (13 0-17.2) | 1069 |
| | 03-04 | 2.16 (1.97-2.37) | 2.10 (1 90-2.50) | 4.80 (4.09-5.30) | 8.30 (6.90-10.1) | 12.4 (10 0-14.9) | 945 |
| Females | 99-00 | * | < LOD | < LOD | < LOD | 13.9 (<LOD-16.3) | 1008 |
| | 01-02 | * | < LOD | < LOD | 11.0 (<LOD-12 2) | 15.2 (13 2-17.3) | 1230 |
| | 03-04 | 2.17 (2.02-2.34) | 2.35 (2 04-2.63) | 4.83 (4.47-5.37) | 8.00 (7.04-9.10) | 11.3 (9.95-13.2) | 949 |
| **Race/ethnicity** | | | | | | | |
| Mexican Americans | 99-00 | * | < LOD | < LOD | < LOD | < LOD | 633 |
| | 01-02 | * | < LOD | < LOD | < LOD | < LOD | 567 |
| | 03-04 | .940 (.826-1.07) | .820 (.780-1.00) | 1.74 (1.21-2.60) | 3.31 (2.80-4 00) | 4.60 (3.47-6.00) | 425 |
| Non-Hispanic blacks | 99-00 | * | < LOD | < LOD | 17.0 (13 4-22.9) | 29.8 (20 2-42.2) | 412 |
| | 01-02 | * | < LOD | < LOD | 16.6 (12.8-21.4) | 23.8 (16 9-31.6) | 515 |
| | 03-04 | 2.81 (2.37-3.34) | 2.60 (2 05-3.50) | 7.10 (4.97-8.90) | 16.8 (11.5-23.2) | 28.5 (17 8-41.6) | 463 |
| Non-Hispanic whites | 99-00 | * | < LOD | < LOD | < LOD | < LOD | 723 |
| | 01-02 | * | < LOD | < LOD | 10.8 (<LOD-12 0) | 15.2 (12 8-16.8) | 1054 |
| | 03-04 | 2.25 (2.06-2.45) | 2.35 (2.10-2.60) | 4.82 (4.37-5.41) | 7.76 (6.94-8.70) | 10.5 (9.51-11.3) | 885 |

Limit of detection (LOD, see Data Analysis section) for Survey years 99-00, 01-02, and 03-04 are 12.4, 10 5, and 0.4, respectively.
< LOD means less than the limit of detection, which may vary for some chemicals by year and by individual sample.
* Not calculated: proportion of results below limit of detection was too high to provide a valid result.

## Serum 2,2',3,4',5,5'-Hexachlorobiphenyl (PCB 146) (whole weight)

Geometric mean and selected percentiles of serum concentrations (in ng/g of serum or parts per billion) for the U.S. population from the National Health and Nutrition Examination Survey.

| | Survey years | Geometric mean (95% conf. interval) | 50th | 75th | 90th | 95th | Sample size |
|---|---|---|---|---|---|---|---|
| **Total** | 99-00 | * | < LOD | < LOD | < LOD | .080 (<LOD-.110) | 1923 |
| | 01-02 | * | < LOD | < LOD | .070 (<LOD- 080) | .110 (.090-.120) | 2299 |
| | 03-04 | .013 ( 012- 014) | .014 (.013-.016) | .032 (.028-.035) | .054 ( 047- 062) | .077 (.069-.090) | 1894 |
| **Age group** | | | | | | | |
| 12-19 years | 99-00 | * | < LOD | < LOD | < LOD | < LOD | 667 |
| | 01-02 | * | < LOD | < LOD | < LOD | < LOD | 758 |
| | 03-04 | .003 ( 003- 003) | .003 (.003-.003) | .006 (.004-.007) | .008 ( 007- 010) | .011 (.009-.014) | 594 |
| 20 years and older | 99-00 | * | < LOD | < LOD | < LOD | .090 (<LOD-.120) | 1256 |
| | 01-02 | * | < LOD | < LOD | .080 ( 070- 090) | .110 (.100-.120) | 1541 |
| | 03-04 | .016 ( 015- 018) | .017 (.015-.020) | .035 (.032-.038) | .058 ( 053- 064) | .084 (.073-.099) | 1300 |
| **Gender** | | | | | | | |
| Males | 99-00 | * | < LOD | < LOD | < LOD | .080 (<LOD-.110) | 915 |
| | 01-02 | * | < LOD | < LOD | .070 (<LOD- 090) | .100 (.090-.120) | 1069 |
| | 03-04 | .013 ( 012- 015) | .014 (.012-.016) | .032 (.027-.036) | .054 ( 045- 063) | .074 (.064-.096) | 945 |
| Females | 99-00 | * | < LOD | < LOD | < LOD | .090 (<LOD-.110) | 1008 |
| | 01-02 | * | < LOD | < LOD | .070 (<LOD- 080) | .110 (.090-.120) | 1230 |
| | 03-04 | .013 ( 012- 014) | .015 (.013-.016) | .032 (.028-.036) | .054 ( 047- 065) | .079 (.069-.088) | 949 |
| **Race/ethnicity** | | | | | | | |
| Mexican Americans | 99-00 | * | < LOD | < LOD | < LOD | < LOD | 633 |
| | 01-02 | * | < LOD | < LOD | < LOD | < LOD | 567 |
| | 03-04 | .006 ( 005- 007) | .005 (.004-.007) | .012 (.008-.016) | .024 ( 017- 033) | .034 (.024-.046) | 425 |
| Non-Hispanic blacks | 99-00 | * | < LOD | < LOD | .110 ( 080-.130) | .180 (.120-.270) | 412 |
| | 01-02 | * | < LOD | < LOD | .100 ( 080-.130) | .150 (.110-.200) | 515 |
| | 03-04 | .016 ( 013- 019) | .016 (.012-.019) | .041 (.030-.061) | .100 ( 069-.167) | .180 (.126-.224) | 463 |
| Non-Hispanic whites | 99-00 | * | < LOD | < LOD | < LOD | < LOD | 723 |
| | 01-02 | * | < LOD | < LOD | .070 (<LOD- 080) | .100 (.090-.120) | 1054 |
| | 03-04 | .014 ( 013- 015) | .015 (.013-.018) | .033 (.028-.036) | .053 ( 047- 057) | .069 (.064-.075) | 885 |

< LOD means less than the limit of detection for the lipid adjusted serum level, which may vary for some chemicals by year and by individual sample.
* Not calculated: proportion of results below limit of detection was too high to provide a valid result.

## Serum 2,2',3,4',5',6-Hexachlorobiphenyl (PCB 149) (lipid adjusted)

Geometric mean and selected percentiles of serum concentrations (in ng/g of lipid or parts per billion on a lipid-weight basis) for the U.S. population from the National Health and Nutrition Examination Survey.

| | Survey years | Geometric mean (95% conf. interval) | Selected percentiles ( 95% confidence interval) | | | | Sample size |
|---|---|---|---|---|---|---|---|
| | | | 50th | 75th | 90th | 95th | |
| **Total** | 01-02 | * | < LOD | < LOD | < LOD | < LOD | 2307 |
| | 03-04 | .598 (.556-.642) | .600 (.550-.680) | .900 (.830-1.00) | 1.45 (1.28-1.60) | 1.90 (1.68-2.20) | 1873 |
| **Age group** | | | | | | | |
| 12-19 years | 01-02 | * | < LOD | < LOD | < LOD | < LOD | 758 |
| | 03-04 | .650 (.605-.698) | .640 (.600-.700) | 1.00 (.900-1.10) | 1.70 (1.40-2.15) | 2.40 (1.80-2.98) | 590 |
| 20 years and older | 01-02 | * | < LOD | < LOD | < LOD | < LOD | 1549 |
| | 03-04 | .590 (.546-.638) | .600 (.540-.680) | .900 (.800-1.00) | 1.40 (1.20-1.60) | 1.89 (1.60-2.17) | 1283 |
| **Gender** | | | | | | | |
| Males | 01-02 | * | < LOD | < LOD | < LOD | < LOD | 1075 |
| | 03-04 | .623 (.578-.671) | .650 (.600-.700) | .960 (.880-1.06) | 1.50 (1.30-1.66) | 1.90 (1.60-2.40) | 930 |
| Females | 01-02 | * | < LOD | < LOD | < LOD | < LOD | 1232 |
| | 03-04 | .575 (.521-.634) | .600 (.500-.620) | .890 (.800-.950) | 1.40 (1.20-1.67) | 1.90 (1.69-2.20) | 943 |
| **Race/ethnicity** | | | | | | | |
| Mexican Americans | 01-02 | * | < LOD | < LOD | < LOD | < LOD | 567 |
| | 03-04 | .549 (.496-.608) | .530 (.500-.600) | .900 (.700-1.04) | 1.28 (1.03-1.60) | 1.60 (1.26-2.30) | 408 |
| Non-Hispanic blacks | 01-02 | * | < LOD | < LOD | < LOD | < LOD | 515 |
| | 03-04 | .760 (.678-.853) | .800 (.700-.880) | 1.20 (1.00-1.58) | 1.98 (1.70-2.59) | 2.90 (2.20-4.20) | 463 |
| Non-Hispanic whites | 01-02 | * | < LOD | < LOD | < LOD | < LOD | 1061 |
| | 03-04 | .574 (.524-.628) | .600 (.510-.670) | .880 (.800-.950) | 1.33 (1.19-1.50) | 1.80 (1.50-2.02) | 881 |

Limit of detection (LOD, see Data Analysis section) for Survey years 01-02 and 03-04 are 10.5 and 0.4.
< LOD means less than the limit of detection, which may vary for some chemicals by year and by individual sample.
* Not calculated: proportion of results below limit of detection was too high to provide a valid result.

## Serum 2,2',3,4',5',6-Hexachlorobiphenyl (PCB 149) (whole weight)

Geometric mean and selected percentiles of serum concentrations (in ng/g of serum or parts per billion) for the U.S. population from the National Health and Nutrition Examination Survey.

| | Survey years | Geometric mean (95% conf. interval) | Selected percentiles ( 95% confidence interval) | | | | Sample size |
|---|---|---|---|---|---|---|---|
| | | | 50th | 75th | 90th | 95th | |
| **Total** | 01-02 | * | < LOD | < LOD | < LOD | < LOD | 2307 |
| | 03-04 | .004 (.003-.004) | .004 (.004-.004) | .006 ( 005-.006) | .009 (.008-.009) | .011 (.010- 013) | 1873 |
| **Age group** | | | | | | | |
| 12-19 years | 01-02 | * | < LOD | < LOD | < LOD | < LOD | 758 |
| | 03-04 | .003 (.003-.004) | .003 (.003-.003) | .005 ( 004-.006) | .008 (.007-.009) | .012 (.008- 016) | 590 |
| 20 years and older | 01-02 | * | < LOD | < LOD | < LOD | < LOD | 1549 |
| | 03-04 | .004 (.003-.004) | .004 (.004-.004) | .006 ( 005-.006) | .009 (.007-.010) | .011 (.010- 013) | 1283 |
| **Gender** | | | | | | | |
| Males | 01-02 | * | < LOD | < LOD | < LOD | < LOD | 1075 |
| | 03-04 | .004 (.004-.004) | .004 (.004-.004) | .006 ( 005-.007) | .009 (.008-.010) | .011 (.010- 013) | 930 |
| Females | 01-02 | * | < LOD | < LOD | < LOD | < LOD | 1232 |
| | 03-04 | .003 (.003-.004) | .004 (.003-.004) | .005 ( 005-.006) | .008 (.007-.010) | .011 (.009- 013) | 943 |
| **Race/ethnicity** | | | | | | | |
| Mexican Americans | 01-02 | * | < LOD | < LOD | < LOD | < LOD | 567 |
| | 03-04 | .003 (.003-.004) | .003 (.003-.004) | .005 ( 004-.006) | .007 (.006-.008) | .009 (.007- 014) | 408 |
| Non-Hispanic blacks | 01-02 | * | < LOD | < LOD | < LOD | < LOD | 515 |
| | 03-04 | .004 (.004-.005) | .004 (.004-.005) | .007 ( 006-.008) | .012 (.010-.013) | .019 (.013- 022) | 463 |
| Non-Hispanic whites | 01-02 | * | < LOD | < LOD | < LOD | < LOD | 1061 |
| | 03-04 | .004 (.003-.004) | .004 (.003-.004) | .005 ( 005-.006) | .008 (.007-.009) | .010 (.009- 012) | 881 |

< LOD means less than the limit of detection for the lipid adjusted serum level, which may vary for some chemicals by year and by individual sample.
* Not calculated: proportion of results below limit of detection was too high to provide a valid result.

## Serum 2,2',3,5,5',6-Hexachlorobiphenyl (PCB 151) (lipid adjusted)

Geometric mean and selected percentiles of serum concentrations (in ng/g of lipid or parts per billion on a lipid-weight basis) for the U.S. population from the National Health and Nutrition Examination Survey.

| | Survey years | Geometric mean (95% conf. interval) | Selected percentiles ( 95% confidence interval) | | | | Sample size |
|---|---|---|---|---|---|---|---|
| | | | 50th | 75th | 90th | 95th | |
| **Total** | 01-02 | * | < LOD | < LOD | < LOD | < LOD | 2307 |
| | 03-04 | * | < LOD | .420 (.400-.500) | .700 (.640-.820) | 1.00 ( 840-1.30) | 1870 |
| **Age group** | | | | | | | |
| 12-19 years | 01-02 | * | < LOD | < LOD | < LOD | < LOD | 758 |
| | 03-04 | * | < LOD | .400 (<LOD-.470) | .700 (.510-.820) | .880 (.700-1.10) | 588 |
| 20 years and older | 01-02 | * | < LOD | < LOD | < LOD | < LOD | 1549 |
| | 03-04 | * | < LOD | .440 (.400-.500) | .720 (.650-.850) | 1.02 ( 850-1.40) | 1282 |
| **Gender** | | | | | | | |
| Males | 01-02 | * | < LOD | < LOD | < LOD | < LOD | 1075 |
| | 03-04 | * | < LOD | .430 (.400-.500) | .720 (.620-.900) | 1.10 ( 830-1.50) | 931 |
| Females | 01-02 | * | < LOD | < LOD | < LOD | < LOD | 1232 |
| | 03-04 | * | < LOD | .410 (.400-.500) | .700 (.600-.820) | 1.00 ( 830-1.20) | 939 |
| **Race/ethnicity** | | | | | | | |
| Mexican Americans | 01-02 | * | < LOD | < LOD | < LOD | < LOD | 567 |
| | 03-04 | * | < LOD | < LOD | .500 (.400-.700) | .700 ( 530-.700) | 426 |
| Non-Hispanic blacks | 01-02 | * | < LOD | < LOD | < LOD | < LOD | 515 |
| | 03-04 | * | .400 (<LOD-.500) | .700 (.500-.900) | 1.30 (.900-1 90) | 2.20 (1.40-4.55) | 461 |
| Non-Hispanic whites | 01-02 | * | < LOD | < LOD | < LOD | < LOD | 1061 |
| | 03-04 | * | < LOD | .400 (<LOD-.450) | .650 (.590-.700) | .850 (.750-1.00) | 864 |

Limit of detection (LOD, see Data Analysis section) for Survey years 01-02 and 03-04 are 10.5 and 0.4.
< LOD means less than the limit of detection, which may vary for some chemicals by year and by individual sample.
* Not calculated: proportion of results below limit of detection was too high to provide a valid result.

## Serum 2,2',3,5,5',6-Hexachlorobiphenyl (PCB 151) (whole weight)

Geometric mean and selected percentiles of serum concentrations (in ng/g of serum or parts per billion) for the U.S. population from the National Health and Nutrition Examination Survey.

| | Survey years | Geometric mean (95% conf. interval) | Selected percentiles ( 95% confidence interval) | | | | Sample size |
|---|---|---|---|---|---|---|---|
| | | | 50th | 75th | 90th | 95th | |
| **Total** | 01-02 | * | < LOD | < LOD | < LOD | < LOD | 2307 |
| | 03-04 | * | < LOD | .003 ( 002-.003) | .004 (.004-.005) | .006 (.005- 008) | 1870 |
| **Age group** | | | | | | | |
| 12-19 years | 01-02 | * | < LOD | < LOD | < LOD | < LOD | 758 |
| | 03-04 | * | < LOD | .002 (<LOD-.002) | .003 (.003-.004) | .004 (.003- 006) | 588 |
| 20 years and older | 01-02 | * | < LOD | < LOD | < LOD | < LOD | 1549 |
| | 03-04 | * | < LOD | .003 ( 003-.003) | .004 (.004-.006) | .007 (.005- 010) | 1282 |
| **Gender** | | | | | | | |
| Males | 01-02 | * | < LOD | < LOD | < LOD | < LOD | 1075 |
| | 03-04 | * | < LOD | .003 ( 003-.003) | .005 (.004-.006) | .006 (.005- 010) | 931 |
| Females | 01-02 | * | < LOD | < LOD | < LOD | < LOD | 1232 |
| | 03-04 | * | < LOD | .003 ( 002-.003) | .004 (.004-.005) | .006 (.005- 008) | 939 |
| **Race/ethnicity** | | | | | | | |
| Mexican Americans | 01-02 | * | < LOD | < LOD | < LOD | < LOD | 567 |
| | 03-04 | * | < LOD | < LOD | .003 (.003-.004) | .004 (.003- 005) | 426 |
| Non-Hispanic blacks | 01-02 | * | < LOD | < LOD | < LOD | < LOD | 515 |
| | 03-04 | * | .002 (<LOD- 003) | .004 ( 003-.006) | .008 (.006-.010) | .013 (.008- 028) | 461 |
| Non-Hispanic whites | 01-02 | * | < LOD | < LOD | < LOD | < LOD | 1061 |
| | 03-04 | * | < LOD | .003 (<LOD-.003) | .004 (.004-.004) | .005 (.004- 006) | 864 |

< LOD means less than the limit of detection for the lipid adjusted serum level, which may vary for some chemicals by year and by individual sample.
* Not calculated: proportion of results below limit of detection was too high to provide a valid result.

## Serum 2,2',4,4',5,5'-Hexachlorobiphenyl (PCB 153) (lipid adjusted)

Geometric mean and selected percentiles of serum concentrations (in ng/g of lipid or parts per billion on a lipid-weight basis) for the U.S. population from the National Health and Nutrition Examination Survey.

| | Survey years | Geometric mean (95% conf. interval) | Selected percentiles ( 95% confidence interval) | | | | Sample size |
|---|---|---|---|---|---|---|---|
| | | | 50th | 75th | 90th | 95th | |
| **Total** | 99-00 | * | < LOD | < LOD | 77.8 (70.2-87.3) | 114 (93 0-133) | 1926 |
| | 01-02 | 27.2 (24.7-30.1) | 30.1 (26.1-34 3) | 57.8 (52.1-63.2) | 94.7 (86.5-104) | 126 (109-142) | 2306 |
| | 03-04 | 19.8 (18.8-20 9) | 20.8 (18.4-22 2) | 43.3 (39.1-46.9) | 71.8 (64.4-82.8) | 97.1 (88 8-111) | 1896 |
| **Age group** | | | | | | | |
| 12-19 years | 99-00 | * | < LOD | < LOD | < LOD | < LOD | 668 |
| | 01-02 | * | < LOD | 12.5 (11.1-14.1) | 21.2 (17.4-26.7) | 31.9 (23.1-64.7) | 757 |
| | 03-04 | 5.86 (5.25-6.55) | 5.40 (4.70-6.21) | 8.50 (7.80-9.85) | 15.7 (12.9-18.4) | 20.7 (16 9-28.3) | 596 |
| 20 years and older | 99-00 | * | < LOD | < LOD | 83.2 (75.9-91.8) | 122 (100-139) | 1258 |
| | 01-02 | 32.6 (29.5-36.1) | 35.1 (31.1-39 0) | 62.8 (57.6-68.0) | 99.5 (90.7-110) | 132 (116-146) | 1549 |
| | 03-04 | 23.7 (22.3-25.1) | 24.2 (21.8-27.4) | 47.1 (43.3-50.5) | 77.5 (68.0-87.9) | 101 (92 9-119) | 1300 |
| **Gender** | | | | | | | |
| Males | 99-00 | * | < LOD | < LOD | 75.0 (66.7-86.2) | 111 (87.7-128) | 917 |
| | 01-02 | 28.5 (25.5-32 0) | 31.5 (26.7-35 2) | 57.7 (48.3-66.2) | 97.5 (82.1-110) | 126 (104-150) | 1074 |
| | 03-04 | 20.0 (18.7-21 3) | 19.7 (17.7-21 2) | 42.9 (37.4-47.6) | 72.7 (60.4-88.8) | 107 (86 8-122) | 947 |
| Females | 99-00 | * | < LOD | < LOD | 79.0 (70.2-92.0) | 119 (91.4-142) | 1009 |
| | 01-02 | 26.1 (23.6-28 8) | 29.0 (25.1-33.4) | 57.9 (52.1-62.9) | 94.3 (87.8-98.2) | 128 (105-145) | 1232 |
| | 03-04 | 19.7 (18.4-21.1) | 21.9 (19.0-24.1) | 43.8 (39.4-47.7) | 70.9 (63.0-81.5) | 93.3 (83 8-100) | 949 |
| **Race/ethnicity** | | | | | | | |
| Mexican Americans | 99-00 | * | < LOD | < LOD | < LOD | 67.5 (59 5-71.8) | 634 |
| | 01-02 | 12.5 (10.8-14.4) | 11.1 (<LOD-13.3) | 24.5 (18.2-33.9) | 47.4 (36.2-60.3) | 66.7 (55 2-72.3) | 567 |
| | 03-04 | 8.75 (7.39-10.4) | 7.86 (6.17-9.40) | 15.6 (11.4-22.2) | 30.3 (25.2-34.9) | 37.8 (31.1-45.2) | 425 |
| Non-Hispanic blacks | 99-00 | * | < LOD | 59.4 (<LOD-82 0) | 121 (90.3-159) | 176 (130-287) | 412 |
| | 01-02 | 30.0 (26.2-34.4) | 31.0 (25.8-36.4) | 65.1 (54.2-82.7) | 127 (97.1-152) | 170 (126-246) | 515 |
| | 03-04 | 22.8 (19.1-27 2) | 20.9 (17.0-28.7) | 54.1 (37.3-69.2) | 126 (92.9-158) | 194 (126-294) | 464 |
| Non-Hispanic whites | 99-00 | * | < LOD | < LOD | 76.4 (69.3-83.9) | 102 (87 8-127) | 725 |
| | 01-02 | 29.9 (26.8-33.4) | 33.0 (28.7-37.1) | 61.2 (55.8-66.7) | 96.3 (86.5-109) | 126 (104-142) | 1061 |
| | 03-04 | 21.3 (19.7-23.1) | 22.2 (20.4-25 9) | 44.9 (39.7-49.5) | 70.9 (60.4-82.1) | 91.3 (82.1-103) | 885 |

Limit of detection (LOD, see Data Analysis section) for Survey years 99-00, 01-02, and 03-04 are 55.6, 10 5, and 1.1, respectively.
< LOD means less than the limit of detection, which may vary for some chemicals by year and by individual sample.
* Not calculated: proportion of results below limit of detection was too high to provide a valid result.

## Serum 2,2',4,4',5,5'-Hexachlorobiphenyl (PCB 153) (whole weight)

Geometric mean and selected percentiles of serum concentrations (in ng/g of serum or parts per billion) for the U.S. population from the National Health and Nutrition Examination Survey.

| | Survey years | Geometric mean (95% conf. interval) | Selected percentiles ( 95% confidence interval) | | | | Sample size |
|---|---|---|---|---|---|---|---|
| | | | 50th | 75th | 90th | 95th | |
| **Total** | 99-00 | * | < LOD | < LOD | .530 (.490-.560) | .750 (.610- 840) | 1926 |
| | 01-02 | .167 (.151-.185) | .190 (.170-.210) | .380 ( 340-.410) | .620 (.560-.690) | .860 (.760- 950) | 2306 |
| | 03-04 | .121 (.114-.128) | .135 (.120-.144) | .283 ( 258-.310) | .477 (.439-.518) | .624 (.575-.733) | 1896 |
| **Age group** | | | | | | | |
| 12-19 years | 99-00 | * | < LOD | < LOD | < LOD | < LOD | 668 |
| | 01-02 | * | < LOD | .060 ( 050-.070) | .110 (.080-.140) | .150 (.110- 310) | 757 |
| | 03-04 | .030 (.027-.033) | .027 (.025-.031) | .044 ( 039-.055) | .076 (.062-.098) | .101 (.079-.129) | 596 |
| 20 years and older | 99-00 | * | < LOD | < LOD | .560 (.510-.610) | .790 (.670- 880) | 1258 |
| | 01-02 | .206 (.187-.228) | .220 (.200-.250) | .410 ( 380-.450) | .670 (.600-.740) | .900 (.820-1.04) | 1549 |
| | 03-04 | .148 (.139-.158) | .156 (.141-.179) | .313 ( 283-.339) | .512 (.452-.563) | .671 (.603-.756) | 1300 |
| **Gender** | | | | | | | |
| Males | 99-00 | * | < LOD | < LOD | .530 (.470-.560) | .690 (.580- 850) | 917 |
| | 01-02 | .177 (.159-.198) | .200 (.170-.220) | .380 ( 340-.430) | .610 (.510-.730) | .850 (.700-1.04) | 1074 |
| | 03-04 | .123 (.115-.133) | .127 (.111-.146) | .277 ( 253-.310) | .474 (.413-.522) | .608 (.533-.794) | 947 |
| Females | 99-00 | * | < LOD | < LOD | .530 (.480-.590) | .770 (.610- 880) | 1009 |
| | 01-02 | .158 (.142-.175) | .180 (.150-.210) | .380 ( 340-.400) | .630 (.570-.710) | .860 (.760- 950) | 1232 |
| | 03-04 | .119 (.110-.128) | .138 (.113-.149) | .291 ( 253-.319) | .492 (.439-.541) | .624 (.578- 689) | 949 |
| **Race/ethnicity** | | | | | | | |
| Mexican Americans | 99-00 | * | < LOD | < LOD | < LOD | .470 (.380- 540) | 634 |
| | 01-02 | .075 (.063-.089) | .060 (<LOD- 080) | .150 (.120-.210) | .330 (.270-.420) | .470 (.380- 550) | 567 |
| | 03-04 | .053 (.044-.064) | .047 (.038-.057) | .100 ( 078-.144) | .205 (.164-.241) | .323 (.213-.435) | 425 |
| Non-Hispanic blacks | 99-00 | * | < LOD | .370 (<LOD-.510) | .750 (.620-.890) | 1.27 (.820-1.64) | 412 |
| | 01-02 | .169 (.146-.195) | .180 (.140-.200) | .390 ( 330-.490) | .780 (.580-.950) | 1.05 (.830-1.43) | 515 |
| | 03-04 | .129 (.108-.156) | .126 (.098-.149) | .330 ( 236-.425) | .734 (.562-1.06) | 1.26 (.892-1.60) | 464 |
| Non-Hispanic whites | 99-00 | * | < LOD | < LOD | .520 (.480-.560) | .740 (.580- 850) | 725 |
| | 01-02 | .185 (.165-.207) | .210 (.180-.230) | .390 ( 370-.430) | .640 (.570-.720) | .840 (.740- 990) | 1061 |
| | 03-04 | .131 (.121-.143) | .144 (.127-.170) | .295 ( 268-.329) | .474 (.412-.518) | .600 (.519- 689) | 885 |

< LOD means less than the limit of detection for the lipid adjusted serum level, which may vary for some chemicals by year and by individual sample.
* Not calculated: proportion of results below limit of detection was too high to provide a valid result.

## Serum 2,2',3,3',4,4',5-Heptachlorobiphenyl (PCB 170) (lipid adjusted)

Geometric mean and selected percentiles of serum concentrations (in ng/g of lipid or parts per billion on a lipid-weight basis) for the U.S. population from the National Health and Nutrition Examination Survey.

| | Survey years | Geometric mean (95% conf. interval) | Selected percentiles ( 95% confidence interval) | | | | Sample size |
|---|---|---|---|---|---|---|---|
| | | | 50th | 75th | 90th | 95th | |
| **Total** | 99-00 | * | < LOD | < LOD | 23.6 (22.0-25.4) | 30.9 (28.1-35.1) | 1798 |
| | 01-02 | * | < LOD | 17.5 (15.7-19.3) | 26.7 (24.9-29.0) | 35.0 (32.4-37.3) | 2301 |
| | 03-04 | 5.46 (5.22-5.71) | 6.30 (5 96-7.10) | 12.9 (12.3-13.9) | 21.7 (19.2-23.5) | 28.2 (25 8-29.8) | 1888 |
| **Age group** | | | | | | | |
| 12-19 years | 99-00 | * | < LOD | < LOD | < LOD | < LOD | 645 |
| | 01-02 | * | < LOD | < LOD | < LOD | < LOD | 756 |
| | 03-04 | 1.12 (.974-1.30) | 1.12 (1 00-1.30) | 1.90 (1.70-2.50) | 4.00 (3.53-4 37) | 5.60 (4.35-6.69) | 592 |
| 20 years and older | 99-00 | * | < LOD | < LOD | 24.9 (23.3-26.4) | 33.9 (29 6-37.5) | 1153 |
| | 01-02 | 10.5 (<LOD-11.3) | 11.1 (<LOD-12.2) | 19.1 (17.3-20.9) | 28.4 (26.2-30.9) | 36.8 (33.4-39.4) | 1545 |
| | 03-04 | 6.86 (6.48-7.26) | 7.83 (6 87-8.70) | 14.2 (13.1-14.9) | 22.7 (20.7-24.9) | 29.5 (26.7-32.2) | 1296 |
| **Gender** | | | | | | | |
| Males | 99-00 | * | < LOD | < LOD | 24.1 (22.0-27.0) | 32.6 (28.1-37.0) | 863 |
| | 01-02 | * | 10.9 (<LOD-11.9) | 18.4 (16.3-20.9) | 28.1 (24.7-31.9) | 36.1 (32.1-38.3) | 1073 |
| | 03-04 | 5.81 (5.43-6.22) | 6.40 (5 61-7.68) | 13.8 (12.4-14.4) | 23.4 (20.4-25.6) | 29.4 (26 0-32.7) | 942 |
| Females | 99-00 | * | < LOD | < LOD | 22.4 (20.7-25.4) | 29.7 (25 8-36.3) | 935 |
| | 01-02 | * | < LOD | 16.4 (15.0-18.0) | 25.9 (24.0-28.4) | 34.0 (30 6-38.4) | 1228 |
| | 03-04 | 5.14 (4.82-5.48) | 6.28 (5 81-7.18) | 12.5 (11.5-13.8) | 19.2 (17.9-21.7) | 26.1 (24 0-29.8) | 946 |
| **Race/ethnicity** | | | | | | | |
| Mexican Americans | 99-00 | * | < LOD | < LOD | < LOD | 23.2 (20 3-26.5) | 606 |
| | 01-02 | * | < LOD | < LOD | 15.4 (11.4-18.7) | 21.1 (17.1-25.1) | 565 |
| | 03-04 | 2.34 (1.91-2.86) | 2.20 (1 54-3.20) | 4.91 (3.40-8.17) | 10.4 (8.40-13.5) | 13.9 (10 8-20.1) | 423 |
| Non-Hispanic blacks | 99-00 | * | < LOD | < LOD | 30.9 (23.1-36.3) | 41.9 (33.7-59.1) | 382 |
| | 01-02 | * | < LOD | 19.0 (14.9-23.2) | 32.5 (25.5-43.9) | 44.4 (32 5-61.7) | 514 |
| | 03-04 | 5.42 (4.63-6.35) | 6.28 (5.11-7.75) | 14.3 (10.7-18.3) | 31.7 (23.1-40.7) | 48.5 (32.1-66.1) | 461 |
| Non-Hispanic whites | 99-00 | * | < LOD | < LOD | 24.1 (22.1-25.9) | 31.0 (26 8-37.3) | 658 |
| | 01-02 | * | 10.9 (<LOD-12.0) | 18.4 (16.8-20.4) | 27.7 (25.4-30.2) | 35.0 (32 3-38.1) | 1059 |
| | 03-04 | 6.13 (5.74-6.56) | 7.40 (6.40-8.18) | 13.8 (12.6-14.6) | 21.7 (19.2-24.2) | 27.0 (24 9-29.5) | 882 |

Limit of detection (LOD, see Data Analysis section) for Survey years 99-00, 01-02, and 03-04 are 17.2, 10 5, and 0.4, respectively.
< LOD means less than the limit of detection, which may vary for some chemicals by year and by individual sample.
* Not calculated: proportion of results below limit of detection was too high to provide a valid result.

## Serum 2,2',3,3',4,4',5-Heptachlorobiphenyl (PCB 170) (whole weight)

Geometric mean and selected percentiles of serum concentrations (in ng/g of serum or parts per billion) for the U.S. population from the National Health and Nutrition Examination Survey.

| | Survey years | Geometric mean (95% conf. interval) | Selected percentiles ( 95% confidence interval) | | | | Sample size |
|---|---|---|---|---|---|---|---|
| | | | 50th | 75th | 90th | 95th | |
| **Total** | 99-00 | * | < LOD | < LOD | .160 (.140-.180) | .210 (.200- 230) | 1798 |
| | 01-02 | * | < LOD | .110 (.110-.120) | .180 (.170-.200) | .250 (.210- 270) | 2301 |
| | 03-04 | .033 (.032-.035) | .041 (.037-.045) | .087 ( 080-.092) | .144 (.134-.149) | .188 (.173- 202) | 1888 |
| **Age group** | | | | | | | |
| 12-19 years | 99-00 | * | < LOD | < LOD | < LOD | < LOD | 645 |
| | 01-02 | * | < LOD | < LOD | < LOD | < LOD | 756 |
| | 03-04 | .006 (.005-.006) | .006 (.005-.007) | .010 ( 009-.012) | .020 (.017-.022) | .029 (.022- 033) | 592 |
| 20 years and older | 99-00 | * | < LOD | < LOD | .170 (.150-.190) | .220 (.200- 250) | 1153 |
| | 01-02 | .067 (<LOD- 072) | .070 (<LOD- 080) | .120 (.110-.130) | .200 (.180-.210) | .250 (.230- 290) | 1545 |
| | 03-04 | .043 (.040-.046) | .051 (.045-.054) | .093 ( 089-.099) | .149 (.141-.160) | .199 (.180- 223) | 1296 |
| **Gender** | | | | | | | |
| Males | 99-00 | * | < LOD | < LOD | .170 (.140-.200) | .220 (.200- 250) | 863 |
| | 01-02 | * | .070 (<LOD- 080) | .120 (.110-.130) | .190 (.170-.210) | .250 (.210- 280) | 1073 |
| | 03-04 | .036 (.033- 039) | .043 (.036-.051) | .089 ( 080-.093) | .148 (.132-.164) | .200 (.173- 225) | 942 |
| Females | 99-00 | * | < LOD | < LOD | .150 (.130-.170) | .210 (.190- 230) | 935 |
| | 01-02 | * | < LOD | .110 (.100-.120) | .180 (.160-.200) | .250 (.210- 280) | 1228 |
| | 03-04 | .031 (.029-.033) | .040 (.034-.044) | .083 ( 075-.092) | .140 (.121-.149) | .176 (.160-.194) | 946 |
| **Race/ethnicity** | | | | | | | |
| Mexican Americans | 99-00 | * | < LOD | < LOD | < LOD | .170 (.130-.190) | 606 |
| | 01-02 | * | < LOD | < LOD | .110 (.080-.130) | .150 (.120-.190) | 565 |
| | 03-04 | .014 (.012-.018) | .015 (.010-.018) | .032 ( 025-.047) | .073 (.054-.113) | .119 (.078-.134) | 423 |
| Non-Hispanic blacks | 99-00 | * | < LOD | < LOD | .190 (.150-.210) | .260 (.190- 370) | 382 |
| | 01-02 | * | < LOD | .110 ( 090-.140) | .210 (.150-.270) | .290 (.210- 390) | 514 |
| | 03-04 | .031 (.026-.037) | .038 (.027-.044) | .087 ( 069-.117) | .210 (.136-.280) | .338 (.221- 380) | 461 |
| Non-Hispanic whites | 99-00 | * | < LOD | < LOD | .160 (.140-.200) | .210 (.200- 240) | 658 |
| | 01-02 | * | .070 (<LOD- 080) | .120 (.110-.130) | .190 (.170-.210) | .250 (.210- 280) | 1059 |
| | 03-04 | .038 (.035-.041) | .046 (.042-.052) | .091 ( 083-.096) | .145 (.132-.151) | .180 (.164- 207) | 882 |

< LOD means less than the limit of detection for the lipid adjusted serum level, which may vary for some chemicals by year and by individual sample.
* Not calculated: proportion of results below limit of detection was too high to provide a valid result.

## Serum 2,2',3,3',4,5,5'-Heptachlorobiphenyl (PCB 172) (lipid adjusted)

Geometric mean and selected percentiles of serum concentrations (in ng/g of lipid or parts per billion on a lipid-weight basis) for the U.S. population from the National Health and Nutrition Examination Survey.

| | Survey years | Geometric mean (95% conf. interval) | Selected percentiles ( 95% confidence interval) | | | | Sample size |
|---|---|---|---|---|---|---|---|
| | | | 50th | 75th | 90th | 95th | |
| **Total** | 99-00 | * | < LOD | < LOD | < LOD | < LOD | 1901 |
| | 01-02 | * | < LOD | < LOD | < LOD | < LOD | 2199 |
| | 03-04 | .647 (.606- 691) | .900 (.800-1.00) | 1.80 (1.69-1.90) | 2.98 (2.70-3 30) | 4.16 (3.65-4.55) | 1878 |
| **Age group** | | | | | | | |
| 12-19 years | 99-00 | * | < LOD | < LOD | < LOD | < LOD | 660 |
| | 01-02 | * | < LOD | < LOD | < LOD | < LOD | 679 |
| | 03-04 | * | < LOD | < LOD | .610 (.460-.840) | 1.10 (.700-1.43) | 585 |
| 20 years and older | 99-00 | * | < LOD | < LOD | < LOD | < LOD | 1241 |
| | 01-02 | * | < LOD | < LOD | < LOD | < LOD | 1520 |
| | 03-04 | .805 (.746- 869) | 1.08 (1 00-1.16) | 1.95 (1.80-2.10) | 3.20 (2.87-3 60) | 4.38 (3.79-5.00) | 1293 |
| **Gender** | | | | | | | |
| Males | 99-00 | * | < LOD | < LOD | < LOD | < LOD | 911 |
| | 01-02 | * | < LOD | < LOD | < LOD | < LOD | 1027 |
| | 03-04 | .668 (.612-.730) | .900 (.800-1.01) | 1.82 (1.70-2.00) | 3.30 (2.80-3 80) | 4.43 (3.76-5.50) | 937 |
| Females | 99-00 | * | < LOD | < LOD | < LOD | < LOD | 990 |
| | 01-02 | * | < LOD | < LOD | < LOD | < LOD | 1172 |
| | 03-04 | .627 (.581- 678) | .900 (.800-1.03) | 1.72 (1.51-1.90) | 2.80 (2.50-3.11) | 3.70 (3.37-4.26) | 941 |
| **Race/ethnicity** | | | | | | | |
| Mexican Americans | 99-00 | * | < LOD | < LOD | < LOD | < LOD | 630 |
| | 01-02 | * | < LOD | < LOD | < LOD | < LOD | 519 |
| | 03-04 | * | < LOD | .700 (.470-1.20) | 1.40 (1.20-1 95) | 2.00 (1.40-2.91) | 423 |
| Non-Hispanic blacks | 99-00 | * | < LOD | < LOD | < LOD | < LOD | 409 |
| | 01-02 | * | < LOD | < LOD | < LOD | < LOD | 494 |
| | 03-04 | .688 (.579- 818) | .900 (.700-1.10) | 2.20 (1.70-2.60) | 5.00 (3.38-6 53) | 7.60 (5.00-11.3) | 458 |
| Non-Hispanic whites | 99-00 | * | < LOD | < LOD | < LOD | < LOD | 706 |
| | 01-02 | * | < LOD | < LOD | < LOD | < LOD | 1027 |
| | 03-04 | .720 (.665-.781) | 1.00 (.870-1.10) | 1.80 (1.69-2.00) | 2.94 (2.70-3 20) | 3.90 (3.53-4.20) | 877 |

Limit of detection (LOD, see Data Analysis section) for Survey years 99-00, 01-02, and 03-04 are 12.5, 10 5, and 0.4, respectively.
< LOD means less than the limit of detection, which may vary for some chemicals by year and by individual sample.
* Not calculated: proportion of results below limit of detection was too high to provide a valid result.

## Serum 2,2',3,3',4,5,5'-Heptachlorobiphenyl (PCB 172) (whole weight)

Geometric mean and selected percentiles of serum concentrations (in ng/g of serum or parts per billion) for the U.S. population from the National Health and Nutrition Examination Survey.

| | Survey years | Geometric mean (95% conf. interval) | 50th | 75th | 90th | 95th | Sample size |
|---|---|---|---|---|---|---|---|
| **Total** | 99-00 | * | < LOD | < LOD | < LOD | < LOD | 1901 |
| | 01-02 | * | < LOD | < LOD | < LOD | < LOD | 2199 |
| | 03-04 | .004 (.004-.004) | .006 (.005-.006) | .012 (.011-.012) | .021 (.019-.022) | .027 (.024-.031) | 1878 |
| **Age group** | | | | | | | |
| 12-19 years | 99-00 | * | < LOD | < LOD | < LOD | < LOD | 660 |
| | 01-02 | * | < LOD | < LOD | < LOD | < LOD | 679 |
| | 03-04 | * | < LOD | < LOD | .003 (.002-.004) | .005 (.004-.009) | 585 |
| 20 years and older | 99-00 | * | < LOD | < LOD | < LOD | < LOD | 1241 |
| | 01-02 | * | < LOD | < LOD | < LOD | < LOD | 1520 |
| | 03-04 | .005 (.005-.005) | .007 (.006-.007) | .013 (.012-.014) | .022 (.020-.024) | .028 (.025-.033) | 1293 |
| **Gender** | | | | | | | |
| Males | 99-00 | * | < LOD | < LOD | < LOD | < LOD | 911 |
| | 01-02 | * | < LOD | < LOD | < LOD | < LOD | 1027 |
| | 03-04 | .004 (.004-.005) | .006 (.005-.007) | .012 (.011-.013) | .021 (.018-.024) | .029 (.024-.036) | 937 |
| Females | 99-00 | * | < LOD | < LOD | < LOD | < LOD | 990 |
| | 01-02 | * | < LOD | < LOD | < LOD | < LOD | 1172 |
| | 03-04 | .004 (.003-.004) | .006 (.005-.006) | .012 (.010-.012) | .019 (.017-.021) | .026 (.023-.028) | 941 |
| **Race/ethnicity** | | | | | | | |
| Mexican Americans | 99-00 | * | < LOD | < LOD | < LOD | < LOD | 630 |
| | 01-02 | * | < LOD | < LOD | < LOD | < LOD | 519 |
| | 03-04 | * | < LOD | .005 (.003-.007) | .010 (.007-.015) | .017 (.011-.022) | 423 |
| Non-Hispanic blacks | 99-00 | * | < LOD | < LOD | < LOD | < LOD | 409 |
| | 01-02 | * | < LOD | < LOD | < LOD | < LOD | 494 |
| | 03-04 | .004 (.003-.005) | .006 (.004-.006) | .013 (.010-.017) | .030 (.020-.048) | .052 (.028-.067) | 458 |
| Non-Hispanic whites | 99-00 | * | < LOD | < LOD | < LOD | < LOD | 706 |
| | 01-02 | * | < LOD | < LOD | < LOD | < LOD | 1027 |
| | 03-04 | .004 (.004-.005) | .006 (.005-.007) | .012 (.011-.013) | .020 (.018-.022) | .026 (.023-.029) | 877 |

< LOD means less than the limit of detection for the lipid adjusted serum level, which may vary for some chemicals by year and by individual sample.
* Not calculated: proportion of results below limit of detection was too high to provide a valid result.

## Serum 2,2',3,3',4,5',6'-Heptachlorobiphenyl (PCB 177) (lipid adjusted)

Geometric mean and selected percentiles of serum concentrations (in ng/g of lipid or parts per billion on a lipid-weight basis) for the U.S. population from the National Health and Nutrition Examination Survey.

| | Survey years | Geometric mean (95% conf. interval) | Selected percentiles ( 95% confidence interval) | | | | Sample size |
|---|---|---|---|---|---|---|---|
| | | | 50th | 75th | 90th | 95th | |
| **Total** | 99-00 | * | < LOD | < LOD | < LOD | < LOD | 1873 |
| | 01-02 | * | < LOD | < LOD | < LOD | < LOD | 2287 |
| | 03-04 | 1.13 (1.07-1.20) | 1.30 (1 20-1.40) | 2.77 (2.50-3.09) | 5.30 (4.70-5 90) | 7.20 (6.38-8.50) | 1882 |
| **Age group** | | | | | | | |
| 12-19 years | 99-00 | * | < LOD | < LOD | < LOD | < LOD | 653 |
| | 01-02 | * | < LOD | < LOD | < LOD | < LOD | 756 |
| | 03-04 | * | < LOD | .600 (.500-.720) | 1.04 (.800-1.40) | 1.70 (1.20-1.95) | 588 |
| 20 years and older | 99-00 | * | < LOD | < LOD | < LOD | < LOD | 1220 |
| | 01-02 | * | < LOD | < LOD | < LOD | < LOD | 1531 |
| | 03-04 | 1.40 (1.30-1.50) | 1.50 (1.40-1.71) | 3.10 (2.80-3.44) | 5.70 (4.99-6 22) | 7.80 (6.50-9.50) | 1294 |
| **Gender** | | | | | | | |
| Males | 99-00 | * | < LOD | < LOD | < LOD | < LOD | 887 |
| | 01-02 | * | < LOD | < LOD | < LOD | < LOD | 1065 |
| | 03-04 | 1.12 (1.03-1.21) | 1.30 (1.17-1.41) | 2.70 (2.40-3.00) | 5.30 (4.72-5 80) | 7.82 (6.22-9.50) | 940 |
| Females | 99-00 | * | < LOD | < LOD | < LOD | < LOD | 986 |
| | 01-02 | * | < LOD | < LOD | < LOD | < LOD | 1222 |
| | 03-04 | 1.15 (1.06-1.23) | 1.30 (1.18-1.49) | 2.80 (2.57-3.19) | 5.30 (4.50-6 06) | 6.97 (6.15-7.92) | 942 |
| **Race/ethnicity** | | | | | | | |
| Mexican Americans | 99-00 | * | < LOD | < LOD | < LOD | < LOD | 622 |
| | 01-02 | * | < LOD | < LOD | < LOD | < LOD | 562 |
| | 03-04 | .500 (<LOD-.649) | .550 (.400-.700) | 1.36 (1.00-1.63) | 2.40 (1.86-3 30) | 3.40 (2.33-4.63) | 423 |
| Non-Hispanic blacks | 99-00 | * | < LOD | < LOD | < LOD | < LOD | 399 |
| | 01-02 | * | < LOD | < LOD | < LOD | 10.6 (<LOD-12.4) | 515 |
| | 03-04 | 1.52 (1.25-1.84) | 1.56 (1 29-2.05) | 4.40 (3.20-5.70) | 9.80 (6.30-13.3) | 15.8 (10 0-25.7) | 458 |
| Non-Hispanic whites | 99-00 | * | < LOD | < LOD | < LOD | < LOD | 698 |
| | 01-02 | * | < LOD | < LOD | < LOD | < LOD | 1048 |
| | 03-04 | 1.16 (1.08-1.25) | 1.34 (1 20-1.50) | 2.74 (2.41-3.09) | 5.00 (4.57-5 56) | 6.50 (5.98-7.40) | 880 |

Limit of detection (LOD, see Data Analysis section) for Survey years 99-00, 01-02, and 03-04 are 12.5, 10 5, and 0.4, respectively.
< LOD means less than the limit of detection, which may vary for some chemicals by year and by individual sample.
* Not calculated: proportion of results below limit of detection was too high to provide a valid result.

## Serum 2,2',3,3',4,5',6'-Heptachlorobiphenyl (PCB 177) (whole weight)

Geometric mean and selected percentiles of serum concentrations (in ng/g of serum or parts per billion) for the U.S. population from the National Health and Nutrition Examination Survey.

| | Survey years | Geometric mean (95% conf. interval) | Selected percentiles ( 95% confidence interval) | | | | Sample size |
|---|---|---|---|---|---|---|---|
| | | | 50th | 75th | 90th | 95th | |
| **Total** | 99-00 | * | < LOD | < LOD | < LOD | < LOD | 1873 |
| | 01-02 | * | < LOD | < LOD | < LOD | < LOD | 2287 |
| | 03-04 | .007 (.007-.007) | .008 (.008-.009) | .018 ( 016-.021) | .034 (.031-.037) | .047 (.043- 056) | 1882 |
| **Age group** | | | | | | | |
| 12-19 years | 99-00 | * | < LOD | < LOD | < LOD | < LOD | 653 |
| | 01-02 | * | < LOD | < LOD | < LOD | < LOD | 756 |
| | 03-04 | * | < LOD | .003 ( 003-.004) | .006 (.005-.007) | .007 (.006- 011) | 588 |
| 20 years and older | 99-00 | * | < LOD | < LOD | < LOD | < LOD | 1220 |
| | 01-02 | * | < LOD | < LOD | < LOD | < LOD | 1531 |
| | 03-04 | .009 (.008-.009) | .010 (.009-.011) | .021 ( 018-.023) | .036 (.033-.041) | .053 (.045- 058) | 1294 |
| **Gender** | | | | | | | |
| Males | 99-00 | * | < LOD | < LOD | < LOD | < LOD | 887 |
| | 01-02 | * | < LOD | < LOD | < LOD | < LOD | 1065 |
| | 03-04 | .007 (.006-.007) | .009 (.008-.009) | .018 ( 016-.021) | .032 (.030-.036) | .045 (.039- 062) | 940 |
| Females | 99-00 | * | < LOD | < LOD | < LOD | < LOD | 986 |
| | 01-02 | * | < LOD | < LOD | < LOD | < LOD | 1222 |
| | 03-04 | .007 (.006-.008) | .008 (.007-.009) | .018 ( 017-.021) | .035 (.032-.042) | .051 (.043- 056) | 942 |
| **Race/ethnicity** | | | | | | | |
| Mexican Americans | 99-00 | * | < LOD | < LOD | < LOD | < LOD | 622 |
| | 01-02 | * | < LOD | < LOD | < LOD | < LOD | 562 |
| | 03-04 | .003 (<LOD- 004) | .003 (.002-.005) | .008 ( 006-.011) | .018 (.012-.025) | .025 (.018- 032) | 423 |
| Non-Hispanic blacks | 99-00 | * | < LOD | < LOD | < LOD | < LOD | 399 |
| | 01-02 | * | < LOD | < LOD | < LOD | .070 (<LOD-.100) | 515 |
| | 03-04 | .009 (.007-.011) | .009 (.007-.012) | .026 ( 018-.036) | .057 (.044-.090) | .105 (.058-.143) | 458 |
| Non-Hispanic whites | 99-00 | * | < LOD | < LOD | < LOD | < LOD | 698 |
| | 01-02 | * | < LOD | < LOD | < LOD | < LOD | 1048 |
| | 03-04 | .007 (.007-.008) | .009 (.008-.010) | .018 ( 016-.021) | .032 (.029-.036) | .044 (.040- 052) | 880 |

< LOD means less than the limit of detection for the lipid adjusted serum level, which may vary for some chemicals by year and by individual sample.
* Not calculated: proportion of results below limit of detection was too high to provide a valid result.

## Serum 2,2',3,3',5,5',6-Heptachlorobiphenyl (PCB 178) (lipid adjusted)

Geometric mean and selected percentiles of serum concentrations (in ng/g of lipid or parts per billion on a lipid-weight basis) for the U.S. population from the National Health and Nutrition Examination Survey.

| | Survey years | Geometric mean (95% conf. interval) | Selected percentiles ( 95% confidence interval) | | | | Sample size |
|---|---|---|---|---|---|---|---|
| | | | 50th | 75th | 90th | 95th | |
| **Total** | 99-00 | * | < LOD | < LOD | < LOD | < LOD | 1932 |
| | 01-02 | * | < LOD | < LOD | < LOD | < LOD | 2299 |
| | 03-04 | .933 (.894- 974) | 1.20 (1.10-1.30) | 2.50 (2.30-2.67) | 4.24 (3.90-4.47) | 6.10 (5.13-7.10) | 1887 |
| **Age group** | | | | | | | |
| 12-19 years | 99-00 | * | < LOD | < LOD | < LOD | < LOD | 669 |
| | 01-02 | * | < LOD | < LOD | < LOD | < LOD | 758 |
| | 03-04 | * | < LOD | .400 (<LOD-.480) | .850 (.620-1 04) | 1.12 (1.00-1.32) | 590 |
| 20 years and older | 99-00 | * | < LOD | < LOD | < LOD | < LOD | 1263 |
| | 01-02 | * | < LOD | < LOD | < LOD | < LOD | 1541 |
| | 03-04 | 1.18 (1.11-1.25) | 1.46 (1 30-1.60) | 2.74 (2.60-2.90) | 4.41 (4.10-4 80) | 6.50 (5.69-7.58) | 1297 |
| **Gender** | | | | | | | |
| Males | 99-00 | * | < LOD | < LOD | < LOD | < LOD | 919 |
| | 01-02 | * | < LOD | < LOD | < LOD | < LOD | 1069 |
| | 03-04 | .991 (.918-1.07) | 1.20 (1.10-1.37) | 2.66 (2.45-2.80) | 4.50 (3.80-5.10) | 6.40 (5.30-7.70) | 940 |
| Females | 99-00 | * | < LOD | < LOD | < LOD | < LOD | 1013 |
| | 01-02 | * | < LOD | < LOD | < LOD | < LOD | 1230 |
| | 03-04 | .881 (.835- 930) | 1.20 (1.10-1.30) | 2.30 (2.20-2.59) | 4.01 (3.71-4 34) | 5.40 (4.47-6.70) | 947 |
| **Race/ethnicity** | | | | | | | |
| Mexican Americans | 99-00 | * | < LOD | < LOD | < LOD | < LOD | 635 |
| | 01-02 | * | < LOD | < LOD | < LOD | < LOD | 567 |
| | 03-04 | * | < LOD | .900 (.600-1.34) | 1.99 (1.37-2 60) | 3.10 (2.00-3.60) | 424 |
| Non-Hispanic blacks | 99-00 | * | < LOD | < LOD | < LOD | < LOD | 415 |
| | 01-02 | * | < LOD | < LOD | < LOD | < LOD | 515 |
| | 03-04 | 1.09 (.911-1.30) | 1.30 (.910-1.65) | 3.10 (2.30-4.21) | 7.10 (5.13-10.1) | 11.4 (6.80-16.5) | 460 |
| Non-Hispanic whites | 99-00 | * | < LOD | < LOD | < LOD | < LOD | 724 |
| | 01-02 | * | < LOD | < LOD | < LOD | < LOD | 1054 |
| | 03-04 | 1.03 (.963-1.10) | 1.30 (1.19-1.50) | 2.61 (2.40-2.80) | 4.20 (3.80-4.40) | 5.33 (4.58-6.30) | 882 |

Limit of detection (LOD, see Data Analysis section) for Survey years 99-00, 01-02, and 03-04 are 12.4, 10 5, and 0.4, respectively.
< LOD means less than the limit of detection, which may vary for some chemicals by year and by individual sample.
* Not calculated: proportion of results below limit of detection was too high to provide a valid result.

## Serum 2,2',3,3',5,5',6-Heptachlorobiphenyl (PCB 178) (whole weight)

Geometric mean and selected percentiles of serum concentrations (in ng/g of serum or parts per billion) for the U.S. population from the National Health and Nutrition Examination Survey.

| | Survey years | Geometric mean (95% conf. interval) | 50th | 75th | 90th | 95th | Sample size |
|---|---|---|---|---|---|---|---|
| **Total** | 99-00 | * | < LOD | < LOD | < LOD | < LOD | 1932 |
| | 01-02 | * | < LOD | < LOD | < LOD | < LOD | 2299 |
| | 03-04 | .006 (.005-.006) | .008 (.007-.008) | .016 (.015-.018) | .029 (.026-.032) | .041 (.035-.045) | 1887 |
| **Age group** | | | | | | | |
| 12-19 years | 99-00 | * | < LOD | < LOD | < LOD | < LOD | 669 |
| | 01-02 | * | < LOD | < LOD | < LOD | < LOD | 758 |
| | 03-04 | * | < LOD | .002 (<LOD-.002) | .004 (.003-.005) | .006 (.004-.007) | 590 |
| 20 years and older | 99-00 | * | < LOD | < LOD | < LOD | < LOD | 1263 |
| | 01-02 | * | < LOD | < LOD | < LOD | < LOD | 1541 |
| | 03-04 | .007 (.007-.008) | .009 (.008-.010) | .018 (.017-.019) | .031 (.028-.034) | .043 (.038-.048) | 1297 |
| **Gender** | | | | | | | |
| Males | 99-00 | * | < LOD | < LOD | < LOD | < LOD | 919 |
| | 01-02 | * | < LOD | < LOD | < LOD | < LOD | 1069 |
| | 03-04 | .006 (.006-.007) | .008 (.007-.009) | .017 (.016-.018) | .030 (.025-.034) | .042 (.034-.050) | 940 |
| Females | 99-00 | * | < LOD | < LOD | < LOD | < LOD | 1013 |
| | 01-02 | * | < LOD | < LOD | < LOD | < LOD | 1230 |
| | 03-04 | .005 (.005-.006) | .008 (.006-.008) | .016 (.014-.017) | .028 (.025-.031) | .040 (.034-.045) | 947 |
| **Race/ethnicity** | | | | | | | |
| Mexican Americans | 99-00 | * | < LOD | < LOD | < LOD | < LOD | 635 |
| | 01-02 | * | < LOD | < LOD | < LOD | < LOD | 567 |
| | 03-04 | * | < LOD | .005 (.004-.008) | .013 (.009-.020) | .022 (.014-.028) | 424 |
| Non-Hispanic blacks | 99-00 | * | < LOD | < LOD | < LOD | < LOD | 415 |
| | 01-02 | * | < LOD | < LOD | < LOD | < LOD | 515 |
| | 03-04 | .006 (.005-.008) | .008 (.006-.008) | .019 (.016-.027) | .044 (.032-.061) | .077 (.045-.089) | 460 |
| Non-Hispanic whites | 99-00 | * | < LOD | < LOD | < LOD | < LOD | 724 |
| | 01-02 | * | < LOD | < LOD | < LOD | < LOD | 1054 |
| | 03-04 | .006 (.006-.007) | .008 (.007-.010) | .017 (.015-.018) | .028 (.025-.031) | .037 (.033-.045) | 882 |

< LOD means less than the limit of detection for the lipid adjusted serum level, which may vary for some chemicals by year and by individual sample.
* Not calculated: proportion of results below limit of detection was too high to provide a valid result.

## Serum 2,2',3,4,4',5,5'-Heptachlorobiphenyl (PCB 180) (lipid adjusted)

Geometric mean and selected percentiles of serum concentrations (in ng/g of lipid or parts per billion on a lipid-weight basis) for the U.S. population from the National Health and Nutrition Examination Survey.

| | Survey years | Geometric mean (95% conf. interval) | Selected percentiles ( 95% confidence interval) | | | | Sample size |
|---|---|---|---|---|---|---|---|
| | | | 50th | 75th | 90th | 95th | |
| **Total** | 99-00 | * | < LOD | 37.5 (32.7-41.8) | 62.0 (56.6-66.6) | 79.3 (72.1-89.2) | 1924 |
| | 01-02 | 19.2 (17.4-21.1) | 21.8 (19.0-24 6) | 42.2 (38.3-47.5) | 69.7 (63.7-75.9) | 87.3 (83 3-93.0) | 2302 |
| | 03-04 | 15.1 (14.5-15.7) | 18.0 (16.4-18 9) | 37.1 (34.9-39.5) | 63.7 (56.2-68.2) | 81.5 (75 8-89.9) | 1896 |
| **Age group** | | | | | | | |
| 12-19 years | 99-00 | * | < LOD | < LOD | < LOD | < LOD | 667 |
| | 01-02 | * | < LOD | < LOD | 12.2 (<LOD-14 8) | 21.3 (14 2-26.0) | 755 |
| | 03-04 | 3.06 (2.65-3.54) | 2.97 (2 57-3.41) | 5.00 (4.20-5.80) | 11.1 (8.70-13.0) | 14.7 (13 0-18.8) | 598 |
| 20 years and older | 99-00 | * | < LOD | 41.1 (37.6-45.2) | 65.6 (60.6-69.4) | 84.8 (75 6-96.1) | 1257 |
| | 01-02 | 23.0 (20.8-25 5) | 26.5 (22.7-28 6) | 46.7 (41.4-51.3) | 74.5 (66.7-79.8) | 91.4 (85 0-99.5) | 1547 |
| | 03-04 | 19.0 (17.9-20.1) | 21.5 (18.9-24 3) | 40.4 (37.9-42.8) | 66.7 (61.0-70.1) | 88.0 (77 8-96.7) | 1298 |
| **Gender** | | | | | | | |
| Males | 99-00 | * | < LOD | 40.6 (34.5-45.0) | 65.1 (58.6-71.4) | 83.8 (75 8-96.3) | 919 |
| | 01-02 | 21.1 (18.8-23.7) | 25.1 (21.2-30 0) | 46.7 (39.8-51.8) | 73.8 (63.2-79.8) | 86.9 (78 0-99.4) | 1073 |
| | 03-04 | 16.1 (14.8-17.4) | 18.5 (15.8-21 3) | 39.6 (35.8-41.7) | 68.6 (63.7-75.0) | 88.3 (76 8-96.7) | 947 |
| Females | 99-00 | * | < LOD | 34.4 (29.8-39.3) | 56.7 (52.2-62.6) | 74.6 (66 6-90.5) | 1005 |
| | 01-02 | 17.5 (15.9-19 3) | 18.5 (16.0-21 6) | 39.7 (34.8-43.9) | 64.3 (58.0-74.8) | 87.9 (79.1-98.1) | 1229 |
| | 03-04 | 14.2 (13.4-15 0) | 17.8 (15.8-19 2) | 35.4 (31.8-38.5) | 55.7 (51.2-59.9) | 74.3 (64 8-87.6) | 949 |
| **Race/ethnicity** | | | | | | | |
| Mexican Americans | 99-00 | * | < LOD | < LOD | 41.7 (33.2-50.5) | 57.8 (49.7-63.8) | 633 |
| | 01-02 | * | < LOD | 18.0 (11.5-22.7) | 36.9 (28.2-45.7) | 54.2 (42 2-60.0) | 566 |
| | 03-04 | 6.14 (4.91-7.67) | 5.80 (3 80-7.50) | 12.6 (8.97-21.5) | 27.2 (22.3-35.4) | 38.8 (27 2-60.7) | 427 |
| Non-Hispanic blacks | 99-00 | * | < LOD | 39.3 (32.2-48.4) | 78.4 (64 3-93.7) | 117 (89 6-144) | 414 |
| | 01-02 | 19.5 (16.5-23.1) | 21.0 (16.9-23 8) | 48.4 (36.7-57.9) | 90.5 (73.7-101) | 116 (96.1-167) | 514 |
| | 03-04 | 15.1 (12.8-17.7) | 18.1 (12.6-20 8) | 39.0 (29.7-51.1) | 89.9 (64.4-122) | 137 (91.4-206) | 464 |
| Non-Hispanic whites | 99-00 | * | < LOD | 39.9 (34.5-45.3) | 62.3 (56.5-68.6) | 79.0 (71 3-91.4) | 719 |
| | 01-02 | 21.4 (19.1-23 9) | 24.8 (21.5-28.1) | 45.6 (40.2-51.0) | 72.4 (63.8-78.0) | 87.9 (83 8-94.3) | 1059 |
| | 03-04 | 16.9 (15.9-18 0) | 19.8 (18.4-23.1) | 39.3 (35.8-42.0) | 63.7 (55.0-69.1) | 79.8 (70.1-89.3) | 883 |

Limit of detection (LOD, see Data Analysis section) for Survey years 99-00, 01-02, and 03-04 are 28.2, 10 5, and 0.4, respectively.
< LOD means less than the limit of detection, which may vary for some chemicals by year and by individual sample.
* Not calculated: proportion of results below limit of detection was too high to provide a valid result.

## Serum 2,2',3,4,4',5,5'-Heptachlorobiphenyl (PCB 180) (whole weight)

Geometric mean and selected percentiles of serum concentrations (in ng/g of serum or parts per billion) for the U.S. population from the National Health and Nutrition Examination Survey.

| | Survey years | Geometric mean (95% conf. interval) | 50th | 75th | 90th | 95th | Sample size |
|---|---|---|---|---|---|---|---|
| **Total** | 99-00 | * | < LOD | .250 ( 220-.270) | .410 (.370-.450) | .540 (.490- 600) | 1924 |
| | 01-02 | .118 (.106-.130) | .140 (.120-.160) | .280 ( 250-.300) | .460 (.400-.510) | .610 (.540- 690) | 2302 |
| | 03-04 | .092 (.088-.096) | .114 (.102-.127) | .246 ( 230-.253) | .409 (.386-.438) | .534 (.495- 598) | 1896 |
| **Age group** | | | | | | | |
| 12-19 years | 99-00 | * | < LOD | < LOD | < LOD | < LOD | 667 |
| | 01-02 | * | < LOD | < LOD | .060 (<LOD-.080) | .090 (.070-.140) | 755 |
| | 03-04 | .016 (.014-.018) | .015 (.013-.017) | .025 ( 022-.030) | .050 (.046-.056) | .076 (.056- 096) | 598 |
| 20 years and older | 99-00 | * | < LOD | .270 ( 240-.300) | .440 (.410-.480) | .560 (.500- 620) | 1257 |
| | 01-02 | .146 (.131-.162) | .170 (.150-.190) | .300 ( 280-.340) | .490 (.430-.560) | .640 (.570-.740) | 1547 |
| | 03-04 | .119 (.112-.126) | .138 (.125-.151) | .270 ( 249-.284) | .433 (.402-.474) | .572 (.511- 635) | 1298 |
| **Gender** | | | | | | | |
| Males | 99-00 | * | < LOD | .260 ( 220-.300) | .460 (.370-.510) | .570 (.500- 650) | 919 |
| | 01-02 | .131 (.117-.147) | .170 (.140-.200) | .300 ( 260-.340) | .480 (.410-.550) | .620 (.530-.720) | 1073 |
| | 03-04 | .099 (.091- 108) | .117 (.098-.148) | .250 ( 231-.274) | .422 (.388-.495) | .596 (.499- 654) | 947 |
| Females | 99-00 | * | < LOD | .230 ( 200-.270) | .380 (.340-.410) | .510 (.430- 560) | 1005 |
| | 01-02 | .106 (.096-.117) | .120 (.100-.140) | .260 ( 230-.280) | .420 (.380-.470) | .610 (.520-.700) | 1229 |
| | 03-04 | .085 (.080-.092) | .110 (.094-.123) | .230 ( 209- 252) | .386 (.349-.421) | .494 (.459- 541) | 949 |
| **Race/ethnicity** | | | | | | | |
| Mexican Americans | 99-00 | * | < LOD | < LOD | .280 (.200-.320) | .390 (.320-.450) | 633 |
| | 01-02 | * | < LOD | .110 ( 080-.160) | .260 (.200-.310) | .360 (.280-.420) | 566 |
| | 03-04 | .037 (.030-.047) | .035 (.024-.051) | .086 ( 059-.118) | .191 (.138-.313) | .343 (.191-.405) | 427 |
| Non-Hispanic blacks | 99-00 | * | < LOD | .250 (.190-.300) | .500 (.350-.660) | .730 (.530-1.04) | 414 |
| | 01-02 | .110 (.092-.131) | .120 (.090-.140) | .290 ( 220-.350) | .580 (.440-.650) | .720 (.520-1.01) | 514 |
| | 03-04 | .086 (.072-.102) | .098 (.070-.126) | .248 (.194-.327) | .580 (.373-.824) | .919 (.592-1.12) | 464 |
| Non-Hispanic whites | 99-00 | * | < LOD | .260 ( 240-.300) | .430 (.380-.470) | .540 (.480- 600) | 719 |
| | 01-02 | .132 (.118-.148) | .160 (.140-.180) | .290 ( 260-.330) | .470 (.410-.530) | .620 (.530-.730) | 1059 |
| | 03-04 | .104 (.097-.112) | .132 (.115-.151) | .253 ( 235-.280) | .409 (.382-.449) | .512 (.478- 572) | 883 |

< LOD means less than the limit of detection for the lipid adjusted serum level, which may vary for some chemicals by year and by individual sample.
* Not calculated: proportion of results below limit of detection was too high to provide a valid result.

## Serum 2,2',3,4,4',5',6-Heptachlorobiphenyl (PCB 183) (lipid adjusted)

Geometric mean and selected percentiles of serum concentrations (in ng/g of lipid or parts per billion on a lipid-weight basis) for the U.S. population from the National Health and Nutrition Examination Survey.

| | Survey years | Geometric mean (95% conf. interval) | Selected percentiles ( 95% confidence interval) | | | | Sample size |
|---|---|---|---|---|---|---|---|
| | | | 50th | 75th | 90th | 95th | |
| **Total** | 99-00 | * | < LOD | < LOD | < LOD | < LOD | 1928 |
| | 01-02 | * | < LOD | < LOD | < LOD | < LOD | 2306 |
| | 03-04 | 1.45 (1.38-1.54) | 1.60 (1 50-1.77) | 3.29 (3.15-3.54) | 5.86 (5.50-6 29) | 7.90 (7.50-8.74) | 1886 |
| **Age group** | | | | | | | |
| 12-19 years | 99-00 | * | < LOD | < LOD | < LOD | < LOD | 668 |
| | 01-02 | * | < LOD | < LOD | < LOD | < LOD | 757 |
| | 03-04 | * | .440 (<LOD-.500) | .730 (.660-.840) | 1.30 (.990-1 62) | 1.91 (1.50-2.24) | 590 |
| 20 years and older | 99-00 | * | < LOD | < LOD | < LOD | < LOD | 1260 |
| | 01-02 | * | < LOD | < LOD | < LOD | < LOD | 1549 |
| | 03-04 | 1.77 (1.67-1.88) | 1.88 (1.73-2.09) | 3.70 (3.34-4.00) | 6.25 (5.71-6 83) | 8.40 (7.70-9.55) | 1296 |
| **Gender** | | | | | | | |
| Males | 99-00 | * | < LOD | < LOD | < LOD | < LOD | 919 |
| | 01-02 | * | < LOD | < LOD | < LOD | < LOD | 1074 |
| | 03-04 | 1.47 (1.34-1.61) | 1.54 (1.40-1.77) | 3.29 (3.10-3.54) | 5.80 (5.30-6 50) | 7.90 (7.20-9.20) | 940 |
| Females | 99-00 | * | < LOD | < LOD | < LOD | < LOD | 1009 |
| | 01-02 | * | < LOD | < LOD | < LOD | < LOD | 1232 |
| | 03-04 | 1.44 (1.34-1.55) | 1.69 (1 50-1.82) | 3.30 (3.05-3.80) | 5.88 (5.21-6 30) | 7.90 (7.31-9.24) | 946 |
| **Race/ethnicity** | | | | | | | |
| Mexican Americans | 99-00 | * | < LOD | < LOD | < LOD | < LOD | 635 |
| | 01-02 | * | < LOD | < LOD | < LOD | < LOD | 567 |
| | 03-04 | .703 (.579- 854) | .700 (.600-.890) | 1.40 (1.19-1.90) | 2.62 (2.20-3.47) | 3.73 (2.60-5.60) | 423 |
| Non-Hispanic blacks | 99-00 | * | < LOD | < LOD | < LOD | 12.7 (<LOD-23.1) | 413 |
| | 01-02 | * | < LOD | < LOD | < LOD | 13.0 (<LOD-14.9) | 514 |
| | 03-04 | 1.64 (1.41-1.90) | 1.60 (1 20-2.00) | 4.31 (3.25-5.63) | 11.0 (6.69-13.7) | 14.8 (11 3-17.4) | 459 |
| Non-Hispanic whites | 99-00 | * | < LOD | < LOD | < LOD | < LOD | 722 |
| | 01-02 | * | < LOD | < LOD | < LOD | < LOD | 1061 |
| | 03-04 | 1.56 (1.43-1.69) | 1.74 (1 55-1.90) | 3.30 (3.14-3.73) | 5.71 (5.20-6 29) | 7.59 (6.70-8.04) | 883 |

Limit of detection (LOD, see Data Analysis section) for Survey years 99-00, 01-02, and 03-04 are 12.4, 10 5, and 0.4, respectively.
< LOD means less than the limit of detection, which may vary for some chemicals by year and by individual sample.
* Not calculated: proportion of results below limit of detection was too high to provide a valid result.

## Serum 2,2',3,4,4',5',6-Heptachlorobiphenyl (PCB 183) (whole weight)

Geometric mean and selected percentiles of serum concentrations (in ng/g of serum or parts per billion) for the U.S. population from the National Health and Nutrition Examination Survey.

| | Survey years | Geometric mean (95% conf. interval) | Selected percentiles ( 95% confidence interval) | | | | Sample size |
|---|---|---|---|---|---|---|---|
| | | | 50th | 75th | 90th | 95th | |
| **Total** | 99-00 | * | < LOD | < LOD | < LOD | < LOD | 1928 |
| | 01-02 | * | < LOD | < LOD | < LOD | < LOD | 2306 |
| | 03-04 | .009 (.008-.009) | .010 (.009-.011) | .021 ( 019-.024) | .039 (.036-.042) | .054 (.048- 059) | 1886 |
| **Age group** | | | | | | | |
| 12-19 years | 99-00 | * | < LOD | < LOD | < LOD | < LOD | 668 |
| | 01-02 | * | < LOD | < LOD | < LOD | < LOD | 757 |
| | 03-04 | * | .002 (<LOD- 003) | .004 ( 004-.004) | .007 (.005-.009) | .009 (.007- 010) | 590 |
| 20 years and older | 99-00 | * | < LOD | < LOD | < LOD | < LOD | 1260 |
| | 01-02 | * | < LOD | < LOD | < LOD | < LOD | 1549 |
| | 03-04 | .011 (.010-.012) | .012 (.011-.014) | .024 ( 022-.027) | .042 (.038-.045) | .057 (.052- 064) | 1296 |
| **Gender** | | | | | | | |
| Males | 99-00 | * | < LOD | < LOD | < LOD | < LOD | 919 |
| | 01-02 | * | < LOD | < LOD | < LOD | < LOD | 1074 |
| | 03-04 | .009 (.008-.010) | .010 (.009-.011) | .022 ( 019-.025) | .038 (.035-.042) | .052 (.043- 064) | 940 |
| Females | 99-00 | * | < LOD | < LOD | < LOD | < LOD | 1009 |
| | 01-02 | * | < LOD | < LOD | < LOD | < LOD | 1232 |
| | 03-04 | .009 (.008-.009) | .010 (.009-.012) | .021 ( 019-.023) | .042 (.036-.044) | .055 (.049- 061) | 946 |
| **Race/ethnicity** | | | | | | | |
| Mexican Americans | 99-00 | * | < LOD | < LOD | < LOD | < LOD | 635 |
| | 01-02 | * | < LOD | < LOD | < LOD | < LOD | 567 |
| | 03-04 | .004 (.003-.005) | .005 (.004-.006) | .009 ( 007-.013) | .019 (.013-.029) | .029 (.017- 044) | 423 |
| Non-Hispanic blacks | 99-00 | * | < LOD | < LOD | < LOD | .070 (<LOD-.150) | 413 |
| | 01-02 | * | < LOD | < LOD | < LOD | .080 (<LOD-.110) | 514 |
| | 03-04 | .009 (.008-.011) | .009 (.008-.012) | .027 ( 019-.037) | .065 (.043-.084) | .090 (.058-.120) | 459 |
| Non-Hispanic whites | 99-00 | * | < LOD | < LOD | < LOD | < LOD | 722 |
| | 01-02 | * | < LOD | < LOD | < LOD | < LOD | 1061 |
| | 03-04 | .010 (.009-.010) | .011 (.010-.012) | .022 ( 019-.025) | .038 (.035-.042) | .049 (.046- 055) | 883 |

< LOD means less than the limit of detection for the lipid adjusted serum level, which may vary for some chemicals by year and by individual sample.
* Not calculated: proportion of results below limit of detection was too high to provide a valid result.

## Serum 2,2',3,4',5,5',6-Heptachlorobiphenyl (PCB 187) (lipid adjusted)

Geometric mean and selected percentiles of serum concentrations (in ng/g of lipid or parts per billion on a lipid-weight basis) for the U.S. population from the National Health and Nutrition Examination Survey.

| | Survey years | Geometric mean (95% conf. interval) | Selected percentiles ( 95% confidence interval) | | | | Sample size |
|---|---|---|---|---|---|---|---|
| | | | 50th | 75th | 90th | 95th | |
| **Total** | 99-00 | * | < LOD | < LOD | 17.7 (15.6-20.4) | 24.8 (22 0-27.7) | 1930 |
| | 01-02 | * | < LOD | 12.2 (10.6-13.8) | 21.7 (19.6-23.7) | 28.1 (26 8-29.7) | 2307 |
| | 03-04 | 4.23 (3.96-4.50) | 4.60 (4 20-5.23) | 10.1 (9.42-10.5) | 17.2 (16.1-18.1) | 24.3 (20 5-27.8) | 1889 |
| **Age group** | | | | | | | |
| 12-19 years | 99-00 | * | < LOD | < LOD | < LOD | < LOD | 667 |
| | 01-02 | * | < LOD | < LOD | < LOD | < LOD | 758 |
| | 03-04 | 1.00 (.859-1.17) | 1.00 (.880-1.10) | 1.66 (1.50-1.99) | 3.20 (2.50-4 34) | 5.00 (3.70-6.07) | 594 |
| 20 years and older | 99-00 | * | < LOD | < LOD | 19.3 (16.8-21.8) | 26.0 (24.1-29.0) | 1263 |
| | 01-02 | * | < LOD | 13.3 (12.0-15.2) | 23.0 (20.9-24.7) | 29.2 (27 3-32.0) | 1549 |
| | 03-04 | 5.20 (4.83-5.60) | 5.71 (5 01-6.19) | 10.9 (10.3-11.7) | 18.1 (16.9-19.5) | 25.9 (22.1-32.1) | 1295 |
| **Gender** | | | | | | | |
| Males | 99-00 | * | < LOD | < LOD | 17.8 (15.8-19.6) | 25.9 (21 6-29.8) | 917 |
| | 01-02 | * | < LOD | 12.7 (<LOD-15 8) | 22.5 (19.4-24.1) | 27.7 (25 2-30.3) | 1075 |
| | 03-04 | 4.34 (3.97-4.75) | 4.50 (4 00-5.40) | 10.4 (9.21-10.9) | 17.9 (16.1-19.5) | 25.1 (20.4-30.9) | 939 |
| Females | 99-00 | * | < LOD | < LOD | 17.7 (15.1-21.7) | 24.2 (21 6-27.0) | 1013 |
| | 01-02 | * | < LOD | 11.9 (<LOD-13 0) | 21.3 (18.5-23.5) | 28.5 (26 2-31.3) | 1232 |
| | 03-04 | 4.12 (3.84-4.41) | 4.67 (4.10-5.30) | 9.85 (8.83-10.5) | 16.4 (15.3-17.9) | 24.2 (19.1-27.8) | 950 |
| **Race/ethnicity** | | | | | | | |
| Mexican Americans | 99-00 | * | < LOD | < LOD | < LOD | 17.6 (15.1-19.1) | 636 |
| | 01-02 | * | < LOD | < LOD | 10.8 (<LOD-13.4) | 15.7 (12.7-18.2) | 567 |
| | 03-04 | 1.79 (1.47-2.20) | 1.58 (1 26-2.00) | 3.96 (2.70-5.90) | 7.86 (5.96-10.3) | 11.6 (9.41-14.9) | 426 |
| Non-Hispanic blacks | 99-00 | * | < LOD | 15.5 (<LOD-21.1) | 31.6 (26.0-39.0) | 47.1 (36 6-72.1) | 412 |
| | 01-02 | * | < LOD | 16.5 (12.3-21.0) | 30.3 (22.9-40.6) | 44.8 (30 3-61.9) | 515 |
| | 03-04 | 5.09 (4.39-5.90) | 5.40 (4 20-6.21) | 13.9 (10.6-17.7) | 31.7 (22.7-46.4) | 51.5 (31.7-76.5) | 458 |
| Non-Hispanic whites | 99-00 | * | < LOD | < LOD | 16.8 (14.9-18.6) | 22.0 (19.1-25.2) | 727 |
| | 01-02 | * | < LOD | 12.5 (10.8-14.6) | 21.7 (18.9-23.7) | 27.4 (25 2-29.5) | 1061 |
| | 03-04 | 4.47 (4.17-4.79) | 5.00 (4.40-5.70) | 10.1 (9.26-10.8) | 16.5 (15.3-17.9) | 21.1 (19.1-24.2) | 884 |

Limit of detection (LOD, see Data Analysis section) for Survey years 99-00, 01-02, and 03-04 are 12.4, 10 5, and 0.4, respectively.
< LOD means less than the limit of detection, which may vary for some chemicals by year and by individual sample.
* Not calculated: proportion of results below limit of detection was too high to provide a valid result.

## Serum 2,2',3,4',5,5',6-Heptachlorobiphenyl (PCB 187) (whole weight)

Geometric mean and selected percentiles of serum concentrations (in ng/g of serum or parts per billion) for the U.S. population from the National Health and Nutrition Examination Survey.

| | Survey years | Geometric mean (95% conf. interval) | 50th | 75th | 90th | 95th | Sample size |
|---|---|---|---|---|---|---|---|
| **Total** | 99-00 | * | < LOD | < LOD | .120 (.110-.130) | .170 (.140-.180) | 1930 |
| | 01-02 | * | < LOD | .080 ( 070-.090) | .140 (.130-.160) | .200 (.180- 220) | 2307 |
| | 03-04 | .026 (.024-.028) | .029 (.027-.032) | .065 ( 061-.069) | .115 (.106-.125) | .167 (.139-.197) | 1889 |
| **Age group** | | | | | | | |
| 12-19 years | 99-00 | * | < LOD | < LOD | < LOD | < LOD | 667 |
| | 01-02 | * | < LOD | < LOD | < LOD | < LOD | 758 |
| | 03-04 | .005 (.004-.006) | .005 (.004-.006) | .009 ( 007-.010) | .016 (.013-.019) | .023 (.016- 029) | 594 |
| 20 years and older | 99-00 | * | < LOD | < LOD | .130 (.110-.140) | .180 (.160-.190) | 1263 |
| | 01-02 | * | < LOD | .090 ( 080-.100) | .150 (.130-.180) | .210 (.190- 230) | 1549 |
| | 03-04 | .033 (.030-.035) | .036 (.032-.040) | .071 ( 067-.075) | .124 (.112-139) | .172 (.143- 215) | 1295 |
| **Gender** | | | | | | | |
| Males | 99-00 | * | < LOD | < LOD | .120 (.100-.140) | .180 (.140- 200) | 917 |
| | 01-02 | * | < LOD | .080 (<LOD-.100) | .150 (.130-.160) | .190 (.170- 230) | 1075 |
| | 03-04 | .027 (.024-.030) | .030 (.026-.035) | .067 ( 061-.072) | .116 (.102-137) | .160 (.137- 215) | 939 |
| Females | 99-00 | * | < LOD | < LOD | .120 (.110-.130) | .160 (.140-.180) | 1013 |
| | 01-02 | * | < LOD | .080 (<LOD-.090) | .140 (.120-.150) | .200 (.180- 220) | 1232 |
| | 03-04 | .025 (.023-.027) | .029 (.026-.033) | .063 ( 056-.070) | .115 (.104-.125) | .168 (.141-.191) | 950 |
| **Race/ethnicity** | | | | | | | |
| Mexican Americans | 99-00 | * | < LOD | < LOD | < LOD | .120 (.100-.130) | 636 |
| | 01-02 | * | < LOD | < LOD | .080 (<LOD-.100) | .100 (.090-.120) | 567 |
| | 03-04 | .011 (.009-.013) | .010 (.007-.015) | .025 ( 018-.038) | .057 (.042-.079) | .094 (.059-.110) | 426 |
| Non-Hispanic blacks | 99-00 | * | < LOD | .090 (<LOD-.130) | .200 (.160-.230) | .290 (.210- 530) | 412 |
| | 01-02 | * | < LOD | .100 ( 070-.120) | .190 (.150-.260) | .290 (.190- 380) | 515 |
| | 03-04 | .029 (.025-.034) | .032 (.024-.037) | .083 ( 070-.109) | .191 (.140-.273) | .330 (.228-.468) | 458 |
| Non-Hispanic whites | 99-00 | * | < LOD | < LOD | .110 (.100-.130) | .150 (.130-.170) | 727 |
| | 01-02 | * | < LOD | .080 ( 070-.090) | .140 (.120-.160) | .190 (.170- 220) | 1061 |
| | 03-04 | .028 (.026-.030) | .032 (.029-.036) | .065 ( 061-.071) | .111 (.101-.124) | .153 (.132-.172) | 884 |

< LOD means less than the limit of detection for the lipid adjusted serum level, which may vary for some chemicals by year and by individual sample.
* Not calculated: proportion of results below limit of detection was too high to provide a valid result.

## Serum 2,2',3,3',4,4',5,5'-Octachlorobiphenyl (PCB 194) (lipid adjusted)

Geometric mean and selected percentiles of serum concentrations (in ng/g of lipid or parts per billion on a lipid-weight basis) for the U.S. population from the National Health and Nutrition Examination Survey.

| | Survey years | Geometric mean (95% conf. interval) | Selected percentiles ( 95% confidence interval) | | | | Sample size |
|---|---|---|---|---|---|---|---|
| | | | 50th | 75th | 90th | 95th | |
| **Total** | 01-02 | * | < LOD | 11.1 (<LOD-11 9) | 18.2 (16.5-19.5) | 23.7 (21 0-27.0) | 2279 |
| | 03-04 | 2.69 (2.53-2.85) | 4.19 (3 55-4.70) | 8.47 (7.79-9.06) | 14.3 (13.3-16.0) | 19.1 (17 6-20.8) | 1835 |
| **Age group** | | | | | | | |
| 12-19 years | 01-02 | * | < LOD | < LOD | < LOD | < LOD | 746 |
| | 03-04 | * | < LOD | 1.11 (.700-1.57) | 2.40 (1.70-3 57) | 5.18 (2.80-6.81) | 572 |
| 20 years and older | 01-02 | * | < LOD | 12.0 (11.0-13.3) | 19.1 (17.7-20.5) | 25.3 (22.7-28.0) | 1533 |
| | 03-04 | 3.64 (3.40-3.89) | 4.95 (4 56-5.42) | 9.30 (8.62-9.90) | 15.3 (13.9-17.1) | 20.1 (18.1-21.9) | 1263 |
| **Gender** | | | | | | | |
| Males | 01-02 | * | < LOD | 12.3 (10.6-14.1) | 19.2 (17.2-21.2) | 25.2 (21.7-29.0) | 1059 |
| | 03-04 | 2.95 (2.61-3.35) | 4.47 (3 55-5.20) | 9.60 (8.30-10.9) | 17.1 (14.2-18.8) | 21.8 (19 8-25.6) | 913 |
| Females | 01-02 | * | < LOD | < LOD | 17.0 (14.7-18.8) | 21.9 (19 3-26.2) | 1220 |
| | 03-04 | 2.45 (2.28-2.64) | 4.00 (3 39-4.49) | 7.50 (7.01-8.39) | 12.7 (11.2-13.6) | 16.6 (13.7-18.6) | 922 |
| **Race/ethnicity** | | | | | | | |
| Mexican Americans | 01-02 | * | < LOD | < LOD | < LOD | 14.3 (10 5-17.6) | 561 |
| | 03-04 | .845 (.582-1.23) | .900 (.640-1.49) | 2.90 (1.79-4.76) | 7.21 (4.80-8 90) | 9.50 (7.40-15.0) | 410 |
| Non-Hispanic blacks | 01-02 | * | < LOD | 12.3 (<LOD-15 3) | 22.6 (18.0-27.5) | 29.8 (23.7-41.1) | 508 |
| | 03-04 | 2.45 (1.94-3.08) | 3.62 (2.70-4.49) | 8.83 (6.80-11.2) | 18.1 (13.0-23.2) | 28.3 (18 9-35.6) | 450 |
| Non-Hispanic whites | 01-02 | * | < LOD | 11.9 (10.9-13.1) | 18.8 (17.1-20.2) | 24.1 (20 9-28.0) | 1048 |
| | 03-04 | 3.25 (2.97-3.56) | 4.90 (4.19-5.42) | 9.08 (8.36-9.80) | 14.7 (13.5-16.6) | 19.1 (17.4-21.2) | 861 |

Limit of detection (LOD, see Data Analysis section) for Survey years 01-02 and 03-04 are 10.5 and 0.4.
< LOD means less than the limit of detection, which may vary for some chemicals by year and by individual sample.
* Not calculated: proportion of results below limit of detection was too high to provide a valid result.

## Serum 2,2',3,3',4,4',5,5'-Octachlorobiphenyl (PCB 194) (whole weight)

Geometric mean and selected percentiles of serum concentrations (in ng/g of serum or parts per billion) for the U.S. population from the National Health and Nutrition Examination Survey.

| | Survey years | Geometric mean (95% conf. interval) | Selected percentiles ( 95% confidence interval) | | | | Sample size |
|---|---|---|---|---|---|---|---|
| | | | 50th | 75th | 90th | 95th | |
| **Total** | 01-02 | * | < LOD | .070 (<LOD- 080) | .120 (.110-.140) | .160 (.150-.190) | 2279 |
| | 03-04 | .016 (.015- 017) | .026 (.022-.028) | .056 (.052-.060) | .096 (.091-.103) | .129 (.116-.139) | 1835 |
| **Age group** | | | | | | | |
| 12-19 years | 01-02 | * | < LOD | < LOD | < LOD | < LOD | 746 |
| | 03-04 | * | < LOD | .006 (.004-.008) | .013 (.009-.020) | .023 ( 013-.035) | 572 |
| 20 years and older | 01-02 | * | < LOD | .080 (.070-.090) | .130 (.110-.150) | .170 (.150-.200) | 1533 |
| | 03-04 | .023 (.021- 024) | .031 (.027-.035) | .061 (.057-.065) | .103 (.094-.113) | .133 (.122-.145) | 1263 |
| **Gender** | | | | | | | |
| Males | 01-02 | * | < LOD | .080 (.070-.090) | .140 (.110-.160) | .170 (.150-.210) | 1059 |
| | 03-04 | .018 (.016- 021) | .027 (.023-.034) | .061 (.054-.069) | .106 (.095-.121) | .142 (.129-.166) | 913 |
| Females | 01-02 | * | < LOD | < LOD | .110 (.090-.130) | .150 (.130-.180) | 1220 |
| | 03-04 | .015 (.014- 016) | .024 (.020-.027) | .051 (.047-.056) | .088 (.080-.096) | .112 (.103-.117) | 922 |
| **Race/ethnicity** | | | | | | | |
| Mexican Americans | 01-02 | * | < LOD | < LOD | < LOD | .100 ( 080-.110) | 561 |
| | 03-04 | .005 (.004- 008) | .006 (.004-.010) | .019 (.012-.031) | .049 (.033-.064) | .081 ( 051-.118) | 410 |
| Non-Hispanic blacks | 01-02 | * | < LOD | .080 (<LOD- 090) | .150 (.100-.180) | .200 (.140-.250) | 508 |
| | 03-04 | .014 (.011- 018) | .020 (.014-.026) | .054 (.045-.063) | .120 (.081-.155) | .172 (.123-.202) | 450 |
| Non-Hispanic whites | 01-02 | * | < LOD | .080 (.070-.090) | .130 (.110-.150) | .170 (.150-.190) | 1048 |
| | 03-04 | .020 (.018- 022) | .029 (.026-.034) | .061 (.056-.066) | .099 (.090-.106) | .132 (.116-.143) | 861 |

< LOD means less than the limit of detection for the lipid adjusted serum level, which may vary for some chemicals by year and by individual sample.
* Not calculated: proportion of results below limit of detection was too high to provide a valid result.

## Serum 2,2',3,3',4,4',5,6-Octachlorobiphenyl (PCB 195) (lipid adjusted)

Geometric mean and selected percentiles of serum concentrations (in ng/g of lipid or parts per billion on a lipid-weight basis) for the U.S. population from the National Health and Nutrition Examination Survey.

| | Survey years | Geometric mean (95% conf. interval) | Selected percentiles ( 95% confidence interval) | | | | Sample size |
|---|---|---|---|---|---|---|---|
| | | | 50th | 75th | 90th | 95th | |
| Total | 01-02 | * | < LOD | < LOD | < LOD | < LOD | 2230 |
| | 03-04 | * | .900 (<LOD-1.01) | 1.98 (1.80-2.10) | 3.40 (3.10-3.60) | 4.51 (3.90-5.18) | 1820 |
| **Age group** | | | | | | | |
| 12-19 years | 01-02 | * | < LOD | < LOD | < LOD | < LOD | 716 |
| | 03-04 | * | < LOD | < LOD | < LOD | 1.74 (.720-3.82) | 567 |
| 20 years and older | 01-02 | * | < LOD | < LOD | < LOD | < LOD | 1514 |
| | 03-04 | .800 (.721-.888) | 1.10 (.980-1 20) | 2.10 (2.00-2.30) | 3.53 (3.20-3.74) | 4.68 (4.12-5.19) | 1253 |
| **Gender** | | | | | | | |
| Males | 01-02 | * | < LOD | < LOD | < LOD | < LOD | 1035 |
| | 03-04 | * | .800 (<LOD-1.00) | 2.08 (1.82-2.20) | 3.50 (3.12-3.70) | 4.60 (3.82-5.40) | 904 |
| Females | 01-02 | * | < LOD | < LOD | < LOD | < LOD | 1195 |
| | 03-04 | * | .970 (<LOD-1.10) | 1.85 (1.64-2.09) | 3.30 (2.86-3.60) | 4.50 (3.57-5.25) | 916 |
| **Race/ethnicity** | | | | | | | |
| Mexican Americans | 01-02 | * | < LOD | < LOD | < LOD | < LOD | 544 |
| | 03-04 | * | < LOD | < LOD | 1.80 (1.11-2.40) | 2.40 (1.80-3.50) | 407 |
| Non-Hispanic blacks | 01-02 | * | < LOD | < LOD | < LOD | < LOD | 490 |
| | 03-04 | .709 (<LOD- 870) | .820 (<LOD-1.14) | 2.00 (1.65-2.57) | 4.18 (3.16-5.30) | 6.90 (4.18-8.10) | 444 |
| Non-Hispanic whites | 01-02 | * | < LOD | < LOD | < LOD | < LOD | 1037 |
| | 03-04 | .749 (<LOD- 850) | 1.00 (.800-1.18) | 2.10 (1.90-2.30) | 3.40 (3.10-3.61) | 4.44 (3.80-5.19) | 856 |

Limit of detection (LOD, see Data Analysis section) for Survey years 01-02 and 03-04 are 28.1 and 0.7.
< LOD means less than the limit of detection, which may vary for some chemicals by year and by individual sample.
* Not calculated: proportion of results below limit of detection was too high to provide a valid result.

## Serum 2,2',3,3',4,4',5,6-Octachlorobiphenyl (PCB 195) (whole weight)

Geometric mean and selected percentiles of serum concentrations (in ng/g of serum or parts per billion) for the U.S. population from the National Health and Nutrition Examination Survey.

| | Survey years | Geometric mean (95% conf. interval) | Selected percentiles ( 95% confidence interval) | | | | Sample size |
|---|---|---|---|---|---|---|---|
| | | | 50th | 75th | 90th | 95th | |
| Total | 01-02 | * | < LOD | < LOD | < LOD | < LOD | 2230 |
| | 03-04 | * | .005 (<LOD- 006) | .012 ( 012-.013) | .022 (.020-.025) | .031 (.027- 034) | 1820 |
| **Age group** | | | | | | | |
| 12-19 years | 01-02 | * | < LOD | < LOD | < LOD | < LOD | 716 |
| | 03-04 | * | < LOD | < LOD | < LOD | .007 (.004- 017) | 567 |
| 20 years and older | 01-02 | * | < LOD | < LOD | < LOD | < LOD | 1514 |
| | 03-04 | .005 (.004-.006) | .007 (.006-.007) | .014 ( 012-.015) | .023 (.021-.026) | .032 (.028- 035) | 1253 |
| **Gender** | | | | | | | |
| Males | 01-02 | * | < LOD | < LOD | < LOD | < LOD | 1035 |
| | 03-04 | * | .005 (<LOD- 006) | .013 ( 012-.014) | .022 (.020-.025) | .031 (.025- 035) | 904 |
| Females | 01-02 | * | < LOD | < LOD | < LOD | < LOD | 1195 |
| | 03-04 | * | .006 (<LOD- 007) | .012 ( 011-.013) | .021 (.019-.025) | .031 (.026- 035) | 916 |
| **Race/ethnicity** | | | | | | | |
| Mexican Americans | 01-02 | * | < LOD | < LOD | < LOD | < LOD | 544 |
| | 03-04 | * | < LOD | < LOD | .012 (.008-.018) | .018 (.013- 025) | 407 |
| Non-Hispanic blacks | 01-02 | * | < LOD | < LOD | < LOD | < LOD | 490 |
| | 03-04 | .004 (<LOD- 005) | .004 (<LOD- 006) | .012 ( 010-.016) | .027 (.019-.034) | .041 (.029- 048) | 444 |
| Non-Hispanic whites | 01-02 | * | < LOD | < LOD | < LOD | < LOD | 1037 |
| | 03-04 | .005 (<LOD- 005) | .006 (.005-.007) | .013 ( 012-.014) | .022 (.020-.025) | .030 (.027- 033) | 856 |

< LOD means less than the limit of detection for the lipid adjusted serum level, which may vary for some chemicals by year and by individual sample.
* Not calculated: proportion of results below limit of detection was too high to provide a valid result.

## Serum 2,2',3,3',4,4',5,6' and 2,2',3,4,4',5,5',6-Octachlorobiphenyl (PCB 196 & 203) (lipid adjusted)

Geometric mean and selected percentiles of serum concentrations (in ng/g of lipid or parts per billion on a lipid-weight basis) for the U.S. population from the National Health and Nutrition Examination Survey.

| | Survey years | Geometric mean (95% conf. interval) | Selected percentiles ( 95% confidence interval) | | | | Sample size |
|---|---|---|---|---|---|---|---|
| | | | 50th | 75th | 90th | 95th | |
| **Total** | 01-02 | * | < LOD | < LOD | 14.2 (13.0-15.7) | 19.2 (17.4-20.9) | 2299 |
| | 03-04 | 2.61 (2.44-2.79) | 3.40 (3 01-3.80) | 6.70 (6.16-7.23) | 11.8 (10.8-12.7) | 15.0 (13 2-17.4) | 1878 |
| **Age group** | | | | | | | |
| 12-19 years | 01-02 | * | < LOD | < LOD | < LOD | < LOD | 755 |
| | 03-04 | .437 (<LOD-.546) | .520 (.400-.700) | 1.10 (.900-1.42) | 2.41 (1.86-3.19) | 3.59 (2.93-4.20) | 587 |
| 20 years and older | 01-02 | * | < LOD | < LOD | 15.0 (13.7-17.0) | 19.9 (18 2-21.4) | 1544 |
| | 03-04 | 3.37 (3.15-3.61) | 4.07 (3.74-4.46) | 7.30 (6.79-8.20) | 12.4 (11.5-13.2) | 15.9 (13.4-19.5) | 1291 |
| **Gender** | | | | | | | |
| Males | 01-02 | * | < LOD | < LOD | 14.6 (13.3-16.5) | 19.4 (16 3-21.2) | 1071 |
| | 03-04 | 2.77 (2.49-3.08) | 3.45 (3 07-3.98) | 6.92 (6.12-7.71) | 12.5 (11.2-13.7) | 16.3 (13.7-23.1) | 935 |
| Females | 01-02 | * | < LOD | < LOD | 13.8 (11.9-15.9) | 19.1 (17 0-21.3) | 1228 |
| | 03-04 | 2.46 (2.27-2.66) | 3.32 (2 83-3.80) | 6.68 (6.12-7.20) | 11.1 (9.74-12.3) | 13.4 (12 8-14.9) | 943 |
| **Race/ethnicity** | | | | | | | |
| Mexican Americans | 01-02 | * | < LOD | < LOD | < LOD | 11.1 (<LOD-12.5) | 565 |
| | 03-04 | .947 (.689-1.30) | 1.00 (.700-1.50) | 2.80 (1.60-4.30) | 5.90 (4.30-7.40) | 8.35 (6.00-12.3) | 424 |
| Non-Hispanic blacks | 01-02 | * | < LOD | < LOD | 17.6 (14.2-21.0) | 23.1 (19 6-30.2) | 513 |
| | 03-04 | 2.45 (2.06-2.90) | 2.90 (2 33-3.80) | 7.18 (5.80-9.00) | 13.8 (11.5-16.8) | 21.6 (14 0-32.3) | 453 |
| Non-Hispanic whites | 01-02 | * | < LOD | < LOD | 14.7 (13.6-16.5) | 19.6 (18.1-21.3) | 1058 |
| | 03-04 | 3.01 (2.76-3.27) | 3.88 (3.44-4.20) | 7.10 (6.32-8.20) | 11.8 (10.8-13.1) | 15.4 (12 9-19.0) | 882 |

Limit of detection (LOD, see Data Analysis section) for Survey years 01-02 and 03-04 are 10.5 and 0.4.
< LOD means less than the limit of detection, which may vary for some chemicals by year and by individual sample.
* Not calculated: proportion of results below limit of detection was too high to provide a valid result.

## Serum 2,2',3,3',4,4',5,6' and 2,2',3,4,4',5,5',6-Octachlorobiphenyl (PCB 196 & 203) (whole weight)

Geometric mean and selected percentiles of serum concentrations (in ng/g of serum or parts per billion) for the U.S. population from the National Health and Nutrition Examination Survey.

| | Survey years | Geometric mean (95% conf. interval) | Selected percentiles ( 95% confidence interval) | | | | Sample size |
|---|---|---|---|---|---|---|---|
| | | | 50th | 75th | 90th | 95th | |
| **Total** | 01-02 | * | < LOD | < LOD | .100 (.090-.110) | .130 (.110-.140) | 2299 |
| | 03-04 | .016 (.015-.017) | .022 (.019-.025) | .044 (.042-.048) | .082 (.071-.087) | .101 ( 091-.112) | 1878 |
| **Age group** | | | | | | | |
| 12-19 years | 01-02 | * | < LOD | < LOD | < LOD | < LOD | 755 |
| | 03-04 | .002 (<LOD-.003) | .003 (.002-.004) | .006 (.005-.007) | .013 (.009-.016) | .016 ( 014-.025) | 587 |
| 20 years and older | 01-02 | * | < LOD | < LOD | .100 (.090-.110) | .130 (.120-.150) | 1544 |
| | 03-04 | .021 (.020-.023) | .026 (.024-.028) | .049 (.045-.052) | .084 (.077-.090) | .104 ( 092-.123) | 1291 |
| **Gender** | | | | | | | |
| Males | 01-02 | * | < LOD | < LOD | .100 (.090-.120) | .130 (.110-.150) | 1071 |
| | 03-04 | .017 (.015-.019) | .023 (.020-.026) | .045 (.042-.050) | .084 (.077-.091) | .106 ( 093-.127) | 935 |
| Females | 01-02 | * | < LOD | < LOD | .090 (.080-.100) | .130 (.110-.140) | 1228 |
| | 03-04 | .015 (.014-.016) | .020 (.017-.023) | .043 (.038-.047) | .076 (.066-.084) | .093 ( 085-.111) | 943 |
| **Race/ethnicity** | | | | | | | |
| Mexican Americans | 01-02 | * | < LOD | < LOD | < LOD | .070 (<LOD-.090) | 565 |
| | 03-04 | .006 (.004-.008) | .007 (.004-.010) | .017 (.011-.026) | .038 (.028-.054) | .058 ( 035-.087) | 424 |
| Non-Hispanic blacks | 01-02 | * | < LOD | < LOD | .110 (.090-.140) | .150 (.110-.210) | 513 |
| | 03-04 | .014 (.012-.017) | .017 (.012-.022) | .046 (.038-.054) | .090 (.065-.111) | .141 ( 094-.209) | 453 |
| Non-Hispanic whites | 01-02 | * | < LOD | < LOD | .100 (.090-.110) | .130 (.110-.140) | 1058 |
| | 03-04 | .019 (.017-.020) | .025 (.022-.028) | .048 (.043-.052) | .084 (.070-.090) | .100 ( 090-.120) | 882 |

< LOD means less than the limit of detection for the lipid adjusted serum level, which may vary for some chemicals by year and by individual sample.
* Not calculated: proportion of results below limit of detection was too high to provide a valid result.

## Serum 2,2',3,3',4,5,5',6-Octachlorobiphenyl (PCB 199) (lipid adjusted)

Geometric mean and selected percentiles of serum concentrations (in ng/g of lipid or parts per billion on a lipid-weight basis) for the U.S. population from the National Health and Nutrition Examination Survey.

| | Survey years | Geometric mean (95% conf. interval) | Selected percentiles ( 95% confidence interval) | | | | Sample size |
|---|---|---|---|---|---|---|---|
| | | | 50th | 75th | 90th | 95th | |
| **Total** | 01-02 | * | < LOD | < LOD | 17.0 (15.4-18.1) | 22.4 (19.9-25 9) | 2292 |
| | 03-04 | 2.81 (2.64-3.00) | 3.80 (3.26-4 26) | 8.30 (7.70-9.08) | 14.9 (13.8-15.7) | 18.9 (17.9-21 3) | 1861 |
| **Age group** | | | | | | | |
| 12-19 years | 01-02 | * | < LOD | < LOD | < LOD | < LOD | 756 |
| | 03-04 | .416 (<LOD- 522) | .500 (<LOD-.700) | 1.17 ( 890-1.59) | 2.43 (2.02-2.73) | 3.92 (2.90-4.10) | 579 |
| 20 years and older | 01-02 | * | < LOD | 10.6 (<LOD-11.8) | 17.9 (16.2-19.2) | 24.4 (20.7-27.4) | 1536 |
| | 03-04 | 3.71 (3.41-4.02) | 4.60 (4.10-5 08) | 9.40 (8.73-10.0) | 15.7 (14.7-16.9) | 20.6 (18.3-23 6) | 1282 |
| **Gender** | | | | | | | |
| Males | 01-02 | * | < LOD | < LOD | 17.3 (15.4-18.7) | 21.3 (19.3-24 6) | 1066 |
| | 03-04 | 3.01 (2.68-3.39) | 3.95 (3.30-4 67) | 9.10 (7.60-9.94) | 16.6 (14.0-17.3) | 22.1 (18.1-27.4) | 925 |
| Females | 01-02 | * | < LOD | < LOD | 16.2 (14.5-17.9) | 22.9 (19.4-27 3) | 1226 |
| | 03-04 | 2.63 (2.49-2.79) | 3.70 (3.20-4 00) | 7.70 (6.92-8.81) | 14.0 (11.6-15.3) | 17.0 (15.7-18 9) | 936 |
| **Race/ethnicity** | | | | | | | |
| Mexican Americans | 01-02 | * | < LOD | < LOD | < LOD | 12.3 (<LOD-14.2) | 565 |
| | 03-04 | .943 (.664-1.34) | 1.00 (.600-1 50) | 3.35 (1.50-5.33) | 7.37 (5.10-10.2) | 10.2 (7.40-13 5) | 418 |
| Non-Hispanic blacks | 01-02 | * | < LOD | 12.5 (<LOD-15.3) | 21.9 (17.0-28.1) | 30.7 (22.4-37.4) | 513 |
| | 03-04 | 3.03 (2.46-3.74) | 3.60 (2.70-4.70) | 10.0 (7.70-13.7) | 21.3 (15.9-30.4) | 35.1 (21.3-43 3) | 452 |
| Non-Hispanic whites | 01-02 | * | < LOD | < LOD | 17.3 (15.9-18.9) | 22.7 (19.8-26 3) | 1051 |
| | 03-04 | 3.24 (3.03-3.47) | 4.19 (3.78-4 69) | 9.08 (7.88-9.86) | 14.8 (13.5-16.3) | 18.6 (16.9-21.7) | 871 |

Limit of detection (LOD, see Data Analysis section) for Survey years 01-02 and 03-04 are 10.5 and 0.4.
< LOD means less than the limit of detection, which may vary for some chemicals by year and by individual sample.
* Not calculated: proportion of results below limit of detection was too high to provide a valid result.


## Serum 2,2',3,3',4,5,5',6-Octachlorobiphenyl (PCB 199) (whole weight)

Geometric mean and selected percentiles of serum concentrations (in ng/g of serum or parts per billion) for the U.S. population from the National Health and Nutrition Examination Survey.

| | Survey years | Geometric mean (95% conf. interval) | Selected percentiles ( 95% confidence interval) | | | | Sample size |
|---|---|---|---|---|---|---|---|
| | | | 50th | 75th | 90th | 95th | |
| **Total** | 01-02 | * | < LOD | < LOD | .110 (.100-.130) | .150 (.140-.170) | 2292 |
| | 03-04 | .017 (.016-.018) | .023 (.020-.027) | .056 ( 053-.060) | .100 (.091-.106) | .127 (.119-.144) | 1861 |
| **Age group** | | | | | | | |
| 12-19 years | 01-02 | * | < LOD | < LOD | < LOD | < LOD | 756 |
| | 03-04 | .002 (<LOD- 003) | .002 (<LOD- 003) | .006 ( 005-.008) | .012 (.009-.015) | .016 (.015- 019) | 579 |
| 20 years and older | 01-02 | * | < LOD | .070 (<LOD-.080) | .120 (.110-.140) | .160 (.140-.180) | 1536 |
| | 03-04 | .023 (.021-.025) | .029 (.026-.033) | .062 ( 058-.067) | .106 (.097-.113) | .135 (.120-.158) | 1282 |
| **Gender** | | | | | | | |
| Males | 01-02 | * | < LOD | < LOD | .110 (.100-.130) | .150 (.130-.180) | 1066 |
| | 03-04 | .019 (.016-.021) | .025 (.020-.030) | .059 ( 053-.068) | .105 (.090-.113) | .138 (.120-.162) | 925 |
| Females | 01-02 | * | < LOD | < LOD | .110 (.100-.130) | .150 (.130-.170) | 1226 |
| | 03-04 | .016 (.015-.017) | .022 (.019-.025) | .054 ( 047-.058) | .094 (.085-.105) | .120 (.108-.133) | 936 |
| **Race/ethnicity** | | | | | | | |
| Mexican Americans | 01-02 | * | < LOD | < LOD | < LOD | .090 (<LOD-.110) | 565 |
| | 03-04 | .006 (.004-.008) | .007 (.004-.010) | .019 ( 011-.031) | .051 (.029-.079) | .079 (.051- 093) | 418 |
| Non-Hispanic blacks | 01-02 | * | < LOD | .070 (<LOD-.090) | .140 (.100-.180) | .190 (.130- 300) | 513 |
| | 03-04 | .017 (.014-.021) | .021 (.015-.026) | .064 ( 054-.073) | .135 (.102-.173) | .207 (.147- 297) | 452 |
| Non-Hispanic whites | 01-02 | * | < LOD | < LOD | .120 (.100-.130) | .150 (.130-.180) | 1051 |
| | 03-04 | .020 (.019-.022) | .027 (.023-.030) | .059 ( 054-.065) | .101 (.087-.108) | .125 (.108-.144) | 871 |

< LOD means less than the limit of detection for the lipid adjusted serum level, which may vary for some chemicals by year and by individual sample.
* Not calculated: proportion of results below limit of detection was too high to provide a valid result.

## Serum 2,2',3,3',4,4',5,5',6-Nonachlorobiphenyl (PCB 206) (lipid adjusted)

Geometric mean and selected percentiles of serum concentrations (in ng/g of lipid or parts per billion on a lipid-weight basis) for the U.S. population from the National Health and Nutrition Examination Survey.

| | Survey years | Geometric mean (95% conf. interval) | Selected percentiles ( 95% confidence interval) | | | | Sample size |
| --- | --- | --- | --- | --- | --- | --- | --- |
| | | | 50th | 75th | 90th | 95th | |
| **Total** | 01-02 | * | < LOD | < LOD | < LOD | < LOD | 2208 |
| | 03-04 | 2.13 (1.97-2.31) | 2.34 (2 00-2.60) | 5.00 (4.69-5.50) | 9.20 (8.55-9.79) | 13.7 (11 5-15.6) | 1867 |
| **Age group** | | | | | | | |
| 12-19 years | 01-02 | * | < LOD | < LOD | < LOD | < LOD | 723 |
| | 03-04 | * | < LOD | .900 (.750-1.20) | 1.75 (1.23-2 92) | 3.12 (1.60-6.91) | 585 |
| 20 years and older | 01-02 | * | < LOD | < LOD | < LOD | < LOD | 1485 |
| | 03-04 | 2.59 (2.37-2.83) | 2.80 (2.42-3.06) | 5.53 (5.10-6.10) | 9.61 (9.03-11.0) | 14.2 (12 2-17.1) | 1282 |
| **Gender** | | | | | | | |
| Males | 01-02 | * | < LOD | < LOD | < LOD | < LOD | 1033 |
| | 03-04 | 2.23 (2.03-2.45) | 2.30 (1 90-2.70) | 5.10 (4.78-5.53) | 9.31 (8.18-10.8) | 13.8 (10 8-15.7) | 933 |
| Females | 01-02 | * | < LOD | < LOD | < LOD | < LOD | 1175 |
| | 03-04 | 2.05 (1.86-2.25) | 2.34 (1 95-2.78) | 5.00 (4.30-5.70) | 9.00 (8.00-9.79) | 13.6 (11 2-16.5) | 934 |
| **Race/ethnicity** | | | | | | | |
| Mexican Americans | 01-02 | * | < LOD | < LOD | < LOD | < LOD | 533 |
| | 03-04 | .861 (<LOD-1.15) | .730 (<LOD-1.10) | 1.70 (1.00-3.14) | 4.40 (2.61-6 20) | 6.20 (4.40-8.40) | 421 |
| Non-Hispanic blacks | 01-02 | * | < LOD | < LOD | < LOD | < LOD | 483 |
| | 03-04 | 2.27 (1.98-2.60) | 2.26 (1 85-2.51) | 5.60 (4.30-7.40) | 11.5 (9.49-16.5) | 20.9 (12.1-31.7) | 456 |
| Non-Hispanic whites | 01-02 | * | < LOD | < LOD | < LOD | < LOD | 1034 |
| | 03-04 | 2.40 (2.19-2.63) | 2.70 (2 37-3.01) | 5.37 (4.88-6.06) | 9.20 (8.65-10.1) | 13.8 (11 2-16.6) | 872 |

Limit of detection (LOD, see Data Analysis section) for Survey years 01-02 and 03-04 are 28.1 and 0.7.
< LOD means less than the limit of detection, which may vary for some chemicals by year and by individual sample.
* Not calculated: proportion of results below limit of detection was too high to provide a valid result.

## Serum 2,2',3,3',4,4',5,5',6-Nonachlorobiphenyl (PCB 206) (whole weight)

Geometric mean and selected percentiles of serum concentrations (in ng/g of serum or parts per billion) for the U.S. population from the National Health and Nutrition Examination Survey.

| | Survey years | Geometric mean (95% conf. interval) | Selected percentiles ( 95% confidence interval) | | | | Sample size |
| --- | --- | --- | --- | --- | --- | --- | --- |
| | | | 50th | 75th | 90th | 95th | |
| **Total** | 01-02 | * | < LOD | < LOD | < LOD | < LOD | 2208 |
| | 03-04 | .013 (.012- 014) | .015 (.012-.017) | .034 (.031-.037) | .060 (.054-.068) | .086 ( 077-.104) | 1867 |
| **Age group** | | | | | | | |
| 12-19 years | 01-02 | * | < LOD | < LOD | < LOD | < LOD | 723 |
| | 03-04 | * | < LOD | .005 (.004-.006) | .010 (.006-.013) | .014 ( 008-.035) | 585 |
| 20 years and older | 01-02 | * | < LOD | < LOD | < LOD | < LOD | 1485 |
| | 03-04 | .016 (.015- 018) | .017 (.016-.020) | .038 (.034-.042) | .066 (.059-.074) | .090 ( 081-.112) | 1282 |
| **Gender** | | | | | | | |
| Males | 01-02 | * | < LOD | < LOD | < LOD | < LOD | 1033 |
| | 03-04 | .014 (.012- 015) | .015 (.012-.018) | .034 (.032-.038) | .060 (.051-.070) | .082 ( 070-.097) | 933 |
| Females | 01-02 | * | < LOD | < LOD | < LOD | < LOD | 1175 |
| | 03-04 | .012 (.011- 014) | .014 (.012-.016) | .035 (.029-.038) | .061 (.054-.069) | .088 ( 078-.118) | 934 |
| **Race/ethnicity** | | | | | | | |
| Mexican Americans | 01-02 | * | < LOD | < LOD | < LOD | < LOD | 533 |
| | 03-04 | .005 (<LOD-.007) | .005 (<LOD-.007) | .011 (.008-.018) | .031 (.019-.044) | .044 ( 030-.062) | 421 |
| Non-Hispanic blacks | 01-02 | * | < LOD | < LOD | < LOD | < LOD | 483 |
| | 03-04 | .013 (.011- 015) | .012 (.010-.014) | .035 (.028-.045) | .078 (.052-.107) | .128 ( 080-.213) | 456 |
| Non-Hispanic whites | 01-02 | * | < LOD | < LOD | < LOD | < LOD | 1034 |
| | 03-04 | .015 (.013- 016) | .017 (.015-.020) | .036 (.033-.040) | .063 (.058-.069) | .088 ( 077-.107) | 872 |

< LOD means less than the limit of detection for the lipid adjusted serum level, which may vary for some chemicals by year and by individual sample.
* Not calculated: proportion of results below limit of detection was too high to provide a valid result.

## Serum 2,2',3,3',4,4',5,5',6,6'-Decachlorobiphenyl (PCB 209) (lipid adjusted)

Geometric mean and selected percentiles of serum concentrations (in ng/g of lipid or parts per billion on a lipid-weight basis) for the U.S. population from the National Health and Nutrition Examination Survey.

| | Survey years | Geometric mean (95% conf. interval) | Selected percentiles ( 95% confidence interval) | | | | Sample size |
|---|---|---|---|---|---|---|---|
| | | | 50th | 75th | 90th | 95th | |
| Total | 03-04 | 1.40 (1.21-1.61) | 1.18 (1.00-1.48) | 3.20 (2.67-4.01) | 7.58 (6.20-8.81) | 11.1 (9.00-15.7) | 1854 |
| Age group | | | | | | | |
| 12-19 years | 03-04 | * | < LOD | < LOD | 1.12 (.800-4.60) | 3.49 (1.12-6.64) | 578 |
| 20 years and older | 03-04 | 1.63 (1.42-1.88) | 1.40 (1.18-1.70) | 3.80 (3.04-4.44) | 8.09 (6.60-9.30) | 12.3 (9.05-18.0) | 1276 |
| Gender | | | | | | | |
| Males | 03-04 | 1.37 (1.18-1.60) | 1.15 (1.00-1.50) | 3.00 (2.70-3.58) | 6.22 (4.97-8.20) | 9.10 (7.09-13.0) | 925 |
| Females | 03-04 | 1.42 (1.22-1.66) | 1.20 (1.00-1.50) | 3.46 (2.45-4.61) | 8.78 (7.45-9.47) | 13.9 (10 0-18.7) | 929 |
| Race/ethnicity | | | | | | | |
| Mexican Americans | 03-04 | * | < LOD | 1.10 (.770-1.60) | 2.40 (1.60-3.60) | 3.71 (2.40-4.97) | 416 |
| Non-Hispanic blacks | 03-04 | 1.56 (1.37-1.78) | 1.35 (1.10-1.52) | 3.40 (2.62-4.82) | 9.83 (6.70-13.6) | 18.0 (11 8-27.7) | 455 |
| Non-Hispanic whites | 03-04 | 1.53 (1.31-1.79) | 1.30 (1.09-1.70) | 3.89 (3.04-4.50) | 7.95 (6.49-9.09) | 11.3 (9.07-16.3) | 864 |

Limit of detection (LOD, see Data Analysis section) for Survey year 03-04 is 0.7.
< LOD means less than the limit of detection, which may vary for some chemicals by year and by individual sample.
* Not calculated: proportion of results below limit of detection was too high to provide a valid result.

## Serum 2,2',3,3',4,4',5,5',6,6'-Decachlorobiphenyl (PCB 209) (whole weight)

Geometric mean and selected percentiles of serum concentrations (in ng/g of serum or parts per billion) for the U.S. population from the National Health and Nutrition Examination Survey.

| | Survey years | Geometric mean (95% conf. interval) | Selected percentiles ( 95% confidence interval) | | | | Sample size |
|---|---|---|---|---|---|---|---|
| | | | 50th | 75th | 90th | 95th | |
| Total | 03-04 | .009 ( 007-.010) | .008 (.006-.009) | .021 (.017-.026) | .049 (.040- 058) | .073 (.059-.097) | 1854 |
| Age group | | | | | | | |
| 12-19 years | 03-04 | * | < LOD | < LOD | .006 (.004- 018) | .017 (.005-.033) | 578 |
| 20 years and older | 03-04 | .010 ( 009-.012) | .009 (.008-.011) | .024 (.020-.028) | .053 (.044- 063) | .077 (.065-.105) | 1276 |
| Gender | | | | | | | |
| Males | 03-04 | .008 ( 007-.010) | .008 (.006-.010) | .019 (.017-.023) | .039 (.032- 051) | .063 (.042-.077) | 925 |
| Females | 03-04 | .009 ( 007-.010) | .008 (.006-.009) | .024 (.016-.032) | .057 (.049- 064) | .092 (.068-.134) | 929 |
| Race/ethnicity | | | | | | | |
| Mexican Americans | 03-04 | * | < LOD | .007 (.005-.010) | .018 (.010- 023) | .024 (.018-.035) | 416 |
| Non-Hispanic blacks | 03-04 | .009 ( 008-.010) | .008 (.006-.009) | .022 (.018-.027) | .065 (.039- 077) | .097 (.065-.144) | 455 |
| Non-Hispanic whites | 03-04 | .009 ( 008-.011) | .009 (.007-.011) | .024 (.020-.029) | .053 (.044- 061) | .076 (.063-.099) | 864 |

< LOD means less than the limit of detection for the lipid adjusted serum level, which may vary for some chemicals by year and by individual sample.
* Not calculated: proportion of results below limit of detection was too high to provide a valid result.

## References

Agency for Toxic Substances and Disease Registry (ATSDR). Toxicological profile for polychlorinated biphenyls. 2000 [online]. Available from URL: http://www.atsdr.cdc.gov/toxprofiles/tp17.html. 03/17/05

Apostoli P, Magoni M, Bergonzi R, Carasi S, Indelicato A, Scarcella C, et al. Assessment of reference values for polychlorinated biphenyl concentration in human blood. Chemosphere 2005;61(3):413-21.

Arulmozhiraja S, Shiraishi F, Okumura T, Iida M, Takigami H, Edmonds JS, et al. Structural requirements for the interaction of 91 hydroxylated polychlorinated biphenyls with estrogen and thyroid hormone receptors. Toxicol Sci 2005;84(1):49-62.

Barr DB, Weihe P, Davis MD, Needham LL, Grandjean P. Serum polychlorinated biphenyl and organochlorine insecticide concentrations in a Faroese birth cohort. Chemosphere 2006;62(7):1167-1182.

Bates MN, Buckland SJ, Garrett N, Ellis H, Needham LL, Patterson DG Jr, et al. Persistent organochlorines in the serum of the non-occupationally exposed New Zealand population. Chemosphere 2004;54:1431-1443.

Carpenter DO, DeCaprio AP, O'Hehir D, Akhtar F, Johnson G, Scrudato RJ, et al. Polychlorinated biphenyls in serum of the Siberian Yupik people from St. Lawrence Island, Alaska. Int J Circumpolar Health 2005;64(4):322-335.

Carpenter DO. Polychlorinated biphenyls (PCBs): routes of exposure and effects on human health. Rev Environ Health 2006;21(1):1-23.

Centers for Disease Control and Prevention (CDC). Third National Report on Human Exposure to Environmental Chemicals. Atlanta (GA). 2005.

Charles MJ, Schell MJ, Willman E, Gross HB, Lin Y, Sonnenberg S, et al. Organochlorines and 8-hydroxy-2-deoxyguanosine in cancerous and noncancerous breast tissue: do the data support the hypothesis that oxidative DNA damage caused by organochlorines affects breast cancer? Arch Environ Contam Toxicol 2001;41:386-395.

De Roos AJ, Hartge P, Lubin JH, Colt JS, Davis S, Cerhan JR, et al. Persistent organochlorine chemicals in plasma and risk of non-Hodgkin's lymphoma. Cancer Res 2005;65(23):11214-11226.

DeCaprio AP, Johnson GW, Tarbell AM, Carpenter DO, Chiarenzelli JR, Morse GS, et al. Polychlorinated biphenyl (PCB) exposure assessment by multivariate statistical analysis of serum congener profiles in an adult Native American population. Environ Res 2005;98(3):284-302.

DeCastro BR, Korrick SA, Spengler JD, Soto AM. Estrogenic activity of polychlorinated biphenyls present in human tissue and the environment. Environ Sci Technol 2006;40(8):2819-2825.

Engel LS, Laden F, Andersen A, Strickland PT, Blair A, Needham LL, et al. Polychlorinated biphenyl levels in peripheral blood and non-Hodgkin's lymphoma: a report from three cohorts. Cancer Res 2007;67(11):5545-5552.

Giwercman AH, Rignell-Hydbom A, Toft G, Rylander L, Hagmar L, Lindh C, et al. Reproductive hormone levels in men exposed to persistent organohalogen pollutants: a study of Inuit and three European cohorts. Environ Health Perspect 2006;114(9):1348-1353.

Gladen BC, Rogan WJ. Effects of perinatal polychlorinated biphenyls and dichlorodiphenyl dichloroethene on later development. J Pediatr 1991;119(1 ( Pt 1)):58-63.

Glynn A, Aune M, Darnerud PO, Cnattingius S, Bjerselius R, Becker W, et al. Determinants of serum concentrations of organochlorine compounds in Swedish pregnant women: a cross-sectional study. Environ Health. 2007;6:2.

Glynn AW, Wolk A, Aune M, Atuma S, Zettermark S, Maehle-Schmid M, et al. Serum concentrations of organochlorines in men: a search for markers of exposure. Sci Total Environ 2000; 263(1-3):197-208.

Gray KA, Klebanoff MA, Brock JW, Zhou H, Darden R, Needham L, Longnecker MP. In utero exposure to background levels of polychlorinated biphenyls and cognitive functioning among school-age children. Am J Epidemiol 2005;162(1):17-26.

Hagmar L, Wallin E, Vessby B, Jonsson BA, Bergman A, Rylander L. Intra-individual variations and time trends 1991-2001 in human serum levels of PCB, DDE and hexachlorobenzene. Chemosphere 2006;64(9):1507-1513.

Hertz-Picciotto I, Charles MJ, James RA, Keller JA, Willman E, Teplin S. In utero polychlorinated biphenyl exposures in relation to fetal and early childhood growth. Epidemiology 2005;16(5):648-656.

Heudorf U, Angerer J, Drexler H. Polychlorinated biphenyls in the blood plasma: current exposure of the population in Germany. Rev Environ Health 2002;17(2):123-134.

Hsu JF, Guo YL, Yang SY, Liao PC. Congener profiles of PCBs and PCDD/Fs in Yucheng victims fifteen years after exposure to toxic rice-bran oils and their implications for epidemiologic studies. Chemosphere 2005;61(9):1231-1243.

Jacobson JL, Jacobson SW. Intellectual impairment in children exposed to polychlorinated biphenyls in utero. N Engl J Med 1996;335:783-789.

Johansson N, Hanber A, Wingfors H, Tysklind M. PCB in building sealant is influencing PCB levels in blood of residents. Organohalogen Compounds, Volumes 60-65, Dioxin 2003. Boston, MA.

Jursa S, Chovancova J, Petrik J, Loksa J. Dioxin-like and non-dioxin-like PCBs in human serum of Slovak population. Chemosphere. 2006;64(4):686-691.

Kimbrough RD, Doemland ML, Mandel JS. A mortality update of male and female capacitor workers exposed to polychlorinated biphenyls. J Occup Environ Med 2003;45(3):271-282.

Kimura-Kuroda J, Nagata I, Kuroda Y. Disrupting effects of hydroxy-polychlorinated biphenyl (PCB) congeners on neuronal development of cerebellar Purkinje cells: a possible causal factor for developmental brain disorders? Chemosphere 2007;67(9):S412-S420.

Kitamura S, Jinno N, Suzuki T, Sugihara K, Ohta S, Kuroki H, et al. Thyroid hormone-like and estrogenic activity of hydroxylated PCBs in cell culture. Toxicology 2005 Mar 30;208(3):377-387.

Kohler M, Tremp J, Zennegg M, Seiler C, Minder-Kohler S, Beck M, et al. Joint sealants: an overlooked diffuse source of polychlorinated biphenyls in buildings. Environ Sci Technol 2005;39(7):1967-1973.

Knerr S, Schrenk D. Carcinogenicity of "non-dioxinlike" polychlorinated biphenyls. Crit Rev Toxicol. 2006;36(9):663-694.

Koopman-Esseboom C, Weisglas-Kuperus N, de Ridder MA, Van der Paauw CG, Tuinstra LG, Sauer PJ. Effects of polychlorinated biphenyl/dioxin exposure and feeding type on infants' mental and psychomotor development. Pediatrics 1996;97(5):700-706.

Langer P, Kocan A, Tajtakova M, Petrik J, Chovancova J, Drobna B, et al. Human thyroid in the population exposed to high environmental pollution by organochlorinated pollutants for several decades. Endocr Regul 2005;39(1):13-20.

Langer P, Tajtakova M, Kocan A, Petrik J, Koska J, Ksinantova L, et al. Thyroid ultrasound volume, structure and function after long-term high exposure of large population to polychlorinated biphenyls, pesticides and dioxin. Chemosphere. 2007a;69(1):118.

Langer P, Kocan A, Tajtakova M, Petrik J, Chovancova J, Drobna B, et al. Fish from industrially polluted freshwater as the main source of organochlorinated pollutants and increased frequency of thyroid disorders and dysglycemia. Chemosphere 2007b;67(9):S379-S385.

Link B, Gabrio T, Zoellner I, Piechotowski I, Paepke O, Herrmann T, et al. Biomonitoring of persistent organochlorine pesticides, PCDD/PCDFs and dioxin-like PCBs in blood of children from South West Germany (Baden-Wuerttemberg) from 1993 to 2003. Chemosphere 2005;58(9):1185-1201.

Longnecker MP, Ryan JJ, Gladen BC, Schecter AJ. Correlations among human plasma levels of dioxin-like compounds and polychlorinated biphenyls (PCBs) and implications for epidemiologic studies. Arch Environ Health 2000;55(3):195-200.

Longnecker MP, Wolff MS, Gladen BC, Brock JW, Grandjean P, Jacobson JL, et al. Comparison of polychlorinated biphenyl levels across studies of human neurodevelopment. Environ Health Perspect 2003;111(1):65-70.

Lundqvist C, Zuurbier M, Leijs M, Johansson C, Ceccatelli S, Saunders M, et al. The effects of PCBs and dioxins on child health. Acta Paediatr Suppl 2006;95(453):55-64.

Meeker JD, Altshul L, Hauser R. Serum PCBs, p,p(')-DDE and HCB predict thyroid hormone levels in men. Environ Res 2007;104(2):296-304.

Negri E, Bosetti C, Fattore E, La Vecchia C. Environmental exposure to polychlorinated biphenyls (PCBs) and breast cancer: a systemic review of the epidemiological evidence. Eur J Cancer Prev 2003;12:509-516.

Needham LL, Barr DB, Caudill SP, Pirkle JL, Turner WE, Osterloh J, et al. Concentrations of environmental chemicals associated with neurodevelopmental effects in U.S. population. Neurotoxicology 2005;26(4):531-545.

Nguon K, Baxter MG, Sajdel-Sulkowska EM. Perinatal exposure to polychlorinated biphenyls differentially affects cerebellar development and motor functions in male and female rat neonates. Cerebellum 2005;4(2):112-122.

Otake T, Yoshinaga J, Enomoto T, Matsuda M, Wakimoto T, Ikegami M, et al. Thyroid hormone status of newborns in relation to in utero exposure to PCBs and hydroxylated PCB metabolites. Environ Res 2007;105(2):240-246.

Park H, Lee SJ, Kang JH, Chang YS. Congener-specific approach to human PCB concentrations by serum analysis. Chemosphere 2007;68(9):1699-1706.

Patterson DG Jr, Todd GD, Turner WE, Maggio V, Alexander LR, Needham LL. Levels of non-ortho-substituted (coplanar), mono- and di-ortho-substituted polychlorinated biphenyls, dibenzo-p-dioxins, and dibenzofurans in human serum and adipose tissue. Environ Health Perspect 1994;102 (Suppl 1):195-204.

Patterson DG Jr, Wong LY, Turner WE, Caudill SP, Dipietro ES, McClure PC, et al. Levels in the U.S. population of those persistent organic pollutants (2003-2004) included in the Stockholm Convention or in other long range transboundary air pollution agreements. Environ Sci Technol 2009;43(4):1211-1218.

Petrik J, Drobna B, Pavuk M, Jursa S, Wimmerova S, Chovancova J. Serum PCBs and organochlorine pesticides in Slovakia:

age, gender, and residence as determinants of organochlorine concentrations. Chemosphere 2006;65(3):410-418.

Porta M, Zumeta E. Implementing the Stockholm treaty on persistent organic pollutants. Occup Environ Med 2002;59:651-653.

Prince MM, Ruder AM, Hein MJ, Waters MA, Whelan EA, Nilsen N, et al. Mortality and exposure response among 14,458 electrical capacitor manufacturing workers exposed to polychlorinated biphenyls (PCBs). Environ Health Perspect 2006;114(10):1508-1514.

Purkey HE, Palaninathan SK, Kent KC, Smith C, Safe SH, Sacchettini JC, et al. Hydroxylated polychlorinated biphenyls selectively bind transthyretin in blood and inhibit amyloidogenesis: rationalizing rodent PCB toxicity. Chem Biol 2004;11(12):1719-1728.

Rignell-Hydbom A, Rylander L, Elzanaty S, Giwercman A, Lindh CH, Hagmar L. Exposure to persistent organochlorine pollutants and seminal levels of markers of epididymal and accessory sex gland functions in Swedish men. Hum Reprod 2005;20(7):1910-1914.

Roegge CS, Morris JR, Villareal S, Wang VC, Powers BE, Klintsova AY, et al. Purkinje cell and cerebellar effects following developmental exposure to PCBs and/or MeHg. Neurotoxicol Teratol 2006;28(1):74-85.

Ross G. The public health implications of polychlorinated biphenyls (PCBs) in the environment. Ecotoxicol Environ Saf 2004;59(3):275-291.

Sagiv SK, Tolbert PE, Altshul LM, Korrick SA. Organochlorine exposures during pregnancy and infant size at birth. Epidemiology 2007;18(1):120-129.

Sala M, Ribas-Fito N, Cardo E, de Muga ME, Marco E, Mazon C, et al. Levels of hexachlorobenzene and other organochlorine compounds in cord blood: exposure across placenta. Chemosphere 2001;43:895-901.

Toft G, Rignell-Hydbom A, Tyrkiel E, Shvets M, Giwercman A, Lindh CH, et al. Semen quality and exposure to persistent organochlorine pollutants. Epidemiology 2006;17(4):450-548.

Turci R, Finozzi E, Catenacci G, Marinaccio A, Balducci C, Minoia C. Reference values of coplanar and non-coplanar PCBs in serum samples from two Italian population groups. Toxicol Lett 2006;162(2-3):250-255.

Turyk M, Anderson HA, Hanrahan LP, Falk C, Steenport DN, Needham LL, et al. Relationship of serum levels of individual PCB, dioxin, and furan congeners and DDE with Great Lakes sport-caught fish consumption. Environ Res. 2006;100(2):173-183.

United States Environmental Protection Agency (U.S.EPA). Health Effects of PCBs. August 8, 2008 [online]. Available at URL: http://www.epa.gov/epawaste/hazard/tsd/pcbs/pubs/effects.htm. 7/8/09

Wang SL, Su PH, Jong SB, Guo YL, Chou WL, Papke O. In utero exposure to dioxins and polychlorinated biphenyls and its relations to thyroid function and growth hormone in newborns. Environ Health Perspect 2005;113(11):1645-1650.

Wolff MS, Engel S, Berkowitz G, Teitelbaum S, Siskind J, Barr DB, et al. Prenatal pesticide and PCB exposures and birth outcomes. Pediatr Res 2007;61(2):243-250.

You SH, Gauger KJ, Bansal R, Zoeller RT. 4-Hydroxy-PCB106 acts as a direct thyroid hormone receptor agonist in rat GH3 cells. Mol Cell Endocrinol 2006;257-258:26-34.

# Dioxin-Like Chemicals: Polychlorinated Dibenzo-*p*-dioxins, Polychlorinated Dibenzofurans, and Coplanar and Mono-*ortho*-substituted Polychlorinated Biphenyls

## General Information

Polychlorinated dibenzo-*p*-dioxins and dibenzofurans are two similar classes of chlorinated aromatic chemicals that are produced as contaminants or by-products. They have no known commercial or natural use. Dioxins are produced primarily during the incineration or burning of waste; the bleaching processes used in pulp and paper mills; and the chemical syntheses of trichlorophenoxyacetic acid, hexachlorophene, vinyl chloride, trichlorophenol, and

pentachlorophenol. Both the synthesis and heat-related degradation of polychlorinated biphenyls (PCBs) will produce dibenzofuran byproducts. Releases from industrial sources have decreased approximately 80% since the 1980s (U.S. EPA, 2004). Today, the largest release of these chemicals occurs as a result of the open burning of household and municipal trash, landfill fires, and agricultural and forest fires. When advanced analytical techniques are used, most soil and water samples will reveal trace amounts of polychlorinated dibenzo-*p*-dioxins and dibenzofurans.

The coplanar and mono-*ortho*-substituted PCBs are chlorinated aromatic hydrocarbon chemicals that belong to the general class PCBs which were once synthesized for use as heat-exchanger, transformer, and hydraulic fluids, and also used as additives to paints, oils, window caulking, and floor tiles. Production of PCBs peaked in the early 1970s and was banned in the United States after 1979. Together

## Dioxin-like Chemicals in this *Report*

| Polychlorinated dibenzo-*p*-dioxins | CAS number |
|---|---|
| 1,2,3,4,6,7,8-Heptachlorodibenzo-*p*-dioxin (HpCDD) | 35822-46-9 |
| 1,2,3,4,7,8-Hexachlorodibenzo-*p*-dioxin (HxCDD) | 39227-28-6 |
| 1,2,3,6,7,8-Hexachlorodibenzo-*p*-dioxin (HxCDD) | 57653-85-7 |
| 1,2,3,7,8,9-Hexachlorodibenzo-*p*-dioxin (HxCDD) | 19408-74-3 |
| 1,2,3,4,6,7,8,9-Octachlorodibenzo-*p*-dioxin (OCDD) | 3268-87-9 |
| 1,2,3,7,8-Pentachlorodibenzo-*p*-dioxin (PeCDD) | 40321-76-4 |
| 2,3,7,8-Tetrachlorodibenzo-*p*-dioxin (TCDD) | 1746-01-6 |

| Polychlorinated dibenzofurans | CAS number |
|---|---|
| 1,2,3,4,6,7,8-Heptachlorodibenzofuran (HpCDF) | 67562-39-4 |
| 1,2,3,4,7,8,9-Heptachlorodibenzofuran (HpCDF) | 55673-89-7 |
| 1,2,3,4,7,8-Hexachlorodibenzofuran (HxCDF) | 70648-26-9 |
| 1,2,3,6,7,8-Hexachlorodibenzofuran (HxCDF) | 57117-44-9 |
| 1,2,3,7,8,9-Hexachlorodibenzofuran (HxCDF) | 72918-21-9 |
| 2,3,4,6,7,8-Hexchlorodibenzofuran (HxCDF) | 60851-34-5 |
| 1,2,3,4,6,7,8,9-Octachlorodibenzofuran (OCDF) | 39001-02-0 |
| 1,2,3,7,8-Pentachlorodibenzofuran (PeCDF) | 57117-41-6 |
| 2,3,4,7,8-Pentachlorodibenzofuran (PeCDF) | 57117-31-4 |
| 2,3,7,8-Tetrachlorodibenzofuran (TCDF) | 51207-31-9 |

| Coplanar polychlorinated biphenyls (IUPAC number) | CAS number |
|---|---|
| 3,4,4',5-Tetrachlorobiphenyl (PCB 81) | 70362-50-4 |
| 3,3',4,4',5-Pentachlorobiphenyl (PCB 126) | 57465-28-8 |
| 3,3',4,4',5,5'-Hexachlorobiphenyl (PCB 169) | 32774-16-6 |

| Mono-*ortho*-substituted polychlorinated biphenyls (IUPAC number) | CAS number |
|---|---|
| 2,3,3',4,4'-Pentachlorobiphenyl (PCB 105) | 32598-14-4 |
| 2,3',4,4',5-Pentachlorobiphenyl (PCB 118) | 31508-00-6 |
| 2,3,3',4,4',5-Hexachlorobiphenyl (PCB 156) | 38380-08-4 |
| 2,3,3',4,4',5'-Hexachlorobiphenyl (PCB 157) | 69782-90-7 |
| 2,3',4,4',5,5'-Hexachlorobiphenyl (PCB 167) | 52663-72-6 |
| 2,3,3',4,4',5,5'-Heptachlorobiphenyl (PCB 189) | 39635-31-9 |

with the polychlorinated dioxins and furans, these two special classes of PCBs are often referred to as "dioxin-like" chemicals because they act in the body through a similar mechanism. Structural nomenclature is available at: http://www.epa.gov/oswer/riskassessment/pdf/1340-erasc-003.pdf. Commonly measured polychlorinated dibenzo-*p*-dioxins, polychlorinated dibenzofurans, and coplanar and mono-*ortho*-substituted PCBs are listed in the table.

In the environment, these dioxin-like chemicals are persistent and usually occur as a mixture of congeners (i.e., compounds that differ by the numbers and positions of chlorine atoms attached to the dibenzo-*p*-dioxin, dibenzofuran, or biphenyl structures). The general population is exposed to low levels of polychlorinated dibenzo-*p*-dioxins and dibenzofurans primarily through ingestion of high-fat foods such as dairy products, eggs, and animal fats, and some fish and wildlife. Dioxin-like chemicals are measurable in U.S. meats and poultry (Hoffman et al., 2006) as a result of the

accumulation of these substances in the food chain. Breast milk is a substantial source of exposure for infants (Beck et al., 1994; Lundqvist et al., 2006), though breast milk levels have been decreasing in recent years (Arisawa et al., 2005). The lesser chlorinated PCBs, including some dioxin-like PCBs, are more volatile. These PCBs can enter air of buildings containing joint sealants made with PCBs prior to 1980 and can increase background serum levels via inhalational exposure (Johansson et al., 2003; Kohler et al., 2005). Volatilization of PCBs from nearby hazardous waste sites may also contribute to human inhalational exposure. Exposure to high levels of these chemicals has occurred in the past as a result of industrial accidents (e.g., after an explosion in a factory in Seveso, Italy); the use of accidentally contaminated cooking oils (e.g., as occurred in Yusho in Japan and Yucheng in Taiwan); the spraying of herbicides contaminated with 2,3,7,8-tetrachlorodibenzo-*p*-dioxin (TCDD) (e.g., as Agent Orange in Vietnam); and the burning of PCBs producing polychlorinated dibenzofurans

## Serum 1,2,3,4,6,7,8-Heptachlorodibenzo-*p*-dioxin (HpCDD) (lipid adjusted)

Geometric mean and selected percentiles of serum concentrations (in pg/g lipid or parts per trillion on a lipid-weight basis) for the U.S. population from the National Health and Nutrition Examination Survey.

| | Survey years | Geometric mean (95% conf. interval) | Selected percentiles ( 95% confidence interval) | | | | Sample size |
|---|---|---|---|---|---|---|---|
| | | | 50th | 75th | 90th | 95th | |
| **Total** | 99-00 | * | < LOD | 58.2 (<LOD-63 6) | 86.0 (75.5-96.7) | 112 (101-131) | 1894 |
| | 01-02 | 39.0 (33.7-45 0) | 40.2 (34.9-46 9) | 68.7 (56.7-82.2) | 115 (88.2-138) | 147 (126-181) | 1220 |
| | 03-04 | 25.3 (23.4-27 3) | 24.9 (22.8-26 9) | 42.5 (38.8-48.1) | 70.4 (62.7-80.1) | 91.3 (73 5-117) | 1874 |
| **Age group** | | | | | | | |
| 12-19 years | 99-00 | * | < LOD | < LOD | < LOD | 63.6 (<LOD-75.6) | 657 |
| | 01-02 | † | † | † | † | † | † |
| | 03-04 | 16.7 (15.1-18.4) | 16.4 (15.1-18 3) | 23.6 (21.5-25.8) | 33.4 (28.6-36.8) | 46.7 (34 5-78.1) | 586 |
| 20 years and older | 99-00 | * | < LOD | 62.0 (57.1-66.7) | 92.9 (81.2-101) | 120 (102-139) | 1237 |
| | 01-02 | 39.0 (33.7-45 0) | 40.2 (34.9-46 9) | 68.7 (56.7-82.2) | 115 (88.2-138) | 147 (126-181) | 1220 |
| | 03-04 | 26.8 (24.6-29 2) | 27.3 (24.6-29 0) | 45.6 (41.3-53.2) | 73.7 (64.1-88.6) | 95.0 (76.1-126) | 1288 |
| **Gender** | | | | | | | |
| Males | 99-00 | * | < LOD | < LOD | 73.6 (69.0-80.8) | 94.7 (83.1-103) | 910 |
| | 01-02 | 36.6 (31.7-42 3) | 39.0 (33.3-42 6) | 62.1 (49.7-75.0) | 102 (75.8-132) | 138 (103-169) | 553 |
| | 03-04 | 24.2 (21.7-27 0) | 23.2 (21.1-25 6) | 40.6 (35.3-46.9) | 64.2 (58.8-73.7) | 85.0 (65 8-113) | 920 |
| Females | 99-00 | * | < LOD | 62.7 (<LOD-69.1) | 102 (86.0-118) | 131 (111-164) | 984 |
| | 01-02 | 41.2 (34.9-48.7) | 43.6 (35.3-52.4) | 76.0 (59.5-90.1) | 125 (93.4-150) | 158 (130-191) | 667 |
| | 03-04 | 26.3 (24.4-28 3) | 26.8 (24.3-28 3) | 44.4 (41.1-50.2) | 76.1 (65.3-89.1) | 95.7 (80.7-128) | 954 |
| **Race/ethnicity** | | | | | | | |
| Mexican Americans | 99-00 | * | < LOD | 61.4 (<LOD-69 0) | 97.7 (82.8-111) | 132 (108-159) | 621 |
| | 01-02 | 39.6 (35.7-43 9) | 39.7 (33.6-47.4) | 64.0 (55.8-74.7) | 107 (82.4-128) | 149 (111-171) | 262 |
| | 03-04 | 25.8 (22.6-29.4) | 26.1 (20.9-30 9) | 41.9 (36.7-44.7) | 61.0 (49.7-71.9) | 80.1 (65 0-89.1) | 424 |
| Non-Hispanic blacks | 99-00 | * | < LOD | 58.1 (<LOD-71.1) | 95.0 (75.1-110) | 125 (102-183) | 408 |
| | 01-02 | 43.7 (35.4-54 0) | 42.8 (32.2-59 8) | 80.6 (60.9-106) | 134 (101-166) | 167 (130-230) | 218 |
| | 03-04 | 25.8 (22.6-29.4) | 23.7 (20.7-27.1) | 41.2 (32.6-56.4) | 69.2 (54.6-115) | 115 (67.1-164) | 454 |
| Non-Hispanic whites | 99-00 | * | < LOD | 59.0 (<LOD-64 8) | 84.9 (72.0-97.0) | 106 (96.7-122) | 709 |
| | 01-02 | 39.3 (33.0-46 8) | 40.5 (34.0-50.1) | 71.0 (56.3-87.5) | 117 (87.1-147) | 147 (125-186) | 657 |
| | 03-04 | 25.0 (22.6-27.7) | 24.6 (22.3-27.4) | 42.6 (39.4-48.5) | 73.5 (60.4-86.7) | 93.7 (71 6-127) | 875 |

Limit of detection (LOD, see Data Analysis section) for Survey years 99-00, 01-02, and 03-04 are 55.9, 10 3, and 13.0, respectively.
† Data not collected for this age group for Survey year 01-02.
< LOD means less than the limit of detection, which may vary for some chemicals by year and by individual sample.
* Not calculated: proportion of results below limit of detection was too high to provide a valid result.

(e.g., such as from electrical transformer fires). Workplace exposures are infrequent today, but incineration plant workers and chemical synthesis workers can be exposed via inhalation and dust exposures. The dioxin-like chemicals are easily absorbed, tend to distribute into body fat, have limited metabolism, and slow elimination from the body. Serum levels may be influenced by both past (stored in body fat) and recent exposures, though the current intakes for most people are now low. Half-lives of the dioxins and furans in the body vary from three to 19 years, with the half-life of TCDD estimated at around seven years (Geyer et al., 2002).

Because exposure to these chemicals includes a mixture of varying congeners, congener-specific effects are difficult to determine (Masuda, 2001; Masuda et al., 1998). However, these four groups of chemicals (polychlorinated dibenzo-p-dioxins, polychlorinated dibenzofurans, and the coplanar and mono-ortho- substituted PCBs) are considered to act

through a similar mechanism to produce toxic effects. These dioxin-like effects are thought to result from interaction with the aryl hydrocarbon receptor (AhR), particularly in the induction of gene expression for cytochromes P450, CYP1A1 and CYP1A2. Dioxins and furans have a planar configuration and require four lateral chlorine atoms (2,3,7,8 positions) on the dibenzo-p-dioxin or dibenzofuran backbone to bind this receptor. The rank order of interaction with the AhR receptor by degree and position of chlorination is roughly similar for both the dioxin and furan series. The coplanar polychlorinated biphenyls (unsubstituted at ortho positions) and the mono-ortho-substituted polychlorinated biphenyls (which contain a chlorine atom at one of the ortho positions) can achieve a planar configuration and also interact with the AhR receptor. The variation in the effect on AhR among the dioxin-like chemicals is 10,000-fold, with TCDD and 1,2,3,7,8-pentachlorodibenzo-p-dioxin being the most potent. To compare potency, each of these congeners has been assigned a potency value relative to

## Serum 1,2,3,4,6,7,8-Heptachlorodibenzo-p-dioxin (HpCDD) (whole weight)

Geometric mean and selected percentiles of serum concentrations (in fg/g of serum or parts per quadrillion) for the U.S. population from the National Health and Nutrition Examination Survey.

| | Survey years | Geometric mean (95% conf. interval) | Selected percentiles ( 95% confidence interval) | | | | Sample size |
|---|---|---|---|---|---|---|---|
| | | | 50th | 75th | 90th | 95th | |
| **Total** | 99-00 | * | < LOD | 354 (<LOD384) | 564 (501-617) | 749 (646-869) | 1894 |
| | 01-02 | 252 (219-289) | 267 (232-305) | 440 (376-529) | 779 (591-989) | 1030 (840-1290) | 1220 |
| | 03-04 | 155 (143-167) | 150 (134-163) | 288 (242-319) | 465 (399-550) | 618 (516-787) | 1874 |
| **Age group** | | | | | | | |
| 12-19 years | 99-00 | * | < LOD | < LOD | < LOD | 289 (<LOD340) | 657 |
| | 01-02 | † | † | † | † | † | † |
| | 03-04 | 84.6 (77.4-92.5) | 83.9 (76.1-92.0) | 118 (106-131) | 165 (139-185) | 210 (176-319) | 586 |
| 20 years and older | 99-00 | * | < LOD | 385 (354-418) | 610 (534-677) | 802 (681-936) | 1237 |
| | 01-02 | 252 (219-289) | 267 (232-305) | 440 (376-529) | 779 (591-989) | 1030 (840-1290) | 1220 |
| | 03-04 | 169 (155-184) | 170 (150-186) | 314 (267-348) | 506 (419-576) | 628 (546-810) | 1288 |
| **Gender** | | | | | | | |
| Males | 99-00 | * | < LOD | < LOD | 489 (436-543) | 613 (535-681) | 910 |
| | 01-02 | 243 (211-279) | 245 (213-291) | 422 (349-527) | 766 (536-976) | 983 (766-1260) | 553 |
| | 03-04 | 150 (135-167) | 144 (129-161) | 273 (236-305) | 424 (365-516) | 554 (440-667) | 920 |
| Females | 99-00 | * | < LOD | 373 (<LOD428) | 637 (562-802) | 907 (806-1040) | 984 |
| | 01-02 | 260 (221-306) | 281 (236-324) | 466 (386-551) | 795 (621-997) | 1140 (849-1330) | 667 |
| | 03-04 | 159 (147-172) | 158 (138-170) | 303 (249-345) | 520 (429-591) | 623 (545-848) | 954 |
| **Race/ethnicity** | | | | | | | |
| Mexican Americans | 99-00 | * | < LOD | 372 (<LOD404) | 598 (546-657) | 849 (657-1020) | 621 |
| | 01-02 | 254 (232-278) | 249 (229-286) | 403 (360-521) | 791 (643-929) | 988 (817-1240) | 262 |
| | 03-04 | 158 (139-180) | 159 (138-193) | 274 (241-299) | 414 (349-469) | 556 (451-592) | 424 |
| Non-Hispanic blacks | 99-00 | * | < LOD | 323 (<LOD391) | 567 (422-716) | 778 (574-1130) | 408 |
| | 01-02 | 258 (208-319) | 262 (180-339) | 478 (343-600) | 852 (578-1170) | 1170 (821-1660) | 218 |
| | 03-04 | 148 (128-170) | 137 (117-156) | 247 (188-344) | 434 (345-599) | 715 (405-1090) | 454 |
| Non-Hispanic whites | 99-00 | * | < LOD | 370 (<LOD401) | 565 (491-634) | 733 (637-816) | 709 |
| | 01-02 | 255 (216-302) | 277 (228-328) | 442 (374-547) | 782 (551-1020) | 1020 (803-1290) | 657 |
| | 03-04 | 155 (140-170) | 152 (131-171) | 292 (248-325) | 492 (390-571) | 621 (506-810) | 875 |

† Data not collected for this age group for Survey year 01-02
< LOD means less than the limit of detection for the lipid adjusted serum level, which may vary for some chemicals by year and by individual sample.
* Not calculated: proportion of results below limit of detection was too high to provide a valid result.

TCDD (toxic equivalency factor [TEF]). When each TEF is multiplied by the concentration of the congener, a toxic equivalency (TEQ) value is obtained. Thus, the dioxin-like toxicity contributed by each of the polychlorinated dibenzo-p-dioxins, dibenzofurans, and PCBs can then be compared. The sum of all congener TEQs in a specimen (total TEQ) can be used to compare dioxin-like activity among specimens. Many of the dioxin-like PCBs have lower potency but are found at higher concentrations than TCDD (Kang et al., 1997; Patterson et al., 1994, Van den Berg et al., 2006), so these less potent chemicals may still contribute substantially to the total TEQ.

In animal studies, TCDD and dioxin-like chemicals have demonstrated many effects including: altered transcription of genes; induction of various enzymes; wasting syndrome; hepatotoxicity; altered immune function; testicular atrophy; altered thyroid function; chloracne; porphyria; neurotoxicity; teratogenicity; and carcinogenicity (EPA, 2004). Since animal species differ dramatically in sensitivity to these chemicals, it is difficult to predict human health effects though animal studies have provided support to observations of effects in human populations. Health effects of exposure to dioxin-like chemicals in people have been observed as a result of industrial or accidental exposures

involving large doses of these chemicals. Chloracne, biochemical liver test abnormalities, elevated blood lipids, fetal injury, and porphyria cutanea tarda have been reported in episodes of high exposure. Developmental effects in humans are of concern since congenital anomalies and intrauterine growth retardation were observed in offspring of Yucheng mothers exposed to cooking oil contaminated with electrical oil containing very high levels of PCB and polychlorinated dibenzofurans. Environmental serum levels of primarily non-dioxin-like PCBs, and some dioxin-like chemicals, have been associated with altered psychomotor development in newborns and children (Arisawa et al., 2005; Jacobsen and Jacobsen, 1996; Koopman-Esseboom et al., 1996; Longnecker et al., 2003; Lundqvist et al., 2006; U.S. EPA, 2004; also see section on Non-Dioxin-Like Polychlorinated Biphenyls).

Cross-sectional associations of type II diabetes or markers of insulin resistance with serum levels of TCDD, other dioxin-like chemicals, non-dioxin-like PCBs and organochlorine pesticides have been reported in both highly exposed and environmentally exposed human populations, though some studies have not found an association (Calvert et al., 1999; Everett et al., 2007; Fierens et al., 2003; Fujiyoshi et al., 2006; Henriksen et al., 1997; Kang et al., 2006; Kern et al.,

### Serum 1,2,3,4,7,8-Hexachlorodibenzo-p-dioxin (HxCDD) (lipid adjusted)

Geometric mean and selected percentiles of serum concentrations (in pg/g lipid or parts per trillion on a lipid-weight basis) for the U.S. population from the National Health and Nutrition Examination Survey.

| | Survey years | Geometric mean (95% conf. interval) | 50th | 75th | 90th | 95th | Sample size |
|---|---|---|---|---|---|---|---|
| **Total** | 01-02 | * | < LOD | < LOD | 10.7 (<LOD-13 9) | 14.9 (11.7-20.0) | 1239 |
| | 03-04 | * | < LOD | < LOD | < LOD | < LOD | 1861 |
| **Age group** | | | | | | | |
| 12-19 years | 01-02 | † | † | † | † | † | † |
| | 03-04 | * | < LOD | < LOD | < LOD | < LOD | 582 |
| 20 years and older | 01-02 | * | < LOD | < LOD | 10.7 (<LOD-13 9) | 14.9 (11.7-20.0) | 1239 |
| | 03-04 | * | < LOD | < LOD | < LOD | < LOD | 1279 |
| **Gender** | | | | | | | |
| Males | 01-02 | * | < LOD | < LOD | 10.9 (<LOD-14 3) | 14.7 (11 5-17.6) | 566 |
| | 03-04 | * | < LOD | < LOD | < LOD | < LOD | 914 |
| Females | 01-02 | * | < LOD | < LOD | 10.7 (<LOD-14.1) | 15.6 (11.1-23.0) | 673 |
| | 03-04 | * | < LOD | < LOD | < LOD | < LOD | 947 |
| **Race/ethnicity** | | | | | | | |
| Mexican Americans | 01-02 | * | < LOD | < LOD | < LOD | 9.20 (<LOD-11.8) | 263 |
| | 03-04 | * | < LOD | < LOD | < LOD | < LOD | 421 |
| Non-Hispanic blacks | 01-02 | * | < LOD | < LOD | 13.9 (<LOD-17 6) | 18.3 (13 9-23.0) | 220 |
| | 03-04 | * | < LOD | < LOD | < LOD | < LOD | 450 |
| Non-Hispanic whites | 01-02 | * | < LOD | < LOD | 11.3 (<LOD-14.4) | 15.1 (12 0-20.5) | 672 |
| | 03-04 | * | < LOD | < LOD | < LOD | < LOD | 870 |

Limit of detection (LOD, see Data Analysis section) for Survey years 01-02 and 03-04 are 9.0 and 11.9.
† Data not collected for this age group for Survey year 01-02.
< LOD means less than the limit of detection, which may vary for some chemicals by year and by individual sample.
* Not calculated: proportion of results below limit of detection was too high to provide a valid result.

2004; Lee et al., 2006; Michalek et al., 1999, and 2003; ) and *in vitro* and *in vivo* animal studies have provided possible mechanistic plausibility. Immune effects of dioxin-like chemicals and non-dioxin-like PCBs have been reported in animal studies (Carpenter, 2006; U.S.EPA, 2004), but few or consistent effects in humans have been observed (Baccarelli et al., 2002; Halperin et al., 1998; Jung et al., 1998; IARC, 1997).

Similar to some other organochlorine-type chemicals, the dioxin-like chemicals weakly mimic or interfere with the action of estrogen; for instance, dioxin-like chemicals may decrease the effect of estrogen through induction of its metabolism. This action contrasts with the non-dioxin-like PCBs and their metabolites, which may have direct estrogenic action (Carpenter, 2006; Wang et al., 2006; Yoshida et al., 2005). Dioxin and other organochlorine chemicals have been shown to interfere with male and female reproductive development in experimental and wild animals, particularly during gestational exposure (Gao et al., 1999; Grey and Ostby, 1995; Roman et al., 1998; Sonne et al., 2006; Theobald et al., 1997). In studies of women with environmental or accidental exposures, associations between dioxin-like chemical exposures and various reproductive endpoints (Eskenazi et al., 2003; Lawson et al., 2004; Schnorr et al., 2001; Warner et al., 2004 and

2007) and endometriosis (Eskenazi et al., 2002; Fierens et al., 2003; Heilier et al., 2005; Hoffman et al., 2007) have been either absent or of unknown significance, though animal studies have demonstrated reproductive effects at high doses (Arisawa et al., 2005; U.S. EPA, 2004). In men, lowered levels of testosterone have been associated with environmental and occupational exposures to dioxin-like chemicals (Dhooge et al., 2006; Egeland et al., 1994; Gupta et al., 2006; Henriksen et al., 1996; Johnson et al., 2001; Sweeney et al., 1998) and gonadal atrophy and lowered testosterone levels have been observed in animal studies.

TCDD is classified separately by the IARC and NTP as a known human carcinogen. The U.S. EPA (2004) and IARC (1997) concluded that the aggregate evidence supports an association between high-dose TCDD exposure (e.g., encountered in contaminated occupational settings or massive unintentional releases) and increases in the all-cancer category (Steenland et al., 2004). The Institute of Medicine (2005) concluded that human epidemiologic evidence is sufficient for a positive association of herbicides contaminated with TCDD and an increased risk for non-Hodgkin's lymphoma, Hodgkin's lymphoma, chronic lymphocytic leukemia, and soft tissue sarcoma. Other individual polychlorinated dibenzo-*p*-dioxins and dibenzofurans have not been studied sufficiently for IARC

### Serum 1,2,3,4,7,8-Hexachlorodibenzo-*p*-dioxin (HxCDD) (whole weight)

Geometric mean and selected percentiles of serum concentrations (in fg/g of serum or parts per quadrillion) for the U.S. population from the National Health and Nutrition Examination Survey.

| | Survey years | Geometric mean (95% conf. interval) | Selected percentiles (95% confidence interval) | | | | Sample size |
|---|---|---|---|---|---|---|---|
| | | | 50th | 75th | 90th | 95th | |
| Total | 01-02 | * | < LOD | < LOD | 74.7 (<LOD-90.7) | 105 (81.2-139) | 1239 |
| | 03-04 | * | < LOD | < LOD | < LOD | < LOD | 1861 |
| **Age group** | | | | | | | |
| 12-19 years | 01-02 | † | † | † | † | † | † |
| | 03-04 | * | < LOD | < LOD | < LOD | < LOD | 582 |
| 20 years and older | 01-02 | * | < LOD | < LOD | 74.7 (<LOD-90.7) | 105 (81.2-139) | 1239 |
| | 03-04 | * | < LOD | < LOD | < LOD | < LOD | 1279 |
| **Gender** | | | | | | | |
| Males | 01-02 | * | < LOD | < LOD | 73.6 (<LOD-90.7) | 105 (77.9-134) | 566 |
| | 03-04 | * | < LOD | < LOD | < LOD | < LOD | 914 |
| Females | 01-02 | * | < LOD | < LOD | 74.7 (<LOD-90.7) | 102 (78.0-152) | 673 |
| | 03-04 | * | < LOD | < LOD | < LOD | < LOD | 947 |
| **Race/ethnicity** | | | | | | | |
| Mexican Americans | 01-02 | * | < LOD | < LOD | < LOD | 71.2 (<LOD-118) | 263 |
| | 03-04 | * | < LOD | < LOD | < LOD | < LOD | 421 |
| Non-Hispanic blacks | 01-02 | * | < LOD | < LOD | 82.1 (<LOD-130) | 130 (75.7-184) | 220 |
| | 03-04 | * | < LOD | < LOD | < LOD | < LOD | 450 |
| Non-Hispanic whites | 01-02 | * | < LOD | < LOD | 77.5 (<LOD-97.1) | 105 (78.8-143) | 672 |
| | 03-04 | * | < LOD | < LOD | < LOD | < LOD | 870 |

† Data not collected for this age group for Survey year 01-02.
< LOD means less than the limit of detection for the lipid adjusted serum level, which may vary for some chemicals by year and by individual sample.
* Not calculated: proportion of results below limit of detection was too high to provide a valid result.

to classify their human potential for carcinogenicity, although EPA considers these other chemicals as likely human carcinogens (U.S.EPA, 2004). Both IARC and NTP consider polychlorinated biphenyls as likely and probable human carcinogens. Additional information about external exposure (i.e., environmental levels) and health effects is available from ATSDR at: http://www.atsdr.cdc.gov/toxpro2.html and from U.S. EPA at: http://www.epa.gov/ncea/pdfs/dioxin/nas-review/.

## Biomonitoring Information

Serum levels of the dioxin-like chemicals reflect accumulated exposure due to their storage in body fat and slow elimination. Observed differences between people in the levels of these chemicals are due in part to differences in environmental exposure. For instance, eating fish from the Great Lakes region can contain higher levels of certain dioxin-like chemicals, particularly coplanar PCBs and therefore can result in mean lipid adjusted serum concentrations that are several times background values in the U.S. population (Anderson et al., 1998; Falk et al., 1999; Hanrahan et al., 1999; Turyk et al., 2006). Observed differences between people may also be due to longer periods of accumulation of these persistent chemicals. Several studies have shown that levels of the more highly chlorinated dioxins, furans, and PCBs in serum or fat will increase with the age of the population studied (Falk et al., 1999; Geyer et al., 2002; Kang et al., 1997; Luotamo et al., 1991; Patterson et al., 1986). Many of the dioxins, furans and PCBs measured in a representative New Zealand population pooled sampling showed an increasing trend with age (Bates et al., 2004). Also, in a U.S. representative sample from NHANES 1999-2000, participants aged 20 years and older had higher levels than participants aged 12-19 years when levels at the higher percentiles of the more

## Serum 1,2,3,6,7,8-Hexachlorodibenzo-*p*-dioxin (HxCDD) (lipid adjusted)

Geometric mean and selected percentiles of serum concentrations (in pg/g lipid or parts per trillion on a lipid-weight basis) for the U.S. population from the National Health and Nutrition Examination Survey.

| | Survey years | Geometric mean (95% conf. interval) | 50th | 75th | 90th | 95th | Sample size |
|---|---|---|---|---|---|---|---|
| **Total** | 99-00 | * | < LOD | 32.6 (28.3-38.2) | 56.9 (47.4-67.3) | 74.0 (68 3-82.4) | 1885 |
| | 01-02 | 34.6 (29.6-40 6) | 39.2 (32.7-44.7) | 60.8 (50.3-74.2) | 95.2 (76.2-120) | 128 (99.4-153) | 1234 |
| | 03-04 | 17.2 (15.7-18 9) | 20.0 (17.8-22 9) | 36.5 (32.2-40.0) | 53.0 (48.1-59.6) | 68.5 (59 6-74.9) | 1871 |
| **Age group** | | | | | | | |
| 12-19 years | 99-00 | * | < LOD | < LOD | < LOD | 26.7 (20 2-29.6) | 648 |
| | 01-02 | † | † | † | † | † | † |
| | 03-04 | * | < LOD | < LOD | 16.1 (14.3-18.1) | 19.4 (16.4-27.7) | 584 |
| 20 years and older | 99-00 | * | < LOD | 36.2 (31.5-40.7) | 62.8 (53.6-69.1) | 75.6 (70 5-84.2) | 1237 |
| | 01-02 | 34.6 (29.6-40 6) | 39.2 (32.7-44.7) | 60.8 (50.3-74.2) | 95.2 (76.2-120) | 128 (99.4-153) | 1234 |
| | 03-04 | 19.7 (17.8-21 8) | 23.8 (20.7-26.4) | 39.3 (35.4-42.2) | 56.6 (49.7-63.8) | 70.8 (60.7-82.2) | 1287 |
| **Gender** | | | | | | | |
| Males | 99-00 | * | < LOD | 31.5 (23.7-38.2) | 55.0 (45.7-64.2) | 71.3 (59.4-79.4) | 908 |
| | 01-02 | 34.1 (28.3-41.1) | 38.9 (32.1-44.7) | 61.9 (50.0-79.5) | 94.9 (70.8-131) | 130 (88 5-181) | 564 |
| | 03-04 | 17.5 (15.5-19 8) | 19.8 (17.8-21 6) | 35.5 (29.8-40.3) | 52.9 (45.4-63.2) | 70.2 (57 5-88.7) | 920 |
| Females | 99-00 | * | < LOD | 34.9 (29.1-39.7) | 61.2 (51.0-69.2) | 74.9 (68.4-92.2) | 977 |
| | 01-02 | 35.1 (29.9-41 2) | 40.1 (32.4-46 3) | 59.8 (49.8-72.3) | 97.6 (77.1-114) | 126 (108-142) | 670 |
| | 03-04 | 16.9 (15.3-18 6) | 20.5 (17.8-24 6) | 36.9 (33.2-41.0) | 53.6 (48.3-59.6) | 65.6 (60 0-73.4) | 951 |
| **Race/ethnicity** | | | | | | | |
| Mexican Americans | 99-00 | * | < LOD | 21.3 (<LOD-27 6) | 43.3 (34.1-52.3) | 58.0 (49 5-64.8) | 624 |
| | 01-02 | 18.3 (15.6-21.4) | 21.2 (19.4-25 0) | 31.9 (27.5-40.3) | 51.5 (40.3-69.9) | 68.3 (48 0-111) | 260 |
| | 03-04 | * | < LOD | 21.1 (16.3-26.5) | 32.2 (24.5-47.4) | 43.0 (31 5-65.3) | 424 |
| Non-Hispanic blacks | 99-00 | * | < LOD | 31.9 (26.6-41.2) | 56.7 (44.9-74.6) | 81.6 (72 2-91.7) | 402 |
| | 01-02 | 38.9 (33.6-45 0) | 40.3 (33.5-47 3) | 63.5 (54.6-76.9) | 93.9 (78.7-133) | 136 (92 6-185) | 219 |
| | 03-04 | 16.2 (12.9-20.4) | 18.1 (14.4-21 6) | 34.9 (28.4-42.9) | 54.5 (44.4-69.4) | 74.0 (54 3-122) | 454 |
| Non-Hispanic whites | 99-00 | * | < LOD | 35.5 (29.7-40.0) | 60.9 (51.4-68.3) | 74.3 (68 3-83.0) | 703 |
| | 01-02 | 37.8 (31.5-45.4) | 42.8 (33.9-51 2) | 65.0 (52.3-82.9) | 99.6 (78.4-130) | 131 (103-165) | 671 |
| | 03-04 | 18.7 (17.0-20 6) | 22.9 (19.9-26 2) | 38.0 (35.2-41.5) | 56.6 (48.7-63.8) | 69.0 (60 6-74.9) | 872 |

Limit of detection (LOD, see Data Analysis section) for Survey years 99-00, 01-02, and 03-04 are 20.1, 9.1, and 12.3, respectively.
† Data not collected for this age group for Survey year 01-02.
< LOD means less than the limit of detection, which may vary for some chemicals by year and by individual sample.
* Not calculated: proportion of results below limit of detection was too high to provide a valid result.

highly chlorinated congeners were compared (CDC, 2005). Similarly, the TEQ increased with age in an analysis of the NHANES 2003-2004 subsample (Patterson et al., 2009). Other factors also explain differences in levels observed between people. In a TEQ analysis of the NHANES 2001-2002 subsample, the total TEQ increased with age, was lower for Mexican Americans than non-Hispanic whites or blacks, and was higher in smokers than nonsmokers older than 60 years of age (Ferriby et al., 2007). Body mass is also a factor associated with increasing levels of some polychlorinated dibenzo-p-dioxins (Collins et al., 2007; Michalek et al., 1999). Gender is another predictor of levels of some dioxin-like chemicals. Compared with Japanese men, women had higher levels of octachlorodibenzo-p-dioxin, 1,2,3,4,6,7,8-heptachlorodibenzo-p-dioxin, and 1,2,3,7,8,9-hexachlorodibenzo-p-dioxin, but men had higher levels of PCBs 169, 156, and 189 (Arisawa et al., 2003). In the NHANES 2001-2002 subsample, females had higher adjusted geometric mean levels

than males for 1,2,3,4,6,7,8-heptachlorodibenzo-p-dioxin, and 3,3',4,4',5-pentachlorobiphenyl (PCB 126). However, males had higher levels than females for 3,3',4,4',5,5'-hexachlorobiphenyl (PCB 169) (CDC, 2005).

The generally low lipid-adjusted levels observed in the U.S. representative NHANES subsamples of 1999-2000, 2001-2002, and 2003-2004 support the observation that human serum levels of polychlorinated dibenzo-p-dioxins, dibenzofurans, and PCBs have decreased by more than 80% since the 1980s (Aylward and Hays, 2002; Lorber, 2002; Patterson et al., 2009). Levels of some dioxin-like chemicals, such as the hexachlordibenzo-p-dioxins, were shown to decrease gradually from 1993 to 2003 in pooled samples from children in selected regions of Germany, whereas the hexachlordibenzofuran levels showed little change (Link et al., 2005). The levels of polychlorinated dibenzo-p-dioxins, dibenzofurans, and coplanar and mono-ortho-substituted biphenyls seen in the U.S. population

## Serum 1,2,3,6,7,8-Hexachlorodibenzo-p-dioxin (HxCDD) (whole weight)

Geometric mean and selected percentiles of serum concentrations (in fg/g of serum or parts per quadrillion) for the U.S. population from the National Health and Nutrition Examination Survey.

| | Survey years | Geometric mean (95% conf. interval) | 50th | 75th | 90th | 95th | Sample size |
|---|---|---|---|---|---|---|---|
| **Total** | 99-00 | * | < LOD | 202 (168-239) | 374 (314-426) | 496 (429-571) | 1885 |
| | 01-02 | 224 (192-261) | 247 (219-287) | 412 (347-498) | 663 (549-785) | 870 (696-1100) | 1234 |
| | 03-04 | 105 (95.7-116) | 123 (111-136) | 240 (219-263) | 357 (325-395) | 443 (395-487) | 1871 |
| **Age group** | | | | | | | |
| 12-19 years | 99-00 | * | < LOD | < LOD | < LOD | 126 (93.2-155) | 648 |
| | 01-02 | † | † | † | † | † | † |
| | 03-04 | * | < LOD | < LOD | 77.6 (67.4-84.8) | 94.5 (77.6-122) | 584 |
| 20 years and older | 99-00 | * | < LOD | 232 (196-268) | 403 (349-458) | 521 (458-607) | 1237 |
| | 01-02 | 224 (192-261) | 247 (219-287) | 412 (347-498) | 663 (549-785) | 870 (696-1100) | 1234 |
| | 03-04 | 124 (112-138) | 146 (125-172) | 259 (235-285) | 376 (334-422) | 466 (403-528) | 1287 |
| **Gender** | | | | | | | |
| Males | 99-00 | * | < LOD | 189 (134-239) | 353 (278-417) | 449 (378-526) | 908 |
| | 01-02 | 226 (190-270) | 263 (223-301) | 425 (347-540) | 678 (547-794) | 883 (666-1180) | 564 |
| | 03-04 | 108 (95.4-123) | 123 (108-141) | 231 (206-261) | 351 (286-424) | 450 (374-538) | 920 |
| Females | 99-00 | * | < LOD | 213 (174-263) | 400 (344-467) | 553 (467-651) | 977 |
| | 01-02 | 222 (190-260) | 239 (207-281) | 397 (338-474) | 644 (526-771) | 864 (720-1060) | 670 |
| | 03-04 | 103 (92.8-113) | 121 (101-142) | 249 (225-277) | 363 (336-395) | 429 (395-512) | 951 |
| **Race/ethnicity** | | | | | | | |
| Mexican Americans | 99-00 | * | < LOD | 128 (<LOD-167) | 284 (242-334) | 380 (328-419) | 624 |
| | 01-02 | 117 (99.4-139) | 130 (107-157) | 233 (198-270) | 409 (278-524) | 524 (384-731) | 260 |
| | 03-04 | * | < LOD | 141 (106-188) | 221 (188-337) | 327 (210-426) | 424 |
| Non-Hispanic blacks | 99-00 | * | < LOD | 191 (150-234) | 374 (267-424) | 477 (389-568) | 402 |
| | 01-02 | 229 (199-264) | 229 (190-284) | 371 (333-477) | 643 (480-799) | 821 (596-1260) | 219 |
| | 03-04 | 92.9 (73.3-118) | 106 (77.0-125) | 219 (165-260) | 362 (279-460) | 461 (372-689) | 454 |
| Non-Hispanic whites | 99-00 | * | < LOD | 222 (183-270) | 403 (346-460) | 520 (450-615) | 703 |
| | 01-02 | 246 (206-293) | 275 (233-325) | 443 (365-553) | 684 (549-870) | 897 (718-1150) | 671 |
| | 03-04 | 116 (105-127) | 136 (120-165) | 258 (231-286) | 375 (333-418) | 466 (402-519) | 872 |

† Data not collected for this age group for Survey year 01-02.
< LOD means less than the limit of detection for the lipid adjusted serum level, which may vary for some chemicals by year and by individual sample.
* Not calculated: proportion of results below limit of detection was too high to provide a valid result.

are generally well below the levels associated with occupational or unintentional exposures that have produced health effects. There are no firmly established relationships between concentrations (mainly considering TCDD) and health effects in people. Observations following industrial and accidental exposures have suggested that acute exposures resulting in serum concentrations of about 800 pg/g of lipid might be necessary to induce clinical effects such as chloracne, although levels in the thousands of pg/g of lipid do not always produce this effect (Mocarelli et al., 1991). Such studies of clinical effects in people after large unintentional exposures have measured concentrations ranging from several hundred to the tens of thousands of pg/g of lipid of TCDD or equivalent (Eskenazi et al., 2004; Masuda, 2001; Masuda et al., 1998; Mocarelli et al., 1991). However, it has been suggested that background total TEQ for the general population are about 10-100 times the TEQ levels associated with a possible risk for adaptive

or subclinical adverse effects (e.g., endocrine changes) (U.S.EPA, 2004).

In general, observations of the levels of dioxin-like chemicals across percentiles in the NHANES 2003-2004 subsample appear roughly similar to previous NHANES surveys. Note that for some chemicals, detection rates and percentile values will change over survey periods due to improvements in analytical methods and limitations of sample volume. In keeping with results from reports from Germany (Papke et al., 1998), New Zealand (Bates et al., 2004) and elsewhere, U.S. NHANES subsamples have shown that the highly chlorinated and laterally substituted congeners are detected most often (CDC, 2005, Patterson et al., 2009). The following listed dioxin-like chemicals were detectable in greater than 10% of the NHANES 2003-2004 subsample (those in bold letters were detectable in greater than 60% of the subsample). Many of these contribute to a

## Serum 1,2,3,7,8,9-Hexachlorodibenzo-*p*-dioxin (HxCDD) (lipid adjusted)

Geometric mean and selected percentiles of serum concentrations (in pg/g lipid or parts per trillion on a lipid-weight basis) for the U.S. population from the National Health and Nutrition Examination Survey.

| | Survey years | Geometric mean (95% conf. interval) | Selected percentiles ( 95% confidence interval) | | | | Sample size |
|---|---|---|---|---|---|---|---|
| | | | 50th | 75th | 90th | 95th | |
| **Total** | 99-00 | * | < LOD | < LOD | < LOD | < LOD | 1870 |
| | 01-02 | * | < LOD | < LOD | **12.5** (10.5-15.3) | **17.0** (14 3-20.0) | 1238 |
| | 03-04 | * | < LOD | < LOD | < LOD | < LOD | 1869 |
| **Age group** | | | | | | | |
| 12-19 years | 99-00 | * | < LOD | < LOD | < LOD | < LOD | 642 |
| | 01-02 | † | † | † | † | † | † |
| | 03-04 | * | < LOD | < LOD | < LOD | < LOD | 585 |
| 20 years and older | 99-00 | * | < LOD | < LOD | < LOD | < LOD | 1228 |
| | 01-02 | * | < LOD | < LOD | **12.5** (10.5-15.3) | **17.0** (14 3-20.0) | 1238 |
| | 03-04 | * | < LOD | < LOD | < LOD | < LOD | 1284 |
| **Gender** | | | | | | | |
| Males | 99-00 | * | < LOD | < LOD | < LOD | < LOD | 895 |
| | 01-02 | * | < LOD | < LOD | **12.1** (<LOD-14 8) | **15.1** (12 9-18.5) | 567 |
| | 03-04 | * | < LOD | < LOD | < LOD | < LOD | 918 |
| Females | 99-00 | * | < LOD | < LOD | < LOD | < LOD | 975 |
| | 01-02 | * | < LOD | < LOD | **13.0** (10.7-16.8) | **18.3** (15.7-21.1) | 671 |
| | 03-04 | * | < LOD | < LOD | < LOD | < LOD | 951 |
| **Race/ethnicity** | | | | | | | |
| Mexican Americans | 99-00 | * | < LOD | < LOD | < LOD | < LOD | 618 |
| | 01-02 | * | < LOD | < LOD | **9.60** (<LOD-11 6) | **12.2** (<LOD-20.6) | 262 |
| | 03-04 | * | < LOD | < LOD | < LOD | < LOD | 423 |
| Non-Hispanic blacks | 99-00 | * | < LOD | < LOD | < LOD | < LOD | 396 |
| | 01-02 | * | < LOD | < LOD | **14.6** (11.2-20.0) | **19.9** (14 6-23.9) | 220 |
| | 03-04 | * | < LOD | < LOD | < LOD | < LOD | 454 |
| Non-Hispanic whites | 99-00 | * | < LOD | < LOD | < LOD | < LOD | 701 |
| | 01-02 | * | < LOD | < LOD | **12.9** (9.90-15.9) | **17.3** (14.7-20.6) | 672 |
| | 03-04 | * | < LOD | < LOD | < LOD | < LOD | 871 |

Limit of detection (LOD, see Data Analysis section) for Survey years 99-00, 01-02, and 03-04 are 20.3, 9.3, and 12.3, respectively.
† Data not collected for this age group for Survey year 01-02.
< LOD means less than the limit of detection, which may vary for some chemicals by year and by individual sample.
* Not calculated: proportion of results below limit of detection was too high to provide a valid result.

significant portion of the total TEQ. The total TEQ at the 90th percentile of the U.S. population in NHANES 2003-2004 was 30.0 pg/g of lipid (Patterson et al. 2009).

- **1,2,3,4,6,7,8,9-octachlorodibenzo-*p*-dioxin**
- **1,2,3,4,6,7,8-heptachlorodibenzo-*p*-dioxin**
- **1,2,3,6,7,8-hexachlorodibenzo-*p*-dioxin**
- 1,2,3,7,8-pentachlorodibenzo-*p*-dioxin
- 2,3,7,8-tetachlordibenzo-*p*-dioxin
- **1,2,3,4,6,7,8-heptachlorodibenzofuran**
- 1,2,3,4,7,8-hexachlorodibenzofuran
- 2,3,4,7,8-pentachlorodibenzofuran
- coplanar PCBs **126** and 169
- mono-*ortho* substituted PCBs **105, 118, 156, 157, 167, 189**

## Octachlorodibenzo-*p*-dioxin

Of the dioxins and furans measured in the U.S. representative subsamples of NHANES 1999-2000, 2001-2002, and 2003-2004, octachlorodibenzo-*p*-dioxin typically is present in the highest concentration, but contributes little to the TEQ, with the other commonly detected dioxin and furan congeners being more than eight-fold lower in concentration. Levels of octachlorodibenzo-*p*-dioxin that were similar to slightly higher than those in these NHANES subsamples were seen in a representative pooled sampling New Zealander residents aged 15 years and older obtained during 1997-1998 and also in a small convenience sample of German residents aged 18-71 years in 1996 (Bates et al., 2004; Papke et al., 1998; CDC, 2005). Similar levels were also found in 232 Belgian blood donors in 2000 (Debacker et al., 2007).

## Hexachlorodibenzo-*p*-dioxins

The three major hexachlorodibenzo-*p*-dioxins are assigned equal TEF values, but the 1,2,3,6,7,8-hexachlorodibenzo-*p*-dioxin often demonstrates multifold higher concentrations than the other two hexachlorodibenzo-

### Serum 1,2,3,7,8,9-Hexachlorodibenzo-*p*-dioxin (HxCDD) (whole weight)

Geometric mean and selected percentiles of serum concentrations (in fg/g of serum or parts per quadrillion) for the U.S. population from the National Health and Nutrition Examination Survey.

| | Survey years | Geometric mean (95% conf. interval) | 50th | 75th | 90th | 95th | Sample size |
|---|---|---|---|---|---|---|---|
| **Total** | 99-00 | * | < LOD | < LOD | < LOD | < LOD | 1870 |
| | 01-02 | * | < LOD | < LOD | 86.5 (68.8-108) | 121 (99.5-146) | 1238 |
| | 03-04 | * | < LOD | < LOD | < LOD | < LOD | 1869 |
| **Age group** | | | | | | | |
| 12-19 years | 99-00 | * | < LOD | < LOD | < LOD | < LOD | 642 |
| | 01-02 | † | † | † | † | † | † |
| | 03-04 | * | < LOD | < LOD | < LOD | < LOD | 585 |
| 20 years and older | 99-00 | * | < LOD | < LOD | < LOD | < LOD | 1228 |
| | 01-02 | * | < LOD | < LOD | 86.5 (68.8-108) | 121 (99.5-146) | 1238 |
| | 03-04 | * | < LOD | < LOD | < LOD | < LOD | 1284 |
| **Gender** | | | | | | | |
| Males | 99-00 | * | < LOD | < LOD | < LOD | < LOD | 895 |
| | 01-02 | * | < LOD | < LOD | 84.1 (<LOD-104) | 108 (90.6-142) | 567 |
| | 03-04 | * | < LOD | < LOD | < LOD | < LOD | 918 |
| Females | 99-00 | * | < LOD | < LOD | < LOD | < LOD | 975 |
| | 01-02 | * | < LOD | < LOD | 89.8 (67.9-121) | 123 (102-157) | 671 |
| | 03-04 | * | < LOD | < LOD | < LOD | < LOD | 951 |
| **Race/ethnicity** | | | | | | | |
| Mexican Americans | 99-00 | * | < LOD | < LOD | < LOD | < LOD | 618 |
| | 01-02 | * | < LOD | < LOD | 74.7 (<LOD-104) | 107 (<LOD-167) | 262 |
| | 03-04 | * | < LOD | < LOD | < LOD | < LOD | 423 |
| Non-Hispanic blacks | 99-00 | * | < LOD | < LOD | < LOD | < LOD | 396 |
| | 01-02 | * | < LOD | < LOD | 92.6 (62.8-126) | 123 (82.6-169) | 220 |
| | 03-04 | * | < LOD | < LOD | < LOD | < LOD | 454 |
| Non-Hispanic whites | 99-00 | * | < LOD | < LOD | < LOD | < LOD | 701 |
| | 01-02 | * | < LOD | < LOD | 88.1 (67.9-119) | 124 (96.6-152) | 672 |
| | 03-04 | * | < LOD | < LOD | < LOD | < LOD | 871 |

† Data not collected for this age group for Survey year 01-02.
< LOD means less than the limit of detection for the lipid adjusted serum level, which may vary for some chemicals by year and by individual sample.
* Not calculated: proportion of results below limit of detection was too high to provide a valid result.

*p*-dioxins; about six-fold higher in the NHANES 2001-2002 subsample (CDC, 2005). The unadjusted geometric mean levels of 1,2,3,6,7,8-hexachlorodibenzo-*p*-dioxin in 2003-2004 and in 2001-2002 were 34.6 vs. 17.2 pg/g of lipid, respectively. The geometric mean levels of 1,2,3,6,7,8-hexachlorodibenzo-*p*-dioxin in the 2001-2002 subsample were slightly higher than levels in either German or New Zealand study mentioned above (Bates et al., 2004; Papke et al., 1998). A convenience sample of Japanese men and women aged 20-76 years studied during 1996-1997 also showed lower median levels than levels in the NHANES 2001-2002 subsample (Arisawa et al., 2003; CDC, 2005)

### 1,2,3,7,8-Pentachlorodibenzo-*p*-dioxin

In prior NHANES surveys, 1,2,3,7,8-pentachlorodibenzo-*p*-dioxin concentrations were nearly 60-fold lower than octachlorodibenzo-*p*-dioxin levels (at the comparable

percentiles) (CDC, 2005), but because of a 10,000-fold greater TEF (equal to that of TCDD), the contribution of 1,2,3,7,8-pentachlorodibenzo-*p*-dioxin to the total TEQ would be about 160 times greater than the octachlorodibenzo-*p*-dioxin. Levels of 1,2,3,7,8-pentachlorodibenzo-*p*-dioxin for the total population at the 95th percentile in the NHANES 2001-2002 and 2003-2004 subsamples were 15.8 pg/g and 11.0 pg/g lipid, respectively. In 1996, a convenience sample of German residents aged 18-71 years showed that levels of 1,2,3,7,8-pentachlorodibenzo-*p*-dioxin at the 95th percentile were 9.9 pg/g lipid (Papke et al., 1998). The 95th percentile of a group of workers with distant past trichlorophenol exposure was about twice as high as the 95th percentile for adults in NHANES 2001-2002 (CDC, 2005; Collins et al., 2006)

### 2,3,7,8-Tetrachlorodibenzo-*p*-dioxin

TCDD is considered the most potent of the dioxin-like

## Serum 1,2,3,4,6,7,8,9-Octachlorodibenzo-*p*-dioxin (OCDD) (lipid adjusted)

Geometric mean and selected percentiles of serum concentrations (in pg/g lipid or parts per trillion on a lipid-weight basis) for the U.S. population from the National Health and Nutrition Examination Survey.

| | Survey years | Geometric mean (95% conf. interval) | Selected percentiles ( 95% confidence interval) 50th | 75th | 90th | 95th | Sample size |
|---|---|---|---|---|---|---|---|
| **Total** | 99-00 | * | < LOD | 406 (359-453) | 674 (597-767) | 913 (787-1010) | 1921 |
| | 01-02 | 346 (<LOD-394) | 333 (<LOD-402) | 573 (498-668) | 944 (780-1090) | 1260 (998-1610) | 1171 |
| | 03-04 | * | < LOD | 336 (283-389) | 582 (490-658) | 767 (645-913) | 1851 |
| **Age group** | | | | | | | |
| 12-19 years | 99-00 | * | < LOD | < LOD | < LOD | 421 (363-517) | 667 |
| | 01-02 | † | † | † | † | † | † |
| | 03-04 | * | < LOD | < LOD | 244 (<LOD-330) | 352 (264-458) | 581 |
| 20 years and older | 99-00 | * | < LOD | 445 (389-496) | 710 (624-802) | 948 (822-1080) | 1254 |
| | 01-02 | 346 (<LOD-394) | 333 (<LOD-402) | 573 (498-668) | 944 (780-1090) | 1260 (998-1610) | 1171 |
| | 03-04 | 220 (<LOD-244) | 223 (<LOD-243) | 358 (297-421) | 597 (502-719) | 794 (665-978) | 1270 |
| **Gender** | | | | | | | |
| Males | 99-00 | * | < LOD | < LOD | 517 (447-580) | 704 (563-838) | 919 |
| | 01-02 | * | < LOD | 442 (346-579) | 767 (593-968) | 1030 (837-1240) | 517 |
| | 03-04 | * | < LOD | 270 (244-320) | 457 (377-559) | 668 (501-856) | 910 |
| Females | 99-00 | * | < LOD | 504 (422-579) | 802 (674-928) | 1010 (928-1180) | 1002 |
| | 01-02 | 410 (356-472) | 405 (335-502) | 647 (574-751) | 1020 (858-1360) | 1450 (1060-1780) | 654 |
| | 03-04 | 235 (<LOD-256) | 238 (225-248) | 402 (321-486) | 640 (551-749) | 829 (675-1020) | 941 |
| **Race/ethnicity** | | | | | | | |
| Mexican Americans | 99-00 | * | < LOD | 418 (365-502) | 703 (610-873) | 940 (737-1230) | 632 |
| | 01-02 | * | < LOD | 432 (394-545) | 755 (578-1220) | 1150 (696-1640) | 250 |
| | 03-04 | * | < LOD | 296 (225-356) | 452 (363-540) | 588 (417-861) | 419 |
| Non-Hispanic blacks | 99-00 | * | < LOD | 444 (371-519) | 741 (566-983) | 1120 (799-1560) | 411 |
| | 01-02 | 421 (352-503) | 420 (339-509) | 682 (537-907) | 1110 (956-1520) | 1640 (1130-1900) | 210 |
| | 03-04 | * | < LOD | 345 (276-455) | 642 (513-883) | 926 (636-1310) | 448 |
| Non-Hispanic whites | 99-00 | * | < LOD | 391 (333-452) | 625 (562-754) | 861 (676-1010) | 721 |
| | 01-02 | 349 (<LOD-409) | 335 (<LOD-421) | 574 (496-679) | 945 (764-1170) | 1290 (972-1660) | 632 |
| | 03-04 | * | < LOD | 343 (282-403) | 585 (464-674) | 758 (635-922) | 865 |

Limit of detection (LOD, see Data Analysis section) for Survey years 99-00, 01-02, and 03-04 are 329.0, 319.0, and 218.0, respectively.
† Data not collected for this age group for Survey year 01-02.
< LOD means less than the limit of detection, which may vary for some chemicals by year and by individual sample.
* Not calculated: proportion of results below limit of detection was too high to provide a valid result.

chemicals and environmental exposure usually results in very low serum concentrations. In the NHANES 2003-2004 subsample, the 95th percentile for the total population (12 years and older) was 5.2 picograms/gram (pg/g) of lipid. In 1996, the 95th percentile for lipid adjusted serum TCDD levels in 139 Germans aged 18-71 years was 4.3 pg/g of lipid, with that percentile comprising mainly older individuals (Papke, 1998). In contrast, the most highly exposed females following the Seveso, Italy, factory explosion in 1976 had median lipid adjusted levels of 272 pg/g lipid (Eskenazi et al., 2004). TCDD levels in chemical plant workers with higher exposures have ranged as high as 2,000 pg/g lipid (IARC, 1997). Median serum TCDD levels measured in chemical production workers 15 years after workplace exposure ended were 68 pg/g of lipid (Calvert et al., 1996; Calvert et al., 1999). TCDD levels in the U.S. general population were also lower than workers with past trichlorophenol exposure (Collins et al., 2006) and lower than Vietnam veterans 20 years after duty-related exposure

to Agent Orange (median serum TCDD concentration was 12.2 pg/g of lipid) (Henriksen et al., 1997).

**Polychlorinated dibenzofurans**

Of the polychlorinated dibenzofurans, the following could be characterized at the 95th percentiles (or lower) in the NHANES 1999-2000, 2001-2002 and 2003-2004 subsamples: 1,2,3,4,6,7,8-heptachlorodibenzofuran, 1,2,3,4,7,8-hexachlorodibenzofuran, 1,2,3,6,7,8-hexachlorodibenzofuran, and 2,3,4,7,8-pentachlorodibenzofuran. Generally, these levels are similar to other large population studies. In 237 workers with past exposure to trichlorophenol, where little polychlorinated dibenzofuran exposure would be expected, higher percentiles values were similar to a referent population and to the NHANES 1999-2000 and 2001-2002 subsamples (Collins et al., 2007; CDC, 2005). In 232 Belgian blood donors from the year 2000, the geometric mean level of 1,2,3,4,6,7,8-heptachlorodibenzofuran was several times lower than the geometric mean

### Serum 1,2,3,4,6,7,8,9-Octachlorodibenzo-*p*-dioxin (OCDD) (whole weight)

Geometric mean and selected percentiles of serum concentrations (in fg/g of serum or parts per quadrillion) for the U.S. population from the National Health and Nutrition Examination Survey.

| | Survey years | Geometric mean (95% conf. interval) | Selected percentiles (95% confidence interval) | | | | Sample size |
|---|---|---|---|---|---|---|---|
| | | | 50th | 75th | 90th | 95th | |
| **Total** | 99-00 | * | < LOD | 2530 (2230-2880) | 4260 (3770-4760) | 5950 (5090-6790) | 1921 |
| | 01-02 | 2230 (<LOD-2540) | 2170 (<LOD-2550) | 3860 (3180-4520) | 6460 (5140-8290) | 9110 (6940-11400) | 1171 |
| | 03-04 | * | < LOD | 2180 (1830-2540) | 3760 (3100-4540) | 5020 (4190-6070) | 1851 |
| **Age group** | | | | | | | |
| 12-19 years | 99-00 | * | < LOD | < LOD | < LOD | 1910 (1600-2340) | 667 |
| | 01-02 | † | † | † | † | † | † |
| | 03-04 | * | < LOD | < LOD | 1160 (<LOD1590) | 1780 (1160-2850) | 581 |
| 20 years and older | 99-00 | * | < LOD | 2810 (2480-3110) | 4570 (4100-5020) | 6200 (5340-7300) | 1254 |
| | 01-02 | 2230 (<LOD-2540) | 2170 (<LOD-2550) | 3860 (3180-4520) | 6460 (5140-8290) | 9110 (6940-11400) | 1171 |
| | 03-04 | 1380 (<LOD-1540) | 1360 (<LOD-1470) | 2350 (1970-2900) | 4030 (3370-4700) | 5340 (4490-6370) | 1270 |
| **Gender** | | | | | | | |
| Males | 99-00 | * | < LOD | < LOD | 3160 (2760-3760) | 4160 (3320-5570) | 919 |
| | 01-02 | * | < LOD | 3160 (2410-4070) | 5270 (4070-7140) | 7620 (6020-9760) | 517 |
| | 03-04 | * | < LOD | 1780 (1540-2070) | 3090 (2410-4020) | 4190 (3410-5350) | 910 |
| Females | 99-00 | * | < LOD | 3110 (2680-3560) | 5090 (4610-5740) | 6760 (5870-8710) | 1002 |
| | 01-02 | 2590 (2250-2980) | 2620 (2160-3000) | 4340 (3880-4860) | 6990 (5870-9040) | 10000 (7070-12300) | 654 |
| | 03-04 | 1420 (<LOD-1560) | 1410 (1300-1510) | 2700 (2210-3030) | 4340 (3750-4830) | 5770 (4590-6740) | 941 |
| **Race/ethnicity** | | | | | | | |
| Mexican Americans | 99-00 | * | < LOD | 2470 (2240-2990) | 4350 (3660-5570) | 6560 (5340-7590) | 632 |
| | 01-02 | * | < LOD | 3410 (2760-3860) | 5810 (4250-7670) | 8050 (5760-11800) | 250 |
| | 03-04 | * | < LOD | 1880 (1560-2220) | 3240 (2450-3880) | 3910 (3240-4630) | 419 |
| Non-Hispanic blacks | 99-00 | * | < LOD | 2520 (2090-2950) | 4770 (4040-5740) | 7140 (4740-10700) | 411 |
| | 01-02 | 2480 (2050-3000) | 2460 (2060-2970) | 4170 (3160-5560) | 7250 (5470-9920) | 9920 (7990-12000) | 210 |
| | 03-04 | * | < LOD | 2150 (1780-2880) | 3860 (3080-5640) | 5720 (3750-7830) | 448 |
| Non-Hispanic whites | 99-00 | * | < LOD | 2560 (2160-2910) | 4120 (3580-4780) | 5800 (4740-6790) | 721 |
| | 01-02 | 2270 (<LOD-2660) | 2200 (<LOD-2770) | 3860 (3090-4720) | 6530 (4890-8860) | 9150 (6630-12300) | 632 |
| | 03-04 | * | < LOD | 2220 (1830-2700) | 3770 (3040-4680) | 5050 (4190-6350) | 865 |

† Data not collected for this age group for Survey year 01-02
< LOD means less than the limit of detection for the lipid adjusted serum level, which may vary for some chemicals by year and by individual sample.
* Not calculated: proportion of results below limit of detection was too high to provide a valid result.

value in the NHANES 2001-2002 subsample of adults and the other dibenzofurans examined in the Belgian donors were lower than the limits of detection in NHANES 2000-2001 (CDC, 2005; Debacker et al., 2007). In Yucheng rice oil contamination victims when examined 15 years after their exposure, levels of the polychlorinated dibenzofurans were still hundreds of times higher than in levels for the U.S. population observed in the NHANES subsamples in this *Report* (Hsu et al., 2005).

## Coplanar PCBs

The coplanar PCBs typically contribute less than about 15% to the total TEQ in the U.S. population (Ferriby et al., 2007). In the NHANES 2001-2002 subsample, the geometric mean levels of PCBs 126 and 169 for adults aged 20 years and older were similar or slightly lower than those reported from a representative pooled sample of New Zealanders in 1996-1997 (Bates et al., 2004; CDC,

2005) and from a smaller sample of non-occupationally exposed men and women aged 20-76 years in Japan in 1999 (Arisawa et al., 2003). Higher levels of these PCBs have been reported for persons consuming sport fish caught in the Great Lakes region (Turyk et al., 2006). In 311 residents of northern Italy, serum PCB 126 and 169 were not detectable, though other PCBs tended to be higher than in the recent NHANES subsamples (Apostoli et al., 2005; CDC, 2005).

## Mono-*ortho*-substituted PCBs

Of the mono-*ortho*-substituted PCB congeners, the most frequently detected in general population studies are PCBs 118 and 156. Of these, PCB 118 levels were higher than levels of PCB 156 in the NHANES 1999-2000, 2001-2002, and 2003-2004 subsamples, although PCB 156 contributes more to the TEQ because its TEF is five-fold greater than the TEF of PCB 118. Although these PCBs are relatively less potent (i.e., lower TEFs), their contribution

### Serum 1,2,3,7,8-Pentachlorodibenzo-*p*-dioxin (PeCDD) (lipid adjusted)

Geometric mean and selected percentiles of serum concentrations (in pg/g lipid or parts per trillion on a lipid-weight basis) for the U.S. population from the National Health and Nutrition Examination Survey.

| | Survey years | Geometric mean (95% conf. interval) | 50th | 75th | 90th | 95th | Sample size |
|---|---|---|---|---|---|---|---|
| **Total** | 99-00 | * | < LOD | < LOD | < LOD | < LOD | 1915 |
| | 01-02 | * | < LOD | < LOD | 11.3 (9.30-13.6) | 15.8 (13 3-19.8) | 1236 |
| | 03-04 | * | < LOD | 6.10 (5.50-6.80) | 9.00 (8.30-9.70) | 11.0 (9.90-12.2) | 1878 |
| **Age group** | | | | | | | |
| 12-19 years | 99-00 | * | < LOD | < LOD | < LOD | < LOD | 659 |
| | 01-02 | † | † | † | † | † | † |
| | 03-04 | * | < LOD | < LOD | < LOD | 4.80 (<LOD-5.90) | 588 |
| 20 years and older | 99-00 | * | < LOD | < LOD | < LOD | < LOD | 1256 |
| | 01-02 | * | < LOD | < LOD | 11.3 (9.30-13.6) | 15.8 (13 3-19.8) | 1236 |
| | 03-04 | * | < LOD | 6.60 (5.90-7.20) | 9.30 (8.60-10.1) | 11.3 (10.1-12.7) | 1290 |
| **Gender** | | | | | | | |
| Males | 99-00 | * | < LOD | < LOD | < LOD | < LOD | 920 |
| | 01-02 | * | < LOD | < LOD | 10.8 (9.10-13.3) | 14.5 (11.7-19.4) | 564 |
| | 03-04 | * | < LOD | 5.90 (5.30-6.40) | 8.90 (7.90-9 60) | 11.0 (9.60-12.7) | 923 |
| Females | 99-00 | * | < LOD | < LOD | < LOD | < LOD | 995 |
| | 01-02 | * | < LOD | 6.10 (<LOD-7.80) | 11.8 (9.40-14.3) | 16.6 (13.7-20.8) | 672 |
| | 03-04 | * | < LOD | 6.50 (5.70-7.20) | 9.10 (8.30-10.1) | 11.0 (10 0-12.2) | 955 |
| **Race/ethnicity** | | | | | | | |
| Mexican Americans | 99-00 | * | < LOD | < LOD | < LOD | < LOD | 632 |
| | 01-02 | * | < LOD | < LOD | < LOD | 8.70 (<LOD-12.7) | 262 |
| | 03-04 | * | < LOD | < LOD | 6.50 (5.20-7 90) | 7.80 (6.70-9.20) | 425 |
| Non-Hispanic blacks | 99-00 | * | < LOD | < LOD | < LOD | < LOD | 408 |
| | 01-02 | * | < LOD | 7.70 (<LOD-9.30) | 13.9 (9.60-18.4) | 18.4 (14 2-24.0) | 218 |
| | 03-04 | * | < LOD | 6.40 (5.30-8.20) | 9.90 (8.50-13.4) | 14.4 (9.60-20.1) | 455 |
| Non-Hispanic whites | 99-00 | * | < LOD | < LOD | < LOD | < LOD | 717 |
| | 01-02 | * | < LOD | < LOD | 11.7 (9.50-14.3) | 16.7 (13 6-20.2) | 672 |
| | 03-04 | * | < LOD | 6.50 (5.80-7.10) | 9.30 (8.60-10.0) | 11.1 (10.1-12.2) | 877 |

Limit of detection (LOD, see Data Analysis section) for Survey years 99-00, 01-02, and 03-04 are 14.2, 6.0, and 4.5, respectively.
† Data not collected for this age group for Survey year 01-02.
< LOD means less than the limit of detection, which may vary for some chemicals by year and by individual sample.
* Not calculated: proportion of results below limit of detection was too high to provide a valid result.

to the total TEQ in the U.S. population is about 25% (Ferriby et al., 2007) since they are present in much higher concentrations than are the coplanar PCBs, dioxins, and furans. In a convenience sample of the U.S. population in 1988 (Patterson et al., 1994), levels of PCB 118 were five-fold higher than in the NHANES 1999-2002 subsamples (CDC, 2005). Comparable levels of PCB 156 levels in NHANES 1999-2000 are slightly lower than those reported for a Canadian population study in 1994 (Longnecker et al., 2000). In a referent population of 311 residents in northern Italy during 2001-2003, the 95th percentile levels of PCB 156 and PCB 118 were two to threefold higher than for the NHANES 1999-2002 subsamples (Apostoli et al., 2005; CDC, 2005). Levels of PCB 156 and PCB 118 were slightly higher in a Swedish study of 150 men than in the NHANES 1999-2000 subsample, possibly due to higher fish intake in the Swedish population (Glynn et al., 2000; CDC, 2005). However, in fish-consuming Japanese men and women studied during 1996-1997, PCB 118 levels at the 75th percentile were similar to levels in the NHANES 2001-2002 subsample (Arisawa et al., 2003).

Finding a measurable amount of one or more of the polychlorinated dibenzo-*p*-dioxins, dibenzofurans, coplanar or mono-*ortho*-substituted biphenyls in serum does not mean that the level of one or more of these chemicals causes an adverse health effect. Biomonitoring studies of serum polychlorinated dibenzo-*p*-dioxins, dibenzofurans, coplanar or mono-*ortho*-substituted biphenyls provide physicians and public health officials with reference values so that they can determine whether or not people have been exposed to higher levels of polychlorinated dibenzo-*p*-dioxins, dibenzofurans, coplanar or mono-*ortho*-substituted biphenyls than levels found in the general population. Biomonitoring data can also help scientists plan and conduct research on exposure and health effects.

## Serum 1,2,3,7,8-Pentachlorodibenzo-*p*-dioxin (PeCDD) (whole weight)

Geometric mean and selected percentiles of serum concentrations (in fg/g of serum or parts per quadrillion) for the U.S. population from the National Health and Nutrition Examination Survey.

| | Survey years | Geometric mean (95% conf. interval) | Selected percentiles (95% confidence interval) | | | | Sample size |
|---|---|---|---|---|---|---|---|
| | | | 50th | 75th | 90th | 95th | |
| **Total** | 99-00 | * | < LOD | < LOD | < LOD | < LOD | 1915 |
| | 01-02 | * | < LOD | < LOD | 77.8 (62.8-96.3) | 117 (90.3-133) | 1236 |
| | 03-04 | * | < LOD | 40.7 (37.4-43.0) | 60.3 (53.2-67.4) | 76.1 (66.9-87.4) | 1878 |
| **Age group** | | | | | | | |
| 12-19 years | 99-00 | * | < LOD | < LOD | < LOD | < LOD | 659 |
| | 01-02 | † | † | † | † | † | † |
| | 03-04 | * | < LOD | < LOD | < LOD | 23.8 (<LOD-27.2) | 588 |
| 20 years and older | 99-00 | * | < LOD | < LOD | < LOD | < LOD | 1256 |
| | 01-02 | * | < LOD | < LOD | 77.8 (62.8-96.3) | 117 (90.3-133) | 1236 |
| | 03-04 | * | < LOD | 43.0 (39 2-47.8) | 63.5 (55.6-71.5) | 80.7 (67.9-89 9) | 1290 |
| **Gender** | | | | | | | |
| Males | 99-00 | * | < LOD | < LOD | < LOD | < LOD | 920 |
| | 01-02 | * | < LOD | < LOD | 76.1 (54.7-93.7) | 107 (83.5-133) | 564 |
| | 03-04 | * | < LOD | 39.3 (35.1-43.4) | 57.3 (49.3-66.1) | 67.8 (58.7-90.4) | 923 |
| Females | 99-00 | * | < LOD | < LOD | < LOD | < LOD | 995 |
| | 01-02 | * | < LOD | 37.8 (<LOD-50.2) | 80.4 (62.9-107) | 121 (85.7-167) | 672 |
| | 03-04 | * | < LOD | 41.8 (37.7-45.2) | 63.6 (55.9-72.9) | 80.7 (70.5-88 3) | 955 |
| **Race/ethnicity** | | | | | | | |
| Mexican Americans | 99-00 | * | < LOD | < LOD | < LOD | < LOD | 632 |
| | 01-02 | * | < LOD | < LOD | < LOD | 66.0 (<LOD-111) | 262 |
| | 03-04 | * | < LOD | < LOD | 44.5 (34.2-52.0) | 52.8 (44.5-76 6) | 425 |
| Non-Hispanic blacks | 99-00 | * | < LOD | < LOD | < LOD | < LOD | 408 |
| | 01-02 | * | < LOD | 43.8 (<LOD-53.8) | 81.9 (58.2-117) | 123 (81.9-169) | 218 |
| | 03-04 | * | < LOD | 39.7 (30 6-48.0) | 67.3 (48.0-93.0) | 93.0 (66.7-137) | 455 |
| Non-Hispanic whites | 99-00 | * | < LOD | < LOD | < LOD | < LOD | 717 |
| | 01-02 | * | < LOD | < LOD | 80.8 (61.6-107) | 121 (88.6-142) | 672 |
| | 03-04 | * | < LOD | 42.6 (38 6-45.1) | 63.4 (55.4-67.9) | 78.8 (67.9-84.7) | 877 |

† Data not collected for this age group for Survey year 01-02.
< LOD means less than the limit of detection for the lipid adjusted serum level, which may vary for some chemicals by year and by individual sample.
* Not calculated: proportion of results below limit of detection was too high to provide a valid result.

## Serum 2,3,7,8-Tetrachlorodibenzo-*p*-dioxin (TCDD) (lipid adjusted)

Geometric mean and selected percentiles of serum concentrations (in pg/g lipid or parts per trillion on a lipid-weight basis) for the U.S. population from the National Health and Nutrition Examination Survey.

| | Survey years | Geometric mean (95% conf. interval) | Selected percentiles ( 95% confidence interval) | | | | Sample size |
|---|---|---|---|---|---|---|---|
| | | | 50th | 75th | 90th | 95th | |
| **Total** | 99-00 | * | < LOD | < LOD | < LOD | < LOD | 1898 |
| | 01-02 | * | < LOD | < LOD | < LOD | < LOD | 1228 |
| | 03-04 | * | < LOD | < LOD | 4.10 (<LOD-4.40) | 5.20 (4.30-5.80) | 1876 |
| **Age group** | | | | | | | |
| 12-19 years | 99-00 | * | < LOD | < LOD | < LOD | < LOD | 658 |
| | 01-02 | † | † | † | † | † | † |
| | 03-04 | * | < LOD | < LOD | < LOD | < LOD | 588 |
| 20 years and older | 99-00 | * | < LOD | < LOD | < LOD | < LOD | 1240 |
| | 01-02 | * | < LOD | < LOD | < LOD | < LOD | 1228 |
| | 03-04 | * | < LOD | < LOD | 4.30 (3.90-4 60) | 5.30 (4.50-6.10) | 1288 |
| **Gender** | | | | | | | |
| Males | 99-00 | * | < LOD | < LOD | < LOD | < LOD | 912 |
| | 01-02 | * | < LOD | < LOD | < LOD | < LOD | 559 |
| | 03-04 | * | < LOD | < LOD | < LOD | 4.60 (3.80-5.30) | 921 |
| Females | 99-00 | * | < LOD | < LOD | < LOD | < LOD | 986 |
| | 01-02 | * | < LOD | < LOD | < LOD | 6.40 (<LOD-9.20) | 669 |
| | 03-04 | * | < LOD | < LOD | 4.40 (4.00-4 90) | 5.50 (4.50-6.60) | 955 |
| **Race/ethnicity** | | | | | | | |
| Mexican Americans | 99-00 | * | < LOD | < LOD | < LOD | < LOD | 630 |
| | 01-02 | * | < LOD | < LOD | < LOD | < LOD | 262 |
| | 03-04 | * | < LOD | < LOD | < LOD | 3.80 (<LOD-5.50) | 424 |
| Non-Hispanic blacks | 99-00 | * | < LOD | < LOD | < LOD | < LOD | 404 |
| | 01-02 | * | < LOD | < LOD | < LOD | 7.50 (<LOD-10.0) | 217 |
| | 03-04 | * | < LOD | < LOD | 4.50 (<LOD-6.10) | 6.20 (4.40-10.3) | 454 |
| Non-Hispanic whites | 99-00 | * | < LOD | < LOD | < LOD | < LOD | 709 |
| | 01-02 | * | < LOD | < LOD | < LOD | < LOD | 665 |
| | 03-04 | * | < LOD | < LOD | 4.10 (<LOD-4.50) | 5.20 (4.30-5.90) | 877 |

Limit of detection (LOD, see Data Analysis section) for Survey years 99-00, 01-02, and 03-04 are 12.1, 5.8, and 3.8, respectively.
† Data not collected for this age group for Survey year 01-02.
< LOD means less than the limit of detection, which may vary for some chemicals by year and by individual sample.
* Not calculated: proportion of results below limit of detection was too high to provide a valid result.

## Serum 2,3,7,8-Tetrachlorodibenzo-*p*-dioxin (TCDD) (whole weight)

Geometric mean and selected percentiles of serum concentrations (in fg/g of serum or parts per quadrillion) for the U.S. population from the National Health and Nutrition Examination Survey.

| | Survey years | Geometric mean (95% conf. interval) | Selected percentiles ( 95% confidence interval) | | | | Sample size |
|---|---|---|---|---|---|---|---|
| | | | 50th | 75th | 90th | 95th | |
| **Total** | 99-00 | * | < LOD | < LOD | < LOD | < LOD | 1898 |
| | 01-02 | * | < LOD | < LOD | < LOD | < LOD | 1228 |
| | 03-04 | * | < LOD | < LOD | 27.5 (<LOD-30.1) | 34.1 (30.2-39 6) | 1876 |
| **Age group** | | | | | | | |
| 12-19 years | 99-00 | * | < LOD | < LOD | < LOD | < LOD | 658 |
| | 01-02 | † | † | † | † | † | † |
| | 03-04 | * | < LOD | < LOD | < LOD | < LOD | 588 |
| 20 years and older | 99-00 | * | < LOD | < LOD | < LOD | < LOD | 1240 |
| | 01-02 | * | < LOD | < LOD | < LOD | < LOD | 1228 |
| | 03-04 | * | < LOD | < LOD | 28.6 (26.4-31.2) | 36.4 (31.5-42.7) | 1288 |
| **Gender** | | | | | | | |
| Males | 99-00 | * | < LOD | < LOD | < LOD | < LOD | 912 |
| | 01-02 | * | < LOD | < LOD | < LOD | < LOD | 559 |
| | 03-04 | * | < LOD | < LOD | < LOD | 28.8 (25.4-34 5) | 921 |
| Females | 99-00 | * | < LOD | < LOD | < LOD | < LOD | 986 |
| | 01-02 | * | < LOD | < LOD | < LOD | 50.7 (<LOD-74.3) | 669 |
| | 03-04 | * | < LOD | < LOD | 30.2 (27.4-33.1) | 38.7 (32.3-44 5) | 955 |
| **Race/ethnicity** | | | | | | | |
| Mexican Americans | 99-00 | * | < LOD | < LOD | < LOD | < LOD | 630 |
| | 01-02 | * | < LOD | < LOD | < LOD | < LOD | 262 |
| | 03-04 | * | < LOD | < LOD | < LOD | 23.6 (<LOD-32.5) | 424 |
| Non-Hispanic blacks | 99-00 | * | < LOD | < LOD | < LOD | < LOD | 404 |
| | 01-02 | * | < LOD | < LOD | < LOD | 55.6 (<LOD-72.0) | 217 |
| | 03-04 | * | < LOD | < LOD | 31.1 (<LOD-42.0) | 42.4 (29.5-67 8) | 454 |
| Non-Hispanic whites | 99-00 | * | < LOD | < LOD | < LOD | < LOD | 709 |
| | 01-02 | * | < LOD | < LOD | < LOD | < LOD | 665 |
| | 03-04 | * | < LOD | < LOD | 28.0 (<LOD-30.0) | 33.6 (31.1-38 8) | 877 |

† Data not collected for this age group for Survey year 01-02.
< LOD means less than the limit of detection for the lipid adjusted serum level, which may vary for some chemicals by year and by individual sample.
* Not calculated: proportion of results below limit of detection was too high to provide a valid result.

## Serum 1,2,3,4,6,7,8-Heptachlorodibenzofuran (HpCDF) (lipid adjusted)

Geometric mean and selected percentiles of serum concentrations (in pg/g lipid or parts per trillion on a lipid-weight basis) for the U.S. population from the National Health and Nutrition Examination Survey.

| | Survey years | Geometric mean (95% conf. interval) | Selected percentiles ( 95% confidence interval) | | | | Sample size |
|---|---|---|---|---|---|---|---|
| | | | 50th | 75th | 90th | 95th | |
| **Total** | 99-00 | * | < LOD | < LOD | 14.7 (<LOD-18 0) | 19.5 (17.4-23.0) | 1709 |
| | 01-02 | 9.64 (8.53-10 9) | 10.3 (8 80-11.7) | 14.6 (12.7-16.7) | 21.3 (18.0-25.5) | 27.1 (22 5-32.0) | 1219 |
| | 03-04 | * | < LOD | 10.6 (9.90-11.4) | 14.6 (13.1-16.5) | 18.7 (16 5-24.2) | 1858 |
| **Age group** | | | | | | | |
| 12-19 years | 99-00 | * | < LOD | < LOD | 18.4 (16.2-20.9) | 24.7 (20 9-28.1) | 600 |
| | 01-02 | † | † | † | † | † | † |
| | 03-04 | 9.36 (8.60-10 2) | 8.80 (<LOD-9.80) | 13.4 (12.3-14.6) | 19.3 (16.2-29.6) | 33.2 (21 2-54.2) | 583 |
| 20 years and older | 99-00 | * | < LOD | < LOD | 14.2 (<LOD-17 5) | 18.4 (15 0-23.8) | 1109 |
| | 01-02 | 9.64 (8.53-10 9) | 10.3 (8 80-11.7) | 14.6 (12.7-16.7) | 21.3 (18.0-25.5) | 27.1 (22 5-32.0) | 1219 |
| | 03-04 | * | < LOD | 10.3 (9.60-11.1) | 13.8 (12.5-16.0) | 18.0 (16 0-20.9) | 1275 |
| **Gender** | | | | | | | |
| Males | 99-00 | * | < LOD | < LOD | 16.4 (<LOD-20 0) | 21.0 (18.1-26.8) | 815 |
| | 01-02 | 10.1 (8.74-11 6) | 11.0 (9 30-12 6) | 15.2 (12.9-17.2) | 20.8 (17.2-27.8) | 28.9 (22 0-34.8) | 557 |
| | 03-04 | * | < LOD | 11.3 (10.1-12.9) | 17.1 (14.3-19.1) | 23.9 (18 3-30.9) | 913 |
| Females | 99-00 | * | < LOD | < LOD | < LOD | 17.5 (14 3-20.3) | 894 |
| | 01-02 | 9.28 (8.20-10 5) | 9.40 (8 20-11 2) | 14.1 (12.4-16.6) | 21.3 (17.4-25.5) | 26.5 (22 3-31.9) | 662 |
| | 03-04 | * | < LOD | 9.90 (9.30-10.5) | 13.0 (12.2-14.3) | 16.0 (14 3-18.4) | 945 |
| **Race/ethnicity** | | | | | | | |
| Mexican Americans | 99-00 | * | < LOD | < LOD | < LOD | 19.7 (<LOD-25.4) | 570 |
| | 01-02 | 7.73 (7.19-8.31) | 8.20 (7 80-8.70) | 11.2 (10.6-12.5) | 16.5 (14.5-19.6) | 20.8 (17 2-26.8) | 260 |
| | 03-04 | * | < LOD | 9.10 (<LOD-10 6) | 12.0 (10.1-16.8) | 15.1 (11 6-20.0) | 420 |
| Non-Hispanic blacks | 99-00 | * | < LOD | < LOD | 22.4 (15.2-28.2) | 28.2 (26 5-29.6) | 359 |
| | 01-02 | 12.3 (10.6-14.4) | 12.8 (10.9-15 2) | 17.4 (15.4-21.0) | 25.5 (22.4-31.2) | 32.1 (25.7-37.6) | 214 |
| | 03-04 | * | < LOD | 11.3 (10.7-12.2) | 16.1 (13.4-19.0) | 20.4 (16.7-26.8) | 454 |
| Non-Hispanic whites | 99-00 | * | < LOD | < LOD | < LOD | 17.5 (14 9-18.9) | 636 |
| | 01-02 | 9.50 (8.30-10 9) | 10.1 (8.40-12 0) | 14.4 (12.6-16.6) | 20.5 (16.9-25.5) | 25.8 (20 5-31.7) | 665 |
| | 03-04 | * | < LOD | 10.5 (9.60-11.5) | 14.6 (12.9-17.4) | 19.0 (16 3-26.2) | 864 |

Limit of detection (LOD, see Data Analysis section) for Survey years 99-00, 01-02, and 03-04 are 13.5, 7.0, and 8.6, respectively.
† Data not collected for this age group for Survey year 01-02.
< LOD means less than the limit of detection, which may vary for some chemicals by year and by individual sample.
* Not calculated: proportion of results below limit of detection was too high to provide a valid result.

## Serum 1,2,3,4,6,7,8-Heptachlorodibenzofuran (HpCDF) (whole weight)

Geometric mean and selected percentiles of serum concentrations (in fg/g of serum or parts per quadrillion) for the U.S. population from the National Health and Nutrition Examination Survey.

| | Survey years | Geometric mean (95% conf. interval) | Selected percentiles ( 95% confidence interval) | | | | Sample size |
|---|---|---|---|---|---|---|---|
| | | | 50th | 75th | 90th | 95th | |
| Total | 99-00 | * | < LOD | < LOD | 85.3 (<LOD-95.8) | 108 (95.8-120) | 1709 |
| | 01-02 | 62.2 (55.4-69.9) | 64.5 (58.0-71.6) | 94.1 (82 3-110) | 134 (119-165) | 181 (147-206) | 1219 |
| | 03-04 | * | < LOD | 63.6 (59 9-67.7) | 88.3 (81.0-100) | 116 (101-137) | 1858 |
| **Age group** | | | | | | | |
| 12-19 years | 99-00 | * | < LOD | < LOD | 79.3 (69.5-84.2) | 102 (83.4-120) | 600 |
| | 01-02 | † | † | † | † | † | † |
| | 03-04 | 47.5 (44.0-51.3) | 43.7 (<LOD-49 3) | 63.7 (59.1-72.3) | 102 (85.3-114) | 175 (113-222) | 583 |
| 20 years and older | 99-00 | * | < LOD | < LOD | 85.7 (<LOD-97.7) | 108 (93.6-127) | 1109 |
| | 01-02 | 62.2 (55.4-69.9) | 64.5 (58.0-71.6) | 94.1 (82 3-110) | 134 (119-165) | 181 (147-206) | 1219 |
| | 03-04 | * | < LOD | 63.5 (59 6-67.6) | 86.5 (78.8-100) | 112 (94.9-135) | 1275 |
| **Gender** | | | | | | | |
| Males | 99-00 | * | < LOD | < LOD | 91.4 (<LOD-108) | 112 (99.3-133) | 815 |
| | 01-02 | 66.3 (58.2-75.6) | 70.4 (59.8-81.8) | 99.3 (85 5-120) | 143 (120-181) | 182 (146-237) | 557 |
| | 03-04 | * | < LOD | 69.7 (62 9-76.0) | 100 (85.9-116) | 135 (113-193) | 913 |
| Females | 99-00 | * | < LOD | < LOD | < LOD | 97.8 (86.2-130) | 894 |
| | 01-02 | 58.8 (52.0-66.4) | 60.2 (53.5-67.6) | 89.5 (74.7-107) | 131 (108-165) | 169 (131-225) | 662 |
| | 03-04 | * | < LOD | 58.5 (54 5-62.4) | 83.5 (74.7-87.7) | 102 (87.7-116) | 945 |
| **Race/ethnicity** | | | | | | | |
| Mexican Americans | 99-00 | * | < LOD | < LOD | < LOD | 113 (<LOD-133) | 570 |
| | 01-02 | 49.5 (46.0-53.4) | 50.4 (45.7-57.2) | 76.9 (67.1-82.1) | 99.7 (90.9-124) | 133 (94.8-202) | 260 |
| | 03-04 | * | < LOD | 56.0 (<LOD-64.6) | 74.2 (62.6-91.4) | 90.5 (76.4-107) | 420 |
| Non-Hispanic blacks | 99-00 | * | < LOD | < LOD | 117 (89.0-143) | 153 (109-197) | 359 |
| | 01-02 | 72.6 (61.9-85.2) | 70.9 (62.4-85.2) | 107 (91 5-128) | 147 (131-177) | 193 (154-259) | 214 |
| | 03-04 | * | < LOD | 66.2 (60 2-75.5) | 91.3 (80.3-112) | 119 (102-151) | 454 |
| Non-Hispanic whites | 99-00 | * | < LOD | < LOD | < LOD | 97.7 (89.3-104) | 636 |
| | 01-02 | 61.8 (54.3-70.4) | 65.4 (57.4-72.2) | 94.3 (78.1-112) | 133 (114-166) | 180 (137-222) | 665 |
| | 03-04 | * | < LOD | 63.9 (59 6-69.2) | 87.8 (79.8-100) | 116 (102-139) | 864 |

† Data not collected for this age group for Survey year 01-02.
< LOD means less than the limit of detection for the lipid adjusted serum level, which may vary for some chemicals by year and by individual sample.
* Not calculated: proportion of results below limit of detection was too high to provide a valid result.

## Serum 1,2,3,4,7,8,9-Heptachlorodibenzofuran (HpCDF) (lipid adjusted)

Geometric mean and selected percentiles of serum concentrations (in pg/g lipid or parts per trillion on a lipid-weight basis) for the U.S. population from the National Health and Nutrition Examination Survey.

| | Survey years | Geometric mean (95% conf. interval) | 50th | 75th | 90th | 95th | Sample size |
|---|---|---|---|---|---|---|---|
| **Total** | 01-02 | * | < LOD | < LOD | < LOD | < LOD | 1224 |
| | 03-04 | * | < LOD | < LOD | < LOD | < LOD | 1852 |
| **Age group** | | | | | | | |
| 12-19 years | 01-02 | † | † | † | † | † | † |
| | 03-04 | * | < LOD | < LOD | < LOD | < LOD | 583 |
| 20 years and older | 01-02 | * | < LOD | < LOD | < LOD | < LOD | 1224 |
| | 03-04 | * | < LOD | < LOD | < LOD | < LOD | 1269 |
| **Gender** | | | | | | | |
| Males | 01-02 | * | < LOD | < LOD | < LOD | < LOD | 558 |
| | 03-04 | * | < LOD | < LOD | < LOD | < LOD | 908 |
| Females | 01-02 | * | < LOD | < LOD | < LOD | < LOD | 666 |
| | 03-04 | * | < LOD | < LOD | < LOD | < LOD | 944 |
| **Race/ethnicity** | | | | | | | |
| Mexican Americans | 01-02 | * | < LOD | < LOD | < LOD | < LOD | 262 |
| | 03-04 | * | < LOD | < LOD | < LOD | < LOD | 423 |
| Non-Hispanic blacks | 01-02 | * | < LOD | < LOD | < LOD | < LOD | 217 |
| | 03-04 | * | < LOD | < LOD | < LOD | < LOD | 452 |
| Non-Hispanic whites | 01-02 | * | < LOD | < LOD | < LOD | < LOD | 661 |
| | 03-04 | * | < LOD | < LOD | < LOD | < LOD | 856 |

Limit of detection (LOD, see Data Analysis section) for Survey years 01-02 and 03-04 are 7.0 and 8.6.
† Data not collected for this age group for Survey year 01-02.
< LOD means less than the limit of detection, which may vary for some chemicals by year and by individual sample.
* Not calculated: proportion of results below limit of detection was too high to provide a valid result.

## Serum 1,2,3,4,7,8,9-Heptachlorodibenzofuran (HpCDF) (whole weight)

Geometric mean and selected percentiles of serum concentrations (in fg/g of serum or parts per quadrillion) for the U.S. population from the National Health and Nutrition Examination Survey.

| | Survey years | Geometric mean (95% conf. interval) | Selected percentiles ( 95% confidence interval) | | | | Sample size |
|---|---|---|---|---|---|---|---|
| | | | 50th | 75th | 90th | 95th | |
| Total | 01-02 | * | < LOD | < LOD | < LOD | < LOD | 1224 |
| | 03-04 | * | < LOD | < LOD | < LOD | < LOD | 1852 |
| Age group | | | | | | | |
| 12-19 years | 01-02 | † | † | † | † | † | † |
| | 03-04 | * | < LOD | < LOD | < LOD | < LOD | 583 |
| 20 years and older | 01-02 | * | < LOD | < LOD | < LOD | < LOD | 1224 |
| | 03-04 | * | < LOD | < LOD | < LOD | < LOD | 1269 |
| Gender | | | | | | | |
| Males | 01-02 | * | < LOD | < LOD | < LOD | < LOD | 558 |
| | 03-04 | * | < LOD | < LOD | < LOD | < LOD | 908 |
| Females | 01-02 | * | < LOD | < LOD | < LOD | < LOD | 666 |
| | 03-04 | * | < LOD | < LOD | < LOD | < LOD | 944 |
| Race/ethnicity | | | | | | | |
| Mexican Americans | 01-02 | * | < LOD | < LOD | < LOD | < LOD | 262 |
| | 03-04 | * | < LOD | < LOD | < LOD | < LOD | 423 |
| Non-Hispanic blacks | 01-02 | * | < LOD | < LOD | < LOD | < LOD | 217 |
| | 03-04 | * | < LOD | < LOD | < LOD | < LOD | 452 |
| Non-Hispanic whites | 01-02 | * | < LOD | < LOD | < LOD | < LOD | 661 |
| | 03-04 | * | < LOD | < LOD | < LOD | < LOD | 856 |

† Data not collected for this age group for Survey year 01-02.
< LOD means less than the limit of detection for the lipid adjusted serum level, which may vary for some chemicals by year and by individual sample.
* Not calculated: proportion of results below limit of detection was too high to provide a valid result.

## Serum 1,2,3,4,7,8-Hexachlorodibenzofuran (HxCDF) (lipid adjusted)

Geometric mean and selected percentiles of serum concentrations (in pg/g lipid or parts per trillion on a lipid-weight basis) for the U.S. population from the National Health and Nutrition Examination Survey.

| | Survey years | Geometric mean (95% conf. interval) | Selected percentiles ( 95% confidence interval) | | | | Sample size |
|---|---|---|---|---|---|---|---|
| | | | 50th | 75th | 90th | 95th | |
| **Total** | 99-00 | * | < LOD | < LOD | < LOD | < LOD | 1890 |
| | 01-02 | * | < LOD | 8.00 (6.90-9.60) | 12.1 (9.40-14.9) | 15.4 (12 9-18.6) | 1223 |
| | 03-04 | * | < LOD | < LOD | 7.50 (<LOD-7.90) | 8.90 (7.90-10.2) | 1866 |
| **Age group** | | | | | | | |
| 12-19 years | 99-00 | * | < LOD | < LOD | < LOD | < LOD | 657 |
| | 01-02 | † | † | † | † | † | † |
| | 03-04 | * | < LOD | < LOD | < LOD | < LOD | 583 |
| 20 years and older | 99-00 | * | < LOD | < LOD | < LOD | 12.8 (<LOD-14.5) | 1233 |
| | 01-02 | * | < LOD | 8.00 (6.90-9.60) | 12.1 (9.40-14.9) | 15.4 (12 9-18.6) | 1223 |
| | 03-04 | * | < LOD | < LOD | 7.60 (<LOD-8.20) | 9.50 (8.00-10.5) | 1283 |
| **Gender** | | | | | | | |
| Males | 99-00 | * | < LOD | < LOD | < LOD | < LOD | 908 |
| | 01-02 | * | < LOD | 8.20 (7.10-10.0) | 12.8 (9.50-15.9) | 15.9 (12 2-20.9) | 562 |
| | 03-04 | * | < LOD | < LOD | 7.40 (<LOD-8.00) | 8.50 (7.80-10.0) | 916 |
| Females | 99-00 | * | < LOD | < LOD | < LOD | 12.9 (<LOD-16.4) | 982 |
| | 01-02 | * | < LOD | 7.90 (6.70-9.00) | 11.7 (9.40-13.8) | 14.5 (12 2-18.6) | 661 |
| | 03-04 | * | < LOD | < LOD | 7.50 (<LOD-8.40) | 9.30 (7.80-10.4) | 950 |
| **Race/ethnicity** | | | | | | | |
| Mexican Americans | 99-00 | * | < LOD | < LOD | < LOD | < LOD | 631 |
| | 01-02 | * | < LOD | < LOD | 7.30 (<LOD-8.00) | 8.00 (7.00-10.9) | 261 |
| | 03-04 | * | < LOD | < LOD | < LOD | < LOD | 423 |
| Non-Hispanic blacks | 99-00 | * | < LOD | < LOD | < LOD | 14.3 (<LOD-15.1) | 399 |
| | 01-02 | * | < LOD | 8.90 (7.70-10.1) | 13.6 (11.1-17.1) | 18.6 (14 6-22.6) | 214 |
| | 03-04 | * | < LOD | < LOD | 7.80 (<LOD-10 9) | 10.9 (7.50-19.4) | 453 |
| Non-Hispanic whites | 99-00 | * | < LOD | < LOD | < LOD | < LOD | 703 |
| | 01-02 | * | < LOD | 8.30 (7.10-10.2) | 12.5 (10.0-15.9) | 15.9 (13.1-19.0) | 664 |
| | 03-04 | * | < LOD | < LOD | 7.60 (<LOD-8.10) | 9.40 (8.00-10.2) | 869 |

Limit of detection (LOD, see Data Analysis section) for Survey years 99-00, 01-02, and 03-04 are 12.7, 6.5, and 7.4, respectively.
† Data not collected for this age group for Survey year 01-02.
< LOD means less than the limit of detection, which may vary for some chemicals by year and by individual sample.
* Not calculated: proportion of results below limit of detection was too high to provide a valid result.

## Serum 1,2,3,4,7,8-Hexachlorodibenzofuran (HxCDF) (whole weight)

Geometric mean and selected percentiles of serum concentrations (in fg/g of serum or parts per quadrillion) for the U.S. population from the National Health and Nutrition Examination Survey.

| | Survey years | Geometric mean (95% conf. interval) | Selected percentiles ( 95% confidence interval) | | | | Sample size |
|---|---|---|---|---|---|---|---|
| | | | 50th | 75th | 90th | 95th | |
| Total | 99-00 | * | < LOD | < LOD | < LOD | < LOD | 1890 |
| | 01-02 | * | < LOD | 54.0 (46 5-63.6) | 82.3 (65.5-104) | 108 (88.0-138) | 1223 |
| | 03-04 | * | < LOD | < LOD | 49.1 (<LOD-54.5) | 60.1 (53.4-68 8) | 1866 |
| Age group | | | | | | | |
| 12-19 years | 99-00 | * | < LOD | < LOD | < LOD | < LOD | 657 |
| | 01-02 | † | † | † | † | † | † |
| | 03-04 | * | < LOD | < LOD | < LOD | < LOD | 583 |
| 20 years and older | 99-00 | * | < LOD | < LOD | < LOD | 84.2 (<LOD-97.2) | 1233 |
| | 01-02 | * | < LOD | 54.0 (46 5-63.6) | 82.3 (65.5-104) | 108 (88.0-138) | 1223 |
| | 03-04 | * | < LOD | < LOD | 51.0 (<LOD-57.2) | 62.2 (56.2-72.7) | 1283 |
| Gender | | | | | | | |
| Males | 99-00 | * | < LOD | < LOD | < LOD | < LOD | 908 |
| | 01-02 | * | < LOD | 56.9 (48 6-71.4) | 90.1 (71.1-108) | 108 (87.4-144) | 562 |
| | 03-04 | * | < LOD | < LOD | 49.3 (<LOD-54.9) | 59.3 (52.9-68 8) | 916 |
| Females | 99-00 | * | < LOD | < LOD | < LOD | 82.8 (<LOD-102) | 982 |
| | 01-02 | * | < LOD | 51.6 (43.7-59.6) | 76.1 (62.6-97.0) | 105 (81.6-140) | 661 |
| | 03-04 | * | < LOD | < LOD | 48.9 (<LOD-57.2) | 61.9 (53.3-72.7) | 950 |
| Race/ethnicity | | | | | | | |
| Mexican Americans | 99-00 | * | < LOD | < LOD | < LOD | < LOD | 631 |
| | 01-02 | * | < LOD | < LOD | 48.4 (<LOD-56.3) | 65.3 (48.6-79.4) | 261 |
| | 03-04 | * | < LOD | < LOD | < LOD | < LOD | 423 |
| Non-Hispanic blacks | 99-00 | * | < LOD | < LOD | < LOD | 90.8 (<LOD-105) | 399 |
| | 01-02 | * | < LOD | 52.7 (45 0-62.7) | 87.1 (63.7-108) | 122 (85.2-147) | 214 |
| | 03-04 | * | < LOD | < LOD | 56.9 (<LOD-71.7) | 71.7 (53.8-112) | 453 |
| Non-Hispanic whites | 99-00 | * | < LOD | < LOD | < LOD | < LOD | 703 |
| | 01-02 | * | < LOD | 56.0 (48 6-66.1) | 84.2 (64.5-115) | 112 (88.6-142) | 664 |
| | 03-04 | * | < LOD | < LOD | 50.6 (<LOD-56.3) | 61.4 (54.0-71 8) | 869 |

† Data not collected for this age group for Survey year 01-02.
< LOD means less than the limit of detection for the lipid adjusted serum level, which may vary for some chemicals by year and by individual sample.
* Not calculated: proportion of results below limit of detection was too high to provide a valid result.

## Serum 1,2,3,6,7,8-Hexachlorodibenzofuran (HxCDF) (lipid adjusted)

Geometric mean and selected percentiles of serum concentrations (in pg/g lipid or parts per trillion on a lipid-weight basis) for the U.S. population from the National Health and Nutrition Examination Survey.

| | Survey years | Geometric mean (95% conf. interval) | Selected percentiles ( 95% confidence interval) | | | | Sample size |
|---|---|---|---|---|---|---|---|
| | | | 50th | 75th | 90th | 95th | |
| **Total** | 99-00 | * | < LOD | < LOD | < LOD | < LOD | 1898 |
| | 01-02 | * | < LOD | 7.10 (<LOD-8.20) | 10.4 (9.00-13.1) | 14.0 (11 0-17.1) | 1236 |
| | 03-04 | * | < LOD | < LOD | < LOD | 8.80 (<LOD-9.80) | 1868 |
| **Age group** | | | | | | | |
| 12-19 years | 99-00 | * | < LOD | < LOD | < LOD | < LOD | 656 |
| | 01-02 | † | † | † | † | † | † |
| | 03-04 | * | < LOD | < LOD | < LOD | < LOD | 585 |
| 20 years and older | 99-00 | * | < LOD | < LOD | < LOD | < LOD | 1242 |
| | 01-02 | * | < LOD | 7.10 (<LOD-8.20) | 10.4 (9.00-13.1) | 14.0 (11 0-17.1) | 1236 |
| | 03-04 | * | < LOD | < LOD | < LOD | 9.00 (8.00-10.1) | 1283 |
| **Gender** | | | | | | | |
| Males | 99-00 | * | < LOD | < LOD | < LOD | < LOD | 913 |
| | 01-02 | * | < LOD | 7.10 (<LOD-8.60) | 11.3 (8.50-13.8) | 15.1 (11 3-18.7) | 566 |
| | 03-04 | * | < LOD | < LOD | < LOD | 9.10 (7.90-10.8) | 918 |
| Females | 99-00 | * | < LOD | < LOD | < LOD | < LOD | 985 |
| | 01-02 | * | < LOD | 7.00 (6.20-8.00) | 10.0 (9.20-11.4) | 13.1 (10 5-15.6) | 670 |
| | 03-04 | * | < LOD | < LOD | < LOD | 8.50 (<LOD-9.20) | 950 |
| **Race/ethnicity** | | | | | | | |
| Mexican Americans | 99-00 | * | < LOD | < LOD | < LOD | < LOD | 625 |
| | 01-02 | * | < LOD | < LOD | < LOD | 6.90 (<LOD-11.1) | 262 |
| | 03-04 | * | < LOD | < LOD | < LOD | < LOD | 423 |
| Non-Hispanic blacks | 99-00 | * | < LOD | < LOD | < LOD | < LOD | 408 |
| | 01-02 | * | < LOD | 7.60 (6.10-9.10) | 12.1 (10.0-14.1) | 16.0 (12 3-21.0) | 219 |
| | 03-04 | * | < LOD | < LOD | < LOD | 8.50 (<LOD-12.1) | 453 |
| Non-Hispanic whites | 99-00 | * | < LOD | < LOD | < LOD | < LOD | 708 |
| | 01-02 | * | < LOD | 7.40 (6.20-9.00) | 10.7 (9.20-14.3) | 14.8 (11 6-17.2) | 670 |
| | 03-04 | * | < LOD | < LOD | < LOD | 9.10 (8.00-10.6) | 871 |

Limit of detection (LOD, see Data Analysis section) for Survey years 99-00, 01-02, and 03-04 are 12.6, 6.1, and 7.9, respectively.
† Data not collected for this age group for Survey year 01-02.
< LOD means less than the limit of detection, which may vary for some chemicals by year and by individual sample.
* Not calculated: proportion of results below limit of detection was too high to provide a valid result.

## Serum 1,2,3,6,7,8-Hexachlorodibenzofuran (HxCDF) (whole weight)

Geometric mean and selected percentiles of serum concentrations (in fg/g of serum or parts per quadrillion) for the U.S. population from the National Health and Nutrition Examination Survey.

| | Survey years | Geometric mean (95% conf. interval) | 50th | 75th | 90th | 95th | Sample size |
|---|---|---|---|---|---|---|---|
| **Total** | 99-00 | * | < LOD | < LOD | < LOD | < LOD | 1898 |
| | 01-02 | * | < LOD | 46.2 (<LOD-56.5) | 70.3 (58.4-90.7) | 101 (77.6-120) | 1236 |
| | 03-04 | * | < LOD | < LOD | < LOD | 59.8 (<LOD-65.4) | 1868 |
| **Age group** | | | | | | | |
| 12-19 years | 99-00 | * | < LOD | < LOD | < LOD | < LOD | 656 |
| | 01-02 | † | † | † | † | † | † |
| | 03-04 | * | < LOD | < LOD | < LOD | < LOD | 585 |
| 20 years and older | 99-00 | * | < LOD | < LOD | < LOD | < LOD | 1242 |
| | 01-02 | * | < LOD | 46.2 (<LOD-56.5) | 70.3 (58.4-90.7) | 101 (77.6-120) | 1236 |
| | 03-04 | * | < LOD | < LOD | < LOD | 61.0 (57.6-65.7) | 1283 |
| **Gender** | | | | | | | |
| Males | 99-00 | * | < LOD | < LOD | < LOD | < LOD | 913 |
| | 01-02 | * | < LOD | 47.9 (<LOD-60.5) | 72.3 (57.5-105) | 104 (73.5-133) | 566 |
| | 03-04 | * | < LOD | < LOD | < LOD | 61.0 (54.0-67.7) | 918 |
| Females | 99-00 | * | < LOD | < LOD | < LOD | < LOD | 985 |
| | 01-02 | * | < LOD | 45.0 (37 0-54.3) | 66.2 (58.3-79.1) | 90.7 (71.9-115) | 670 |
| | 03-04 | * | < LOD | < LOD | < LOD | 58.1 (<LOD-65.0) | 950 |
| **Race/ethnicity** | | | | | | | |
| Mexican Americans | 99-00 | * | < LOD | < LOD | < LOD | < LOD | 625 |
| | 01-02 | * | < LOD | < LOD | < LOD | 52.7 (<LOD-65.9) | 262 |
| | 03-04 | * | < LOD | < LOD | < LOD | < LOD | 423 |
| Non-Hispanic blacks | 99-00 | * | < LOD | < LOD | < LOD | < LOD | 408 |
| | 01-02 | * | < LOD | 44.4 (37 2-57.3) | 71.5 (59.8-90.9) | 107 (70.7-142) | 219 |
| | 03-04 | * | < LOD | < LOD | < LOD | 58.4 (<LOD-73.0) | 453 |
| Non-Hispanic whites | 99-00 | * | < LOD | < LOD | < LOD | < LOD | 708 |
| | 01-02 | * | < LOD | 49.6 (41 9-57.9) | 72.8 (58.4-102) | 103 (82.6-121) | 670 |
| | 03-04 | * | < LOD | < LOD | < LOD | 63.4 (57.3-67.7) | 871 |

† Data not collected for this age group for Survey year 01-02.
< LOD means less than the limit of detection for the lipid adjusted serum level, which may vary for some chemicals by year and by individual sample.
* Not calculated: proportion of results below limit of detection was too high to provide a valid result.

## Serum 1,2,3,7,8,9-Hexachlorodibenzofuran (HxCDF) (lipid adjusted)

Geometric mean and selected percentiles of serum concentrations (in pg/g lipid or parts per trillion on a lipid-weight basis) for the U.S. population from the National Health and Nutrition Examination Survey.

| | Survey years | Geometric mean (95% conf. interval) | Selected percentiles ( 95% confidence interval) | | | | Sample size |
|---|---|---|---|---|---|---|---|
| | | | 50th | 75th | 90th | 95th | |
| **Total** | 99-00 | * | < LOD | < LOD | < LOD | < LOD | 1875 |
| | 01-02 | * | < LOD | < LOD | < LOD | < LOD | 1223 |
| | 03-04 | * | < LOD | < LOD | < LOD | < LOD | 1864 |
| **Age group** | | | | | | | |
| 12-19 years | 99-00 | * | < LOD | < LOD | < LOD | < LOD | 645 |
| | 01-02 | † | † | † | † | † | † |
| | 03-04 | * | < LOD | < LOD | < LOD | < LOD | 583 |
| 20 years and older | 99-00 | * | < LOD | < LOD | < LOD | < LOD | 1230 |
| | 01-02 | * | < LOD | < LOD | < LOD | < LOD | 1223 |
| | 03-04 | * | < LOD | < LOD | < LOD | < LOD | 1281 |
| **Gender** | | | | | | | |
| Males | 99-00 | * | < LOD | < LOD | < LOD | < LOD | 894 |
| | 01-02 | * | < LOD | < LOD | < LOD | < LOD | 559 |
| | 03-04 | * | < LOD | < LOD | < LOD | < LOD | 914 |
| Females | 99-00 | * | < LOD | < LOD | < LOD | < LOD | 981 |
| | 01-02 | * | < LOD | < LOD | < LOD | < LOD | 664 |
| | 03-04 | * | < LOD | < LOD | < LOD | < LOD | 950 |
| **Race/ethnicity** | | | | | | | |
| Mexican Americans | 99-00 | * | < LOD | < LOD | < LOD | < LOD | 620 |
| | 01-02 | * | < LOD | < LOD | < LOD | < LOD | 261 |
| | 03-04 | * | < LOD | < LOD | < LOD | < LOD | 423 |
| Non-Hispanic blacks | 99-00 | * | < LOD | < LOD | < LOD | < LOD | 400 |
| | 01-02 | * | < LOD | < LOD | < LOD | < LOD | 216 |
| | 03-04 | * | < LOD | < LOD | < LOD | < LOD | 454 |
| Non-Hispanic whites | 99-00 | * | < LOD | < LOD | < LOD | < LOD | 699 |
| | 01-02 | * | < LOD | < LOD | < LOD | < LOD | 665 |
| | 03-04 | * | < LOD | < LOD | < LOD | < LOD | 866 |

Limit of detection (LOD, see Data Analysis section) for Survey years 99-00, 01-02, and 03-04 are 12.7, 6.0, and 8.3, respectively.
† Data not collected for this age group for Survey year 01-02.
< LOD means less than the limit of detection, which may vary for some chemicals by year and by individual sample.
* Not calculated: proportion of results below limit of detection was too high to provide a valid result.

# Serum 1,2,3,7,8,9-Hexachlorodibenzofuran (HxCDF) (whole weight)

Geometric mean and selected percentiles of serum concentrations (in fg/g of serum or parts per quadrillion) for the U.S. population from the National Health and Nutrition Examination Survey.

| | Survey years | Geometric mean (95% conf. interval) | Selected percentiles ( 95% confidence interval) | | | | Sample size |
|---|---|---|---|---|---|---|---|
| | | | 50th | 75th | 90th | 95th | |
| Total | 99-00 | * | < LOD | < LOD | < LOD | < LOD | 1875 |
| | 01-02 | * | < LOD | < LOD | < LOD | < LOD | 1223 |
| | 03-04 | * | < LOD | < LOD | < LOD | < LOD | 1864 |
| **Age group** | | | | | | | |
| 12-19 years | 99-00 | * | < LOD | < LOD | < LOD | < LOD | 645 |
| | 01-02 | † | † | † | † | † | † |
| | 03-04 | * | < LOD | < LOD | < LOD | < LOD | 583 |
| 20 years and older | 99-00 | * | < LOD | < LOD | < LOD | < LOD | 1230 |
| | 01-02 | * | < LOD | < LOD | < LOD | < LOD | 1223 |
| | 03-04 | * | < LOD | < LOD | < LOD | < LOD | 1281 |
| **Gender** | | | | | | | |
| Males | 99-00 | * | < LOD | < LOD | < LOD | < LOD | 894 |
| | 01-02 | * | < LOD | < LOD | < LOD | < LOD | 559 |
| | 03-04 | * | < LOD | < LOD | < LOD | < LOD | 914 |
| Females | 99-00 | * | < LOD | < LOD | < LOD | < LOD | 981 |
| | 01-02 | * | < LOD | < LOD | < LOD | < LOD | 664 |
| | 03-04 | * | < LOD | < LOD | < LOD | < LOD | 950 |
| **Race/ethnicity** | | | | | | | |
| Mexican Americans | 99-00 | * | < LOD | < LOD | < LOD | < LOD | 620 |
| | 01-02 | * | < LOD | < LOD | < LOD | < LOD | 261 |
| | 03-04 | * | < LOD | < LOD | < LOD | < LOD | 423 |
| Non-Hispanic blacks | 99-00 | * | < LOD | < LOD | < LOD | < LOD | 400 |
| | 01-02 | * | < LOD | < LOD | < LOD | < LOD | 216 |
| | 03-04 | * | < LOD | < LOD | < LOD | < LOD | 454 |
| Non-Hispanic whites | 99-00 | * | < LOD | < LOD | < LOD | < LOD | 699 |
| | 01-02 | * | < LOD | < LOD | < LOD | < LOD | 665 |
| | 03-04 | * | < LOD | < LOD | < LOD | < LOD | 866 |

† Data not collected for this age group for Survey year 01-02.
< LOD means less than the limit of detection for the lipid adjusted serum level, which may vary for some chemicals by year and by individual sample.
* Not calculated: proportion of results below limit of detection was too high to provide a valid result.

## Serum 2,3,4,6,7,8-Hexachlorodibenzofuran (HxCDF) (lipid adjusted)

Geometric mean and selected percentiles of serum concentrations (in pg/g lipid or parts per trillion on a lipid-weight basis) for the U.S. population from the National Health and Nutrition Examination Survey.

| | Survey years | Geometric mean (95% conf. interval) | Selected percentiles ( 95% confidence interval) | | | | Sample size |
|---|---|---|---|---|---|---|---|
| | | | 50th | 75th | 90th | 95th | |
| **Total** | 99-00 | * | < LOD | < LOD | < LOD | < LOD | 1884 |
| | 01-02 | * | < LOD | < LOD | < LOD | < LOD | 1230 |
| | 03-04 | * | < LOD | < LOD | < LOD | < LOD | 1866 |
| **Age group** | | | | | | | |
| 12-19 years | 99-00 | * | < LOD | < LOD | < LOD | < LOD | 652 |
| | 01-02 | † | † | † | † | † | † |
| | 03-04 | * | < LOD | < LOD | < LOD | < LOD | 584 |
| 20 years and older | 99-00 | * | < LOD | < LOD | < LOD | < LOD | 1232 |
| | 01-02 | * | < LOD | < LOD | < LOD | < LOD | 1230 |
| | 03-04 | * | < LOD | < LOD | < LOD | < LOD | 1282 |
| **Gender** | | | | | | | |
| Males | 99-00 | * | < LOD | < LOD | < LOD | < LOD | 900 |
| | 01-02 | * | < LOD | < LOD | < LOD | < LOD | 565 |
| | 03-04 | * | < LOD | < LOD | < LOD | < LOD | 916 |
| Females | 99-00 | * | < LOD | < LOD | < LOD | < LOD | 984 |
| | 01-02 | * | < LOD | < LOD | < LOD | < LOD | 665 |
| | 03-04 | * | < LOD | < LOD | < LOD | < LOD | 950 |
| **Race/ethnicity** | | | | | | | |
| Mexican Americans | 99-00 | * | < LOD | < LOD | < LOD | < LOD | 614 |
| | 01-02 | * | < LOD | < LOD | < LOD | < LOD | 260 |
| | 03-04 | * | < LOD | < LOD | < LOD | < LOD | 422 |
| Non-Hispanic blacks | 99-00 | * | < LOD | < LOD | < LOD | < LOD | 408 |
| | 01-02 | * | < LOD | < LOD | < LOD | < LOD | 218 |
| | 03-04 | * | < LOD | < LOD | < LOD | < LOD | 454 |
| Non-Hispanic whites | 99-00 | * | < LOD | < LOD | < LOD | < LOD | 704 |
| | 01-02 | * | < LOD | < LOD | < LOD | < LOD | 671 |
| | 03-04 | * | < LOD | < LOD | < LOD | < LOD | 869 |

Limit of detection (LOD, see Data Analysis section) for Survey years 99-00, 01-02, and 03-04 are 12.9, 5.8, and 8.2, respectively.
† Data not collected for this age group for Survey year 01-02.
< LOD means less than the limit of detection, which may vary for some chemicals by year and by individual sample.
* Not calculated: proportion of results below limit of detection was too high to provide a valid result.

## Serum 2,3,4,6,7,8-Hexachlorodibenzofuran (HxCDF) (whole weight)

Geometric mean and selected percentiles of serum concentrations (in fg/g of serum or parts per quadrillion) for the U.S. population from the National Health and Nutrition Examination Survey.

| | Survey years | Geometric mean (95% conf. interval) | Selected percentiles ( 95% confidence interval) | | | | Sample size |
|---|---|---|---|---|---|---|---|
| | | | 50th | 75th | 90th | 95th | |
| Total | 99-00 | * | < LOD | < LOD | < LOD | < LOD | 1884 |
| | 01-02 | * | < LOD | < LOD | < LOD | < LOD | 1230 |
| | 03-04 | * | < LOD | < LOD | < LOD | < LOD | 1866 |
| Age group | | | | | | | |
| 12-19 years | 99-00 | * | < LOD | < LOD | < LOD | < LOD | 652 |
| | 01-02 | † | † | † | † | † | † |
| | 03-04 | * | < LOD | < LOD | < LOD | < LOD | 584 |
| 20 years and older | 99-00 | * | < LOD | < LOD | < LOD | < LOD | 1232 |
| | 01-02 | * | < LOD | < LOD | < LOD | < LOD | 1230 |
| | 03-04 | * | < LOD | < LOD | < LOD | < LOD | 1282 |
| Gender | | | | | | | |
| Males | 99-00 | * | < LOD | < LOD | < LOD | < LOD | 900 |
| | 01-02 | * | < LOD | < LOD | < LOD | < LOD | 565 |
| | 03-04 | * | < LOD | < LOD | < LOD | < LOD | 916 |
| Females | 99-00 | * | < LOD | < LOD | < LOD | < LOD | 984 |
| | 01-02 | * | < LOD | < LOD | < LOD | < LOD | 665 |
| | 03-04 | * | < LOD | < LOD | < LOD | < LOD | 950 |
| Race/ethnicity | | | | | | | |
| Mexican Americans | 99-00 | * | < LOD | < LOD | < LOD | < LOD | 614 |
| | 01-02 | * | < LOD | < LOD | < LOD | < LOD | 260 |
| | 03-04 | * | < LOD | < LOD | < LOD | < LOD | 422 |
| Non-Hispanic blacks | 99-00 | * | < LOD | < LOD | < LOD | < LOD | 408 |
| | 01-02 | * | < LOD | < LOD | < LOD | < LOD | 218 |
| | 03-04 | * | < LOD | < LOD | < LOD | < LOD | 454 |
| Non-Hispanic whites | 99-00 | * | < LOD | < LOD | < LOD | < LOD | 704 |
| | 01-02 | * | < LOD | < LOD | < LOD | < LOD | 671 |
| | 03-04 | * | < LOD | < LOD | < LOD | < LOD | 869 |

† Data not collected for this age group for Survey year 01-02.
< LOD means less than the limit of detection for the lipid adjusted serum level, which may vary for some chemicals by year and by individual sample.
* Not calculated: proportion of results below limit of detection was too high to provide a valid result.

## Serum 1,2,3,4,6,7,8,9-Octachlorodibenzofuran (OCDF) (lipid adjusted)

Geometric mean and selected percentiles of serum concentrations (in pg/g lipid or parts per trillion on a lipid-weight basis) for the U.S. population from the National Health and Nutrition Examination Survey.

| | Survey years | Geometric mean (95% conf. interval) | Selected percentiles ( 95% confidence interval) | | | | Sample size |
|---|---|---|---|---|---|---|---|
| | | | 50th | 75th | 90th | 95th | |
| **Total** | 99-00 | * | < LOD | < LOD | < LOD | < LOD | 1884 |
| | 01-02 | * | < LOD | < LOD | < LOD | < LOD | 1202 |
| | 03-04 | * | < LOD | < LOD | < LOD | < LOD | 1849 |
| **Age group** | | | | | | | |
| 12-19 years | 99-00 | * | < LOD | < LOD | < LOD | < LOD | 652 |
| | 01-02 | † | † | † | † | † | † |
| | 03-04 | * | < LOD | < LOD | < LOD | < LOD | 581 |
| 20 years and older | 99-00 | * | < LOD | < LOD | < LOD | < LOD | 1232 |
| | 01-02 | * | < LOD | < LOD | < LOD | < LOD | 1202 |
| | 03-04 | * | < LOD | < LOD | < LOD | < LOD | 1268 |
| **Gender** | | | | | | | |
| Males | 99-00 | * | < LOD | < LOD | < LOD | < LOD | 904 |
| | 01-02 | * | < LOD | < LOD | < LOD | < LOD | 541 |
| | 03-04 | * | < LOD | < LOD | < LOD | < LOD | 905 |
| Females | 99-00 | * | < LOD | < LOD | < LOD | < LOD | 980 |
| | 01-02 | * | < LOD | < LOD | < LOD | < LOD | 661 |
| | 03-04 | * | < LOD | < LOD | < LOD | < LOD | 944 |
| **Race/ethnicity** | | | | | | | |
| Mexican Americans | 99-00 | * | < LOD | < LOD | < LOD | < LOD | 623 |
| | 01-02 | * | < LOD | < LOD | < LOD | < LOD | 257 |
| | 03-04 | * | < LOD | < LOD | < LOD | < LOD | 420 |
| Non-Hispanic blacks | 99-00 | * | < LOD | < LOD | < LOD | < LOD | 404 |
| | 01-02 | * | < LOD | < LOD | < LOD | < LOD | 212 |
| | 03-04 | * | < LOD | < LOD | < LOD | < LOD | 453 |
| Non-Hispanic whites | 99-00 | * | < LOD | < LOD | < LOD | < LOD | 705 |
| | 01-02 | * | < LOD | < LOD | < LOD | < LOD | 653 |
| | 03-04 | * | < LOD | < LOD | < LOD | < LOD | 857 |

Limit of detection (LOD, see Data Analysis section) for Survey years 99-00, 01-02, and 03-04 are 35.6, 21 0, and 12.0, respectively.
† Data not collected for this age group for Survey year 01-02.
< LOD means less than the limit of detection, which may vary for some chemicals by year and by individual sample.
* Not calculated: proportion of results below limit of detection was too high to provide a valid result.

## Serum 1,2,3,4,6,7,8,9-Octachlorodibenzofuran (OCDF) (whole weight)

Geometric mean and selected percentiles of serum concentrations (in fg/g of serum or parts per quadrillion) for the U.S. population from the National Health and Nutrition Examination Survey.

| | Survey years | Geometric mean (95% conf. interval) | Selected percentiles ( 95% confidence interval) | | | | Sample size |
|---|---|---|---|---|---|---|---|
| | | | 50th | 75th | 90th | 95th | |
| Total | 99-00 | * | < LOD | < LOD | < LOD | < LOD | 1884 |
| | 01-02 | * | < LOD | < LOD | < LOD | < LOD | 1202 |
| | 03-04 | * | < LOD | < LOD | < LOD | < LOD | 1849 |
| Age group | | | | | | | |
| 12-19 years | 99-00 | * | < LOD | < LOD | < LOD | < LOD | 652 |
| | 01-02 | † | † | † | † | † | † |
| | 03-04 | * | < LOD | < LOD | < LOD | < LOD | 581 |
| 20 years and older | 99-00 | * | < LOD | < LOD | < LOD | < LOD | 1232 |
| | 01-02 | * | < LOD | < LOD | < LOD | < LOD | 1202 |
| | 03-04 | * | < LOD | < LOD | < LOD | < LOD | 1268 |
| Gender | | | | | | | |
| Males | 99-00 | * | < LOD | < LOD | < LOD | < LOD | 904 |
| | 01-02 | * | < LOD | < LOD | < LOD | < LOD | 541 |
| | 03-04 | * | < LOD | < LOD | < LOD | < LOD | 905 |
| Females | 99-00 | * | < LOD | < LOD | < LOD | < LOD | 980 |
| | 01-02 | * | < LOD | < LOD | < LOD | < LOD | 661 |
| | 03-04 | * | < LOD | < LOD | < LOD | < LOD | 944 |
| Race/ethnicity | | | | | | | |
| Mexican Americans | 99-00 | * | < LOD | < LOD | < LOD | < LOD | 623 |
| | 01-02 | * | < LOD | < LOD | < LOD | < LOD | 257 |
| | 03-04 | * | < LOD | < LOD | < LOD | < LOD | 420 |
| Non-Hispanic blacks | 99-00 | * | < LOD | < LOD | < LOD | < LOD | 404 |
| | 01-02 | * | < LOD | < LOD | < LOD | < LOD | 212 |
| | 03-04 | * | < LOD | < LOD | < LOD | < LOD | 453 |
| Non-Hispanic whites | 99-00 | * | < LOD | < LOD | < LOD | < LOD | 705 |
| | 01-02 | * | < LOD | < LOD | < LOD | < LOD | 653 |
| | 03-04 | * | < LOD | < LOD | < LOD | < LOD | 857 |

† Data not collected for this age group for Survey year 01-02.
< LOD means less than the limit of detection for the lipid adjusted serum level, which may vary for some chemicals by year and by individual sample.
* Not calculated: proportion of results below limit of detection was too high to provide a valid result.

## Serum 1,2,3,7,8-Pentachlorodibenzofuran (PeCDF) (lipid adjusted)

Geometric mean and selected percentiles of serum concentrations (in pg/g lipid or parts per trillion on a lipid-weight basis) for the U.S. population from the National Health and Nutrition Examination Survey.

| | Survey years | Geometric mean (95% conf. interval) | Selected percentiles ( 95% confidence interval) | | | | Sample size |
|---|---|---|---|---|---|---|---|
| | | | 50th | 75th | 90th | 95th | |
| **Total** | 99-00 | * | < LOD | < LOD | < LOD | < LOD | 1922 |
| | 01-02 | * | < LOD | < LOD | < LOD | < LOD | 1235 |
| | 03-04 | * | < LOD | < LOD | < LOD | < LOD | 1867 |
| **Age group** | | | | | | | |
| 12-19 years | 99-00 | * | < LOD | < LOD | < LOD | < LOD | 663 |
| | 01-02 | † | † | † | † | † | † |
| | 03-04 | * | < LOD | < LOD | < LOD | < LOD | 586 |
| 20 years and older | 99-00 | * | < LOD | < LOD | < LOD | < LOD | 1259 |
| | 01-02 | * | < LOD | < LOD | < LOD | < LOD | 1235 |
| | 03-04 | * | < LOD | < LOD | < LOD | < LOD | 1281 |
| **Gender** | | | | | | | |
| Males | 99-00 | * | < LOD | < LOD | < LOD | < LOD | 920 |
| | 01-02 | * | < LOD | < LOD | < LOD | < LOD | 565 |
| | 03-04 | * | < LOD | < LOD | < LOD | < LOD | 917 |
| Females | 99-00 | * | < LOD | < LOD | < LOD | < LOD | 1002 |
| | 01-02 | * | < LOD | < LOD | < LOD | < LOD | 670 |
| | 03-04 | * | < LOD | < LOD | < LOD | < LOD | 950 |
| **Race/ethnicity** | | | | | | | |
| Mexican Americans | 99-00 | * | < LOD | < LOD | < LOD | < LOD | 637 |
| | 01-02 | * | < LOD | < LOD | < LOD | < LOD | 263 |
| | 03-04 | * | < LOD | < LOD | < LOD | < LOD | 423 |
| Non-Hispanic blacks | 99-00 | * | < LOD | < LOD | < LOD | < LOD | 409 |
| | 01-02 | * | < LOD | < LOD | < LOD | < LOD | 217 |
| | 03-04 | * | < LOD | < LOD | < LOD | < LOD | 454 |
| Non-Hispanic whites | 99-00 | * | < LOD | < LOD | < LOD | < LOD | 717 |
| | 01-02 | * | < LOD | < LOD | < LOD | < LOD | 670 |
| | 03-04 | * | < LOD | < LOD | < LOD | < LOD | 869 |

Limit of detection (LOD, see Data Analysis section) for Survey years 99-00, 01-02, and 03-04 are 13.2, 5.8, and 7.1, respectively.
† Data not collected for this age group for Survey year 01-02.
< LOD means less than the limit of detection, which may vary for some chemicals by year and by individual sample.
* Not calculated: proportion of results below limit of detection was too high to provide a valid result.

## Serum 1,2,3,7,8-Pentachlorodibenzofuran (PeCDF) (whole weight)

Geometric mean and selected percentiles of serum concentrations (in fg/g of serum or parts per quadrillion) for the U.S. population from the National Health and Nutrition Examination Survey.

| | Survey years | Geometric mean (95% conf. interval) | Selected percentiles ( 95% confidence interval) | | | | Sample size |
|---|---|---|---|---|---|---|---|
| | | | 50th | 75th | 90th | 95th | |
| Total | 99-00 | * | < LOD | < LOD | < LOD | < LOD | 1922 |
| | 01-02 | * | < LOD | < LOD | < LOD | < LOD | 1235 |
| | 03-04 | * | < LOD | < LOD | < LOD | < LOD | 1867 |
| **Age group** | | | | | | | |
| 12-19 years | 99-00 | * | < LOD | < LOD | < LOD | < LOD | 663 |
| | 01-02 | † | † | † | † | † | † |
| | 03-04 | * | < LOD | < LOD | < LOD | < LOD | 586 |
| 20 years and older | 99-00 | * | < LOD | < LOD | < LOD | < LOD | 1259 |
| | 01-02 | * | < LOD | < LOD | < LOD | < LOD | 1235 |
| | 03-04 | * | < LOD | < LOD | < LOD | < LOD | 1281 |
| **Gender** | | | | | | | |
| Males | 99-00 | * | < LOD | < LOD | < LOD | < LOD | 920 |
| | 01-02 | * | < LOD | < LOD | < LOD | < LOD | 565 |
| | 03-04 | * | < LOD | < LOD | < LOD | < LOD | 917 |
| Females | 99-00 | * | < LOD | < LOD | < LOD | < LOD | 1002 |
| | 01-02 | * | < LOD | < LOD | < LOD | < LOD | 670 |
| | 03-04 | * | < LOD | < LOD | < LOD | < LOD | 950 |
| **Race/ethnicity** | | | | | | | |
| Mexican Americans | 99-00 | * | < LOD | < LOD | < LOD | < LOD | 637 |
| | 01-02 | * | < LOD | < LOD | < LOD | < LOD | 263 |
| | 03-04 | * | < LOD | < LOD | < LOD | < LOD | 423 |
| Non-Hispanic blacks | 99-00 | * | < LOD | < LOD | < LOD | < LOD | 409 |
| | 01-02 | * | < LOD | < LOD | < LOD | < LOD | 217 |
| | 03-04 | * | < LOD | < LOD | < LOD | < LOD | 454 |
| Non-Hispanic whites | 99-00 | * | < LOD | < LOD | < LOD | < LOD | 717 |
| | 01-02 | * | < LOD | < LOD | < LOD | < LOD | 670 |
| | 03-04 | * | < LOD | < LOD | < LOD | < LOD | 869 |

† Data not collected for this age group for Survey year 01-02.
< LOD means less than the limit of detection for the lipid adjusted serum level, which may vary for some chemicals by year and by individual sample.
* Not calculated: proportion of results below limit of detection was too high to provide a valid result.

## Serum 2,3,4,7,8-Pentachlorodibenzofuran (PeCDF) (lipid adjusted)

Geometric mean and selected percentiles of serum concentrations (in pg/g lipid or parts per trillion on a lipid-weight basis) for the U.S. population from the National Health and Nutrition Examination Survey.

| | Survey years | Geometric mean (95% conf. interval) | Selected percentiles ( 95% confidence interval) | | | | Sample size |
|---|---|---|---|---|---|---|---|
| | | | 50th | 75th | 90th | 95th | |
| **Total** | 99-00 | * | < LOD | < LOD | < LOD | 15.9 (13.7-17.1) | 1895 |
| | 01-02 | * | < LOD | 9.20 (7.50-11.1) | 14.3 (12.3-16.2) | 18.1 (16.1-21.1) | 1230 |
| | 03-04 | * | < LOD | 6.80 (<LOD-7.20) | 9.90 (8.90-10.7) | 12.3 (11 0-13.3) | 1871 |
| **Age group** | | | | | | | |
| 12-19 years | 99-00 | * | < LOD | < LOD | < LOD | < LOD | 656 |
| | 01-02 | † | † | † | † | † | † |
| | 03-04 | * | < LOD | < LOD | < LOD | < LOD | 586 |
| 20 years and older | 99-00 | * | < LOD | < LOD | 12.7 (<LOD-13 9) | 16.1 (14.1-17.6) | 1239 |
| | 01-02 | * | < LOD | 9.20 (7.50-11.1) | 14.3 (12.3-16.2) | 18.1 (16.1-21.1) | 1230 |
| | 03-04 | * | < LOD | 7.20 (<LOD-7.70) | 10.3 (9.40-11.2) | 13.0 (11.4-14.7) | 1285 |
| **Gender** | | | | | | | |
| Males | 99-00 | * | < LOD | < LOD | < LOD | 13.9 (12 8-15.4) | 906 |
| | 01-02 | * | < LOD | 9.40 (7.30-11.6) | 14.1 (11.6-16.7) | 16.7 (14 0-22.8) | 560 |
| | 03-04 | * | < LOD | 7.00 (<LOD-7.30) | 9.80 (8.70-10.6) | 12.2 (10.4-14.8) | 920 |
| Females | 99-00 | * | < LOD | < LOD | 13.1 (<LOD-16.1) | 16.7 (14 3-19.2) | 989 |
| | 01-02 | * | < LOD | 9.10 (7.50-10.7) | 14.5 (13.0-16.1) | 18.5 (16.4-21.2) | 670 |
| | 03-04 | * | < LOD | < LOD | 10.3 (8.90-11.0) | 12.6 (11 0-13.7) | 951 |
| **Race/ethnicity** | | | | | | | |
| Mexican Americans | 99-00 | * | < LOD | < LOD | < LOD | < LOD | 632 |
| | 01-02 | * | < LOD | < LOD | 7.80 (6.10-9 80) | 9.80 (7.80-12.5) | 264 |
| | 03-04 | * | < LOD | < LOD | < LOD | 7.90 (<LOD-10.5) | 423 |
| Non-Hispanic blacks | 99-00 | * | < LOD | < LOD | < LOD | 16.3 (13.4-19.0) | 400 |
| | 01-02 | * | < LOD | 8.40 (6.80-9.30) | 14.1 (11.7-16.4) | 19.1 (15.1-23.0) | 216 |
| | 03-04 | * | < LOD | < LOD | 9.80 (8.00-13.9) | 15.9 (9.70-23.9) | 454 |
| Non-Hispanic whites | 99-00 | * | < LOD | < LOD | < LOD | 15.6 (13 8-17.1) | 706 |
| | 01-02 | * | 5.90 (<LOD-6.90) | 10.3 (8.10-12.0) | 15.5 (13.0-17.6) | 18.5 (16 5-22.2) | 665 |
| | 03-04 | * | < LOD | 7.10 (<LOD-7.70) | 10.3 (9.10-11.2) | 12.4 (11 0-13.7) | 873 |

Limit of detection (LOD, see Data Analysis section) for Survey years 99-00, 01-02, and 03-04 are 12.7, 5.5, and 6.8, respectively.
† Data not collected for this age group for Survey year 01-02.
< LOD means less than the limit of detection, which may vary for some chemicals by year and by individual sample.
* Not calculated: proportion of results below limit of detection was too high to provide a valid result.

## Serum 2,3,4,7,8-Pentachlorodibenzofuran (PeCDF) (whole weight)

Geometric mean and selected percentiles of serum concentrations (in fg/g of serum or parts per quadrillion) for the U.S. population from the National Health and Nutrition Examination Survey.

| | Survey years | Geometric mean (95% conf. interval) | Selected percentiles ( 95% confidence interval) | | | | Sample size |
|---|---|---|---|---|---|---|---|
| | | | 50th | 75th | 90th | 95th | |
| Total | 99-00 | * | < LOD | < LOD | < LOD | 103 (96.0-113) | 1895 |
| | 01-02 | * | < LOD | 60.8 (51 3-70.6) | 99.4 (83.4-114) | 134 (113-152) | 1230 |
| | 03-04 | * | < LOD | 44.2 (<LOD-46.9) | 65.7 (60.5-71.1) | 83.9 (74.9-92 9) | 1871 |
| **Age group** | | | | | | | |
| 12-19 years | 99-00 | * | < LOD | < LOD | < LOD | < LOD | 656 |
| | 01-02 | † | † | † | † | † | † |
| | 03-04 | * | < LOD | < LOD | < LOD | < LOD | 586 |
| 20 years and older | 99-00 | * | < LOD | < LOD | 85.2 (<LOD-96.0) | 107 (98.3-125) | 1239 |
| | 01-02 | * | < LOD | 60.8 (51 3-70.6) | 99.4 (83.4-114) | 134 (113-152) | 1230 |
| | 03-04 | * | < LOD | 46.5 (<LOD-50.6) | 69.3 (62.2-74.6) | 86.8 (78.3-99 8) | 1285 |
| **Gender** | | | | | | | |
| Males | 99-00 | * | < LOD | < LOD | < LOD | 95.7 (80.1-101) | 906 |
| | 01-02 | * | < LOD | 62.7 (49 3-76.6) | 98.5 (76.6-134) | 135 (105-160) | 560 |
| | 03-04 | * | < LOD | 43.4 (<LOD-46.3) | 62.0 (56.8-71.9) | 83.2 (72.4-95 0) | 920 |
| Females | 99-00 | * | < LOD | < LOD | 90.0 (<LOD-101) | 111 (97.2-129) | 989 |
| | 01-02 | * | < LOD | 59.8 (52 0-67.6) | 100 (90.5-105) | 126 (107-146) | 670 |
| | 03-04 | * | < LOD | < LOD | 66.9 (59.7-74.3) | 84.4 (74.7-95.7) | 951 |
| **Race/ethnicity** | | | | | | | |
| Mexican Americans | 99-00 | * | < LOD | < LOD | < LOD | < LOD | 632 |
| | 01-02 | * | < LOD | < LOD | 55.8 (48.7-69.7) | 76.3 (61.9-92.4) | 264 |
| | 03-04 | * | < LOD | < LOD | < LOD | 57.1 (<LOD-70.2) | 423 |
| Non-Hispanic blacks | 99-00 | * | < LOD | < LOD | < LOD | 105 (82.7-116) | 400 |
| | 01-02 | * | < LOD | 50.0 (41 3-60.4) | 89.5 (72.3-107) | 121 (92.0-154) | 216 |
| | 03-04 | * | < LOD | < LOD | 66.8 (48.5-93.2) | 97.4 (79.1-129) | 454 |
| Non-Hispanic whites | 99-00 | * | < LOD | < LOD | < LOD | 103 (96.8-122) | 706 |
| | 01-02 | * | 37.5 (<LOD-44.1) | 65.7 (52 9-78.2) | 104 (90.7-118) | 136 (118-154) | 665 |
| | 03-04 | * | < LOD | 45.9 (<LOD-50.6) | 68.3 (61.3-73.6) | 85.0 (74.6-102) | 873 |

† Data not collected for this age group for Survey year 01-02.
< LOD means less than the limit of detection for the lipid adjusted serum level, which may vary for some chemicals by year and by individual sample.
* Not calculated: proportion of results below limit of detection was too high to provide a valid result.

## Serum 2,3,7,8-Tetrachlorodibenzofuran (TCDF) (lipid adjusted)

Geometric mean and selected percentiles of serum concentrations (in pg/g lipid or parts per trillion on a lipid-weight basis) for the U.S. population from the National Health and Nutrition Examination Survey.

| | Survey years | Geometric mean (95% conf. interval) | Selected percentiles ( 95% confidence interval) | | | | Sample size |
|---|---|---|---|---|---|---|---|
| | | | 50th | 75th | 90th | 95th | |
| **Total** | 99-00 | * | < LOD | < LOD | < LOD | < LOD | 1903 |
| | 01-02 | * | < LOD | < LOD | < LOD | < LOD | 1229 |
| | 03-04 | * | < LOD | < LOD | < LOD | < LOD | 1868 |
| **Age group** | | | | | | | |
| 12-19 years | 99-00 | * | < LOD | < LOD | < LOD | < LOD | 660 |
| | 01-02 | † | † | † | † | † | † |
| | 03-04 | * | < LOD | < LOD | < LOD | < LOD | 586 |
| 20 years and older | 99-00 | * | < LOD | < LOD | < LOD | < LOD | 1243 |
| | 01-02 | * | < LOD | < LOD | < LOD | < LOD | 1229 |
| | 03-04 | * | < LOD | < LOD | < LOD | < LOD | 1282 |
| **Gender** | | | | | | | |
| Males | 99-00 | * | < LOD | < LOD | < LOD | < LOD | 912 |
| | 01-02 | * | < LOD | < LOD | < LOD | < LOD | 558 |
| | 03-04 | * | < LOD | < LOD | < LOD | < LOD | 917 |
| Females | 99-00 | * | < LOD | < LOD | < LOD | < LOD | 991 |
| | 01-02 | * | < LOD | < LOD | < LOD | < LOD | 671 |
| | 03-04 | * | < LOD | < LOD | < LOD | < LOD | 951 |
| **Race/ethnicity** | | | | | | | |
| Mexican Americans | 99-00 | * | < LOD | < LOD | < LOD | < LOD | 628 |
| | 01-02 | * | < LOD | < LOD | < LOD | < LOD | 262 |
| | 03-04 | * | < LOD | < LOD | < LOD | < LOD | 423 |
| Non-Hispanic blacks | 99-00 | * | < LOD | < LOD | < LOD | < LOD | 409 |
| | 01-02 | * | < LOD | < LOD | < LOD | < LOD | 217 |
| | 03-04 | * | < LOD | < LOD | < LOD | < LOD | 454 |
| Non-Hispanic whites | 99-00 | * | < LOD | < LOD | < LOD | < LOD | 707 |
| | 01-02 | * | < LOD | < LOD | < LOD | < LOD | 667 |
| | 03-04 | * | < LOD | < LOD | < LOD | < LOD | 870 |

Limit of detection (LOD, see Data Analysis section) for Survey years 99-00, 01-02, and 03-04 are 11.9, 5.2, and 6.0, respectively.
† Data not collected for this age group for Survey year 01-02.
< LOD means less than the limit of detection, which may vary for some chemicals by year and by individual sample.
* Not calculated: proportion of results below limit of detection was too high to provide a valid result.

## Serum 2,3,7,8-Tetrachlorodibenzofuran (TCDF) (whole weight)

Geometric mean and selected percentiles of serum concentrations (in fg/g of serum or parts per quadrillion) for the U.S. population from the National Health and Nutrition Examination Survey.

| | Survey years | Geometric mean (95% conf. interval) | 50th | 75th | 90th | 95th | Sample size |
|---|---|---|---|---|---|---|---|
| Total | 99-00 | * | < LOD | < LOD | < LOD | < LOD | 1903 |
| | 01-02 | * | < LOD | < LOD | < LOD | < LOD | 1229 |
| | 03-04 | * | < LOD | < LOD | < LOD | < LOD | 1868 |
| **Age group** | | | | | | | |
| 12-19 years | 99-00 | * | < LOD | < LOD | < LOD | < LOD | 660 |
| | 01-02 | † | † | † | † | † | † |
| | 03-04 | * | < LOD | < LOD | < LOD | < LOD | 586 |
| 20 years and older | 99-00 | * | < LOD | < LOD | < LOD | < LOD | 1243 |
| | 01-02 | * | < LOD | < LOD | < LOD | < LOD | 1229 |
| | 03-04 | * | < LOD | < LOD | < LOD | < LOD | 1282 |
| **Gender** | | | | | | | |
| Males | 99-00 | * | < LOD | < LOD | < LOD | < LOD | 912 |
| | 01-02 | * | < LOD | < LOD | < LOD | < LOD | 558 |
| | 03-04 | * | < LOD | < LOD | < LOD | < LOD | 917 |
| Females | 99-00 | * | < LOD | < LOD | < LOD | < LOD | 991 |
| | 01-02 | * | < LOD | < LOD | < LOD | < LOD | 671 |
| | 03-04 | * | < LOD | < LOD | < LOD | < LOD | 951 |
| **Race/ethnicity** | | | | | | | |
| Mexican Americans | 99-00 | * | < LOD | < LOD | < LOD | < LOD | 628 |
| | 01-02 | * | < LOD | < LOD | < LOD | < LOD | 262 |
| | 03-04 | * | < LOD | < LOD | < LOD | < LOD | 423 |
| Non-Hispanic blacks | 99-00 | * | < LOD | < LOD | < LOD | < LOD | 409 |
| | 01-02 | * | < LOD | < LOD | < LOD | < LOD | 217 |
| | 03-04 | * | < LOD | < LOD | < LOD | < LOD | 454 |
| Non-Hispanic whites | 99-00 | * | < LOD | < LOD | < LOD | < LOD | 707 |
| | 01-02 | * | < LOD | < LOD | < LOD | < LOD | 667 |
| | 03-04 | * | < LOD | < LOD | < LOD | < LOD | 870 |

† Data not collected for this age group for Survey year 01-02.
< LOD means less than the limit of detection for the lipid adjusted serum level, which may vary for some chemicals by year and by individual sample.
* Not calculated: proportion of results below limit of detection was too high to provide a valid result.

## Serum 3,4,4',5-Tetrachlorobiphenyl (PCB 81) (lipid adjusted)

Geometric mean and selected percentiles of serum concentrations (in pg/g lipid or parts per trillion on a lipid-weight basis) for the U.S. population from the National Health and Nutrition Examination Survey.

| | Survey years | Geometric mean (95% conf. interval) | Selected percentiles ( 95% confidence interval) | | | | Sample size |
|---|---|---|---|---|---|---|---|
| | | | 50th | 75th | 90th | 95th | |
| **Total** | 99-00 | * | < LOD | < LOD | < LOD | < LOD | 1883 |
| | 01-02 | * | < LOD | < LOD | < LOD | < LOD | 1215 |
| | 03-04 | * | < LOD | < LOD | < LOD | 13.4 (<LOD-16.4) | 1860 |
| **Age group** | | | | | | | |
| 12-19 years | 99-00 | * | < LOD | < LOD | < LOD | < LOD | 651 |
| | 01-02 | † | † | † | † | † | † |
| | 03-04 | * | < LOD | < LOD | < LOD | 14.7 (<LOD-16.5) | 579 |
| 20 years and older | 99-00 | * | < LOD | < LOD | < LOD | < LOD | 1232 |
| | 01-02 | * | < LOD | < LOD | < LOD | < LOD | 1215 |
| | 03-04 | * | < LOD | < LOD | < LOD | 13.1 (<LOD-16.5) | 1281 |
| **Gender** | | | | | | | |
| Males | 99-00 | * | < LOD | < LOD | < LOD | < LOD | 900 |
| | 01-02 | * | < LOD | < LOD | < LOD | < LOD | 554 |
| | 03-04 | * | < LOD | < LOD | < LOD | 14.4 (<LOD-17.9) | 913 |
| Females | 99-00 | * | < LOD | < LOD | < LOD | < LOD | 983 |
| | 01-02 | * | < LOD | < LOD | < LOD | < LOD | 661 |
| | 03-04 | * | < LOD | < LOD | < LOD | < LOD | 947 |
| **Race/ethnicity** | | | | | | | |
| Mexican Americans | 99-00 | * | < LOD | < LOD | < LOD | < LOD | 621 |
| | 01-02 | * | < LOD | < LOD | < LOD | < LOD | 259 |
| | 03-04 | * | < LOD | < LOD | < LOD | 18.7 (<LOD-25.2) | 420 |
| Non-Hispanic blacks | 99-00 | * | < LOD | < LOD | < LOD | < LOD | 405 |
| | 01-02 | * | < LOD | < LOD | < LOD | < LOD | 218 |
| | 03-04 | * | < LOD | < LOD | < LOD | < LOD | 453 |
| Non-Hispanic whites | 99-00 | * | < LOD | < LOD | < LOD | < LOD | 699 |
| | 01-02 | * | < LOD | < LOD | < LOD | < LOD | 657 |
| | 03-04 | * | < LOD | < LOD | < LOD | 13.1 (<LOD-16.4) | 867 |

Limit of detection (LOD, see Data Analysis section) for Survey years 99-00, 01-02, and 03-04 are 68.4, 26 8, and 13.1, respectively.
† Data not collected for this age group for Survey year 01-02.
< LOD means less than the limit of detection, which may vary for some chemicals by year and by individual sample.
* Not calculated: proportion of results below limit of detection was too high to provide a valid result.

# Serum 3,4,4',5-Tetrachlorobiphenyl (PCB 81) (whole weight)

Geometric mean and selected percentiles of serum concentrations (in fg/g of serum or parts per quadrillion) for the U.S. population from the National Health and Nutrition Examination Survey.

| | Survey years | Geometric mean (95% conf. interval) | Selected percentiles ( 95% confidence interval) | | | | Sample size |
|---|---|---|---|---|---|---|---|
| | | | 50th | 75th | 90th | 95th | |
| **Total** | 99-00 | * | < LOD | < LOD | < LOD | < LOD | 1883 |
| | 01-02 | * | < LOD | < LOD | < LOD | < LOD | 1215 |
| | 03-04 | * | < LOD | < LOD | < LOD | 80.3 (<LOD-96.2) | 1860 |
| **Age group** | | | | | | | |
| 12-19 years | 99-00 | * | < LOD | < LOD | < LOD | < LOD | 651 |
| | 01-02 | † | † | † | † | † | † |
| | 03-04 | * | < LOD | < LOD | < LOD | 71.4 (<LOD-82.8) | 579 |
| 20 years and older | 99-00 | * | < LOD | < LOD | < LOD | < LOD | 1232 |
| | 01-02 | * | < LOD | < LOD | < LOD | < LOD | 1215 |
| | 03-04 | * | < LOD | < LOD | < LOD | 80.7 (<LOD-99.3) | 1281 |
| **Gender** | | | | | | | |
| Males | 99-00 | * | < LOD | < LOD | < LOD | < LOD | 900 |
| | 01-02 | * | < LOD | < LOD | < LOD | < LOD | 554 |
| | 03-04 | * | < LOD | < LOD | < LOD | 81.1 (<LOD-104) | 913 |
| Females | 99-00 | * | < LOD | < LOD | < LOD | < LOD | 983 |
| | 01-02 | * | < LOD | < LOD | < LOD | < LOD | 661 |
| | 03-04 | * | < LOD | < LOD | < LOD | < LOD | 947 |
| **Race/ethnicity** | | | | | | | |
| Mexican Americans | 99-00 | * | < LOD | < LOD | < LOD | < LOD | 621 |
| | 01-02 | * | < LOD | < LOD | < LOD | < LOD | 259 |
| | 03-04 | * | < LOD | < LOD | < LOD | 103 (<LOD-199) | 420 |
| Non-Hispanic blacks | 99-00 | * | < LOD | < LOD | < LOD | < LOD | 405 |
| | 01-02 | * | < LOD | < LOD | < LOD | < LOD | 218 |
| | 03-04 | * | < LOD | < LOD | < LOD | < LOD | 453 |
| Non-Hispanic whites | 99-00 | * | < LOD | < LOD | < LOD | < LOD | 699 |
| | 01-02 | * | < LOD | < LOD | < LOD | < LOD | 657 |
| | 03-04 | * | < LOD | < LOD | < LOD | 80.5 (<LOD-106) | 867 |

† Data not collected for this age group for Survey year 01-02.
< LOD means less than the limit of detection for the lipid adjusted serum level, which may vary for some chemicals by year and by individual sample.
* Not calculated: proportion of results below limit of detection was too high to provide a valid result.

## Serum 3,3',4,4',5-Pentachlorobiphenyl (PCB 126) (lipid adjusted)

Geometric mean and selected percentiles of serum concentrations (in pg/g lipid or parts per trillion on a lipid-weight basis) for the U.S. population from the National Health and Nutrition Examination Survey.

| | Survey years | Geometric mean (95% conf. interval) | Selected percentiles ( 95% confidence interval) | | | | Sample size |
|---|---|---|---|---|---|---|---|
| | | | 50th | 75th | 90th | 95th | |
| **Total** | 99-00 | * | < LOD | 28.5 (24.9-32.8) | 53.2 (45.7-59.9) | 80.5 (62 8-100) | 1896 |
| | 01-02 | 22.7 (20.9-24.7) | 24.5 (22.2-26 8) | 40.8 (36.1-47.5) | 69.3 (61.6-80.8) | 108 (92.7-116) | 1226 |
| | 03-04 | 16.3 (14.9-17 9) | 14.7 (<LOD-16.5) | 24.8 (22.4-27.4) | 46.7 (41.6-51.9) | 68.7 (58.1-84.4) | 1860 |
| **Age group** | | | | | | | |
| 12-19 years | 99-00 | * | < LOD | < LOD | 24.3 (<LOD-27 5) | 31.1 (26.4-36.4) | 658 |
| | 01-02 | † | † | † | † | † | † |
| | 03-04 | * | < LOD | < LOD | 17.0 (15.2-20.2) | 21.2 (17 3-25.6) | 577 |
| 20 years and older | 99-00 | * | < LOD | 30.8 (27.2-36.3) | 57.1 (50.5-65.8) | 89.5 (66.1-110) | 1238 |
| | 01-02 | 22.7 (20.9-24.7) | 24.5 (22.2-26 8) | 40.8 (36.1-47.5) | 69.3 (61.6-80.8) | 108 (92.7-116) | 1226 |
| | 03-04 | 17.6 (16.0-19 3) | 16.0 (14.2-18 6) | 26.8 (24.2-30.3) | 49.8 (43.5-59.1) | 74.8 (60 2-94.4) | 1283 |
| **Gender** | | | | | | | |
| Males | 99-00 | * | < LOD | 25.8 (<LOD-28 9) | 41.6 (36.1-45.7) | 62.0 (49.7-75.0) | 911 |
| | 01-02 | 20.3 (18.5-22 3) | 23.1 (20.8-25.4) | 36.6 (32.8-39.4) | 52.7 (46.4-62.3) | 81.9 (61 0-101) | 561 |
| | 03-04 | 14.9 (<LOD-16.4) | < LOD | 21.8 (20.1-25.4) | 38.5 (31.0-46.1) | 51.5 (46 5-60.5) | 912 |
| Females | 99-00 | * | < LOD | 33.6 (27.4-41.4) | 59.4 (53.0-78.7) | 98.1 (69 9-120) | 985 |
| | 01-02 | 25.1 (22.9-27 4) | 26.1 (23.0-28 8) | 48.6 (41.4-54.4) | 82.9 (71.1-96.8) | 116 (98 6-128) | 665 |
| | 03-04 | 17.8 (16.0-19.7) | 15.7 (<LOD-18.4) | 27.6 (24.3-33.4) | 57.1 (46.0-67.1) | 82.5 (63 0-109) | 948 |
| **Race/ethnicity** | | | | | | | |
| Mexican Americans | 99-00 | * | < LOD | 23.8 (<LOD-30 3) | 43.2 (37.0-52.6) | 66.1 (52.4-79.2) | 631 |
| | 01-02 | 17.8 (15.5-20.4) | 19.9 (18.3-21 2) | 28.5 (26.5-34.2) | 47.9 (39.7-54.9) | 69.2 (49 3-103) | 262 |
| | 03-04 | 15.5 (<LOD-17.9) | 14.2 (<LOD-17.5) | 22.5 (18.9-26.8) | 31.2 (27.4-37.8) | 42.0 (33 5-48.0) | 420 |
| Non-Hispanic blacks | 99-00 | * | < LOD | 30.6 (25.2-43.1) | 67.4 (45.0-126) | 126 (67.4-224) | 404 |
| | 01-02 | 22.2 (18.2-27 0) | 22.1 (19.6-25.4) | 44.3 (37.9-51.5) | 88.4 (59.0-111) | 115 (96.1-153) | 217 |
| | 03-04 | 16.5 (13.9-19 5) | < LOD | 23.5 (18.9-34.6) | 63.4 (41.5-126) | 142 (52.1-292) | 452 |
| Non-Hispanic whites | 99-00 | * | < LOD | 28.3 (<LOD-34 0) | 50.5 (41.6-57.0) | 67.8 (57 0-94.1) | 704 |
| | 01-02 | 23.1 (20.9-25.4) | 24.7 (22.0-27 6) | 42.0 (35.4-49.6) | 72.3 (63.9-82.9) | 114 (91 0-128) | 663 |
| | 03-04 | 16.0 (14.3-17 8) | 14.5 (<LOD-16.9) | 24.3 (21.4-28.2) | 46.5 (41.6-50.9) | 64.0 (52.1-76.1) | 869 |

Limit of detection (LOD, see Data Analysis section) for Survey years 99-00, 01-02, and 03-04 are 23.2, 10 8, and 13.9, respectively.
† Data not collected for this age group for Survey year 01-02.
< LOD means less than the limit of detection, which may vary for some chemicals by year and by individual sample.
* Not calculated: proportion of results below limit of detection was too high to provide a valid result.

## Serum 3,3',4,4',5-Pentachlorobiphenyl (PCB 126) (whole weight)

Geometric mean and selected percentiles of serum concentrations (in fg/g of serum or parts per quadrillion) for the U.S. population from the National Health and Nutrition Examination Survey.

| | Survey years | Geometric mean (95% conf. interval) | 50th | 75th | 90th | 95th | Sample size |
|---|---|---|---|---|---|---|---|
| **Total** | 99-00 | * | < LOD | 177 (151-212) | 336 (294-404) | 564 (455-663) | 1896 |
| | 01-02 | 147 (135-160) | 158 (143-175) | 270 (249-298) | 482 (436-541) | 738 (625-840) | 1226 |
| | 03-04 | 100 (91.0-110) | 89.8 (<LOD-101) | 159 (146-178) | 308 (273-349) | 475 (378-590) | 1860 |
| **Age group** | | | | | | | |
| 12-19 years | 99-00 | * | < LOD | < LOD | 108 (<LOD-126) | 144 (116-196) | 658 |
| | 01-02 | † | † | † | † | † | † |
| | 03-04 | * | < LOD | < LOD | 88.2 (78.8-106) | 109 (89.2-135) | 577 |
| 20 years and older | 99-00 | * | < LOD | 204 (173-232) | 381 (319-451) | 596 (479-709) | 1238 |
| | 01-02 | 147 (135-160) | 158 (143-175) | 270 (249-298) | 482 (436-541) | 738 (625-840) | 1226 |
| | 03-04 | 111 (100-122) | 100 (88.7-115) | 176 (158-194) | 326 (286-394) | 534 (394-668) | 1283 |
| **Gender** | | | | | | | |
| Males | 99-00 | * | < LOD | 154 (<LOD182) | 260 (241-274) | 382 (308-509) | 911 |
| | 01-02 | 134 (121-149) | 152 (130-169) | 249 (233-267) | 399 (346-467) | 566 (467-693) | 561 |
| | 03-04 | 92.3 (<LOD-102) | < LOD | 148 (131-168) | 245 (203-296) | 360 (296-442) | 912 |
| Females | 99-00 | * | < LOD | 212 (159-250) | 429 (350-531) | 648 (534-744) | 985 |
| | 01-02 | 159 (146-172) | 160 (149-186) | 301 (270-348) | 550 (483-637) | 818 (658-958) | 665 |
| | 03-04 | 108 (96.2-121) | 94.5 (<LOD-110) | 180 (153-212) | 370 (303-455) | 559 (438-843) | 948 |
| **Race/ethnicity** | | | | | | | |
| Mexican Americans | 99-00 | * | < LOD | 146 (<LOD213) | 285 (229-364) | 424 (361-534) | 631 |
| | 01-02 | 114 (97.8-133) | 125 (106-150) | 217 (175-257) | 335 (272-460) | 593 (354-784) | 262 |
| | 03-04 | 95.3 (<LOD-111) | 91.4 (<LOD-99.4) | 145 (116-180) | 238 (172-288) | 298 (238-461) | 420 |
| Non-Hispanic blacks | 99-00 | * | < LOD | 192 (147-258) | 457 (308-691) | 786 (457-1520) | 404 |
| | 01-02 | 131 (106-161) | 128 (110-158) | 266 (214-304) | 532 (361-662) | 779 (585-1060) | 217 |
| | 03-04 | 94.3 (79.0-112) | < LOD | 143 (106-254) | 483 (254-847) | 976 (483-1430) | 452 |
| Non-Hispanic whites | 99-00 | * | < LOD | 175 (<LOD215) | 311 (274-356) | 508 (394-660) | 704 |
| | 01-02 | 150 (136-164) | 160 (146-179) | 276 (249-301) | 486 (431-553) | 746 (600-937) | 663 |
| | 03-04 | 98.4 (87.5-111) | 89.4 (<LOD-104) | 158 (142-182) | 297 (260-346) | 431 (365-541) | 869 |

† Data not collected for this age group for Survey year 01-02.
< LOD means less than the limit of detection for the lipid adjusted serum level, which may vary for some chemicals by year and by individual sample.
* Not calculated: proportion of results below limit of detection was too high to provide a valid result.

## Serum 3,3',4,4',5,5'-Hexachlorobiphenyl (PCB 169) (lipid adjusted)

Geometric mean and selected percentiles of serum concentrations (in pg/g lipid or parts per trillion on a lipid-weight basis) for the U.S. population from the National Health and Nutrition Examination Survey.

| | Survey years | Geometric mean (95% conf. interval) | Selected percentiles ( 95% confidence interval) | | | | Sample size |
|---|---|---|---|---|---|---|---|
| | | | 50th | 75th | 90th | 95th | |
| **Total** | 99-00 | * | < LOD | < LOD | 34.4 (31.0-38.7) | 44.9 (40 6-48.9) | 1888 |
| | 01-02 | 17.9 (16.0-19 9) | 19.0 (17.0-22 0) | 33.1 (27.7-38.6) | 50.0 (43.9-55.0) | 60.9 (56.1-65.8) | 1223 |
| | 03-04 | * | < LOD | 19.5 (16.8-22.7) | 31.0 (27.9-36.0) | 40.6 (36 5-47.3) | 1866 |
| **Age group** | | | | | | | |
| 12-19 years | 99-00 | * | < LOD | < LOD | < LOD | < LOD | 648 |
| | 01-02 | † | † | † | † | † | † |
| | 03-04 | * | < LOD | < LOD | < LOD | < LOD | 581 |
| 20 years and older | 99-00 | * | < LOD | < LOD | 36.4 (33.8-40.3) | 47.8 (42 8-51.0) | 1240 |
| | 01-02 | 17.9 (16.0-19 9) | 19.0 (17.0-22 0) | 33.1 (27.7-38.6) | 50.0 (43.9-55.0) | 60.9 (56.1-65.8) | 1223 |
| | 03-04 | * | < LOD | 21.9 (19.0-24.2) | 32.7 (28.6-37.3) | 43.2 (37 3-49.5) | 1285 |
| **Gender** | | | | | | | |
| Males | 99-00 | * | < LOD | < LOD | 36.2 (31.9-40.1) | 44.3 (39 0-51.3) | 908 |
| | 01-02 | 20.2 (17.8-22 8) | 22.1 (18.5-25 3) | 36.0 (29.5-43.2) | 53.7 (46.5-57.3) | 60.9 (55.7-69.0) | 559 |
| | 03-04 | * | < LOD | 22.3 (17.7-24.8) | 36.3 (29.3-41.1) | 46.1 (38 8-52.0) | 917 |
| Females | 99-00 | * | < LOD | < LOD | 34.0 (29.4-38.6) | 46.5 (37 9-51.1) | 980 |
| | 01-02 | 16.0 (14.2-18.1) | 17.0 (14.7-19 2) | 30.2 (24.5-36.5) | 46.4 (40.7-51.9) | 60.9 (52 2-70.0) | 664 |
| | 03-04 | * | < LOD | 18.4 (<LOD-20.4) | 28.4 (27.2-30.6) | 35.8 (31 0-41.1) | 949 |
| **Race/ethnicity** | | | | | | | |
| Mexican Americans | 99-00 | * | < LOD | < LOD | < LOD | 31.9 (28 8-35.2) | 622 |
| | 01-02 | * | < LOD | 15.0 (11.3-18.3) | 25.4 (18.3-32.3) | 32.5 (26.7-41.9) | 260 |
| | 03-04 | * | < LOD | < LOD | < LOD | 20.9 (16 5-30.2) | 420 |
| Non-Hispanic blacks | 99-00 | * | < LOD | < LOD | 40.3 (28.7-48.6) | 52.2 (44 3-63.6) | 403 |
| | 01-02 | 17.2 (15.4-19.1) | 18.5 (15.7-20 0) | 31.7 (25.8-35.4) | 47.5 (42.0-54.0) | 57.3 (48 3-64.5) | 217 |
| | 03-04 | * | < LOD | 17.3 (<LOD-22 6) | 31.5 (26.8-36.9) | 58.7 (31 5-97.9) | 453 |
| Non-Hispanic whites | 99-00 | * | < LOD | < LOD | 34.6 (31.7-40.1) | 45.3 (40.1-50.9) | 709 |
| | 01-02 | 19.5 (17.2-22 2) | 21.4 (17.4-24.7) | 36.0 (29.8-41.1) | 53.5 (47.0-58.3) | 64.3 (59 2-72.8) | 662 |
| | 03-04 | * | < LOD | 21.2 (17.4-24.5) | 32.6 (27.3-38.8) | 41.1 (35 9-50.2) | 873 |

Limit of detection (LOD, see Data Analysis section) for Survey years 99-00, 01-02, and 03-04 are 27.0, 11 0, and 15.9, respectively.
† Data not collected for this age group for Survey year 01-02.
< LOD means less than the limit of detection, which may vary for some chemicals by year and by individual sample.
* Not calculated: proportion of results below limit of detection was too high to provide a valid result.

# Serum 3,3',4,4',5,5'-Hexachlorobiphenyl (PCB 169) (whole weight)

Geometric mean and selected percentiles of serum concentrations (in fg/g of serum or parts per quadrillion) for the U.S. population from the National Health and Nutrition Examination Survey.

| | Survey years | Geometric mean (95% conf. interval) | Selected percentiles ( 95% confidence interval) | | | | Sample size |
|---|---|---|---|---|---|---|---|
| | | | 50th | 75th | 90th | 95th | |
| **Total** | 99-00 | * | < LOD | < LOD | 230 (219-244) | 287 (274-319) | 1888 |
| | 01-02 | 115 (103-129) | 125 (108-146) | 217 (189-253) | 344 (300-376) | 416 (379-490) | 1223 |
| | 03-04 | * | < LOD | 133 (114-149) | 203 (191-226) | 269 (243-305) | 1866 |
| **Age group** | | | | | | | |
| 12-19 years | 99-00 | * | < LOD | < LOD | < LOD | < LOD | 648 |
| | 01-02 | † | † | † | † | † | † |
| | 03-04 | * | < LOD | < LOD | < LOD | < LOD | 581 |
| 20 years and older | 99-00 | * | < LOD | < LOD | 241 (227-261) | 303 (281-339) | 1240 |
| | 01-02 | 115 (103-129) | 125 (108-146) | 217 (189-253) | 344 (300-376) | 416 (379-490) | 1223 |
| | 03-04 | * | < LOD | 146 (130-160) | 216 (198-242) | 287 (245-325) | 1285 |
| **Gender** | | | | | | | |
| Males | 99-00 | * | < LOD | < LOD | 229 (215-258) | 286 (256-338) | 908 |
| | 01-02 | 133 (117-152) | 151 (130-168) | 244 (198-293) | 363 (309-409) | 449 (372-529) | 559 |
| | 03-04 | * | < LOD | 143 (122-159) | 225 (190-259) | 291 (245-334) | 917 |
| Females | 99-00 | * | < LOD | < LOD | 234 (197-257) | 293 (261-346) | 980 |
| | 01-02 | 102 (90.0-115) | 107 (91.0-123) | 195 (170-234) | 319 (282-368) | 402 (373-462) | 664 |
| | 03-04 | * | < LOD | 120 (<LOD140) | 194 (182-203) | 249 (222-284) | 949 |
| **Race/ethnicity** | | | | | | | |
| Mexican Americans | 99-00 | * | < LOD | < LOD | < LOD | 215 (181-261) | 622 |
| | 01-02 | * | < LOD | 98.1 (79 3-138) | 184 (143-250) | 266 (179-341) | 260 |
| | 03-04 | * | < LOD | < LOD | < LOD | 168 (109-237) | 420 |
| Non-Hispanic blacks | 99-00 | * | < LOD | < LOD | 251 (190-299) | 320 (262-410) | 403 |
| | 01-02 | 101 (91.2-113) | 104 (88.0-118) | 190 (147-234) | 299 (267-335) | 362 (309-423) | 217 |
| | 03-04 | * | < LOD | 110 (<LOD-144) | 216 (162-257) | 338 (221-556) | 453 |
| Non-Hispanic whites | 99-00 | * | < LOD | < LOD | 238 (222-257) | 286 (267-340) | 709 |
| | 01-02 | 127 (112-144) | 145 (124-157) | 229 (195-275) | 368 (317-388) | 438 (388-515) | 662 |
| | 03-04 | * | < LOD | 141 (116-165) | 210 (189-242) | 277 (239-324) | 873 |

† Data not collected for this age group for Survey year 01-02.
< LOD means less than the limit of detection for the lipid adjusted serum level, which may vary for some chemicals by year and by individual sample.
* Not calculated: proportion of results below limit of detection was too high to provide a valid result.

## Serum 2,3,3',4,4'-Pentachlorobiphenyl (PCB 105) (lipid adjusted)

Geometric mean and selected percentiles of serum concentrations (in ng/g of lipid or parts per billion on a lipid-weight basis) for the U.S. population from the National Health and Nutrition Examination Survey.

| | Survey years | Geometric mean (95% conf. interval) | Selected percentiles ( 95% confidence interval) | | | | Sample size |
|---|---|---|---|---|---|---|---|
| | | | 50th | 75th | 90th | 95th | |
| **Total** | 99-00 | * | < LOD | < LOD | < LOD | < LOD | 1915 |
| | 01-02 | * | < LOD | < LOD | < LOD | < LOD | 2307 |
| | 03-04 | 1.20 (1.09-1.31) | 1.09 (1 00-1.20) | 1.90 (1.75-2.20) | 4.04 (3.40-4 89) | 6.24 (5.20-7.79) | 1879 |
| **Age group** | | | | | | | |
| 12-19 years | 99-00 | * | < LOD | < LOD | < LOD | < LOD | 665 |
| | 01-02 | * | < LOD | < LOD | < LOD | < LOD | 758 |
| | 03-04 | .686 (.603-.781) | .700 (.600-.720) | 1.00 (.900-1.11) | 1.50 (1.20-2 00) | 2.26 (1.50-3.50) | 593 |
| 20 years and older | 99-00 | * | < LOD | < LOD | < LOD | < LOD | 1250 |
| | 01-02 | * | < LOD | < LOD | < LOD | < LOD | 1549 |
| | 03-04 | 1.30 (1.18-1.43) | 1.15 (1 04-1.30) | 2.10 (1.86-2.40) | 4.44 (3.80-5 20) | 6.82 (5.70-8.30) | 1286 |
| **Gender** | | | | | | | |
| Males | 99-00 | * | < LOD | < LOD | < LOD | < LOD | 913 |
| | 01-02 | * | < LOD | < LOD | < LOD | < LOD | 1075 |
| | 03-04 | 1.02 (.923-1.12) | .980 (.850-1.08) | 1.60 (1.40-1.80) | 3.20 (2.76-3.42) | 4.70 (3.83-5.50) | 937 |
| Females | 99-00 | * | < LOD | < LOD | < LOD | < LOD | 1002 |
| | 01-02 | * | < LOD | < LOD | < LOD | < LOD | 1232 |
| | 03-04 | 1.40 (1.25-1.57) | 1.20 (1 05-1.40) | 2.30 (2.00-2.79) | 5.17 (4.47-5 90) | 7.70 (6.00-9.55) | 942 |
| **Race/ethnicity** | | | | | | | |
| Mexican Americans | 99-00 | * | < LOD | < LOD | < LOD | < LOD | 635 |
| | 01-02 | * | < LOD | < LOD | < LOD | < LOD | 567 |
| | 03-04 | .719 (.624-829) | .700 (.600-.800) | 1.10 (.900-1.36) | 1.90 (1.80-2 20) | 2.90 (1.98-3.52) | 427 |
| Non-Hispanic blacks | 99-00 | * | < LOD | < LOD | < LOD | 12.8 (<LOD-18.0) | 409 |
| | 01-02 | * | < LOD | < LOD | < LOD | < LOD | 515 |
| | 03-04 | 1.41 (1.15-1.74) | 1.14 (.980-1.32) | 2.47 (1.70-3.90) | 6.70 (4.09-10.1) | 11.9 (6.40-18.1) | 456 |
| Non-Hispanic whites | 99-00 | * | < LOD | < LOD | < LOD | < LOD | 714 |
| | 01-02 | * | < LOD | < LOD | < LOD | < LOD | 1061 |
| | 03-04 | 1.21 (1.08-1.36) | 1.10 (1 00-1.20) | 1.90 (1.74-2.28) | 3.91 (3.22-4 85) | 5.93 (4.98-7.79) | 878 |

Limit of detection (LOD, see Data Analysis section) for Survey years 99-00, 01-02, and 03-04 are 12.4, 10 5, and 0.4, respectively.
< LOD means less than the limit of detection, which may vary for some chemicals by year and by individual sample.
* Not calculated: proportion of results below limit of detection was too high to provide a valid result.

## Serum 2,3,3',4,4'-Pentachlorobiphenyl (PCB 105) (whole weight)

Geometric mean and selected percentiles of serum concentrations (in ng/g of serum or parts per billion) for the U.S. population from the National Health and Nutrition Examination Survey.

| | Survey years | Geometric mean (95% conf. interval) | 50th | 75th | 90th | 95th | Sample size |
|---|---|---|---|---|---|---|---|
| **Total** | 99-00 | * | < LOD | < LOD | < LOD | < LOD | 1915 |
| | 01-02 | * | < LOD | < LOD | < LOD | < LOD | 2307 |
| | 03-04 | .007 (.007-.008) | .007 (.006-.007) | .012 ( 011-.014) | .027 (.023-.031) | .043 (.037- 049) | 1879 |
| **Age group** | | | | | | | |
| 12-19 years | 99-00 | * | < LOD | < LOD | < LOD | < LOD | 665 |
| | 01-02 | * | < LOD | < LOD | < LOD | < LOD | 758 |
| | 03-04 | .003 (.003-.004) | .003 (.003-.004) | .005 ( 005-.006) | .008 (.006-.010) | .011 (.008- 020) | 593 |
| 20 years and older | 99-00 | * | < LOD | < LOD | < LOD | < LOD | 1250 |
| | 01-02 | * | < LOD | < LOD | < LOD | < LOD | 1549 |
| | 03-04 | .008 (.007-.009) | .007 (.006-.008) | .014 ( 012-.015) | .030 (.026-.035) | .047 (.039- 053) | 1286 |
| **Gender** | | | | | | | |
| Males | 99-00 | * | < LOD | < LOD | < LOD | < LOD | 913 |
| | 01-02 | * | < LOD | < LOD | < LOD | < LOD | 1075 |
| | 03-04 | .006 (.006-.007) | .006 (.005-.007) | .010 ( 009-.011) | .019 (.016-.023) | .030 (.027- 039) | 937 |
| Females | 99-00 | * | < LOD | < LOD | < LOD | < LOD | 1002 |
| | 01-02 | * | < LOD | < LOD | < LOD | < LOD | 1232 |
| | 03-04 | .008 (.007-.010) | .007 (.006-.009) | .015 ( 013-.017) | .033 (.029-.040) | .049 (.043- 067) | 942 |
| **Race/ethnicity** | | | | | | | |
| Mexican Americans | 99-00 | * | < LOD | < LOD | < LOD | < LOD | 635 |
| | 01-02 | * | < LOD | < LOD | < LOD | < LOD | 567 |
| | 03-04 | .004 (.004-.005) | .004 (.004-.005) | .007 ( 006-.009) | .014 (.011-.017) | .019 (.015- 023) | 427 |
| Non-Hispanic blacks | 99-00 | * | < LOD | < LOD | < LOD | .090 (<LOD-.110) | 409 |
| | 01-02 | * | < LOD | < LOD | < LOD | < LOD | 515 |
| | 03-04 | .008 (.007-.010) | .007 (.005-.008) | .015 ( 010-.020) | .041 (.027-.067) | .082 (.041-.116) | 456 |
| Non-Hispanic whites | 99-00 | * | < LOD | < LOD | < LOD | < LOD | 714 |
| | 01-02 | * | < LOD | < LOD | < LOD | < LOD | 1061 |
| | 03-04 | .007 (.007-.008) | .007 (.006-.007) | .012 ( 011-.014) | .027 (.022-.031) | .043 (.035- 049) | 878 |

< LOD means less than the limit of detection for the lipid adjusted serum level, which may vary for some chemicals by year and by individual sample.
* Not calculated: proportion of results below limit of detection was too high to provide a valid result.

## Serum 2,3',4,4',5-Pentachlorobiphenyl (PCB 118) (lipid adjusted)

Geometric mean and selected percentiles of serum concentrations (in ng/g of lipid or parts per billion on a lipid-weight basis) for the U.S. population from the National Health and Nutrition Examination Survey.

| | Survey years | Geometric mean (95% conf. interval) | Selected percentiles ( 95% confidence interval) | | | | Sample size |
|---|---|---|---|---|---|---|---|
| | | | 50th | 75th | 90th | 95th | |
| **Total** | 99-00 | * | < LOD | 13.1 (<LOD-15.1) | 27.0 (22.1-30.3) | 40.8 (32 8-48.6) | 1926 |
| | 01-02 | * | < LOD | 15.1 (13.0-17.5) | 29.0 (26.1-33.7) | 44.6 (39 6-48.9) | 2307 |
| | 03-04 | 6.00 (5.54-6.50) | 5.19 (4 80-5.61) | 10.4 (9.70-11.6) | 21.8 (19.3-23.8) | 31.3 (28 2-36.6) | 1887 |
| **Age group** | | | | | | | |
| 12-19 years | 99-00 | * | < LOD | < LOD | < LOD | < LOD | 667 |
| | 01-02 | * | < LOD | < LOD | < LOD | < LOD | 758 |
| | 03-04 | 3.06 (2.76-3.39) | 2.83 (2.70-3.10) | 4.15 (3.60-4.56) | 6.80 (4.70-9 60) | 9.60 (6.80-13.2) | 596 |
| 20 years and older | 99-00 | * | < LOD | 14.9 (12.9-17.4) | 28.1 (24.8-33.8) | 43.8 (35 6-52.3) | 1259 |
| | 01-02 | * | < LOD | 16.9 (15.1-19.0) | 32.4 (28.3-37.3) | 46.5 (41.1-51.0) | 1549 |
| | 03-04 | 6.62 (6.10-7.18) | 5.65 (5 21-6.40) | 11.5 (10.2-12.6) | 22.8 (20.7-25.9) | 34.3 (29 6-39.6) | 1291 |
| **Gender** | | | | | | | |
| Males | 99-00 | * | < LOD | < LOD | 19.6 (16.6-24.4) | 28.0 (24.4-38.1) | 919 |
| | 01-02 | * | < LOD | 12.0 (<LOD-14 9) | 22.0 (17.6-27.1) | 32.7 (25.4-47.5) | 1075 |
| | 03-04 | 5.11 (4.70-5.57) | 4.71 (4.16-5.06) | 8.72 (7.30-9.70) | 16.4 (14.0-18.9) | 23.2 (20.7-25.1) | 940 |
| Females | 99-00 | * | < LOD | 16.7 (13.6-19.7) | 32.0 (27.1-40.3) | 46.8 (41 2-57.8) | 1007 |
| | 01-02 | * | < LOD | 18.7 (16.5-21.0) | 36.4 (31.6-40.9) | 48.9 (44 5-54.3) | 1232 |
| | 03-04 | 6.99 (6.32-7.73) | 6.02 (5 31-6.84) | 12.3 (11.1-14.4) | 27.3 (22.7-30.0) | 37.8 (31 3-45.0) | 947 |
| **Race/ethnicity** | | | | | | | |
| Mexican Americans | 99-00 | * | < LOD | < LOD | 17.3 (14.5-19.6) | 23.7 (20 9-27.1) | 636 |
| | 01-02 | * | < LOD | < LOD | 16.8 (12.5-21.7) | 26.4 (19 3-33.2) | 567 |
| | 03-04 | 3.56 (3.04-4.18) | 3.15 (2 60-3.82) | 5.02 (4.26-6.66) | 9.37 (7.45-11.7) | 14.0 (10 0-17.6) | 426 |
| Non-Hispanic blacks | 99-00 | * | < LOD | 19.0 (13.6-21.7) | 38.7 (28.4-54.4) | 59.7 (45.7-80.8) | 413 |
| | 01-02 | * | < LOD | 15.6 (12.6-19.9) | 37.3 (26.1-46.4) | 54.9 (40 0-66.6) | 515 |
| | 03-04 | 6.70 (5.52-8.14) | 5.25 (4.40-6.10) | 12.7 (8.80-18.0) | 35.1 (21.1-45.0) | 57.8 (33 5-110) | 462 |
| Non-Hispanic whites | 99-00 | * | < LOD | 13.1 (<LOD-15 6) | 25.6 (20.8-32.0) | 40.3 (30.4-46.8) | 720 |
| | 01-02 | * | < LOD | 15.9 (13.6-18.1) | 31.1 (27.1-35.9) | 45.3 (38.7-50.1) | 1061 |
| | 03-04 | 6.19 (5.57-6.87) | 5.46 (4 85-6.20) | 10.9 (9.62-12.1) | 22.0 (19.3-24.4) | 30.7 (26 2-36.6) | 878 |

Limit of detection (LOD, see Data Analysis section) for Survey years 99-00, 01-02, and 03-04 are 12.5, 10 5, and 0.6, respectively.
< LOD means less than the limit of detection, which may vary for some chemicals by year and by individual sample.
* Not calculated: proportion of results below limit of detection was too high to provide a valid result.

## Serum 2,3',4,4',5-Pentachlorobiphenyl (PCB 118) (whole weight)

Geometric mean and selected percentiles of serum concentrations (in ng/g of serum or parts per billion) for the U.S. population from the National Health and Nutrition Examination Survey.

| | Survey years | Geometric mean (95% conf. interval) | 50th | 75th | 90th | 95th | Sample size |
|---|---|---|---|---|---|---|---|
| Total | 99-00 | * | < LOD | .090 (<LOD-.100) | .180 (.150-.200) | .260 (.220- 320) | 1926 |
| | 01-02 | * | < LOD | .100 ( 090-.110) | .190 (.160-.220) | .300 (.270- 320) | 2307 |
| | 03-04 | .037 (.034-.040) | .032 (.029-.036) | .066 ( 061-.073) | .143 (.127-.160) | .216 (.192- 233) | 1887 |
| **Age group** | | | | | | | |
| 12-19 years | 99-00 | * | < LOD | < LOD | < LOD | < LOD | 667 |
| | 01-02 | * | < LOD | < LOD | < LOD | < LOD | 758 |
| | 03-04 | .015 (.014-.017) | .014 (.013-.016) | .021 ( 018-.023) | .036 (.024-.046) | .047 (.035- 076) | 596 |
| 20 years and older | 99-00 | * | < LOD | .100 ( 090-.110) | .190 (.170-.220) | .280 (.230- 360) | 1259 |
| | 01-02 | * | < LOD | .110 (.100-.130) | .210 (.180-.250) | .310 (.280- 370) | 1549 |
| | 03-04 | .041 (.038-.045) | .036 (.032-.041) | .072 ( 066-.081) | .159 (.137-.174) | .226 (.202- 249) | 1291 |
| **Gender** | | | | | | | |
| Males | 99-00 | * | < LOD | < LOD | .130 (.110-.140) | .190 (.160- 220) | 919 |
| | 01-02 | * | < LOD | .080 (<LOD-.100) | .140 (.120-.170) | .210 (.160- 300) | 1075 |
| | 03-04 | .032 (.029-.035) | .030 (.026-.033) | .054 ( 046-.062) | .110 (.083-.125) | .160 (.136-.180) | 940 |
| Females | 99-00 | * | < LOD | .110 ( 090-.130) | .210 (.180-.260) | .320 (.260-.410) | 1007 |
| | 01-02 | * | < LOD | .130 (.100-.140) | .240 (.210-.260) | .360 (.300- 380) | 1232 |
| | 03-04 | .042 (.038-.047) | .036 (.030-.043) | .081 ( 068-.097) | .176 (.152-.206) | .242 (.217- 290) | 947 |
| **Race/ethnicity** | | | | | | | |
| Mexican Americans | 99-00 | * | < LOD | < LOD | .110 (.090-.130) | .140 (.130-.180) | 636 |
| | 01-02 | * | < LOD | < LOD | .120 (.080-.160) | .180 (.130- 220) | 567 |
| | 03-04 | .022 (.018-.026) | .019 (.016-.024) | .034 ( 029-.039) | .069 (.046-.086) | .094 (.075-.117) | 426 |
| Non-Hispanic blacks | 99-00 | * | < LOD | .120 ( 080-.150) | .220 (.180-.320) | .400 (.260- 500) | 413 |
| | 01-02 | * | < LOD | .100 ( 070-.120) | .210 (.170-.270) | .320 (.230-.460) | 515 |
| | 03-04 | .038 (.031-.046) | .030 (.026-.034) | .074 ( 054-.106) | .218 (.133-.277) | .370 (.218- 618) | 462 |
| Non-Hispanic whites | 99-00 | * | < LOD | .090 (<LOD-.100) | .180 (.150-.200) | .250 (.200- 330) | 720 |
| | 01-02 | * | < LOD | .100 ( 090-.120) | .210 (.170-.240) | .300 (.270- 360) | 1061 |
| | 03-04 | .038 (.034-.043) | .034 (.029-.040) | .067 ( 062-.076) | .143 (.127-.165) | .209 (.178- 234) | 878 |

< LOD means less than the limit of detection for the lipid adjusted serum level, which may vary for some chemicals by year and by individual sample.
* Not calculated: proportion of results below limit of detection was too high to provide a valid result.

## Serum 2,3,3',4,4',5-Hexachlorobiphenyl (PCB 156) (lipid adjusted)

Geometric mean and selected percentiles of serum concentrations (in ng/g of lipid or parts per billion on a lipid-weight basis) for the U.S. population from the National Health and Nutrition Examination Survey.

| | Survey years | Geometric mean (95% conf. interval) | Selected percentiles ( 95% confidence interval) | | | | Sample size |
|---|---|---|---|---|---|---|---|
| | | | 50th | 75th | 90th | 95th | |
| **Total** | 99-00 | * | < LOD | < LOD | 12.6 (<LOD-13 8) | 17.0 (15 5-18.0) | 1907 |
| | 01-02 | * | < LOD | < LOD | 14.3 (12.1-16.0) | 18.3 (15 6-21.1) | 2296 |
| | 03-04 | 2.54 (2.36-2.74) | 3.29 (2 90-3.80) | 7.00 (6.20-8.07) | 11.4 (10.4-12.6) | 15.3 (13 8-17.5) | 1880 |
| **Age group** | | | | | | | |
| 12-19 years | 99-00 | * | < LOD | < LOD | < LOD | < LOD | 665 |
| | 01-02 | * | < LOD | < LOD | < LOD | < LOD | 756 |
| | 03-04 | * | .500 (<LOD-.660) | 1.20 (1.00-1.43) | 2.30 (2.06-2.45) | 3.00 (2.37-3.60) | 586 |
| 20 years and older | 99-00 | * | < LOD | < LOD | 13.6 (<LOD-14.7) | 17.5 (16 0-20.1) | 1242 |
| | 01-02 | * | < LOD | < LOD | 15.0 (13.3-17.0) | 19.7 (17 0-22.1) | 1540 |
| | 03-04 | 3.31 (3.05-3.60) | 4.10 (3.40-4.66) | 7.81 (6.80-8.70) | 12.0 (10.9-13.5) | 16.8 (14.7-18.6) | 1294 |
| **Gender** | | | | | | | |
| Males | 99-00 | * | < LOD | < LOD | 12.6 (<LOD-14 0) | 17.0 (14 6-18.0) | 912 |
| | 01-02 | * | < LOD | < LOD | 13.7 (11.3-16.4) | 18.4 (14 3-22.1) | 1069 |
| | 03-04 | 2.57 (2.34-2.82) | 3.10 (2 80-3.80) | 6.92 (5.82-8.00) | 11.8 (9.79-14.2) | 17.1 (14.7-19.3) | 940 |
| Females | 99-00 | * | < LOD | < LOD | 12.8 (<LOD-14.7) | 16.5 (15.4-20.7) | 995 |
| | 01-02 | * | < LOD | < LOD | 14.8 (13.2-15.5) | 18.2 (16 2-21.0) | 1227 |
| | 03-04 | 2.51 (2.28-2.76) | 3.42 (2 80-4.10) | 7.09 (6.35-8.10) | 11.1 (10.4-12.0) | 14.1 (12.7-16.8) | 940 |
| **Race/ethnicity** | | | | | | | |
| Mexican Americans | 99-00 | * | < LOD | < LOD | < LOD | < LOD | 631 |
| | 01-02 | * | < LOD | < LOD | < LOD | < LOD | 566 |
| | 03-04 | .858 (.640-1.15) | 1.00 (.700-1.40) | 2.48 (1.50-3.60) | 4.78 (4.00-5 68) | 6.40 (5.40-7.70) | 423 |
| Non-Hispanic blacks | 99-00 | * | < LOD | < LOD | 14.6 (<LOD-20 5) | 23.1 (17 2-32.1) | 412 |
| | 01-02 | * | < LOD | < LOD | 15.5 (12.7-21.0) | 23.5 (16.4-31.4) | 511 |
| | 03-04 | 2.32 (1.87-2.89) | 3.04 (2.40-3.60) | 7.40 (5.48-9.80) | 14.7 (11.5-18.6) | 24.8 (15 0-33.0) | 456 |
| Non-Hispanic whites | 99-00 | * | < LOD | < LOD | 13.6 (<LOD-15 2) | 17.4 (16 0-18.9) | 711 |
| | 01-02 | * | < LOD | < LOD | 15.0 (13.2-17.5) | 19.4 (16 2-22.1) | 1056 |
| | 03-04 | 3.03 (2.70-3.39) | 4.03 (3.15-4.66) | 7.76 (6.51-8.79) | 11.7 (10.5-13.1) | 15.7 (13 5-18.5) | 880 |

Limit of detection (LOD, see Data Analysis section) for Survey years 99-00, 01-02, and 03-04 are 12.5, 10 5, and 0.4, respectively.
< LOD means less than the limit of detection, which may vary for some chemicals by year and by individual sample.
* Not calculated: proportion of results below limit of detection was too high to provide a valid result.

# Serum 2,3,3',4,4',5-Hexachlorobiphenyl (PCB 156) (whole weight)

Geometric mean and selected percentiles of serum concentrations (in ng/g of serum or parts per billion) for the U.S. population from the National Health and Nutrition Examination Survey.

| | Survey years | Geometric mean (95% conf. interval) | Selected percentiles ( 95% confidence interval) | | | | Sample size |
|---|---|---|---|---|---|---|---|
| | | | 50th | 75th | 90th | 95th | |
| **Total** | 99-00 | * | < LOD | < LOD | .090 (<LOD-.090) | .110 (.100-.130) | 1907 |
| | 01-02 | * | < LOD | < LOD | .100 (.080-.110) | .130 (.110-.140) | 2296 |
| | 03-04 | .016 (.014-.017) | .021 (.018-.024) | .048 ( .041-.052) | .075 (.069-.085) | .103 (.094-.112) | 1880 |
| **Age group** | | | | | | | |
| 12-19 years | 99-00 | * | < LOD | < LOD | < LOD | < LOD | 665 |
| | 01-02 | * | < LOD | < LOD | < LOD | < LOD | 756 |
| | 03-04 | * | .003 (<LOD-.003) | .006 ( .005-.007) | .012 (.011-.012) | .015 (.012-.018) | 586 |
| 20 years and older | 99-00 | * | < LOD | < LOD | .090 (<LOD-.100) | .120 (.100-.140) | 1242 |
| | 01-02 | * | < LOD | < LOD | .100 (.090-.120) | .130 (.120-.140) | 1540 |
| | 03-04 | .021 (.019-.023) | .026 (.021-.030) | .051 ( .045-.057) | .082 (.072-.093) | .109 (.098-.121) | 1294 |
| **Gender** | | | | | | | |
| Males | 99-00 | * | < LOD | < LOD | .090 (<LOD-.100) | .110 (.090-.130) | 912 |
| | 01-02 | * | < LOD | < LOD | .090 (.080-.120) | .120 (.110-.150) | 1069 |
| | 03-04 | .016 (.014-.018) | .021 (.017-.025) | .045 ( .037-.054) | .076 (.068-.094) | .108 (.094-.123) | 940 |
| Females | 99-00 | * | < LOD | < LOD | .090 (<LOD-.090) | .110 (.090-.140) | 995 |
| | 01-02 | * | < LOD | < LOD | .100 (.090-.100) | .130 (.110-.140) | 1227 |
| | 03-04 | .015 (.014-.017) | .020 (.017-.025) | .049 ( .044-.052) | .073 (.064-.085) | .101 (.089-.112) | 940 |
| **Race/ethnicity** | | | | | | | |
| Mexican Americans | 99-00 | * | < LOD | < LOD | < LOD | < LOD | 631 |
| | 01-02 | * | < LOD | < LOD | < LOD | < LOD | 566 |
| | 03-04 | .005 (.004-.007) | .007 (.004-.009) | .015 ( .011-.022) | .036 (.025-.041) | .046 (.037-.070) | 423 |
| Non-Hispanic blacks | 99-00 | * | < LOD | < LOD | .090 (<LOD-.120) | .150 (.110-.190) | 412 |
| | 01-02 | * | < LOD | < LOD | .100 (.080-.130) | .150 (.100-.180) | 511 |
| | 03-04 | .013 (.010-.017) | .018 (.014-.022) | .044 ( .032-.056) | .099 (.067-.127) | .166 (.108-.198) | 456 |
| Non-Hispanic whites | 99-00 | * | < LOD | < LOD | .090 (<LOD-.100) | .110 (.100-.130) | 711 |
| | 01-02 | * | < LOD | < LOD | .100 (.090-.120) | .130 (.120-.140) | 1056 |
| | 03-04 | .019 (.017-.021) | .025 (.020-.031) | .051 ( .044-.057) | .078 (.069-.089) | .104 (.094-.119) | 880 |

< LOD means less than the limit of detection for the lipid adjusted serum level, which may vary for some chemicals by year and by individual sample.
* Not calculated: proportion of results below limit of detection was too high to provide a valid result.

## Serum 2,3,3',4,4',5'-Hexachlorobiphenyl (PCB 157) (lipid adjusted)

Geometric mean and selected percentiles of serum concentrations (in ng/g of lipid or parts per billion on a lipid-weight basis) for the U.S. population from the National Health and Nutrition Examination Survey.

| | Survey years | Geometric mean (95% conf. interval) | Selected percentiles ( 95% confidence interval) | | | | Sample size |
|---|---|---|---|---|---|---|---|
| | | | 50th | 75th | 90th | 95th | |
| **Total** | 99-00 | * | < LOD | < LOD | < LOD | < LOD | 1897 |
| | 01-02 | * | < LOD | < LOD | < LOD | < LOD | 2294 |
| | 03-04 | .605 (.554- 661) | .800 (.700-.940) | 1.73 (1.47-1.93) | 2.80 (2.50-3.10) | 3.80 (3.36-4.30) | 1858 |
| **Age group** | | | | | | | |
| 12-19 years | 99-00 | * | < LOD | < LOD | < LOD | < LOD | 654 |
| | 01-02 | * | < LOD | < LOD | < LOD | < LOD | 755 |
| | 03-04 | * | < LOD | < LOD | .690 (.540-.760) | .980 (.750-1.12) | 580 |
| 20 years and older | 99-00 | * | < LOD | < LOD | < LOD | < LOD | 1243 |
| | 01-02 | * | < LOD | < LOD | < LOD | < LOD | 1539 |
| | 03-04 | .743 (.675- 817) | .980 (.800-1.10) | 1.88 (1.69-2.05) | 2.98 (2.68-3 30) | 3.97 (3.51-4.59) | 1278 |
| **Gender** | | | | | | | |
| Males | 99-00 | * | < LOD | < LOD | < LOD | < LOD | 901 |
| | 01-02 | * | < LOD | < LOD | < LOD | < LOD | 1068 |
| | 03-04 | .594 (.541- 653) | .750 (.700-.900) | 1.65 (1.38-1.88) | 2.90 (2.39-3 50) | 4.00 (3.57-4.87) | 928 |
| Females | 99-00 | * | < LOD | < LOD | < LOD | < LOD | 996 |
| | 01-02 | * | < LOD | < LOD | < LOD | < LOD | 1226 |
| | 03-04 | .615 (.552- 685) | .890 (.700-1.00) | 1.79 (1.60-1.99) | 2.70 (2.50-2 91) | 3.40 (3.20-3.93) | 930 |
| **Race/ethnicity** | | | | | | | |
| Mexican Americans | 99-00 | * | < LOD | < LOD | < LOD | < LOD | 622 |
| | 01-02 | * | < LOD | < LOD | < LOD | < LOD | 566 |
| | 03-04 | * | < LOD | .600 (<LOD- 820) | 1.12 (.960-1 32) | 1.59 (1.20-1.80) | 422 |
| Non-Hispanic blacks | 99-00 | * | < LOD | < LOD | < LOD | < LOD | 405 |
| | 01-02 | * | < LOD | < LOD | < LOD | < LOD | 510 |
| | 03-04 | .568 (.488- 662) | .720 (.600-.930) | 1.80 (1.39-2.26) | 3.55 (3.10-4.40) | 5.35 (3.60-8.80) | 448 |
| Non-Hispanic whites | 99-00 | * | < LOD | < LOD | < LOD | < LOD | 716 |
| | 01-02 | * | < LOD | < LOD | < LOD | < LOD | 1055 |
| | 03-04 | .713 (.635- 801) | .980 (.760-1.12) | 1.81 (1.58-2.06) | 2.86 (2.54-3 27) | 3.80 (3.27-4.73) | 869 |

Limit of detection (LOD, see Data Analysis section) for Survey years 99-00, 01-02, and 03-04 are 12.5, 10 5, and 0.4, respectively.
< LOD means less than the limit of detection, which may vary for some chemicals by year and by individual sample.
* Not calculated: proportion of results below limit of detection was too high to provide a valid result.

## Serum 2,3,3',4,4',5'-Hexachlorobiphenyl (PCB 157) (whole weight)

Geometric mean and selected percentiles of serum concentrations (in ng/g of serum or parts per billion) for the U.S. population from the National Health and Nutrition Examination Survey.

| | Survey years | Geometric mean (95% conf. interval) | 50th | 75th | 90th | 95th | Sample size |
|---|---|---|---|---|---|---|---|
| **Total** | 99-00 | * | < LOD | < LOD | < LOD | < LOD | 1897 |
| | 01-02 | * | < LOD | < LOD | < LOD | < LOD | 2294 |
| | 03-04 | .004 (.003-.004) | .005 (.004-.006) | .011 ( 010-.013) | .018 (.016-.021) | .024 (.022-027) | 1858 |
| **Age group** | | | | | | | |
| 12-19 years | 99-00 | * | < LOD | < LOD | < LOD | < LOD | 654 |
| | 01-02 | * | < LOD | < LOD | < LOD | < LOD | 755 |
| | 03-04 | * | < LOD | < LOD | .004 (.003-.004) | .005 (.004- 005) | 580 |
| 20 years and older | 99-00 | * | < LOD | < LOD | < LOD | < LOD | 1243 |
| | 01-02 | * | < LOD | < LOD | < LOD | < LOD | 1539 |
| | 03-04 | .005 (.004-.005) | .006 (.005-.007) | .012 ( 011-.014) | .019 (.017-.022) | .026 (.023- 031) | 1278 |
| **Gender** | | | | | | | |
| Males | 99-00 | * | < LOD | < LOD | < LOD | < LOD | 901 |
| | 01-02 | * | < LOD | < LOD | < LOD | < LOD | 1068 |
| | 03-04 | .004 (.003-.004) | .005 (.004-.006) | .011 ( 009-.012) | .018 (.016-.022) | .025 (.022-.027) | 928 |
| Females | 99-00 | * | < LOD | < LOD | < LOD | < LOD | 996 |
| | 01-02 | * | < LOD | < LOD | < LOD | < LOD | 1226 |
| | 03-04 | .004 (.003-.004) | .005 (.004-.006) | .012 ( 010-.013) | .017 (.016-.020) | .024 (.021- 027) | 930 |
| **Race/ethnicity** | | | | | | | |
| Mexican Americans | 99-00 | * | < LOD | < LOD | < LOD | < LOD | 622 |
| | 01-02 | * | < LOD | < LOD | < LOD | < LOD | 566 |
| | 03-04 | * | < LOD | .004 (<LOD-.006) | .008 (.006-.009) | .011 (.009-014) | 422 |
| Non-Hispanic blacks | 99-00 | * | < LOD | < LOD | < LOD | < LOD | 405 |
| | 01-02 | * | < LOD | < LOD | < LOD | < LOD | 510 |
| | 03-04 | .003 (.003-.004) | .004 (.003-.006) | .011 ( 008-.014) | .025 (.016-.031) | .040 (.026- 050) | 448 |
| Non-Hispanic whites | 99-00 | * | < LOD | < LOD | < LOD | < LOD | 716 |
| | 01-02 | * | < LOD | < LOD | < LOD | < LOD | 1055 |
| | 03-04 | .004 (.004-.005) | .006 (.005-.008) | .012 ( 010-.014) | .018 (.016-.021) | .025 (.022- 027) | 869 |

< LOD means less than the limit of detection for the lipid adjusted serum level, which may vary for some chemicals by year and by individual sample.
* Not calculated: proportion of results below limit of detection was too high to provide a valid result.

## Serum 2,3',4,4',5,5'-Hexachlorobiphenyl (PCB 167) (lipid adjusted)

Geometric mean and selected percentiles of serum concentrations (in ng/g of lipid or parts per billion on a lipid-weight basis) for the U.S. population from the National Health and Nutrition Examination Survey.

| | Survey years | Geometric mean (95% conf. interval) | Selected percentiles ( 95% confidence interval) | | | | Sample size |
|---|---|---|---|---|---|---|---|
| | | | 50th | 75th | 90th | 95th | |
| **Total** | 99-00 | * | < LOD | < LOD | < LOD | < LOD | 1908 |
| | 01-02 | * | < LOD | < LOD | < LOD | < LOD | 2298 |
| | 03-04 | .494 (.441- 553) | .700 (.560-.800) | 1.60 (1.40-1.70) | 2.99 (2.74-3 36) | 4.10 (3.80-4.47) | 1864 |
| **Age group** | | | | | | | |
| 12-19 years | 99-00 | * | < LOD | < LOD | < LOD | < LOD | 666 |
| | 01-02 | * | < LOD | < LOD | < LOD | < LOD | 758 |
| | 03-04 | * | < LOD | < LOD | .640 (.500-.770) | .870 (.700-1.10) | 584 |
| 20 years and older | 99-00 | * | < LOD | < LOD | < LOD | < LOD | 1242 |
| | 01-02 | * | < LOD | < LOD | < LOD | < LOD | 1540 |
| | 03-04 | .592 (.521- 673) | .860 (.700-1.00) | 1.72 (1.55-2.03) | 3.30 (2.90-3 60) | 4.30 (3.90-4.81) | 1280 |
| **Gender** | | | | | | | |
| Males | 99-00 | * | < LOD | < LOD | < LOD | < LOD | 908 |
| | 01-02 | * | < LOD | < LOD | < LOD | < LOD | 1069 |
| | 03-04 | .423 (<LOD-.471) | .500 (.440-.600) | 1.33 (1.16-1.60) | 2.70 (2.25-3 50) | 3.80 (3.50-4.70) | 931 |
| Females | 99-00 | * | < LOD | < LOD | < LOD | < LOD | 1000 |
| | 01-02 | * | < LOD | < LOD | < LOD | < LOD | 1229 |
| | 03-04 | .573 (.492- 669) | .880 (.660-1.06) | 1.71 (1.51-2.10) | 3.21 (2.82-3 62) | 4.30 (3.80-4.70) | 933 |
| **Race/ethnicity** | | | | | | | |
| Mexican Americans | 99-00 | * | < LOD | < LOD | < LOD | < LOD | 627 |
| | 01-02 | * | < LOD | < LOD | < LOD | < LOD | 564 |
| | 03-04 | * | < LOD | .600 (.400-.800) | 1.20 (.960-1.44) | 1.70 (1.30-1.94) | 419 |
| Non-Hispanic blacks | 99-00 | * | < LOD | < LOD | < LOD | < LOD | 411 |
| | 01-02 | * | < LOD | < LOD | < LOD | < LOD | 515 |
| | 03-04 | .521 (.432- 628) | .560 (.460-.800) | 1.95 (1.25-2.40) | 4.30 (3.27-6.79) | 7.90 (4.70-11.8) | 451 |
| Non-Hispanic whites | 99-00 | * | < LOD | < LOD | < LOD | < LOD | 715 |
| | 01-02 | * | < LOD | < LOD | < LOD | < LOD | 1056 |
| | 03-04 | .538 (.458- 632) | .800 (.600-.990) | 1.66 (1.42-1.90) | 2.98 (2.70-3.45) | 3.94 (3.62-4.47) | 875 |

Limit of detection (LOD, see Data Analysis section) for Survey years 99-00, 01-02, and 03-04 are 12.4, 10 5, and 0.4, respectively.
< LOD means less than the limit of detection, which may vary for some chemicals by year and by individual sample.
* Not calculated: proportion of results below limit of detection was too high to provide a valid result.

## Serum 2,3',4,4',5,5'-Hexachlorobiphenyl (PCB 167) (whole weight)

Geometric mean and selected percentiles of serum concentrations (in ng/g of serum or parts per billion) for the U.S. population from the National Health and Nutrition Examination Survey.

| | Survey years | Geometric mean (95% conf. interval) | 50th | 75th | 90th | 95th | Sample size |
|---|---|---|---|---|---|---|---|
| **Total** | 99-00 | * | < LOD | < LOD | < LOD | < LOD | 1908 |
| | 01-02 | * | < LOD | < LOD | < LOD | < LOD | 2298 |
| | 03-04 | .003 (.003-.003) | .004 (.003-.005) | .010 ( 009-.012) | .020 (.018-.022) | .026 (.024-027) | 1864 |
| **Age group** | | | | | | | |
| 12-19 years | 99-00 | * | < LOD | < LOD | < LOD | < LOD | 666 |
| | 01-02 | * | < LOD | < LOD | < LOD | < LOD | 758 |
| | 03-04 | * | < LOD | < LOD | .004 (.003-.004) | .005 (.004- 005) | 584 |
| 20 years and older | 99-00 | * | < LOD | < LOD | < LOD | < LOD | 1242 |
| | 01-02 | * | < LOD | < LOD | < LOD | < LOD | 1540 |
| | 03-04 | .004 (.003-.004) | .005 (.004-.006) | .012 ( 010-.013) | .021 (.019-.023) | .027 (.025- 030) | 1280 |
| **Gender** | | | | | | | |
| Males | 99-00 | * | < LOD | < LOD | < LOD | < LOD | 908 |
| | 01-02 | * | < LOD | < LOD | < LOD | < LOD | 1069 |
| | 03-04 | .003 (<LOD- 003) | .003 (.003-.004) | .009 ( 008-.010) | .018 (.015-.021) | .023 (.021- 026) | 931 |
| Females | 99-00 | * | < LOD | < LOD | < LOD | < LOD | 1000 |
| | 01-02 | * | < LOD | < LOD | < LOD | < LOD | 1229 |
| | 03-04 | .003 (.003-.004) | .005 (.004-.006) | .012 ( 010-.013) | .022 (.019-.024) | .027 (.025- 031) | 933 |
| **Race/ethnicity** | | | | | | | |
| Mexican Americans | 99-00 | * | < LOD | < LOD | < LOD | < LOD | 627 |
| | 01-02 | * | < LOD | < LOD | < LOD | < LOD | 564 |
| | 03-04 | * | < LOD | .004 ( 003-.004) | .009 (.007-.011) | .013 (.010- 015) | 419 |
| Non-Hispanic blacks | 99-00 | * | < LOD | < LOD | < LOD | < LOD | 411 |
| | 01-02 | * | < LOD | < LOD | < LOD | < LOD | 515 |
| | 03-04 | .003 (.002-.004) | .003 (.003-.005) | .012 ( 008-.015) | .028 (.019-.042) | .051 (.030- 072) | 451 |
| Non-Hispanic whites | 99-00 | * | < LOD | < LOD | < LOD | < LOD | 715 |
| | 01-02 | * | < LOD | < LOD | < LOD | < LOD | 1056 |
| | 03-04 | .003 (.003-.004) | .005 (.004-.006) | .011 ( 009-.013) | .020 (.018-.022) | .025 (.023- 027) | 875 |

< LOD means less than the limit of detection for the lipid adjusted serum level, which may vary for some chemicals by year and by individual sample.
* Not calculated: proportion of results below limit of detection was too high to provide a valid result.

# Serum 2,3,3',4,4',5,5'-Heptachlorobiphenyl (PCB 189) (lipid adjusted)

Geometric mean and selected percentiles of serum concentrations (in ng/g of lipid or parts per billion on a lipid-weight basis) for the U.S. population from the National Health and Nutrition Examination Survey.

| | Survey years | Geometric mean (95% conf. interval) | Selected percentiles ( 95% confidence interval) | | | | Sample size |
|---|---|---|---|---|---|---|---|
| | | | 50th | 75th | 90th | 95th | |
| **Total** | 01-02 | * | < LOD | < LOD | < LOD | < LOD | 2298 |
| | 03-04 | * | < LOD | < LOD | .900 (.700-1.16) | 1.47 (1.10-2.18) | 1817 |
| **Age group** | | | | | | | |
| 12-19 years | 01-02 | * | < LOD | < LOD | < LOD | < LOD | 752 |
| | 03-04 | * | < LOD | < LOD | < LOD | 1.00 (<LOD-3.09) | 570 |
| 20 years and older | 01-02 | * | < LOD | < LOD | < LOD | < LOD | 1546 |
| | 03-04 | * | < LOD | < LOD | 1.00 (.760-1 20) | 1.50 (1.10-2.14) | 1247 |
| **Gender** | | | | | | | |
| Males | 01-02 | * | < LOD | < LOD | < LOD | < LOD | 1070 |
| | 03-04 | * | < LOD | < LOD | 1.00 (.800-1 20) | 1.54 (1.20-2.23) | 903 |
| Females | 01-02 | * | < LOD | < LOD | < LOD | < LOD | 1228 |
| | 03-04 | * | < LOD | < LOD | .830 (.600-1.14) | 1.39 ( 890-2.18) | 914 |
| **Race/ethnicity** | | | | | | | |
| Mexican Americans | 01-02 | * | < LOD | < LOD | < LOD | < LOD | 564 |
| | 03-04 | * | < LOD | < LOD | < LOD | .700 (<LOD-1.00) | 406 |
| Non-Hispanic blacks | 01-02 | * | < LOD | < LOD | < LOD | < LOD | 514 |
| | 03-04 | * | < LOD | < LOD | 1.20 (.840-1 60) | 1.85 (1.20-2.83) | 444 |
| Non-Hispanic whites | 01-02 | * | < LOD | < LOD | < LOD | < LOD | 1057 |
| | 03-04 | * | < LOD | < LOD | .900 (.700-1 26) | 1.51 (1.04-2.19) | 851 |

Limit of detection (LOD, see Data Analysis section) for Survey years 01-02 and 03-04 are 10.5 and 0.4.
< LOD means less than the limit of detection, which may vary for some chemicals by year and by individual sample.
* Not calculated: proportion of results below limit of detection was too high to provide a valid result.

## Serum 2,3,3',4,4',5,5'-Heptachlorobiphenyl (PCB 189) (whole weight)

Geometric mean and selected percentiles of serum concentrations (in ng/g of serum or parts per billion) for the U.S. population from the National Health and Nutrition Examination Survey.

| | Survey years | Geometric mean (95% conf. interval) | Selected percentiles ( 95% confidence interval) | | | | Sample size |
|---|---|---|---|---|---|---|---|
| | | | 50th | 75th | 90th | 95th | |
| **Total** | 01-02 | * | < LOD | < LOD | < LOD | < LOD | 2298 |
| | 03-04 | * | < LOD | < LOD | .006 (.005-.008) | .010 (.007- 014) | 1817 |
| **Age group** | | | | | | | |
| 12-19 years | 01-02 | * | < LOD | < LOD | < LOD | < LOD | 752 |
| | 03-04 | * | < LOD | < LOD | < LOD | .005 (<LOD-.017) | 570 |
| 20 years and older | 01-02 | * | < LOD | < LOD | < LOD | < LOD | 1546 |
| | 03-04 | * | < LOD | < LOD | .006 (.005-.008) | .010 (.007- 014) | 1247 |
| **Gender** | | | | | | | |
| Males | 01-02 | * | < LOD | < LOD | < LOD | < LOD | 1070 |
| | 03-04 | * | < LOD | < LOD | .006 (.005-.009) | .011 (.008- 014) | 903 |
| Females | 01-02 | * | < LOD | < LOD | < LOD | < LOD | 1228 |
| | 03-04 | * | < LOD | < LOD | .005 (.004-.008) | .009 (.006- 014) | 914 |
| **Race/ethnicity** | | | | | | | |
| Mexican Americans | 01-02 | * | < LOD | < LOD | < LOD | < LOD | 564 |
| | 03-04 | * | < LOD | < LOD | < LOD | .005 (<LOD-.007) | 406 |
| Non-Hispanic blacks | 01-02 | * | < LOD | < LOD | < LOD | < LOD | 514 |
| | 03-04 | * | < LOD | < LOD | .008 (.005-.010) | .012 (.007- 016) | 444 |
| Non-Hispanic whites | 01-02 | * | < LOD | < LOD | < LOD | < LOD | 1057 |
| | 03-04 | * | < LOD | < LOD | .006 (.005-.008) | .010 (.007- 014) | 851 |

< LOD means less than the limit of detection for the lipid adjusted serum level, which may vary for some chemicals by year and by individual sample.
* Not calculated: proportion of results below limit of detection was too high to provide a valid result.

## References

Anderson HA, Falk C, Hanrahan L, Olson J, Burse VW, Needham LL, et al. Profiles of Great Lakes critical pollutants: a sentinel analysis of human blood and urine. The Great Lakes Consortium. Environ Health Perspect 1998;106(5):279-289.

Apostoli P, Magoni M, Bergonzi R, Carasi S, Indelicato A, Scarcella C, et al. Assessment of reference values for polychlorinated biphenyl concentration in human blood. Chemosphere 2005;61(3):413-421.

Arisawa K, Takeda H, Mikasa H. Background exposure to PCDDs/PCDFs/PCBs and its potential health effects: a review of epidemiologic studies. J Med Invest. 2005;52(1-2):10-21.

Arisawa K, Matsumura T, Tohyama C, Saito H, Satoh H, Nagai M, et al. Fish intake, plasma omega-3 polyunsaturated fatty acids, and polychlorinated dibenzo-*p*-dioxins/polychlorinated dibenzo-furans and co-planar polychlorinated biphenyls in the blood of the Japanese population. Int Arch Occup Environ Health 2003;76(3):205-215.

Aylward LL, Hays SM. Temporal trends in human TCDD body burden: decreases over three decades and implications for exposure levels. J Expo Anal Environ Epidemiol. 2002;12(5):319-328.

Baccarelli A, Mocarelli P, Patterson DG Jr, Bonzini M, Pesatori AC, Caporaso N, et al. Immunologic effects of dioxin: new results from Seveso and comparison with other studies. Environ Health Perspect 2002;110:1169-1173.

Bates MN, Buckland SJ, Garrett N, Ellis H, Needham LL, Patterson DG Jr, et al. Persistent organochlorines in the serum of the non-occupationally exposed New Zealand population. Chemosphere 2004;54:1431-1443.

Beck H, Dross A, Mathar W. PCDD and PCDF exposure and levels in humans in Germany. Environ Health Perspect 1994;102 Suppl 1:173-185.

Calvert GM, Willie KK, Sweeney MH, Fingerhut MA, Halperin WE. Evaluation of serum lipid concentrations among U.S. workers exposed to 2,3,7,8-tetrachlorodibenzo-*p* dioxin. Arch Environ Health 1996;51(2):100-107.

Calvert GM, Sweeney MH, Deddens J, Wall DK. Evaluation of diabetes mellitus, serum glucose, and thyroid function among United States workers exposed to 2,3,7,8-tetrachlorodibenzo-*p*-dioxin. Occup Environ Med 1999;56(4):270-276.

Carpenter DO. Polychlorinated biphenyls (PCBs): routes of exposure and effects on human health. Rev Environ Health 2006;21(1):1-23.

Centers for Disease Control and Prevention (CDC). Third National Report on Human Exposure to Environmental Chemicals. Atlanta (GA). 2005.

Collins JJ, Bodner K, Burns CJ, Budinsky RA, Lamparski LL, Wilken M, et al. Body mass index and serum chlorinated dibenzo-*p*-dioxin and dibenzofuran levels. Chemosphere 2007;66(6):1079-1085.

Collins JJ, Budinsky RA, Burns CJ, Lamparski LL, Carson ML, Martin GD, et al. Serum dioxin levels in former chlorophenol workers. J Expo Sci Environ Epidemiol 2006;16(1):76-84.

Debacker N, Sasse A, van Wouwe N, Goeyens L, Sartor F, van Oyen H. PCDD/F levels in plasma of a belgian population before and after the 1999 Belgian PCB/DIOXIN incident. Chemosphere 2007;67(9):S217-223.

Dhooge W, van Larebeke N, Koppen G, Nelen V, Schoeters G, Vlietinck R, et al. Serum dioxin-like activity is associated with reproductive parameters in young men from the general Flemish population. Environ Health Perspect 2006;114(11):1670-1676.

Egeland GM, Sweeney MH, Fingerhut MA, Wille KK, Schnorr TM, Halperin WE. Total serum testosterone and gonadotropins in workers exposed to dioxin. Am J Epidemiol 1994;139(3):272-281.

Eskenazi B, Mocarelli P, Warner M, Chee WY, Gerthoux PM, Samuels S, et al. Maternal serum dioxin levels and birth outcomes in women of Seveso, Italy. Environ Health Perspect 2003;111(7):947-953.

Eskenazi B, Mocarelli P, Warner M, Needham L, Patterson DG Jr, Samuels S, et al. Relationship of serum TCDD concentrations and age at exposure of female residents of Seveso, Italy. Environ Health Perspect 2004;112(1):22-27.

Eskenazi B, Mocarelli P, Warner M, Samuels S, Vercellini P, Olive D, et al. Serum dioxin concentrations and endometriosis: a cohort study in Seveso, Italy. Environ Health Perspect 2002;110(7):629-634.

Everett CJ, Frithsen IL, Diaz VA, Koopman RJ, Simpson WM Jr, Mainous AG 3rd. Association of a polychlorinated dibenzo-*p*-dioxin, a polychlorinated biphenyl, and DDT with diabetes in the 1999-2002 National Health and Nutrition Examination Survey. Environ Res 2007;103(3):413-418.

Falk C, Hanrahan L, Anderson HA, Kanarek MS, Draheim L, Needham LL. Body burden levels of dioxin, furans, and PCBs among frequent consumers of Great Lakes sport fish. The Great Lakes Consortium. Environ Res 1999;80(2 Pt 2):S19-S25.

Ferriby LL, Knutsen JS, Harris M, Unice KM, Scott P, Nony P, et al. Evaluation of PCDD/F and dioxin-like PCB serum concentration data from the 2001-2002 National Health and Nutrition Examination Survey of the United States population. J Expo Sci Environ Epidemiol 2007;17(4):358-371.

Fierens S, Mairesse H, Heilier JF, De Burbure C, Focant JF, Eppe G, et al. Dioxin/polychlorinated biphenyl body burden, diabetes and endometriosis: findings in a population-based study in Belgium. Biomarkers 2003;8(6):529-534.

Fujiyoshi PT, Michalek JE, Matsumura F. Molecular epidemiologic evidence for diabetogenic effects of dioxin exposure in U.S. Air Force veterans of the Vietnam war. Environ Health Perspect 2006;114(11):1677-1683.

Gao X, Son DS, Terranova PF, Rozman KK. Toxic equivalency factors of polychlorinated dibenzo-p-dioxins in an ovulation model: validation of the toxic equivalency concept for one aspect of endocrine disruption. Toxicol Appl Pharmacol 1999;157(2):107-16.

Geyer HJ, Schramm KW, Feicht EA, Behechti A, Steinberg C, Bruggemann R, et al. Half-lives of tetra-, penta-, hexa-, hepta-, and octachlorodibenzo-p-dioxin in rats, monkeys, and humans—a critical review. Chemosphere 2002;48(6):631-644.

Glynn AW, Wolk A, Aune M, Atuma S, Zettermark S, Maehle-Schmid M, et al. Serum concentrations of organochlorines in men: a search for markers of exposure. Sci Total Environ 2000; 263(1-3):197-208.

Gray LE Jr, Ostby JS. In utero 2,3,7,8-tetrachlorodibenzo-p-dioxin (TCDD) alters reproductive morphology and function in female rat offspring. Toxicol Appl Pharmacol 1995;133(2):285-294.

Gupta A, Ketchum N, Roehrborn CG, Schecter A, Aragaki CC, Michalek JE. Serum dioxin, testosterone, and subsequent risk of benign prostatic hyperplasia: a prospective cohort study of Air Force veterans. Environ Health Perspect 2006;114(11):1649-1654.

Halperin W, Vogt R, Sweeney MH, Shopp G, Fingerhut M, Petersen M. Immunological markers among workers exposed to 2,3,7,8-tetrachlorodibenzo-p-dioxin. Occup Environ Med 1998;55(11):742-749.

Hanrahan LP, Falk C, Anderson HA, Draheim L, Kanarek MS, Olson J. Serum PCB and DDE levels of frequent Great Lakes sport fish consumers—a first look. The Great Lakes Consortium. Environ Res 1999;80(2 Pt 2):S26-S37.

Heilier JF, Nackers F, Verougstraete V, Tonglet R, Lison D, Donnez J. Increased dioxin-like compounds in the serum of women with peritoneal endometriosis and deep endometriotic (adenomyotic) nodules. Fertil Steril 2005;84(2):305-312.

Henriksen GL, Ketchum NS, Michalek JE, Swaby JA. Serum dioxin and diabetes mellitus in veterans of Operation Ranch Hand. Epidemiology 1997;8(3):252-258.

Henriksen GL, Michalek JE, Swaby JA, Rahe AJ. Serum dioxin, testosterone, and gonadotropins in veterans of Operation Ranch Hand. Epidemiology 1996;7(4):352-357.

Hoffman MK, Huwe J, Deyrup CL, Lorentzsen M, Zaylskie R, Clinch NR, et al. Statistically designed survey of polychlorinated dibenzo-p-dioxins, polychlorinated dibenzofurans, and co-planar polychlorinated biphenyls in U. S. meat and poultry, 2002 2003: results, trends, and implications. Environ Sci Technol 2006;40(17):5340-5346.

Hoffman CS, Small CM, Blanck HM, Tolbert P, Rubin C, Marcus M. Endometriosis among women exposed to polybrominated biphenyls. Ann Epidemiol. 2007;17(7):503-510.

Hsu JF, Guo YL, Yang SY, Liao PC. Congener profiles of PCBs and PCDD/Fs in Yucheng victims fifteen years after exposure to toxic rice-bran oils and their implications for epidemiologic studies. Chemosphere 2005;61(9):1231-1243.

International Agency for Research in Cancer (IARC). Working Group on the Evaluation of Carcinogenic Risks to Humans: Polychlorinated Dibenzo-Para-Dioxins and Polychlorinated Dibenzofurans. Lyon, France, 4-11 February 1997. IARC Monogr Eval Carcinog Risks Hum. 1997;69:1-631.

Institute of Medicine (IOM). Veterans and Agent Orange: Update 2004. Committee to Review the Health Effects in Vietman Veterans of Exposure to Herbicides (Fifth Biennial Update). Division of Health Promotion and Disease Prevention. Washington (DC): National Academy Press; 2005. Available at URL: http://www. nap.edu/catalog.php?record_id=11242. 11/28/08

Jacobson JL, Jacobson SW. Intellectual impairment in children exposed to polychlorinated biphenyls in utero. N Engl J Med 1996;335:783-789.

Johansson N, Hanber A, Wingfors H, Tysklind M. PCB in building sealant is influencing PCB levels in blood of residents. Organohalogen Compounds, Volumes 60-65, Dioxin 2003. Boston, MA.

Johnson E, Shorter C, Bestervelt L, Patterson D, Needham L, Piper W, Lucier G, et al. Serum hormone levels in humans with low serum concentrations of 2,3,7,8 TCDD. Toxicol Ind Health 2001;17(4):105-12.

Jung D, Berg PA, Edler L, Ehrenthal W, Fenner D, Flesch-Janys D, et al. Immunologic findings in workers formerly exposed to 2,3,7,8-tetrachlorodibenzo-p-dioxin and its congeners. Environ Health Perspect 1998;106(Suppl 2):689-695.

Kang HK, Dalager NA, Needham LL, Patterson DG Jr, Lees PS, Yates K, Matanoski GM. Health status of Army Chemical Corps Vietnam veterans who sprayed defoliant in Vietnam. Am J Ind Med 2006;49(11):875-884.

Kang D, Tepper A, Patterson DG Jr. Coplanar PCBs and the relative contribution of coplanar PCBs, PCDDs, and PCDFs to the total 2,3,7,8-TCDD toxicity equivalents in human serum.

Chemosphere 1997;35(3):503-511.

Kern PA, Said S, Jackson WG Jr, Michalek JE. Insulin sensitivity following agent orange exposure in Vietnam veterans with high blood levels of 2,3,7,8-tetrachlorodibenzo-*p* dioxin. J Clin Endocrinol Metab 2004;89(9):4665-4672.

Kohler M, Tremp J, Zennegg M, Seiler C, Minder-Kohler S, Beck M, et al. Joint sealants: an overlooked diffuse source of polychlorinated biphenyls in buildings. Environ Sci Technol 2005 Apr 1;39(7):1967-73.

Koopman-Esseboom C, Weisglas-Kuperus N, de Ridder MA, Van der Paauw CG, Tuinstra LG, Sauer PJ. Effects of polychlorinated biphenyl/dioxin exposure and feeding type on infants' mental and psychomotor development. Pediatrics. 1996;97(5):700-6.

Lawson CC, Schnorr TM, Whelan EA, Deddens JA, Dankovic DA, Piacitelli LA, et al. Paternal occupational exposure to 2,3,7,8-tetrachlorodibenzo-*p*-dioxin and birth outcomes of offspring: birth weight, preterm delivery, and birth defects. Environ Health Perspect 2004;112(14):1403-1408.

Lee DH, Lee IK, Song K, Steffes M, Toscano W, Baker BA, Jacobs DR Jr. A strong dose-response relation between serum concentrations of persistent organic pollutants and diabetes: results from the National Health and Examination Survey 1999-2002. Diabetes Care 2006;29(7):1638-1644.

Link B, Gabrio T, Zoellner I, Piechotowski I, Paepke O, Herrmann T, et al. Biomonitoring of persistent organochlorine pesticides, PCDD/PCDFs and dioxin-like PCBs in blood of children from South West Germany (Baden-Wuerttemberg) from 1993 to 2003. Chemosphere 2005;58(9):1185-1201.

Longnecker MP, Ryan JJ, Gladen BC, Schecter AJ. Correlations among human plasma levels of dioxin-like compounds and polychlorinated biphenyls (PCBs) and implications for epidemiologic studies. Arch Environ Health 2000;55(3):195-200.

Longnecker MP, Wolff MS, Gladen BC, Brock JW, Grandjean P, Jacobson JL, et al. Comparison of polychlorinated biphenyl levels across studies of human neurodevelopment. Environ Health Perspect 2003;111(1):65-70.

Lorber M. A pharmacokinetic model for estimating exposure of Americans to dioxin-like compounds in the past, present, and future. Sci Total Environ. 2002;288(1-2):81-95.

Lundqvist C, Zuurbier M, Leijs M, Johansson C, Ceccatelli S, Saunders M, et al. The effects of PCBs and dioxins on child health. Acta Paediatr Suppl 2006;95(453):55-64.

Luotamo M, Jarvisalo J, Aitio A. Assessment of exposure to polychlorinated biphenyls: analysis of selected isomers in blood and adipose tissue. Environ Res 1991;54(2):121-134.

Masuda Y. Fate of PCDF/PCB congeners and change of clinical symptoms in patients with Yusho PCB poisoning for 30 years. Chemosphere 2001:43(4-7):925-930.

Masuda Y, Schecter A, Papke O. Concentrations of PCBs, PCDFs and PCDDs in the blood of Yusho patients and their toxic equivalent contribution. Chemosphere 1998;37(9-12):1773-1780.

Michalek JE, Akhtar FZ, Kiel JL. Serum dioxin, insulin, fasting glucose, and sex hormone-binding globulin in veterans of Operation Ranch Hand. J Clin Endocrinol Metab 1999;84(5):1540-1543.

Michalek JE, Ketchum NS, Tripathi RC. Diabetes mellitus and 2,3,7,8 tetrachlorodibenzo-*p*-dioxin elimination in veterans of Operation Ranch Hand. J Toxicol Environ Health A. 2003;66(3):211-221.

Mocarelli P, Needham LL, Marocchi A, Patterson DG Jr, Brambilla P, Gerthoux PM, et al. Serum concentrations of 2,3,7,8-tetrachlorodibenzo-*p*-dioxin and test results from selected residents of Seveso, Italy. J Toxicol Environ Health 1991;32(4):357-366.

Papke O. PCDD/PCDD: human background data for Germany, a 10-year experience. Environ Health Perspect 1998;106 (Suppl 2):723-731.

Patterson DG Jr, Todd GD, Turner WE, Maggio V, Alexander LR, Needham LL. Levels of non-*ortho*-substituted (coplanar), mono- and di-*ortho*-substituted polychlorinated biphenyls, dibenzo-*p*-dioxins, and dibenzofurans in human serum and adipose tissue. Environ Health Perspect 1994;102 (Suppl 1):195-204.

Patterson DG Jr, Hoffman RE, Needham LL, Roberts DW, Bagby JR, Pirkle JL, et al. 2,3,7,8-Tetrachlorodibenzo-*p*-dioxin levels in adipose tissue of exposed and control persons in Missouri. An interim report. JAMA 1986;21;256(19):2683-2686.

Patterson DG Jr, Wong LY, Turner WE, Caudill SP, Dipietro ES, McClure PC, et al. Levels in the U.S. population of those persistent organic pollutants (2003-2004) included in the Stockholm Convention or in other long range transboundary air pollution agreements. Environ Sci Technol 2009;43(4):1211-1218.

Roman BL, Timms BG, Prins GS, Peterson RE. In utero and lactational exposure of the male rat to 2,3,7,8-tetrachlorodibenzo-*p*-dioxin impairs prostate development. 2. Effects on growth and cytodifferentiation. Toxicol Appl Pharmacol 1998;150(2):254-270.

Schnorr TM, Lawson CC, Whelan EA, Dankovic DA, Deddens JA, Piacitelli LA, et al. Spontaneous abortion, sex ratio, and paternal occupational exposure to 2,3,7,8-tetrachlorodibenzo-*p*-dioxin. Environ Health Perspect 2001;109(11):1127-1132.

Sonne C, Leifsson PS, Dietz R, Born EW, Letcher RJ, Hyldstrup

L, et al. Xenoendocrine pollutants may reduce size of sexual organs in East Greenland polar bears (Ursus maritimus). Environ Sci Technol 2006;40(18):5668-74.

Steenland K, Bertazzi P, Baccarelli A, Kogevinas M. Dioxin revisited: developments since the 1997 IARC classification of dioxin as a human carcinogen. Environ Health Perspect 2004;112(13):1265-1268.

Sweeney MH, Calvert GM, Egeland GA, Fingerhut MA, Halperin WE, et al. Review and update of the results of the NIOSH medical study of workers exposed to chemicals contaminated with 2,3,7,8-tetrachlorodibenzodioxin. Teratog Carcinog Mutagen 1997-1998;17(4-5):241-247.

Theobald HM, Peterson RE. In utero and lactational exposure to 2,3,7,8-tetrachlorodibenzo-rho-dioxin: effects on development of the male and female reproductive system of the mouse. Toxicol Appl Pharmacol 1997;145(1):124-135.

Turyk M, Anderson HA, Hanrahan LP, Falk C, Steenport DN, Needham LL, et al. Relationship of serum levels of individual PCB, dioxin, and furan congeners and DDE with Great Lakes sport-caught fish consumption. Environ Res 2006;100(2):173-183.

United States Environmental Protection Agency (U.S.EPA). Exposure and Human Health Reassessment of 2,3,7,8-Tetrachlorodibenzo-p-Dioxin (TCDD) and Related Compounds National Academy Sciences (NAS) Review Draft. 2004. Available at URL: http://www.epa.gov/ncea/pdfs/dioxin/nas-review/. 5/11/07

Van den Berg M, Birnbaum LS, Denison M, De Vito M, Farland W, Feeley M, et al. The 2005 World Health Organization reevaluation of human and Mammalian toxic equivalency factors for dioxins and dioxin-like compounds. Toxicol Sci 2006;93(2):223-241.

Wang SL, Chang YC, Chao HR, Li CM, Li LA, Lin LY, et al. Body burdens of polychlorinated dibenzo-p-dioxins, dibenzofurans, and biphenyls and their relations to estrogen metabolism in pregnant women. Environ Health Perspect 2006;114(5):740-745.

Warner M, Eskenazi B, Olive DL, Samuels S, Quick-Miles S, Vercellini P, et al. Serum dioxin concentrations and quality of ovarian function in women of Seveso. Environ Health Perspect 2007;115(3):336-340.

Warner M, Samuels S, Mocarelli P, Gerthoux PM, Needham L, Patterson DG Jr, et al. Serum dioxin concentrations and age at menarche. Environ Health Perspect 2004;112(13):1289-1292.

Yoshida J, Kumagai S, Tabuchi T, Kosaka H, Akasaka S, Oda H. Effects of dioxin on metabolism of estrogens in waste incinerator workers. Arch Environ Occup Health 2005;60(4):215-222.

# Polycyclic Aromatic Hydrocarbons

## General Information

Polycyclic aromatic hydrocarbons (PAHs) are a class of more than 100 chemicals generally produced during the incomplete burning of organic materials, including coal, oil, gas, wood, garbage, and tobacco. PAHs are composed of up to six benzene rings fused together such that any two adjacent benzene rings share two carbon bonds. Examples include phenanthrenes, naphthalene, and pyrene. Important PAH sources include motor vehicle exhaust, residential and industrial heating sources, coal, crude oil and natural gas processing, waste incineration, and tobacco smoke. The emitted PAHs can form or bind to particles in the air, and particle size depends in part on the source of the PAHs. The smaller or fine particulates (e.g., PM2.5 or smaller) have higher concentrations of PAHs than the larger or coarse particulates (Bostrom et al., 2002; Rehwagen et al., 2005). Ambient air PAH concentrations show seasonal variation (IPCS, 1998; Rehwagen et al., 2005). Smoking, grilling, broiling, or other high temperature processing leads to PAH formation in meat and in other foods, as well. Uncooked foods and vegetables generally contain low levels of PAHs but can be contaminated by airborne particle deposition or growth in contaminated soil. With the exception of naphthalene, the PAHs described here are not produced commercially in the U.S.

Human exposure usually occurs to PAH mixtures rather than to individual chemicals, and PAH mixture composition varies with the combustion source and temperature (ATSDR, 1995). For persons without occupational exposure, important sources of PAHs include ambient air pollution (especially motor vehicle exhaust), smoke from wood or fossil fuels, tobacco smoke, and foods. PAH exposure can occur in workplaces where petroleum products are burned or coked, such as coke production, coal gasification and gas refining, iron or steel production, roofing tar and asphalt application, waste incineration, and aluminum smelting. Coal tar ointments containing PAHs are used to treat several inflammatory skin conditions.

PAHs are lipid soluble and can be absorbed through the skin, respiratory tract, and gastrointestinal tract. PAH metabolism is complex and occurs primarily in the liver, and to a lesser extent, in other tissues. PAH elimination occurs via urine and feces, and urinary metabolites are eliminated within a few days (Ramesh et al., 2004). PAHs and their urinary hydroxylated metabolites that are measured in this *Report* are shown in the table. The metabolic pathways and enzyme-inducing effects of specific PAHs, such as benz[a]pyrene, have been actively studied to elucidate cancer potential and causal mechanisms (Ramesh et al., 2004). Although immunologic, kidney and brain toxicity have been seen in animals after high doses were administered, it is unclear if similar effects may occur in humans. Lung, bladder, and skin cancers have been reported in occupational settings following high PAH exposures (Bosetti et al., 2007; Bostrom et al., 2002; Lloyd, 1971). Exposure to fine particulates has been associated with fetal growth retardation, respiratory disorders, and cardiovascular disease, but it is unknown whether PAHs contained within fine particulates are etiologic (ATSDR, 1995; Choi, 2006).

IARC classifies naphthalene as a possible human carcinogen. NTP determined that naphthalene is reasonably anticipated to be a human carcinogen. Many other PAHs are considered to be probable or possible human carcinogens. IARC and NTP have classified specific PAH-containing chemical mixtures (e.g., soot, coke oven emissions, coal tars and coal tar pitches) as human carcinogens. OSHA has developed

### Polycyclic Aromatic Hydrocarbon Metabolites in this *Report*

| Polycyclic Aromatic Hydrocarbon (CAS number) | Urinary hydroxylated metabolite (CAS number) |
|---|---|
| Fluorene (86-73-7) | 2-Hydroxyfluorene (2443-58-5)<br>3-Hydroxyfluorene (6344-67-8)<br>9-Hydroxyfluorene (484-17-3) |
| Naphthalene (91-20-3) | 1-Hydroxynapthalene (90-15-3)<br>2-Hydroxynapthalene (135-19-3) |
| Phenanthrene (85-01-8) | 1-Hydroxyphenanthrene (2433-56-9)<br>2-Hydroxyphenanthrene<br>3-Hydroxyphenanthrene (605-87-8)<br>4-Hydroxyphenanthrene (7651-86-7) |
| Pyrene (129-00-0) | 1-Hydroxypyrene (5315-79-7) |

criteria on the allowable levels of these chemicals in the workplace.

Information about external exposure (i.e., environmental levels) and health effects is available in reviews (Bosetti et al., 2007; Bostrom et al., 2002; Brandt and Watson 2003) and from ATSDR at: http://www.atsdr.cdc.gov/toxpro2.html.

## Biomonitoring Information

Measurement of urinary metabolites reflects recent exposure to PAHs. Some of the parent PAHs can produce more than one measurable urinary metabolite, as shown in the Table. The hydroxylated metabolites of PAHs are excreted in human urine both as free hydroxylated metabolites and as hydroxylated metabolites conjugated to glucuronic acid and sulfate. Urine metabolite profiles can vary depending on the PAH source(s), but also have been found to vary between individuals experiencing similar exposures within the same workplace (Grimmer et al., 1997; Jacob and Seidel 2002).

Finding a measurable amount of one or more metabolites in the urine does not mean that the levels of the PAH metabolites or the parent PAH cause an adverse health effect. Biomonitoring studies of urinary PAHs provide physicians and public health officials with reference values so that they can determine whether or not people have been exposed to higher levels of PAHs than are found in the general population. Biomonitoring data can also help scientists plan and conduct research on exposure and health effects.

## References

Agency for Toxic Substances and Disease Registry (ATSDR). Toxicological profile for polycyclic aromatic hydrocarbons 1995 [online]. Available at URL: http://www.atsdr.cdc.gov/toxprofiles/tp69 html. 5/26/09

Bosetti C, Boffetta P, La Vecchia C. Occupational exposures to polycyclic aromatic hydrocarbons, and respiratory and urinary tract cancers: a quantitative review to 2005. Ann Oncol 2007;18:431-446.

Bostrom CE, Gerde P, Hanberg A, Jernstrom B, Johansson C, Kyrklund T, et al. Cancer risk assessment, indicators, and guidelines for polycyclic aromatic hydrocarbons in the ambient air. Environ Health Perspect 2002;110Suppl 3:451-488.

Brandt HCA, Watson WP. Monitoring human occupational and environmental exposures to polycyclic aromatic compounds. Ann Occup Hyg 2003;47(5):349-378.

Choi H, Jedrychowski W, Spengler J, Camann DE, Whyatt RM, Rauh V, et al., International studies of prenatal exposure to polycyclic aromatic hydrocarbons and fetal growth. Environ Health Perspect 2006;114(11):1744-1750.

Grimmer G, Jacob J, Dettbarn G, Naujack K-W. Determination of urinary metabolites of polycyclic aromatic hydrocarbons (PAH) for the risk assessment of PAH-exposed workers. Int Arch Occup Environ Health 1997;69:231-239.

International Programme on Chemical Safety (IPCS). Selected non-heterocyclic policyclic aromatic hydrocarbons. Environmental Health Criteria 202. 1998 [online].Available at URL: http://www.inchem.org/documents/ehc/ehc/ehc202.htm. 5/26/09

Jacob J, Seidel A. Biomonitoring of polycyclic aromatic hydrocarbons in human urine. J Chromatogr B 2002;778(1-2):31-47.

Lloyd J. Long-term mortality study of steelworkers. V. Respiratory cancer in coke plant workers. J Occup Med 1971;13:53-68.

Ramesh A, Walker SA, Hood DB, Guillen MD, Schneider K, Weyand EH. Bioavailability and risk assessment of orally ingested polycyclic aromatic hydrocarbons. Int J Toxicol 2004;23(5):301-333.

Rehwagen M, Muller A, Massolo L, Herbarth O, Ronco A. Polycyclic aromatic hydrocarbons associated with particles in ambient air from urban and industrial areas. Sci Tot Environ 2005;348:199-210.

# Fluorene
CAS No. 86-73-7

Fluorene can be an intermediate in several chemical processes, and it is used to form polyradicals for resins and in manufacturing dyestuffs. Fluorene is frequently detected in the vapor phase of various PAH emission sources, including coal tar pitch, petroleum refineries, diesel exhaust fumes, and tobacco smoke, where it is the second most abundant PAH (Ding et al., 2005). Fluorene is present in air particulates resulting from vehicle emissions and combustion of coal and petroleum-based fuels (Fang et al., 2006). IARC determined that fluorene was not classifiable with respect to human carcinogenicity.

## Biomonitoring Information

Urinary levels of 2-hydroxyfluorene, 3-hydroxyfluorene, and 9-hydroxyfluorene reflect recent exposure. Mean levels of 2-hydroxyfluorene were significantly higher in Japanese smokers than non-smokers in one small study (Toriba et al., 2003). By comparison, geometric mean and median urinary 2-hydroxyfluorene levels in adults in this *Report* were similar to the mean levels in the smokers and somewhat higher than those in the non-smokers.

Finding a measurable amount of one or more urinary fluorene metabolites does not mean that the level causes an adverse health effect. Biomonitoring studies of urinary fluorene metabolites can provide physicians and public health officials with reference values so that they can

determine whether or not people have been exposed to higher levels of fluorene than levels found in the general population. Biomonitoring data can also help scientists plan and conduct research on exposure and health effects.

## Urinary 2-Hydroxyfluorene

*Metabolite of Fluorene*

Geometric mean and selected percentiles of urine concentrations (in ng/L) for the U.S. population from the National Health and Nutrition Examination Survey.

| | Survey years | Geometric mean (95% conf. interval) | Selected percentiles ( 95% confidence interval) | | | | Sample size |
|---|---|---|---|---|---|---|---|
| | | | 50th | 75th | 90th | 95th | |
| Total | 03-04 | 304 (262-354) | 280 (242-319) | 679 (561-815) | 1850 (1430-2190) | 2670 (2230-3130) | 2521 |
| Age group | | | | | | | |
| 6-11 years | 03-04 | 209 (183-239) | 228 (189-259) | 341 (295-411) | 576 (423-728) | 763 (613-827) | 338 |
| 12-19 years | 03-04 | 281 (245-321) | 292 (259-323) | 502 (445-601) | 1000 (753-1320) | 1480 (1320-1930) | 707 |
| 20 years and older | 03-04 | 323 (272-383) | 290 (247-334) | 832 (653-1020) | 2090 (1680-2460) | 2920 (2410-3650) | 1476 |
| Gender | | | | | | | |
| Males | 03-04 | 385 (333-446) | 338 (300-415) | 900 (739-1150) | 2120 (1770-2450) | 2930 (2490-3390) | 1213 |
| Females | 03-04 | 243 (204-290) | 226 (184-269) | 490 (405-617) | 1400 (907-1930) | 2310 (1740-3070) | 1308 |
| Race/ethnicity | | | | | | | |
| Mexican Americans | 03-04 | 248 (215-286) | 235 (203-293) | 502 (412-580) | 1100 (771-1330) | 1640 (1250-2240) | 629 |
| Non-Hispanic blacks | 03-04 | 432 (361-516) | 381 (317-462) | 856 (702-1270) | 2200 (1830-2610) | 2960 (2350-4460) | 684 |
| Non-Hispanic whites | 03-04 | 308 (255-372) | 280 (233-332) | 728 (554-898) | 1940 (1540-2390) | 2920 (2400-3500) | 1045 |

Limit of detection (LOD, see Data Analysis section) for Survey year 03-04 is 5.0.

## Urinary 2-Hydroxyfluorene (creatinine corrected)

*Metabolite of Fluorene*

Geometric mean and selected percentiles of urine concentrations (in ng/g of creatinine) for the U.S. population from the National Health and Nutrition Examination Survey.

| | Survey years | Geometric mean (95% conf. interval) | Selected percentiles ( 95% confidence interval) | | | | Sample size |
|---|---|---|---|---|---|---|---|
| | | | 50th | 75th | 90th | 95th | |
| Total | 03-04 | 286 (256-320) | 221 (200-249) | 495 (429-629) | 1510 (1150-1800) | 2070 (1850-2390) | 2521 |
| Age group | | | | | | | |
| 6-11 years | 03-04 | 221 (199-246) | 217 (188-238) | 305 (270-356) | 462 (370-535) | 695 (465-807) | 338 |
| 12-19 years | 03-04 | 213 (189-240) | 189 (172-211) | 310 (275-377) | 649 (512-778) | 937 (762-1320) | 707 |
| 20 years and older | 03-04 | 310 (274-350) | 233 (203-269) | 659 (494-835) | 1730 (1420-1940) | 2310 (1930-2590) | 1476 |
| Gender | | | | | | | |
| Males | 03-04 | 302 (271-337) | 242 (218-272) | 635 (494-758) | 1510 (1200-1700) | 1940 (1700-2310) | 1213 |
| Females | 03-04 | 271 (235-314) | 208 (183-244) | 415 (352-521) | 1530 (991-1890) | 2220 (1730-2590) | 1308 |
| Race/ethnicity | | | | | | | |
| Mexican Americans | 03-04 | 224 (197-255) | 198 (178-227) | 370 (306-432) | 745 (562-1030) | 1200 (745-1730) | 629 |
| Non-Hispanic blacks | 03-04 | 308 (259-365) | 249 (210-305) | 609 (430-803) | 1430 (939-1870) | 1880 (1430-2500) | 684 |
| Non-Hispanic whites | 03-04 | 304 (266-349) | 226 (199-261) | 581 (449-796) | 1630 (1410-1940) | 2310 (1940-2540) | 1045 |

## Urinary 3-Hydroxyfluorene

*Metabolite of Fluorene*

Geometric mean and selected percentiles of urine concentrations (in ng/L) for the U.S. population from the National Health and Nutrition Examination Survey.

| | Survey years | Geometric mean (95% conf. interval) | 50th | 75th | 90th | 95th | Sample size |
|---|---|---|---|---|---|---|---|
| | | | \_\_\_\_\_ Selected percentiles ( 95% confidence interval) \_\_\_\_\_ | | | | |
| **Total** | 01-02 | **134** (115-155) | **111** (96.0-126) | **253** (207-349) | **959** (666-1300) | **1620** (1390-1900) | 2745 |
| | 03-04 | **126** (108-148) | **103** (90.4-118) | **302** (231-404) | **1090** (934-1270) | **1740** (1400-2070) | 2502 |
| **Age group** | | | | | | | |
| 6-11 years | 01-02 | **106** (94.8-119) | **106** (91.0-124) | **174** (145-200) | **287** (235-358) | **385** (306-455) | 387 |
| | 03-04 | **89.2** (77.3-103) | **92.3** (79.7-103) | **151** (113-172) | **238** (184-331) | **343** (241-423) | 336 |
| 12-19 years | 01-02 | **129** (103-161) | **113** (97.0-137) | **222** (177-266) | **542** (325-1070) | **1210** (680-2130) | 733 |
| | 03-04 | **116** (100-134) | **114** (94.7-133) | **214** (181-269) | **476** (317-748) | **924** (609-1410) | 701 |
| 20 years and older | 01-02 | **138** (119-161) | **111** (94.0-129) | **311** (228-429) | **1130** (823-1400) | **1850** (1470-2080) | 1625 |
| | 03-04 | **134** (112-160) | **105** (86.5-125) | **408** (300-537) | **1240** (1050-1480) | **1910** (1620-2290) | 1465 |
| **Gender** | | | | | | | |
| Males | 01-02 | **163** (137-194) | **134** (115-155) | **352** (242-481) | **1110** (721-1600) | **1850** (1390-2190) | 1346 |
| | 03-04 | **165** (140-194) | **133** (108-162) | **458** (313-681) | **1270** (1030-1530) | **1920** (1580-2120) | 1205 |
| Females | 01-02 | **111** (95.0-130) | **94.0** (83.0-108) | **204** (169-250) | **796** (498-1040) | **1390** (1250-1670) | 1399 |
| | 03-04 | **98.2** (81.2-119) | **80.5** (66.7-101) | **195** (163-272) | **842** (530-1200) | **1590** (1180-1800) | 1297 |
| **Race/ethnicity** | | | | | | | |
| Mexican Americans | 01-02 | **108** (87.1-134) | **99.0** (81.0-119) | **190** (144-255) | **476** (302-641) | **718** (476-1140) | 662 |
| | 03-04 | **93.4** (79.6-110) | **83.4** (67.0-96 9) | **190** (150-252) | **520** (388-726) | **1030** (688-1320) | 622 |
| Non-Hispanic blacks | 01-02 | **203** (169-244) | **162** (135-188) | **449** (308-830) | **1420** (1130-1780) | **2350** (1520-3000) | 692 |
| | 03-04 | **195** (157-242) | **160** (124-187) | **482** (303-827) | **1460** (1070-1800) | **2110** (1580-2830) | 683 |
| Non-Hispanic whites | 01-02 | **130** (108-157) | **108** (93.0-127) | **246** (202-352) | **948** (621-1320) | **1620** (1320-1990) | 1207 |
| | 03-04 | **129** (106-155) | **105** (87.6-124) | **313** (237-464) | **1200** (1010-1410) | **1870** (1430-2220) | 1035 |

Limit of detection (LOD, see Data Analysis section) for Survey years 01-02 and 03-04 are 2.0 and 5 0.

## Urinary 3-Hydroxyfluorene (creatinine corrected)

*Metabolite of Fluorene*

Geometric mean and selected percentiles of urine concentrations (in ng/g of creatinine) for the U.S. population from the National Health and Nutrition Examination Survey.

| | Survey years | Geometric mean (95% conf. interval) | Selected percentiles ( 95% confidence interval) | | | | Sample size |
|---|---|---|---|---|---|---|---|
| | | | 50th | 75th | 90th | 95th | |
| Total | 01-02 | 125 (108-144) | 94.4 (83.3-106) | 220 (174-303) | 754 (622-873) | 1060 (909-1290) | 2745 |
| | 03-04 | 119 (106-134) | 86.6 (76.8-97.3) | 256 (201-337) | 856 (668-1060) | 1330 (1130-1590) | 2502 |
| **Age group** | | | | | | | |
| 6-11 years | 01-02 | 119 (103-137) | 110 (96.7-121) | 153 (135-197) | 265 (206-377) | 382 (254-631) | 387 |
| | 03-04 | 94.6 (84.3-106) | 92.4 (83.1-98.5) | 130 (115-154) | 202 (168-282) | 311 (197-435) | 336 |
| 12-19 years | 01-02 | 99.3 (81.6-121) | 81.9 (74.2-92.6) | 144 (109-197) | 390 (214-700) | 711 (372-1380) | 733 |
| | 03-04 | 88.1 (78.0-99.6) | 79.0 (72.5-83.2) | 137 (114-170) | 319 (225-440) | 586 (356-880) | 701 |
| 20 years and older | 01-02 | 131 (113-151) | 94.4 (81.0-108) | 279 (195-367) | 862 (727-923) | 1210 (1010-1350) | 1625 |
| | 03-04 | 128 (113-146) | 88.2 (76.8-104) | 364 (242-484) | 1020 (828-1240) | 1500 (1290-1710) | 1465 |
| **Gender** | | | | | | | |
| Males | 01-02 | 132 (111-156) | 100 (88.5-117) | 260 (194-361) | 745 (560-914) | 1130 (862-1380) | 1346 |
| | 03-04 | 129 (114-147) | 95.8 (82.5-111) | 338 (226-456) | 833 (672-1010) | 1220 (980-1510) | 1205 |
| Females | 01-02 | 119 (104-136) | 88.9 (78.6-103) | 179 (156-227) | 777 (604-888) | 1030 (923-1270) | 1399 |
| | 03-04 | 110 (93.4-129) | 81.7 (69.5-91.5) | 183 (132-285) | 920 (488-1270) | 1460 (1130-1750) | 1297 |
| **Race/ethnicity** | | | | | | | |
| Mexican Americans | 01-02 | 101 (84.2-121) | 84.0 (74.8-97.2) | 159 (124-214) | 364 (227-598) | 604 (357-1230) | 662 |
| | 03-04 | 84.8 (73.1-98.4) | 68.8 (60.0-80.2) | 170 (119-213) | 353 (319-435) | 668 (353-1050) | 622 |
| Non-Hispanic blacks | 01-02 | 143 (118-173) | 110 (90.7-133) | 316 (186-525) | 849 (622-1230) | 1240 (882-1430) | 692 |
| | 03-04 | 139 (113-169) | 106 (93.1-118) | 328 (211-488) | 961 (580-1310) | 1310 (961-1770) | 683 |
| Non-Hispanic whites | 01-02 | 128 (108-152) | 94.7 (83.4-109) | 223 (171-323) | 816 (642-914) | 1150 (910-1410) | 1207 |
| | 03-04 | 127 (110-146) | 89.8 (79.1-104) | 311 (212-418) | 980 (768-1180) | 1460 (1270-1700) | 1035 |

## Urinary 9-Hydroxyfluorene
*Metabolite of Fluorene*

Geometric mean and selected percentiles of urine concentrations (in ng/L) for the U.S. population from the National Health and Nutrition Examination Survey.

| | Survey years | Geometric mean (95% conf. interval) | Selected percentiles ( 95% confidence interval) | | | | Sample size |
|---|---|---|---|---|---|---|---|
| | | | 50th | 75th | 90th | 95th | |
| Total | 03-04 | 267 (234-305) | 269 (233-313) | 541 (463-620) | 929 (839-1060) | 1390 (1130-1600) | 2504 |
| Age group | | | | | | | |
| 6-11 years | 03-04 | 209 (184-238) | 216 (173-240) | 331 (267-458) | 594 (446-809) | 853 (553-1500) | 333 |
| 12-19 years | 03-04 | 253 (216-297) | 271 (215-324) | 506 (413-560) | 894 (773-988) | 1210 (929-1510) | 698 |
| 20 years and older | 03-04 | 277 (240-320) | 279 (237-335) | 583 (476-656) | 979 (842-1140) | 1490 (1140-1770) | 1473 |
| Gender | | | | | | | |
| Males | 03-04 | 330 (291-374) | 330 (285-372) | 632 (583-709) | 1090 (898-1370) | 1720 (1360-2250) | 1208 |
| Females | 03-04 | 218 (188-253) | 226 (191-253) | 439 (357-521) | 833 (697-973) | 1100 (955-1310) | 1296 |
| Race/ethnicity | | | | | | | |
| Mexican Americans | 03-04 | 229 (200-261) | 232 (197-274) | 435 (362-492) | 773 (561-1010) | 1030 (849-1170) | 614 |
| Non-Hispanic blacks | 03-04 | 380 (311-465) | 357 (291-475) | 709 (559-825) | 1260 (1080-1600) | 1880 (1560-2330) | 679 |
| Non-Hispanic whites | 03-04 | 266 (226-313) | 266 (228-324) | 558 (453-659) | 939 (824-1130) | 1450 (1090-1770) | 1048 |

Limit of detection (LOD, see Data Analysis section) for Survey year 03-04 is 5.0.

## Urinary 9-Hydroxyfluorene (creatinine corrected)
*Metabolite of Fluorene*

Geometric mean and selected percentiles of urine concentrations (in ng/g of creatinine) for the U.S. population from the National Health and Nutrition Examination Survey.

| | Survey years | Geometric mean (95% conf. interval) | Selected percentiles ( 95% confidence interval) | | | | Sample size |
|---|---|---|---|---|---|---|---|
| | | | 50th | 75th | 90th | 95th | |
| Total | 03-04 | 252 (230-276) | 233 (205-266) | 412 (371-461) | 729 (609-905) | 1100 (918-1390) | 2504 |
| Age group | | | | | | | |
| 6-11 years | 03-04 | 223 (200-247) | 208 (176-264) | 343 (299-389) | 548 (433-689) | 866 (533-958) | 333 |
| 12-19 years | 03-04 | 192 (172-215) | 182 (161-200) | 323 (286-360) | 484 (412-696) | 738 (571-1110) | 698 |
| 20 years and older | 03-04 | 267 (242-294) | 243 (219-280) | 446 (392-490) | 788 (641-994) | 1280 (991-1560) | 1473 |
| Gender | | | | | | | |
| Males | 03-04 | 260 (238-283) | 236 (209-269) | 429 (382-480) | 739 (591-952) | 1300 (916-1800) | 1208 |
| Females | 03-04 | 244 (217-275) | 227 (198-269) | 396 (342-467) | 717 (569-905) | 1020 (905-1280) | 1296 |
| Race/ethnicity | | | | | | | |
| Mexican Americans | 03-04 | 209 (188-232) | 195 (181-209) | 335 (293-379) | 541 (447-722) | 793 (569-1440) | 614 |
| Non-Hispanic blacks | 03-04 | 272 (226-326) | 258 (208-307) | 463 (349-568) | 777 (628-920) | 1040 (863-1300) | 679 |
| Non-Hispanic whites | 03-04 | 263 (235-295) | 244 (211-287) | 439 (387-490) | 773 (607-1020) | 1290 (967-1700) | 1048 |

## References

Ding YS, Trommel JS, Yan Xj, Ashley D, Watson CH. Determination of 14 polycyclic aromatic hydrocarbons in mainstream smoke from domestic cigarettes. Environ Sci Technol 2005;39:471-478.

Fang G-C, Wu Y-S, Chen J-C, Chang C-N, Ho T-T. characteristic of polycyclic aromatic hydrocarbon concentrations and source identification for fine and coarse particulates at Taichung Harbor near Taiwan Strait during 2004-2005. Sci Tot Environ 2006;366:729-738.

Toriba A, Chetiyanukornkul T, Kizu R, Hayakawa K. Quantification of 2-hydroxyfluorene in human urine by column-switching high performance liquid chromatography with fluorescence detection. Analyst 2003;128(6):605-610.

# Naphthalene
CAS No. 91-20-3

Naphthalene is produced commercially from coal tar and petroleum. It is used in producing an assortment of chemicals: phthalate plasticizers, naphthalene sulfonates and dyes, the insecticide carbaryl, and synthetic leather tanning chemicals. Naphthalene is an intermediate in manufacturing several pharmaceuticals. Crystalline naphthalene has been used as a moth repellent. Naphthalene is the most abundant PAH in cigarette smoke (Ding et al., 2005), and it is present in fossil fuel smoke and exhaust fumes, especially from diesel and jet fuels. Non-occupational exposure typically occurs through inhaling ambient and indoor air, and cigarette smoke. Naphthalene can be absorbed through the skin as a result of handling moth repellent or wearing clothes stored with moth repellent. Workers may be exposed via inhalation or dermal absorption in settings such as naphthalene production, coal coking operations, and wood treatment with creosote.

In the body, naphthalene metabolism is complex, leading to biologically reactive metabolites and other metabolites that are excreted in the urine. In studies of workers, naphthalene air concentrations were correlated with 1- and 2-hydroxynaphthalene urine concentrations (Bieniek 1994; 1997). Both naphthalene and the insecticide carbaryl are metabolized to 1-hydroxynaphthalene, making it difficult to distinguish between these exposures in the general population (Meeker et al., 2007). In contrast, only

naphthalene metabolism results in 2-hydroxynaphthalene in urine.

Humans can develop hemolytic anemia and jaundice after high dose naphthalene exposure by either inhalation or ingestion, or from skin exposure to clothing and bedding treated with naphthalene moth repellents (ATSDR, 2005). Exposure to naphthalene vapor can irritate the eyes and respiratory tract. High dose and chronic exposure in occupational settings can result in cataracts or lens opacities (ATSDR, 2005). OSHA has established a workplace standard. IARC considers naphthalene to be a possible human carcinogen, and NTP considers that it is reasonably anticipated to be a human carcinogen.

## Biomonitoring Information

Urinary levels of 1-hydroxynaphthalene and 2-hydroxynaphthalene (1-naphthol and 2-naphthol, respectively) reflect recent exposure. Levels similar to those reported in NHANES 2001-2002 and 2003-2004 subsamples have been found in small studies of pre-school children, adolescents and non-occupationally exposed adults (Kang et al., 2002; Kim et al., 2003; Kuusimaki et al., 2004; Wilson et al., 2003). Smokers typically have urinary 1- and 2-hydroxynaphthalene levels that are about 2 to 3 times higher than nonsmokers in both occupationally exposed and general populations (Campo et al., 2006; Nan et al., 2001; Serdar et al., 2003a, 2003b). Depending on the intensity of exposure, workers exposed to naphthalene have been found to have geometric mean urinary 1- and

## Urinary 1-Hydroxynaphthalene (1-Naphthol)
*Metabolite of Naphthalene*
Geometric mean and selected percentiles of urine concentrations (in ng/L) for the U.S. population from the National Health and Nutrition Examination Survey.

| | Survey years | Geometric mean (95% conf. interval) | 50th | 75th | 90th | 95th | Sample size |
|---|---|---|---|---|---|---|---|
| Total | 03-04 | 2680 (2360-3050) | 2260 (1980-2650) | 7660 (6270-9420) | 18500 (15500-20900) | 26100 (23000-33600) | 2595 |
| **Age group** | | | | | | | |
| 6-11 years | 03-04 | 1540 (1360-1750) | 1330 (1110-1680) | 2790 (2180-3520) | 5770 (4110-8200) | 10500 (5870-17000) | 340 |
| 12-19 years | 03-04 | 1960 (1680-2280) | 1670 (1500-1970) | 4190 (3100-5400) | 10500 (8430-14300) | 20900 (13500-26100) | 727 |
| 20 years and older | 03-04 | 3020 (2580-3520) | 2650 (2200-3200) | 9420 (7320-11500) | 20500 (16500-23400) | 29400 (23400-37400) | 1528 |
| **Gender** | | | | | | | |
| Males | 03-04 | 3170 (2820-3560) | 2840 (2370-3390) | 8790 (7130-11000) | 19600 (16100-22200) | 25800 (22500-30600) | 1243 |
| Females | 03-04 | 2290 (1940-2720) | 1840 (1500-2310) | 6380 (4450-8810) | 17900 (14000-21500) | 28500 (21500-37400) | 1352 |
| **Race/ethnicity** | | | | | | | |
| Mexican Americans | 03-04 | 1950 (1720-2190) | 1650 (1370-2040) | 4380 (3520-5300) | 11600 (9040-15500) | 20100 (14900-22500) | 651 |
| Non-Hispanic blacks | 03-04 | 3340 (2800-3990) | 2650 (2190-3460) | 7840 (6520-10800) | 20800 (17000-28600) | 34700 (25400-48900) | 695 |
| Non-Hispanic whites | 03-04 | 2800 (2410-3250) | 2310 (1930-2840) | 8630 (6820-11000) | 19900 (15900-22600) | 27600 (23400-35100) | 1084 |

Limit of detection (LOD, see data analysis section) for Survey period 03-04 is 46.7.

2-hydroxynaphthalene levels that range from around 2 to 100 times higher than the levels in this *Report* (Bieniek 1997; Elovaara et al., 2006; Nan et al., 2001; Serdar et al., 2003*a*).

Finding a measurable amount of 1- or 2-hydroxynaphthalene in the urine does not mean that the level causes an adverse health effect. Biomonitoring studies on levels of 1- and 2-naphthalene provide physicians and public health officials with reference values so that they can determine whether people have been exposed to higher levels of naphthalene than are found in the general population. Biomonitoring data can also help scientists plan and conduct research on exposure and health effects.

## Urinary 1-Hydroxynaphthalene (1-Naphthol) (creatinine corrected)

*Metabolite of Naphthalene*

Geometric mean and selected percentiles of urine concentrations (in ng/g of creatinine) for the U.S. population from the National Health and Nutrition Examination Survey.

| | Survey years | Geometric mean (95% conf. interval) | Selected percentiles ( 95% confidence interval) | | | | Sample size |
|---|---|---|---|---|---|---|---|
| | | | 50th | 75th | 90th | 95th | |
| Total | 03-04 | 2520 (2280-2790) | 2100 (1870-2400) | 6560 (5430-8180) | 15100 (13500-17400) | 21800 (18200-25400) | 2595 |
| **Age group** | | | | | | | |
| 6-11 years | 03-04 | 1630 (1430-1860) | 1360 (1180-1740) | 2770 (2260-3200) | 5690 (3990-8950) | 10200 (5690-16400) | 340 |
| 12-19 years | 03-04 | 1470 (1260-1710) | 1200 (1020-1390) | 2840 (2490-4080) | 7560 (5470-9120) | 10800 (9120-13400) | 727 |
| 20 years and older | 03-04 | 2900 (2590-3250) | 2520 (2120-3060) | 8210 (6450-9810) | 16900 (14400-19800) | 24200 (20000-27200) | 1528 |
| **Gender** | | | | | | | |
| Males | 03-04 | 2490 (2250-2750) | 2140 (1860-2590) | 6560 (5500-8010) | 13500 (12300-14400) | 18300 (16600-20700) | 1243 |
| Females | 03-04 | 2560 (2220-2950) | 2040 (1730-2440) | 6680 (5000-8850) | 17500 (13500-21700) | 24700 (19800-30600) | 1352 |
| **Race/ethnicity** | | | | | | | |
| Mexican Americans | 03-04 | 1750 (1590-1930) | 1500 (1260-1690) | 3240 (2900-4250) | 8550 (7150-12000) | 17500 (13500-21400) | 651 |
| Non-Hispanic blacks | 03-04 | 2370 (2020-2780) | 2000 (1560-2420) | 5900 (4440-7070) | 13800 (8930-18700) | 21100 (17100-27800) | 695 |
| Non-Hispanic whites | 03-04 | 2770 (2460-3120) | 2350 (1940-2900) | 8030 (6330-9260) | 16600 (14400-18500) | 23600 (20000-26600) | 1084 |

# Urinary 2-Hydroxynaphthalene (2-Naphthol)

*Metabolite of Naphthalene*

Geometric mean and selected percentiles of urine concentrations (in ng/L) for the U.S. population from the National Health and Nutrition Examination Survey.

| | Survey years | Geometric mean (95% conf. interval) | Selected percentiles ( 95% confidence interval) | | | | Sample size |
|---|---|---|---|---|---|---|---|
| | | | 50th | 75th | 90th | 95th | |
| **Total** | 01-02 | 2470 (2110-2890) | 2280 (1930-2670) | 5680 (4580-6830) | 14700 (12800-19500) | 26000 (22500-29700) | 2748 |
| | 03-04 | 3180 (2760-3670) | 2960 (2500-3500) | 7500 (6190-9690) | 17300 (14500-22100) | 25800 (22600-27700) | 2575 |
| **Age group** | | | | | | | |
| 6-11 years | 01-02 | 1690 (1560-1840) | 1700 (1400-1950) | 3010 (2580-3470) | 5410 (3890-6700) | 7720 (6300-9540) | 387 |
| | 03-04 | 2110 (1800-2470) | 2140 (1790-2590) | 3570 (3140-4380) | 5580 (5050-6380) | 9710 (5230-20000) | 339 |
| 12-19 years | 01-02 | 2220 (1700-2900) | 2150 (1740-2530) | 4390 (3150-6110) | 11000 (6990-20400) | 22500 (13900-28400) | 735 |
| | 03-04 | 3040 (2680-3460) | 2910 (2510-3500) | 5290 (4670-6590) | 12400 (8530-16800) | 17600 (15100-25900) | 721 |
| 20 years and older | 01-02 | 2620 (2220-3100) | 2440 (1940-2950) | 6380 (5110-8110) | 17600 (14000-21100) | 28100 (23300-33700) | 1626 |
| | 03-04 | 3360 (2860-3960) | 3180 (2590-3960) | 8770 (7210-11300) | 19200 (16000-23200) | 26600 (23400-28800) | 1515 |
| **Gender** | | | | | | | |
| Males | 01-02 | 2750 (2360-3210) | 2510 (2090-2970) | 6060 (4820-7810) | 16900 (11900-23000) | 28100 (20800-35600) | 1349 |
| | 03-04 | 3520 (3090-4010) | 3370 (2910-3880) | 8520 (6960-10500) | 18400 (15300-22600) | 26100 (22200-27900) | 1233 |
| Females | 01-02 | 2220 (1860-2660) | 2060 (1650-2480) | 5240 (3890-6440) | 13900 (12300-17700) | 25300 (19700-28300) | 1399 |
| | 03-04 | 2890 (2420-3450) | 2600 (2140-3160) | 6800 (5140-9210) | 16600 (12700-21300) | 23900 (22100-27600) | 1342 |
| **Race/ethnicity** | | | | | | | |
| Mexican Americans | 01-02 | 2700 (2360-3080) | 2710 (2350-3260) | 5140 (4360-6150) | 9640 (8150-10600) | 14300 (10400-18700) | 665 |
| | 03-04 | 3130 (2710-3630) | 3110 (2570-3850) | 6740 (5600-8280) | 14500 (10400-15600) | 18000 (15500-20500) | 648 |
| Non-Hispanic blacks | 01-02 | 3970 (3470-4540) | 3460 (3100-4020) | 9290 (6820-13200) | 22800 (16000-29100) | 33000 (25900-38700) | 692 |
| | 03-04 | 4690 (3830-5750) | 4290 (3250-5540) | 10300 (7670-13100) | 21200 (17300-26100) | 30100 (22300-40600) | 690 |
| Non-Hispanic whites | 01-02 | 2190 (1760-2720) | 1910 (1610-2420) | 4970 (3710-6780) | 14100 (10700-20200) | 25900 (20700-30000) | 1207 |
| | 03-04 | 3080 (2580-3670) | 2660 (2200-3530) | 7640 (5890-10400) | 18000 (14600-22900) | 26100 (22900-27900) | 1072 |

Limit of detection (LOD see data analysis section) for Survey periods 01-02 and 03-04 are 2.4 and 31.1.

## Urinary 2-Hydroxynaphthalene (2-Naphthol) (creatinine corrected)

*Metabolite of Naphthalene*

Geometric mean and selected percentiles of urine concentrations (in ng/g of creatinine) for the U.S. population from the National Health and Nutrition Examination Survey.

| | Survey years | Geometric mean (95% conf. interval) | 50th | 75th | 90th | 95th | Sample size |
|---|---|---|---|---|---|---|---|
| **Total** | 01-02 | 2310 (1980-2680) | 1940 (1670-2300) | 4730 (3820-5860) | 11500 (9980-13100) | 16700 (14100-19200) | 2748 |
| | 03-04 | 2990 (2670-3340) | 2560 (2200-2970) | 6340 (5010-7870) | 14100 (11800-16300) | 19900 (16000-23800) | 2575 |
| **Age group** | | | | | | | |
| 6-11 years | 01-02 | 1890 (1740-2070) | 1830 (1720-1940) | 3110 (2510-3470) | 5040 (4380-5540) | 6490 (5270-12400) | 387 |
| | 03-04 | 2240 (1890-2650) | 2040 (1660-2440) | 3540 (2840-3910) | 5950 (4140-8510) | 8720 (7560-12000) | 339 |
| 12-19 years | 01-02 | 1720 (1350-2190) | 1510 (1340-1830) | 2750 (2080-4070) | 7180 (4070-10900) | 11100 (7860-17400) | 735 |
| | 03-04 | 2280 (2060-2520) | 2030 (1770-2350) | 3780 (3200-4470) | 7840 (6130-9110) | 10500 (9100-12500) | 721 |
| 20 years and older | 01-02 | 2480 (2130-2880) | 2080 (1680-2600) | 5630 (4460-6940) | 12400 (10900-13900) | 17700 (15200-20600) | 1626 |
| | 03-04 | 3230 (2870-3640) | 2910 (2360-3410) | 7540 (6200-9100) | 15600 (13100-17900) | 21800 (17200-24000) | 1515 |
| **Gender** | | | | | | | |
| Males | 01-02 | 2230 (1900-2610) | 1860 (1630-2100) | 4790 (3510-6120) | 11400 (8950-14300) | 15800 (13100-19200) | 1349 |
| | 03-04 | 2770 (2500-3060) | 2360 (2130-2810) | 6300 (5080-7360) | 12800 (11300-14600) | 16400 (14600-18300) | 1233 |
| Females | 01-02 | 2380 (2050-2770) | 1990 (1660-2560) | 4730 (3790-6000) | 11500 (10300-12800) | 17400 (13700-21500) | 1399 |
| | 03-04 | 3210 (2760-3730) | 2680 (2200-3260) | 6430 (4740-8580) | 16000 (11500-19900) | 22500 (18100-25000) | 1342 |
| **Race/ethnicity** | | | | | | | |
| Mexican Americans | 01-02 | 2520 (2230-2850) | 2350 (2010-2950) | 4650 (3970-5210) | 7320 (6050-8090) | 12000 (7820-15300) | 665 |
| | 03-04 | 2830 (2440-3280) | 2570 (2200-3230) | 5000 (4100-5940) | 10300 (6790-13000) | 13300 (11000-15500) | 648 |
| Non-Hispanic blacks | 01-02 | 2790 (2390-3270) | 2410 (2040-2770) | 5980 (4840-6980) | 11600 (9090-15300) | 17400 (12200-23400) | 692 |
| | 03-04 | 3320 (2700-4090) | 3060 (2310-3860) | 7050 (5140-9410) | 12800 (10200-16500) | 19000 (15700-23400) | 690 |
| Non-Hispanic whites | 01-02 | 2160 (1780-2620) | 1740 (1440-2180) | 4340 (3320-6090) | 11900 (9930-14300) | 16900 (13800-20600) | 1207 |
| | 03-04 | 3040 (2660-3460) | 2480 (2110-3020) | 7170 (5100-8950) | 15500 (13300-17600) | 21800 (17100-24000) | 1072 |

## References

Agency for Toxic Substances and Disease Registry (ATSDR). Toxicological profile for naphthalene, 1-methylnaphthalene, and 2-methylnaphthalene. August 2005 (update) [online] Available at URL: http://www.atsdr.cdc.gov/toxprofiles/tp67.html. 5/26/09

Bieniek G. The presence of 1-naphthol in the urine of industrial workers exposed to naphthalene. Occup Environ Med 1994;51(5):357-359.

Bieniek G. Urinary napthols as an indicator of exposure to naphthalene. Scand J Work Environ Health 1997;23:414-420.

Campo L, Buratti M, Fustinoni S, Cirla PE, Martinotti I, Longhi O, et al. Evaluation of exposure to PAHs in asphalt workers by environmental and biological monitoring. Ann NY Acad Sci 2006;1076:405-420.

Ding YS, Trommel JS, Yan Xj, Ashley D, Watson CH. Determination of 14 polycyclic aromatic hydrocarbons in mainstream smoke from domestic cigarettes. Environ Sci Technol 2005;39:471-478.

Elovaara E, Mikkola J, Makela M, Paldanius B, Priha E. Assessment of soil remediation workers' exposure to polycyclic aromatic hydrocarbons (PAH): Biomonitoring of naphthols, phenanthrols, and 1-hydroxypyrene in urine. Toxicol Lett 2006;162:158-163.

Kang JW, Cho SH, Kim H, Lee CH. Correlation of urinary 1-hydroxypyrene and 2-naphthol with total suspended particulates in ambient air in municipal middle-school students in Korea. Arch Environ Health 2002;57(4):377-382.

Kim YD, Lee CH, Nan HM, Kang JW, Kim H. Effects of genetic polymorphisms in metabolic enzymes on the relationships between 8-hydroxydeoxyguanosine levels in human leukocytes and urinary 1-hydroxypyrene and 2-naphthol concentrations. J Occup Health 2003;45(3):160-167.

Kuusimaki L, Peltonen Y, Mutanen P, Peltonen K, Savela K. Urinary hydroxy-metabolites of naphthalene, phenanthrene and pyrene as markers of exposure to diesel exhaust. Int Arch Occup Environ Health 2004;77(1):23-30.

Meeker JD, Barr DB, Serbar B, Rappaport SM, Hauser R. Utility of urinary 1-naphthol and 2-naphthol levels to assess environmental carbaryl and naphthalene exposure in an epidemiology study. J Expo Sci Eviron Epidemiol 2007;17(4):314-320.

Nan HM, Kim H, Lim HS, Choi JK, Kawamoto T, Kang JW, et al. Effects of occupation, lifestyle and genetic polymorphisms of CYP1A1, CYP2E1, GSTM1 and GSTT1 on urinary 1-hydroxypyrene and 2-naphthol concentrations. Carcinogenesis 2001;22(5):787-793.

Serdar B, Egeghy PP, Waidyanatha S, Gibson R, Rappaport SM. Urinary biomarkers of exposure to jet fuel (JP-8). Environ Health Perspect 2003a;111(14):1760-1764.

Serdar B, Waidyanatha S, Zheng Y, Rappaport SM. Simultaneous determination of urinary 1- and 2-naphthols, 3- and 9-phenanthrols, and 1-pyrenol in coke oven workers. Biomarkers 2003b;8(2):93-109.

# Phenanthrene
CAS No. 85-01-8

Phenanthrene is used in manufacturing dyestuffs and explosives and in biological research. Sources of phenanthrene include diesel fuel exhaust, coal tar pitch and tobacco smoke. Phenanthrene has been found in particle emissions from natural gas combustion and municipal incinerator waste, and in the particulates present in ambient air pollution near high vehicular traffic and industrial or urban areas (ATSDR, 1995; Fang et al., 2006; Rehwagen et al., 2005). IARC determined that phenanthrene was not classifiable with respect to human carcinogenicity.

## Biomonitoring Information

Urinary levels of 1-hydroxyphenanthrene, 2-hydroxyphenanthrene, 3-hydroxyphenanthrene, and 4-hydroxyphenanthrene reflect recent exposure. Geometric mean and median urine concentrations of 1- and 3-hydroxyphenanthrene in a 1998 sample of German adults were about 2-fold higher than levels in the NHANES 2001-2002 and 2003-2004 subsamples (Becker et al.,

2003). Children and adults in housing where coal tar flooring glue was applied had similar urinary 1-, 2-, 3-, and 4-hydroxyphenanthrene levels compared to residents in houses without the glue; mean levels of these metabolites were higher than levels for similar age groups in this *Report* (Heudorf and Angerer, 2001a). Smoking increases levels of urinary 2-, 3-, and 4-hydroxyphenanthrene (Becker et al., 2003; Elovaara et al., 2006; Heudorf and Angerer 2001b; Jacob et al., 1999). Occupational PAH exposures have been associated with median urinary phenanthrene metabolite concentrations that range from 10 to 100 times higher than median values in the general population (Elovaara et al., 2006; Gundel et al., 2000).

Finding a measurable amount of one or more urinary phenanthrene metabolites does not mean that the level causes an adverse health effect. Biomonitoring studies on levels of phenanthrene metabolites provide physicians and public health officials with reference values so that they can determine whether people have been exposed to higher levels of phenanthrene than are found in the general population. Biomonitoring data can also help scientists plan and conduct research on exposure and health effects.

### Urinary 1-Hydroxyphenanthrene
*Metabolite of Phenanthrene*
Geometric mean and selected percentiles of urine concentrations (in ng/L) for the U.S. population from the National Health and Nutrition Examination Survey.

| | Survey years | Geometric mean (95% conf. interval) | 50th | 75th | 90th | 95th | Sample size |
|---|---|---|---|---|---|---|---|
| Total | 01-02 | 140 (125-158) | 141 (130-154) | 266 (229-312) | 476 (426-539) | 684 (581-763) | 2741 |
| | 03-04 | 156 (140-173) | 166 (150-179) | 287 (263-321) | 464 (423-508) | 625 (538-745) | 2496 |
| **Age group** | | | | | | | |
| 6-11 years | 01-02 | 119 (104-137) | 121 (98.0-142) | 228 (182-249) | 357 (265-501) | 501 (367-661) | 387 |
| | 03-04 | 138 (124-154) | 131 (111-161) | 222 (200-275) | 397 (304-500) | 615 (384-916) | 328 |
| 12-19 years | 01-02 | 133 (110-162) | 131 (110-153) | 238 (198-303) | 431 (376-546) | 579 (439-820) | 733 |
| | 03-04 | 158 (141-178) | 171 (138-193) | 300 (262-333) | 470 (437-537) | 654 (563-745) | 692 |
| 20 years and older | 01-02 | 145 (127-164) | 145 (133-164) | 274 (237-329) | 499 (440-565) | 713 (595-819) | 1621 |
| | 03-04 | 157 (141-176) | 167 (152-182) | 296 (264-337) | 469 (430-513) | 625 (534-783) | 1476 |
| **Gender** | | | | | | | |
| Males | 01-02 | 150 (133-169) | 145 (132-164) | 284 (235-348) | 501 (424-593) | 713 (575-845) | 1344 |
| | 03-04 | 176 (161-194) | 182 (167-198) | 321 (283-363) | 492 (459-536) | 662 (541-929) | 1196 |
| Females | 01-02 | 132 (115-152) | 137 (121-151) | 254 (221-297) | 464 (390-520) | 654 (538-769) | 1397 |
| | 03-04 | 138 (122-156) | 144 (126-164) | 263 (240-294) | 430 (404-469) | 589 (489-680) | 1300 |
| **Race/ethnicity** | | | | | | | |
| Mexican Americans | 01-02 | 117 (90.8-152) | 116 (88.0-147) | 214 (157-306) | 369 (254-583) | 549 (342-847) | 664 |
| | 03-04 | 138 (120-158) | 152 (129-175) | 246 (213-291) | 413 (311-492) | 518 (352-896) | 611 |
| Non-Hispanic blacks | 01-02 | 150 (127-179) | 145 (126-170) | 287 (243-327) | 493 (423-629) | 713 (568-975) | 690 |
| | 03-04 | 182 (152-217) | 178 (149-212) | 346 (274-418) | 552 (459-645) | 797 (606-1050) | 679 |
| Non-Hispanic whites | 01-02 | 144 (125-166) | 144 (131-162) | 276 (241-330) | 489 (436-552) | 661 (550-793) | 1204 |
| | 03-04 | 159 (140-180) | 168 (151-186) | 296 (265-330) | 475 (421-539) | 641 (528-843) | 1046 |

Limit of detection (LOD, see Data Analysis section) for Survey years 01-02 and 03-04 are 3 5 and 5.0.

## Urinary 1-Hydroxyphenanthrene (creatinine corrected)

*Metabolite of Phenanthrene*

Geometric mean and selected percentiles of urine concentrations (in ng/g of creatinine) for the U.S. population from the National Health and Nutrition Examination Survey.

| | Survey years | Geometric mean (95% conf. interval) | Selected percentiles ( 95% confidence interval) | | | | Sample size |
|---|---|---|---|---|---|---|---|
| | | | 50th | 75th | 90th | 95th | |
| Total | 01-02 | 132 (118-147) | 125 (113-141) | 210 (191-231) | 344 (310-385) | 464 (404-539) | 2741 |
| | 03-04 | 146 (138-155) | 141 (133-150) | 222 (205-244) | 352 (330-384) | 487 (416-546) | 2496 |
| **Age group** | | | | | | | |
| 6-11 years | 01-02 | 133 (116-153) | 126 (110-147) | 188 (165-225) | 344 (245-437) | 467 (364-598) | 387 |
| | 03-04 | 145 (129-163) | 138 (121-155) | 205 (169-240) | 315 (244-456) | 477 (313-803) | 328 |
| 12-19 years | 01-02 | 103 (87.9-121) | 97.3 (81.4-117) | 158 (131-192) | 240 (198-322) | 354 (235-531) | 733 |
| | 03-04 | 119 (108-130) | 115 (101-131) | 176 (157-197) | 275 (230-331) | 345 (269-496) | 692 |
| 20 years and older | 01-02 | 137 (122-153) | 132 (117-145) | 223 (200-243) | 351 (319-395) | 476 (421-541) | 1621 |
| | 03-04 | 151 (142-161) | 147 (134-157) | 237 (212-254) | 365 (335-397) | 500 (422-580) | 1476 |
| **Gender** | | | | | | | |
| Males | 01-02 | 122 (108-137) | 116 (104-131) | 194 (173-218) | 321 (262-395) | 455 (348-642) | 1344 |
| | 03-04 | 138 (131-146) | 130 (117-143) | 201 (187-227) | 335 (301-391) | 437 (392-550) | 1196 |
| Females | 01-02 | 142 (125-160) | 136 (118-156) | 226 (199-256) | 355 (323-399) | 473 (421-541) | 1397 |
| | 03-04 | 154 (142-168) | 150 (138-160) | 241 (212-269) | 364 (323-425) | 505 (418-635) | 1300 |
| **Race/ethnicity** | | | | | | | |
| Mexican Americans | 01-02 | 110 (88.6-136) | 101 (85.5-131) | 162 (138-203) | 275 (187-452) | 400 (268-755) | 664 |
| | 03-04 | 124 (111-140) | 122 (107-136) | 183 (159-242) | 304 (246-392) | 392 (318-437) | 611 |
| Non-Hispanic blacks | 01-02 | 106 (88.7-127) | 102 (92.4-111) | 172 (141-203) | 274 (224-356) | 384 (308-598) | 690 |
| | 03-04 | 129 (112-148) | 126 (108-143) | 199 (173-242) | 337 (272-400) | 428 (374-522) | 679 |
| Non-Hispanic whites | 01-02 | 142 (126-161) | 137 (119-153) | 228 (206-247) | 363 (321-406) | 476 (411-552) | 1204 |
| | 03-04 | 157 (146-168) | 150 (140-159) | 241 (216-256) | 372 (335-424) | 515 (426-658) | 1046 |

## Urinary 2-Hydroxyphenanthrene

*Metabolite of Phenanthrene*

Geometric mean and selected percentiles of urine concentrations (in ng/L) for the U.S. population from the National Health and Nutrition Examination Survey.

| | Survey years | Geometric mean (95% conf. interval) | 50th | 75th | 90th | 95th | Sample size |
|---|---|---|---|---|---|---|---|
| | | | \multicolumn{4}{c}{Selected percentiles (95% confidence interval)} | | |
| **Total** | 01-02 | 54.0 (46.0-63.5) | 58.0 (50.0-68.0) | 117 (102-140) | 240 (201-271) | 332 (299-377) | 2742 |
| | 03-04 | 59.3 (52.5-66.9) | 62.2 (55.4-69.7) | 117 (105-129) | 206 (180-235) | 291 (252-336) | 2512 |
| **Age group** | | | | | | | |
| 6-11 years | 01-02 | 40.5 (34.3-47.7) | 46.0 (37.0-57.0) | 87.0 (71.0-101) | 170 (133-207) | 257 (195-320) | 387 |
| | 03-04 | 45.3 (40.0-51.3) | 48.1 (41.9-56.8) | 72.7 (63.2-89.4) | 135 (104-176) | 225 (136-299) | 337 |
| 12-19 years | 01-02 | 49.5 (37.3-65.7) | 52.0 (41.0-68.0) | 108 (93.0-122) | 210 (145-270) | 281 (214-524) | 733 |
| | 03-04 | 58.0 (50.7-66.2) | 62.5 (54.5-71.6) | 104 (88.8-132) | 198 (166-215) | 258 (199-318) | 707 |
| 20 years and older | 01-02 | 56.8 (48.1-66.9) | 60.0 (52.0-73.0) | 126 (104-152) | 249 (207-292) | 342 (308-398) | 1622 |
| | 03-04 | 61.5 (53.7-70.4) | 64.9 (57.2-73.5) | 125 (111-138) | 216 (187-250) | 310 (259-389) | 1468 |
| **Gender** | | | | | | | |
| Males | 01-02 | 62.1 (53.3-72.5) | 67.0 (58.0-80.0) | 136 (109-161) | 274 (245-303) | 367 (329-414) | 1345 |
| | 03-04 | 72.3 (64.4-81.3) | 71.6 (65.8-83.3) | 138 (123-150) | 240 (200-279) | 337 (279-428) | 1211 |
| Females | 01-02 | 47.4 (39.1-57.5) | 50.0 (41.0-60.0) | 105 (88.0-129) | 200 (171-240) | 294 (236-357) | 1397 |
| | 03-04 | 49.0 (42.4-56.6) | 52.5 (45.3-58.7) | 95.4 (84.1-110) | 166 (146-202) | 247 (202-291) | 1301 |
| **Race/ethnicity** | | | | | | | |
| Mexican Americans | 01-02 | 46.8 (32.7-66.8) | 51.0 (36.0-73.0) | 97.0 (72.0-140) | 191 (122-332) | 303 (187-652) | 665 |
| | 03-04 | 53.9 (46.7-62.1) | 60.1 (50.8-68.6) | 104 (89.5-115) | 164 (144-187) | 200 (187-219) | 627 |
| Non-Hispanic blacks | 01-02 | 71.1 (58.0-87.1) | 74.0 (66.0-90.0) | 152 (124-182) | 262 (217-311) | 374 (284-560) | 690 |
| | 03-04 | 81.2 (68.1-96.7) | 73.4 (61.8-101) | 158 (125-199) | 280 (219-374) | 390 (289-574) | 678 |
| Non-Hispanic whites | 01-02 | 53.1 (43.6-64.6) | 57.0 (48.0-68.0) | 117 (99.0-144) | 242 (199-286) | 333 (303-385) | 1204 |
| | 03-04 | 58.2 (50.1-67.7) | 60.7 (52.5-71.0) | 115 (97.9-133) | 209 (172-255) | 299 (251-351) | 1044 |

Limit of detection (LOD, see Data Analysis section) for Survey years 01-02 and 03-04 are 3 2 and 5.0.

## Urinary 2-Hydroxyphenanthrene  (creatinine corrected)

*Metabolite of Phenanthrene*

Geometric mean and selected percentiles of urine concentrations (in ng/g of creatinine) for the U.S. population from the National Health and Nutrition Examination Survey.

| | Survey years | Geometric mean (95% conf. interval) | Selected percentiles ( 95% confidence interval) | | | | Sample size |
|---|---|---|---|---|---|---|---|
| | | | 50th | 75th | 90th | 95th | |
| **Total** | 01-02 | 50.6 (43.3-59 2) | 52.5 (46.4-59 6) | 91.4 (78.7-108) | 164 (138-200) | 233 (206-275) | 2742 |
| | 03-04 | 55.4 (51.1-60 0) | 52.3 (48.8-55 8) | 85.8 (79.4-97 0) | 150 (128-174) | 212 (180-252) | 2512 |
| **Age group** | | | | | | | |
| 6-11 years | 01-02 | 45.3 (38.8-52 8) | 50.0 (40.0-57 8) | 85.9 (69.6-100) | 144 (105-217) | 234 (138-397) | 387 |
| | 03-04 | 47.9 (43.6-52.7) | 46.6 (41.0-51.4) | 66.3 (60.3-72 8) | 106 (81.0-125) | 183 (108-295) | 337 |
| 12-19 years | 01-02 | 38.4 (29.6-49.7) | 38.5 (30.6-48.7) | 64.9 (52.4-84 0) | 117 (86.7-167) | 173 (128-305) | 733 |
| | 03-04 | 43.6 (39.3-48 5) | 40.8 (37.7-45 0) | 70.6 (55.8-84.7) | 106 (88.2-123) | 127 (115-176) | 707 |
| 20 years and older | 01-02 | 53.7 (46.2-62.4) | 55.6 (49.4-62.7) | 94.6 (84.1-112) | 173 (145-201) | 241 (209-287) | 1622 |
| | 03-04 | 58.7 (53.6-64 2) | 54.8 (50.7-60 9) | 91.6 (83.5-105) | 164 (139-182) | 227 (183-291) | 1468 |
| **Gender** | | | | | | | |
| Males | 01-02 | 50.4 (43.3-58 5) | 52.5 (47.2-59 2) | 91.4 (78.6-103) | 176 (140-208) | 245 (206-349) | 1345 |
| | 03-04 | 56.6 (52.5-61 0) | 52.3 (48.1-57.1) | 84.7 (79.2-96.4) | 157 (132-180) | 227 (184-284) | 1211 |
| Females | 01-02 | 50.9 (42.7-60.7) | 52.8 (45.5-61 0) | 91.6 (75.0-115) | 158 (133-183) | 214 (200-245) | 1397 |
| | 03-04 | 54.3 (48.7-60 5) | 52.3 (47.0-57 2) | 88.1 (76.4-101) | 146 (118-179) | 202 (175-246) | 1301 |
| **Race/ethnicity** | | | | | | | |
| Mexican Americans | 01-02 | 43.7 (31.9-59 8) | 44.0 (34.3-58 8) | 80.8 (59.8-115) | 146 (103-245) | 245 (144-394) | 665 |
| | 03-04 | 48.8 (42.5-55 9) | 50.1 (42.4-58 8) | 79.5 (68.2-86.1) | 124 (96.2-149) | 155 (127-206) | 627 |
| Non-Hispanic blacks | 01-02 | 50.2 (40.5-62 2) | 49.7 (44.3-56 0) | 87.7 (72.6-103) | 174 (127-224) | 257 (178-459) | 690 |
| | 03-04 | 57.6 (49.8-66.7) | 53.1 (45.7-63 5) | 90.3 (77.9-117) | 152 (128-186) | 218 (173-348) | 678 |
| Non-Hispanic whites | 01-02 | 52.5 (43.8-62 9) | 54.8 (47.7-61 9) | 92.7 (80.5-113) | 170 (140-204) | 233 (202-293) | 1204 |
| | 03-04 | 57.1 (51.7-63 0) | 52.9 (49.1-57 2) | 88.5 (79.2-102) | 159 (128-187) | 237 (180-295) | 1044 |

# Urinary 3-Hydroxyphenanthrene

*Metabolite of Phenanthrene*

Geometric mean and selected percentiles of urine concentrations (in ng/L) for the U.S. population from the National Health and Nutrition Examination Survey.

| | Survey years | Geometric mean (95% conf. interval) | 50th | 75th | 90th | 95th | Sample size |
|---|---|---|---|---|---|---|---|
| **Total** | 01-02 | 105 (92.5-118) | 105 (92.0-118) | 200 (179-225) | 401 (336-480) | 649 (542-747) | 2741 |
| | 03-04 | 115 (104-128) | 118 (107-129) | 219 (201-237) | 424 (351-487) | 647 (509-788) | 2426 |
| **Age group** | | | | | | | |
| 6-11 years | 01-02 | 105 (91.1-122) | 109 (82.0-138) | 195 (160-231) | 298 (245-346) | 412 (319-545) | 387 |
| | 03-04 | 116 (99.9-134) | 107 (93.0-135) | 205 (170-223) | 333 (241-435) | 472 (322-881) | 325 |
| 12-19 years | 01-02 | 104 (87.3-125) | 107 (90.0-122) | 201 (165-231) | 329 (255-445) | 459 (331-631) | 733 |
| | 03-04 | 120 (103-141) | 127 (107-149) | 221 (195-262) | 366 (327-424) | 564 (391-730) | 677 |
| 20 years and older | 01-02 | 105 (91.7-119) | 105 (89.0-118) | 201 (180-231) | 433 (366-515) | 683 (597-806) | 1621 |
| | 03-04 | 114 (103-128) | 118 (105-130) | 221 (203-243) | 450 (353-505) | 696 (511-885) | 1424 |
| **Gender** | | | | | | | |
| Males | 01-02 | 122 (107-138) | 117 (106-132) | 224 (188-278) | 474 (372-597) | 734 (597-1010) | 1344 |
| | 03-04 | 137 (122-154) | 135 (119-157) | 251 (221-287) | 487 (398-579) | 754 (606-913) | 1167 |
| Females | 01-02 | 90.8 (77.7-106) | 93.0 (80.0-108) | 184 (155-207) | 328 (291-399) | 518 (434-649) | 1397 |
| | 03-04 | 97.7 (86.5-110) | 100 (86.6-114) | 193 (170-210) | 351 (287-445) | 531 (447-647) | 1259 |
| **Race/ethnicity** | | | | | | | |
| Mexican Americans | 01-02 | 83.5 (64.1-109) | 84.0 (64.0-111) | 144 (117-198) | 259 (193-430) | 454 (253-1140) | 664 |
| | 03-04 | 92.7 (81.3-106) | 92.8 (84.1-111) | 164 (133-204) | 317 (236-374) | 436 (338-501) | 576 |
| Non-Hispanic blacks | 01-02 | 145 (122-172) | 135 (120-163) | 281 (228-346) | 516 (414-684) | 957 (609-1410) | 690 |
| | 03-04 | 166 (141-195) | 159 (137-193) | 313 (249-399) | 542 (458-670) | 798 (579-1200) | 686 |
| Non-Hispanic whites | 01-02 | 104 (90.8-120) | 106 (92.0-120) | 199 (177-224) | 401 (331-495) | 649 (518-747) | 1204 |
| | 03-04 | 114 (100-129) | 117 (104-128) | 220 (201-237) | 440 (332-509) | 702 (505-915) | 1010 |

Limit of detection (LOD, see Data Analysis section) for Survey years 01-02 and 03-04 are 3 6 and 5.0.

## Urinary 3-Hydroxyphenanthrene (creatinine corrected)

*Metabolite of Phenanthrene*

Geometric mean and selected percentiles of urine concentrations (in ng/g of creatinine) for the U.S. population from the National Health and Nutrition Examination Survey.

| | Survey years | Geometric mean (95% conf. interval) | Selected percentiles ( 95% confidence interval) | | | | Sample size |
|---|---|---|---|---|---|---|---|
| | | | 50th | 75th | 90th | 95th | |
| Total | 01-02 | 98.0 (87.4-110) | 86.5 (78.8-97.1) | 158 (142-174) | 299 (252-342) | 428 (365-621) | 2741 |
| | 03-04 | 108 (101-115) | 99.5 (91.9-106) | 172 (158-189) | 321 (273-363) | 497 (406-566) | 2426 |
| **Age group** | | | | | | | |
| 6-11 years | 01-02 | 118 (103-135) | 114 (94.9-131) | 173 (150-201) | 289 (238-368) | 410 (308-544) | 387 |
| | 03-04 | 124 (110-138) | 119 (110-129) | 165 (145-202) | 283 (231-402) | 484 (269-710) | 325 |
| 12-19 years | 01-02 | 81.1 (70.1-93 8) | 78.0 (66.7-89.4) | 116 (96.5-144) | 205 (153-275) | 283 (198-511) | 733 |
| | 03-04 | 90.3 (81.5-100) | 84.9 (76.1-93 9) | 139 (116-160) | 212 (193-231) | 295 (225-429) | 677 |
| 20 years and older | 01-02 | 98.9 (88.3-111) | 85.3 (78.3-96 6) | 164 (147-183) | 320 (273-356) | 488 (379-774) | 1621 |
| | 03-04 | 109 (102-117) | 99.1 (91.7-106) | 180 (161-198) | 343 (282-385) | 523 (417-608) | 1424 |
| **Gender** | | | | | | | |
| Males | 01-02 | 98.6 (87.7-111) | 87.1 (79.5-98 2) | 159 (138-188) | 310 (245-368) | 505 (356-761) | 1344 |
| | 03-04 | 107 (98.2-116) | 99.2 (87.4-109) | 169 (154-184) | 305 (261-343) | 491 (383-592) | 1167 |
| Females | 01-02 | 97.5 (84.9-112) | 86.4 (76.9-100) | 158 (139-178) | 292 (245-333) | 410 (352-583) | 1397 |
| | 03-04 | 109 (99.6-119) | 100 (88.9-110) | 176 (155-202) | 328 (265-398) | 497 (380-594) | 1259 |
| **Race/ethnicity** | | | | | | | |
| Mexican Americans | 01-02 | 78.2 (62.4-98 0) | 70.8 (56.2-87.4) | 130 (92.9-171) | 224 (173-321) | 333 (224-656) | 664 |
| | 03-04 | 83.8 (75.1-93 6) | 79.5 (72.9-87 0) | 137 (111-165) | 224 (188-274) | 305 (247-406) | 576 |
| Non-Hispanic blacks | 01-02 | 102 (85.8-122) | 91.9 (79.8-108) | 160 (133-202) | 296 (234-475) | 673 (347-1260) | 690 |
| | 03-04 | 118 (103-135) | 106 (90.5-126) | 186 (156-219) | 357 (257-439) | 505 (384-772) | 686 |
| Non-Hispanic whites | 01-02 | 103 (91.5-117) | 89.4 (80.2-102) | 167 (148-193) | 324 (272-368) | 447 (365-738) | 1204 |
| | 03-04 | 112 (104-121) | 103 (96.9-108) | 183 (160-200) | 346 (278-402) | 544 (417-656) | 1010 |

## Urinary 4-Hydroxyphenanthrene

*Metabolite of Phenanthrene*

Geometric mean and selected percentiles of urine concentrations (in ng/L) for the U.S. population from the National Health and Nutrition Examination Survey.

| | Survey years | Geometric mean (95% conf. interval) | 50th | 75th | 90th | 95th | Sample size |
|---|---|---|---|---|---|---|---|
| Total | 03-04 | 25.1 (22.6-27.9) | 25.9 (22.5-29.6) | 53.7 (47.4-59.7) | 96.8 (85.0-116) | 152 (118-176) | 2443 |
| **Age group** | | | | | | | |
| 6-11 years | 03-04 | 25.2 (22.3-28.4) | 26.3 (22.8-30.0) | 45.7 (38.6-53.3) | 95.5 (61.7-137) | 138 (95.1-202) | 321 |
| 12-19 years | 03-04 | 23.7 (20.3-27.6) | 25.8 (20.5-31.4) | 49.9 (45.2-53.0) | 77.4 (67.2-95.1) | 123 (94.6-142) | 683 |
| 20 years and older | 03-04 | 25.3 (22.4-28.6) | 25.8 (22.4-29.5) | 54.8 (48.6-61.9) | 101 (87.1-120) | 163 (117-197) | 1439 |
| **Gender** | | | | | | | |
| Males | 03-04 | 30.0 (26.5-34.0) | 29.6 (25.5-35.1) | 60.4 (53.4-68.7) | 110 (90.6-130) | 169 (118-211) | 1180 |
| Females | 03-04 | 21.1 (18.7-23.8) | 21.3 (18.3-25.3) | 46.5 (41.6-53.3) | 88.4 (73.5-103) | 136 (106-157) | 1263 |
| **Race/ethnicity** | | | | | | | |
| Mexican Americans | 03-04 | 23.5 (20.9-26.3) | 24.4 (21.4-29.4) | 46.1 (40.1-53.0) | 80.5 (60.9-94.1) | 99.7 (80.2-154) | 607 |
| Non-Hispanic blacks | 03-04 | 35.4 (29.6-42.3) | 37.1 (29.8-46.1) | 71.4 (60.3-83.3) | 123 (104-145) | 167 (133-215) | 657 |
| Non-Hispanic whites | 03-04 | 24.4 (21.5-27.7) | 25.2 (21.8-29.1) | 51.5 (45.1-58.5) | 97.9 (77.4-127) | 163 (113-202) | 1021 |

Limit of detection (LOD, see Data Analysis section) for Survey year 03-04 is 5 0.

## Urinary 4-Hydroxyphenanthrene (creatinine corrected)

*Metabolite of Phenanthrene*

Geometric mean and selected percentiles of urine concentrations (in ng/g of creatinine) for the U.S. population from the National Health and Nutrition Examination Survey.

| | Survey years | Geometric mean (95% conf. interval) | 50th | 75th | 90th | 95th | Sample size |
|---|---|---|---|---|---|---|---|
| Total | 03-04 | 23.3 (21.7-25.0) | 22.7 (20.5-24.9) | 42.0 (38.6-44.6) | 74.3 (66.3-85.4) | 114 (102-130) | 2443 |
| **Age group** | | | | | | | |
| 6-11 years | 03-04 | 26.3 (23.7-29.2) | 24.8 (21.6-28.6) | 43.3 (35.2-48.8) | 72.9 (56.3-113) | 126 (79.3-173) | 321 |
| 12-19 years | 03-04 | 17.7 (15.9-19.8) | 16.7 (15.7-18.4) | 31.4 (26.0-37.1) | 47.9 (40.7-54.1) | 61.7 (51.7-86.0) | 683 |
| 20 years and older | 03-04 | 24.0 (22.0-26.2) | 23.3 (21.1-25.4) | 43.5 (39.4-48.1) | 79.0 (66.8-100) | 121 (104-138) | 1439 |
| **Gender** | | | | | | | |
| Males | 03-04 | 23.4 (21.6-25.4) | 22.7 (20.3-24.9) | 40.9 (35.9-45.7) | 72.7 (61.5-86.8) | 112 (100-126) | 1180 |
| Females | 03-04 | 23.2 (21.2-25.5) | 22.8 (19.7-26.0) | 42.5 (38.3-46.2) | 75.1 (63.4-94.0) | 119 (93.1-139) | 1263 |
| **Race/ethnicity** | | | | | | | |
| Mexican Americans | 03-04 | 21.2 (18.8-23.8) | 20.7 (19.1-22.9) | 35.9 (29.8-40.7) | 59.0 (43.3-87.5) | 83.4 (60.9-139) | 607 |
| Non-Hispanic blacks | 03-04 | 25.0 (21.6-28.9) | 25.3 (23.1-28.8) | 42.0 (37.4-51.4) | 75.0 (61.6-87.9) | 102 (79.2-137) | 657 |
| Non-Hispanic whites | 03-04 | 23.7 (21.5-26.2) | 22.4 (19.4-25.4) | 43.6 (38.8-47.3) | 82.2 (68.5-101) | 126 (103-143) | 1021 |

## References

Agency for Toxic Substances and Disease Registry (ATSDR). Toxicological profile for polycyclic aromatic hydrocarbons [online] 1995. Available at URL: http://www.atsdr.cdc.gov/toxprofiles/tp69.html. 5/26/09

Becker K, Schulz C, Kaus S, Seiwert M, Seifert B. German environmental survey 1998 (GerES III): environmental pollutants in the urine of the German population. Int J Hyg Environ Health 2003; 206:15-24.

Elovaara E, Mikkola J, Makela M, Paldanius B, Priha E. Assessment of soil remediation workers' exposure to polycyclic aromatic hydrocarbons (PAH): Biomonitoring of naphthols, phenanthrols, and 1-hydroxypyrene in urine. Toxicol Lett 2006;162:158-163.

Fang G-C, Wu Y-S, Chen J-C, Chang C-N, Ho T-T. characteristic of polycyclic aromatic hydrocarbon concentrations and source identification for fine and coarse particulates at Taichung Harbor near Taiwan Strait during 2004-2005. Sci Tot Environ 2006;366:729-738.

Gundel J, Schaller KH, Angerer J. Occupational exposure to polycyclic aromatic hydrocarbons in a fireproof stone producing plant: biological monitoring of 1-hydroxypyrene, 1-, 2-, 3- and 4-hydroxyphenanthrene, 3-hydroxybenz(a)anthracene and 3-hydroxybenzo-(a)-pyrene. Int Arch Occup Environ Health 2000;73(4):270-274.

Heudorf U, Angerer J. Internal exposure to PAHs of children and adults living in homes with parquet flooring containing high levels of PAHs in the parquet glue. Int Arch Occup Environ Health 2001*a*;74(2):91-101.

Heudorf U, Angerer J. Urinary monohydroxylated phenanthrenes and hydroxypyrene--the effects of smoking habits and changes induced by smoking on monooxygenase-mediated metabolism. Int Arch Occup Environ Health. 2001*b* 74(3):177-83.

Jacob J, Grimmer G, Dettbarn G. Profile of urinary phenanthrene metabolites in smokers and non-smokers. Biomarkers 1999;4(5):319-327.

# Pyrene

CAS No. 129-00-0

Pyrene has been used as a starting material for producing optical brighteners and dyes. Notable pyrene sources include domestic heating sources, particularly wood burning; gasoline fuel exhaust; coal tar and asphalt; and cigarette smoke. Pyrene is commonly found in PAH mixtures, and its urinary metabolite, 1-hydroxypyrene, has been used widely as an indicator of exposure to PAH chemicals, particularly in occupational exposure studies. IARC determined that pyrene was not classifiable as to its human carcinogenicity.

**Biomonitoring Information**

Urinary levels of 1-hydroxypyrene reflect recent exposure. The overall geometric mean of 1-hydroxypyrene levels in the NHANES 2003-2004 subsample was similar to that of general populations in other industrialized countries (Becker et al., 2003; Chuang et al., 1999; Goen et al., 1995; Heudorf and Angerer 2001a, 2001b; Yang et al., 2003). Higher levels have been noted in residents of industrialized and high traffic urban areas compared with rural or suburban settings, and the mean urinary 1-hydroxypyrene levels from the former group were somewhat higher than in the NHANES 2003-2004 subsample (Kanoh et al., 1993; Kuo et al., 2004; Yang et al., 2003). Variation also has been noted in the mean 1-hydroxypyrene urine levels between different industrialized countries (for example, South Korea or China, compared to the U.S.), which is attributable to such factors as ambient air pollution and residential heating and cooking sources (Huang et al., 2004; Kuo et al., 2004; Roggi et al., 1997; Siwinska et al., 1999; Yang et al., 2003). In general, smokers have about 2 to 4-fold higher urinary 1-hydroxypyrene levels than non-smokers (Goen et al., 1995; Heudorf and Angerer 2001b; Jacob et al., 1999). Environmental tobacco smoke may contribute to higher urinary 1-hydroxypyrene levels in exposed children (Chuang et al., 1999; Siwinska et al., 1999; Tsai et al., 2003).

Numerous studies of workers with occupational exposure to excessive vehicular exhaust have found increased urinary 1-hydroxypyrene levels compared to non-exposed individuals (Kuusimaki et al., 2004; Merlo et al., 1998; Tsai et al., 2004). The highest urinary levels of 1-hydroxypyrene measured in occupational studies have been found in aluminum smelter and coke oven workers exposed to heated tar and coal tar products (Alexandrie et al., 2000; Goen et al., 1995; Jacob and Seidel, 2002; Lu et al., 2002; Serdar et al., 2003). Results in these workers have ranged from about 100 to more than 1000 times greater than non-

exposed levels and the geometric mean values found in this *Report*. Tobacco smoking also was associated with levels about double those in nonsmoking workers (Campo et al., 2006; Merlo et al., 1998; Mukherjee et al., 2004).

Finding a measurable amount of urinary 1-hydroxypyrene does not mean that the level of 1-hydroxypyrene causes an adverse health effect. Biomonitoring studies on levels of 1-hydroxypyrene provide physicians and public health officials with reference values so that they can determine whether people have been exposed to higher levels of pyrene than are found in the general population. Biomonitoring data can also help scientists plan and conduct research on exposure and health effects.

## Urinary 1-Hydroxypyrene
*Metabolite of Pyrene*
Geometric mean and selected percentiles of urine concentrations (in ng/L) for the U.S. population from the National Health and Nutrition Examination Survey.

| | Survey years | Geometric mean (95% conf. interval) | 50th | 75th | 90th | 95th | Sample size |
|---|---|---|---|---|---|---|---|
| Total | 03-04 | 89.2 (79.8-99.7) | 91.3 (83.5-98 8) | 189 (168-208) | 389 (345-459) | 569 (493-676) | 2515 |
| **Age group** | | | | | | | |
| 6-11 years | 03-04 | 112 (96.9-130) | 119 (99.0-143) | 193 (163-229) | 351 (233-484) | 514 (336-680) | 333 |
| 12-19 years | 03-04 | 119 (103-137) | 115 (98.0-145) | 244 (213-274) | 506 (359-608) | 705 (636-788) | 705 |
| 20 years and older | 03-04 | 82.8 (73.0-93 8) | 83.8 (75.6-92.4) | 177 (155-203) | 387 (337-437) | 553 (483-644) | 1477 |
| **Gender** | | | | | | | |
| Males | 03-04 | 108 (96.0-122) | 111 (98.7-121) | 227 (197-265) | 459 (387-518) | 644 (526-811) | 1214 |
| Females | 03-04 | 74.0 (64.3-85.1) | 75.3 (66.3-83 9) | 158 (143-173) | 334 (258-407) | 502 (389-604) | 1301 |
| **Race/ethnicity** | | | | | | | |
| Mexican Americans | 03-04 | 89.4 (78.6-102) | 92.4 (79.8-113) | 173 (153-191) | 331 (281-415) | 495 (404-548) | 623 |
| Non-Hispanic blacks | 03-04 | 128 (105-155) | 126 (108-153) | 296 (226-355) | 553 (400-669) | 699 (564-935) | 681 |
| Non-Hispanic whites | 03-04 | 84.8 (73.5-97 9) | 85.4 (75.6-97 3) | 182 (156-214) | 386 (336-462) | 566 (470-749) | 1050 |

Limit of detection (LOD, see Data Analysis section) for Survey year 03-04 is 5.0.

## Urinary 1-Hydroxypyrene (creatinine corrected)
*Metabolite of Pyrene*
Geometric mean and selected percentiles of urine concentrations (in ng/g of creatinine) for the U.S. population from the National Health and Nutrition Examination Survey.

| | Survey years | Geometric mean (95% conf. interval) | 50th | 75th | 90th | 95th | Sample size |
|---|---|---|---|---|---|---|---|
| Total | 03-04 | 83.4 (77.4-90 0) | 79.9 (72.6-86 9) | 149 (133-167) | 279 (236-343) | 424 (352-474) | 2515 |
| **Age group** | | | | | | | |
| 6-11 years | 03-04 | 119 (102-138) | 112 (98.2-137) | 185 (156-225) | 336 (227-440) | 475 (336-566) | 333 |
| 12-19 years | 03-04 | 89.4 (77.7-103) | 81.6 (74.3-93 0) | 146 (123-187) | 269 (196-364) | 364 (251-611) | 705 |
| 20 years and older | 03-04 | 79.1 (73.2-85.4) | 73.5 (66.7-82 3) | 142 (127-160) | 278 (236-331) | 424 (349-472) | 1477 |
| **Gender** | | | | | | | |
| Males | 03-04 | 84.8 (77.3-93.1) | 82.8 (72.7-91 0) | 163 (145-175) | 290 (241-352) | 416 (353-513) | 1214 |
| Females | 03-04 | 82.1 (73.5-91.7) | 78.3 (69.2-86 8) | 137 (119-165) | 274 (215-350) | 440 (313-479) | 1301 |
| **Race/ethnicity** | | | | | | | |
| Mexican Americans | 03-04 | 81.2 (73.9-89 2) | 80.9 (70.4-91.7) | 146 (122-167) | 247 (221-301) | 372 (321-460) | 623 |
| Non-Hispanic blacks | 03-04 | 91.0 (77.7-107) | 92.4 (76.6-106) | 173 (145-211) | 315 (227-433) | 451 (301-680) | 681 |
| Non-Hispanic whites | 03-04 | 83.3 (75.4-92 0) | 77.9 (69.1-86 8) | 148 (127-174) | 287 (241-360) | 438 (360-506) | 1050 |

# References

Alexandrie AK, Warholm M, Carstensen U, Axmon A, Hagmar L, Levin JO, et al. CYP1A1 and GSTM1 polymorphisms affect urinary 1-hydroxypyrene levels after PAH exposure. Carcinogenesis 2000;21(4):669-676.

Becker K, Schulz C, Kaus S, Seiwert M, Seifert B. German environmental survey 1998 (GerES III): environmental pollutants in the urine of the German population. Int J Hyg Environ Health 2003; 206:15-24.

Campo L, Buratti M, Fustinoni S, Cirla PE, Martinotti I, Longhi O, et al. Evaluation of exposure to PAHs in asphalt workers by environmental and biological monitoring. Ann NY Acad Sci 2006;1076:405-420.

Chuang JC, Callahan PJ, Lyu CW, Wilson NK. Polycyclic aromatic hydrocarbon exposures of children in low-income families. J Expo Anal Environ Epidemiol 1999;9(2):85-98.

Goen T, Gundel J, Schaller KH, Angerer J. The elimination of 1-hydroxypyrene in the urine of the general population and workers with different occupational exposures to PAH. Sci Total Environ 1995;163(1-3):195-201.

Heudorf U, Angerer J. Internal exposure to PAHs of children and adults living in homes with parquet flooring containing high levels of PAHs in the parquet glue. Int Arch Occup Environ Health 2001a;74(2):91-101.

Heudorf U, Angerer J. Urinary monohydroxylated phenanthrenes and hydroxypyrene--the effects of smoking habits and changes induced by smoking on monooxygenase-mediated metabolism. Int Arch Occup Environ Health. 2001b 74(3):177-183.

Huang W, Grainger J, Patterson DG, Turner WE, Caudill SP, Needham LL, et al. Comparison of 1-hydroxypyrene exposure in the US population with that in occupational exposure studies. Int Arch Occup Environ Health 2004;77:491-498.

Jacob J, Grimmer G, Dettbarn G. Profile of urinary phenanthrene metabolites in smokers and non-smokers. Biomarkers 1999;4(5):319-327.

Jacob J, Seidel A. Biomonitoring of polycyclic aromatic hydrocarbons in human urine. J Chromatogr B 2002;778(1-2):31-47.

Kanoh T, Fukuda M, Onozuka H, Kinouchi T, Ohnishi Y. Urinary 1-hydroxypyrene as a marker of exposure to polycyclic aromatic hydrocarbons in environment. Environ Res 1993;62(2):230-241.

Kuo CT, Chen HW, Chen JL. Determination of 1-hydroxypyrene in children urine using column-switching liquid chromatography and fluorescence detection. J Chromatogr B 2004;805(2):187-193.

Kuusimaki L, Peltonen Y, Mutanen P, Peltonen K, Savela K. Urinary hydroxy-metabolites of naphthalene, phenanthrene and pyrene as markers of exposure to diesel exhaust. Int Arch Occup Environ Health 2004;77(1):23-30.

Lu PL, Chen ML, Mao IF. Urinary 1-hydroxypyrene levels in workers exposed to coke oven emissions at various locations in a coke oven plant. Arch Environ Health 2002;57(3):255-261.

Merlo F, Andreassen A, Weston A, Pan CF, Haugen A, Valerio F, et al. Urinary excretion of 1-hydroxypyrene as a marker for exposure to urban air levels of polycyclic aromatic hydrocarbons. Cancer Epidemiol Biomarkers Prev 1998;7(2):147-155.

Mukherjee S, Palmer LJ, Kim JY, Aeschliman DB, Houk RS, Woodin MA, et al. Smoking status and occupational exposure affects oxidative DNA injury in boilermakers exposed to metal fume and residual oil fly ash. Cancer Epidemiol Biomarkers Prev 2004;13(3):454-460.

Roggi C, Minoia C, Sciarra GF, Apostoli P, Maccarini L, Magnaghi S, et al. Urinary 1-hydroxypyrene as a marker of exposure to pyrene: an epidemiological survey on a general population group. Sci Total Environ 1997;199(3):247-254.

Serdar B, Waidyanatha S, Zheng Y, Rappaport SM. Simultaneous determination of urinary 1- and 2-naphthols, 3- and 9-phenanthrols, and 1-pyrenol in coke oven workers. Biomarkers 2003;8(2):93-109.

Siwinska E, Mielzynska D, Bubak A, Smolik E. The effect of coal stoves and environmental tobacco smoke on the level of urinary 1-hydroxypyrene. Mutat Res 1999;445(2):147-153.

Tsai HT, Wu MT, Hauser R, Rodrigues E, Ho CK, Liu CL, et al. Exposure to environmental tobacco smoke and urinary 1-hydroxypyrene levels in preschool children. Kaohsiung J Med Sci 2003;19(3):97-104.

Tsai PJ, Shih TS, Chen HL, Lee WJ, Lai CH, Liou SH. Urinary 1-hydroxypyrene as an indicator for assessing the exposures of booth attendants of a highway toll station to polycyclic aromatic hydrocarbons. Environ Sci Technol 2004;38(1):56-61.

Yang M, Kim S, Lee E, Cheong HK, Chang SS, Kang D, et al. Sources of polycyclic aromatic hydrocarbon exposure in non-occupationally exposed Koreans. Environ Mol Mutagen 2003;42(4):250-257.

# Benzene
CAS No. 71-43-2

## General Information

Benzene is a volatile chemical that is produced commercially from coal and petroleum sources. It is among the most abundantly produced chemicals in the U.S. and is used extensively as an industrial solvent, in the synthesis of numerous chemicals, and as an additive in unleaded gasoline (ATSDR, 2007).

Human exposure occurs primarily by inhaling benzene in ambient air (Hattemer-Frey et al., 1990; Wallace, 1996). Sources of benzene in the air may result from either natural (e.g., forest fires) or industrial sources. Among industrial sources, automobile emissions and vapor around gasoline filling stations contribute to benzene in air (ATSDR, 2007). Tobacco smoke contributes to benzene in indoor air (Duarte-Davidson, et al., 2001), and tobacco smoke is estimated to account for about half of the total estimated exposure to benzene (ATSDR, 2007). Indoor sources for benzene, which include the offgassing of building materials, account for a significant portion of a non-smoker's benzene exposure (Wallace, 1996; Wallace et al., 1987). The consumption of food, drinking water, and beverages are considered negligible sources of exposure unless benzene contamination has occurred, such as from leaking underground fuel storage tanks (ATSDR, 2007; Wallace, 1996). In recent years, less than five percent of domestic wells used for drinking water in the U.S. have been found to contain detectable amounts of benzene (Rowe et al., 2007). Workplace exposure to benzene may result from production, use, or transportation of petroleum products.

Benzene is well absorbed after inhalational, oral, or dermal exposure. In the blood, benzene is distributed rapidly throughout the body, especially into the brain and fatty tissues, and can cross the placenta. Benzene is metabolized in the liver, and some metabolites may be distributed to the bone marrow, where additional metabolism may result in toxic effects on hematopoietic cells (ATSDR, 2007; Ross, 2000). The primary benzene metabolites are phenol, catechol, hydroquinone, 1,2,4-benzenetriol, and to a lesser extent, *trans, trans*-muconic acid, which are eliminated in urine as glucuronide and sulfate conjugates (Ross, 2000). Urinary S-phenylmercapturic and *t,t*-muconic acids are used for monitoring workplace exposure. A very small amount of unchanged benzene is eliminated in the breath.

## Blood Benzene

Geometric mean and selected percentiles of blood concentrations (in ng/mL) for the U.S. population from the National Health and Nutrition Examination Survey.

| | Survey years# | Geometric mean (95% conf. interval) | Selected percentiles ( 95% confidence interval) | | | | Sample size |
|---|---|---|---|---|---|---|---|
| | | | 50th | 75th | 90th | 95th | |
| **Total** | 01-02 | * | .030 (<LOD-.050) | .100 (.060-.140) | .190 (.140-.290) | .320 (.190-.480) | 837 |
| | 03-04 | * | .027 (.025-.031) | .064 (.050-.084) | .170 (.150-.190) | .260 (.210-.320) | 1345 |
| **Age group** | | | | | | | |
| 20-59 years | 01-02 | * | .030 (<LOD-.050) | .100 (.060-.140) | .190 (.140-.290) | .320 (.190-.480) | 837 |
| | 03-04 | * | .027 (.025-.031) | .064 (.050-.084) | .170 (.150-.190) | .260 (.210-.320) | 1345 |
| **Gender** | | | | | | | |
| Males | 01-02 | * | .030 (<LOD-.050) | .110 (.060-.160) | .230 (.150-.370) | .370 (.210-.510) | 403 |
| | 03-04 | .039 (.035-.043) | .030 (.027-.035) | .069 (.053-.084) | .160 (.140-.180) | .240 (.190-.320) | 654 |
| Females | 01-02 | * | .030 (<LOD-.050) | .100 (.060-.130) | .180 (.120-.240) | .250 (.170-.330) | 434 |
| | 03-04 | * | .025 (<LOD-.029) | .057 (.040-.090) | .180 (.150-.220) | .290 (.220-.420) | 691 |
| **Race/ethnicity** | | | | | | | |
| Mexican Americans | 01-02 | * | .030 (<LOD-.070) | .070 (.030-.170) | .140 (.060-.360) | .230 (.130-.370) | 227 |
| | 03-04 | * | .027 (<LOD-.035) | .041 (.034-.057) | .077 (.058-.110) | .130 (.084-.320) | 254 |
| Non-Hispanic blacks | 01-02 | * | < LOD | .060 (<LOD-.160) | .180 (.090-.300) | .250 (.160-.480) | 137 |
| | 03-04 | .043 (.033-.058) | .029 (<LOD-.054) | .092 (.055-.140) | .210 (.140-.290) | .320 (.240-.460) | 302 |
| Non-Hispanic whites | 01-02 | * | .030 (<LOD-.060) | .110 (.070-.160) | .210 (.140-.340) | .330 (.190-.510) | 411 |
| | 03-04 | * | .028 (.025-.033) | .068 (.053-.088) | .180 (.150-.200) | .280 (.210-.330) | 687 |

Limits of detection (LOD, see Data Analysis section) for Survey years 01-02 and 03-04 are 0.024 and 0.024.
# Survey period 2001-2002 is a one-third subsample of 20-59 year olds; Survey period 2003-2004 is a one-half subsample of 20-59 year olds.
< LOD means less than the limit of detection, which may vary for some chemicals by year and by individual sample.
* Not calculated: proportion of results below limit of detection was too high to provide a valid result.

Accidental and intentional exposures to high concentrations of benzene vapor can lead rapidly to euphoria, central nervous system depression, cardiac arrhythmias, followed by unconsciousness and death (ATSDR, 2007). Workers have developed skin irritation following repeated dermal exposure and mucous membrane irritation following repeated vapor inhalation (ATSDR, 2007). Epidemiologic studies of workers in industries involving benzene have found that benzene exposure can cause bone marrow suppression and increases the risk of various leukemias (Savitz and Andrews, 1997). Supportive evidence for benzene carcinogenicity comes from animal studies and from *in vitro* studies demonstrating the clastogenic properties of benzene on blood forming cells (NTP, 1986; Ross, 2000). The background exposure levels for the general population have been estimated to be much lower than the estimated lowest effect level for benzene at which leukemia risk is increased (Duarte-Davidson, et al., 2001).

Workplace standards and guidelines for benzene have been established by OSHA and ACGIH, respectively. The U.S. EPA has established environmental and drinking water standards for benzene, and the FDA has established a bottled water standard. Benzene is classified as a known human carcinogen by IARC and by NTP. Information about external exposure (ie., environmental levels) and health effects is available from ATSDR at: http://www.atsdr.cdc.gov/toxpro2.html.

## Biomonitoring Information

Levels of blood benzene reflect recent exposure. The median level of blood benzene observed in the NHANES 2003-2004 subsample appear slightly lower than the median level in a nonrepresentative subsample of adults in NHANES III (1988-1994) (Ashley et al., 1994), as well for other previous studies of the U.S. general population (Bonanno et al., 2001; Buckley et al., 1997; Sexton et al., 2005 and 2006; Lin et al., 2008), and studies from other countries (Brugnone et al., 1994; Navasumrit et al., 2005).

Smoking, residing, or working in urban areas and exposure to gasoline and petroleum products can result in blood benzene levels that are higher than those in the nonsmoking general population (Ashley et al., 1995; Carrer et al., 2000; Backer et al., 1997). The amount and duration of cigarette smoking increases the likelihood of higher blood benzene levels (Bonanno et al., 2001; Churchill et al., 2001; Lin et al., 2008). Workers exposed to gasoline fumes, such as garage mechanics, drivers, and street vendors, and workers exposed to solvent fumes have been found to have blood benzene levels as much as tenfold higher than levels in

the general population (Brugnone, et al., 1994 and 1999; Moolenaar et al., 1997; Perbellini et al., 2002; Romieu et al., 1999).

Finding a measurable amount of benzene in blood does not mean that the level of benzene causes an adverse health effect. Biomonitoring studies of blood benzene can provide physicians and public health officials with reference values so that they can determine whether or not people have been exposed to higher levels of benzene than levels found in the general population. Biomonitoring data can also help scientists plan and conduct research on exposure and health effects.

## References

Agency for Toxic Substances and Disease Registry (ATSDR). Toxicological profile for benzene update. 2007 [online]. Available at URL: http://www.atsdr.cdc.gov/toxprofiles/tp3.html. 4/20/09

Ashley DL, Bonin MA, Cardinali FL, McCraw JM, Wooten JV. Blood concentrations of volatile organic compounds in a nonoccupationally exposed US population and in groups with suspected exposure. Clin Chem 1994;40(7 Pt 2):1401-1404.

Ashley DL, Bonin MA, Hamar B, McGeehin MA. Removing the smoking confounder from blood volatile organic compounds measurements. Environ Res 1995;71:39-45.

Backer LC, Egeland GM, Ashley DL, Lawryk NJ, Weisel CP, White MC, et al. Exposure to regular gasoline and ethanol oxyfuel during refueling in Alaska. Environ Health Perspect 1997;105(8):850-855.

Bonanno LJ, Freeman NCG, Greenberg M, Lioy PJ. Multivariate analysis on levels of selected metals, particulate matter, VOC, and household characteristics and activities from the Midwestern states NHEXAS. Appl Occup Environ Hyg 2001;6(9):859-874.

Brugnone F. Benzene in blood as a biomarker of low level occupational exposure. Sci Tot Environ. 1999;235:247.

Brugnone F, Perbellini L, Giuliari C, Cerpelloni M, Soave M. Blood and urine concentrations of chemical pollutants in the general population. Med Lav 1994;85(5):370-389.

Buckley TJ, Liddle J, Ashley DL, Paschal DC, Burse VW, Needham LL. Environmental and biomarker measurements in nine homes in the lower Rio Grande Valley: multimedia results for pesticides, metals, PAHs and VOCs. Environ Int 1997;23(5):705-732.

Carrer P, Maroni M, Alcini D, Cavallo D, Fustinoni S, Lovato L, et al. Assessment through environmental and biological measurements of total daily exposure to volatile organic compounds of office workers in Milan, Italy. Indoor Air

2000;10:258-268.

Churchill JE, Ashley DL, Kaye WE. Recent chemical exposures and blood volatile organic compound levels in a large population-based sample. Arch Environ Health 2001;56(2):157-166.

Duarte-Davidson R, Courage C, Rushton L, Levy L. Benzene in the environment: an assessment of the potential risks to the health of the population. Occup Environ Med 2001;58(1):2-13.

Hattemer-Frey HA, Travis CC, Land ML. Benzene: Environmental partitioning and human exposure. Environ Res 1990;53:221-232.

Lin YS, Egeghy PP, Rappaport SM. Relationships between levels of volatile organic compounds in air and blood from the general population. J Expo Sci Environ Epidemiol 2008;18(4):421-9.

Moolenaar RL, Brockton JH, Ashley DL, Middauth JP, Etzel RA. Blood benzene concentrations in workers exposed to oxygenated fuel in Fairbanks, Alaska. Int Arch Occup Environ Health 1997;69:139-143.

National Toxicology Program (NTP). Toxicology and carcinogenesis studies of benzene (CAS No. 71-43-2) in F344/N rats and B6C3F1 mice (gavage studies). National Toxicology Program Tech Rep Series No. 289. 1986 [online]. Available at URL: http://ntp.niehs.nih.gov/go/reports. 4/20/09

Navasumrit P, Chanvaivit S, Intarasunanont P, Arayasiri M, Lauhareungpanya N, Parnlob V, et al. Environmental and occupational exposure to benzene in Thailand. Chem Biol Interact. 2005;153-154:75-83.

Perbellini L, Pasini F, Romani S, Princivalle A, Brugnone F. Analysis of benzene, toluene, ethylbenzene and m-xylene in biological samples from the general population. J Chromat B 2002;778:198-210.

Romieu I, Ramirez M, Meneses F, Ashley DL, Lemire S, Colome S, et al. Environmental exposure to volatile organic compounds among workers in Mexico City as assessed by personal monitors and blood concentrations. Environ Health Perspect 1999;107(7):511-515.

Ross D. The role of metabolism and specific metabolites in benzene-induced toxicity: evidence and issues. J Toxicol Environ Health A 2000;61(5-6):357-372.

Rowe BL, Toccalino PL, Moran MJ, Zogorski JS, Price CV. occurrence and potential human-health relevance of colatile organic compounds in drinking water from domestic wells in the United States. Environ Health Perspect 2007;115(11):1539-1546.

Savitz DA, Andrews KW. Review of epidemiologic evidence on benzene and lymphatic and hematopoietic cancers. Am J Ind Med 1997 Mar;31(3):287-95.

Sexton K, Adgate JL, Church TR, Ashley DL, Needham LL,

Ramachandran G, et al. Children's exposure to volatile organic compounds as determined by longitudinal measurements in blood. Environ Health Perspect 2005;113(3):342-349.

Sexton K, Adgate JL, Fredrickson AL, Ryan AD, Needham LL, Ashley DL. Using biologic markers in blood to assess exposure to multiple environmental chemicals for inner-city children 3-6 years of age. Environ Health Perspect 2006;114(3):453-459.

Wallace L. Environmental exposure to benzene: an update. Environ Health Perspect 1996;104 Suppl 6:1129-1136.

Wallace L, Pellizzari E, Leaderer B, Zelon H, Sheldon L. Emissions of volatile organic compounds from building materials and consumer products. Atmos Environ 1987;21:385-393.

# Chlorobenzenes

**Chlorobenzene (Monochlorobenzene)**
CAS No. 108-90-7

**1,2-Dichlorobenzene (*o*-dichlorobenzene)**
CAS No. 95-50-1

**1,3-Dichlorobenzene (*m*-dichlorobenzene)**
CAS No. 541-73-1

**1,4-Dichlorobenzene (*p*-dichlorobenzene,
Paradichlorobenzene)** CAS No. 106-46-7

## General Information

Chlorobenzene (monochlorobenzene) and the three dichlorobenzenes are halogenated aromatic hydrocarbons pirmarily used in industrial and chemical synthetic processes. Chlorobenzene has been used to produce DDT, phenol, and nitrobenzene. The dichlorobenzenes are also chemical intermediates in synthesis of dyes, pesticides, and other industrial products. The chlorobenzenes have sometimes been used as solvents for pesticides and auto parts degreasers (ATSDR, 2007). 1,4-Dichlorobenzene (1,4-DCB; para-dichlorobenzene) is used also as a moth repellent and as a deodorizer (ATSDR, 2007).

Ambient air is the primary source of chlorobenzene exposure for the general population. Indoor air levels of 1,4-DCB may exceed outdoor levels when moth repellents or deodorizers

are in use (Wallace et al., 1987, 1991). Dietary sources are negligible (Schaum et al., 2003), and chlorobenzenes generally are not detected in drinking water or groundwater in the United States (USGS, 2006), but may be detected where industrial waste containing these chemicals has been discharged (IPCS, 2004). Chlorobenzenes volatilize from soil and water (ATSDR, 2007, 2008). People involved in the production or use of chlorobenzenes may be exposed by inhalation or dermal contact. Chlorobenzenes are well absorbed after inhalation and ingestion. 1,4-DCB is not appreciably absorbed through intact skin. Within a few hours following exposure, these chemicals are eliminated from tissues via oxidative hepatic metabolism followed by conjugation or oxidation. The major urinary metabolites are dichlorophenols (ATSDR, 2007, 2006).

Human health effects from chlorobenzenes at low environmental doses or at biomonitored levels from low environmental exposures are unknown. In humans, high air levels of 1,2- or 1,4-dichlorobenzenes cause eye and nasal irritation, and prolonged or repeated contact with concentrated solutions of either chemical may cause skin irritation or sensitization (Elovaara, 1998). Asthma and reduced pulmonary function have been associated with recent exposure to aromatic chemicals, including 1,4-DCB, but causation is unclear (Arif and Shah, 2007; Elliott et al., 2006). Laboratory animals exposed to high levels of chlorobenzene may demonstrate liver enlargement and serum transaminase elevations, renal tubular cell damage, and central nervous system depression. High doses of 1,2- or 1,3-dichlorbenzenes can result in centrilobular liver necrosis and decreased thyroid hormone levels and, among

## Blood Chlorobenzene (Monochlorobenzene)

Geometric mean and selected percentiles of blood concentrations (in ng/mL) for the U.S. population from the National Health and Nutrition Examination Survey.

| | Survey years# | Geometric mean (95% conf. interval) | Selected percentiles ( 95% confidence interval) | | | | Sample size |
|---|---|---|---|---|---|---|---|
| | | | 50th | 75th | 90th | 95th | |
| **Total** | 03-04 | * | < LOD | < LOD | < LOD | < LOD | 1366 |
| **Age group** | | | | | | | |
| 20-59 years | 03-04 | * | < LOD | < LOD | < LOD | < LOD | 1366 |
| **Gender** | | | | | | | |
| Males | 03-04 | * | < LOD | < LOD | < LOD | < LOD | 669 |
| Females | 03-04 | * | < LOD | < LOD | < LOD | < LOD | 697 |
| **Race/ethnicity** | | | | | | | |
| Mexican Americans | 03-04 | * | < LOD | < LOD | < LOD | < LOD | 267 |
| Non-Hispanic blacks | 03-04 | * | < LOD | < LOD | < LOD | < LOD | 300 |
| Non-Hispanic whites | 03-04 | * | < LOD | < LOD | < LOD | < LOD | 694 |

Limit of detection (LOD, see Data Analysis section) for Survey year 03-04 is 0.011.
# Survey period 2003-2004 is a one-half subsample of 20-59 year olds.
< LOD means less than the limit of detection, which may vary for some chemicals by year and by individual sample.
* Not calculated: proportion of results below limit of detection was too high to provide a valid result.

male animals, renal tubular degeneration (ATSDR, 2007; Elovaara, 1998; NTP, 1987). 1,4-DCB is not as acutely hepatotoxic or thyrotoxic as the other dichlorobenzene isomers (den Besten et al., 1991, 1992; Stine et al., 1991). In animal studies, 1,4-DCB is not considered to be a reproductive or developmental toxicant (ATSDR, 2007, 2008; Elovaara, 1998). Animals fed high doses of 1,4-DCB demonstrated an increased incidence of renal and hepatic tumors, but no evidence was found of mutagenicity or genotoxicity *in vitro* (NTP, 1987).

The U.S. EPA and the FDA regulate the levels of 1,2- or 1,4-dichlorobenzene in air and water and in bottled drinking water, respectively. U.S. EPA regulates the monochlorobenzene level in drinking water. NIOSH and ACGIH provide workplace guidelines for 1,2- and 1,4-dichlorobenzenes and monochlorobenzene levels in air. IARC classified 1,4-dichlorobenze as a possible human carcinogen and NTP determined that it was reasonably anticipated to be a human carcinogen. However, IARC determined that the human carcinogenicity of 1,2-dichlorobenzene and 1,3-dichlorobenzene was unclassifiable. Additional information about external exposure (i.e., environmental levels) and health effects is available from ATSDR at: http://www.atsdr.cdc.gov/toxpro2.html.

## Biomonitoring Information

Levels of chlorobenzene, 1,2-dichlorobenzene, 1,3-dichlorobenzene, and 1,4-dichlorobenzene in blood reflect recent exposure. Data from the NHANES 2003-2004 subsample are shown in the tables for all the chlorobenzenes. In addition, the table for 1,4-dichlorobenzene shows data from the NHANES 2001-2002 subsample.

Generally, blood levels of chlorobenzene, 1,2-dichlorobenzene, 1,3-dichlorobenzene were not detected in NHANES 2003-2004 and were detected in only less than 10% of the U.S. general population samples in earlier surveys (Ashley et al., 1994; Elliott et al., 2006). For 1,4-dichlorobenzene, a nonrepresentative sample of adults from the National Health and Nutrition Examination Survey (NHANES) III (1988–1994) demonstrated a median level of 1,4-DCB level of 0.33 μg/L (Hill et al., 1995), or equivalent to the 75th percentile of the NHANES 2003-2004 subsample, and about three times higher than levels found in a sample of Midwestern adults and children (Bonanno et al., 2001). A small study of urban, low-income children monitored over a two year period reported that median 1,4-DCB blood levels were slightly lower than NHANES III (Sexton et al., 2005, 2006). Ambient air and blood levels have been shown to correlate reasonably well (Lin et al., 2008; Sexton et al., 2005). Residential construction and cleaning activities, including the recent use of toilet bowl deodorants, may contribute to elevated indoor air and blood levels of 1,4-DCB (Bonanno et al., 2001; Churchill et al., 2001).

Finding a measurable amount of chlorobenzenes in the urine does not mean that the level of chlorobenzene causes an adverse health effect. Biomonitoring studies of urinary chlorobenzenes can provide physicians and public health officials with reference values so that they can determine

## Blood 1,2-Dichlorobenzene (*o*-Dichlorobenzene)

Geometric mean and selected percentiles of blood concentrations (in ng/mL) for the U.S. population from the National Health and Nutrition Examination Survey.

| | Survey years# | Geometric mean (95% conf. interval) | Selected percentiles ( 95% confidence interval) | | | | Sample size |
|---|---|---|---|---|---|---|---|
| | | | 50th | 75th | 90th | 95th | |
| **Total** | 03-04 | * | < LOD | < LOD | < LOD | < LOD | 1327 |
| **Age group** | | | | | | | |
| 20-59 years | 03-04 | * | < LOD | < LOD | < LOD | < LOD | 1327 |
| **Gender** | | | | | | | |
| Males | 03-04 | * | < LOD | < LOD | < LOD | < LOD | 647 |
| Females | 03-04 | * | < LOD | < LOD | < LOD | < LOD | 680 |
| **Race/ethnicity** | | | | | | | |
| Mexican Americans | 03-04 | * | < LOD | < LOD | < LOD | < LOD | 250 |
| Non-Hispanic blacks | 03-04 | * | < LOD | < LOD | < LOD | < LOD | 291 |
| Non-Hispanic whites | 03-04 | * | < LOD | < LOD | < LOD | < LOD | 682 |

Limit of detection (LOD, see Data Analysis section) for Survey year 03-04 is 0.1.
# Survey period 2003-2004 is a one-half subsample of 20-59 year olds.
< LOD means less than the limit of detection, which may vary for some chemicals by year and by individual sample.
* Not calculated: proportion of results below limit of detection was too high to provide a valid result.

whether people have been exposed to higher levels of chlorobenzenes than are found in the general population. Biomonitoring data can also help scientists plan and conduct research on exposure and health effects.

## Blood 1,3-Dichlorobenzene (*m*-Dichlorobenzene)

Geometric mean and selected percentiles of blood concentrations (in ng/mL) for the U.S. population from the National Health and Nutrition Examination Survey.

| | Survey years# | Geometric mean (95% conf. interval) | 50th | 75th | 90th | 95th | Sample size |
|---|---|---|---|---|---|---|---|
| | | | **Selected percentiles** ( 95% confidence interval) | | | | |
| Total | 03-04 | * | < LOD | < LOD | < LOD | < LOD | 1334 |
| **Age group** | | | | | | | |
| 20-59 years | 03-04 | * | < LOD | < LOD | < LOD | < LOD | 1334 |
| **Gender** | | | | | | | |
| Males | 03-04 | * | < LOD | < LOD | < LOD | < LOD | 659 |
| Females | 03-04 | * | < LOD | < LOD | < LOD | < LOD | 675 |
| **Race/ethnicity** | | | | | | | |
| Mexican Americans | 03-04 | * | < LOD | < LOD | < LOD | < LOD | 266 |
| Non-Hispanic blacks | 03-04 | * | < LOD | < LOD | < LOD | < LOD | 279 |
| Non-Hispanic whites | 03-04 | * | < LOD | < LOD | < LOD | < LOD | 686 |

Limit of detection (LOD, see Data Analysis section) for Survey year 03-04 is 0.05.
# Survey period 2003-2004 is a one-half subsample of 20-59 year olds.
< LOD means less than the limit of detection, which may vary for some chemicals by year and by individual sample.
* Not calculated: proportion of results below limit of detection was too high to provide a valid result.

## Blood 1,4-Dichlorobenzene (Paradichlorobenzene)

Geometric mean and selected percentiles of blood concentrations (in ng/mL) for the U.S. population from the National Health and Nutrition Examination Survey.

| | Survey years# | Geometric mean (95% conf. interval) | 50th | 75th | 90th | 95th | Sample size |
|---|---|---|---|---|---|---|---|
| | | | **Selected percentiles** ( 95% confidence interval) | | | | |
| Total | 01-02 | * | < LOD | .300 (.190-.550) | 1.19 (.610-2.90) | 4.10 (1.40-7.60) | 807 |
| | 03-04 | * | < LOD | .320 (.250-.400) | 1.10 (.710-1.60) | 3.30 (1.70-5.10) | 1322 |
| **Age group** | | | | | | | |
| 20-59 years | 01-02 | * | < LOD | .300 (.190-.550) | 1.19 (.610-2.90) | 4.10 (1.40-7.60) | 807 |
| | 03-04 | * | < LOD | .320 (.250-.400) | 1.10 (.710-1.60) | 3.30 (1.70-5.10) | 1322 |
| **Gender** | | | | | | | |
| Males | 01-02 | * | < LOD | .270 (.180-.530) | .900 (.570-2.90) | 3.60 (1.10-7.20) | 390 |
| | 03-04 | * | < LOD | .320 (.250-.380) | .770 (.580-1.20) | 1.90 (1.20-4.00) | 651 |
| Females | 01-02 | * | < LOD | .360 (.190-.620) | 1.20 (.620-3.90) | 4.10 (1.68-8.30) | 417 |
| | 03-04 | * | < LOD | .350 (.220-.450) | 1.40 (.810-2.10) | 4.10 (2.20-5.90) | 671 |
| **Race/ethnicity** | | | | | | | |
| Mexican Americans | 01-02 | .331 (.246-.446) | .180 (<LOD-.260) | .790 (.400-1.30) | 6.00 (1.30-16.0) | 16.0 (6.20-33.0) | 217 |
| | 03-04 | .381 (.256-.566) | .210 (.140-.400) | .730 (.370-2.90) | 6.20 (2.90-9.30) | 10.0 (6.30-19.0) | 262 |
| Non-Hispanic blacks | 01-02 | .558 (.376-.827) | .360 (.260-.560) | 1.80 (.710-3.90) | 6.30 (1.40-29.0) | 15.0 (3.60-51.0) | 136 |
| | 03-04 | .423 (.292-.613) | .340 (.200-.480) | .980 (.550-1.50) | 4.10 (1.60-9.20) | 11.0 (2.50-19.0) | 297 |
| Non-Hispanic whites | 01-02 | * | < LOD | .200 (<LOD-.380) | .570 (.300-1.20) | 1.19 (.570-3.70) | 396 |
| | 03-04 | * | < LOD | .200 (.160-.260) | .490 (.370-.720) | .940 (.690-2.00) | 658 |

Limits of detection (LOD, see Data Analysis section) for Survey years 01-02 and 03-04 are 0.12 and 0.12.
# Survey period 2001-2002 is a one-third subsample of 20-59 year olds; Survey period 2003-2004 is a one-half subsample of 20-59 year olds.
< LOD means less than the limit of detection, which may vary for some chemicals by year and by individual sample.
* Not calculated: proportion of results below limit of detection was too high to provide a valid result.

# References

Agency for Toxic Substances and Disease Registry (ATSDR). Toxicological profile for chlorobenzene. Atlanta GA [updated 2008 August 08] Available at URL: http://www.atsdr.cdc.gov/toxprofiles/tp131.html. 4/13/09

Agency for Toxic Substances and Disease Registry (ATSDR). Toxicological profile for dichlorobenzenes update. Atlanta GA [updated 2007 October 19] Available at URL: http://www.atsdr.cdc.gov/toxprofiles/tp10 html#bookmark09. 4/13/09

Arif AA, Shah SM. Association between personal exposure to volatile organic compounds and asthma among US adult population. Int Arch Occup Environ Health 2007;80(8):711-719.

Ashley DL, Bonin MA, Cardinali FL, McCraw JM, Wooten JV. Blood concentrations of volatile organic compounds in a nonoccupationally exposed US population and in groups with suspected exposure. Clin Chem 1994;40(7 Pt 2):1401-1404.

Bonanno LJ, Freeman NCG, Greenberg M, Lioy PJ. Multivariate analysis on levels of selected metals, particulate matter, VOC, and household characteristics and activities from the Midwestern states NHEXAS. Appl Occup Environ Hyg 2001;16(9):859-874.

Churchill JE, Ashley DL, Kaye WE. Recent chemical exposures and blood volatile organic compound levels in a large population-based sample. Arch Environ Health 2001;56(2):157-166.

Den Besten C, Ellenbroek M, van der Ree MAE, Rietjens IMCM, van Bladeren PJ. The involvement of primary and secondary metabolism in the covalent bainding of 1,2- and 1,4-dichlorobenzenes. Chem Biol Interact 1992;84:259-275.

Den Besten C, Vet JJRM, Besselink HT, Kiel FS, van Berke BJM, Beems R, et al. The liver, kidney, and thyroid toxicity of chlorinated benzenes. Toxicol Appl Pharmacol 1991;111:69-81.

Elliott L, Longnecker MP, Kissling GE, London SJ. Volatile organic compounds and pulmonary function in the Third National Health and Nutrition Examination Survey, 1988-1994. Environ Health Perspect 2006;114(8):1210-1214.

Elovaara E. 122. Dichlorobenzenes, The Nordic Expert Group for Criteria Documentation of Health Risks from Chemicals. The National Institute for Working Life. Stockholm, Sweden. 1998. Availableat URL: https://gupea.ub.gu.se/dspace/bitstream/2077/4199/1/ah1998_04.pdf . 4/13/09

Hill RH Jr, Ashley DL, Head SL, Needham LL, Pirkle JL. p-Dichlorobenzene exposure among 1,000 adults in the United States. Arch Environ Health 1995;50(4):277-280.

International Programme on Chemical Safety (IPCS). Chlorobenzenes other than hexachlorobenzene: environmental aspects (Cicads 60). Geneva, Switzerland. 2004. Available at URL: http://www.inchem.org/documents/cicads/cicads/cicad60.htm. 4/13/09

Lin YS, Egeghy PP, Rappaport SM. Relationships between levels of volatile organic compounds in air and blood from the general population. J Expo Sci Environ Epidemiol. 2008 Jul;18(4):421-429.

National Toxicology Program (NTP). Toxicology and carcinogenesis studies of 1,4-dichlorobenzene in F344/N rats and B6C3F1 mice (gavage studies), NTP TR 319, NIH Publication No. 87-2575 . Research Triangle Park NC. 1987. Available from: http://ntp niehs.nih.gov:8080/cs.html?charset=iso-8859-1&url=http%3A//ntp.niehs.nih.gov/ntp/htdocs/LT_rpts/tr319.pdf&qt=1%2C4-dichlorobenzene&col=020rpt&n=2&la=en. 4/13/09

Schaum J, Schuda L, Wu C, Sears R, Ferrario J, Andrews K. A national survey of persistent, bioaccumulative, and toxic (PBT) pollutants in the United States milk supply. J Exp Anal Environ Epidemiol 2003;13:177-186.

Sexton K, Adgate JL, Church TR, Ashley DL, Needham LL, Ramachandran, et al. Children's exposure to volatile organic compounds as determined by longitudinal measurements in blood. Environ Health Perspect 2005;113(3):342-349.

Sexton K, Adgate JL, Fredrickson AL, Ryan AD, Needham LL, Ashley DL. Using biologic markers in blood to assess exposure to multiple environmental chemicals for inner-city children 3-6 years of age. Environ Health Perspect 2006;114(3):453-459.

Stine ER, Gunawardhana L, Sipes IG. The acute hepatotoxicity of the isomers of dichlorobenzene in Fischer-344 and Sprague-Dawley rats: isomer-specific and strain-specific differential toxicity. Toxicol Appl Pharmacol 1991;42:197-208.

United States Geological Survey (USGS). Volatile organic compounds in the nation's ground water and drinking-water supply wells. Reston VA [updated 2006 August 28] Available from: http://pubs.usgs.gov/circ/circ1292/. 4/13/09

Wallace L, Pellizzari E, Hartwell T, et al. The TEAM study: personal exposures to toxic substances in air, drinking water, and breath of 400 residents of New Jersey, North Carolina, and North Dakota. Environ Res 1987;43:290–307.

Wallace L, Nelson W, Ziegenfus R, et al. The Los Angeles team study: personal exposures, indoor-outdoor air concentrations, and breath concentrations of 25 volatile organic compounds. J Exposure Anal Environ Epidemiol 1991;1:157–192.

# 1,2-Dibromo-3-Chloropropane (DBCP)

CAS No. 96-12-8

## General Information

1,2-Dibromo-3-chloropropane (DBCP) is a liquid soil fumigant used until 1985 when the U.S. Environmental Protection Agency (U.S. EPA) banned applications (ATSDR, 1992). DBCP volatilizes from soil into the air after application. Recent surveys of U.S. public drinking water supplies have not detected DBCP (USGS, 2006).

Exposure to the general population is rare. In the past, inhalational and dermal exposure occurred primarily in formulators and applicators. DBCP can be absorbed by ingestion, inhalation, and dermal routes. After absorption, DBCP is shown in animal studies to distribute widely into most tissues. Metabolites are excreted in urine, feces, and, to a limited extent, exhaled air (ATSDR, 1992; MacFarland et al., 1984).

In animal studies, large acute doses of DBCP produce lethargy, ataxia, and convulsions. High chronic doses in laboratory animals demonstrate kidney toxicity, testicular injury and reduced sperm production, and altered estrus cycles and infertility (ATSDR, 1992; Lag et al., 1989; Rao et al., 1982). Male workers exposed during DBCP production have demonstrated oligospermia or azoospermia; sperm count recovery occurred generally with less than 3 years of workplace exposure (Potashnik, 1983; Potashnik and Yani-Inbar, 1987; Whorton et al., 1979; Lipschultz et al., 1980). In general populations, epidemiologic investigations found no association between exposure to previously contaminated drinking water and birth rates, birth outcomes, gastric cancer, or leukemia (Whorton et al., 1989; Wong et al., 1988).

An increased risk for certain cancers was found in several studies of workers exposed to DBCP (Olsen et al., 1995; Wesseling et al., 1996); however, these studies may have been confounded by other unmeasured exposures. Rodents that were administered DBCP developed tumors in the nasal cavity, lungs, and forestomach (NCI, 1978; NTP, 1982). The International Agency for Research on Cancer classified DBCP as a possible human carcinogen; the National Toxicology Program determined that DBCP was reasonably anticipated to be a human carcinogen. U.S. EPA established drinking water and other environmental standards and the Occupational Safety and Health Administration established workplace standards for DBCP. Information about external exposure (i.e., environmental levels) and health effects is available from ATSDR at: http://www.atsdr.cdc.gov/toxpro2.html.

## Biomonitoring Information

Levels of DBCP in blood reflect recent exposure. In the general population, DBCP was not detected in the NHANES 2003-2004 subsample, similar to other studies (Ashley et al. 1994; Churchill et al., 2001). Finding a measurable amount of DBCP in the blood does not mean that the level of DBCP causes an adverse health effect. Biomonitoring studies of DBCP in the blood can provide physicians and

## Blood 1,2-Dibromo-3-chloropropane (DBCP)

Geometric mean and selected percentiles of blood concentrations (in ng/mL) for the U.S. population from the National Health and Nutrition Examination Survey.

| | Survey years# | Geometric mean (95% conf. interval) | Selected percentiles ( 95% confidence interval) | | | | Sample size |
|---|---|---|---|---|---|---|---|
| | | | 50th | 75th | 90th | 95th | |
| Total | 03-04 | * | < LOD | < LOD | < LOD | < LOD | 1170 |
| **Age group** | | | | | | | |
| 20-59 years | 03-04 | * | < LOD | < LOD | < LOD | < LOD | 1170 |
| **Gender** | | | | | | | |
| Males | 03-04 | * | < LOD | < LOD | < LOD | < LOD | 568 |
| Females | 03-04 | * | < LOD | < LOD | < LOD | < LOD | 602 |
| **Race/ethnicity** | | | | | | | |
| Mexican Americans | 03-04 | * | < LOD | < LOD | < LOD | < LOD | 234 |
| Non-Hispanic blacks | 03-04 | * | < LOD | < LOD | < LOD | < LOD | 239 |
| Non-Hispanic whites | 03-04 | * | < LOD | < LOD | < LOD | < LOD | 603 |

Limit of detection (LOD, see Data Analysis section) for Survey year 03-04 is 0.1.
# Survey period 2003-2004 is a one-half subsample of 20-59 year olds.
< LOD means less than the limit of detection, which may vary for some chemicals by year and by individual sample.
* Not calculated: proportion of results below limit of detection was too high to provide a valid result.

public health officials with reference values so that they can determine whether people have been exposed to higher levels of DBCP than are found in the general population. Biomonitoring data can also help scientists plan and conduct research on exposure and health effects.

## References

Agency for Toxic Substances and Disease Registry (ATSDR). Toxicological profile for 1,2-dibromo-3-chloropropane. 1992 [online]. Available at URL: http://www.atsdr.cdc.gov/toxprofiles/tp36.html. 7/3/08

Ashley DL, Bonin MA, Cardinali FL, McCraw JM, Wooten JV. Blood concentrations of volatile organic compounds in a nonoccupationally exposed US population and in groups with suspected exposure. Clin Chem 1994;40(7 Pt 2):1401-1404.

Churchill JE, Ashley DL, Kaye WE. Recent chemical exposures and blood volatile organic compound levels in a large population-based sample. Arch Environ Health 2001;56(2):157-166.

Lag M, Omichinski JG, Soderlund EJ, Brunborg G, Holme JA, Dahl JE, et al. Role of P-450 activity and glutathione levels in 1,2-dibromo-3-chloropropane tissue distribution, renal necrosis and in vivo DNA damage. Toxicology 1989;56:273-288.

Lipshultz LI, Ross CE, Ehorton D, Milby T, Samith R, Joyner RE. Dibromochloropropane and its effect on testicular function in man. J Urol 1980;124:464-468.

MacFarland RT, Gandolfi AT, Sipes IC. Extra-hepatic GSH-dependent metabolism of 1,2-dibromoethane (DBE) and 1,2-dibromo-3-chloropropane (DBCP) in the rat and mouse. Drug Chem Toxicol 1984;7:213-227.

National Cancer Institute (NCI). Bioassay of dibromochloropropane for possible carcinogenicity (CAS no. 96-12-8). Technical Report Series No. 28. 1978 [online]. Available at URL: http://ntp.niehs.nih.gov/ntp/htdocs/LT_rpts/tr028.pdf. 7/3/08

National Toxicology Program (NTP). Carcinogenesis bioassay of 1,2-dibromo-3-chloro-propane (CAS no. 96-12-8) inF344/N rats and B6C31F mice (inhalation studies). Technical Report Series No. 206. 1982 [online]. Available at URL: http://ntp.niehs.nih.gov/ntp/htdocs/LT_rpts/tr206.pdf. 7/3/08

Olsen GW, Bodner KM, Stafford BA, Cartmill JB, Gondek MR. Update of the mortality experience of employees with occupational exposure to 1,2-dibromo-3-chloropropane (DBCP). Am J Ind Med 1995;28(3):399-410.

Potashnik G. A four-year reassessment of workers with dibromochloropropane-induced testicular dysfunction. Andrologia 1983;15(2):164-170.

Potashnik G, Yanai-Inbar I. Dibromochloropropane (DBCP): an 8-year reevaluation of testicular function and reproductive performance. Fertil Steril 1987;47(2):317-323.

Rao, K.S., J.D. Burek, F. Murray, John JA, Schwetz BA, Beyer JE, Parker CM. Toxicologic and reproductive effects of inhaled 1,2-dibromo-3-chloropropane in male rabbits. Fund Appl Toxicol 1982;2(5): 241-251.

United States Geological Survey (USGS). Volatile Organic Compounds in the Nation's Ground Water and Drinking-Water Supply Wells. 2006 [online]. Available at URL: http://pubs.usgs.gov/circ/circ1292/. 7/3/08

Wesseling C, Ahlbom A, Antich D, Rodriguez AC, Castro R. Cancer in banana plantation workers in Costa Rica. Int J Epidemiol 1996;25(6):1125-1131.

Whorton D, Milby TH, Krauss RM, Stubbs HA. Testicular function in DBCP exposed pesticide workers. J Occup Med 1979;21(3):161-166.

Whorton DM, Wong O, Morgan RW, Gordon N. An epidemiologic investigation of birth outcomes in relation to dibromochloropropane contamination in drinking water in Fresno County, California, USA. Int Arch Occup Environ Health 1989;61:403-407.

Wong O, Whorton MD, Gordon N, Morgan RW. An epidemiologic investigation of the relationship between DBCP contamination in drinking water and birth rates in Fresno County, California. Am J Public Health 1988;78:43-46.

# 2,5-Dimethylfuran

CAS No. 625-86-5

## General Information

2,5-Dimethylfuran is a volatile chemical found in tobacco smoke (Baggett et al., 1974) and in roasted coffee aroma (Wang et al., 1983). Exposure among the general population may occur through inhaling cigarette smoke and coffee aroma. 2,5-Dimethylfuran in blood and exhaled air has been used to determine smoking status (Ashley et al., 1996; Gordon et al., 2002; Perbellini et al., 2003). In addition, levels of 2,5-dimethylfuran found in blood provide a rough estimate of the number of cigarettes smoked per day (Ashley et al., 1995, 1996). After a person smokes cigarettes, 2,5-dimethylfuran is absorbed from the respiratory tract and then rapidly eliminated from the blood (Egle and Gochberg, 1979; Gordon et al., 2002). 2,5-Dimethylfuran is also a human urinary metabolite of n-hexane. Workers exposed to n-hexane will eliminate 2,5-dimethylfuran, along with other metabolites, in their urine (ATSDR, 2007; Iwata et al., 1983; Mutti et al., 1984; Perbellini et al., 1981).

Human health effects from 2,5-dimethylfuran at low environmental doses or at biomonitored levels from low environmental exposures are unknown. Neither IARC or NTP has evaluated 2,5-dimethylfuran's human carcinogenicity. 2,5-Dimethylfuran is not mutagenic by *in vitro* testing (Zeiger et al., 1992).

## Biomonitoring Information

Levels of 2,5-dimethylfuran in blood reflect recent exposure and are generally undetectable among nonsmoking adults and in the general population. Ashley et al. (1995) and Perbellini et al. (2003) reported median blood 2,5-dimethylfuran levels of 0.13 µg/L in smokers which were similar values to the 95th percentile in participants of NHANES 2003-2004 reflecting the U.S. population mix of nonsmokers and smokers. Levels of 2,5-dimethylfuran in blood increase generally with the number of cigarettes smoked per day (Ashley et al., 1995, 1996).

Finding a measurable amount of 2,5-dimethylfuran in blood does not mean that the level of 2,5-dimethylfuran causes an adverse health effect. Biomonitoring studies of 2,5-dimethylfuran in blood can provide physicians and public health officials with reference values so that they can determine whether people have been exposed to higher levels of 2,5-dimethylfuran than are found in the general population. Biomonitoring data can also help scientists plan and conduct research on exposure and health effects.

## Blood 2,5-Dimethylfuran

Geometric mean and selected percentiles of blood concentrations (in ng/mL) for the U.S. population from the National Health and Nutrition Examination Survey.

| | Survey years# | Geometric mean (95% conf. interval) | Selected percentiles ( 95% confidence interval) | | | | Sample size |
|---|---|---|---|---|---|---|---|
| | | | 50th | 75th | 90th | 95th | |
| Total | 03-04 | * | < LOD | .015 (<LOD-.031) | .100 (.083-.110) | .140 (.120-.180) | 1221 |
| Age group | | | | | | | |
| 20-59 years | 03-04 | * | < LOD | .015 (<LOD-.031) | .100 (.083-.110) | .140 (.120-.180) | 1221 |
| Gender | | | | | | | |
| Males | 03-04 | * | < LOD | .019 (<LOD-.031) | .094 (.071-.110) | .130 (.110-.190) | 602 |
| Females | 03-04 | * | < LOD | < LOD | .110 (.074-.120) | .150 (.120-.210) | 619 |
| Race/ethnicity | | | | | | | |
| Mexican Americans | 03-04 | * | < LOD | < LOD | .012 (<LOD-.020) | .038 (.013-.054) | 237 |
| Non-Hispanic blacks | 03-04 | * | < LOD | .041 (.018-.063) | .110 (.079-.160) | .170 (.099-.220) | 261 |
| Non-Hispanic whites | 03-04 | * | < LOD | .020 (<LOD-.041) | .110 (.087-.120) | .150 (.120-.210) | 628 |

Limit of detection (LOD, see Data Analysis section) for Survey year 03-04 is 0.012.
# Survey period 2003-2004 is a one-half subsample of 20-59 year olds.
< LOD means less than the limit of detection, which may vary for some chemicals by year and by individual sample.
* Not calculated: proportion of results below limit of detection was too high to provide a valid result.

## References

Agency for Toxic Substances and Disease Registry (ATSDR). Toxicological profile for *n*-hexane. 1999 [online]. Available at URL: http://www.atsdr.cdc.gov/toxprofiles/tp113.html. 4/14/09

Agency for Toxic Substances and Disease Registry (ATSDR). Toxicological profile for *n*-hexane. Atlanta GA 2007 [online]. Available at URL: http://www.atsdr.cdc.gov/toxprofiles/tp113.html. 4/14/09

Ashley DL, Bonin MA, Hamar B, McGeehin MA. Removing the smoking confounder from blood volatile organic compounds measurements. Environ Res 1995;71(1):39-45.

Ashley DL, Bonin MA, Hamar B, McGeehin M. Using the blood concentration of 2,5-dimethylfuran as a marker for smoking. Int Arch Occup Environ Health 1996;68(3):183-187.

Baggett MS, Morie GP, Simmons MW, Lewis JS. Quantitative determination of semivolatile compounds in cigarette smoke. J Chromatogr 1974;97(1):79-82.

Egle JL Jr, Gochberg BJ. Retention of inhaled 2-methylfuran and 2,5-dimethylfuran. Am Ind Hyg Assoc J 1979;40(10):866-869.

Gordon SM, Wallace LA, Brinkman MC, Callahan PJ, Kenny DV. Volatile organic compounds as breath biomarkers for active and passive smoking. Environ Health Perspect 2002;110(7):689-698.

Iwata M, Takeuchi Y, Hisanaga N, Ono Y. A study on biological monitoring of n-hexane exposure. Int Arch Occup Environ Health 1983;51(3):253-260.

Mutti A, Falzoi M, Lucertini S, Arfini G, Zignani M, Lombardi S, Franchini I. *n*-Hexane metabolism in occupationally exposed workers. Br J Ind Med 1984;41(4):533-538.

Perbellini L, Brugnone F, Faggionato G. Urinary excretion of the metabolites of n-hexane and its isomers during occupational exposure. Br J Ind Med 1981;38:20-26.

Perbellini L, Princivalle A, Cerpelloni M, Pasini F, Brugnone f. Comparison of breath, blood and urine concentrations in the biomonitoring of environmental exposure to 1,3-butadiene, 2,5-dimethylfuran, and benzene. Int Arch Occup Environ Health 2003;76:461-466.

Wang TH, Shanfield, Zlatkis A. Analysis of trace volatile organic compounds in coffee by headspace concentration and gas chromatography-mass spectrometry. Chromatographia 1983;17:411-417.

Zeiger E, Anderson B, Haworth S, Lawlor T, Mortelmans K. Salmonella mutagenicity tests: V. Results from the testing of 311 chemicals. Environ Mol Mutagen 1992;19 supp. 21:2-141.

# Ethylbenzene
CAS No. 100-41-4

## General Information

Ethylbenzene is a flammable hydrocarbon found in crude oil. It is a high production chemical used largely to synthesize styrene and also as a solvent and an additive to automobile and aviation fuels. Automobile emission contributes a significant amount of ethylbenzene to outdoor air. Indoor sources of ethylbenzene include carpet adhesives and tobacco smoke. Ethylbenzene is ubiquitous in ambient air, with higher concentrations in areas with greater vehicular traffic. It undergoes biodegradation or photooxidation in air, water, and soil, and it does not bioaccumulate in aquatic food chains (ATSDR, 2007). Producing and using petroleum products are potential sources of workplace exposure to ethylbenzene.

The general population may be exposed to ethylbenzene through inhalation, particularly from motor vehicle emissions, self-service gasoline pump vapors, and cigarette smoke. Drinking water is contaminated rarely by leaking underground storage tanks containing petroleum products. Ethylbenzene is well absorbed by inhalation, oral, or dermal exposure routes. After absorption, ethylbenzene is metabolized rapidly by the liver. Mandelic and phenylglyoxylic acids are the predominant urinary metabolites and have been used to monitor workplace exposure (Knecht et al., 2000).

Human health effects from ethylbenzene at low environmental doses or at biomonitored levels from low environmental exposures are unknown. Ethylbenzene can cause respiratory tract and eye irritation and dizziness at air concentrations that exceed workplace standards (Cometto-Muniz and Cain, 1995). Much higher levels occurring with accidental exposures can produce central nervous system depression. Laboratory animals exposed to ethylbenzene for several weeks to months at air concentrations several times higher than occupational standards have shown respiratory irritation, increased liver weight, liver microsomal enzyme induction, and increased leukocyte counts (ATSDR, 2007). Chronic animal exposure studies have also demonstrated renal tubular, alveolar, and hepatic tumors with some evidence of gender-specific susceptibility (NTP, 1999).

The IARC classified ethylbenzene as a possible human carcinogen. OSHA and ACGIH established workplace standards and guidelines, respectively, for ethylbenzene.

## Blood Ethylbenzene

Geometric mean and selected percentiles of blood concentrations (in ng/mL) for the U.S. population from the National Health and Nutrition Examination Survey.

| | Survey years# | Geometric mean (95% conf. interval) | Selected percentiles ( 95% confidence interval) 50th | 75th | 90th | 95th | Sample size |
|---|---|---|---|---|---|---|---|
| **Total** | 01-02 | .034 (.029-.039) | .030 (.030-.040) | .050 (.050-.070) | .090 (.070-.120) | .140 (.090-.180) | 879 |
| | 03-04 | .035 (.033-.037) | .032 (.030-.036) | .053 (.048-.057) | .083 (.077-.088) | .110 (.098-.120) | 1299 |
| **Age group** | | | | | | | |
| 20-59 years | 01-02 | .034 (.029-.039) | .030 (.030-.040) | .050 (.050-.070) | .090 (.070-.120) | .140 (.090-.180) | 879 |
| | 03-04 | .035 (.033-.037) | .032 (.030-.036) | .053 (.048-.057) | .083 (.077-.088) | .110 (.098-.120) | 1299 |
| **Gender** | | | | | | | |
| Males | 01-02 | .035 (.029-.041) | .030 (<LOD-.040) | .060 (.040-.070) | .100 (.070-.150) | .150 (.090-.220) | 419 |
| | 03-04 | .037 (.034-.041) | .036 (.031-.040) | .057 (.051-.065) | .086 (.078-.099) | .110 (.094-.130) | 625 |
| Females | 01-02 | .033 (.028-.038) | .030 (.030-.040) | .050 (.040-.060) | .080 (.060-.120) | .130 (.070-.180) | 460 |
| | 03-04 | .032 (.030-.034) | .030 (.027-.033) | .048 (.041-.053) | .081 (.071-.089) | .100 (.091-.120) | 674 |
| **Race/ethnicity** | | | | | | | |
| Mexican Americans | 01-02 | * | .030 (<LOD-.040) | .040 (.040-.060) | .070 (.050-.110) | .120 (.070-.210) | 220 |
| | 03-04 | .031 (.027-.036) | .029 (<LOD-.035) | .044 (.035-.048) | .064 (.051-.074) | .091 (.066-.170) | 253 |
| Non-Hispanic blacks | 01-02 | .032 (.027-.038) | .030 (<LOD-.040) | .050 (.030-.070) | .080 (.060-.130) | .130 (.070-.240) | 159 |
| | 03-04 | .032 (.027-.038) | .030 (<LOD-.037) | .050 (.037-.066) | .079 (.065-.100) | .110 (.084-.130) | 281 |
| Non-Hispanic whites | 01-02 | .035 (.029-.043) | .030 (<LOD-.040) | .060 (.050-.070) | .090 (.070-.140) | .150 (.090-.190) | 432 |
| | 03-04 | .036 (.034-.038) | .034 (.030-.038) | .055 (.050-.061) | .087 (.081-.092) | .110 (.098-.130) | 669 |

Limits of detection (LOD, see Data Analysis section) for Survey years 01-02 and 03-04 are 0.024 and 0 024.
# Survey period 2001-2002 is a one-third subsample of 20-59 year olds; Survey period 2003-2004 is a one-half subsample of 20-59 year olds.
< LOD means less than the limit of detection, which may vary for some chemicals by year and by individual sample.

The U.S. EPA established environmental and drinking water standards for ethylbenzene. Information about external exposure (i.e., environmental levels) and health effects is available from ATSDR at: http://www.atsdr.cdc.gov/toxpro2.html.

## Biomonitoring Information

Levels of ethylbenzene in blood reflect recent exposure. In a nonrepresentative subsample of adults in the National Health and Nutrition Examination Survey (NHANES) III (1988-1994), the median ethylbenzene level in blood was 0.060 µg/L (Ashley et al., 1994), which is similar to the geometric mean value reported for nonsmokers in the NHANES 1999-2000 subsample (Lin et al., 2008). The geometric mean level in participants 20 years and older in the NHANES 2001-2002 and 2003-2004 subsamples appear similar or slightly below these previously reported values, though differences in methodology and sampled populations may account for slight differences in levels. Also, approximately similar levels were observed in sample of southwestern U.S. residents (Buckley et al., 1997), but such levels were about two to three times higher than levels reported among low-income children in a Midwestern U.S. city (Sexton et al., 2005, 2006).

Smoking cigarettes increases blood ethylbenzene levels, but environmental tobacco smoke exposure appears not to increase blood ethylbenzene (Lin et al., 2008; Perbellini et al., 2002). Residents in high density urban areas and commuters may have ethylbenzene levels up to two times higher than the nonsmoking general population (Lemire et al., 2004). Street vendors and workers exposed to gasoline fumes can have blood ethylbenzene levels up to ten times higher than levels found in the general population (Mannino et al., 1995; Romieu et al., 1999). Workers in the petroleum industry and those with solvent exposure can have blood ethylbenzene levels that are several hundred times higher than those in the general population (Angerer and Wulf, 1985; Kawai et al., 1992).

Finding a measurable amount of ethylbenzene in the blood does not mean that the level of ethylbenzene causes an adverse health effect. Biomonitoring studies of ethylbenzene in blood can provide physicians and public health officials with reference values so that they can determine whether people have been exposed to higher levels of ethylbenzene than are found in the general population. Biomonitoring data can also help scientists plan and conduct research on exposure and health effects.

## References

Agency for Toxic Substances and Disease Registry (ATSDR). Toxicological profile for ethylbenzene, draft. September 2007 [online]. Available at URL: http://www.atsdr.cdc.gov/toxprofiles/tp110 html#bookmark08. 4/15/09

Angerer J, Wulf H. Occupational chronic exposure to organic solvents.XI. Alkylbenzene exposure of varnish workers: Effects on hematopoietic system. Int Arch Occup Environ Health 1985;56:307-321.

Ashley DL, Bonin MA, Cardinali FL, McCraw JM, Wooten JV. Blood concentrations of volatile organic compounds in a nonoccupationally exposed US population and in groups with suspected exposure. Clin Chem 1994;40(7 Pt 2):1401-1404.

Buckley TJ, Liddle J, Ashley DL, Paschal DC, Burse VW, Needham LL. Environmental and biomarker measurements in nine homes in the lower Rio Grande Valley: multimedia results for pesticides, metals, PAHs and VOCs. Environ Int 1997;23(5):705-732.

Cometto-Muniz JE, Cain WS. Relative sensitivity of the ocular trigeminal, nasal trigeminal and olfactory systems to airborne chemicals. Chemical Senses 1995;20(2):191-198.

Kawai T, Yasugi T, Mizunuma K, Horiguchi SI, Iguchi H, Uchida Y, et al. Comparative evaluation of urinalysis and blood analysis as means of detecting exposure to organic solvents at low concentrations. Int Arch Occup Environ Health 1992;64(4):223-234.

Knecht U, Reske A, Woitowitz HJ. Biological monitoring of standardized exposure to ethylbenzene: evaluation of a biological tolerance (BAT) value. Arch Toxicol 2000;73(12):632-640.

Lemire S, Ashley D, Olaya P, Romieu I, Welch S, Meneses-Gonzalez F, Hernandez-Avila M. Environmental exposure of commuters in Mexico City to volatile organic compounds as assessed by blood concentrations, 1998. Salud Publica Mex 004;46:32-38.

Lin YS, Egeghy PP, Rappaport SM.Relationships between levels of volatile organic compounds in air and blood from the general population. J Expo Sci Environ Epidemiol 2008 Jul;18(4):421-9. Epub 2007 Dec 5.

Mannino DM, Schreiber J, Aldous K, Ashley D, Moolenaar R, Almaguer D. Human exposure to volatile organic compounds: a comparison of organic vapor monitoring badge levels with blood levels. Int Arch Occp Environ Health 1995;67:59-64.

National Toxicology Program (NTP). Toxicology and Carcinogenesis Studies of Ethylbenzene (CAS No. 100-41-4) in F344/N Rats and B6C3F1 Mice (Inhalation Studies). 1999 [online]. Available at URL: http://ntp.niehs.nih.gov/ntp/htdocs/LT_rpts/tr466.pdf. 4/15/09

Perbellini L, Pasini F, Romani S, Princivalle A, Brugnone F. Analysis of benzene, toluene, ethylbenzene and *m*-xylene in biological samples from the general population. J Chromat B 2002;778:198-210.

Romieu I, Ramirez M, Meneses F, Ashley DL, Lemire S, Colome S, et al. Environmental exposure to volatile organic compounds among workers in Mexico City as assessed by personal monitors and blood concentrations. Environ Health Perspect 1999;107(7):511-515.

Sexton K, Adgate JL, Church TR, Ashley DL, Needham LL, Ramachandran, et al. Children's exposure to volatile organic compounds as determined by longitudinal measurements in blood. Environ Health Perspect 2005;113(3):342-349.

Sexton K, Adgate JL, Fredrickson AL, Ryan AD, Needham LL, Ashley DL. Using biologic markers in blood to assess exposure to multiple environmental chemicals for inner-city children 3-6 years of age. Environ Health Perspect 2006;114(3):453-459.

# Halogenated Solvents

**Dichloromethane (Methylene chloride)**
CAS No. 75-09-2

**Trichloroethene (Trichloroethylene)** CAS No. 79-01-6

**Tetrachloroethene (Tetrachloroethylene, Perchloro-ethylene)** CAS No. 127-18-4

## General Information

Dichloromethane, trichloroethene, and tetrachloroethene are volatile halogenated short-chain hydrocarbons. Dichloromethane is used principally as a solvent in paint removers and thinners, as well as in other household products (cleaners, glues, and adhesives), and also as a degreasing agent. Trichloroethene is used primarily as an industrial degreaser, solvent, and in the synthesis of other chemicals. In the past, it was used in dry cleaning, food processing, household cleaners, and as a general anesthetic. Tetrachloroethene is used in dry cleaning, metal cleaning, the synthesis of other chemicals, and household products such as water repellants, silicone lubricants, and spot removers. All three of these halogenated solvents are produced and used in high volumes in the U.S., and have been detected in urban and ambient air and occasionally, soils, and drinking water most likely contaminated by industrial discharge (Moran et al., 2007; Rowe et al., 2007). Because of their volatility, these solvents do not persist in the soil or water following the discontinuation of contamination.

Inhalation is the most common exposure route for the general population including indoor sources from paints, adhesives, and cleaning solutions. Volatilization from contaminated water (eg., shower water) as well as the use of household products containing these solvents can result in higher indoor than outdoor air concentrations (ATSDR, 1997b; Martin et al., 2005). Nearby dry cleaning establishments, industries producing these solvents, and contaminated waste disposal sites can also contribute to human exposure (Armstrong and Green, 2004; ATSDR, 1997a, 1997b, and 2000; Schreiber et al., 1993; Wallace et al., 1991). Drinking water may contribute to exposure when underground drinking water supplies have been contaminated. Workers in industries such as dry cleaning, aircraft maintenance, electronics manufacturing, and chemical production may be exposed by inhalation or by dermal contact with the liquid solvents. The U.S. EPA has established drinking water standards and other environmental standards for all three solvents, and the FDA regulates tetrachloroethene and trichloroethene as indirect food additives. For all three solvents, workplace standards have been established by OSHA, and ACGIH has recommended occupational guidelines and biological exposure indices for monitoring workers.

All three solvents are well absorbed by ingestion and inhalation, and animal studies have demonstrated that liquid forms can be dermally absorbed. Following absorption, part of the solvent dose is excreted into expired air; for tetrachloroethene, about 97-99% of the dose is eliminated unmetabolized into expired air, though it has an elimination half-life of several days (ATSDR1997a; Monster et

## Blood Dichloromethane (Methylene chloride)

Geometric mean and selected percentiles of blood concentrations (in ng/mL) for the U.S. population from the National Health and Nutrition Examination Survey.

| | Survey years# | Geometric mean (95% conf. interval) | Selected percentiles ( 95% confidence interval) | | | | Sample size |
|---|---|---|---|---|---|---|---|
| | | | 50th | 75th | 90th | 95th | |
| Total | 03-04 | * | < LOD | < LOD | < LOD | < LOD | 1165 |
| Age group | | | | | | | |
| 20-59 years | 03-04 | * | < LOD | < LOD | < LOD | < LOD | 1165 |
| Gender | | | | | | | |
| Males | 03-04 | * | < LOD | < LOD | < LOD | < LOD | 568 |
| Females | 03-04 | * | < LOD | < LOD | < LOD | < LOD | 597 |
| Race/ethnicity | | | | | | | |
| Mexican Americans | 03-04 | * | < LOD | < LOD | < LOD | < LOD | 225 |
| Non-Hispanic blacks | 03-04 | * | < LOD | < LOD | < LOD | < LOD | 245 |
| Non-Hispanic whites | 03-04 | * | < LOD | < LOD | < LOD | < LOD | 607 |

Limit of detection (LOD, see Data Analysis section) for Survey year 03-04 is 0.07.
# Survey period 2003-2004 is a one-half subsample of 20-59 year olds.
< LOD means less than the limit of detection, which may vary for some chemicals by year and by individual sample.
* Not calculated: proportion of results below limit of detection was too high to provide a valid result.

al., 1986). The retained solvent can undergo hepatic metabolism. Trichloroethene and tetrachloroethene are metabolized to trichloroacetic acid and tricholoroethanol, which are eliminated in the urine. Dichloromethane is partially metabolized to carbon monoxide and carbon dioxide. Elevated carboxyhemoglobin levels in blood have been reported following intentional dichloromethane overdose or exposure to air concentrations greatly exceeding occupational standards (ATSDR, 2000; Hughes and Tracy, 1993).

Human health effects from dichloromethane, tetrachloroethene, and trichloroethene at low environmental doses or at biomonitored levels from low environmental exposures are unknown. Accidental or intentional high dose acute exposure by ingestion or inhalation of any of these solvents can result in loss of motor coordination, somnolence, and unconsciousness. Inhaling high doses of trichloroethene and tetrachloroethene may also produce cardiac arrhythmias attributed to enhanced sensitivity to catecholamines. High dose acute exposure to tetrachloroethene has resulted in reversible kidney impairment, and prolonged, low level exposure to either tetrachloroethene or trichloroethene has been associated with altered renal enzyme excretion and liver enlargement

(ATSDR, 1997a, b). Chronic occupational exposure to any of these three solvents may be associated with mild degrees of neurological impairments, including reaction times, verbal skills, cognitive ability and motor function (Armstrong and Green, 2004).

Various epidemiologic studies of chronic tetrachloroethene exposure in dry cleaning workers found increased incidences of esophageal and cervical cancers and non-Hodgkins lymphoma, but confounding exposures (e.g., other solvents and trichloroethene) were likely (IPCS, 2006). In animals studies, tetrachloroethene and trichloroethene each induced kidney and liver tumors; tetrachloroethene also caused leukemia, and trichloroethene caused lung and testicular tumors (IARC, 1995). Animal studies of inhaled dichloromethane have reported increased incidences of lung and hepatocellular cancers, and in female animals, mammary gland tumors (NTP, 2004). Trichloroethene and tetrachloroethene are classified as probable human carcinogens by IARC, and dichloromethane is classified as a possible human carcinogen by IARC. All three are classified as reasonably anticipated to be human carcinogens by NTP. Additional information about these solvents is available from ATSDR at: http://www.atsdr.cdc.gov/toxpro2.html.

## Blood Trichloroethene (Trichloroethylene)

Geometric mean and selected percentiles of blood concentrations (in ng/mL) for the U.S. population from the National Health and Nutrition Examination Survey.

| | Survey years# | Geometric mean (95% conf. interval) | Selected percentiles ( 95% confidence interval) | | | | Sample size |
|---|---|---|---|---|---|---|---|
| | | | 50th | 75th | 90th | 95th | |
| **Total** | 01-02 | * | < LOD | < LOD | < LOD | < LOD | 922 |
| | 03-04 | * | < LOD | < LOD | < LOD | < LOD | 1228 |
| **Age group** | | | | | | | |
| 20-59 years | 01-02 | * | < LOD | < LOD | < LOD | < LOD | 922 |
| | 03-04 | * | < LOD | < LOD | < LOD | < LOD | 1228 |
| **Gender** | | | | | | | |
| Males | 01-02 | * | < LOD | < LOD | < LOD | < LOD | 434 |
| | 03-04 | * | < LOD | < LOD | < LOD | < LOD | 604 |
| Females | 01-02 | * | < LOD | < LOD | < LOD | < LOD | 488 |
| | 03-04 | * | < LOD | < LOD | < LOD | < LOD | 624 |
| **Race/ethnicity** | | | | | | | |
| Mexican Americans | 01-02 | * | < LOD | < LOD | < LOD | < LOD | 228 |
| | 03-04 | * | < LOD | < LOD | < LOD | < LOD | 224 |
| Non-Hispanic blacks | 01-02 | * | < LOD | < LOD | < LOD | < LOD | 191 |
| | 03-04 | * | < LOD | < LOD | < LOD | < LOD | 266 |
| Non-Hispanic whites | 01-02 | * | < LOD | < LOD | < LOD | < LOD | 441 |
| | 03-04 | * | < LOD | < LOD | < LOD | < LOD | 644 |

Limits of detection (LOD, see Data Analysis section) for Survey years 01-02 and 03-04 are 0.012 and 0.012.
# Survey period 2001-2002 is a one-third subsample of 20-59 year olds; Survey period 2003-2004 is a one-half subsample of 20-59 year olds.
< LOD means less than the limit of detection, which may vary for some chemicals by year and by individual sample.
* Not calculated: proportion of results below limit of detection was too high to provide a valid result.

## Biomonitoring Information

Levels of halogenated solvents in blood reflect recent exposure. In the NHANES 2003-2004 subsample, the level of blood tetrachloroethene for adults at the 75th percentile of the U.S. population appear similar to the levels at the 75th percentile reported for non-smoking adults in a subsample of NHANES 1999-2000 participants (Lin et al., 2008) and were similar or slightly less that levels reported in a nonrepresentative subsample of the earlier NHANES III (1988-1994) (Ashley et al., 1994; Churchill et al., 2001). A recent study of low income, urban children in the Midwest reported slightly lower median tetrachloroethene levels (Sexton et al., 2005; Sexton et al., 2006) than the NHANES III levels (Ashley et al., 1994; Churchill et al., 2001). Other population studies have reported similarly low tetrachloroethene levels (Begerow et al., 1996; Bonanno et al., 2001). Population studies in Italy and Germany have reported multifold higher tetrachloroethene and trichloroethene blood levels than the U.S. surveys (Brugnone et al., 1994; Hajimiragha et al., 1986). Blood levels of trichloroethene and dichloromethane were detected infrequently in previous U.S. surveys and were generally not detected in the NHANES 2003-2004 subsample.

Comparatively higher blood levels of tetrachloroethene and trichloroethene have been noted for urban and industrial residential settings than for rural settings (Barkley et al., 1980; Begerow et al., 1996; Brugnone et al., 1994). Residing near dry-cleaning facilities or storing recently dry-cleaned clothes at home can contribute to increased blood tetrachloroethene levels (Begerow et al., 1996; Popp et al., 1992). In contrast, tetrachloroethene blood levels in occupationally exposed workers have been reported to be many thousand times higher than the unexposed general population (Begerow et al., 1996; Furuki et al., 2000; Monster et al., 1983). The occupational biological exposure index associated with an 8-hour exposure of 25 ppm is 500 µg/L tetrachloroethene in blood (ACGIH, 2007). Non-occupational exposures are usually well below this level.

Finding a measurable amount of any of these solvents in blood does not mean that the level of the solvent causes an adverse health effect. Biomonitoring studies of blood halogenated solvents can provide physicians and public health officials with reference values so that they can determine whether or not people have been exposed to higher levels of halogenated solvents than levels found in the general population. Biomonitoring data can also help scientists plan and conduct research on exposure and health effects.

## Blood Tetrachloroethene (Perchloroethylene)

Geometric mean and selected percentiles of blood concentrations (in ng/mL) for the U.S. population from the National Health and Nutrition Examination Survey.

| | Survey years# | Geometric mean (95% conf. interval) | Selected percentiles ( 95% confidence interval) | | | | Sample size |
|---|---|---|---|---|---|---|---|
| | | | 50th | 75th | 90th | 95th | |
| **Total** | 01-02 | * | < LOD | .050 (<LOD-.060) | .100 (.070-.150) | .190 (.130-.260) | 978 |
| | 03-04 | * | < LOD | < LOD | .076 (.060-.097) | .140 (.091-.300) | 1317 |
| **Age group** | | | | | | | |
| 20-59 years | 01-02 | * | < LOD | .050 (<LOD-.060) | .100 (.070-.150) | .190 (.130-.260) | 978 |
| | 03-04 | * | < LOD | < LOD | .076 (.060-.097) | .140 (.091-.300) | 1317 |
| **Gender** | | | | | | | |
| Males | 01-02 | * | < LOD | .050 (<LOD-.060) | .110 (.070-.170) | .210 (.170-.340) | 457 |
| | 03-04 | * | < LOD | < LOD | .082 (.060-.140) | .230 (.097-.410) | 639 |
| Females | 01-02 | * | < LOD | .050 (<LOD-.060) | .100 (.070-.140) | .150 (.100-.220) | 521 |
| | 03-04 | * | < LOD | < LOD | .069 (.050-.091) | .120 (.085-.180) | 678 |
| **Race/ethnicity** | | | | | | | |
| Mexican Americans | 01-02 | * | < LOD | < LOD | .060 (<LOD-.070) | .070 (.060-.230) | 226 |
| | 03-04 | * | < LOD | < LOD | .049 (<LOD-.097) | .100 (.054-.180) | 248 |
| Non-Hispanic blacks | 01-02 | * | < LOD | < LOD | .070 (.050-.110) | .110 (.060-.190) | 195 |
| | 03-04 | * | < LOD | < LOD | .086 (.050-.220) | .220 (.082-.360) | 284 |
| Non-Hispanic whites | 01-02 | * | < LOD | .050 (<LOD-.070) | .110 (.090-.170) | .210 (.150-.260) | 487 |
| | 03-04 | * | < LOD | < LOD | .072 (.060-.091) | .140 (.085-.330) | 686 |

Limits of detection (LOD, see Data Analysis section) for Survey years 01-02 and 03-04 are 0.048 and 0.048.
# Survey period 2001-2002 is a one-third subsample of 20-59 year olds; Survey period 2003-2004 is a one-half subsample of 20-59 year olds.
< LOD means less than the limit of detection, which may vary for some chemicals by year and by individual sample.
* Not calculated: proportion of results below limit of detection was too high to provide a valid result.

## References

ACGIH. TLVs and BEIs Based on the documentation of the threshold limit values for chemical substances and physical agents and biological exposure indices. 2007. Signature Publications. Cincinnati OH. p.104.

Agency for Toxic Substances and Disease Registry (ATSDR). Toxicological profile for trichloroethylene update. 1997*b* [online]. Available at URL: http://www.atsdr.cdc.gov/toxprofiles/tp19.html. 4/22/09

Agency for Toxic Substances and Disease Registry (ATSDR). Toxicological profile for tetrachloroethylene update. 1997*a* [online]. Available at URL: http://www.atsdr.cdc.gov/toxprofiles/tp18.html. 4/22/09

Agency for Toxic Substances and Disease Registry (ATSDR). Toxicological profile for Methylene chloride update. 2000 [online]. Available at URL: http://www.atsdr.cdc.gov/toxprofiles/tp14.html. 4/22/09

Armstrong SR, Green LC. Chlorinated hydrocarbon solvents. Clin Occup Environ Med 2004;4(3):481-496.

Ashley DL, Bonin MA, Cardinali FL, McCraw JM, Wooten JV. Blood concentrations of volatile organic compounds in a nonoccupationally exposed US population and in groups with suspected exposure. Clin Chem 1994;40(7 Pt 2):1401-1404.

Barkley J, Bunch J, Bursey JT, Castillo N, Cooper SD, Davis JM, et al. Gas chromatography mass spectrometry computer analysis of volatilie halogenated hydrocarbons in man and his environment—a multimedia environmental study. Biomed Mass Spectrom 1980;7(4):139-147.

Begerow J, Jermann E, Keles T, Freier I, Ranft U, Dunemann L. Internal and external tetrachloroethene exposure of persons living in differently polluted areas of Northrhine-Westphalia (Germany). Zentralbl Hyg Umweltmed. 1996;198(5):394-406.

Bonanno LJ, Freeman NCG, Greenberg M, Lioy PJ. Multivariate analysis on levels of selected metals, particulate matter, VOC, and household characteristics and activities from the Midwestern states NHEXAS. Appl Occup Environ Hyg 2001;16(9):859-874.

Brugnone F, Perbellini L, Guiliari C, Cerpelloni M, Soave M. Blood and urine concentrations of chemical pollutants in the general population. Med Lav 1994;8(5):370-389.

Churchill JA, Ashley DL, Kaye WE. Recent chemical exposures and blood volatile organic compound levels in a large population-based sample. Arch Environ Health 2001;56(2):157-166.

Furuki K, Ukai H, Okamoto S, Takada S, Kawai T, Miyama Y, Mitsuyoshi K, et al. Monitoring of occupational exposure to tetrachloroethene by analysis for unmetabolized tetrachloroethene in blood and urine in comparison with urinalysis for trichloroacetic acid. Int Arch Occup Environ Health. 2000;73(4):221-227.

Hughes NJ, Tracey JA. A case of methylene chloride (nitromors) poisoning, effects on carboxyhaemoglobin levels. Hum Exp Toxicol 1993;12(2):159-60.

International Programme on Chemical Safety (IPCS). Concise International Chemical Assessment Document 68-Tetrachloroethene. 2006 [online]. Available at URL: http://www.inchem.org/documents/cicads/cicads/cicad68.htm. 4/22/09

Lin YS, Egeghy PP, Rappaport SM. Relationships between levels of volatile organic compounds in air and blood from the general population. J Exp Sci Environ Epidemiol 2008;18:421-429.

Martin SA, Simmons MB, Ortiz-Serrano M, Kendrick C, Gallo A, Campbell J, et al. Environmental exposure of a community to airborne trichloroethylene. Arch Environ Occup Health 2005;60(6):341-316.

Monster AC. Biological monitoring of chlorinated hydrocarbon solvents. J Occup Med 1986;28:583-588.

Monster AC, Regouin-Peeters W, Van Schijndel A, van der Tuin J. Biological monitoring of occupational exposure to tetrachloroethene. Scand J Work Environ Health 1983;9:273-281.

Moran MJ, Zogorski JS, Squillace PJ. Chlorinated solvents in groundwater of the United States. Environ Sci Technol 2007;41:74-81.

National Toxicology Program (NTP). Report on Carcinogens, 11th ed. 2004. [online]. Available at URL: http://ntp niehs.nih.gov/ntp/roc/eleventh/profiles/s066dich.pdf. 4/22/09

Popp W, Muller G, Baltes-Schmitz B, Wehner B, Vahrenholz C, Schmieding W, et al. concentrations of tetrachloroethene in blood and trichloroacetic acid in urine in workers and neighbours of dry-cleaning shops. Int Arch Occup Environ Health 1992;63:393-395.

Rowe BL, Toccalino PL, Moran MJ, Zogorski JS, Price CV. Occurrence and potential human-health relevance of volatile organic compounds in drinking water from domestic wells in the United States. Environ Health Perspect 2007;115(11):1539-1546.

Schreiber JS, House S, Prohonic E, Smead G, Hudson C, Styk M, et al. An investigation of indoor air contamination in residences above dry cleaners. Risk Anal 1993;13(3):335-344.

Sexton K, Adgate JL, Church TR, Ashley DL, Needham LL, Ramachandran, et al. Children's exposure to volatile organic compounds as determined by longitudinal measurements in blood. Environ Health Perspect 2005;113(3):342-349.

Sexton K, Adgate JL, Fredrickson AL, Ryan AD, Needham LL, Ashley DL. Using biologic markers in blood to assess exposure to multiple environmental chemicals for inner-city children 3-6 years of age. Environ Health Perspect 2006;114(3):453-459.

Wallace L, Nelson W, Ziegenfus R, Pellizzari E, Michael L, Whitmore R, et al. The Los Angeles TEAM Study: Personal exposures, indoor-outdoor air concentrations, and breath concentrations of 25 volatile organic compounds. J Exp Anal Environ Epidemiol 1991;1(2):157-192.

# Other Halogenated Solvents

**Dibromomethane** CAS No. 74-95-3

**1,1-Dichloroethane**
CAS No. 75-34-3

**1,2-Dichloroethane (Ethylene dichloride)**
CAS No. 107-06-2

**1,1-Dichloroethene (Vinylidene chloride)**
CAS No. 75-34-3

*cis*-**1,2-Dichloroethene** CAS No. 156-59-2

*trans*-**1,2-Dichloroethene** CAS No. 156-60-5

**1,2-Dichloropropane** CAS No. 78-87-5

**1,1,1-Trichloroethane (Methyl chloroform)**
CAS No. 71-55-6

**1,1,2-Trichloroethane** CAS No. 79-00-5

**1,1,2,2-Tetrachloroethane** CAS No. 79-34-5

**Tetrachloromethane (Carbon tetrachloride)**
CAS No. 56-23-5

## General Information

The halogenated solvents are volatile organic chemicals consisting of a hydrocarbon chain or one hydrocarbon substituted with one or more chlorine or bromine atoms. Most of these chemicals are used as degreasers and solvents in various products such as paints. In the past, 1,1,1-trichloroethane was used as a dry cleaning agent, insect fumigant, and solvent in consumer products; more recently, its U.S. production has been restricted because of its principal use in manufacturing hydrofluorocarbons (Armstrong, et al., 2004; ATSDR, 2006b). Production of 1,1,2,2-tetrachloroethane in the U.S. has ceased, and currently, it is only used as a chemical intermediate in the production of several other halogenated solvents (ATSDR, 2006a). 1,1,2-trichloroethane, 1,2-dichloroethane and 1,1-dichloroethene are used in the synthesis of other chemicals, such as polyvinylidene. Tetrachloromethane use as a solvent and fumigant has been discontinued due to toxicity concerns, and its other major use, production of chlorofluorocarbon refrigerants, has been restricted as a result of regulations of ozone-depleting chemicals (ATSDR, 2005).

These volatile halogenated solvents may be released into the air from facilities that produce or use them, from contaminated waste water, or from hazardous waste sites. In surveys of U.S. drinking water, 1,1,1-trichloroethane was one of the most frequently detected chlorinated solvents; detected in less than 10 percent of domestic wells (Moran et al., 2007; Rowe et al., 2007). When 1,1,1-trichlorethane was available in consumer products, indoor air concentrations

## Blood Dibromomethane

Geometric mean and selected percentiles of blood concentrations (in ng/mL) for the U.S. population from the National Health and Nutrition Examination Survey.

| | Survey years# | Geometric mean (95% conf. interval) | Selected percentiles ( 95% confidence interval) | | | | Sample size |
|---|---|---|---|---|---|---|---|
| | | | 50th | 75th | 90th | 95th | |
| **Total** | 03-04 | * | < LOD | < LOD | < LOD | < LOD | 1355 |
| **Age group** | | | | | | | |
| 20-59 years | 03-04 | * | < LOD | < LOD | < LOD | < LOD | 1355 |
| **Gender** | | | | | | | |
| Males | 03-04 | * | < LOD | < LOD | < LOD | < LOD | 666 |
| Females | 03-04 | * | < LOD | < LOD | < LOD | < LOD | 689 |
| **Race/ethnicity** | | | | | | | |
| Mexican Americans | 03-04 | * | < LOD | < LOD | < LOD | < LOD | 267 |
| Non-Hispanic blacks | 03-04 | * | < LOD | < LOD | < LOD | < LOD | 292 |
| Non-Hispanic whites | 03-04 | * | < LOD | < LOD | < LOD | < LOD | 693 |

Limit of detection (LOD, see Data Analysis section) for Survey year 03-04 is 0.03.
# Survey period 2003-2004 is a one-half subsample of 20-59 year olds.
< LOD means less than the limit of detection, which may vary for some chemicals by year and by individual sample.
* Not calculated: proportion of results below limit of detection was too high to provide a valid result.

could exceed outdoor air concentrations (Wallace, et al., 1991). Because of their volatility, these halogenated solvents generally do not persist in soil or water. Workers involved in the production or use of these solvents may be exposed by inhalation or by dermal contact with the liquid solvents.

Inhalation is the most common exposure route for the general population, including indoor sources from such as paints, adhesives, cleaning solutions, and aerosolized insecticide sprays; from industries producing these solvents; and from contaminated waste disposal sites (Armstrong et al., 2004; ATSDR, 2006a and 2001). Drinking water may contribute to exposure due to contaminated underground drinking water supplies. In general, these solvents are well absorbed by inhalation, dermal, or oral exposure. After absorption, small amounts may be exhaled in expired air, and the remaining amount rapidly distributed to tissues. 1,1,1-Trichloroethane is exceptional in that most of a dose is exhaled unchanged in expired air and less than 10 percent of a dose is metabolized (Monster, et al., 1979). Fatty tissues can transiently accumulate these solvents, which are slowly released back into the blood stream. Many of these halogenated solvents are metabolized to more water soluble metabolites that can be excreted in the urine. Hepatic transformation of tetrachloromethane may lead to the generation of reactive intermediate metabolites which may be responsible for liver toxicity (Weber et al., 2003). Other halogenated solvents may undergo similar metabolism to reactive intermediates that contribute to toxicity (Casciola and Ivanetich, 1984; IPCS, 2003; Raucy et al., 1993).

Human health effects from these solvents at low environmental doses or at biomonitored levels from low environmental exposures are unknown. Acute exposure to massive doses by either inhalation or ingestion can cause central nervous system depression and unconsciousness, cardiac dysrhythmias, and hepatic and renal injury. Eye and respiratory tract irritation may occur with exposure to high vapor concentrations of most of these solvents, and allergic contact dermatitis has been reported following 1, 2-dichloroethane dermal exposure (Baruffini et al., 1989). Exposures to vapor concentrations exceeding occupational standards have been associated with fatigue, headache, delayed reactions, and neuropsychological impairment (ATSDR, 2001; Bowler et al., 2003). Epidemiologic studies of workers exposed to various halogenated solvents have found occasional associations between exposure and reduced fertility and spontaneous abortion in women (Figa-Talamanca, 2006). In animal studies, reproductive toxicity has not been consistently demonstrated in the absence of maternal toxicity (IPCS, 1990, 1992, and 1993).

Experimental animals exposed chronically to high doses of each of these solvents developed tumors of the liver, lung, and kidney. In addition, lymphoid and hematopoietic tumors were observed with 1,2-dichloroethane and 1,1,1-trichloroethane; mammary gland tumors were observed with tetrachloromethane, 1,2-dichloroethane, and 1,1-dichloroethene. IARC has determined that the dichloroethanes and tetrachloromethane are possible human carcinogens; the other halogenated solvents in this section are not classifiable regarding human carcinogenicity. NTP has determined that tetrachloromethane and

## Blood 1,1-Dichloroethane

Geometric mean and selected percentiles of blood concentrations (in ng/mL) for the U.S. population from the National Health and Nutrition Examination Survey.

| | Survey years# | Geometric mean (95% conf. interval) | Selected percentiles ( 95% confidence interval) | | | | Sample size |
|---|---|---|---|---|---|---|---|
| | | | 50th | 75th | 90th | 95th | |
| Total | 03-04 | * | < LOD | < LOD | < LOD | < LOD | 1367 |
| Age group | | | | | | | |
| 20-59 years | 03-04 | * | < LOD | < LOD | < LOD | < LOD | 1367 |
| Gender | | | | | | | |
| Males | 03-04 | * | < LOD | < LOD | < LOD | < LOD | 670 |
| Females | 03-04 | * | < LOD | < LOD | < LOD | < LOD | 697 |
| Race/ethnicity | | | | | | | |
| Mexican Americans | 03-04 | * | < LOD | < LOD | < LOD | < LOD | 267 |
| Non-Hispanic blacks | 03-04 | * | < LOD | < LOD | < LOD | < LOD | 300 |
| Non-Hispanic whites | 03-04 | * | < LOD | < LOD | < LOD | < LOD | 695 |

Limit of detection (LOD, see Data Analysis section) for Survey year 03-04 is 0.01.
# Survey period 2003-2004 is a one-half subsample of 20-59 year olds.
< LOD means less than the limit of detection, which may vary for some chemicals by year and by individual sample.
* Not calculated: proportion of results below limit of detection was too high to provide a valid result.

1,2-dichloroethane are reasonably anticipated to be human carcinogens. With the exception of dibromomethane, the U.S. EPA has established drinking water standards and other environmental criteria. The FDA regulates several of these solvents in bottled water and as indirect food additives. Occupational standards and guidelines are available for most of these chemicals from OSHA and ACGIH, respectively. Further information on the halogenated solvents is available from ATSDR at: http://www.atsdr.cdc. gov/toxpro2.html.

## Biomonitoring Information

Levels of halogenated solvents in blood reflect recent exposure. Except for tetrachloromethane in the NHANES 2003-2004 subsample, the other ten halogenated solvents were detectable in less that a few percent of the participants. In a non-representative sample of adults in NHANES III (1988-1994), blood levels were also non-detectable or detected in <10% of samples, except for 1,1,1-trichloroethane which was detected in a majority of samples with a median of 0.13 µg/L (Ashley et al., 1994; Churchill et al., 2001). 1,1,1-Trichloroethane was not detected in children who underwent periodic blood testing as part of an environmental exposure study (Sexton et al., 2005 and 2006). In a study of German residents, 1,1,1-trichloroethane levels were of similar magnitude to the NHANES III study (Hajimiragha et al., 1986).

Finding a measurable amount of any of these halogenated solvents in blood does not mean that the level of the solvent causes an adverse health effect. Biomonitoring studies of blood halogenated solvents can provide physicians and public health officials with reference values so that they can determine whether or not people have been exposed to higher levels of halogenated solvents than levels found in the general population. Biomonitoring data can also help scientists plan and conduct research on exposure and health effects.

## Blood 1,2-Dichloroethane (Ethylene dichloride)

Geometric mean and selected percentiles of blood concentrations (in ng/mL) for the U.S. population from the National Health and Nutrition Examination Survey.

| | Survey years# | Geometric mean (95% conf. interval) | Selected percentiles ( 95% confidence interval) | | | | Sample size |
|---|---|---|---|---|---|---|---|
| | | | 50th | 75th | 90th | 95th | |
| Total | 03-04 | * | < LOD | < LOD | < LOD | < LOD | 1346 |
| Age group | | | | | | | |
| 20-59 years | 03-04 | * | < LOD | < LOD | < LOD | < LOD | 1346 |
| Gender | | | | | | | |
| Males | 03-04 | * | < LOD | < LOD | < LOD | < LOD | 661 |
| Females | 03-04 | * | < LOD | < LOD | < LOD | < LOD | 685 |
| Race/ethnicity | | | | | | | |
| Mexican Americans | 03-04 | * | < LOD | < LOD | < LOD | < LOD | 267 |
| Non-Hispanic blacks | 03-04 | * | < LOD | < LOD | < LOD | < LOD | 289 |
| Non-Hispanic whites | 03-04 | * | < LOD | < LOD | < LOD | < LOD | 689 |

Limit of detection (LOD, see Data Analysis section) for Survey year 03-04 is 0.01.
# Survey period 2003-2004 is a one-half subsample of 20-59 year olds.
< LOD means less than the limit of detection, which may vary for some chemicals by year and by individual sample.
* Not calculated: proportion of results below limit of detection was too high to provide a valid result.

## Blood 1,1-Dichloroethene (Vinylidene chloride)

Geometric mean and selected percentiles of blood concentrations (in ng/mL) for the U.S. population from the National Health and Nutrition Examination Survey.

| | Survey years# | Geometric mean (95% conf. interval) | Selected percentiles ( 95% confidence interval) | | | | Sample size |
|---|---|---|---|---|---|---|---|
| | | | 50th | 75th | 90th | 95th | |
| Total | 03-04 | * | < LOD | < LOD | < LOD | < LOD | 1367 |
| Age group | | | | | | | |
| 20-59 years | 03-04 | * | < LOD | < LOD | < LOD | < LOD | 1367 |
| Gender | | | | | | | |
| Males | 03-04 | * | < LOD | < LOD | < LOD | < LOD | 670 |
| Females | 03-04 | * | < LOD | < LOD | < LOD | < LOD | 697 |
| Race/ethnicity | | | | | | | |
| Mexican Americans | 03-04 | * | < LOD | < LOD | < LOD | < LOD | 267 |
| Non-Hispanic blacks | 03-04 | * | < LOD | < LOD | < LOD | < LOD | 300 |
| Non-Hispanic whites | 03-04 | * | < LOD | < LOD | < LOD | < LOD | 695 |

Limit of detection (LOD, see Data Analysis section) for Survey year 03-04 is 0.009.
# Survey period 2003-2004 is a one-half subsample of 20-59 year olds.
< LOD means less than the limit of detection which may vary for some chemicals by year and by individual sample.
* Not calculated: proportion of results below limit of detection was too high to provide a valid result.

## Blood *cis*-1,2-Dichloroethene

Geometric mean and selected percentiles of blood concentrations (in ng/mL) for the U.S. population from the National Health and Nutrition Examination Survey.

| | Survey years# | Geometric mean (95% conf. interval) | Selected percentiles ( 95% confidence interval) | | | | Sample size |
|---|---|---|---|---|---|---|---|
| | | | 50th | 75th | 90th | 95th | |
| Total | 03-04 | * | < LOD | < LOD | < LOD | < LOD | 1366 |
| Age group | | | | | | | |
| 20-59 years | 03-04 | * | < LOD | < LOD | < LOD | < LOD | 1366 |
| Gender | | | | | | | |
| Males | 03-04 | * | < LOD | < LOD | < LOD | < LOD | 669 |
| Females | 03-04 | * | < LOD | < LOD | < LOD | < LOD | 697 |
| Race/ethnicity | | | | | | | |
| Mexican Americans | 03-04 | * | < LOD | < LOD | < LOD | < LOD | 267 |
| Non-Hispanic blacks | 03-04 | * | < LOD | < LOD | < LOD | < LOD | 300 |
| Non-Hispanic whites | 03-04 | * | < LOD | < LOD | < LOD | < LOD | 694 |

Limit of detection (LOD see Data Analysis section) for Survey year 03-04 is 0.01.
# Survey period 2003-2004 is a one-half subsample of 20-59 year olds.
< LOD means less than the limit of detection, which may vary for some chemicals by year and by individual sample.
* Not calculated: proportion of results below limit of detection was too high to provide a valid result.

## Blood *trans*-1,2-Dichloroethene

Geometric mean and selected percentiles of blood concentrations (in ng/mL) for the U.S. population from the National Health and Nutrition Examination Survey.

| | Survey years# | Geometric mean (95% conf. interval) | Selected percentiles ( 95% confidence interval) | | | | Sample size |
|---|---|---|---|---|---|---|---|
| | | | 50th | 75th | 90th | 95th | |
| Total | 03-04 | * | < LOD | < LOD | < LOD | < LOD | 1367 |
| Age group | | | | | | | |
| 20-59 years | 03-04 | * | < LOD | < LOD | < LOD | < LOD | 1367 |
| Gender | | | | | | | |
| Males | 03-04 | * | < LOD | < LOD | < LOD | < LOD | 670 |
| Females | 03-04 | * | < LOD | < LOD | < LOD | < LOD | 697 |
| Race/ethnicity | | | | | | | |
| Mexican Americans | 03-04 | * | < LOD | < LOD | < LOD | < LOD | 267 |
| Non-Hispanic blacks | 03-04 | * | < LOD | < LOD | < LOD | < LOD | 300 |
| Non-Hispanic whites | 03-04 | * | < LOD | < LOD | < LOD | < LOD | 695 |

Limit of detection (LOD, see Data Analysis section) for Survey year 03-04 is 0.01.
# Survey period 2003-2004 is a one-half subsample of 20-59 year olds.
< LOD means less than the limit of detection, which may vary for some chemicals by year and by individual sample.
* Not calculated: proportion of results below limit of detection was too high to provide a valid result.

## Blood 1,2-Dichloropropane

Geometric mean and selected percentiles of blood concentrations (in ng/mL) for the U.S. population from the National Health and Nutrition Examination Survey.

| | Survey years# | Geometric mean (95% conf. interval) | Selected percentiles ( 95% confidence interval) | | | | Sample size |
|---|---|---|---|---|---|---|---|
| | | | 50th | 75th | 90th | 95th | |
| Total | 03-04 | * | < LOD | < LOD | < LOD | < LOD | 1364 |
| Age group | | | | | | | |
| 20-59 years | 03-04 | * | < LOD | < LOD | < LOD | < LOD | 1364 |
| Gender | | | | | | | |
| Males | 03-04 | * | < LOD | < LOD | < LOD | < LOD | 667 |
| Females | 03-04 | * | < LOD | < LOD | < LOD | < LOD | 697 |
| Race/ethnicity | | | | | | | |
| Mexican Americans | 03-04 | * | < LOD | < LOD | < LOD | < LOD | 267 |
| Non-Hispanic blacks | 03-04 | * | < LOD | < LOD | < LOD | < LOD | 300 |
| Non-Hispanic whites | 03-04 | * | < LOD | < LOD | < LOD | < LOD | 692 |

Limit of detection (LOD  see Data Analysis section) for Survey year 03-04 is 0.008.
# Survey period 2003-2004 is a one-half subsample of 20-59 year olds.
< LOD means less than the limit of detection, which may vary for some chemicals by year and by individual sample.
* Not calculated: proportion of results below limit of detection was too high to provide a valid result.

## Blood 1,1,1-Trichloroethane (Methyl chloroform)

Geometric mean and selected percentiles of blood concentrations (in ng/mL) for the U.S. population from the National Health and Nutrition Examination Survey.

| | Survey years# | Geometric mean (95% conf. interval) | Selected percentiles ( 95% confidence interval) | | | | Sample size |
|---|---|---|---|---|---|---|---|
| | | | 50th | 75th | 90th | 95th | |
| Total | 03-04 | * | < LOD | < LOD | < LOD | < LOD | 1345 |
| Age group | | | | | | | |
| 20-59 years | 03-04 | * | < LOD | < LOD | < LOD | < LOD | 1345 |
| Gender | | | | | | | |
| Males | 03-04 | * | < LOD | < LOD | < LOD | < LOD | 660 |
| Females | 03-04 | * | < LOD | < LOD | < LOD | < LOD | 685 |
| Race/ethnicity | | | | | | | |
| Mexican Americans | 03-04 | * | < LOD | < LOD | < LOD | < LOD | 267 |
| Non-Hispanic blacks | 03-04 | * | < LOD | < LOD | < LOD | < LOD | 289 |
| Non-Hispanic whites | 03-04 | * | < LOD | < LOD | < LOD | < LOD | 688 |

Limit of detection (LOD, see Data Analysis section) for Survey year 03-04 is 0.048.
# Survey period 2003-2004 is a one-half subsample of 20-59 year olds.
< LOD means less than the limit of detection which may vary for some chemicals by year and by individual sample.
* Not calculated: proportion of results below limit of detection was too high to provide a valid result.

## Blood 1,1,2-Trichloroethane

Geometric mean and selected percentiles of blood concentrations (in ng/mL) for the U.S. population from the National Health and Nutrition Examination Survey.

| | Survey years# | Geometric mean (95% conf. interval) | Selected percentiles ( 95% confidence interval) | | | | Sample size |
|---|---|---|---|---|---|---|---|
| | | | 50th | 75th | 90th | 95th | |
| Total | 03-04 | * | < LOD | < LOD | < LOD | < LOD | 1354 |
| Age group | | | | | | | |
| 20-59 years | 03-04 | * | < LOD | < LOD | < LOD | < LOD | 1354 |
| Gender | | | | | | | |
| Males | 03-04 | * | < LOD | < LOD | < LOD | < LOD | 664 |
| Females | 03-04 | * | < LOD | < LOD | < LOD | < LOD | 690 |
| Race/ethnicity | | | | | | | |
| Mexican Americans | 03-04 | * | < LOD | < LOD | < LOD | < LOD | 267 |
| Non-Hispanic blacks | 03-04 | * | < LOD | < LOD | < LOD | < LOD | 297 |
| Non-Hispanic whites | 03-04 | * | < LOD | < LOD | < LOD | < LOD | 686 |

Limit of detection (LOD  see Data Analysis section) for Survey year 03-04 is 0.01.
# Survey period 2003-2004 is a one-half subsample of 20-59 year olds.
< LOD means less than the limit of detection, which may vary for some chemicals by year and by individual sample.
* Not calculated: proportion of results below limit of detection was too high to provide a valid result.

## Blood 1,1,2,2-Tetrachloroethane

Geometric mean and selected percentiles of blood concentrations (in ng/mL) for the U.S. population from the National Health and Nutrition Examination Survey.

| | Survey years# | Geometric mean (95% conf. interval) | 50th | 75th | 90th | 95th | Sample size |
|---|---|---|---|---|---|---|---|
| | | | Selected percentiles (95% confidence interval) | | | | |
| Total | 03-04 | * | < LOD | < LOD | < LOD | < LOD | 1235 |
| **Age group** | | | | | | | |
| 20-59 years | 03-04 | * | < LOD | < LOD | < LOD | < LOD | 1235 |
| **Gender** | | | | | | | |
| Males | 03-04 | * | < LOD | < LOD | < LOD | < LOD | 613 |
| Females | 03-04 | * | < LOD | < LOD | < LOD | < LOD | 622 |
| **Race/ethnicity** | | | | | | | |
| Mexican Americans | 03-04 | * | < LOD | < LOD | < LOD | < LOD | 250 |
| Non-Hispanic blacks | 03-04 | * | < LOD | < LOD | < LOD | < LOD | 282 |
| Non-Hispanic whites | 03-04 | * | < LOD | < LOD | < LOD | < LOD | 606 |

Limit of detection (LOD, see Data Analysis section) for Survey year 03-04 is 0.01.
# Survey period 2003-2004 is a one-half subsample of 20-59 year olds.
< LOD means less than the limit of detection which may vary for some chemicals by year and by individual sample.
* Not calculated: proportion of results below limit of detection was too high to provide a valid result.

## Blood Tetrachloromethane (Carbon tetrachloride)

Geometric mean and selected percentiles of blood concentrations (in ng/mL) for the U.S. population from the National Health and Nutrition Examination Survey.

| | Survey years# | Geometric mean (95% conf. interval) | 50th | 75th | 90th | 95th | Sample size |
|---|---|---|---|---|---|---|---|
| | | | Selected percentiles (95% confidence interval) | | | | |
| Total | 01-02 | * | < LOD | .010 (<LOD-.010) | .010 (<LOD-.140) | .020 (.010-.050) | 742 |
| | 03-04 | * | < LOD | < LOD | < LOD | < LOD | 1362 |
| **Age group** | | | | | | | |
| 20-59 years | 01-02 | * | < LOD | .010 (<LOD-.010) | .010 (<LOD-.140) | .020 (.010-.050) | 742 |
| | 03-04 | * | < LOD | < LOD | < LOD | < LOD | 1362 |
| **Gender** | | | | | | | |
| Males | 01-02 | * | < LOD | .010 (<LOD-.010) | .010 (<LOD-.140) | .010 (.010-.040) | 364 |
| | 03-04 | * | < LOD | < LOD | < LOD | < LOD | 667 |
| Females | 01-02 | * | < LOD | .010 (<LOD-.010) | .010 (<LOD-.090) | .040 (.010-.080) | 378 |
| | 03-04 | * | < LOD | < LOD | < LOD | < LOD | 695 |
| **Race/ethnicity** | | | | | | | |
| Mexican Americans | 01-02 | * | < LOD | < LOD | .010 (<LOD-.750) | .020 (.010-.050) | 193 |
| | 03-04 | * | < LOD | < LOD | < LOD | < LOD | 266 |
| Non-Hispanic blacks | 01-02 | * | < LOD | .010 (<LOD-.010) | .010 (<LOD-.020) | .010 (<LOD-.020) | 132 |
| | 03-04 | * | < LOD | < LOD | < LOD | < LOD | 299 |
| Non-Hispanic whites | 01-02 | * | < LOD | .010 (<LOD-.010) | .010 (<LOD-.140) | .030 (.010-.080) | 366 |
| | 03-04 | * | < LOD | < LOD | < LOD | < LOD | 692 |

Limits of detection (LOD, see Data Analysis section) for Survey years 01-02 and 03-04 are 0.01 and 0.005.
# Survey period 2001-2002 is a one-third subsample of 20-59 year olds  Survey period 2003-2004 is a one-half subsample of 20-59 year olds.
< LOD means less than the limit of detection, which may vary for some chemicals by year and by individual sample.
* Not calculated: proportion of results below limit of detection was too high to provide a valid result.

# References

Agency for Toxic Substances and Disease Registry (ATSDR). Toxicological profile for carbon tetrachloride. Atlanta GA. 2005 [online]. Available at URL: http://www.atsdr.cdc.gov/toxprofiles/tp30 html. 4/21/09

Agency for Toxic Substances and Disease Registry (ATSDR). Toxicological profile for 1,2-dichloroethane update. Atlanta GA. 2001 [online]. Available at URL: http://www.atsdr.cdc.gov/toxprofiles/tp38.html. 4/21/09

Agency for Toxic Substances and Disease Registry (ATSDR). Toxicological profile for 1,1,1-trichloroethane update. Atlanta GA. 2006b [online}. Available at URL: http://www.atsdr.cdc.gov/toxprofiles/tp70.html. 4/21/09

Agency for Toxic Substances and Disease Registry (ATSDR). Toxicological profile for 1,1,2,2-tetracholoroethane draft. Atlanta GA. 2006a [online]. Available at URL: http://www.atsdr.cdc.gov/toxprofiles/tp93.html#bookmark08. 4/21/09

Armstrong SR, Green LC. Chlorinated hydrocarbon solvents. Clin Occup Environ Med 2004;4(3):481-496, vi.

Baruffini A, Cirla AM, Pisati G, Ratti R, Zedda S. Allergic contact dermatitis from 1,2-dichloropropane. Contact Dermatitis 1989;20(5):379-380.

Bell BP, Franks P, Hildreth N, et al. Methylene chloride exposure and birthweight in Monroe County, New York. Environ Res 1991:55:31-39.

Bove FJ, Fulcomer MC, Klotz JB, Esmart J, Dufficy EM, Savrin JE. Public drinking water contamination and birth outcomes.Am J Epidemiol 1995 May 1;141(9):850-62.

Bowler RM, Gysens S, Hartney C. Neuropsychological effects of ethylene dichloride exposure. Neurotoxicology 2003;24(4-5):553-562.

Casciola LA, Ivanetich KM. Metabolism of chloroethanes by rat liver nuclear cytochrome P-450. Carcinogenesis 1984;5(5):543-548.

Costas K, Knorr RS, Condon SK. A case-control study of childhood leukemia in Woburn, Massachusetts: the relationship between leukemia incidence and exposure to public drinking water. Sci Total Environ 2002;300(1-3):23-35.

Croen LA, Shaw GM, Sanbonmatsu L, et al. 1997. Maternal residential proximity to hazardous waste sites and risk for selected congenital malformations. Epidemiology 1997;8:347-354.

Eskenazi B, Fenster L, Hudes M, Wyrobek AJ, Katz DF, Gerson J, et al. A study of the effect of perchloroethylene exposure on the reproductive outcomes of wives of dry cleaning workers. Am J Ind Med 1991a; 20:593-600.

Eskenazi B, Wyrobek AJ, Fenster L, Katz DF, Sadler M, Lee J, et al. A study of the effect of perchloroethylene exposure on semen quality in dry cleaning workers. Am J Ind Med 1991b;20:575-591.

Figa-Telemanca I. Occupational risk factors and reproductive health of women. Occup Med (Lond) 2006;56(8):521-531.

Hajimiragha H, Ewers U, Jansen-Rosseck R, Brockhaus A. Human exposure to volatile halogenated hydrocarbons from the general environment. Int Arch Occup Environ Health. 1986;58(2):141-150.

Hill RH Jr, Ashley DL, Head SL, Needham LL, Pirkle JL. p-Dichlorobenzene exposure among 1,000 adults in the United States. Arch Environ Health 1995;50(4):277-280.

International Programme on Chemical Safety (IPCS). Concise International Chemical Assessment Document 51. 1,1-Dicholoroethene (vinylidene chloride). 2003 [online]. Available at URL: http://www.inchem.org/documents/cicads/cicads/cicad51.htm. 4/21/09

International Programme on Chemical Safety (IPCS). Environmental Health Criteria 146. 1,3-Dichloropropene, 1,2-Dichloropropane & Mixtures. 1993 [online]. Available at URL: http://www.intox.org/databank/documents/chemical/dichlorp/ehc146 htm. 4/21/09

International Programme on Chemical Safety (IPCS). Environmental Health Criteria 136. 1,1,1-Trichloroethane. 1992 [online]. Available at URL: http://www.inchem.org/documents/ehc/ehc/ehc136 htm. 4/21/09

International Programme on Chemical Safety (IPCS). Environmental Health Criteria 100. Vinylidene chloride. 1990 [online]. Available at URL: http://www.inchem.org/documents/ehc/ehc/ehc100 htm. 4/21/09

Monster AC, Boersma G, Steenweg H. Kinetics of tetrachloroethylene in volunteers: influence of exposure concentration and work load. Int Arch Occup Environ Health 1979;42:303-309.

Moran MJ, Zogorski JS, Squillace PJ. Chlorinated solvents in groundwater of the United States. Environ Sci Technol 2007;41:74-81.

Raucy JL, Kraner JC, Lasker JM. Bioactivation of halogenated hydrocarbons by cytochrome P4502E1. Crit Rev Toxicol 1993;23(1):1-20.

Rodenbeck SE, Sanderson LM, Rene A. Maternal exposure to trichloroethylene in drinking water and birth-weight outcomes. Arch Environ Health 2000;55(3):188-194.

Rowe BL, Toccalino PL, Moran MJ, Zogorski JS, Price CV.

Occurrence and potential human-health relevance of volatile organic compounds in drinking water from domestic wells in the United States. Environ Health Perspect 2007;115(11):1539-1546.

Sexton K, Adgate JL, Church TR, Ashley DL, Needham LL, Ramachandran G, et al. Children's exposure to volatile organic compounds as determined by longitudinal measurements in blood. Environ Health Perspect 2005;113(3):342-349.

Sexton K, Adgate JL, Fredrickson AL, Ryan AD, Needham LL, Ashley DL. Using biologic markers in blood to assess exposure to multiple environmental chemicals for inner-city children 3-6 years of age. Environ Health Perspect 2006;114(3):453-459.

Weber LW, Boll M, Stampfl A. Hepatotoxicity and mechanism of action of haloalkanes: carbon tetrachloride as a toxicological model. Crit Rev Toxicol 2003;33(2):105-136.

Windham GC, Shusterman D, Swan SH, Fenster L, Eskenazi B. Exposure to organic solvents and adverse pregnancy outcome. Am J Ind Med. 1991;20(2):241-259.

# Hexachloroethane
CAS No. 67-72-1

## General Information

Hexachloroethane is a solid that sublimates at room temperature. It is primarily used in combination with zinc or titanium oxides in military pyrotechnic or smoke generating devices, as an agent to degas or purify molten ores, as an ignition and explosive suppressant, and as a vulcanizing agent. Hexachloroethane is no longer produced in the U. S., and usage has declined since the 1970's (ATSDR, 1997). In the past, hexachloroethane was used as an ingredient in some pesticides, in fire extinguisher fluids, and as a veterinary antihelminthic (ATSDR, 1997). Hexachloroethane can enter the atmosphere from emissions during its production and use, or as a byproduct from the chlorination of other hydrocarbons. Hexachloroethane is relatively persistent in the environment and has been detected a low levels in ambient air and rarely in drinking water systems (USGS, 2006).

For the general population, hexachloroethane exposure is infrequent and occurs by inhaling contaminated air. A less common pathway is the ingestion of contaminated drinking water. Workers in metal and alloy refining or pyrotechnic and smoke device production may be exposed to larger amounts. Hexachloroethane is absorbed by inhalation, dermal and ingestion routes, and it is preferentially distributed to fat, kidney and liver. Metabolism in the liver results in formation of trichloroacetic acid and trichloroethanol, which are excreted in urine (ATSDR,

1997). A small portion of unmetabolized hexachloroethane is excreted in the feces.

Human health effects from hexachloroethane at low environmental doses or at biomonitored levels from low environmental exposures are unknown. Workers exposed to hexachloroethane reported irritation of the skin and mucous membranes, but no changes were noted in pulmonary function tests or in serum tests of renal, pancreatic, and liver function (Selden et al., 1994, Selden et al., 1997). Animals exposed to high air levels of hexachloroethane developed ataxia, facial twitching, tremors, and pneumonitis (Weeks et al., 1979). In feeding studies, animals developed dose-related abnormalities of the liver (enlargement, transaminase elevation, centrilobular necrosis) and kidney (tubular nephrosis and nephrocalcinosis) (ATSDR, 1997). Animal carcinogenicity studies show inconsistent evidence of hepatocellular carcinomas (NCI, 1978), an increased incidence of renal tumors in males (NTP, 1989), and no clear evidence of mutagenicity or genotoxicity. Hexachloroethane does not appear to be a reproductive or developmental toxicant in animal studies (ATSDR, 1997).

Hexachloroethane is classified as a possible human carcinogen by IARC and is reasonably anticipated to be a human carcinogen by NTP. The U.S. EPA has established drinking water and other environmental regulations for hexachloroethane. Workplace standards and guidelines for hexachloroethane have been established by OSHA and ACGIH, respectively. Information about external exposure (ie., environmental levels) and health effects is available from ATSDR at: http://www.atsdr.cdc.gov/toxpro2.html.

## Blood Hexachloroethane

Geometric mean and selected percentiles of blood concentrations (in ng/mL) for the U.S. population from the National Health and Nutrition Examination Survey.

| | Survey years# | Geometric mean (95% conf. interval) | 50th | 75th | 90th | 95th | Sample size |
|---|---|---|---|---|---|---|---|
| Total | 03-04 | * | < LOD | < LOD | < LOD | < LOD | 1366 |
| **Age group** | | | | | | | |
| 20-59 years | 03-04 | * | < LOD | < LOD | < LOD | < LOD | 1366 |
| **Gender** | | | | | | | |
| Males | 03-04 | * | < LOD | < LOD | < LOD | < LOD | 669 |
| Females | 03-04 | * | < LOD | < LOD | < LOD | < LOD | 697 |
| **Race/ethnicity** | | | | | | | |
| Mexican Americans | 03-04 | * | < LOD | < LOD | < LOD | < LOD | 267 |
| Non-Hispanic blacks | 03-04 | * | < LOD | < LOD | < LOD | < LOD | 300 |
| Non-Hispanic whites | 03-04 | * | < LOD | < LOD | < LOD | < LOD | 694 |

Limit of detection (LOD, see Data Analysis section) for Survey year 03-04 is 0.011.
# Survey period 2003-2004 is a one-half subsample of 20-59 year olds.
< LOD means less than the limit of detection, which may vary for some chemicals by year and by individual sample.
* Not calculated: proportion of results below limit of detection was too high to provide a valid result.

## Biomonitoring Information

Levels of hexachloroethane in the blood reflect recent exposure. Blood levels were not detectable in the NHANES 2003-2004 subsample as has been the case in several other general population studies (Ashley et al., 1994; Buckley et al., 1997; Foster, 1995; Selden et al., 1993).

Finding a measureable amount of hexachloroethane in blood does not mean that the level of hexachloroethane causes an adverse health effect. Biomonitoring studies of blood hexachloroethane can provide physicians and public health officials with reference values so that they can determine whether or not people have been exposed to higher levels of hexachloroethane than levels found in the general population. Biomonitoring data can also help scientists plan and conduct research on exposure and health effects.

## References

Agency for Toxic Substances and Disease Registry (ATSDR). Toxicological profile for hexachloroethane. 1997 [online]. Available from URL: http://www.atsdr.cdc.gov/toxprofiles/tp97.html. 4/21/09

Ashley DL, Bonin MA, Cardinali FL, McCraw JM, Wooten JV. Blood concentrations of volatile organic compounds in a nonoccupationally exposed US population and in groups with suspected exposure. Clin Chem 1994;40(7 Pt 2):1401-1404.

Buckley TJ, Liddle J, Ashley DL, Paschal DC, Burse VW, Needham LL, Akland G. Environmental and biomarker measurements in nine homes in the lower Rio Grande Valley: multimedia results for pesticides, metals, PAHs, and VOCs. Environ Int 1997;23:705-732.

Foster WG. The reproductive toxicology of Great Lakes contaminants. Environ Health Perspect 1995;103 Suppl 9:63-9.

National Cancer Institute (NCI). Bioassay of hexachloroethane for possible carcinogenicity (CAS No. 67-72-1). NCI-CG-TR-68. Tech Report Ser No. 68. U.S. DHEW. Publ. No. (NIH) 78-1318. Bethesda MD. 1978. Available at URL: http://ntp.niehs.nih.gov/ntp/htdocs/LT_rpts/tr068.pdf. 4/21/09

National Toxicology Program (NTP). Toxicology and carcinogenesis studies of hexachloroethane (CAS No.67-72-1) in F344/N rats (gavage studies). Tech Report Ser No. 361. NIH Publication No. 89-2816. Research Triangle Part, NC: National Toxicology Program. Research Triangle Park NC, 1989 [online]. Available at URL: http://ntp.niehs.nih.gov/ntp/htdocs/LT_rpts/tr361.pdf. 4/21/09

Selden A, Kvamlof A, Bodin L, et al. Health effects of low level occupational exposure to hexachloroethane. J Occup Med Toxicol 1994;3(10):73-79.

Selden A, Nygren M, Kvarnlof A, Sundell K, Spangberg O. Biological monitoring of hexachloroethane. Int Arch Occup Environ Health 1993;65(1 Suppl):S111-S114.

Selden AI, Nygren Y, Westberg HB, Bodin LS. Hexachlorobenzene and octachlorostyrene in plasma of aluminium foundry workers using hexachloroethane for degassing. Occup Environ Med 1997;54(8):613-618.

United States Geological Survey (USGS). Volatile organic compounds in the nation's ground water and drinking-water supply wells. Reston VA. 2006 [online]. Available at URL: http://pubs.usgs.gov/circ/circ1292/. 4/21/09

Weeks MH, Angerhofer RA, Bishop R, Thomasino J, Pope CR. The toxicity of hexachloroethane in laboratory animals. Am Ind Hyg Assoc J 1979;40:187-199.

# Methyl *tert*-Butyl Ether (MTBE)
CAS No. 1634-04-4

## General Information

Methyl *tert*-butyl ether (MTBE) was added to reformulated gasoline to boost octane and to reduce carbon monoxide exhaust emissions in high smog areas of the United States in the1980s. Because of concerns for groundwater contamination and water quality, MTBE was banned or its usage was limited in several states. Ethanol has replaced MTBE as an additive to reformulated gasoline (U.S. DOE, 2003 and 2006; U.S. EPA, 2000). MTBE contamination of groundwater has been more common in urban areas (Squillace et al., 2004) and in areas near leaking underground storage tanks (Rowe et al., 2007). MTBE also has been detected in ambient air near blending facilities, in cities where MTBE is used in reformulated gasoline, and in the breathing zone during consumer refueling at service stations (IPCS, 1998). MBTE is also used in small amounts as a laboratory solvent and as a pharmaceutical agent (ATSDR, 1996).

The general population is exposed to MBTE primarily by inhalation of contaminated air. Contaminated water is a less common source though exposure can occur by ingestion or inhalation of vaporized MTBE from water (IPCS, 1998). Workplace exposure to MTBE may occur in the production, transportation, and use of petrochemicals. MTBE is well absorbed after inhalational, oral, or dermal exposure and is rapidly cleared from the blood with an estimated half-life of several hours (Dekant et al., 2001). Most MTBE absorbed by the body is metabolized by the liver and then eliminated in urine, primarily as 2-hydroxyisobutyrate with *tert*-butyl alcohol and 2-methyl-1,2-propanediol as minor urinary metabolites (Amberg et al., 1999; Amberg et al., 2001). Depending upon the dose, more than one third of inhaled MTBE may be excreted in exhaled air (ATSDR, 1996; Nihlen et al., 1998).

Human health effects from MTBE at low environmental doses or at biomonitored levels from low environmental exposures are unknown. Following the introduction of MTBE reformulated gasoline, complaints of respiratory tract irritation, headache, nausea, and dizziness prompted several population surveys, epidemiologic studies, and experimental human volunteer studies that provided little evidence of an association between MTBE exposure and health complaints (ATSDR, 1996). Based upon high dose animal studies, MTBE has been considered to be a skin and

## Blood Methyl *tert*-butyl ether (MTBE)

Geometric mean and selected percentiles of blood concentrations (in pg/mL) for the U.S. population from the National Health and Nutrition Examination Survey.

| | Survey years# | Geometric mean (95% conf. interval) | Selected percentiles ( 95% confidence interval) | | | | Sample size |
|---|---|---|---|---|---|---|---|
| | | | 50th | 75th | 90th | 95th | |
| Total | 01-02 | 16.4 (4.77-56.7) | 27.7 (7.29-64.9) | 73.8 (35.5-127) | 132 (64.0-278) | 188 (109-339) | 672 |
| | 03-04 | 11.0 (5.98-20.1) | 10.0 (4.60-25.1) | 45.0 (16.0-98.0) | 110 (70.0-180) | 170 (110-340) | 1307 |
| Age group | | | | | | | |
| 20-59 years | 01-02 | 16.4 (4.77-56.7) | 27.7 (7.29-64.9) | 73.8 (35.5-127) | 132 (64.0-278) | 188 (109-339) | 672 |
| | 03-04 | 11.0 (5.98-20.1) | 10.0 (4.60-25.1) | 45.0 (16.0-98.0) | 110 (70.0-180) | 170 (110-340) | 1307 |
| Gender | | | | | | | |
| Males | 01-02 | 16.9 (4.96-57.7) | 27.9 (6.82-64.6) | 75.0 (35.5-131) | 132 (54.9-307) | 167 (109-417) | 334 |
| | 03-04 | 12.2 (6.29-23.6) | 11.0 (4.80-29.0) | 55.0 (18.0-110) | 130 (79.0-200) | 200 (110-470) | 641 |
| Females | 01-02 | 16.0 (4.12-61.8) | 26.6 (5.93-74.6) | 72.7 (32.6-132) | 142 (73.5-255) | 194 (92.3-336) | 338 |
| | 03-04 | 9.88 (5.62-17.4) | 8.90 (4.30-23.0) | 38.0 (14.0-85.0) | 94.0 (58.0-160) | 140 (90.0-250) | 666 |
| Race/ethnicity | | | | | | | |
| Mexican Americans | 01-02 | 23.3 (4.96-110) | 33.4 (2.92-187) | 91.3 (26.1-255) | 225 (80.6-339) | 273 (182-358) | 166 |
| | 03-04 | 11.6 (5.35-25.3) | 12.0 (3.80-29.0) | 32.0 (14.0-80.0) | 80.0 (38.0-190) | 160 (74.0-220) | 245 |
| Non-Hispanic blacks | 01-02 | 14.9 (6.11-36.4) | 26.4 (3.11-55.6) | 52.6 (30.0-86.8) | 87.4 (38.6-155) | 120 (70.0-155) | 119 |
| | 03-04 | 9.63 (4.83-19.2) | 10.0 (3.50-28.0) | 32.8 (11.0-85.0) | 77.0 (36.0-160) | 140 (61.0-210) | 285 |
| Non-Hispanic whites | 01-02 | 16.0 (4.13-62.4) | 27.9 (4.71-74.6) | 72.7 (33.3-132) | 132 (59.6-249) | 165 (92.8-366) | 333 |
| | 03-04 | 11.5 (5.51-23.8) | 11.0 (4.00-33.5) | 59.0 (14.0-120) | 120 (73.0-230) | 180 (110-430) | 673 |

Limits of detection (LOD, see Data Analysis section) for Survey years 01-02 and 03-04 are 0.232 and 2.0.
# Survey period 2001-2002 is a one-third subsample of 20-59 year olds; Survey period 2003-2004 is a one-half subsample of 20-59 year olds.

eye irritant (IPCS, 1998). Animal studies of carcinogenicity have been inconclusive (ATSDR, 1996). MTBE does not appear to be a reproductive or developmental in animal studies (IPCS, 1998). Methyl *tert*-butyl ether is unclassifiable as a human carcinogen by IARC. The U.S. EPA has established standards and guidelines for MTBE in water and air, and ACGIH has adopted guidelines for workplace air exposure. Information about external exposure (i.e., environmental levels) and health effects is available from ATSDR at: http://www.atsdr.cdc.gov/toxpro2.html.

## Biomonitoring Information

Levels of MTBE in blood reflect recent exposure. In the NHANES 2003-2004 subsample, MTBE was detectable in most of the population; the geometric mean was 11.0 pg/mL for the total population. In a subsample of adults in NHANES 1999-2000, Lin et al. (2008) found geometric mean blood levels of MTBE to be 17 and 15 pg/mL in smokers and non-smokers, respectively. In a small study of U.S. automobile drivers when MTBE was used as a fuel additive, blood levels were about 100 times higher than those in the NHANES subsamples (White et al., 1995). Commuters in urban areas with high vehicular traffic had median blood MTBE blood levels that were more than tenfold higher than those in the U.S. general population (Lemire et al., 2004). Workers exposed to oxygenated gasoline fumes and vehicle exhaust had levels that were by 10 to 100 times higher than general population levels (Mannino et al., 1995; Moolenaar et al., 1994; Romieu et al., 1999; White et al., 1995), depending in part on the concentration of MTBE in the gasoline.

Finding a measurable amount of MTBE in blood does not mean that the level of MTBE causes an adverse health effect. Biomonitoring studies of blood MTBE can provide physicians and public health officials with reference values so that they can determine whether or not people have been exposed to higher levels of MTBE than levels found in the general population. Biomonitoring data can also help scientists plan and conduct research on exposure and health effects.

## References

Agency for Toxic Substances and Disease Registry (ATSDR). Toxicological profile for methyl *tert*-butyl ether. 1996 [online]. Available at URL: http://www.atsdr.cdc.gov/toxprofiles/tp91.html#bookmark07. 4/21/09

Amberg A, Rosner E, Dekant W. Biotransformation and kinetics of excretion of methyl-*tert*-butyl ether in rats and humans. Toxicol Sci 1999;51(1):1-8.

Amberg A, Rosner E, Dekant W. Toxicokinetics of methyl *tert*-butyl ether and its metabolites in humans after oral exposure. Toxicol Sci 2001;61(1):62-67.

Dekant W, Bernauer U, Rosner E, Amberg A. Biotransformation of MTBE, ETBE, and TAME after inhalation or ingestion in rats and humans. Res Rep Health Eff Inst 2001;102:29-71.

International Programme on Chemical Safety (IPCS). Environmental Health Criteria 206. Methyl Tertiary-Butyl Ether. Geneva, Switzerland.1998 [online]. Available at URL: http://www.inchem.org/documents/ehc/ehc/ehc206 htm. 4/21/09

Lemire S, Ashley D, Olaya P, Romieu I, Welch S, Meneses-Gonzalez F, Hernandez-Avila M. Environmental exposure of commuters in Mexico City to volatile organic compounds as assessed by blood concentrations, 1998. Salud Publica Mex 2004;46:32-38.

Lin YS, Egeghy PP, Rappaport SM. Relationships between levels of volatile organic compounds in air and blood from the general population. J Expo Sci Environ Epidemiol 2008;18(4):421-429.

Mannino DM, Schreiber J, Aldous K, Ashley D, Moolenaar R, Almaguer D. Human exposure to volatile organic compounds: a comparison of organic vapor monitoring badge levels with blood levels. Int Arch Occup Environ Health. 1995;67(1):59-64.

Moolenaar RL, Heffline BJ, Ashley DL, Middaugh JP, Etzel RA. Methyl tertiary butly ether in human blood after exposure to oxygenated fuel in Fairbanks, Alaska. Arch Environ Health 1994;49(5):402-409.

Nihlen A, Lof A, Johanson G. Experimental exposure to methyl *tertiary*-butyl ether. I. Toxicokinetics in humans. Toxicol Appl Pharmacol 1998;148:274-280.

Romieu I, Ramirez M, Meneses F, Ashley D, Lemire S, Colome S, et al. Environmental exposure to volatile organic compounds among workers in Mexico City as assessed by personal monitors and blood concentrations. Environ Health Perspect 1999;107(7):511-515.

Rowe BL, Toccalino PL, Moran MJ, Zogorski JS, Price CV. Occurrence and potential human-health relevance of volatile organic compounds in drinking water from domestic wells in the United States. Environ Health Perspect 2007;115(11):1539-1546.

Squillace PJ, Moran MJ, Price CV. VOCs in shallow groundwater in new residential/commercial areas of the United States. Environ Sci Technol 2004;38(20):5327-5338.

United States Environmental Protection Agency (U.S. EPA). Advance notice of proposed rulemaking to control MTBE in gasoline. Regulatory Announcement. Office of Transportation and Air Quality. Federal Register: March 24, 2000 (Volume 65,

Number 58) [online]. Available at URL: http://www.epa.gov/EPA-TOX/2000/March/Day-24/t7323 htm. 4/21/09

United States Department of Energy (U.S. DOE). Status and impact of state MTBE ban. 2003 [online]. Available at URL: http://www.eia.doe.gov/oiaf/servicerpt/mtbeban/. 4/21/09

United States Department of Energy (U.S. DOE). Eliminating MTBE in gasoline in 2006. 2006 [online]. Available at URL: http://www.eia.doe.gov/pub/oil_gas/petroleum/feature_articles/2006/mtbe2006/mtbe2006.pdf. 4/21/09

White MC, Johnson CA, Ashley DL, Buchta TM, Pelletier DJ. Exposure to methyl tertiary-butyl ether from oxygenated gasoline in Stamford, Connecticut. Arch Environ Health. 1995;50(3):183-189.

# Nitrobenzene

CAS No. 98-95-3

## General Information

Nitrobenzene is a synthetic aromatic chemical made from benzene and used to manufacture aniline, which is in turn, is used to make some types of polyurethanes. Nitrobenzene is also used in the synthesis of other chemicals, including pesticides, dyes, and explosives and as a solvent in petroleum refining. Less common or discontinued applications include use in shoe polish, special lubricating oils, and as an almond flavoring. Environmental sources for nitrobenzene include emissions from its production or use and the atmospheric chemical reaction of benzene with nitrogen oxides. Nitrobenzene was detected infrequently at low levels in ambient air taken in urban, rural and waste disposal areas in the 1970s and 1980s (IPCS, 2003). Nitrobenzene was rarely detected in surface and industrial effluent water and was not detected in soil and sediment specimens obtained from selected locations in the United States (IPCS, 2003).

The general population can be exposed infrequently to nitrobenzene in contaminated air and water. Workers may be exposed to nitrobenzene during its use or production. Nitrobenzene is absorbed after dermal, inhalational, or oral exposure and then metabolized to various intermediates. About 10 to 20 percent of a dose is eliminated in the urine as $p$-nitrophenol, which is used in biological monitoring of occupational exposures. A smaller fraction of a dose is eliminated in urine as $p$-aminophenol (Astier, 1992; IARC, 1996). The nitroreduced metabolites of nitrobenzene may mediate some toxic effects (e.g., methemoglobinemia or carcinogenicity) (IPCS, 2003).

Human health effects from nitrobenzene at low environmental doses or at biomonitored levels from low environmental exposures are unknown. People having accidental exposures to large amounts of nitrobenzene have developed methemoglobinemia, hemolytic anemia, and toxic hepatitis (IARC, 1996). In animals treated with high doses of nitrobenzene, methemoglobinemia, testicular atrophy and reduced sperm counts, and increased liver and kidney weights were observed (NTP, 2002). In animals exposed to high concentrations of nitrobenzene in air, multiple tumors were observed, depending on gender, including lung, thyroid, mammary gland, liver, and kidney tumors (Cattley et al., 1994; NTP, 2002). Nitrobenzene is classified by IARC as a possible human carcinogen and by NTP as reasonably anticipated to be human carcinogen. The U.S. EPA has established environmental standards for nitrobenzene. Workplace standards and guidelines for nitrobenzene have been established by OSHA and ACGIH, respectively. The ACGIH recommends biological exposure indices to monitor workplace exposure. Information about external exposure (ie., environmental levels) and health effects is available from ATSDR at: http://www.atsdr.cdc.gov/toxpro2.html.

## Biomonitoring Information

Levels of nitrobenzene in blood reflect recent exposure. In

## Blood Nitrobenzene

Geometric mean and selected percentiles of blood concentrations (in ng/mL) for the U.S. population from the National Health and Nutrition Examination Survey.

| | Survey years# | Geometric mean (95% conf. interval) | 50th | 75th | 90th | 95th | Sample size |
|---|---|---|---|---|---|---|---|
| **Total** | 03-04 | * | < LOD | < LOD | < LOD | < LOD | 1066 |
| **Age group** | | | | | | | |
| 20-59 years | 03-04 | * | < LOD | < LOD | < LOD | < LOD | 1066 |
| **Gender** | | | | | | | |
| Males | 03-04 | * | < LOD | < LOD | < LOD | < LOD | 529 |
| Females | 03-04 | * | < LOD | < LOD | < LOD | < LOD | 537 |
| **Race/ethnicity** | | | | | | | |
| Mexican Americans | 03-04 | * | < LOD | < LOD | < LOD | < LOD | 206 |
| Non-Hispanic blacks | 03-04 | * | < LOD | < LOD | < LOD | < LOD | 205 |
| Non-Hispanic whites | 03-04 | * | < LOD | < LOD | < LOD | < LOD | 564 |

Limit of detection (LOD, see Data Analysis section) for Survey year 03-04 is 0.3.
# Survey period 2003-2004 is a one-half subsample of 20-59 year olds.
< LOD means less than the limit of detection, which may vary for some chemicals by year and by individual sample.
* Not calculated: proportion of results below limit of detection was too high to provide a valid result.

the NHANES 2003-2004 subsample, nitrobenzene was not detected. Finding a measureable amount of nitrobenzene in blood does not mean that the level of nitrobenzene causes an adverse health effect. Biomonitoring studies of blood nitrobenzene can provide physicians and public health officials with reference values so that they can determine whether or not people have been exposed to higher levels of nitrobenzene than levels found in the general population. Biomonitoring data can also help scientists plan and conduct research on exposure and health effects.

### References

Astier A. Simultaneous high-performance liquid chromatographic determination of urinary metabolites of benzene, nitrobenzene, toluene, xylene and styrene. J Chromatogr 1992;573(2):318-22.

Cattley RC, Everitt JI, Gross EA, Moss OR, Hamm TE Jr, Popp JA. Carcinogenicity and toxicity of inhaled nitrobenzene in B6C3F1 mice and F344 and CD rats. Fundam Appl Toxicol 1994;22(3):328-40. Erratum in: Fundam Appl Toxicol 1995;25(1):159.

International Agency for Research on Cancer (IARC). IARC Monographs on the Evaluation of Carcinogenic Risks to Humans. Volume 65. Printing Processes and Printing inks, Carbon black and Some Nitro Compounds. Summary of Data Reported and Evaluation 1996 [online]. Available at URL: http://monographs. iarc fr/ENG/Monographs/vol65/volume65.pdf. 4/21/09

International Programme on Chemical Safety-INCHEM (IPCS). Environmental Health Criteria 230. Nitrobenzene. 2003 [online]. Available at URL: http://www.inchem.org/documents/ehc/ehc/ehc230 htm. 4/21/09

National Toxicology Program (NTP). Report on Carcinogens Background Document for Nitrobenzene. 2002 [online]. Available at URL: http://ntp niehs nih.gov/ntp/newhomeroc/roc11/NBPub.pdf. 4/21/09

# Styrene
CAS No. 100425

## General Information

Styrene is a high production, hydrocarbon chemical used to manufacture of polystyrene resins, which are widely used in plastic packaging, disposal cups and containers, insulation, adhesives, and in composite materials such as fiberglass. It is also used to produce synthetic rubber and latex. Because styrene is synthesized largely from ethylbenzene, it may be present in products made from styrene. Styrene is commonly detected in urban air, especially near industrial sites where it is produced and used, and in high motor vehicle traffic areas. Air concentrations of styrene may be greater indoors than outdoors, as a result of emissions from photocopiers and laser printers, cigarette smoke, and consumer products in the home (ATSDR, 2007; Wallace et al., 1987). Styrene does not persist in the aquatic or soil environments because of its volatility and is rarely detected in U.S. groundwater or drinking water supplies (USGS, 2006).

For the general population, inhalation of styrene is the primary exposure route. Trace amounts can be ingested when styrene migrates from packaging into foods. Styrene is well absorbed by inhalation, ingestion or dermal routes. Workplace exposure may occur during the production of styrene or products derived from styrene. After absorption, styrene is metabolized within hours by the liver. The main urinary excretion products are mandelic acid and phenylglyoxylic acid, which have been used in monitoring workplace exposure (ATSDR, 2007; Brugnone et al., 1993; Ramsey et al., 1980). The U.S. EPA has established a drinking water and other environmental standards for styrene. Workplace standards and guidelines for styrene have been established by OSHA and ACGIH, respectively. The ACGIH recommends biological exposure indices to monitor workplace exposure.

Human health effects from styrene at low environmental doses or at biomonitored levels from low environmental exposures are unknown. Eye and upper respiratory tract irritation occur after several hours of exposure to air concentrations that exceed the occupational standard for workers. Several studies of chronic occupational exposure to styrene reported neurological effects, including altered color vision, vestibular dysfunction, impaired hearing and altered performance on neuropsychological and neurophysiological tests (ATSDR, 2007). Various studies of workers with styrene exposure have not provided

## Blood Styrene

Geometric mean and selected percentiles of blood concentrations (in ng/mL) for the U.S. population from the National Health and Nutrition Examination Survey.

| | Survey years# | Geometric mean (95% conf. interval) | Selected percentiles (95% confidence interval) | | | | Sample size |
|---|---|---|---|---|---|---|---|
| | | | 50th | 75th | 90th | 95th | |
| **Total** | 01-02 | * | < LOD | .080 (.050-.100) | .130 (.090-.200) | .200 (.140-.260) | 950 |
| | 03-04 | * | < LOD | .050 (.044-.061) | .089 (.081-.097) | .120 (.110-.130) | 1245 |
| **Age group** | | | | | | | |
| 20-59 years | 01-02 | * | < LOD | .080 (.050-.100) | .130 (.090-.200) | .200 (.140-.260) | 950 |
| | 03-04 | * | < LOD | .050 (.044-.061) | .089 (.081-.097) | .120 (.110-.130) | 1245 |
| **Gender** | | | | | | | |
| Males | 01-02 | * | < LOD | .080 (.050-.110) | .140 (.100-.230) | .220 (.140-.340) | 445 |
| | 03-04 | * | < LOD | .056 (.045-.068) | .089 (.081-.100) | .120 (.095-.150) | 608 |
| Females | 01-02 | * | < LOD | .070 (.050-.100) | .120 (.090-.180) | .180 (.120-.260) | 505 |
| | 03-04 | * | < LOD | .048 (.040-.060) | .090 (.074-.100) | .110 (.097-.140) | 637 |
| **Race/ethnicity** | | | | | | | |
| Mexican Americans | 01-02 | * | < LOD | .050 (.030-.070) | .090 (.070-.110) | .120 (.090-.470) | 225 |
| | 03-04 | * | < LOD | < LOD | .049 (.033-.066) | .062 (.048-.100) | 241 |
| Non-Hispanic blacks | 01-02 | * | .040 (<LOD-.080) | .100 (.040-.180) | .180 (.110-.350) | .300 (.170-1.00) | 192 |
| | 03-04 | * | < LOD | .060 (.047-.077) | .100 (.077-.130) | .130 (.110-.160) | 264 |
| Non-Hispanic whites | 01-02 | * | .030 (<LOD-.050) | .080 (.050-.110) | .130 (.090-.210) | .200 (.130-.260) | 462 |
| | 03-04 | * | < LOD | .056 (.046-.067) | .096 (.083-.110) | .130 (.110-.140) | 646 |

Limits of detection (LOD, see Data Analysis section) for Survey years 01-02 and 03-04 are 0.03 and 0.03.
# Survey period 2001-2002 is a one-third subsample of 20-59 year olds; Survey period 2003-2004 is a one-half subsample of 20-59 year olds.
< LOD means less than the limit of detection, which may vary for some chemicals by year and by individual sample.
* Not calculated: proportion of results below limit of detection was too high to provide a valid result.

clear evidence of an increased risk for reproductive or developmental effects, or cancer (ATSDR, 2007), but increased serum prolactin levels have been correlated with levels of its urinary metabolite (Mutti et al., 1984) and levels of styrene in blood (Luderer et al., 2004) in both male and female workers.

Animal carcinogenicity studies have shown variable results, including lung tumors in mice and no increase in tumor incidence in rats (IARC, 2002). Styrene-7, 8-oxide, a biological metabolite of styrene and also a chemical used in making fragrances and epoxy resins, is classified as a probable human carcinogen by IARC and is reasonably anticipated to be human carcinogen by NTP. Styrene is classified as a possible human carcinogen by IARC. Additional information about external exposure (ie., environmental levels) and health effects is available from ATSDR at: http://www.atsdr.cdc.gov/toxpro2.html.

## Biomonitoring Information

Levels of styrene in blood reflect recent exposure. In NHANES 2003-2004 subsample, levels of styrene in blood are of a similar range to those found in a non-representative sample of adults in NHANES III (1988-1994) (Ashley et al., 1994; Churchill et al., 2001). Other small studies of the U.S. general population have reported similar or slightly higher blood styrene levels (Bonanno et al., Buckley, et al., 1997; Sexton et al., 2005 and 2006). Blood styrene levels can be three to fourfold higher in smokers than nonsmokers (Ashley et al., 1995; Bonanno et al., 2001), but exposure to environmental tobacco smoke or vehicle exhaust in urban areas has not been associated with higher blood styrene levels (Bonanno et al., 2001; Romieu et al., 1999). Workers exposed to styrene can have blood levels that are 25 times higher than those in the general population (Brugnone et al., 1993; Triebig et al., 1985).

Finding a measureable amount of styrene in blood does not mean that the level of styrene causes an adverse health effect. Biomonitoring studies of blood styrene can provide physicians and public health officials with reference values so that they can determine whether or not people have been exposed to higher levels of styrene than levels found in the general population. Biomonitoring data can also help scientists plan and conduct research on exposure and health effects.

## References

Agency for Toxic Substances and Disease Registry (ATSDR). Toxicological profile for styrene draft. Atlanta GA. September 2007 [online]. Available at URL: http://www.atsdr.cdc.gov/toxprofiles/tp53.html. 4/15/08

Ashley DL, Bonin MA, Cardinali FL, McCraw JM, Wooten JV. Blood concentrations of volatile organic compounds in a nonoccupationally exposed US population and in groups with suspected exposure. Clin Chem 1994;40(7 Pt 2):1401-1404.

Ashley DL, Bonin MA, Hamar B, McGeehin MA. Removing the smoking confounder from blood volatile organic compounds measurements. Environ Res 1995;71:39-45.

Bonanno LJ, Freeman NCG, Greenberg M, Lioy PJ. Multivariate analysis on levels of selected metals, particulate matter, VOC, and household characteristics and activities from the Midwestern states NHEXAS. Appl Occup Environ Hyg 2001;6(9):859-874.

Brugnone F, Perbellini L, Wang GZ, Maranelli G, Raineri E, De Rosa E, et al. Blood styrene concentrations in a "normal" population and in exposed workers 16 hours after the end of the workshift. Int Arch Occup Environ Health 1993;65(2):125-130.

Buckley TJ, Liddle J, Ashley DL, Paschal DC, Burse VW, Needham LL. Environmental and biomarker measurements in nine homes in the lower Rio Grande Valley: multimedia results for pesticides, metals, PAHs and VOCs. Environ Int 1997;23(5):705-732.

Churchill JE, Ashley DL, Kaye WE. Recent chemical exposures and blood volatile organic compound levels in a large population-based sample. Arch Environ Health 2001;56(2):157-166.

International Agency for Research on Cancer (IARC). IARC Monographs on the Evaluation of Carcinogenic Risks to Humans. Volume 82. Some Traditional Herbal Medicines, Some Mycotoxins, Naphthalene and Styrene Summary of Data Reported and Evaluation. Lyon, France. 2002 [online]. Available at URL: http://monographs.iarc.fr/ENG/Monographs/vol82/volume82.pdf. 4/15/08

Luderer U, Tornero-Velez R, Shay T, Rappaport S, Heyer N, Echeverria D. Temporal association between serum prolactin concentration and exposure to styrene. Occup Environ Med. 2004:61(4):325-333.

Mutti A, Vescovi PP, Falzoi M, Arfini G, Valenti G, Franchini I. Neuroendocrine effects of styrene on occupationally exposed workers. Scand J Work Environ Health. 1984;10(4):225-228.

Ramsey JC, Young JD, Karbowski RJ, Chenoweth MB, McCarty LP, Braun WH. Pharmacokinetics of inhaled styrene in human volunteers. Toxicol Appl Pharmacol 1980;53:54-63.

Romieu I, Ramirez M, Meneses F, Ashley D, Lemire S, Colome S, et al. Environmental exposure to volatile organic compounds among workers in Mexico City as assessed by personal monitors and blood concentrations. Environ Health Perspect 1999;107(7):511-515.

Sexton K, Adgate JL, Church TR, Ashley DL, Needham LL, Ramachandran G, et al. Children's exposure to volatile organic compounds as determined by longitudinal measurements in blood. Environ Health Perspect 2005;113(3):342-349.

Sexton K, Adgate JL, Fredrickson AL, Ryan AD, Needham LL, Ashley DL. Using biologic markers in blood to assess exposure to multiple environmental chemicals for inner-city children 3-6 years of age. Environ Health Perspect 2006;114(3):453-459.

Triebig G, Schaller K-H, Valentin H. Investigations on neurotoxicity of chemical substances at the workplace. VII. Longitudinal study with determination of nerve conductions velocities in persons occupationally exposed to styrene. Int Arch Occup Environ Health. 1985;56:239-247.

United States Geological Survey (USGS). Volatile organic compounds in the nation's ground water and drinking-water supply wells. Reston VA. 2006 [online]. Available at URL: http://pubs.usgs.gov/circ/circ1292/. 4/15/08

Wallace LA, Pellizzari ED, Hartwell TD, Sparacino C, Whitmore R, Sheldon L, et al. The TEAM study: personal exposures to toxic substances in air, drinking water, and breath of 400 residents of New Jersey, North Carolina, and North Dakota. Environ Res 1987;43:290-307.

# Toluene

CAS No. 108-88-3

## General Information

Toluene (methylbenzene) is a flammable, liquid, aromatic hydrocarbon. It is a high production chemical isolated from crude oil. Toluene is used widely as a solvent and to synthesize chemicals such as benzene, trinitrotoluene, and toluene diisocyanate. As with other aromatic solvents, it is a minor component of gasoline, and additives containing toluene are used as octane boosters. Toluene is detected frequently in urban air, especially in high motor traffic areas and near industrial areas or hazardous waste sites (ATSDR, 2000; Mukund et al., 1996). Indoor air levels of toluene can exceed outdoor levels, largely due to consumer products (e.g., nail polish solvent, adhesive glues, paints, and paint thinner) and cigarette smoke (ATSDR, 2000; Gordon et al., 1999). Toluene does not persist in soil due to its volatility and is not detected commonly in U.S. groundwater and drinking water supplies (USGS, 2006).

The general population is exposed to toluene mainly by breathing contaminated air. Workplace exposure to toluene may occur during the production and use of petrochemicals and solvents. Toluene is well absorbed by inhalation, dermal, and oral exposure routes. After absorption, toluene is metabolized rapidly by hepatic microsomal enzymes, and the major urinary excretion product is hippuric acid. Other urinary metabolites include *ortho*- and *para*-cresol, S-benzylmercapturic acid, and S-*para*-toluylmercapturic acid.

Human health effects from toluene at low environmental doses or at biomonitored levels from low environmental exposures are unknown. Humans exposed to high levels of toluene in air for a short time can show central nervous system depression (lassitude, stupor, and coma). Persons with short term exposures to toluene at levels higher than workplace air standards have shown poor performance on cognitive tests, neurobehavioral impairment, and eye and upper respiratory tract irritation (ATSDR, 2000). Its distinctive aromatic smell is detectable well below workplace air standards. Chronic solvent inhalant abuse, usually involving toluene and other volatile hydrocarbons, has resulted in permanent brain damage with dementia (Filley et al., 2004). Chronic occupational exposures at levels exceeding workplace standards have damaged hearing and possibly color vision (Lomax et al., 2004). In animal studies, prenatal toluene exposure impaired fetal

## Blood Toluene

Geometric mean and selected percentiles of blood concentrations (in ng/mL) for the U.S. population from the National Health and Nutrition Examination Survey.

| | Survey years# | Geometric mean (95% conf. interval) | Selected percentiles ( 95% confidence interval) | | | | Sample size |
|---|---|---|---|---|---|---|---|
| | | | 50th | 75th | 90th | 95th | |
| Total | 01-02 | .156 (.122-.198) | .160 (.120-.220) | .340 (.260-.430) | .670 (.480-.950) | 1.06 (.700-1.43) | 954 |
| | 03-04 | .114 (.100-.129) | .096 (.087-.110) | .220 (.180-.260) | .430 (.380-.550) | .680 (.560-.880) | 1336 |
| Age group | | | | | | | |
| 20-59 years | 01-02 | .156 (.122-.198) | .160 (.120-.220) | .340 (.260-.430) | .670 (.480-.950) | 1.06 (.700-1.43) | 954 |
| | 03-04 | .114 (.100-.129) | .096 (.087-.110) | .220 (.180-.260) | .430 (.380-.550) | .680 (.560-.880) | 1336 |
| Gender | | | | | | | |
| Males | 01-02 | .165 (.130-.209) | .170 (.120-.230) | .360 (.260-.520) | .780 (.580-1.06) | 1.22 (.850-1.43) | 450 |
| | 03-04 | .128 (.112-.148) | .110 (.096-.130) | .250 (.190-.310) | .500 (.380-.660) | .730 (.590-1.10) | 647 |
| Females | 01-02 | .147 (.114-.190) | .150 (.110-.220) | .320 (.240-.390) | .550 (.400-.740) | .810 (.530-1.63) | 504 |
| | 03-04 | .101 (.086-.118) | .085 (.070-.100) | .190 (.150-.230) | .410 (.340-.500) | .580 (.480-.750) | 689 |
| Race/ethnicity | | | | | | | |
| Mexican Americans | 01-02 | .136 (.106-.176) | .140 (.080-.210) | .270 (.210-.340) | .550 (.400-.980) | .990 (.500-1.30) | 219 |
| | 03-04 | .084 (.074-.096) | .076 (.064-.091) | .120 (.100-.170) | .280 (.170-.410) | .400 (.310-.620) | 253 |
| Non-Hispanic blacks | 01-02 | .137 (.089-.210) | .150 (.070-.200) | .310 (.200-.460) | .690 (.390-1.19) | 1.15 (.660-1.69) | 194 |
| | 03-04 | .105 (.077-.144) | .095 (.070-.130) | .200 (.130-.330) | .440 (.290-.620) | .620 (.480-.710) | 297 |
| Non-Hispanic whites | 01-02 | .165 (.125-.217) | .170 (.120-.240) | .350 (.270-.450) | .710 (.450-1.12) | 1.14 (.710-1.63) | 467 |
| | 03-04 | .123 (.110-.139) | .100 (.092-.120) | .240 (.210-.280) | .500 (.400-.590) | .750 (.590-.940) | 685 |

Limits of detection (LOD, see Data Analysis section) for Survey years 01-02 and 03-04 are 0.025 and 0.025.
\# Survey period 2001-2002 is a one-third subsample of 20-59 year olds; Survey period 2003-2004 is a one-half subsample of 20-59 year olds.

growth and skeletal development, and altered behavioral development in the offspring (ADSDR, 2000; Jones and Balster, 1997). Evidence for human reproductive effects is inconclusive, and reports of developmental effects have been reported mainly in children exposed *in utero* by maternal solvent abuse (Bukowski, 2001). Epidemiologic studies of workers exposed to toluene (or toluene together with other solvents) have not demonstrated increased risks for cancer, and animal studies have not demonstrated an increased incidence of tumors (IARC, 1999). IARC determined that toluene was not classifiable with regard to human carcinogenicity. The U.S. EPA has established a drinking water and other environmental standards for toluene. The FDA has established a bottle water standard and level for toluene as an indirect food additive. OSHA and ACGIH established workplace standards and guidelines, respectively, for toluene. Information about external exposure (i.e., environmental levels) and health effects is available from ATSDR at: http://www.atsdr.cdc.gov/toxpro2.html.

## Biomonitoring Information

Levels of blood toluene reflect recent exposure. A nonrepresentative sample of adults in NHANES III (1988-1994) had geometric mean and median blood toluene levels, respectively, of 0.52 and 0.28 µg/L (Ashley et al., 1994; Churchill et al., 2001), generally higher than comparable levels in NHANES 2001-2002 and 2003-2004. Similar median blood toluene levels have been reported in U.S. children (Sexton et al., 2005, 2006) and in studies of adults without occupational exposure (Backer et al., 1997; Bonanno et al., 2001; Buckley et al., 1997). Population studies in Italy and Mexico have reported median blood toluene levels that were about twice as high as those in the U.S. (Brugnone et al., 1994; Carrer et al., 2000; Lemire et al., 2004; Perbellini et al., 2002). Geometric mean blood toluene levels were 0.191 and 0.669 ng/mL in non-smoking and smoking adults, respectively, from a subsample of NHANES 1999-2000 participants (Lin et al., 2008). Other studies have reported blood toluene levels that were approximately four times higher in smokers than non-smokers (Ashley et al., 1995; Bonanno et al., 2001; Brugnone et al., 1994; Perbellini et al., 2002), but environmental tobacco smoke exposure has not been associated with elevated blood toluene levels (Carrer et al., 2000; Sexton et al., 2005). Exposure to gasoline fumes can increase blood toluene levels during self-service refueling (Backer et al., 1997). Vehicle exhaust and gasoline fumes in such occupational settings as gas stations, automobile repair shops, and street vending can result in blood toluene levels that are two to three times higher than background levels (Mannino et al., 1995; Romieu et al., 1999).

Finding a measureable amount of toluene in blood does not mean that the level of toluene causes an adverse health effect. Biomonitoring studies of blood toluene can provide physicians and public health officials with reference values so that they can determine whether or not people have been exposed to higher levels of toluene than levels found in the general population. Biomonitoring data can also help scientists plan and conduct research on exposure and health effects.

## References

Agency for Toxic Substances and Disease Registry (ATSDR). Toxicological profile for toluene update. September 2000 [online]. Available at URL: http://www.atsdr.cdc.gov/toxprofiles/tp56.html. 4/26/09

Ashley DL, Bonin MA, Cardinali FL, McCraw JM, Wooten JV. Blood concentrations of volatile organic compounds in a nonoccupationally exposed US population and in groups with suspected exposure. Clin Chem 1994;40(7 Pt 2):1401-1404.

Ashley DL, Bonin MA, Hamar B, McGeehin MA. Removing the smoking confounder from blood volatile organic compounds measurements. Environ Res 1995;71:39-45.

Backer LC, Egeland GM, Ashley DL, Lawryk NJ, Weisel CP, White MC, et al. Exposure to regular gasoline and ethanol oxyfuel during refueling in Alaska. Environ Health Perspect 1997;105(8):850-855.

Bonanno LJ, Freeman NCG, Greenberg M, Lioy PJ. Multivariate analysis on levels of selected metals, particulate matter, VOC, and household characteristics and activities from the Midwestern states NHEXAS. Appl Occup Environ Hyg 2001;6(9):859-874.

Brugnone F, Perbellini L, Giuliari C, Cerpelloni M, Soave M. Blood and urine concentrations of chemical pollutants in the general population. Med Lav 1994;85(5):370-389.

Buckley TJ, Liddle J, Ashley DL, Paschal DC, Burse VW, Needham LL. Environmental and biomarker measurements in nine homes in the lower Rio Grande Valley: multimedia results for pesticides, metals, PAHs and VOCs. Environ Int 1997;23(5):705-732.

Bukowski JA. Review of the epidemiological evicdence relating toluene to reproductive outcomes. Regul Toxicol Pharmacol 2001;33(2):147-156.

Carrer P, Marconi M, Alcini D, Cavallo D, Fustinoni S, Lovato L, et al., Assessment through environmental and biological measurements of total daily exposure to volatile organic compounds of office workers in Milan, Italy. Indoor Air 2000;10:258-268.

Churchill JE, Ashley DL, Kaye WE. Recent chemical exposures

and blood volatile organic compound levels in a large population-based sample. Arch Environ Health 2001;56(2):157-166.

Filley CM, Halliday W, Kleinschmidt-DeMasters BK. The effects of toluene on the central nervous system. J Neuropathol Exp Neurol 2004;63(1):1-12.

Gordon SM, Callahan PJ, Nishioka MG, Brinkman MC, O'Rourke MK, Lebowitz MD, et al. Residential environmental measurements in the National Human Exposure Assessment Survey (NHEXAS) pilot study in Arizona: preliminary results for pesticides and VOCs. J Exp Anal Environ Epidemiol 1999;9:456-470.

International Agency for Research on Cancer (IARC). IARC Monographs on the Evaluation of Carcinogenic Risks to Humans. Volume 71. Re-Evaluation of Some Organic Chemicals, Hydrazine and Hydrogen Peroxide. Summary of Data Reported and Evaluation 1999 [online]. Available at URL: http://monographs.iarc.fr/ENG/Monographs/vol71/volume71.pdf. 4/27/09

Jones HE, Balster RL. Neurobehavioral consequences of intermittent prenatal exposure to high concentrations of toluene. Neurotoxicol Teratol 1997;19(4):305-313.

Lemire S, Ashley D, Olaya P, Romieu I, Welch S, Meneses-Gonzalez F, et al. Environmental exposure of commuters in Mexico City to volatile organic compounds as assessed by blood concentrations, 1998. Salud Publica Mex 2004;46:32-38.

Lin YS, Egeghy PP, Rappaport SM. Relationships between levels of volatile organic compounds in air and blood from the general population. J Expo Sci Environ Epidemiol 2008;18(4):421-429.

Lomax FB, Ridgway P, Meldrum M. Does occupational exposure to organic solvents affect colour discrimination? Toxicol Rev 2004;23(2):91-121.

Mannino DM, Schreiber J, Aldous K, Ashley D, Moolenaar R, Almaguer D. Human exposure to volatile organic compounds: a comparison of organic vapor monitoring badge levels with blood levels. Int Arch Occup Environ Health 1995;67:59-64.

Mukund R, Kelly TJ, Spicer CW. Source attribution of ambient air toxic and other VOCs in Columbus, Ohio. Atmospheric Environment 1996;30(20):3457-3470.

Perbellini L, Pasini F, Romani S, Princivalle A, Brugnone F. Analysis of benzene, toluene, ethylbenzene and *m*-xylene in biological samples from the general population. J Chromat B 2002;778:198-210.

Romieu I, Ramirez M, Meneses F, Ashley DL, Lemire S, Colome S, et al. Environmental exposure to volatile organic compounds among workers in Mexico City as assessed by personal monitors and blood concentrations. Environ Health Perspect 1999;107(7):511-515.

Sexton K, Adgate JL, Church TR, Ashley DL, Needham LL, Ramachandran G, et al. Children's exposure to volatile organic compounds as determined by longitudinal measurements in blood. Environ Health Perspect 2005;113(3):342-349.

Sexton K, Adgate JL, Fredrickson AL, Ryan AD, Needham LL, Ashley DL. Using biologic markers in blood to assess exposure to multiple environmental chemicals for inner-city children 3-6 years of age. Environ Health Perspect 2006;114(3):453-459.

United States Geological Survey (USGS). Volatile organic compounds in the nation's ground water and drinking-water supply wells. 2006 [online]. Available at URL: http://pubs.usgs.gov/circ/circ1292/. 4/26/09

# Xylenes
CAS No. 1330-20-7

*o*-xylene CAS No. 95-47-6

*m*-xylene CAS No. 108-38-3

*p*-xylene CAS No. 106-42-3

## General Information

Xylenes are aromatic chemicals that exist in three isomeric forms: *o*-, *m*-, and *p*-xylene. Commercial production results in mixed xylenes, which contain these three isomers, in addition to ethylbenzene and trace amounts of several non-xylene hydrocarbons. Specific xylene isomers are produced from mixed xylene and are used to synthesize other chemicals. Mixed xylenes are used widely as gasoline additives; as solvents in manufacturing and laboratory processes; in glues, adhesives, printing inks, paint thinners, and sealants; and as carrier solvents for delivery of some pesticides. Indoor air sources of xylene include building and consumer products, such as adhesives and paints, and also tobacco smoke (ATSDR, 2007). The most important route of exposure for the general population is inhaling volatized xylenes, although dermal contact with liquids containing xylene may also contribute. Workplace exposure to xylenes may occur when producing, transporting, and using petrochemicals and industrial solvents.

Following inhalational, dermal, or oral exposure, xylenes are well absorbed and then rapidly and widely distributed throughout the body tissues, especially adipose tissue. A fraction of an absorbed xylene dose is excreted unchanged in exhaled air, and about 90% of a dose is metabolized by the liver and then eliminated in urine over several days. Methylhippuric acids are the predominant urinary metabolites and have been used to monitor workplace exposures.

Human health effects from xylenes at low environmental doses or at biomonitored levels from low environmental exposures are unknown. Among humans, accidental exposure to high levels of xylene in air can cause eye and mucous membrane irritation, dyspnea, and central nervous system effects, such as headaches, dizziness, forgetfulness, delayed reaction times, and poor coordination (ATSDR, 2007). Epidemiologic studies of cancer and xylene exposure have been inconclusive and are limited by small numbers, lack of exposure measurements, and the concomitant

## Blood *o*-Xylene

Geometric mean and selected percentiles of blood concentrations (in ng/mL) for the U.S. population from the National Health and Nutrition Examination Survey.

| | Survey years# | Geometric mean (95% conf. interval) | Selected percentiles ( 95% confidence interval) | | | | Sample size |
|---|---|---|---|---|---|---|---|
| | | | 50th | 75th | 90th | 95th | |
| **Total** | 01-02 | * | < LOD | .070 (.050-.080) | .100 (.080-.130) | .130 (.110-.180) | 981 |
| | 03-04 | * | < LOD | .051 (<LOD-.057) | .072 (.066-.079) | .090 (.081-.097) | 1365 |
| **Age group** | | | | | | | |
| 20-59 years | 01-02 | * | < LOD | .070 (.050-.080) | .100 (.080-.130) | .130 (.110-.180) | 981 |
| | 03-04 | * | < LOD | .051 (<LOD-.057) | .072 (.066-.079) | .090 (.081-.097) | 1365 |
| **Gender** | | | | | | | |
| Males | 01-02 | * | < LOD | .070 (.050-.090) | .110 (.080-.140) | .150 (.110-.180) | 465 |
| | 03-04 | * | < LOD | .057 (.050-.060) | .074 (.068-.084) | .096 (.084-.110) | 667 |
| Females | 01-02 | * | < LOD | .060 (.050-.080) | .100 (.070-.130) | .120 (.100-.180) | 516 |
| | 03-04 | * | < LOD | < LOD | .067 (.059-.076) | .085 (.074-.095) | 698 |
| **Race/ethnicity** | | | | | | | |
| Mexican Americans | 01-02 | * | < LOD | .060 (<LOD-.080) | .090 (.080-.110) | .120 (.090-.270) | 227 |
| | 03-04 | * | < LOD | .052 (<LOD-.067) | .074 (.067-.080) | .100 (.075-.130) | 265 |
| Non-Hispanic blacks | 01-02 | * | < LOD | .050 (<LOD-.070) | .100 (.080-.110) | .110 (.100-.160) | 197 |
| | 03-04 | * | < LOD | < LOD | .065 (.055-.078) | .084 (.068-.100) | 301 |
| Non-Hispanic whites | 01-02 | * | < LOD | .070 (.050-.090) | .110 (.080-.140) | .140 (.110-.180) | 483 |
| | 03-04 | * | < LOD | .052 (<LOD-.058) | .073 (.066-.082) | .090 (.081-.100) | 694 |

Limits of detection (LOD, see Data Analysis section) for Survey years 01-02 and 03-04 are 0.049 and 0 049.
# Survey period 2001-2002 is a one-third subsample of 20-59 year olds; Survey period 2003-2004 is a one-half subsample of 20-59 year olds.
< LOD means less than the limit of detection, which may vary for some chemicals by year and by individual sample.
* Not calculated: proportion of results below limit of detection was too high to provide a valid result.

exposure to other solvents (IARC, 1999). Animal studies involving high doses showed hepatic enzyme induction, liver enlargement, increased kidney weight and renal cytochrome P450 content, as well as neurobehavioral effects and altered catecholamine levels in the brain (ATSDR 2007). Pregnant animals that inhaled high doses had increased fetal resorptions and offspring with skeletal abnormalities and decreased body weight (ATSDR 2007). Neurobehavioral effects resulted in laboratory animals exposed during gestation to xylene concentrations in the air that were about five times higher than U.S. occupational standards (Hass et al., 1997,1995). Animals exposed to high doses of technical grade xylene by gavage did not demonstrate an increase in the incidence of tumors (NTP, 1986).

Workplace standards for xylene levels in air have been established by OSHA, and ACGIH recommends a biological exposure index to monitor workplace exposure. The U.S. EPA has established a drinking water standard and other environmental standards for xylene. FDA has established a bottled drinking water standard. IARC has determined that xylene is not classifiable with regard to its human carcinogenicity. Information about external exposure (i.e., environmental levels) and health effects is available from ATSDR at: http://www.atsdr.cdc.gov/toxpro2.html.

## Biomonitoring Information

Levels of blood xylenes reflect recent exposure. The *m*- and *p*- xylene isomers usually are measured together and reported as *m/p*-xylene; the *o*-xylene isomer is measured and reported separately. In the NHANES 2001-2002 and 2003-2004 subsamples, blood *o*-xylene was nondetectable in a majority of the participants, whereas the median blood *m/p*-xylene levels were similar to the earlier NHANES III results. In a nonrepresentative subsample of adults in NHANES III (1988-1994), the median blood levels of *o*-xylene and *m/p*-xylene were 0.11 µg/L and 0.19 µg/L, respectively (Ashley et al., 1994). These results were roughly similar to geometric mean levels of nonsmokers reported in a subsample of NHANES 1999-2000 (Lin et al., 2008) and in other studies of the U.S. general population (Bonanno et al., 2001; Buckley et al., 1997; Hamar et al., 1996), and to levels in adults in other countries (Lemire et al., 2002). Blood *o*-xylene levels in U.S. children were two to three times lower than adult levels (Sexton et al., 2005, 2006). Smokers can have blood *o*- and *m/p*-xylene levels that are each about twice as high as those for nonsmokers (Ashley et al., 1995; Bonanno et al., 2001; Lin et al., 2008).

## Blood *m*- and *p*-Xylene

Geometric mean and selected percentiles of blood concentrations (in ng/mL) for the U.S. population from the National Health and Nutrition Examination Survey.

| | Survey years# | Geometric mean (95% conf. interval) | 50th | 75th | 90th | 95th | Sample size |
|---|---|---|---|---|---|---|---|
| | | | Selected percentiles (95% confidence interval) | | | | |
| **Total** | 01-02 | .156 (.124-.198) | .150 (.110-.200) | .280 (.190-.430) | .500 (.370-.690) | .670 (.500-.890) | 962 |
| | 03-04 | .136 (.123-.150) | .130 (.120-.150) | .200 (.190-.210) | .280 (.260-.300) | .340 (.310-.400) | 1346 |
| **Age group** | | | | | | | |
| 20-59 years | 01-02 | .156 (.124-.198) | .150 (.110-.200) | .280 (.190-.430) | .500 (.370-.690) | .670 (.500-.890) | 962 |
| | 03-04 | .136 (.123-.150) | .130 (.120-.150) | .200 (.190-.210) | .280 (.260-.300) | .340 (.310-.400) | 1346 |
| **Gender** | | | | | | | |
| Males | 01-02 | .155 (.121-.200) | .140 (.110-.190) | .280 (.180-.440) | .510 (.350-.700) | .700 (.500-.890) | 455 |
| | 03-04 | .149 (.134-.166) | .140 (.130-.170) | .220 (.200-.230) | .290 (.270-.320) | .380 (.300-.490) | 654 |
| Females | 01-02 | .157 (.124-.199) | .150 (.110-.220) | .270 (.190-.410) | .480 (.360-.650) | .650 (.460-.890) | 507 |
| | 03-04 | .124 (.112-.138) | .130 (.110-.140) | .180 (.160-.200) | .270 (.240-.300) | .340 (.290-.390) | 692 |
| **Race/ethnicity** | | | | | | | |
| Mexican Americans | 01-02 | .134 (.097-.184) | .130 (.090-.180) | .240 (.150-.370) | .400 (.290-.540) | .540 (.380-1.10) | 223 |
| | 03-04 | .132 (.109-.160) | .120 (.110-.150) | .180 (.140-.230) | .250 (.220-.320) | .360 (.260-.490) | 257 |
| Non-Hispanic blacks | 01-02 | .147 (.107-.202) | .140 (.090-.220) | .280 (.160-.460) | .470 (.330-.850) | .590 (.420-1.08) | 198 |
| | 03-04 | .117 (.094-.146) | .120 (.099-.140) | .170 (.140-.220) | .270 (.210-.330) | .330 (.260-.450) | 297 |
| Non-Hispanic whites | 01-02 | .163 (.124-.214) | .160 (.110-.220) | .300 (.190-.480) | .520 (.370-.740) | .700 (.510-.960) | 468 |
| | 03-04 | .141 (.128-.155) | .140 (.130-.150) | .210 (.190-.220) | .290 (.270-.310) | .350 (.330-.400) | 690 |

Limits of detection (LOD, see Data Analysis section) for Survey years 01-02 and 03-04 are 0.034 and 0.034.
# Survey period 2001-2002 is a one-third subsample of 20-59 year olds; Survey period 2003-2004 is a one-half subsample of 20-59 year olds.

Workers who are exposed to vehicle exhaust can have *o*- and *m/p*-xylene blood levels that are each about two to three times higher than levels in the general population (Backer et al., 1997; Mannino et al., 1995; Romieu et al., 1999).

Finding a measurable amount of any of the xylenes in blood does not mean that the level of xylene causes an adverse health effect. Biomonitoring studies of blood xylenes can provide physicians and public health officials with reference values so that they can determine whether or not people have been exposed to higher levels of xylenes than levels found in the general population. Biomonitoring data can also help scientists plan and conduct research on exposure and health effects.

## References

Agency for Toxic Substances and Disease Registry (ATSDR). Toxicological profile for xylene. 2007 [online]. Available at URL: http://www.atsdr.cdc.gov/toxprofiles/tp71 html#bookmark07. 7/1/08

Ashley DL, Bonin MA, Cardinali FL, McCraw JM, Wooten JV. Blood concentrations of volatile organic compounds in a nonoccupationally exposed US population and in groups with suspected exposure. Clin Chem 1994;40(7 Pt 2):1401-1404.

Ashley DL, Bonin MA, Hamar B, McGeehin MA. Removing the smoking confounder from blood volatile organic compounds measurements. Environ Res 1995;71:39-45.

Backer LC, Egeland GM, Ashley DL, Lawryk NJ, Weisel CP, White MC, et al. Exposure to regular gasoline and ethanol oxyfuel during refueling in Alaska. Environ Health Perspect 1997;105(8):850-855.

Bonanno LJ, Freeman NCG, Greenberg M, Lioy PJ. Multivariate analysis on levels of selected metals, particulate matter, VOC, and household characteristics and activities from the Midwestern states NHEXAS. Appl Occup Environ Hyg 2001;6(9):859-874.

Buckley TJ, Liddle J, Ashley DL, Paschal DC, Burse VW, Needham LL. Environmental and biomarker measurements in nine homes in the lower Rio Grande Valley: multimedia results for pesticides, metals, PAHs and VOCs. Environ Int 1997;23(5):705-732.

Hamar GB, McGeehin MA, Phifer BL, Ashley DL. Volatile organic compound testing of a population living near a hazardous waste site. J Exp Anal Environ Epidemiol 1996;6(2):247-255.

Hass U, Lund SP, Simonsen L. Long-lasting neurobehavioral effects of prenatal exposure to xylene in rats. Neurotoxicology 1997;18(2):547-551.

Hass U, Lund SP, Simonsen L, Fries AS. Effects of prenatal

exposure to xylene on postnatal development and behavior in rats. Neurotoxicol Teratol 1995;17(3):341-349.

International Agency for Research on Cancer (IARC). Volume 71.Re-Evaluation of Some Organic Chemicals, Hydrazine and Hydrogen Peroxide. 1999 [online]. Available at URL: http://monographs.iarc fr/ENG/Monographs/vol71/volume71.pdf. 7/1/08

Lemire S, Ashley D, Olaya P, Romieu I, Welch S, Meneses-Gonzalez F, Hernandez-Avila M. Environmental exposure of commuters in Mexico City to volatile orgnic compounds as assessed by blood concentrations, 1998. Salud Publica Mex 004;46:32-38.

Lin YS, Egeghy PP, Rappaport SM. Relationships between levels of volatile organic compounds in air and blood from the general population. J Expo Sci Environ Epidemiol 2008;18(4):421-429.

Mannino DM, Schreiber J, Aldous K, Ashley D, Moolenaar R, Almaguer D. Human exposure to volatile organic compounds: a comparison of organic vapor monitoring badge levels with blood levels. Int Arch Occp Environ Health 1995;67:59-64.

National Toxicology Program (NTP). Toxicology and carcinogenesis studies of xylenes (mixed) (60% m-xylene, 14% p-xylene, 9% o-xylene, and 17% ethylbenzene) (CAS No. 1330-20-7) in F344/N rats and B6C3Fl mice (gavage studies). 1986 [online]. Available at URL: http://ntp.niehs.nih.gov/ntp/htdocs/LT_rpts/tr327.pdf. 7/1/08

Romieu I, Ramirez M, Meneses F, Ashley DL, Lemire S, Colome S, et al. Environmental exposure to volatile organic compounds among workers in Mexico City as assessed by personal monitors and blood concentrations. Environ Health Perspect 1999;107(7):511-515.

Sexton K, Adgate JL, Church TR, Ashley DL, Needham LL, Ramachandran G, et al. Children's exposure to volatile organic compounds as determined by longitudinal measurements in blood. Environ Health Perspect 2005;113(3):342-349.

Sexton K, Adgate JL, Fredrickson AL, Ryan AD, Needham LL, Ashley DL. Using biologic markers in blood to assess exposure to multiple environmental chemicals for inner-city children 3-6 years of age. Environ Health Perspect 2006;114(3):453-459.

# Appendix A. Procedure to Estimate Percentiles

## Including percentiles whose estimate falls on a value that is repeated multiple times in the dataset

A common practice to calculate confidence intervals from survey data is to use large-sample normal approximations. Ninety-five percent confidence intervals on point estimates of percentiles are often computed by adding and subtracting from the point estimate a quantity equal to twice its standard error. This normal approximation method may not be adequate, however, when estimating the proportion of subjects above or below a selected value, especially when the proportion is near 0.0 or 1.0 or when the effective sample size is small. In addition, confidence intervals on proportions deviating from 0.5 are not theoretically expected to be symmetric around the point estimate. Further, adding and subtracting a multiple of the standard error to an estimate near 0.0 or 1.0 can lead to impossible confidence limits (i.e., proportion estimates below 0.0 or above 1.0). The approach used for the *Report* data tables (and for previous *Reports*) produces asymmetric confidence intervals consistent with skewed (nonnormal) biologic data distributions.

The method we use to estimate percentiles and their confidence limits for the *Report* data tables and for previous reports is adapted from a method proposed by Woodruff (1952) for percentile estimation and a method described by Korn and Graubard (1998) for estimating confidence intervals for proportions. This method essentially involves first obtaining an empirical point estimate of the desired percentile by creating a rank ordered listing of the sampled observations along with their sampling weights. From this listing and the sampling weights, it is possible to determine an empirical percentile estimate for the target population. After this point estimate of the percentile has been obtained, the fraction of results below the estimate is calculated. The fraction below the point estimate should be very close to the proportion corresponding to the desired percentile, but can deviate from this proportion depending on the frequency of non-unique sampled observations in the vicinity of the empirical percentile estimate and depending on the sampling weight associated with the sampled observation. For example, when measuring some compounds as part of NHANES there may be multiple results below a common limit of detection (LOD) or multiple results with identical measured values due to the reporting limitations of the instrument. This phenomenon coupled with the sampling weight assigned to each measured result and with the limitations of statistical software can lead to difficulties in accurately estimating some percentiles and their corresponding confidence limits because an exact percentile may fall within a large group of results with identical measured values. We circumvented this potential problem for the *Report* data tables by adding a unique, negligibly small number to each measured result. This small number was later subtracted from the percentile estimate without affecting the percentile estimate and without altering any of the original measured results.

By adding a unique, negligibly small number to each sampled observation, it was possible to associate a single sampled observation with the percentile estimate and thus to minimize the difference between the fraction below the point estimate and the proportion corresponding to the desired percentile. However, due to sample weighting, it is still possible to obtain a different point estimate (which will only differ by the difference between numerically adjacent analyte values) depending on how the data are sorted before adding the unique number to each result. We circumvented this potential problem by replacing actual sample weights with an average sample weight where the average is computed across subjects in the same demographic domain who have identical measured results. We computed standard error estimates in a separate step using the original (unaltered) data. Clopper-Pearson 95% confidence intervals around the estimated proportion are obtained using the method described by Korn and Graubard (1998).

We describe below how SAS Proc Univariate and SUDAAN can be used to carry out this method of percentile and confidence interval estimation. SAS code for calculating these confidence intervals can be downloaded from http://www.cdc.gov/exposurereport. In the narrative that follows, the term 'demographic domain' refers to a demographic group of interest, for example non-Hispanic blacks. The term 'set of subsample weights' refers to the sampling weights that correspond to the variable for which percentiles will be estimated, for example the set of subsample weights associated with total blood mercury measurements. The term 'analyte' refers to the biological or chemical compound measured in a group of subjects and for which percentiles are to be estimated.

**Procedure to calculate percentile estimates and their confidence intervals**

**Step 1:** Obtain a percentile estimate using the original (unaltered data):

Create a separate file with original data (ORIG_DATA). Use SAS (SAS Institute Inc. 1999) Proc Univariate (with default percentile definition equivalent to option PCTLDEF = 5 and with the Freq option variable equal to the original subsample sampling weight) to obtain a point estimate of the percentile (PTLE_ORIG) of an analyte's original results for the demographic domain of interest, for example, the 90th percentile of blood lead results for children aged 1-5 years.

**Step 2:** Obtain a percentile estimate using the altered data:

Create a separate file for use with altered data (ALTR_DATA). Sort the data by analyte measured value separately for each particular demographic domain and set of subsample weights. Use SAS Proc Means to compute the average sampling weight ($WT_{AVE}$) for each unique measured result. For each unique measured result, use a counter from 1 to the total number of subjects with identical values to create a unique integer to associate with each measured observation. Each of these numbers should then be divided by 1,000,000,000 and added to the corresponding measured observation. This will result in each measured observation having an additional fractional amount beyond the fourth decimal as long as there are less than 10,000 subjects with the same measured result. Use SAS Proc Univariate (again with default percentile definition equivalent to option PCTLDEF = 5 but now with the Freq option variable equal to $WT_{AVE}$) to obtain a point estimate of the percentile (PTLE_ALTR) of an analyte's altered results for the demographic domain of interest.

**Step 3:** Sort the data in the ORIG_DATA file by the stratum (sdmvstra) and primary sampling unit (sdmvpsu) variables. Use SUDAAN (SUDAAN Users Manual, 2001) Proc Descript with Taylor Linearization DESIGN = WR (i.e., sampling with replacement), with proper NEST statement, and with the original subsample sampling weight variable to estimate the proportion (P_ORIG) of subjects with results below the percentile estimate (PTLE_ORIG) obtained in Step 1 and discard P_ORIG but retain the standard error (SEMEAN_ORIG) associated with PTLE_ORIG.

**Step 4:** Sort the data in the ALTR_DATA file by the stratum (sdmvstra) and primary sampling unit (sdmvpsu) variables. Use SUDAAN (SUDAAN Users Manual, 2001) Proc Descript with Taylor Linearization DESIGN = WR (i.e., sampling with replacement), with proper NEST statement, and with the average sampling weight variable ($WT_{AVE}$) to estimate the proportion (P_ALTR) of subjects with results below the percentile estimate (PTLE_ALTR) obtained in Step 2 and keep P_ALTR but discard the standard error (SEMEAN_ALTR) associated with PTLE_ALTR. Compute the degrees-of-freedom adjusted effective sample size.

(1) $n_{df} = ((t_{num}/t_{denom})^2) P\_ALTR(1 - P\_ALTR)/(SEMEAN\_ORIG^2)$

where $t_{num}$ and $t_{denom}$ are 0.975 critical values of the Student's t distribution with degrees of freedom equal to the actual sample size minus 1 and the number of primary sampling units (PSUs) minus the number of strata, respectively. Note: the degrees of freedom for $t_{denom}$ can vary with the demographic domain of interest (e.g., males).

**Step 5:** After obtaining an estimate of P_ALTR (i.e., the proportion obtained in Step 4), compute the Clopper-Pearson 95% confidence interval ($P_L(x, n_{df})$, $P_U(x, n_{df})$) as follows:

(2) $P_L(x, n_{df}) = v_1 F_{v1,v2}(0.025)/(v_2 + v_1 F_{v1,v2}(0.025))$ & $P_U(x, n_{df}) = v_3 F_{v3,v4}(0.975)/(v_4 + v_3 F_{v3,v4}(0.975))$

where x is equal to P_ALTR times $n_{df}$, $v_1 = 2x$, $v_2 = 2(n_{df} - x + 1)$, $v_3 = 2(x + 1)$, $v_4 = 2(n_{df} - x)$, and $F_{d1,d2}(\beta)$ is the β quantile of an F distribution with $d_1$ and $d_2$ degrees of freedom. (Note: If $n_{df}$ is greater than the actual sample size or if P_ALTR is equal to zero, then the actual sample size should be used.) This step will produce a lower and an upper limit for the estimated proportion obtained in Step 4.

**Step 6:** Use SAS Proc Univariate (again with default percentile definition equivalent to option PCTLDEF = 5 and with the Freq option variable equal to $WT_{AVE}$) to determine the analyte values that correspond to the desired percentile (proportion) and the lower and upper proportion limits obtained in Step 5. Round these results to 2 or 3 decimals depending on the significant figures associated with the original measured values.

**Example:**

To estimate the 75th percentile of blood lead in children age 1-5 years in the 2003-2004 survey, create two separate files: name one ORIG_DATA and the other ALTR_DATA. For the ORIG_DATA file use SAS Proc Univariate with the Freq option and the subsample sampling weight (or in this case the full sample sampling weight because blood lead is the analyte of interest) to get a weighted point estimate of the analyte value that corresponds to the 75th percentile (PTLE_ ORIG). For this example the value is 2.5 µg/dL.

Sort the results in the ALTR_DATA file by analyte measured value. Use SAS Proc Means to compute the average sampling weight ($WT_{AVE}$) for each unique analyte measured value. For each unique measured result, use a counter from 1 to the total number of subjects with identical values to create a unique integer to associate with each measured observation. Divide each counter value by 1,000,000,000 and add this amount to the corresponding measured observation. For this altered data file (ALTR_DATA) use SAS Proc Univariate with the Freq option and $WT_{AVE}$ to get a weighted point estimate of the analyte value that corresponds to the 75th percentile (PTLE_ALTR). For this example the value is also 2.5 µg/dL.

For the ORIG_DATA file use SUDAAN to estimate the weighted proportion (P_ORIG) of subjects with results below the value of PTLE_ORIG (which can differ from 0.75 depending on the number of results with identical values; for this example the proportion is 0.7374) and the standard error (SEMEAN_ORIG) associated with P_ORIG (for this example SEMEAN_ORIG = 0.0237).

For the ALTR_DATA file use SUDAAN to estimate the weighted proportion of subjects (P_ALTR) with results below the value of PTLE_ALTR (which should also be very close to 0.75 regardless of the number of original results with identical values; for this example the proportion is 0.7497). Then obtain a confidence interval on P_ALTR by computing the weighted Clopper-Pearson 95% confidence limits (equation 2 above) using the degrees-of-freedom adjusted effective sample size as described in equation 1 above. For this example the effective sample size is 283.911 resulting in lower and upper confidence limits of 0.6951 and 0.7990, respectively. Then use SAS Proc Univariate (with the Freq option variable equal to $WT_{AVE}$) to determine the analyte values corresponding to the weighted 69.5[th] and 79.9[th] percentiles. These point estimates are the lower and upper confidence limits on the 75th percentile estimate. Round the 75th percentile estimate and its confidence limits to 2 or 3 decimals depending on the significant figures associated with the original measured values. For this example the rounded point estimate is 2.5 µg/dL with lower and upper confidence limits of 2.3 and 2.8 µg/dL, respectively.

Note: Previous reports of the analyses of 1999-2000 data (in the *Second National Report on Human Exposure to Environmental Chemicals*) used a jackknife method (available within SUDAAN) for variance estimation that was based on replicate weights. To better address multiple 2-year data sets and to combine 2-year data sets into 4-year data sets, NCHS developed a new approach based on masked variance units that uses a Taylor series (linearization) method that is also available in SUDAAN. The two methods produce very similar, but not identical, variance estimates. In the *Third National Report on Human Exposure to Environmental Chemicals* and in the current *Report* data tables, all variance estimates (1999-2000, 2001-2002, 2003-2004) were calculated using the Taylor series (linearization) method within SUDAAN.

# Appendix B. Changes and Edits to Results Released in the *Third Report*

Some biomonitoring results from earlier NHANES survey periods require corrections due to analytical issues. Corrections can include changes in specific data tables or the removal of data tables in this *Report*, as compared to the previous *Third National Report on Human Exposure to Environmental Chemicals*. The following chemical tables are affected:

1. The data for *beta*-hexachlorocyclohexane serum levels (lipid adjusted and whole weight) in the *Third National Report on Human Exposure to Environmental Chemicals* for the NHANES survey period 2001-2002 should have been adjusted by multiplying each data point by a factor of 1.5528. The data for this chemical in the current *Report* have had this adjustment applied. This adjustment was needed due to a misassignment of the concentration of a purchased standard material.

2. Urinary 2,4-dichlorophenol and 2,5-dichlorophenol were presented in the *Third National Report on Human Exposure to Environmental Chemicals* for the years 1999-2002 and have been removed from this *Report* due to matrix-based calibration biases. Data Tables for these two chemicals in the 2003-2004 survey period will be included in the next release of the *Report*.

3. Improvements in analytical methods have resulted in dropping data for some urinary Polycyclic Aromatic Hydrocarbon (PAH) metabolites. For the 1999-2000 survey period, urinary data for 2-hydroxyfluorene, 3-hydroxyfluorene, 1-hydroxyphenanthrene, 2-hydroxyphenanthrene, 3-hydroxyphenanthrene, and 1-hydroxypyrene have been removed from the Data Tables in the current *Report*. The data from 1999-2000 for these specific analytes are not in agreement with current methods -- specifically interferences in some analytical peaks have been detected with newer analytic methods and newer techniques have shown that deconjugation in the analytical method was not complete for some PAHs. For the 1999-2002 period, data for urinary metabolites of 1-Hydroxybenz[a]anthracene, 3-hydroxybenz[a]anthracene, 9-Hydroxybenz[a]anthracene, 1-Hydroxybenzo[c]phenanthrene, 2-Hydroxybenzo[c]phenanthrene, 3-Hydroxybenzo[c]phenanthrene, 1-Hydroxychrysene, 2-Hydroxychrysene, 3-Hydroxychrysene, 4-Hydroxychrysene, 6-Hydroxychrysene and 3-Hydroxybenzo[a]pyrene have been removed and are not planned for future *Reports*. Improvements in analytical methods have found uncertainties due to interferences in accurate mass detection in the previous method. In addition, data for 3-Hydroxybenzo[a]

pyrene in the 2001-2002 survey period has been removed due to an interference in a purchased reagent used in the deconjugation step of the analytical method.

Data for three additional PAH urinary metabolites have been removed for the 1999-2002 survey period. Urinary 9-hydroxyphenanthrene has been removed due to degradation during the deconjugation step of the analytical method. Urinary 9-hydroxyphenanthrene will not be reported in future survey periods. Urinary 9-hydroxyfluorene has been removed due to an incomplete deconjugation step revealed by improved methods. Data for urinary 9-hydroxyfluorene *is* reported in the 2003-2004 survey period. Urinary 4-hydroxyphenanthrene has been removed as a result of infrequent interferences in the analytical method, which were detected by an improved analytical method. Urinary 4-Hydroxyphenanthrene *is* reported in the 2003-2004 survey period.

Data for three urinary PAH metabolites from the 2001-2002 survey are under current evaluation and do not appear in this release of the *Report*: 1-hydroxynaphthalene, 2-hydroxyfluorene, and 1-hydroxypyrene.

# Appendix C. References for Biomonitoring Analytical Methods

## Acrylamide Adducts

Vesper HW, Bernert JT, Ospina M, Meyers T, Ingham L, Smith A, et al. Assessment of the relation between biomarkers for smoking and biomarkers for acrylamide exposure in humans. Cancer Epidemiol Biomarkers Prev 2007;16(11):2471-2478.

Vesper HW, Slimani N, Hallmans G, Tjonneland A, Agudo A, Benetou V, et al. Cross-sectional study on acrylamide hemoglobin adducts in subpopulations from the European Prospective Investigation into Cancer and Nutrition (EPIC) study. J Agric Food Chem 2008; 56 (15):6046–6053.

## Cotinine

Bernert JT, McGuffey JE, Morrison MA, Pirkle JL. Comparison of serum and salivary cotinine measurements by a sensitive high-performance liquid chromatography/ tandem mass spectrometry method as an indicator of exposure to tobacco smoke among smokers and nonsmokers. J Anal Toxicol 2000;24:333-339.

Bernert JT, Turner WE, Pirkle JL, Sosnoff CS, Akins JR, Waldrep MK, et al. Development and validation of a sensitive measurement of serum cotinine in both smokers and nonsmokers by liquid chromatography/atmospheric pressure ionization tandem mass spectrometry. Clin Chem 1997;43:2281-2291.

## N,N-Diethyl-meta-toluamide (DEET)

Olsson AO, Baker SE, Nguyen JV, Romanoff LC, Udunka SO, Walker RD, et al. A liquid chromatography-tandem mass spectrometry multiresidue method for quantification of specific metabolites of organophosphorus pesticides, synthetic pyrethroids, selected herbicides, and DEET in human urine. Anal Chem 2004;76(9):2453-2461.

## Disinfection By-Products (Trihalomethanes)

Blount BC, Kobelski RJ, McElprang DO, Ashley DL, Morrow JC, Chambers DM, et al. Quantification of 31 volatile organic compounds in whole blood using solid-phase microextraction and gas chromatography-mass spectrometry. J Chromatogr B Analyt Technol Biomed Life Sci 2006;832: 292-301.

## Environmental Phenols

Ye X, Kuklenyik Z, Needham LL, Calafat AM. Automated on-line column-switching HPLC-MS/MS method with peak focusing for the determination of nine environmental phenols in urine. Anal Chem 2005;77:5407-5413.

## Fungicides

Hill RH Jr, Shealy DB, Head SL, Williams CC, Bailey SL, Gregg M, et al. Determination of pesticide metabolites in human urine using isotope dilution technique and tandem mass spectrometry. J Anal Toxicol 1995;19(5):323-329.

Bravo R, Caltabiano LM, Fernandez C, Smith KD, Gallegos M, Whitehead RD, et al. Quantification of phenolic metabolites of environmental chemicals in human urine using gas chromatography-tandem mass spectrometry and isotope dilution quantification. J Chromatog B 2005;820(2):229-236.

## Herbicides

Bravo R, Caltabiano LM, Fernandez C, Smith KD, Gallegos M, Whitehead RD, et al. Quantification of phenolic metabolites of environmental chemicals in human urine using gas chromatography-tandem mass spectrometry and isotope dilution quantification. J Chromatog B 2005;820(2):229-236.

Hill RH Jr, Shealy DB, Head SL, Williams CC, Bailey SL, Gregg M, et al. Determination of pesticide metabolites in human urine using isotope dilution technique and tandem mass spectrometry. J Anal Toxicol 1995;19(5):323-329.

Olsson AO, Baker SE, Nguyen JV, Romanoff LC, Udunka SO, Walker RD, et al. A liquid chromatography-tandem mass spectrometry multiresidue method for quantification of specific metabolites of organophosphorus pesticides, synthetic pyrethroids, selected herbicides, and DEET in human urine. Anal Chem 2004;76(9):2453-2461.

## Insecticides and Pesticides

### Carbamate Insecticides

Bravo R, Caltabiano LM, Fernandez C, Smith KD, Gallegos M, Whitehead RD, et al. Quantification of phenolic metabolites of environmental chemicals in human urine using gas chromatography-tandem mass spectrometry and isotope dilution quantification. J Chromatog B 2005;820(2):229-236.

Hill RH Jr, Shealy DB, Head SL, Williams CC, Bailey SL, Gregg M, et al. Determination of pesticide metabolites in human urine using isotope dilution technique and tandem mass spectrometry. J Anal Toxicol 1995;19(5):323-329.

## Organochlorines Pesticides

Barr JB, Maggio VL, Barr DB, Turner WE, Sjödin A, Sandau CD, et al. New high-resolution mass spectrometric approach for the measurement of polychlorinated biphenyls and organochlorine pesticides in human serum. J Chromatog B 2003;794:137-148.

Hill RH Jr, Shealy DB, Head SL, Williams CC, Bailey SL, Gregg M, et al. Determination of pesticide metabolites in human urine using isotope dilution technique and tandem mass spectrometry. J Anal Toxicol 1995;19(5):323-329.

Turner WE, DiPietro E, Lapeza CR, Jr., Green V, Gill J, Patterson DG Jr., et al. Universal automated cleanup system for the isotope-dilution high-resolution mass spectrometric analysis of PCDDs, PCDFs, coplanar PCBs, PCB congeners, and persistent pesticides from the same serum sample. Organohalogen Compounds 1997;31:26-31.

## Organophosphate Insecticides: Dialkyl Phosphate Metabolites

Bravo R, Caltabiano LM, Weerasekera G, Whitehead RD, Fernandez C, Needham LL, et al. Measurement of dialkyl phosphate metabolites of organophosphorus pesticides in human urine using lyophilization with gas chromatography-tandem mass spectrometry and isotope dilution quantification. J Expo Anal Environ Epidemiol 2004;14:249-259.

Bravo R, Driskell WJ, Whitehead RD Jr, Needham LL, Barr DB. Quantitation of dialkyl phosphate metabolites of organophosphate pesticides in human urine using GC-MS-MS with isotopic internal standards. J Anal Toxicol 2002;26:245-252.

## Organophosphate Insecticides: Specific Metabolites

Bravo R, Caltabiano LM, Fernandez C, Smith KD, Gallegos M, Whitehead RD, et al. Quantification of phenolic metabolites of environmental chemicals in human urine using gas chromatography-tandem mass spectrometry and isotope dilution quantification. J Chromatog B 2005;820(2):229-236.

Hill RH Jr, Shealy DB, Head SL, Williams CC, Bailey SL, Gregg M, et al. Determination of pesticide metabolites in human urine using isotope dilution technique and tandem mass spectrometry. J Anal Toxicol 1995;19(5):323-329.

Olsson AO, Baker SE, Nguyen JV, Romanoff LC, Udunka SO, Walker RD, et al. A liquid chromatography-tandem mass spectrometry multiresidue method for quantification of specific metabolites of organophosphorus pesticides, synthetic pyrethroids, selected herbicides, and DEET in human urine. Anal Chem 2004;76(9):2453-2461.

## Pyrethroid Pesticides

Olsson AO, Baker SE, Nguyen JV, Romanoff LC, Udunka SO, Walker RD, et al. A liquid chromatography-tandem mass spectrometry multiresidue method for quantification of specific metabolites of organophosphorus pesticides, synthetic pyrethroids, selected herbicides, and DEET in human urine. Anal Chem 2004;76(9):2453-2461.

## Metals

Caldwell KL, Hartel J, Jarrett J, Jones RL. Inductively coupled plasma mass spectrometry to measure multiple toxic elements in urine in NHANES 1999-2000. Atomic Spectroscopy. 2005;26(1):1-7.

Chen HP, Paschal DC, Miller DT, Morrow JC. Determination of total and inorganic mercury in whole blood by on-line digestion with flow injection. Atomic Spectroscopy 1998;19:176-179.

Jarrett JM, Jones RL, Caldwell KL, Verdon CP. Total urine arsenic measurements using inductively coupled plasma mass spectrometry with a dynamic reaction cell. Atomic Spectroscopy 2007;28(4):113-122.

Miller, DT, Paschal DC, Gunter EW, Stroud PE, D'Angelo J. Determination of lead in blood using electrothermal atomization atomic absorption spectrometry with a L'vov platform and matrix modifier. Analyst 1987;112:1701-1704.

Paschal DC, Ting BG, Morrow JC, Pirkle JL, Jackson RJ, Sampson EJ, et al. Trace metals in urine of United States residents: reference range concentrations. Environ Res 1998;76:53-59.

Stoeppler M, Brandt K. Determination of cadmium in whole blood and urine by electrothermal atomic-absorption spectrophotometry. Fresnius A Anal Chem 1980;300:372-380.

Verdon CP, Caldwell KL, Fresques MR, Jones RL. Determination of seven arsenic compounds in urine by HPLC-ICP-DRC-MS: a CDC population biomonitoring method. Anal Bioanal Chem 2008;393(3):939-947.

## Perchlorate

Valentin-Blasini L, Blount BC, Delinsky A. Quantification of iodide and sodium-iodide symporter inhibitors in human urine using ion chromatography tandem mass spectrometry. J Chrom A 2007;1155(1):40-46.

Valentin-Blasini L, Mauldin JP, Maple D and Blount BC. Analysis of perchlorate in human urine using ion chromatography and electrospray tandem mass spectrometry. Anal Chem 2005;77(8):2475-2481.

## Perfluorochemicals

Kuklenyik Z, Needham LL, Calafat AM. Measurement of 18 perfluorinated organic acids and amides in human serum using on-line solid-phase extraction. Anal Chem 2005;77:6085-6091.

## Phthalates

Blount BC, Milgram KE, Silva M, Malek N, Reidy J, Needham LL, et al. Quantitative detection of eight phthalate metabolites in human urine using HPLC-APCI-MS/MS. Anal Chem 2000;72:4127-4134.

Silva MJ, Malek NA, Hodge CC, Reidy JA, Kato K, Barr DB, et al. Improved quantitative detection of 11 urinary phthalate metabolites in humans using liquid chromatography-atmospheric pressure chemical ionization tandem mass spectrometry. J Chromatog B 2003;789:393-404.

Silva MJ, Slakman AR, Reidy JA, Preau JLJ, Herbert AR, Samandar E, et al. Analysis of human urine for 15 phthalate metabolites using automated solid-phase extraction. J Chromatog B 2004;805:161-167.

## Phytoestrogens

Valentin-Blasini L, Blount BC, Rogers HS, Needham LL. HPLC-MS/MS method for the measurement of seven phytoestrogens in human serum and urine. J Expo Anal Environ Epidemiol 2000;10:799-807.

Kuklenyik Z, Ye X, Reich JA, Needham LL, Calafat AM. Automated on-line and off-line solid phase extraction methods for measuring isoflavones and lignans in urine. J Chromatogr Sci 2004; 42:495-500.

## Polybrominated Diphenyl Ethers and 2,2',4,4',5,5'-Hexabromobiphenyl

Sjödin A, Jones RS, Lapeza CR, Focant J-F, McGahee EE III, Patterson DG. Semiautomated high-throughput extraction and cleanup method for the measurement of polybrominated diphenyl ethers, polybrominated biphenyls, and polychlorinated biphenyls in human serum. Anal Chem 2004;76:1921-1927.

## Polychlorinated Biphenyls, Polychlorinated Dibenzo-*p*-dioxins, Dibenzofurans

Barr JB, Maggio VL, Barr DB, Turner WE, Sjödin A, Sandau CD, et al. New high-resolution mass spectrometric approach for the measurement of polychlorinated biphenyls and organochlorine pesticides in human serum. J Chromatog B 2003;794:137-148.

Patterson DG Jr., Alexander LR, Turner WE, Isaacs SG, Needham LL. The development and application of a high resolution mass spectrometry method for measuring polychlorinated dibenzo-p-dioxins and dibenzofurans in serum. In: Clement RE, Sui KM, Hill HH Jr., eds. Instrumentation for trace organic monitoring. Chelsea, MI: Lewis Publishers; 1990. pp. 119-53.

Patterson DG Jr., Hampton L, Lapeza CR Jr., Belser WT, Green V, Alexander L, et al. High resolution gas chromatographic/high resolution mass spectrometric analysis of human serum on a whole weight and lipid basis for 2,3,7,8 TCDD. Anal Chem 1987;59:2000-2005.

Patterson, DG Jr., Wong L-Y, Turner WE, Caudill SP, DiPietro ES, McClure PC, et al. Levels in the U.S. population of those persistent organic pollutants (2003-2004) included in the Stockholm Convention or in other Long-Range Tran boundary Air Pollution Agreements. Environ Sci Technol 2009;43(4):1211-1218.

Turner WE, DiPietro E, Cash TP, McClure PC, Patterson DG Jr., Shirkhan H. An improved SPE extraction and automated sample cleanup method for serum PCDDs, PCDFs, and coplanar PCBs. Organohalogen Compounds 1994;19:31-35.

Turner WE, DiPietro E, Lapeza CR, Jr., Green V, Gill J, Patterson DG Jr., et al. Universal automated cleanup system for the isotope-dilution high-resolution mass spectrometric analysis of PCDDs, PCDFs, coplanar PCBs, PCB congeners, and persistent pesticides from the same serum sample. Organohalogen Compounds 1997;31:26-31.

## Polycyclic Aromatic Hydrocarbons

Li Z, Romanoff LC, Young KJ, Blakely NC III, Wei RW, Needham LL, et al. Biomonitoring of human exposure to polycyclic aromatic hydrocarbons (PAH) and diesel exhaust by measurement of urinary biomarkers. Epidemiology 2004;15(4):S75.

Romanoff LC, Li Z, Young KJ, Blakely NC III, Patterson DG, Sandau CD. Automated solid-phase extraction method for measuring urinary polycyclic aromatic hydrocarbon metabolites in human biomonitoring using isotope-dilution gas chromatography high-resolution mass spectrometry. J Chromatog B 2006;835:47-54.

Smith CJ, Huang WL, Walcott CJ, Turner WE, Grainger J, Patterson DG Jr. Quantification of monohydroxy-PAH metabolites in urine by solid-phase extraction with isotope dilution GC-HRMS. Anal Bioanal Chem 2002;372:216-220.

**Volatile Organic Compounds**

Blount B.C, Kobelski R.J, McElprang D.O, Ashley D.L, Morrow J.C, Chambers D.M, et al. Quantification of 31 volatile organic compounds in whole blood using solid-phase microextraction and gas chromatography-mass spectrometry. J Chromatogr B Analyt Technol Biomed Life Sci 2006;832: 292-301.

# Appendix D. Limit of Detection Table

The analytical limit of detection (LOD) for each of the different chemical measurements is presented in the table below. The LOD is the level at which the measurement has a 95% probability of being greater than zero (Taylor, 1987). For most chemicals, the LOD is constant for each sample analyzed. However, for dioxins, furans, PCBs, organochlorine insecticides, and some other pesticides, each individual sample has its own LOD. These analyses have an individual LOD for each sample, mostly because the sample volume available for analysis differed for each sample. A higher sample volume results in a lower LOD and a better ability to detect low levels.

For chemicals with sample-specific LODs, we report in the table the maximum LOD among the samples analyzed. In general, the average LOD for these samples is about 40-50% of the maximum LOD. If a geometric mean or percentile estimate is less than the maximum LOD, it is noted in the results tables, and we do not report a number for that estimate. This conservative approach is to assure high confidence in all number reported in the results tables.

As analytical methods improve, LODs will often change. For this reason, LOD results are reported by survey periods (e.g., 1999-2000, 2001-2002, 2003-2004).

Reference: Taylor JK. *Quality Assurance of Chemical Measurements*. Chelsea (MI): Lewis Publishing. 1987.

| Chemical | Matrix | Units | 1999-2000 | 2001-2002 | 2003-2004 |
|---|---|---|---|---|---|
| **Acrylamide Adducts** | | | | | |
| Acrylamide | blood | pmol/g hemoglobin | | | 3.0 |
| Glycidamide | blood | pmol/g hemoglobin | | | 4.0 |
| Cotinine | serum | ng/mL | 0.05 | 0.05 | 0.015 |
| N,N-Diethyl-*meta*-toluamide (DEET) | urine | µg/L | 0.449 | 0.1 | |
| **Disinfection By-Products (Trihalomethanes)** | | | | | |
| Bromodichloromethane | blood | pg/mL | | 0.233 | 0.62 |
| Dibromochloromethane (Chlorodibromomethane) | blood | pg/mL | | 0.271 | 0.62 |
| Tribromomethane (Bromoform) | blood | pg/mL | | 0.596 | 1.5 |
| Trichloromethane (Chloroform) | blood | pg/mL | | 2.37 | 2.11 |

| Chemical | Matrix | Units | 1999-2000 | 2001-2002 | 2003-2004 |
|---|---|---|---|---|---|
| **Environmental Phenols** | | | | | |
| Bisphenol A (2,2-bis[4-Hydroxyphenyl] propane) | urine | µg/L | | | 0.4 |
| Benzophenone-3 (2-Hydroxy-4-methoxybenzophenone) | urine | µg/L | | | 0.3 |
| 4-tert-Octylphenol (4-[1,1,3,3-Tetramethylbutyl] phenol) | urine | µg/L | | | 0.2 |
| Triclosan (2,4,4'-Trichloro-2'-hydroxyphenyl ether) | urine | µg/L | | | 2.3 |
| **Fungicides and Metabolites** | | | | | |
| Pentachlorophenol | urine | µg/L | 0.25 | 0.5 | |
| ortho-Phenylphenol | urine | µg/L | 0.3 | 0.3 | |
| **Herbicides and Metabolites** | | | | | |
| Acetochlor mercapturate | urine | µg/L | | 0.1 | |
| Alachlor mercapturate | urine | µg/L | 1.18 | | |
| Atrazine mercapturate | urine | µg/L | 0.791 | 0.3 | |
| 2,4-Dichlorophenoxyacetic acid | urine | µg/L | 0.952 | 0.2 | |
| Metolachlor mercapturate | urine | µg/L | | 0.2 | |
| 2,4,5-Trichlorophenoxyacetic acid | urine | µg/L | 1.2 | 0.1 | |
| **Insecticides and Metabolites** | | | | | |
| **Carbamates** | | | | | |
| Carbofuranphenol | urine | µg/L | 0.4 | 0.4 | |
| 2-Isopropoxyphenol | urine | µg/L | 1.1 | 0.4 | |
| **Organochlorines and Metabolites** | | | | | |
| Aldrin | serum | ng/g of lipid | | 5.94 | 7.8 |
| o,p'-Dichlorodiphenyltrichloroethane | serum | ng/g of lipid | 20.7 | 17.4 | 7.8 |
| p,p'-Dichlorodiphenyltrichloroethane (DDT) | serum | ng/g of lipid | 20.7 | 17.4 | 7.8 |
| p,p'-Dichlorodiphenyldichloroethene (DDE) | serum | ng/g of lipid | 18.6 | 8.3 | 7.8 |
| Dieldrin | serum | ng/g of lipid | | 10.5 | 7.8 |
| Endrin | serum | ng/g of lipid | | 5.09 | 7.8 |
| Hexachlorobenzene | serum | ng/g of lipid | 118 | 31.4 | 7.8 |
| beta-Hexachlorocyclohexane | serum | ng/g of lipid | 9.36 | 6.76 | 7.8 |
| gamma-Hexachlorocyclohexane (Lindane) | serum | ng/g of lipid | 14.5 | 10.5 | 7.8 |
| Heptachlor epoxide | serum | ng/g of lipid | 14.6 | 10.5 | 7.8 |
| Mirex | serum | ng/g of lipid | 14.6 | 10.5 | 7.8 |
| trans-Nonachlor | serum | ng/g of lipid | 14.5 | 10.5 | 7.8 |
| Oxychlordane | serum | ng/g of lipid | 14.5 | 10.5 | 7.8 |
| 2,4,5-Trichlorophenol | urine | µg/L | 0.9 | 0.9 | |
| 2,4,6-Trichlorophenol | urine | µg/L | 1 | 1.3 | |

| Chemical | Matrix | Units | 1999-2000 | 2001-2002 | 2003-2004 |
|---|---|---|---|---|---|
| **Organophosphorus Insecticides: Dialkyl Phosphate Metabolites** | | | | | |
| Diethylphosphate (DEP) | urine | µg/L | 0.2 | 0.2 | 0.1 |
| Dimethylphosphate (DMP) | urine | µg/L | 0.58 | 0.5 | 0.5 |
| Diethylthiophosphate (DETP) | urine | µg/L | 0.09 | 0.1 | 0.2 |
| Dimethylthiophosphate (DMTP) | urine | µg/L | 0.18 | 0.4 | 0.5 |
| Diethyldithiophosphate (DEDTP) | urine | µg/L | 0.05 | 0.1 | 0.1 |
| Dimethyldithiophosphate (DMDTP) | urine | µg/L | 0.08 | 0.1 | 0.1 |
| **Organophosphorus Insecticides: Specific Insecticides and Metabolites** | | | | | |
| 3-Chloro-7-hydroxy-4-methyl-2H-chromen-2-one/ol | urine | µg/L | | | |
| 2-(Diethylamino)-6-methylpyrimidin-4-ol/one | urine | µg/L | | 0.2 | |
| 2-Isopropyl-4-methyl-6-hydroxypyrimidine | urine | µg/L | 7.2 | 0.2 | |
| Malathion dicarboxylic acid | urine | µg/L | 2.64 | 0.7 | |
| para-Nitrophenol | urine | µg/L | 0.8 | 0.1 | |
| 3,5,6-Trichloro-2-pyridinol | urine | µg/L | 0.4 | 0.4 | |
| **Pyrethroid Pesticide Metabolites** | | | | | |
| cis-3-(2,2-Dibromovinyl)-2,2-dimethylcyclopropane carboxylic acid | urine | µg/L | 0.1 | 0.1 | |
| cis-3-(2,2-Dichlorovinyl)-2,2-dimethylcyclopropane carboxylic acid | urine | µg/L | 0.1 | 0.1 | |
| trans-3-(2,2-Dichlorovinyl)-2,2-dimethylcyclopropane carboxylic acid | urine | µg/L | 0.4 | 0.4 | |
| 4-Fluoro-3-phenoxybenzoic acid | urine | µg/L | 0.2 | 0.2 | |
| 3-Phenoxybenzoic acid | urine | µg/L | 0.1 | 0.1 | |
| **Metals** | | | | | |
| Antimony | urine | µg/L | 0.04 | 0.04 | 0.07 |
| Arsenic, Total | urine | µg/L | | | 0.74 |
| Arsenic (V) Acid | urine | µg/L | | | 1.0 |
| Arsenobetaine | urine | µg/L | | | 0.4 |
| Arsenocholine | urine | µg/L | | | 0.6 |
| Arsenous (III) Acid | urine | µg/L | | | 1.2 |
| Dimethylarsinic Acid | urine | µg/L | | | 1.7 |
| Monomethylarsonic Acid | urine | µg/L | | | 0.9 |
| Trimethylarsine oxide | urine | µg/L | | | 1.0 |
| Barium | urine | µg/L | 0.12 | 0.12 | 0.31 |

| Chemical | Matrix | Units | 1999-2000 | 2001-2002 | 2003-2004 |
|---|---|---|---|---|---|
| **Metals (continued)** | | | | | |
| Beryllium | urine | µg/L | 0.13 | 0.13 | 0.13 |
| Cadmium | blood | µg/L | 0.3 | 0.3 | 0.14 |
| Cadmium | urine | µg/L | 0.06 | 0.06 | 0.06 |
| Cesium | urine | µg/L | 0.14 | 0.14 | 0.2 |
| Cobalt | urine | µg/L | 0.07 | 0.07 | 0.08 |
| Lead | blood | µg/dL | 0.3 | 0.3 | 0.28 |
| Lead | urine | µg/L | 0.1 | 0.1 | 0.33 |
| Mercury, Inorganic | blood | µg/L | | | 0.42 |
| Mercury, Total | blood | µg/L | 0.14 | 0.14 | 0.2 |
| Mercury | urine | µg/L | 0.14 | 0.14 | 0.14 |
| Molybdenum | urine | µg/L | 0.8 | 0.8 | 1.5 |
| Platinum | urine | µg/L | 0.04 | 0.04 | 0.07 |
| Thallium | urine | µg/L | 0.02 | 0.02 | 0.02 |
| Tungsten | urine | µg/L | 0.04 | 0.04 | 0.04 |
| Uranium | urine | µg/L | 0.004 | 0.004 | 0.005 |
| **Perchlorate** | urine | µg/L | | 0.05 | 0.05 |
| **Perfluorinated Compounds** | | | | | |
| Perfluorobutane sulfonic acid (PFBuS) | serum | µg/L | | | 0.4 |
| Perfluorodecanoic acid (PFDeA) | serum | µg/L | | | 0.3 |
| Perfluorododecanoic acid (PFDoA) | serum | µg/L | | | 1.0 |
| Perfluoroheptanoic acid (PFHpA) | serum | µg/L | | | 0.3 |
| Perfluorohexane sulfonic acid (PFHxS) | serum | µg/L | | | 0.3 |
| Perfluorononanoic acid (PFNA) | serum | µg/L | | | 0.1 |
| Perfluorooctanoic acid (PFOA) | serum | µg/L | | | 0.1 |
| Perfluorooctane sulfonic acid (PFOS) | serum | µg/L | | | 0.4 |
| Perfluorooctane sulfonamide (PFOSA) | serum | µg/L | | | 0.2 |
| 2-(N-Ethyl-perfluorooctane sulfonamido) acetic acid (Et-PFOSA-AcOH) | serum | µg/L | | | 0.4 |
| 2-(N-Methyl-perfluorooctane sulfonamido) acetic acid (Me-PFOSA-AcOH) | serum | µg/L | | | 0.6 |
| Perfluoroundecanoic acid (PFUA) | serum | µg/L | | | 0.3 |
| **Phthalate Metabolites** | | | | | |
| Mono-benzyl phthalate (MBzP) | urine | µg/L | 0.8 | 0.3 | 0.1 |
| Mono-isobutyl phthalate (MiBP) | urine | µg/L | 1.0 | 1.0 | 0.3 |
| Mono-n-butyl phthalate (MnBP) | urine | µg/L | 0.9 | 1.1 | 0.4 |
| Mono-cyclohexyl phthalate (MCHP) | urine | µg/L | 0.9 | 0.3 | 0.2 |

| Chemical | Matrix | Units | 1999-2000 | 2001-2002 | 2003-2004 |
|---|---|---|---|---|---|
| **Phthalate Metabolites (continued)** | | | | | |
| Mono-ethyl phthalate (MEP) | urine | µg/L | 1.2 | 0.9 | 0.4 |
| Mono-2-ethylhexyl phthalate (MEHP) | urine | µg/L | 1.2 | 1.0 | 0.9 |
| Mono-(2-ethyl-5-hydroxyhexyl) phthalate (MEHHP) | urine | µg/L | | 1.0 | 0.3 |
| Mono-(2-ethyl-5-oxohexyl) phthalate (MEOHP) | urine | µg/L | | 1.1 | 0.5 |
| Mono-(2-ethyl-5-carboxypentyl) phthalate (MECPP) | urine | µg/L | | | 0.3 |
| Mono-isononyl phthalate (MiNP) | urine | µg/L | 0.8 | 0.8 | 1.0 |
| Mono-methyl phthalate (MMP) | urine | µg/L | | 0.2 | 1.0 |
| Mono-(3-carboxypropyl) phthalate (MCPP) | urine | µg/L | | 0.4 | 0.2 |
| Mono-n-octyl phthalate (MOP) | urine | µg/L | 0.9 | 1.0 | 1.0 |
| **Phytoestrogens and Metabolites** | | | | | |
| Daidzein | urine | µg/L | 0.5 | 1.6 | 1.6 |
| O-Desmethylangolensin | urine | µg/L | 0.2 | 0.4 | 0.4 |
| Enterodiol | urine | µg/L | 0.8 | 1.5 | 1.5 |
| Enterolactone | urine | µg/L | 0.6 | 1.9 | 1.9 |
| Equol | urine | µg/L | 3.0 | 3.3 | 3.3 |
| Genistein | urine | µg/L | 0.3 | 0.8 | 0.8 |
| **Polybrominated Diphenyl Ethers and Polybrominated Biphenyl** | | | | | |
| 2,2',4-Tribromodiphenyl ether (BDE 17) | serum | ng/g of lipid | | | 1.0 |
| 2,4,4'-Tribromodiphenyl ether (BDE 28) | serum | ng/g of lipid | | | 0.8 |
| 2,2',4,4'-Tetrabromodiphenyl ether (BDE 47) | serum | ng/g of lipid | | | 4.2 |
| 2,3',4,4'-Tetrabromodiphenyl ether (BDE 66) | serum | ng/g of lipid | | | 1.0 |
| 2,2',3,4,4'-Pentabromodiphenyl ether (BDE 85) | serum | ng/g of lipid | | | 2.4 |
| 2,2',4,4',5-Pentabromodiphenyl ether (BDE 99) | serum | ng/g of lipid | | | 5.0 |
| 2,2',4,4',6-Pentabromodiphenyl ether (BDE 100) | serum | ng/g of lipid | | | 1.4 |
| 2,2',4,4',5,5'-Hexabromodiphenyl ether (BDE 153) | serum | ng/g of lipid | | | 2.2 |
| 2,2',4,4',5,6'-Hexabromodiphenyl ether (BDE 154) | serum | ng/g of lipid | | | 0.8 |
| 2,2',3,4,4',5',6-Heptabromodiphenyl ether (BDE 183) | serum | ng/g of lipid | | | 1.7 |
| 2,2',4,4',5,5'-Hexabromobiphenyl (BB 153) | serum | ng/g of lipid | | | 0.8 |
| **Polychlorinated Biphenyls, Non-Dioxin-Like** | | | | | |
| 2,4,4'-Trichlorobiphenyl (PCB 28) | serum | ng/g of lipid | 32.4 | | 1.7 |
| 2,2'3,5'-Tetrachlorobiphenyl (PCB 44) | serum | ng/g of lipid | | | 0.4 |
| 2,2',4,5'-Tetrachlorobiphenyl (PCB 49) | serum | ng/g of lipid | | | 0.4 |
| 2,2',5,5'-Tetrachlorobiphenyl (PCB 52) | serum | ng/g of lipid | 12.5 | 12.4 | 0.8 |
| 2,3',4,4'-Tetrachlorobiphenyl (PCB 66) | serum | ng/g of lipid | 12.4 | 12.4 | 0.8 |
| 2,4,4',5-Tetrachlorobiphenyl (PCB 74) | serum | ng/g of lipid | 12.4 | 10.5 | 0.8 |
| 2,2',3,4,5'-Pentachlorobiphenyl (PCB 87) | serum | ng/g of lipid | | 10.5 | 0.4 |

## Polychlorinated Biphenyls, Non-Dioxin-Like (continued)

| Chemical | Matrix | Units | 1999-2000 | 2001-2002 | 2003-2004 |
|---|---|---|---|---|---|
| 2,2',4,4',5-Pentachlorobiphenyl (PCB 99) | serum | ng/g of lipid | 12.5 | 10.5 | 0.6 |
| 2,2',4,5,5'-Pentachlorobiphenyl (PCB 101) | serum | ng/g of lipid | 25.7 | 10.5 | 0.6 |
| 2,3,3',4',6-Pentachlorobiphenyl (PCB 110) | serum | ng/g of lipid | | 10.5 | 0.8 |
| 2,2',3,3',4,4'-Hexachlorobiphenyl (PCB 128) | serum | ng/g of lipid | 12.4 | 10.5 | 0.4 |
| 2,2',3,4,4',5' and 2,3,3',4,4',6-Hexachlorobiphenyl (PCB 138 & 158) | serum | ng/g of lipid | 41.1 | 10.5 | 0.4 |
| 2,2',3,4,5,5'-Hexachlorobiphenyl (PCB 146) | serum | ng/g of lipid | 12.4 | 10.5 | 0.4 |
| 2,2',3,4',5',6-Hexachlorobiphenyl (PCB 149) | serum | ng/g of lipid | | 10.5 | 0.4 |
| 2,2',3,5,5',6-Hexachlorobiphenyl (PCB 151) | serum | ng/g of lipid | | 10.5 | 0.4 |
| 2,2',4,4',5,5'-Hexachlorobiphenyl (PCB 153) | serum | ng/g of lipid | 55.6 | 10.5 | 1.1 |
| 2,2',3,3',4,4',5-Heptachlorobiphenyl (PCB 170) | serum | ng/g of lipid | 17.2 | 10.5 | 0.4 |
| 2,2',3,4,5,5'-Heptachlorobiphenyl (PCB 172) | serum | ng/g of lipid | 12.5 | 10.5 | 0.4 |
| 2,2',3,4,5',6'-Heptachlorobiphenyl (PCB 177) | serum | ng/g of lipid | 12.5 | 10.5 | 0.4 |
| 2,2',3,3',5,5',6-Heptachlorobiphenyl (PCB 178) | serum | ng/g of lipid | 12.4 | 10.5 | 0.4 |
| 2,2',3,4,4',5,5'-Heptachlorobiphenyl (PCB 180) | serum | ng/g of lipid | 28.2 | 10.5 | 0.4 |
| 2,2',3,4,4',5',6-Heptachlorobiphenyl (PCB 183) | serum | ng/g of lipid | 12.4 | 10.5 | 0.4 |
| 2,2',3,4',5,5',6-Heptachlorobiphenyl (PCB 187) | serum | ng/g of lipid | 12.4 | 10.5 | 0.4 |
| 2,2',3,3',4,4',5,5'-Octachlorobiphenyl (PCB 194) | serum | ng/g of lipid | | 10.5 | 0.4 |
| 2,2',3,3',4,4',5,6-Octachlorobiphenyl (PCB 195) | serum | ng/g of lipid | | 28.1 | 0.7 |
| 2,2',3,3',4,4',5,6' and 2,2',3,4,4',5,5',6-Octachlorobiphenyl (PCB 196 & 203) | serum | ng/g of lipid | | 10.5 | 0.4 |
| 2,2',3,3',4,5,5',6-Octachlorobiphenyl (PCB 199) | serum | ng/g of lipid | | 10.5 | 0.4 |
| 2,2',3,3',4,4',5,5',6-Nonachlorobiphenyl (PCB 206) | serum | ng/g of lipid | | 28.1 | 0.7 |
| 2,2',3,3',4,4',5,5',6,6'-Decachlorobiphenyl (PCB 209) | serum | ng/g of lipid | | | 0.7 |

## Polychlorinated Dibenzo-p-dioxins, Dibenzofurans, and Dioxin-Like Polychlorinated Biphenyls

### Coplanar Polychlorinated Biphenyls

| Chemical | Matrix | Units | 1999-2000 | 2001-2002 | 2003-2004 |
|---|---|---|---|---|---|
| 3,4,4',5-Tetrachlorobiphenyl (PCB 81) | serum | pg/g of lipid | 68.4 | 26.8 | 13.1 |
| 3,3',4,4',5-Pentachlorobiphenyl (PCB 126) | serum | pg/g of lipid | 23.2 | 10.8 | 13.9 |
| 3,3',4,4',5,5'-Hexachlorobiphenyl (PCB 169) | serum | pg/g of lipid | 27.0 | 11.0 | 15.9 |

### Mono-ortho-substituted Polychlorinated Biphenyls

| Chemical | Matrix | Units | 1999-2000 | 2001-2002 | 2003-2004 |
|---|---|---|---|---|---|
| 2,3,3',4,4'-Pentachlorobiphenyl (PCB 105) | serum | ng/g of lipid | 12.4 | 10.5 | 0.4 |
| 2,3',4,4',5-Pentachlorobiphenyl (PCB 118) | serum | ng/g of lipid | 12.5 | 10.5 | 0.6 |
| 2,3,3',4,4',5-Hexachlorobiphenyl (PCB 156) | serum | ng/g of lipid | 12.5 | 10.5 | 0.4 |
| 2,3,3',4,4',5'-Hexachlorobiphenyl (PCB 157) | serum | ng/g of lipid | 12.5 | 10.5 | 0.4 |
| 2,3',4,4',5,5'-Hexachlorobiphenyl (PCB 167) | serum | ng/g of lipid | 12.4 | 10.5 | 0.4 |
| 2,3,3',4,4',5,5'-Heptachlorobiphenyl (PCB 189) | serum | ng/g of lipid | | 10.5 | 0.4 |

| Chemical | Matrix | Units | 1999-2000 | 2001-2002 | 2003-2004 |
|---|---|---|---|---|---|
| **Polychlorinated Dibenzofurans** | | | | | |
| 1,2,3,4,6,7,8-Heptachlorodibenzofuran (HpCDF) | serum | pg/g of lipid | 13.5 | 7.0 | 8.6 |
| 1,2,3,4,7,8,9-Heptachlorodibenzofuran (HpCDF) | serum | pg/g of lipid | | 7.0 | 8.6 |
| 1,2,3,4,7,8-Hexachlorodibenzofuran (HxCDF) | serum | pg/g of lipid | 12.7 | 6.5 | 7.4 |
| 1,2,3,6,7,8-Hexachlorodibenzofuran (HxCDF) | serum | pg/g of lipid | 12.6 | 6.1 | 7.9 |
| 1,2,3,7,8,9-Hexachlorodibenzofuran (HxCDF) | serum | pg/g of lipid | 12.7 | 6.0 | 8.3 |
| 2,3,4,6,7,8-Hexachlorodibenzofuran (HxCDF) | serum | pg/g of lipid | 12.9 | 5.8 | 8.2 |
| 1,2,3,4,6,7,8,9-Octachlorodibenzofuran (OCDF) | serum | pg/g of lipid | 35.6 | 21.0 | 12.0 |
| 1,2,3,7,8-Pentachlorodibenzofuran (PeCDF) | serum | pg/g of lipid | 13.2 | 5.8 | 7.1 |
| 2,3,4,7,8-Pentachlorodibenzofuran (PeCDF) | serum | pg/g of lipid | 12.7 | 5.5 | 6.8 |
| 2,3,7,8-Tetrachlorodibenzofuran (TCDF) | serum | pg/g of lipid | 11.9 | 5.2 | 6.0 |
| **Polychlorinated Dibenzo-p-dioxins** | | | | | |
| 1,2,3,4,6,7,8-Heptachlorodibenzo-p-dioxin (HpCDD) | serum | pg/g of lipid | 55.9 | 10.3 | 13.0 |
| 1,2,3,4,7,8-Hexachlorodibenzo-p-dioxin (HxCDD) | serum | pg/g of lipid | | 9.0 | 11.9 |
| 1,2,3,6,7,8-Hexachlorodibenzo-p-dioxin (HxCDD) | serum | pg/g of lipid | 20.1 | 9.1 | 12.3 |
| 1,2,3,7,8,9-Hexachlorodibenzo-p-dioxin (HxCDD) | serum | pg/g of lipid | 20.3 | 9.3 | 12.3 |
| 1,2,3,4,6,7,8,9-Octachlorodibenzo-p-dioxin (OCDD) | serum | pg/g of lipid | 329.0 | 319.0 | 218.0 |
| 1,2,3,7,8-Pentachlorodibenzo-p-dioxin (PeCDD) | serum | pg/g of lipid | 14.2 | 6.0 | 4.5 |
| 2,3,7,8-Tetrachlorodibenzo-p-dioxin (TCDD) | serum | pg/g of lipid | 12.1 | 5.8 | 3.8 |
| **Polycyclic Aromatic Hydrocarbon Metabolites** | | | | | |
| 2-Hydroxyfluorene | urine | ng/L | | | 5.0 |
| 3-Hydroxyfluorene | urine | ng/L | | 2.0 | 5.0 |
| 9-Hydroxyfluorene | urine | ng/L | | | 5.0 |
| 1-Hydroxynaphthalene (1-Naphthol) | urine | ng/L | | | 46.7 |
| 2-Hydroxynaphthalene (2-Naphthol) | urine | ng/L | | 2.4 | 31.1 |
| 1-Hydroxyphenanthrene | urine | ng/L | | 3.5 | 5.0 |
| 2-Hydroxyphenanthrene | urine | ng/L | | 3.2 | 5.0 |
| 3-Hydroxyphenanthrene | urine | ng/L | | | 5.0 |
| 4-Hydroxyphenanthrene | urine | ng/L | | 3.6 | 5.0 |
| 1-Hydroxypyrene | urine | ng/L | | | 5.0 |

| Chemical | Matrix | Units | 1999-2000 | 2001-2002 | 2003-2004 |
|---|---|---|---|---|---|
| Volatile Organic Compounds (VOCs) | | | | | |
| Benzene | blood | ng/mL | | 0.024 | 0.024 |
| Chlorobenzene (Monochlorobenzene) | blood | ng/mL | | | 0.011 |
| 1,2-Dibromo-3-chloropropane (DBCP) | blood | ng/mL | | | 0.1 |
| Dibromomethane | blood | ng/mL | | | 0.03 |
| 1,2-Dichlorobenzene (o-Dichlorobenzene) | blood | ng/mL | | | 0.1 |
| 1,3-Dichlorobenzene (m-Dichlorobenzene) | blood | ng/mL | | | 0.05 |
| 1,4-Dichlorobenzene (Paradichlorobenzene) | blood | ng/mL | | 0.12 | 0.12 |
| 1,1-Dichloroethane | blood | ng/mL | | | 0.01 |
| 1,2-Dichloroethane (Ethylene dichloride) | blood | ng/mL | | | 0.01 |
| 1,1-Dichloroethene (Vinylidene chloride) | blood | ng/mL | | | 0.009 |
| cis-1,2-Dichloroethene | blood | ng/mL | | | 0.01 |
| trans-1,2-Dichloroethene | blood | ng/mL | | | 0.01 |
| Dichloromethane (Methylene chloride) | blood | ng/mL | | | 0.07 |
| 1,2-Dichloropropane | blood | ng/mL | | | 0.008 |
| 2,5-Dimethylfuran | blood | ng/mL | | | 0.012 |
| Ethylbenzene | blood | ng/mL | | 0.024 | 0.024 |
| Hexachloroethane | blood | ng/mL | | | 0.011 |
| Methyl tert-butyl ether (MTBE) | blood | pg/mL | | 0.232 | 2.0 |
| Nitrobenzene | blood | ng/mL | | | 0.3 |
| Styrene | blood | ng/mL | | 0.03 | 0.03 |
| 1,1,2,2-Tetrachloroethane | blood | ng/mL | | | 0.01 |
| Tetrachloroethene (Perchloroethylene) | blood | ng/mL | | 0.048 | 0.048 |
| Tetrachloromethane (Carbon tetrachloride) | blood | ng/mL | | 0.01 | 0.005 |
| Toluene | blood | ng/mL | | 0.025 | 0.025 |
| 1,1,1-Trichloroethane (Methyl chloroform) | blood | ng/mL | | | 0.048 |
| 1,1,2-Trichloroethane | blood | ng/mL | | | 0.01 |
| Trichloroethene (Trichloroethylene) | blood | ng/mL | | 0.012 | 0.012 |
| o-Xylene | blood | ng/mL | | 0.049 | 0.049 |
| m- and p-Xylene | blood | ng/mL | | 0.034 | 0.034 |

# Appendix E. Abbreviations Used in Text

| | |
|---|---|
| **ACGIH** | American Conference of Governmental Industrial Hygienists |
| **ATSDR** | Agency for Toxic Substances and Disease Registry |
| **CDC** | Centers for Disease Control and Prevention |
| **DHHS** | Department of Health and Human Services |
| **FAO/WHO** | Food and Agriculture Organization of the United Nations |
| **FDA** | Food and Drug Administration |
| **IARC** | International Agency for Research on Cancer |
| **IOM** | Institute of Medicine |
| **IPCS** | International Programme on Chemical Safety |
| **NAS** | National Academy of Sciences |
| **NCEH** | National Center of Environmental Health |
| **NCHS** | National Center for Health Statistics |
| **NHANES** | National Health and Nutrition Examination Survey |
| **NIOSH** | National Institute of Occupational Safety and Health |
| **NRC** | National Research Council of the NAS |
| **NTP** | National Toxicology Program |
| **OSHA** | Occupational Safety and Health Administration |
| **U.S.** | United States |
| **USDA** | U.S. Department of Agriculture |
| **U.S.EPA** | U.S. Environmental Protection Agency |
| **USGS** | U.S. Geological Survey |
| **WHO** | World Health Organization |

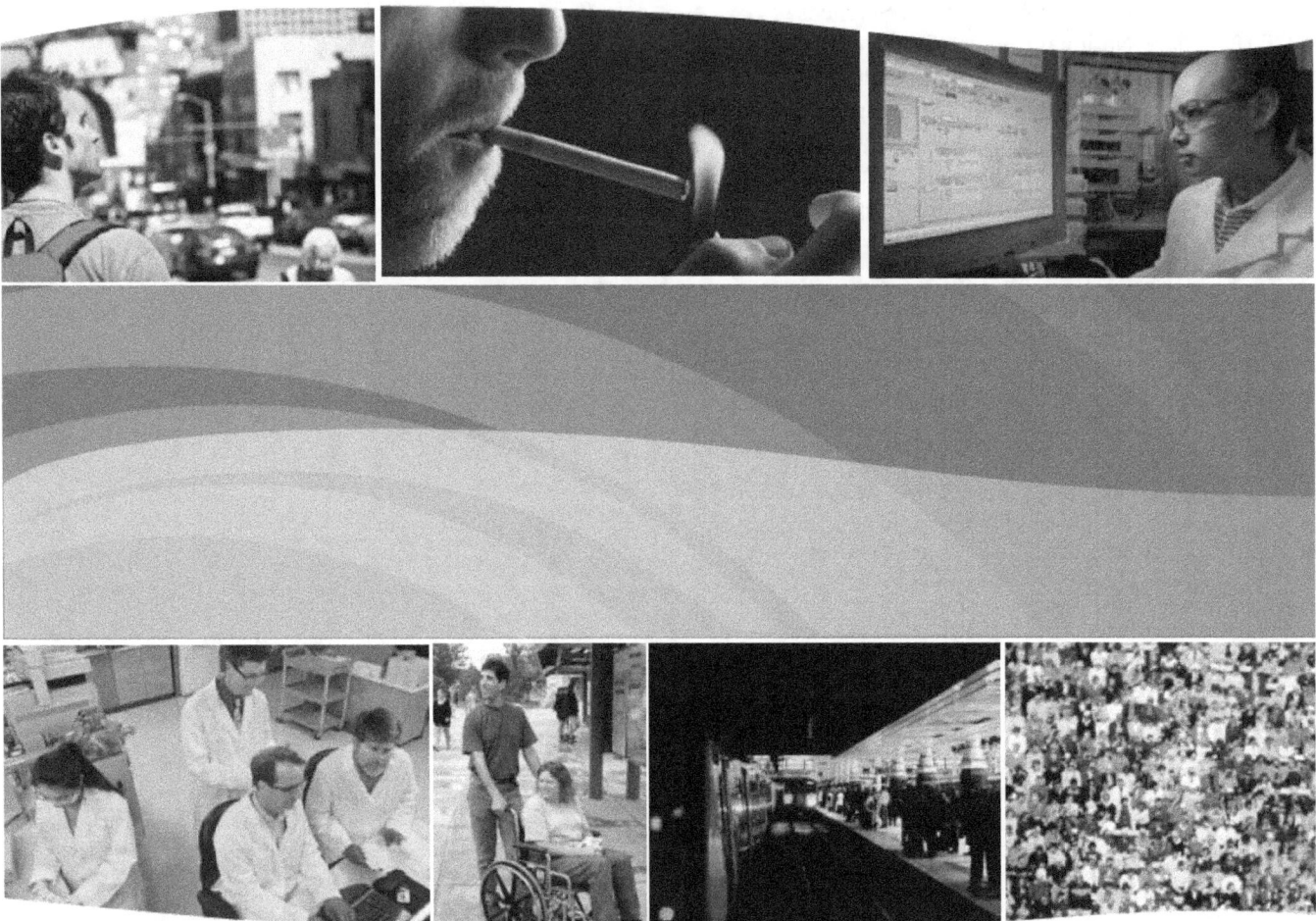

Centers for Disease Control and Prevention
National Center for Environmental Health
Division of Laboratory Sciences
Mail Stop F-20
4770 Buford Highway, NE
Atlanta, GA 30341-3724

Telephone: (toll free) 1-800-CDC-INFO (1-800-232-4636)
Email: CDCINFO@cdc.gov
Website: http://www.cdc.gov/exposurereport

www.ingramcontent.com/pod-product-compliance
Lightning Source LLC
Chambersburg PA
CBHW080227180526
45167CB00006B/2237